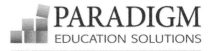
PARADIGM
EDUCATION SOLUTIONS
A DIVISION OF KENDALL HUNT

Seventh Edition

Pharmacology
for Technicians

Skye A. McKennon

Sara Burda Alvarez

Jen Danielson

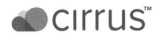

Care has been taken to verify the accuracy of information presented in this book. However, the authors, editors, and publisher cannot accept responsibility for Web, e-mail, newsgroup, or chat room subject matter or content, or for consequences from application of the information in this book, and make no warranty, expressed or implied, with respect to its content.

Trademarks: Some of the product names and company names included in this book have been used for identification purposes only and may be trademarks or registered trade names of their respective manufacturers and sellers. The authors, editors, and publisher disclaim any affiliation, association, or connection with, or sponsorship or endorsement by, such owners.

Photo Credits: Following the index.

We have made every effort to trace the ownership of all copyrighted material and to secure permission from copyright holders. In the event of any question arising as to the use of any material, we will be pleased to make the necessary corrections in future printings. Thanks are due to the authors, publishers, and agents listed in the Photo Credits for permission to use the materials therein indicated.

978-0-76389-302-6

Brief Contents

Preface   xiii

Unit 1   Introduction to Pharmacology   1

Chapter 1   Introduction to Pharmacology and Medications in the Body   3
Chapter 2   Pharmaceutical Development   21
Chapter 3   Pharmacology Study for the Pharmacy Technician   43
Chapter 4   Prescription Orders and Medication Safety   59

Unit 2   Body Systems and Corresponding Drug Therapies   85

Chapter 5   The Integumentary System and Drug Therapy   87
Chapter 6   The Musculoskeletal System and Drug Therapy   119
Chapter 7   The Nervous System and Drug Therapy   161
Chapter 8   The Nervous System, Mental Health, and Drug Therapy   211
Chapter 9   The Sensory System and Drug Therapy   263
Chapter 10   The Cardiovascular System and Drug Therapy   283
Chapter 11   The Respiratory System and Drug Therapy   343
Chapter 12   The Gastrointestinal System and Drug Therapy   405
Chapter 13   The Endocrine System and Drug Therapy   463
Chapter 14   The Reproductive System and Drug Therapy   497
Chapter 15   The Renal System and Drug Therapy   537

Unit 3   Pharmacology and Multisystems   579

Chapter 16   The Immune System, Bacterial Infections, Fungal Infections, and Drug Therapy   581
Chapter 17   The Immune System, Viral Infections, and Drug Therapy   631
Chapter 18   Pain, Anesthesia, and Drug Therapy   677
Chapter 19   Nutrition, Fluids, Electrolytes, and Drug Therapy   731
Chapter 20   Cancer and Drug Therapy   767

Appendix A   Common Pharmacy Abbreviations and Acronyms   815
Appendix B   Common Look-Alike and Sound-Alike Medication   821
Appendix C   ASHP/ACPE Accreditation Standards   823
Glossary   825
Index   861
Photo Credits   895

Contents

Preface xiii

Unit 1
Introduction to Pharmacology 1

Chapter 1
Introduction to Pharmacology and Medications in the Body 3
1.1 **Medicinal Drugs** 4
    Drug Origins and Sources 4
    Drug Names 5
1.2 **Drug Actions** 5
    Pharmacodynamics 6
    Pharmacokinetics 7
    Pharmacokinetic Parameters 10
    Pharmacokinetic Modeling 12
1.3 **Drug Effects** 13
    Beneficial Responses 13
    Adverse Effects or Side Effects 13
    Drug Interactions 14
1.4 **Complementary and Alternative Medicine** 15
    Dietary Supplements 16
    Homeopathy 17

Chapter 2
Pharmaceutical Development 21
2.1 **History of Medicinal Drugs** 21
    Early Remedies 22
    Chinese and Indian Medicine 22
    Drugs in the Middle Ages 23
    Drugs in the Modern Age 24
    Early North American Pharmacology 24
    19th- and 20th-Century Pharmacology . . . 25
2.2 **Contemporary Pharmacy Practice** 25
    The Pharmacist and Pharmacy Technician . . 26
    Pharmacy Technician Certification 28
2.3 **Drug Regulation** 29
    The Food and Drug Administration 29
    Drug Approval Process 29
    Medication Guides 32
    FDA Recalls 33
    Boxed or Black Box Warnings 33
    Controlled Substances 34
    Generic Drugs 36

    Biosimilar Medications 36
    Over-the-Counter Drugs 37

Chapter 3
Pharmacology Study for the Pharmacy Technician 43
3.1 **Evidence-Based Study Methods** 43
    Spacing as a Study Method 44
    Interleaving versus Blocking as a Study Method 44
    Self-Testing as a Study Method 45
    Contiguity Principle Study Method 45
    Eliminating Distractions 46
    Adopting a Growth Mindset 46
3.2 **Pharmacy-Specific Study Aids** 47
    Learning by Drug Class 47
    Identifying Drugs Using Generic Drug Stems 48
    Using Mnemonic Devices 50
3.3 **Drug Information Resources** 52
    Package Inserts 52
    FDA Orange, Purple, and Green Books . . . 52
    Electronic and Drug Resource Apps 53
3.4 **Health Information Resources** 54
    Government Healthcare Websites 54
    Medical Dictionaries and Encyclopedias . . 55

Chapter 4
Prescription Orders and Medication Safety 59
4.1 **The Prescription** 59
    Abbreviations in the Pharmacy 62
    Medication Orders in the Institutional Setting 63
4.2 **Correct Drug Administration Rights** . . . 64
4.3 **Dosage Forms and Routes of Administration** 65
    Oral Routes 66
    Parenteral Routes 67
    Topical Routes 68
4.4 **Factors That Influence Drug Action** 69
    Special Considerations in Older Adults . . . 69
    Special Considerations in Children 72
    Allergic Response 73

4.5 Teaching Patients Medication
Management. **74**
4.6 **Medication Safety** **76**
Technician Role 77
E-Prescribing. 77
Physician Order Entry. 77
Dispensing Cautions. 78
Tamper-Resistant Prescription Pads 79
Medication Reconciliation 79
Medication Error Reporting Systems 79
REMS Programs. 79
4.7 **Understanding the Profession** **80**

Unit 2
Body Systems and Corresponding
Drug Therapies **85**

Chapter 5
The Integumentary System
and Drug Therapy. 87
5.1 **Anatomy and Physiology of the**
Integumentary System **87**
5.2 **Sun Exposure and Drug Treatments.** . . . **88**
Drug Therapies for Sun Exposure 90
5.3 **Acne, Wrinkles, Rosacea,**
and Drug Treatments **91**
Topical Antibiotics 92
Retinoids 94
Miscellaneous Agents 95
5.4 **Dermatitis, Eczema, Psoriasis,**
Dandruff, and Drug Treatments **96**
Topical Corticosteroids 98
Calcineurin Inhibitors 100
Vitamin D Analogs 101
Calamine 101
Selenium Sulfide and Pyrithione Zinc . . . 102
5.5 **Skin Infections and Drug Treatments** . **102**
Topical Antibacterials. 104
Topical Antifungals. 105
Topical Antivirals. 107
5.6 **External Parasites and**
Drug Treatments **108**
5.7 **Antiseptics and Disinfectants.** **111**
Topical Antiseptics and Disinfectants . . . 112
Miscellaneous Products 113
5.8 **Complementary and**
Alternative Therapies. **113**

Chapter 6
The Musculoskeletal System
and Drug Therapy. 119
6.1 **Anatomy of the Musculoskeletal**
System **120**
6.2 **Physiology of the**
Musculoskeletal System. **121**

6.3 **Osteoarthritis and Drug**
Treatments **123**
Analgesics. 123
Conventional Nonsteroidal
Anti-Inflammatory Drugs 126
COX-2 Inhibitor. 129
6.4 **Rheumatoid Arthritis and Drug**
Treatments **130**
Disease-Modifying Antirheumatic
Drugs (DMARDs) 131
6.5 **Gouty Arthritis and Drug**
Treatments **137**
Uricosuric Agents, Xanthine Oxidase
Inhibitors, and Antigout Agents 138
6.6 **Osteoporosis and Drug Treatments** . . . **140**
Bisphosphonates 142
Selective Estrogen Receptor Modulators . 143
Other Osteoporosis Medications. 144
6.7 **Muscle Spasms and Drug Treatments** . **145**
Skeletal Muscle Relaxants 146
6.8 **Inflammation and Swelling and Drug**
Treatments **151**
Salicylates. 151
6.9 **Complementary and Alternative**
Therapies for Disorders of the
Musculoskeletal System. **154**

Chapter 7
The Nervous System
and Drug Therapy. 161
7.1 **Anatomy and Physiology of the**
Nervous System **161**
Anatomical Divisions 162
Functional Divisions. 162
Neurons and Neurotransmitters 163
Neurotransmitter Mechanism of
Action 165
7.2 **Seizure Disorders and**
Drug Treatments **166**
Focal Seizures 167
Generalized Seizures 168
Antiepileptic Therapy 169
Sodium Channel Blockers 171
Calcium Channel Blockers 177
GABA Enhancers 178
Glutamate Inhibitors 180
Synaptic Vesicle Protein Binders 182
7.3 **Parkinson's Disease and**
Drug Treatments **183**
Levodopa / Carbidopa and Dopamine
Agonists 186
Anticholinergics. 188
Catechol-O-Methyltransferase
Inhibitors. 189

Monoamine Oxidase Inhibitors......... 189
Other Agents for Parkinson's
Disease 191

**7.4 Multiple Sclerosis and
Drug Treatments....................191**
Beta Interferons 191
Other Disease-Modifying Therapies..... 193

**7.5 Alzheimer's Disease and
Drug Treatments....................195**
Acetylcholinesterase Inhibitors 196
NMDA Antagonist..................... 197

**7.6 Attention Deficit Hyperactivity
Disorder and Drug Treatments 197**
Central Nervous System
Stimulants 198
Nonstimulant Drugs 200

**7.7 Other Central Nervous System
Disorders and Drug Treatments 201**
Myasthenia Gravis..................... 201
Amyotrophic Lateral Sclerosis 203
Huntington's Disease 203
Restless Legs Syndrome and
Fibromyalgia 204

**7.8 Complementary and Alternative
Therapies..........................204**

Chapter 8
The Nervous System, Mental Health, and Drug Therapy..................... 211

**8.1 Depression, Mood Disorders, and
Drug Treatments...................212**
Selective Serotonin Reuptake
Inhibitors........................... 214
Serotonin-Norepinephrine Reuptake
Inhibitors........................... 218
Cyclic Antidepressants 220
Monoamine Oxidase Inhibitors........ 222
Other Antidepressant Drugs........... 223

**8.2 Bipolar Disorder and Drug
Treatments 225**

**8.3 Schizophrenia, Psychosis, and
Drug Treatments...................228**
Typical Antipsychotics 230
Atypical Antipsychotics 232

8.4 Anxiety and Drug Treatments 240
Benzodiazepines...................... 242
Other Antianxiety Agents 243

**8.5 Sleep Disorders and Drug
Treatments 244**
Non-Benzodiazepine Hypnotics
(Z-Drugs) 246
Stimulants for Narcolepsy............. 248
Miscellaneous Hypnotic Agent......... 250
Benzodiazepines for Insomnia 250

**8.6 Alcohol Dependence and Drug
Treatments 251**
Dependence on and Withdrawal
from Alcohol........................ 252
Drugs Used for Alcohol Dependence 253

**8.7 Complementary and Alternative
Therapies.........................255**

Chapter 9
The Sensory System and Drug Therapy... 263
9.1 Anatomy and Physiology of the Eyes ..263
9.2 Glaucoma and Drug Treatments......265
**9.3 Chronic Dry Eye and Drug
Treatments 267**
9.4 Conjunctivitis and Drug Treatments ..270
9.5 Anatomy and Physiology of the Ears ..274
**9.6 Otitis (Media and Externa) and
Drug Treatments...................275**
Oral and Otic Antibiotics............... 276
Topical Otic Preparations 277
**9.7 Complementary and Alternative
Therapies.........................278**

Chapter 10
The Cardiovascular System and Drug Therapy.........................283
**10.1 Anatomy and Physiology of the
Cardiovascular System...............283**
Cardiac Contractility................... 286
Blood Pressure 287
10.2 Hypertension and Drug Treatments...288
Angiotensin-Converting Enzyme
(ACE) Inhibitors...................... 291
Angiotensin Receptor Blockers
(ARBs).............................. 292
Calcium Channel Blockers 293
Beta-Blockers 294
Direct Renin Inhibitors 296
Alpha-Blockers 297
Thiazide Diuretics.................... 297
Vasodilators......................... 297
**10.3 Cardiac Arrhythmias and
Drug Treatments...................297**
Membrane-Stabilizing Agents/Sodium
Channel Blockers (Class I
Antiarrhythmics) 301
Beta-Blockers (Class II
Antiarrhythmics) 302
Potassium Channel Blockers
(Class III Antiarrhythmics) 302
Calcium Channel Blockers
(Class IV Antiarrhythmics) 304
Other Agents Used to Treat
Arrhythmias......................... 304

10.4 Angina, Myocardial Infarction, and Corresponding Drug Treatments 306
    Nitrates 308
    Metabolic Modifiers 310
    ACE Inhibitors 310
    Anticoagulants 310
    Beta-Blockers 310
    Calcium Channel Blockers 311

10.5 Heart Failure and Drug Treatments . . . 311
    ACE Inhibitors 311
    Angiotensin Receptor Blockers 312
    Angiotensin Receptor–Neprilysin Inhibitors 312
    Beta-Blockers 312
    Loop Diuretics 312
    Aldosterone Antagonists 313
    Digoxin 313
    Combination Vasodilators 313

10.6 Dyslipidemia, Hypercholesterolemia, Hyperlipidemia, and Drug Treatments . . 313
    HMG-CoA Reductase Inhibitors (Statins) . . 316
    Fibric Acid Derivatives (Fibrates) 317
    Bile Acid Sequestrants 318
    ATP Citrate Lyase (ACL) Inhibitors 319
    Other Cholesterol-Lowering Agents 319

10.7 Clotting Disorders, Stroke, and Drug Treatments 320
    Direct Thrombin Inhibitors 325
    Heparin and Low-Molecular-Weight Heparins 326
    Factor Xa Inhibitors 327
    Vitamin K Antagonists 329
    Antiplatelet Agents 331
    Glycoprotein Antagonists 333
    Thrombolytic Agents 333

10.8 Complementary and Alternative Therapies 334

Chapter 11
The Respiratory System and Drug Therapy 343

11.1 Anatomy of the Respiratory System . . . 343
11.2 Asthma and Drug Treatments 345
    Asthma Management and Drug Therapy . . 346
    Short-Acting Beta-2 Agonists 351
    Corticosteroids 352
    Leukotriene Inhibitors 353
    Mast Cell Stabilizer 355
    Monoclonal Antibodies 355
    Xanthine Derivative 356

11.3 Chronic Obstructive Pulmonary Disease and Drug Treatments 356
    Anticholinergics 361
    Antitrypsin Deficiency Agent 364
    Long-Acting Beta-2 Agonists 364

    Mucolytics 365
    Phosphodiesterase-4 Enzyme Inhibitor . . 366
    Combination Products for Asthma and COPD 366

11.4 Cystic Fibrosis and Drug Treatments . . 368
    Antibiotics for Cystic Fibrosis 368
    Mucolytics for Cystic Fibrosis 370
    Pancreatic Enzymes for Cystic Fibrosis . . 370
    CFTR Modulators 370

11.5 Other Lung Diseases and Drug Treatments 371
    Pneumonia 372
    Respiratory Distress Syndrome 373
    Tuberculosis 374
    Histoplasmosis 376

11.6 Cough, Cold, and Allergy and Corresponding Drug Treatments 377
    Antitussives 378
    Expectorants 384
    Decongestants 384
    Antihistamines 387
    First-Generation Antihistamines 388
    Second-Generation Antihistamines 389
    Nasal Corticosteroids 390

11.7 Tobacco Use, Smoking Cessation, and Corresponding Drug Treatment . . 391
    Quitting Nicotine 393
    Smoking Cessation Agents 394

11.8 Complementary and Alternative Therapies 396

Chapter 12
The Gastrointestinal System and Drug Therapy 405

12.1 Anatomy and Physiology of the Gastrointestinal System 405
12.2 Gastroesophageal Reflux Disease and Drug Treatments 408
    Antacids 410
    Histamine H_2 Receptor Antagonists 412
    Proton Pump Inhibitors 413
    Coating Agents 415
    Prostaglandin E_1 Analogs 415

12.3 Peptic Disease and Drug Treatment . . . 416
    H. Pylori Agents 417

12.4 Ulcerative Colitis, Crohn's Disease, and Drug Treatments 419
    Corticosteroids 420
    Aminosalicylates 421
    Biologic Therapies 422
    Immunosuppressants 423

12.5 Gallstones and Drug Treatments 424
    Gallstone Dissolution Agent 424

12.6 Diarrhea and Drug Treatments 425
    Adsorbents 426

Antimotility Drugs 427
Drugs for Infectious Diarrhea 429

12.7 Constipation and Flatulence and Drug Treatments 430
Fiber and Fiber Supplementation 432
Bulk-Forming Laxatives 435
Stool Softeners/Surfactant Laxatives 436
Osmotic Laxatives 436
Stimulant Laxatives.................... 437
Miscellaneous Constipation Agents 438
Antiflatulent Agents 439
Bowel Evacuants..................... 439

12.8 Other Gastrointestinal Diseases That May Accompany Constipation and Drug Treatments 440
Diverticular Disease 440
Hiatal Hernia 441
Irritable Bowel Syndrome 441
Hemorrhoids......................... 442

12.9 Nausea and Vomiting and Drug Treatments 443
Antihistamines and Anticholinergics 445
Serotonin Receptor Antagonists 446
Dopamine Receptor Antagonists........ 447
Neurokinin-1 Receptor Antagonists..... 448

12.10 Hepatitis and Drug Treatments...... 449
Hepatitis B and Hepatitis C Agents...... 449

12.11 Complementary and Alternative Therapies................ 456

Chapter 13
The Endocrine System and Drug Therapy 463

13.1 Anatomy and Physiology of the Endocrine System 463
Thyroid Gland 465
Adrenal Glands and Corticosteroids 466
Pancreas 467

13.2 Thyroid Disorders and Drug Treatments 467
Hypothyroidism and Thyroid Replacement Therapy.................. 468
Hyperthyroidism 470

13.3 Adrenal Glands and Drug Treatments 471
Cushing's Syndrome 472
Addison's Disease..................... 472
Corticosteroid Therapy 472

13.4 Diabetes and Drug Treatments 473
Types of Diabetes and Treatment 474
Insulin.............................. 478
Glucagon-Like Peptide 1 (GLP-1) Receptor Agonists 484
Dipeptidyl Peptidase-4 (DPP-4) Inhibitors............................ 485

Metformin (Biguanide)................. 485
Sodium-Glucose Linked Transporter-2 (SGLT-2) Inhibitors 487
Insulin Secretagogues.................. 487
Thiazolidinediones (TZDs) 488
Miscellaneous Products 489

13.5 Complementary and Alternative Therapies......................... 490

Chapter 14
The Reproductive System and Drug Therapy....................... 497

14.1 The Reproductive System and Related Hormones 497
Androgen 498
Estrogen 499
Progesterone 499

14.2 Hormone Replacement Therapy 499
Male Hypogonadism................... 501
Female Hypogonadism and Menopause 503
Gender-Affirming Hormone Therapy.... 506

14.3 Sexual Dysfunction and Drug Treatments 507
Erectile Dysfunction 508
Sexual Dysfunction 510

14.4 Contraception and Drug Treatments 511
Barrier Contraception................. 511
Hormonal Contraceptives 513
Heavy Menstrual Bleeding............. 523

14.5 Pregnancy, Childbirth, and Drug Treatments.................... 524
Pregnancy Tests and Pregnancy 525
Drugs Used to Slow Labor.............. 526
Drugs Used to Induce Labor............ 526

14.6 Growth Disorders and Drug Treatments 527
Growth Hormone 528
Growth Hormone Deficiency 528

14.7 Complementary and Alternative Therapies................ 529

Chapter 15
The Renal System and Drug Therapy..... 537

15.1 Anatomy and Physiology of the Renal System 538
Kidneys.............................. 539
Ureters and Urinary Bladder............ 541

15.2 Renal Function and Pharmacokinetics 542
Renal System Dysfunction 542
Assessment of Renal Function 542
Nephrotoxicity and Renal Dosing....... 543

15.3 Urinary Tract Infection and
Drug Treatments .543
    Antibiotics 544
    Urinary Analgesics 544

15.4 Urinary Incontinence and
Drug Treatments .545
    Anticholinergics (Antimuscarinics) 546
    Beta-3 Adrenergic Agonists 547

15.5 Benign Prostatic Hyperplasia and
Drug Treatments .548
    Alpha-Blockers 549
    5-Alpha-Reductase Inhibitors 550

15.6 Chronic Kidney Disease and
Drug Treatments .551
    Carbonic Anhydrase Inhibitors 554
    Loop Diuretics 554
    Potassium-Sparing Diuretics 556
    Thiazide and Thiazide-Related
    Diuretics 558

15.7 Anemia and Drug Treatments 559
    Erythropoietin-Stimulating Agents 560
    Oral and Parenteral Iron Supplements . . . 561
    B Vitamins 563

15.8 Advanced Chronic Kidney Disease
and Dialysis Therapies 564
    Phosphate Binders 566
    Vitamin D Supplements 566
    Calcimimetics 567

15.9 End-Stage Chronic Kidney Disease
and Kidney Transplantation 568
    Immunosuppressants 569

15.10 Complementary and Alternative
Therapies 571

Unit 3
Pharmacology and Multisystems 579

Chapter 16
The Immune System, Bacterial Infections,
Fungal Infections, and Drug Therapy 581

16.1 Anatomy and Physiology of the
Immune System .582
    The Innate Immune System 583
    The Adaptive Immune System 583

16.2 Bacterial Infections 584
    Types of Bacteria 584
    Antibiotic Selection 586
    Antibiotic Side Effects and
    Dispensing Issues 588
    Antimicrobial Resistance 588

16.3 Antibiotic Drugs and Their
Mechanisms of Action 589
    Sulfonamides and Nitrofurantoin 593
    Penicillins 595
    Cephalosporins 597

    Carbapenems and Monobactams 599
    Lincosamides and Macrolides 600
    Aminoglycosides 602
    Tetracyclines 604
    Fluoroquinolones (Quinolones) 605
    Miscellaneous Antibiotics 606

16.4 Storage of Liquid Antibiotics 609

16.5 Ophthalmic Antibiotics 610

16.6 Sexually Transmitted Infections
and Drug Treatments 611
    Chlamydia 611
    Gonorrhea 612
    Syphilis 612
    Other Sexually Transmitted Infections . . 613
    Agents for Treating Sexually
    Transmitted Infections 613

16.7 Fungi, Fungal Diseases, and
Drug Treatments .614
    Azoles 618
    Echinocandins 619
    Polyenes 620
    Miscellaneous Antifungals 621

16.8 Complementary and Alternative
Therapies 622

Chapter 17
The Immune System, Viral Infections,
and Drug Therapy 631

17.1 Viruses and Viral Infections 631
    Stages of Viral Infection 632
    Significant Viral Infections 632
    Classification of Viral Infections 634
    Latent Viruses 634
    Virus and Host-Cell Interaction 634

17.2 Antiviral Agents (Nonretroviral) 635
    Therapeutic Uses of Antiviral Agents 635
    Antiherpes Agents 637
    Anti-Influenza Agents 639
    Other Antiviral Agents 641

17.3 HIV/AIDS and Antiretroviral
Agents 642
    Nucleoside Reverse Transcriptase
    Inhibitors 643
    Nonnucleoside Reverse Transcriptase
    Inhibitors 648
    Protease Inhibitors 651
    Entry Inhibitors: Fusion Inhibitors,
    Post-Attachment Inhibitors, and
    CCR5 Antagonists 655
    Integrase Strand Transfer Inhibitors 657
    Combining Antiretroviral Medications . . 659
    HIV Regimens 661
    Treatment as Prevention 661
    Responding to Accidental Exposure 662

Preexposure Prophylaxis (PrEP) 662
17.4 Immunity and Immunization. 662
Immunizations. 663
Immunization Schedule. 665
Common Vaccines 665
**17.5 Complementary and Alternative
Therapy 670**

Chapter 18
Pain, Anesthesia, and Drug Therapy 677
18.1 Physiology of Pain. 677
Pain Mechanisms. 678
Timing of Pain 679
Response to Pain 680
18.2 Opioids and Pain Management 681
Opioid Analgesics 681
Dosing and Administering Opioids 683
Opioid Side Effects 685
Opioid Cautions and Considerations. . . . 685
Mu Opioid Agonists 686
Mixed Opioid Agonists 692
**18.3 Opioid Use Disorder and
Treatments 694**
Opioid Antagonists. 696
18.4 Anesthesia. 697
General Anesthetics: Inhaled Agents. 702
General Anesthetics: Injectable
Agents. 704
Anesthesia Induction Agents 707
Neuromuscular Blocking Agents. 709
Drugs Used to Reverse Anesthesia or
Overdose. 710
General Anesthetics and Malignant
Hyperthermia 713
Local Anesthetics 714
**18.5 Migraine Headaches and
Drug Treatments 715**
5HT Agonists 718
Ergot Derivatives 719
Calcitonin Gene-Related Peptide
(CGRP) Receptor Antagonists 720
Antiemetic Agents 721
Combination Agents 722
**18.6 Complementary and Alternative
Therapies. 722**

Chapter 19
Nutrition, Fluids, Electrolytes,
and Drug Therapy 731
19.1 Vitamins 732
Fat-Soluble Vitamins. 732
Water-Soluble Vitamins 735
**19.2 Fluids, Electrolytes, and Acid-Base
Balance. 738**
Fluids 738

Fluids and Solutions. 739
Electrolytes, Electrolyte Deficiency,
and Electrolyte Replacement. 742
Acidifying and Alkalinizing Agents. 748
19.3 Obesity and Drug Therapy 750
Lipase Inhibitor 752
Sympathomimetic Drugs 753
Opioid Antagonist and Bupropion. 754
**19.4 Malnutrition and Drug
Therapy 754**
Enteral Nutrition. 755
Parenteral Nutrition 757
**19.5 Complementary and Alternative
Therapies. 760**

Chapter 20
Cancer and Drug Therapy 767
20.1 Cancer and Its Development. 768
Pathophysiology of Cancer 768
Tumor Cell Proliferation and
Tumor Burden 770
20.2 Cancer Stages and Treatments 770
Surgery 771
Radiation Therapy. 771
Immunotherapy. 772
Chemotherapy 772
20.3 Chemotherapy Drugs 773
Cell Cycle and Mechanism of
Action 773
Cytotoxic Drugs and Side Effects 774
Combination Chemotherapy 780
Alkylating Agents. 781
Antimetabolites 782
Topoisomerase Inhibitors 784
Antimicrotubule Agents. 786
Miscellaneous Chemotherapy
Drugs 788
20.4 Hormonal Drug Therapies 789
Antiestrogens 790
Antiandrogens 791
Luteinizing Hormone–Releasing
Hormone Agonists. 792
Cyclin-Dependent Kinase (CDK 4/6)
Inhibitors. 792
20.5 Targeted Anticancer Therapies 793
Angiogenesis Inhibitors 795
Monoclonal Antibodies 796
Signal Transduction Inhibitors 798
Bruton's Tyrosine Kinase Inhibitors. 799
PI3K/AKT/mTOR Pathway Agents. 800
20.6 Immunotherapy. 800
Immune Checkpoints. 800
Cytotoxic T-Lymphocyte-Associated
Protein 4 (CTLA-4) 801

Programmed Death Pathway 801
Immune Checkpoint Inhibitors 802
20.7 Handling Hazardous Agents 804
Personal Protective Equipment 805
Spill Kit 806
Hazardous Drug Communication
Program 806
Preventing Chemotherapy-Related
Medication Errors 807
**20.8 Complementary and Alternative
Therapies 808**

Appendix A
Common Pharmacy Abbreviations and
Acronyms 815

Appendix B
Common Look-Alike
and Sound-Alike Medication 821

Appendix C
ASHP/ACPE Accreditation Standards 823

Glossary 825

Index 861

Photo Credits 895

Pharmacology for Technicians: What Makes This New Edition Exciting?

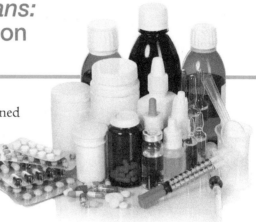

Pharmacology for Technicians, Seventh Edition, is cutting edge and up-to-date courseware designed to help students achieve success in the workplace. Using an accessible and student-friendly approach, this courseware supports a comprehensive pharmacology course for students preparing to become a certified pharmacy technicians. *Pharmacology for Technicians*, Seventh Edition, helps students develop a commitment to the pharmacy field so that, as pharmacy technicians, they remain challenged by this swiftly changing field and motivated to continue to learn about the drugs that improve the lives of patients. The seventh edition features include:

- Alignment with new ASHP™/ACPE curriculum standards, covering accreditation topics in a logical order with easy-to-understand language
- The cloud-based Cirrus learning environment to assemble all student and instructor resources in one easy-access location
- A new chapter that explores study strategies for pharmacy technician students

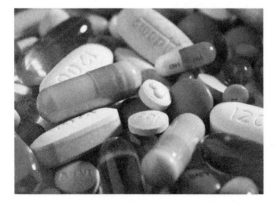

- Restructured content that addresses drugs by major body systems
- Expanded information about drugs, including dosage forms and administration, side effects, contraindications, cautions and considerations, and drug interactions
- Margin features to engage students and assist their learning
- Exploration of complementary and alternative drug therapies
- Coverage of professionalism, soft skills, communication, and cultural awareness

Study Assets: A Visual Walk-Through

Learning Objectives

Each chapter begins with a list of the major concepts students should learn after reading the chapter and completing the exercises.

ASHP/ACPE Accreditation Standards

A mapping of chapter-specific topics to industry standards for pharmacy technician training is provided in Appendix C.

Feature Boxes

Workplace Wisdom and Field Note feature boxes highlight pharmacology concepts and skills that will be important when working as a pharmacy technician.

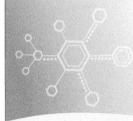

Introduction to Pharmacology and Medications in the Body — 1

Learning Objectives

1 Describe the term *pharmacology*. (Introduction)
2 Explain why the pharmacy technician needs to understand and learn about pharmacology. (Introduction)
3 Describe the role of receptors in the body. (Section 1.2)
4 Compare and contrast the meaning of agonist and antagonist in terms of pharmacology. (Section 1.2)
5 Explain the concepts associated with pharmacodynamics: messengers, receptors, and mechanisms of drug action. (Section 1.2)

6 Describe the four processes of pharmacokinetics: absorption, distribution, metabolism, and elimination. (Section 1.2)
7 Define the terms used to describe the beneficial and harmful effects of drugs. (Section 1.3)
8 Describe the ways through which common drug interactions occur. (Section 1.3)
9 Explain why pharmacy technicians should be familiar with complementary and alternative therapies. (Section 1.4)

ASHP/ACPE Accreditation Standards
To view the *ASHP/ACPE Accreditation Standards* addressed in this chapter, refer to Appendix C.

People have been treating physical and mental ailments with drugs for thousands of years. A **drug**, or medicine, is a substance that changes the way a living organism functions. Tremendous advances have been made in understanding how diseases and disorders are caused and how they are treated with medicine.

Pharmacology is the study of drugs, including their origins, properties, actions, and effects on the body. The goal of drug therapy is to produce a response in the body that cures or controls a specific disease or medical condition. The main concepts (or divisions) of pharmacology—pharmacodynamics, the branch of pharmacology that studies a drug's effects or actions on the body, and pharmacokinetics, the study of what happens to a drug in the body through the ...tion, distribution, metabolism, and elimination—are discussed ...An understanding of these processes enables safe ...ed for various diseases.

FIELD NOTES

Health care is a constantly evolving field. Those in healthcare fields, such as pharmacy technicians, need to stay informed on health-related information. One way to keep informed is to regularly check health information resources, including the websites mentioned in this chapter. Verified social media accounts are another option to help you stay abreast of new and noteworthy health developments. Consider following the CDC and NIH on social media. Both organizations have Facebook, Instagram, and Twitter accounts. The FDA and MedlinePlus have Twitter accounts. If you prefer to watch videos, you can follow the CDC and the NIH on YouTube.

Margin Reminders

Short tips and hints spotlight important information related to chapter content.

Practice Tip

Provides reminders about key elements of pharmacy practice.

Pharm Fact

Highlight interesting trivia and fun facts.

Safety Alert

Serves as warnings to avoid problems in the field.

Put Down Roots

Identifies shared word parts and word origins to make terms memorable.

Work Wise

Gives advice on professionalism, and on-the-job scenarios.

Name Exchange

In practice, the drugs noted in this section will often include "topical" after the brand name to indicate the topical application—for example, Azelex topical and Finacea topical.

Visually Engaging Study Tools

Photographs, figures, and tables enhance visual learning and aid retention of course content.

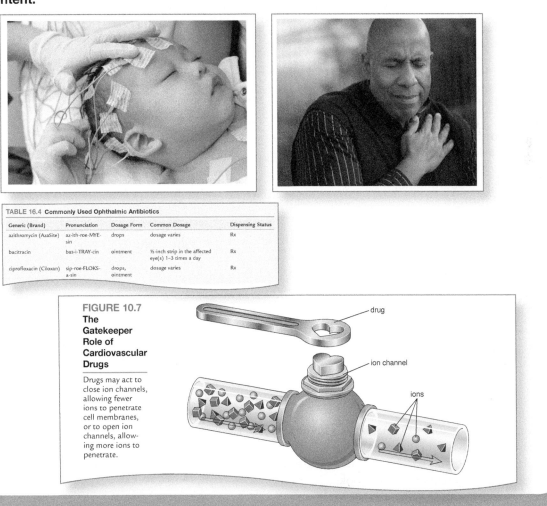

TABLE 16.4 Commonly Used Ophthalmic Antibiotics

Generic (Brand)	Pronunciation	Dosage Form	Common Dosage	Dispensing Status
azithromycin (AzaSite)	az-ith-roe-MYE-sin	drops	dosage varies	Rx
bacitracin	bas-i-TRAY-cin	ointment	½-inch strip in the affected eye(s) 1–3 times a day	Rx
ciprofloxacin (Ciloxan)	sip-roe-FLOKS-a-sin	drops, ointment	dosage varies	Rx

FIGURE 10.7
The Gatekeeper Role of Cardiovascular Drugs

Drugs may act to close ion channels, allowing fewer ions to penetrate cell membranes, or to open ion channels, allowing more ions to penetrate.

drug

ion channel

ions

Review and Assessment

Each chapter ends with a set of resources that includes a summary of key concepts, a list of chapter-specific drugs, a quick quiz to check understanding of course content, and critical thinking challenges.

Appendices

Additional resources support student learning with succinct, at-a-glance reference materials. These include:

Appendix A: Common Look-Alike and Sound-Alike Medication

Appendix B: Common Pharmacy Abbreviations and Acronyms

Appendix C: ASHP/ACPE Accreditation Standards Alignment*

Glossary

Chapter key terms are presented in bold and are contextually defined when introduced in each chapter. The terms and their formal definitions are compiled in a course-level glossary. The digital courseware provides the same content in a searchable, filter-enabled format.

Index

The index provides a quick location guide for terms and topics.

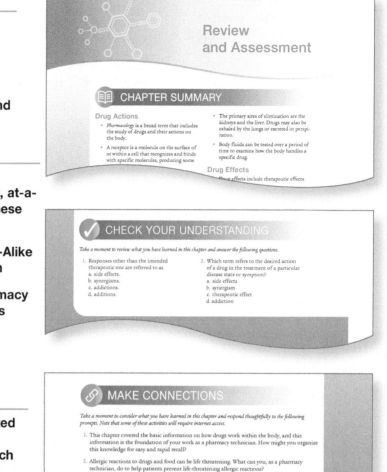

*Appendix C identifies the *ASHP/ACPE Accreditation Standards* associated with the chapter content. This list is meant for guidance purposes only and was created by the author of this text. Neither ASHP nor ACPE has participated in or had any role in creating the list of standards or any other content that is included in this book.

The Cirrus Solution

Elevating student success and instructor efficiency

Powered by Paradigm, Cirrus is the next-generation learning solution for teaching pharmacy technician students the concepts and skills needed to become successful employees valued by patients, colleagues, and supervisors. Cirrus seamlessly delivers complete course content in a cloud-based learning environment that puts students on the fast track to success. Students can access their content from any device, anywhere, through a live internet connection. Because Cirrus is platform-independent, students receive the same learning experience whether they are using PCs, Macs, or Chromebook computers. Cirrus also provides access to all the Pharmacy Technician series content. This content is delivered in a series of scheduled assignments that report to a grade book, thus tracking student progress and achievement. Compatible with Blackboard, Canvas, D2L, and Moodle Cirrus content is exportable through Learning Tools Interoperability (LTI) for flexible learning using a school's learning management system (LMS).

Cirrus courseware provides a complete, digitally delivered training and assessment solution for a pharmacology course.

Watch and Learn Lessons

Providing chapter-specific eContent, videos, and quizzes, Watch and Learn Lessons ensure that students have multiple ways to consume the course content. Each chapter includes eContent for all sections of the chapter and a corresponding video. These lessons also include chapter summaries, drug lists, and a Check Your Understanding quiz that allows students to check their comprehension of key chapter concepts.

Additional Activities

The Apply the Concept and the Internet Research assignments provide activities for students to apply their understanding of the materials and explore additional materials.

Practice Tests

A practice test for students is available for each chapter to help students prepare for the instructor-controlled chapter exam.

Canadian Pharmacy Technician Supplement

Available only through Cirrus, this supplement assists Canadian students in understanding the differences between US and Canadian pharmacy practice. The supplement has four parts:

- Part 1: Scope of Pharmacy Technicians in Canada
- Part 2: Drug Regulation in Canada
- Part 3: Controlled Substances
- Part 4: Top 100 Drugs Dispensed in Canadian Pharmacies

Instructor Resources

Designed to support *Pharmacology for Technicians*, Seventh Edition, the Instructor Resources include materials to help instructors plan their course, teach the content, and assess student progress and mastery. Accessed through Cirrus and visible only to instructors, these resources include course planning, delivery, and assessment support.

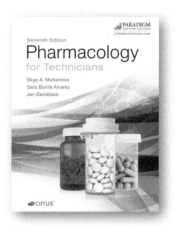

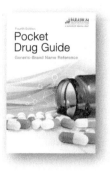

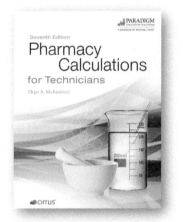

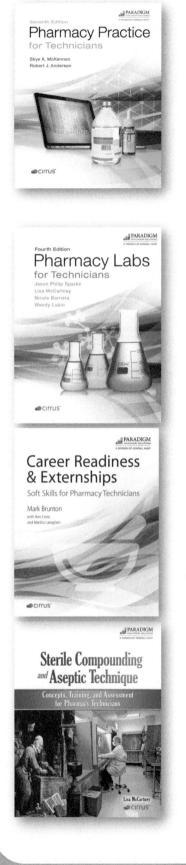

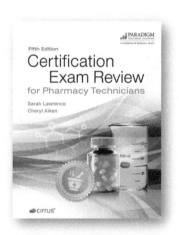

Paradigm's Comprehensive Pharmacy Technician Series

In addition to Pharmacology for Technicians, Seventh Edition, Paradigm Education Solutions offers additional courseware designed specifically for the pharmacy technician curriculum:

- *Pharmacy Practice for Technicians,* Seventh Edition
- *Pocket Drug Guide: Generic Brand Name Reference,* Fourth Edition
- *Pharmacy Labs for Technicians,* Fourth Edition
- *Pharmacy Calculations for Technicians,* Seventh Edition
- *Certification Exam Review for Pharmacy Technicians,* Fifth Edition
- *Career Readiness & Externships: Soft Skills for Pharmacy Technicians*
- *Sterile Compounding and Aseptic Technique*

Additional Health Careers Courseware

The following learning solutions are particularly useful for pharmacy technicians:

- *Medical Terminology: Connecting through Language*
- *Emergency & Disaster Preparedness for Health Professionals*, Second Edition
- *Pharmacology Essentials for Allied Health*
- *What Language Does Your Patient Hurt In?: A Practical Guide to Culturally Competent Care, Third Edition*
- *Exploring Electronic Health Records*
- *Introduction to Health Information Management*

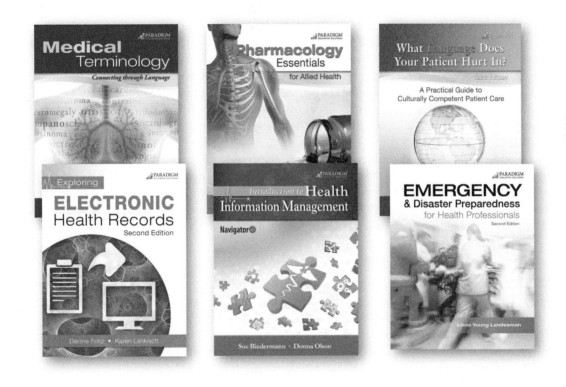

About the Authors

Dr. Skye McKennon

Dr. Skye A. McKennon is a licensed pharmacist, board-certified pharmacotherapy specialist (BCPS), group exercise instructor, certified lifestyle coach, and preventionist. Dr. McKennon completed her bachelor's degree and doctor of pharmacy (PharmD) degree from Washington State University. She completed postdoctoral residency training at the Swedish Medical Center in Seattle, Washington and received a teaching certificate from the University of Washington. Dr. McKennon has practice experience in the community, institutional, and ambulatory pharmacy settings. Her passion for teaching and education led her to faculty positions at the University of Washington School of Pharmacy and at the Washington State University College of Pharmacy, where she has received honors for teaching, mentorship, scholarship, and community service.

Dr. McKennon has published in multiple peer-reviewed journals (including the *American Journal of Pharmacy Education* and *Currents in Pharmacy Teaching and Learning*) and co-authored five pharmacy textbooks. She has presented her work at international and national symposiums such as the Seventh International Conference on Interprofessional Practice and Education, the American Association of Colleges of Pharmacy annual meeting, the Academy of Integrative Health and Medicine annual meeting, and the Pharmacy Technicians Educators Council conference.

Courses designed and directed by Dr. McKennon include applied pharmacotherapeutics, institutional pharmacy practice, diabetes prevention, and evidence-based preventive health. She has been both an instructor and a guest lecturer for various courses for pharmacy and other health science students, including calculations, therapeutics, pharmacotherapy for older adults, global health brigades, and law and ethics.

Dr. Sara Burda Alvarez

Dr. Sara Burda Alvarez is a licensed pharmacist and board-certified pharmacotherapy specialist (BCPS). Dr. Alvarez received her doctor of pharmacy from the University of Nebraska Medical Center and obtained her post-doctoral residency training from The Johns Hopkins Hospital. Additionally, she holds a Master of Science degree in Pharmaceutical Outcomes and Policy from the University of Florida. Dr. Alvarez's experience includes practicing in health system settings in critical care and pharmacy department management; in the managed care setting in clinical program development and pharmacoeconomic evaluations, and in the pharmaceutical industry in health economic outcomes research.

Dr. Alvarez has been adjunct faculty at the University of Washington School of Pharmacy since 2010. Her practice and research interests include health economics and outcomes research, diabetes, obesity, general medicine, leadership, as well as patient and medication safety.

Dr. Jen Danielson

Dr. Jen Danielson has been a pharmacist since 1993 and a recognized leader in pharmacy education since 1996. She has spent most of her academic career serving as Director of Experiential Education at four pharmacy schools (University of Washington, University of Colorado, Campbell University, and Oregon State University). From 2004 to 2006, Dr. Danielson served as chair of the pharmacy technician program at Pikes Peak Community College in

Colorado Springs where she taught pharmacology. It was her work in Colorado that formed the basis for her approach to teaching this topic to pharmacy technician students in both this textbook and her previous book, *Pharmacology Essentials for Technicians*.

Dr. Danielson has presented and published on various topics in pharmacy education on the national, regional, and local levels. Her current teaching and scholarship responsibilities are in interprofessional education and diabetes-related topics. Her practice background in diabetes care in the ambulatory clinic setting provides inspiration for her teaching and writing. Her most recent work at the University of Washington involves the provision of collaborative learning opportunities between pharmacy and allied health students.

Dr. Danielson lives with her family in Mill Creek, Washington.

About the Experts

Several exceptional instructors and content specialists reviewed and contributed to this program's courseware to help ensure accuracy and appropriate instructional approaches. Special thanks are due to these individuals who shared their vast expertise and passion for the profession.

Contributing Writers

Nelly Adel, PharmD, BCOP, BCPS
Chair of Pharmacy Practice
Associate Professor, Oncology
Touro College of Pharmacy

Diana Broome, BS, CPhT, PhTR
Lone Star College

Andrea R.Redman, PharmD, BCPS
Emory Healthcare

Expert Reviewers

Anne LaVance, BS, CPhT
Delgado Community College

Andrea R.Redman, PharmD, BCPS
Emory Healthcare

Writing and Research Support

Angelica Barnhill, PharmD

Stacie Chan, PharmD
University of Washington

Rachel Hansen-Pfaff, PharmD

Sam J. Miller, PharmD

Ailish O'Sullivan, PharmD

Additional Contributors

The quality of this body of work is a testament to the feedback we have received from many instructors, additional contributors, and series survey respondents.

Nicole Barriera, CPhT
Pikes Peak Community College

Mark Brunton, CPhT, MSHE
Northwest Career College

Kevin Hope, RPh
Clinical Pharmacy Education Specialist

Anne LaVance, BS, CPhT
Delgado Community College

Wendy Almeda Lubin BS, CPhT
Front Range Community College

Nader Rassaei, MD, MA, BS, CPhT
El Paso Community College

Andrea Redman, Pharm D, BCPS
Emory Healthcare

Hannah Brooke Stokely, BS, CPhT
Southeastern Institute, Pfeiffer Institute

Veronica Velasquez, BA, PhTR, CPhT
Austin Community College

Irene Villatoro, BS, PhTR, CPhT
San Jacinto College North

Special Thanks

A special thank you to **Don A. Ballington**, **Mary M. Laughlin**, and the many experts and contributors who contributed to earlier editions of this courseware.

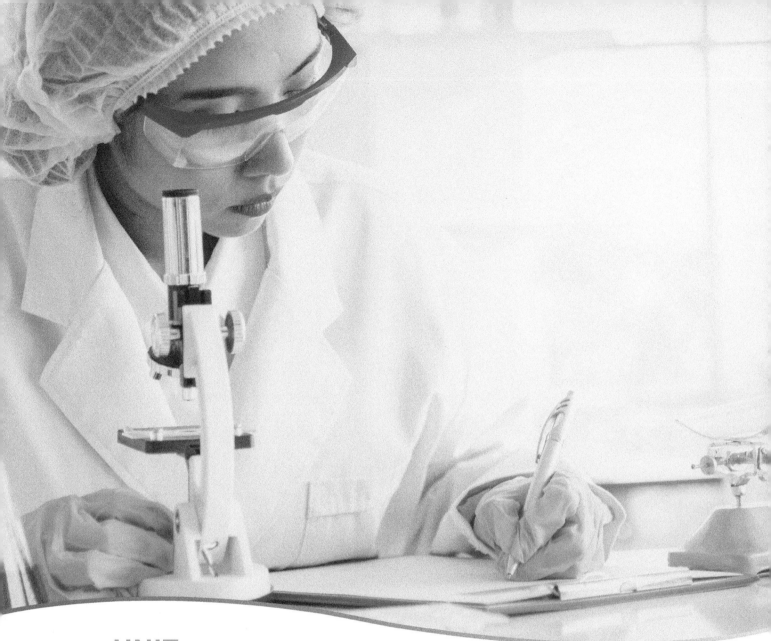

UNIT

1 Introduction to Pharmacology

Chapter 1   Introduction to Pharmacology and Medications in the Body   3

Chapter 2   Pharmaceutical Development   21

Chapter 3   Pharmacology Study for the Pharmacy Technician   43

Chapter 4   Medication Safety and Prescription Orders   59

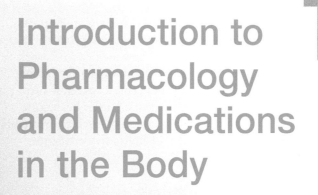

Introduction to Pharmacology and Medications in the Body

1

Learning Objectives

1 Describe the term *pharmacology*. (Introduction)

2 Explain why the pharmacy technician needs to understand and learn about pharmacology. (Introduction)

3 Describe the role of receptors in the body. (Section 1.2)

4 Compare and contrast the meaning of agonist and antagonist in terms of pharmacology. (Section 1.2)

5 Explain the concepts associated with pharmacodynamics: messengers, receptors, and mechanisms of drug action. (Section 1.2)

6 Describe the four processes of pharmacokinetics: absorption, distribution, metabolism, and elimination. (Section 1.2)

7 Define the terms used to describe the beneficial and harmful effects of drugs. (Section 1.3)

8 Describe the ways through which common drug interactions occur. (Section 1.3)

9 Explain why pharmacy technicians should be familiar with complementary and alternative therapies. (Section 1.4)

ASHP/ACPE Accreditation Standards

To view the *ASHP/ACPE Accreditation Standards* addressed in this chapter, refer to Appendix C.

People have been treating physical and mental ailments with drugs for thousands of years. A **drug**, or medicine, is a substance that changes the way a living organism functions. Tremendous advances have been made in understanding how diseases and disorders are caused and how they are treated with medicine.

Pharmacology is the study of drugs, including their origins, properties, actions, and effects on the body. The goal of drug therapy is to produce a response in the body that cures or controls a specific disease or medical condition. The main concepts (or divisions) of pharmacology—pharmacodynamics, the branch of pharmacology that studies a drug's effects or actions on the body, and pharmacokinetics, the study of what happens to a drug in the body through the processes of absorption, distribution, metabolism, and elimination—are discussed more in depth in this chapter. An understanding of these processes enables safe and effective treatments to be developed for various diseases.

Pharmacy technicians are important members of the healthcare team, and understanding pharmacology will help them in several ways. Familiarity with medication properties—how medications work, how they are administered, and for what they are used—can help pharmacy technicians in the preparation and handling of medications. In addition, this knowledge helps pharmacy technicians effectively communicate with patients and other healthcare workers. This chapter will cover foundational pharmacology concepts, such as medicinal drugs, drug actions, drug effects, and complementary and alternative medicine.

1.1 Medicinal Drugs

Recall that a drug is used to change the way a living organism functions. Drug action on a living system is known as **pharmacologic effect**. Medications are used for many reasons, such as relief of symptoms, replacement of missing natural chemicals, supplementation, diagnosis of disease, disease prevention, and healing. Drugs are often classified according to their use. Drugs can be used to treat a disease or relieve symptoms of a disease; this type of drug is a **therapeutic agent**. In some situations a drug can also be used to prevent a disease; this type of drug is known as a **prophylactic drug**.

Drug Origins and Sources

The study and identification of natural sources for drugs is called **pharmacognosy**. Drugs are derived from a variety of sources: plant parts or products, animals, fungi, minerals, chemicals, and recombinant deoxyribonucleic acid (rDNA). **rDNA** is a type of DNA that has been formed in a laboratory by combining two or more different strands of DNA from different organisms.

Various parts of many plants can be used to make drugs. Examples of drugs that are derived from plants include ergotamine (Ergomar) from rye fungi, digoxin (Lanoxin) from foxglove, and morphine from the opium poppy. Drugs from animal products include some thyroid replacement medications that are obtained from porcine (pig) thyroid glands. An example of a drug derived from a mineral is silver nitrate.

Many drugs are produced synthetically from chemical substances and have a low molecular weight. These are known as **small molecules**. Small molecules have been the mainstay of drug development over the years. The majority of drugs available on the market today are small molecules. Many small molecule drugs can be taken orally. Their small size helps them penetrate cell membranes and work inside the body's cells. Examples of small molecule drugs include aspirin, atorvastatin (Lipitor) for cholesterol, and citalopram (Celexa) for depression.

Bioengineered drugs, produced by rDNA technology, are some of the most expensive drugs available. These drugs are also known as **large molecules** or biologics. They are large protein structures that are complex and extremely complicated to develop. Often, biologics are made within a living system like modified cells of bacteria, yeast, or mammalian cells. It can take greater than 1,000 process steps to assemble the final biologic drug. Large molecules or biologic drugs are given through injection or infusion because if they were to be taken by mouth, they would be digested in the stomach and intestines like other proteins. Examples of large molecule drugs are adalimumab (Humira) and etanercept (Enbrel), which are used to treat rheumatoid arthritis. The development of bioengineered drugs has led to treatment options for medical conditions that in the past had no other options. Table 1.1 provides examples of drug sources along with the corresponding drug names and therapeutic effects.

TABLE 1.1 Drug Sources, Drug Names, and Their Therapeutic Effects

Drug Source	Drug Name	Therapeutic Effect
Animal: pig	Armour Thyroid	Thyroid hormone
Bioengineered: adalimuab	Humira	Stimulator of red blood cell formation
Mineral: silver	Silver nitrate	Anti-infective
Plant: foxglove	Digoxin	Cardiac
Synthetic: omeprazole	Prilosec	Gastric acid inhibitor

Drug Names

Drugs are often referred to by either a generic name or brand name. The **generic name** or **nonproprietary name** identifies the drug without regard to who is manufacturing and marketing the drug, such as acetaminophen. Also referred to as a USAN (United States Adopted Name), the generic name is not protected by a trademark. It is often a shortened version of the chemical name or an indicator of the class of drug. The **brand name** (also known as the trade name or proprietary name) is the name under which the manufacturer markets the drug, such as Tylenol. It is a trademark of a particular company, which has the exclusive right to use that brand name.

The generic name for a drug begins with a lowercase letter, as in pantoprazole, whereas the brand name usually begins with a capital letter, as in Protonix. Both terms refer to the same drug. Several different companies can manufacture the drug denoted by a given generic name, but they use different brand names.

Drug names are developed according to principles of safety, consistency, and logic, while considering the drug's intended use and existing brand names. *The USP Dictionary of USAN and International Drug Names* describes the process for giving a name. General considerations include safety in using the name for prescribing, dispensing, ordering, and administering a drug as well as suitability of the name for use in health-related educational programs and publications. Another consideration is the ability to use the name for drug identification and exchange of information internationally. A request for a drug name is made after an investigational new drug application has been submitted to the Food and Drug Administration (FDA).

Pharm Fact

Generic names can offer clues for how the drug works or the condition for which the drug is used. For example, atorva<u>statin</u> and prava<u>statin</u> are statin drugs used to treat high cholesterol.

1.2 Drug Actions

Drugs work by a variety of mechanisms. Although detailed understanding of these mechanisms involves an advanced knowledge of biochemistry (the chemistry of the molecules of living organisms) and is beyond the scope of this book, it is important for the pharmacy technician to have a basic understanding of these processes.

Homeostasis describes the body's constant effort to maintain a state of health and stability. Homeostasis is achieved by a system of control and feedback mechanisms that helps the body to keep its living processes in balance. When the body's own processes cannot maintain a healthy state, drugs can be used to help restore or maintain homeostasis. Many drugs exert powerful and specific actions in the body by working the same way as the chemical components the body itself uses for control and feedback. Understanding these processes, including pharmacodynamics and pharmacokinetics, will help a pharmacy technician better understand the drugs that are dispensed from the pharmacy every day.

Pharmacodynamics

Pharmacodynamics is a branch of pharmacology that studies the drug's molecular, biochemical, and physiologic effects or actions on the body. In other words, it is how the drug acts on the body. All medications produce their effects by interacting with biological targets.

Messengers and Receptors

For the body to maintain healthy control over its processes, cells must perform various tasks and communicate with each other. The principal way in which cells communicate is through the action of chemical messengers. These messengers are chemical substances that cells produce and send out into the extracellular fluids of the body. Histamine, prostaglandin, and bradykinin are some important **endogenous chemical messengers** (ones that originate within the body). Once the messenger has been released, it can diffuse throughout the extracellular fluid and eventually reach its target cell. The messenger recognizes and communicates with the target cell via a specific protein molecule, or receptor, on the surface of or within the cell. A **receptor** is what the drug binds to in the body to cause an effect or reaction. When the messenger molecule binds with the receptor, some effect is produced in the target cell. That effect is the next step in the body's response to the condition that caused the messenger to be produced.

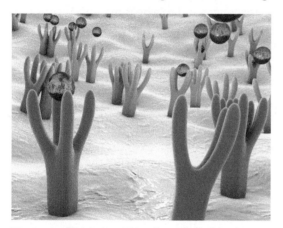

The receptors (depicted in red) are bound by the chemical messengers (in black).

The various types of cells within the body contain different types of receptors, and only certain cell types possess the receptor required to combine with a particular chemical messenger. To bind with a specific cell type, the messenger must have a chemical structure (i.e., the specific geometrical arrangement of atoms) that is complementary to the structure of that cell's receptors. This property of a receptor site is known as **specificity**. For example, the cells involved in immune responses have receptors that are highly specific to molecules on the surfaces of bacteria, viruses, and some cancer cells. Receptors control many important body functions, such as blood clotting and smooth muscle contraction; they also play an important role in protecting the body against injury and infection.

The strength by which a specific messenger binds to its receptor site is referred to as its **affinity** for the site. Affinity is an important concept for understanding how drugs work in the body.

Mechanisms of Drug Action

Drugs act like chemical messengers to perform their specific actions in the body. Like chemical messengers, drugs can also use receptors to bind to the body and cause an effect or reaction. Some drugs bind to a particular receptor and trigger the same cellular response as the body's own chemical messenger. Such a drug is termed an **agonist** of the messenger and enhances the natural reactions of the body.

Other drugs work using a competitive mechanism to block the action of the endogenous messenger. When two substances, such as an endogenous messenger and a drug, have an affinity for the same receptor, they compete for available receptor sites. The number of receptor molecules occupied by each substance depends on the relative concentrations of the two substances as well as their relative affinities for the

Practice Tip

Drugs that are classified as blockers (like beta-blockers) are antagonists. This means beta-blockers prevent stimulation of certain beta-receptors.

receptor. A drug that has a similar structure to the endogenous messenger may have a high affinity for the receptor site. When the drug binds to the receptor site, it prevents the endogenous messenger from binding there. If the drug does not trigger the cell's response itself, it inhibits the natural reaction of the body to the messenger. Such a drug is termed an **antagonist** (see Figure 1.1).

FIGURE 1.1 Antagonist Drugs

Medications typically work as agonists (those that stimulate a receptor site) or antagonists (those that block a receptor site to prevent stimulation).

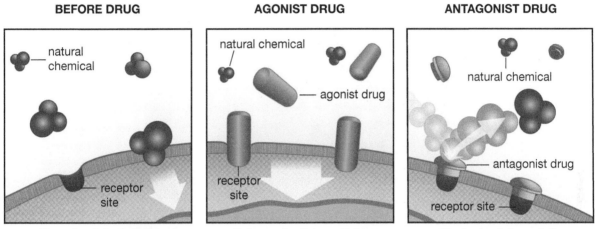

| BEFORE DRUG | AGONIST DRUG | ANTAGONIST DRUG |

Normal cellular activity · Enhanced cellular activity · Blocked cellular activity

Some drugs produce their effects not by interacting with specific receptors but by embedding themselves in cell membranes, which largely consist of chemically nonspecific lipids. A **lipid** is a fatty molecule, which is an important part of the cell membrane. Lipids generally repel water. The effectiveness of these drugs is related to their lipid solubility. **Solubility** is the ability of a substance to dissolve in a fluid, whether a watery one such as blood or a fatty one such as membrane lipids.

Drugs can also combine with specific molecules in the body other than receptors, such as enzymes, transport proteins, and nucleic acids. Some antidepressants, for example, work by binding to the protein that removes the messenger serotonin from nerve terminals.

Other drugs act without any direct interaction with the cell. For example, some drugs can work through an osmotic effect, meaning they can change the amount of water available to flow across a permeable barrier. Mannitol (Osmitrol) is such a drug. It interferes osmotically with water reabsorption by the kidneys.

Work Wise

Some pharmacists and other health-care providers use the term PK as an abbreviation for *pharmacokinetics* and *ADME* for absorption, distribution, metabolism, and elimination.

Pharmacokinetics

The study of the activity of a drug within the body over a period of time is known as **pharmacokinetics**. In other words, pharmacokinetics is the study of how the body affects the drug. Pharmacokinetic research enables scientists to understand how a drug works within the body to affect both normal physiology and disease.

Pharmacokinetics can be described in terms of four processes with the body: absorption, distribution, metabolism, and elimination. These processes are often referred to as **ADME**. An understanding of these processes provides an important framework for researchers who are involved in developing drugs. Figure 1.2 presents a schematic model of these processes.

FIGURE 1.2
The Pharmacokinetic Process

The main phases of drug/body interactions are absorption, distribution, metabolism, and elimination (ADME).

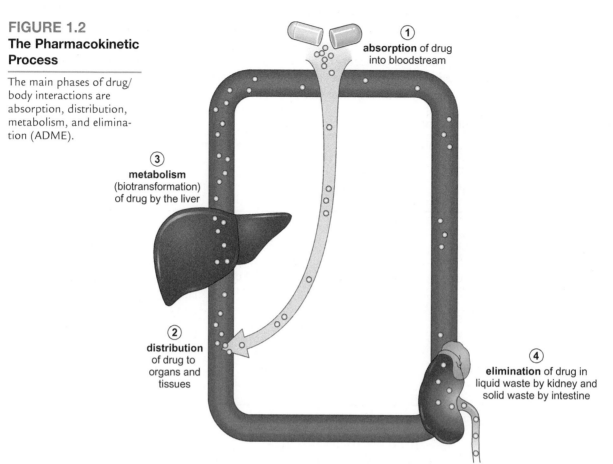

① **absorption** of drug into bloodstream

③ **metabolism** (biotransformation) of drug by the liver

② **distribution** of drug to organs and tissues

④ **elimination** of drug in liquid waste by kidney and solid waste by intestine

Absorption

Absorption is the process whereby a drug enters the circulatory system. That is, the chemical constituents of the drug are absorbed into the bloodstream. The absorption of a drug depends on its route of administration, its solubility in blood or other bodily fluids, and other physical properties. The form of the drug is an important factor controlling its solubility. For example, drugs in liquid solution are already dissolved, so they are absorbed more readily than those in solid form.

Practice Tip

Absorption of certain orally administered drugs depends on food. Some drugs are absorbed better by the body on an empty stomach. Others are better absorbed with food. As a pharmacy technician, you can help patients by placing auxiliary labels on drugs that require special attention to food.

The most common route of administration is oral. Other routes include intramuscular, subcutaneous, rectal, sublingual, transdermal, inhalation, and epicutaneous (topical) routes. Intravenous and intra-arterial administration do not require time for absorption because the drug is immediately present in the systemic blood circulation.

Disintegration and dissolution depend on the physical properties of the drug and its dosage form. Oral medications in the form of tablets or capsules must first disintegrate to release the drug into the gastrointestinal (GI) tract, where it is dissolved; therefore, the rate of absorption is slower with tablets and capsules than with oral solutions. Factors that affect dissolution include the chemistry of the drug as well as manufacturing variables such as the surface area of the drug particles released from the tablet or capsule. Some drugs interact with gastric contents such as food. This effect can reduce the amount of drug available for absorption or, more often, increase the amount of time it takes the drug to be absorbed.

Because of its large surface area, the small intestine is the primary site of absorption for many drugs, just as it is the site of absorption for food. The degree of movement within the GI tract also affects absorption of oral drugs. The faster the rate of gastric emptying, the more rapid the absorption rate of a drug because it reaches the vast absorptive surface of the small intestine more quickly.

In the small intestine, the drug must cross the cell membranes of the epithelial cells. Membranes are composed of lipids, proteins, and carbohydrates. Pores are small openings or empty spaces in the membrane through which low-weight molecules pass freely. Lipid-soluble molecules, small hydrophilic (water-soluble) molecules, and ions readily pass through cell membranes. Some drugs may be metabolized by enzyme action within the epithelial cells before they reach systemic blood.

Distribution

Distribution is the process by which a drug moves from the bloodstream into other body fluids and tissues and ultimately to its sites of action. Blood flow is the most important rate limiting factor for distribution of a drug. Three additional factors affect the rate and degree of distribution.

Binding to Plasma Proteins The biological activity of a drug relates to the concentration of unbound or "free" drug in circulation. If a drug molecule binds to a protein in blood plasma, that drug molecule is essentially inactive. An unbound drug molecule, however, can reach its site of action. Disease states can also affect protein binding. Renal failure, for example, may cause a loss of plasma proteins (with less available for binding) or accumulation of metabolic wastes that could potentially displace some bound drugs. Liver disease may also decrease the number of plasma proteins to transport drugs. These conditions can therefore increase both the therapeutic and the toxic effects of a drug.

Binding to Cellular Constituents Drugs can bind to proteins other than those in blood plasma, such as proteins in tissues. This type of binding usually occurs when the drug has an affinity for some cellular constituent.

Blood-Brain Barrier The capillaries in the central nervous system (CNS) are enveloped by glial cells, which present a barrier to many water-soluble compounds. This **blood-brain barrier** prevents many substances from entering the cerebrospinal fluid from the blood. Therefore, many drugs cannot get to the CNS because they are unable to pass through the blood-brain barrier. Pathologic states such as inflammation will reduce this resistance, and the barrier can become more permeable under such conditions. For example, though general anesthetics easily penetrate this barrier, penicillin cannot penetrate the CNS unless the meninges are swollen.

Metabolism

Metabolism is the process of converting drugs to other biochemical compounds and then excreting them through metabolic pathways. The converted substance is called a **metabolite** of the drug, and the sequence of chemical steps that convert a drug to a metabolite is called a **metabolic pathway**. The liver is the primary site for drug metabolism. The liver is able to metabolize medications through a system of enzymes called **cytochrome P-450**.

Many factors can alter metabolism. Disease states, age, and genetic predisposition all affect the way the body metabolizes drugs. In addition, induction and inhibition of the cytochrome P-450 enzymes are two processes that are important to drug metabolism.

Induction **Induction** refers to an increase in the amount of an enzyme available to metabolize a drug. Drugs, foods, and smoking can affect the concentration of a particular enzyme. Drugs that increase these enzymes can decrease the pharmacologic response to other agents (e.g., phenobarbital increases the metabolism and therefore decreases the effect of warfarin) or to themselves (e.g., carbamazepine (Tegretol) can stimulate self-metabolism).

Inhibition **Inhibition** refers to a decrease in the amount of an enzyme available to metabolize a drug. Some agents can slow or block enzyme activity, which impairs the metabolism of drugs and may increase their concentration. This could result in an increase in the drugs' pharmacologic effects or cause toxicity. For example, alprazolam (Xanax) is a benzodiazepine that can be used for anxiety. When combined with a drug that inhibits its metabolism (such as the antifungal drug ketoconazole), alprazolam concentrations increase. This can lead to undesirable effects such as respiratory depression.

In addition, if given together, two drugs may decrease or enhance each other's metabolism. Some drugs decrease the metabolism of other drugs by competitive inhibition. **Competitive inhibition** is a process whereby one drug blocks enzyme activity and impairs the metabolism of another drug; this can generally be overcome by increasing the dosage. **Noncompetitive inhibition** occurs when a drug completely blocks enzyme activity and impairs the metabolism of another drug. Increasing the dose of the other drug will not overcome the interaction. Often this type of inhibition leads to **complete inhibition** whereby the drug cannot be metabolized by the body.

Elimination

Elimination, the removal of a drug or its metabolites from the body, occurs primarily in the kidneys (through urine) and the liver (through feces), but other routes exist. Drugs may be exhaled by the lungs or excreted in perspiration, saliva, and breast milk. The rate at which a drug is eliminated from a specific volume of blood per unit of time is referred to as its **clearance**.

Pharmacokinetic Parameters

An understanding of the pharmacokinetic processes enables researchers to determine how a drug should be administered to the patient to obtain a specific response. Safe and effective drug therapy requires that a drug is delivered to its target sites in concentrations that will treat the disease state for which it is intended without producing a state of toxicity.

A **dose** is the quantity of a drug administered at one time (e.g., milligrams). **Dosage** refers to the administration of a specific amount, dose number, and dose frequency of drug (e.g., 325 mg every 6 hours). The **dose-response** relationship of a drug is studied in order to maximize the benefit of the medicine and reduce the toxicity. As higher dosages of a drug are given, a greater response will occur. However, a point is reached where no greater benefit is seen or the adverse effects or toxicities of the drug are greater than the benefits. This limitation is called the **ceiling effect**. This relationship can be seen on a **dose-response curve** (see Figure 1.3). Increased dosing beyond the ceiling may result in toxicity, leading to side effects or even death.

FIGURE 1.3
Dose-Response Curve

As greater doses of a drug are given, a greater response is noted until a point is reached when the response no longer improves with increased dosing. This is known as the ceiling effect.

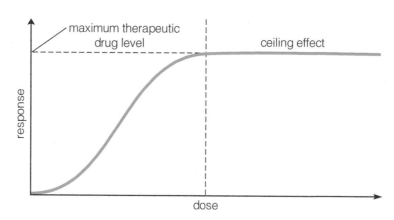

Many dosages are fairly universal from patient to patient. In some cases, however, dosage must be individualized to the patient because of variables such as age, size, weight, sex, race, nutritional state, disease state, kidney function, and pregnancy, as well as other drugs the patient may be taking. A determination of individual patient dose and dosing intervals can be made, if necessary, based on the testing of drug concentrations in body fluids such as blood, plasma, and urine. Typically, only a portion of the dose administered becomes biologically active in the body. The fraction of the administered dose that is available to the target tissue is an expression of the drug's **bioavailability** (see Figure 1.4). Drugs taken orally must pass through the intestinal wall and traverse the liver before entering the blood and reaching systemic sites. Metabolism in the liver before a drug reaches the systemic circulation is referred to as the **first-pass effect** (or first-pass metabolism). If a drug undergoes considerable first-pass metabolism, its bioavailability will be decreased when it is administered orally. Some drugs have such a substantial first-pass effect.

FIGURE 1.4
Furosemide Labels

Oral furosemide is approximately 50% bioavailable. Therefore, only half of the ingested amount is available to the target tissue. Nearly all of a dose of intravenous furosemide is bioavailable. The oral furosemide label shown in the top image is 40 mg while the intravenous furosemide label in the bottom image is 20 mg. Due to the bioavailability of each dosage form, these doses are roughly equivalent in terms of physiologic effect.

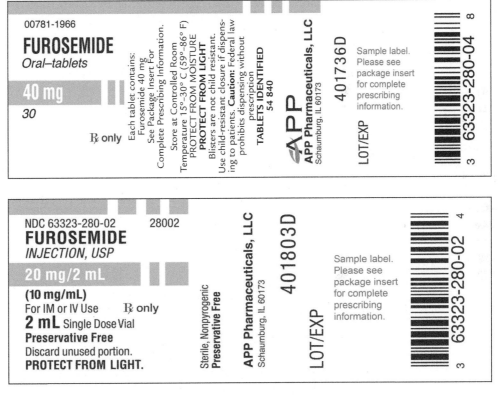

The **therapeutic range**, also called the therapeutic window, is the range of serum concentrations for a particular drug that provides the optimum probability of achieving the desired response with the least probability of toxicity. Figure 1.5 illustrates the concept of therapeutic range. A defined therapeutic range provides the best chance for successful therapy. Some patients may require concentrations of drug below or above the usual therapeutic range.

FIGURE 1.5
Therapeutic Range

An optimum dosage range yields beneficial effects without causing toxic effects, whereas underdosing has little benefit on the healing process, and over-dosing can lead to toxicity and death.

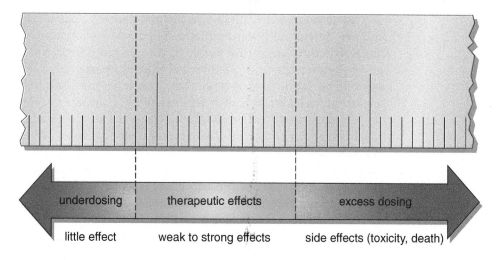

underdosing | therapeutic effects | excess dosing

little effect | weak to strong effects | side effects (toxicity, death)

Doses and dosing intervals are determined by results from clinical trials but may need to be adjusted on an individual basis. Adjustment is often determined based on a blood sample and is particularly beneficial for attaining the desired concentration for a drug with a narrow therapeutic range. When the amount of drug in a patient's blood gives the desired response, it is said to be at the **therapeutic level**.

The length of time a drug is at the therapeutic level is referred to as its **duration of action**. This concept is illustrated by the curve in Figure 1.6.

FIGURE 1.6
Duration of Action

Duration of action is the time when the plasma drug concentration is at the therapeutic level (the time between the onset and termination of drug action).

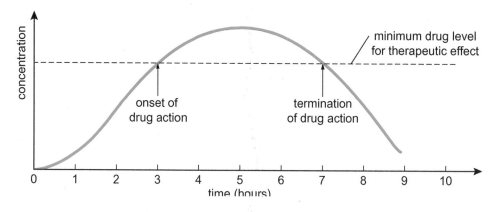

The time required to achieve therapeutic levels of a drug can be shortened by the administration of a **loading dose**—an amount of a drug that will bring the blood concentration rapidly to a therapeutic level. When the drug concentration reaches a therapeutic level, the patient receives a **maintenance dose** at regular intervals to keep the drug at a therapeutic level. The rate of clearance of the drug is important for calculating the maintenance dose.

Pharmacokinetic Modeling

Pharmacokinetic modeling is a method of mathematically describing the process of absorption, distribution, metabolism, and elimination of a drug within the body. For some drugs, elimination is a **zero-order** process; that is, a fixed quantity of drug is eliminated per unit of time. The best example is alcohol. For the majority of drugs, elimination is said to be **first order**; that is, a constant fraction of the remaining drug is eliminated per unit of time. The time it takes the body to eliminate half of such a drug is called the **half-life** of the drug and is written $t_{1/2}$. A longer half-life implies a longer duration of the drug action. It takes about five to seven half-lives to consider the drug "removed" from the body—meaning that only 1%–3% remains. If the $t_{1/2}$ of a drug is two hours, then the majority of the drug will be gone in 10 to 14 hours. If the $t_{1/2}$ is 30 hours, then it will take 150 to 210 hours, or six to nine days, to eliminate most of the drug. A drug with a long half-life may produce effects for days or even weeks after being discontinued.

1.3 Drug Effects

The pharmacokinetics described above provide critical insight for predicting the effects of each specific drug. Some effects are beneficial, while other effects can be detrimental or dangerous. Just as each person is different, each person's reaction to a drug may be different. Thus, monitoring patients closely helps to ensure their response to the drug is appropriate.

Beneficial Responses

The desired action of a drug in the treatment of a disease state or symptom is referred to as a **therapeutic effect**. The therapeutic effect is the action for which the drug is prescribed. Drugs can act locally, or they can act on the body as a whole. A **local effect** is confined to a specific part of the body (e.g., using lidocaine to numb an area for stitches). A **systemic effect**, on the other hand, is a generalized, all-inclusive effect on the entire body (e.g., using lisinopril to lower blood pressure).

Sometimes drugs are prescribed to prevent the occurrence of an infection or disease. In this case, the drug effect is referred to as **prophylaxis**. Patients who will be undergoing surgery often receive prophylactic antibiotics, which aim to prevent the occurrence of infections.

In selecting a drug for an individual patient, the healthcare practitioner considers its medically accepted uses and situations in which it should or should not be given. A disease, symptom, or condition for which a drug is known to be of benefit is termed an **indication** for the drug; that is, if the patient has the condition, use of the drug may be beneficial. A disease, symptom, or condition for which the drug may be beneficial and may do harm is termed a **precaution**. Precautions are situations where the benefit of the medication may still outweigh the risks, but the risks need to be further evaluated by the prescriber. When a drug will cause harm and should not be used due to a specific situation (e.g., disease state, drug interaction, pregnancy), it is called a **contraindication**.

Practice Tip

Over-the-counter (OTC) drugs are medications that may be purchased without a prescription.

Adverse Effects or Side Effects

An **adverse effect** or **side effect** is a secondary response to a drug other than the primary therapeutic effect that the drug was intended to produce. Nausea, rash, and constipation are the most common side effects of many medications and are usually fairly tolerable. Other side effects can be more bothersome and even serious. On occasion, drugs can be prescribed for their side effects. For example, many antihistamines cause drowsiness, and therefore, they are found in many over-the-counter (OTC) insomnia preparations.

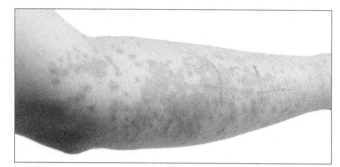

Hives are caused by an allergic reaction.

Allergic Responses

An **allergic response** is a local or general reaction of the immune system to a substance. A substance that produces an allergic response is known as an **allergen**. In general, a molecule that stimulates an immune response, whether allergic or not, is known as an **antigen**.

The first exposure to an allergen may produce little or no observable response. Rather, what is critical about the initial exposure is the resulting "memory storage" that characterizes active immunity. Upon a subsequent exposure, the body recognizes ("remembers") the antigen and responds with a more potent antibody response. This response can elicit reactions that range from uncomfortable to life threatening. Although some responses start within minutes of exposure, others may be delayed.

Exposure to the allergen may be mild, moderate, or, in some cases, severe. Some common allergic reactions to drugs include nasal secretions, swelling, wheezing, an excessively rapid heart rate, **urticaria** (hives), **pruritus** (itching), **angioedema** (abnormal accumulation of fluid in tissue), **wheals** (red, elevated areas on body), and, in rare cases, even death.

An **anaphylactic reaction** is a severe allergic response resulting in immediate, life-threatening respiratory distress, usually followed by vascular collapse and shock and accompanied by hives. An **idiosyncratic reaction** is an unusual or unexpected response to a drug that is unrelated to the dose given.

Other Responses to Drugs

Drug dependence is a state in which a person's body adapts physiologically and psychologically to a drug and cannot function without it. Dependence should not be confused with **drug addiction**, which is a dependence characterized by a perceived need to use a drug to attain the psychological and physical effects of mood-altering substances. One sign of addiction is a decrease in psychological well-being and social or vocational functioning. Patients who are being treated for various disease states may become dependent on medications without exhibiting the signs of addiction.

Drug abuse is the use of a drug for purposes other than those prescribed and/or in amounts that were not directed. Abusive use of drugs can be, but is not always, linked to addiction.

When patients have been taking a drug over a significant period, they may begin to develop a decreased response to the drug. This decrease in response to the effects of a drug with continued administration is referred to as **tolerance**. As tolerance develops, the dosage of the drug may need to be increased to maintain a constant response.

Drug Interactions

Another reaction to drugs involves interaction. One drug can have an effect on the action of another. A **drug interaction** is a change in the action of a drug that is caused by another drug, a food, or a substance such as alcohol or nicotine. A common mechanism in which a substance can interact with a drug is by inducing or inhibiting enzymes that metabolize the drug, as described previously. A system of enzymes called cytochrome P-450 contributes to many drug interactions because it plays a key role in oxidizing drugs and other substances.

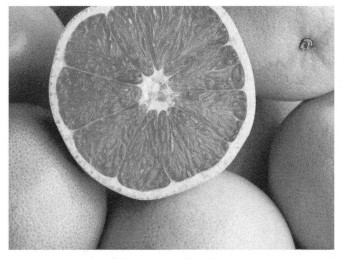

Grapefruit and grapefruit juice interfere with proper absorption of several common drugs.

Grapefruit provides an example of a food-drug interaction. Grapefruit juice contains certain chemicals that inhibit a form of cytochrome P-450 that is found primarily in the intestines. Because of this inhibition, less of the drug undergoes first-pass metabolism, so more active drug is absorbed into the bloodstream, increasing the risk of overdose. The effect of grapefruit juice on intestinal enzymes is partially irreversible; thus, enzyme levels do not return to normal immediately after the juice is cleared from the intestine. Absorption of drugs from the intestines may be affected for up to a day following ingestion of grapefruit juice.

It is important that prescribers and pharmacists have a complete list of all prescription drugs, OTC medications, vitamins, and herbal remedies that a patient is taking so that potential interactions can be recognized and appropriately handled. The pharmacy technician should routinely ask for this information. Table 1.2 lists common drug relationships, including **addition** (the combined effect of two drugs), **potentiation** (when one drug increases or prolongs the effect of another drug), and **synergism** (the combined effect of two drugs is more intense or longer than the sum of their individual effects).

TABLE 1.2 Common Drug Relationships

Drug Relationship	Description
Addition	The combined effect of two drugs is equal to the sum of the effects of each drug taken alone.
Antagonism	The action of one drug negates the action of a second drug.
Potentiation	One drug increases or prolongs the action of another drug, and the total effect is greater than the sum of the effects of each drug used alone. If one drug prescribed alone cannot produce the desired effect, another drug can be prescribed to increase the first drug's potency. This term is used when one of the drugs has little or no action when given alone, and the second drug increases the potency of the first drug.
Synergism	The combined effect of two drugs is more intense or longer in duration than the sum of their individual effects. Drugs that work synergistically are usually prescribed together.

1.4 Complementary and Alternative Medicine

Americans spend billions of dollars each year on many different types of alternative medicine. **Alternative medicine** is a term used to describe medical products and practices that are not part of standard care. It is used in place of conventional medicinal practices and standard care, and it may include homeopathy, herbs, supplements, and acupuncture. An example of alternative medicine could be using acupuncture to treat back pain from a muscle spasm.

Complementary medicine employs similar methods to alternative medicine but is used together with conventional practices. An example of complementary medicine is using an alternative strategy (acupuncture) with a conventional strategy (muscle relaxant medication) to treat back pain from a muscle spasm. However, pharmacy technicians should be aware that the terms *alternative* and *complementary medicine* may be used interchangeably. In fact, the abbreviation CAM stands for **complementary and alternative medicine**.

More than 40% of Americans admit to using CAM. Reasons for popularity include greater availability of information on the internet, increased contact with cultures that use alternative medicine, perceptions of greater safety, and distrust of conventional medicine.

Although interest in CAM is widespread, there are concerns about its use. First, scientific evidence to support the efficacy and safety of CAM is limited and usually does not mirror the strength of evidence available for drugs. Second, many healthcare providers (such as pharmacists and physicians) lack training for, knowledge of, and confidence in CAM. Third, patients frequently do not disclose use of CAM therapies to their healthcare providers. This omission may be dangerous because interactions can occur between CAM (such as herbs) and prescribed drugs.

CAM products do not undergo the same rigorous regulations as medications, which can cause confusion. For example, if a product is made by two different manufacturers, there is no way to know whether one is as strong as the other. Another example of CAM is cannabidiol (CBD), a chemical found in the cannabis plant. Unlike marijuana, CBD does not contain the psychoactive ingredient that produces a high. CBD has been used as a complementary or alternative medicine to treat health issues like anxiety, insomnia, or pain. CBD if often found as an oil, but products like food and beverages with CBD are also available. Like other CAM, CBD is unregulated, and concerns regarding the efficacy, safety, quality, and potency of CBD products exist.

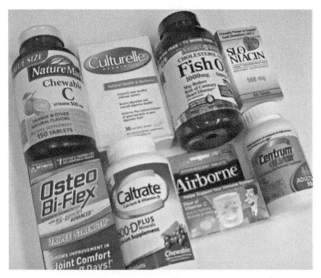

Manufacturers of dietary supplements are not permitted to make claims of curing or treating ailments. They may state only that the products are supplements to support health.

Dietary Supplements

A dietary supplement, especially an herb, exerts a weak pharmacologic effect on the body similar to that of drugs. A **dietary supplement** describes a category of nonprescription drugs that includes vitamins, minerals, and herbs. Glucosamine is an example of a dietary supplement that provides nutrients for bone cartilage to treat mild arthritic symptoms. Consequently, dietary supplements may cause side effects, adverse reactions, and drug interactions. As with OTC drugs, consumers can purchase dietary supplements without a prescription and should read the labels carefully.

Because dietary supplements are considered food supplements that maintain health, consumers should not exceed the recommended daily dose or serving size.

Pharmacy technicians should be aware that dietary supplements do not have the same stringent controls as prescription medications and are regulated by the Dietary Supplement Health and Education Act of 1994. The FDA can regulate dietary supplements only when concerns for patient safety exist, as in the case of weight-loss drugs. Consumers should know that while many of these products are tested by independent consumer laboratories, their quality is questionable.

The use of herbs by patients poses a challenge to healthcare practitioners. Quite often, patients take herbal supplements and fail to disclose that information when asked about their current medications or medication histories. As a result, some patients, particularly older adults, may have an adverse reaction when combining their herbal supplements and their prescription medications. Therefore, pharmacy technicians can help patients avoid adverse reactions by gathering and recording information about the patient's use of herbs or other dietary supplements.

Homeopathy

Another alternative medical practice pharmacy technicians may be asked about is homeopathy. Homeopathic products contain subclinical doses of natural extracts or alcohol tinctures in which the active ingredient is highly diluted from one part per ten (1:10) to greater than one part per thousand (1:1,000). These products can include ingredients from minerals, plants, chemicals, or animal or human sources. A main principle of homeopathy is that "like cures like," meaning that a substance that can produce symptoms in a healthy person can in small doses stimulate the body's own immune system to overcome the targeted symptom in a sick individual. Homeopathic products are available over the counter, and patients may seek their use to treat self-diagnosable conditions such as cold symptoms, headaches, and indigestion.

It is important to understand that homeopathic products are marketed without the FDA evaluating them for safety or effectiveness to diagnose, treat, cure, prevent, or mitigate any disease. The FDA has oversight over the manufacturing and labeling of homeopathic medications to ensure compliance with Current Good Manufacturing Practices.

Drug Facts

Active Ingredients .... Purpose

Conium maculatum 6X ....redness
Graphites 12X...dryness
Sulphur 12X .... tearing, burning

Uses:

According to homeopathic principles, the active ingredients in this medication temporarily relieve minor symptoms associated with styes, such as:
• redness • burning • dryness • tearing

Homeopathic medications contain one or more ingredients in a diluted form to stimulate the immune system.

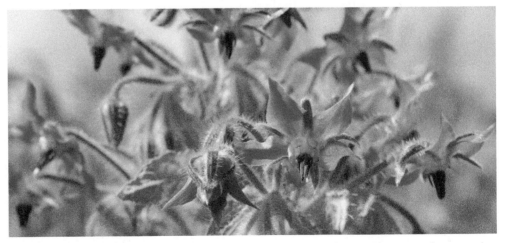

The flowers and leaves of the borage plant are used as a homeopathic remedy to treat fever, cough, and depression. The seed oil of the plant is used to treat skin conditions such as eczema and seborrheic dermatitis.

Review and Assessment

📖 CHAPTER SUMMARY

Drug Actions

- *Pharmacology* is a broad term that includes the study of drugs and their actions on the body.

- A receptor is a molecule on the surface of or within a cell that recognizes and binds with specific molecules, producing some effect in the cell.

- By binding to receptors on or within body cells, drugs can mimic or block the action of chemical messengers to exert powerful and specific actions in the body.

- One drug can compete with another drug for its intended receptor.

- Pharmacokinetics is the study of the time course of absorption, distribution, metabolism, and elimination (ADME) of drugs and their metabolites in relation to the time they are present in the body.

- The primary sites of elimination are the kidneys and the liver. Drugs may also be exhaled by the lungs or excreted in perspiration.

- Body fluids can be tested over a period of time to examine how the body handles a specific drug.

Drug Effects

- Drug effects include therapeutic effects and side effects.

- Drugs can interact with other drugs, herbs, food, and the patient's own body.

- Two drugs may be prescribed together because the combination has fewer or more tolerable side effects than a high dose of either.

✓ CHECK YOUR UNDERSTANDING

Take a moment to review what you have learned in this chapter and answer the following questions.

1. Responses other than the intended therapeutic one are referred to as
   a. side effects.
   b. synergisms.
   c. addictions.
   d. additions.

2. Which term refers to the desired action of a drug in the treatment of a particular disease state or symptom?
   a. side effects
   b. synergism
   c. therapeutic effect
   d. addiction

3. Increasing resistance to the usual effects of an established dosage of a drug as a result of continued use is known as
   a. an idiosyncratic reaction.
   b. an anaphylactic reaction.
   c. tolerance.
   d. dependence.

4. A response that is unusual, unexpected, or opposite from the expected response to a drug is
   a. an idiosyncratic reaction.
   b. an anaphylactic reaction.
   c. tolerance.
   d. dependence.

5. A severe, life-threatening allergic response with breathing difficulty, vascular collapse, and shock is
   a. an idiosyncratic reaction.
   b. an anaphylactic reaction.
   c. tolerance.
   d. dependence.

6. Complete removal of a drug from a specific volume of blood per unit of time is known as
   a. pharmacokinetics.
   b. bioavailability.
   c. volume of distribution.
   d. clearance.

7. A drug that is prescribed to prevent the occurrence of an infection or disease is referred to as
   a. allergic.
   b. localized.
   c. prophylaxis.
   d. systemic.

8. When the action of one drug negates the action of a second drug, it is referred to as a(n)
   a. addition.
   b. antagonism.
   c. potentiation.
   d. synergism.

9. The degree to which a drug becomes available to the target tissue is known as
   a. pharmacokinetics.
   b. bioavailability.
   c. volume of distribution.
   d. clearance.

10. The study of drug behavior in the human body is known as
    a. pharmacokinetics.
    b. bioavailability.
    c. volume of distribution.
    d. clearance.

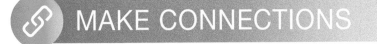

MAKE CONNECTIONS

Take a moment to consider what you have learned in this chapter and respond thoughtfully to the following prompts. Note that some of these activities will require internet access.

1. This chapter covered the basic information on how drugs work within the body, and this information is the foundation of your work as a pharmacy technician. How might you organize this knowledge for easy and rapid recall?

2. Allergic reactions to drugs and food can be life threatening. What can you, as a pharmacy technician, do to help patients prevent life-threatening allergic reactions?

 The online course includes additional review and assessment resources.

Pharmaceutical Development

2

Learning Objectives

1 Recognize the important contributors, events, and resources in pharmacology through the ages. (Section 2.1)

2 Describe various drug sources. (Section 2.2)

3 List the federal laws that regulate drugs and the agencies that administer those laws. (Section 2.3)

4 List the procedure for getting a new drug to market. (Section 2.3)

ASHP/ACPE Accreditation Standards
To view the *ASHP/ACPE Accreditation Standards* addressed in this chapter, refer to Appendix C.

The use of drugs to treat illnesses has changed dramatically since early civilizations first attempted to heal the sick. Pharmacology today is based on science and systematic research rather than conventional wisdom and trial and error. The discovery of many new drugs during the 20th century revolutionized medical care, and a rational system of laws governing drug manufacture and distribution was developed. Today, laws and regulations protect patients and ensure that drugs are effective and safe before they are approved for the market.

2.1 History of Medicinal Drugs

Over the last few centuries, tremendous advances have been made in the understanding of the causes of diseases and their treatments with medicine. The study of ancient documents shows that people have been treating physical and mental ailments with medicines for thousands of years. Clay tablets from Babylonia, from the 18th century BCE, list more than 500 medicinal remedies.

Early humans believed the world was controlled by good and evil spirits. The sick were thought to be victims of evil forces or of a god's anger. Consequently, medical treatment was largely controlled by religious leaders who guarded their healing knowledge closely. At the same time, folk knowledge of the healing properties of natural substances slowly grew through trial and error.

Early Remedies

For thousands of years, only materials like plants and minerals that were located nearby and were easy to gather were used as medicines. With time and experience, ancient people learned to formulate practical recipes for various treatments. Eventually, many of these ancient people began to document their recipes and remedies.

Plants and other naturally occurring substances were administered using some of the same methods used today: topically, orally, through inhalation, and rectally. The *Ebers Papyrus*, an Egyptian medical source compiled in approximately 1550 BCE, lists more than 700 different herbal remedies used by healers. These remedies consisted of botanical drugs drawn from the natural environment and used internally, such as castor bean, garlic, and poppy seed. The most common mixtures were laxatives and enemas. The concept of a drug (or a medication) appears in early Greek records as the word **pharmakon**, which also meant "magic spell," "remedy," or "poison."

The Greek physician Hippocrates (c. 460–377 BCE) was the first to propose that disease was caused by natural rather than supernatural causes. Although he practiced herbal medicine like his contemporaries, he rejected unsupported theory and superstition in favor of observation and classification, or empirical learning. Hippocrates was also the first to dissect the human body to study the functions of specific organs. He is often called the "father of medicine."

Another Greek physician, Galen (c. 130–201 CE), lived in Rome and built on Hippocrates's ideas of *empirical learning*, which means gaining knowledge by observation or experience. Using concepts discussed by Hippocrates and the philosopher Aristotle, Galen believed disease was caused by an imbalance in the blood, phlegm, black bile, or yellow bile (these were known as the four humors). Illnesses were treated using herbal compounds that were meant to bring balance to the body using the opposite quality (moist vs. dry or cold vs. warm). Galen's vast writings about these compounds that involved extraction of healing materials from plants, known as galenicals, influenced medical knowledge for more than 1,000 years. Greek physicians had such a profound effect on the field of medicine that knowledge of the Greek alphabet is vital to an understanding of many medical and pharmacologic terms. Greek letters may be found in some drug names. For example, interferon beta-1a (Rebif) is a medication that may be used to treat multiple sclerosis. Table 2.1 features the Greek alphabet.

De Materia Medica, a text compiled by Dioscorides in the first century CE, was a major influence on European pharmaceutical knowledge until the 16th century. In it, Dioscorides scientifically described and classified 600 plants by substance rather than by the disease they were intended to treat.

Chinese and Indian Medicine

The roots of Chinese traditional medicine rest on the extensive body of knowledge produced by Li Shizhen, a 16th-century Chinese physician who lived during the Ming Dynasty. Li Shizhen compiled a resource called *Bencao Gangmu (Compendium of Materia Medica)* that lists more than 1,000 plants and 8,000 recipes used in the treatment of illnesses. This work, which also describes the causes of various illnesses, is considered the most comprehensive text in traditional Chinese medicine.

In 1000 BCE, a Hindu surgeon named Sushruta wrote a medicinal work called *The Book of Life*. It is divided into 184 chapters and contains descriptions of 1,120 illnesses, 700 medicinal plants, 64 preparations (mixtures) from minerals, and 57 preparations from animal sources.

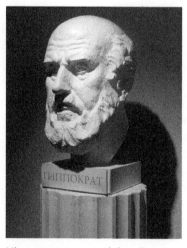

Hippocrates proposed that diseases came from natural rather than supernatural causes, and he was the first to dissect the human body to study the functions of specific organs.

TABLE 2.1 Greek Alphabet

Capital	Lowercase	Greek Name	English
A	α	alpha	a
B	β	beta	b
Γ	γ	gamma	g
Δ	δ	delta	d
E	ε	epsilon	e
Z	ζ	zeta	z
H	η	eta	h
Θ	θ	theta	th
I	ι	iota	i
K	κ	kappa	k
Λ	λ	lambda	l
M	μ	mu	m
N	ν	nu	n
Ξ	ξ	xi	x
O	o	omicron	o
Π	π	pi	p
P	ρ	rho	r
Σ	σ	sigma	s
T	τ	tau	t
Y	υ	upsilon	u
Φ	φ	phi	ph
X	χ	chi	ch
Ψ	ψ	psi	ps
Ω	ω	omega	o

Drugs in the Middle Ages

During the Middle Ages, as the Christian church became a dominating cultural force, the practice of medicine and pharmacy passed again from lay practitioners to religious leaders. Monasteries became centers of treatment and intellectual studies. Monks wrote and copied medical texts and grew medicinal plants in herb gardens.

The Swiss physician Paracelsus (1493–1541) was the first to challenge the teachings of Galen. He denounced the philosophy of humors in medicine and advocated the use of individual drugs rather than mixtures or potions. He reasoned that treating diseases with individual drugs would make it easier to determine which agent helped, which made the patient worse, and how much of a drug was needed. This concept continues to be used in modern pharmacology.

In 1546, Valerius Cordus, a German botanist and physician, published the *Dispensatorium* in Nuremberg, Germany. This was the first official **pharmacopoeia**, or listing of medicinal preparations, that soon became a model for other towns and countries.

Drugs in the Modern Age

The 17th and 18th centuries saw several advances in pharmacy and chemistry. In 1618, London physicians compiled the first English pharmacopoeia. Some drug mixtures introduced at this time, such as tincture of opium, cocoa, and ipecac, are still used today.

In the 19th century, the French physiologist Claude Bernard (1813–1878) advanced the knowledge of how drugs work on the body when he demonstrated that certain drugs (such as curare) have specific sites of action within the body. His use of laboratory methods to study drugs led him to be credited as one of the founders of the field of **pharmacology**, which is the science of drugs and their interactions with the systems of living animals.

Pharm Fact

Note that the term *apothecary* can describe both the profession and a business.

Early North American Pharmacology

Early North American colonies had few medical personnel. As a result, early settlers had to rely on domestic or home remedies. As the colonies grew in the 18th century, they attracted a broader range of immigrants, including physicians and apothecaries. An **apothecary** was the forerunner of today's pharmacist and pharmacy.

Like their European counterparts, most colonial physicians owned a dispensary or pharmacy. They prescribed, prepared, and dispensed drugs imported from Britain. The American Revolution forced American physicians, druggists, and wholesale distributors of drugs to manufacture their own chemically based drugs and to make common preparations of crude drugs. In 1820, the first official listing of drugs in the United States, the *Pharmacopoeia of the United States*, known today as the **US Pharmacopeia (USP)**, was published by the Massachusetts Medical Society, with approval from a national convention of physicians.

During the 19th century, in both the United States and Europe, a division emerged between those medical practitioners who treated patients and those who were primarily interested in preparing medicines. It wasn't until after the American Civil War (1861–1865), however, that the boundaries between the professions of physician and pharmacist were clearly drawn. Practitioners who treated patients supported the growth of the pharmaceutical profession because it released them from the responsibility of compounding medicines and stocking a shop. In 1852, the American Pharmaceutical Association (now called the American Pharmacists Association), or APhA, was formed, partly as a result of encroachment by other medical areas into pharmacy. Through this organization, pharmacists realized the opportunity for individual growth and increased professional stature.

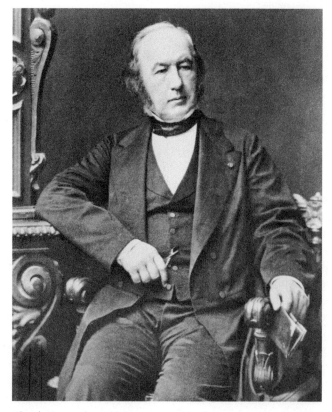
Claude Bernard used laboratory methods to study drugs and demonstrated that certain drugs have specific sites of action within the body.

19th- and 20th-Century Pharmacology

By the second half of the 19th century, pharmacology had become a scientific discipline. Following the lead of Oswald Schmiedeberg (1838–1921) at the University of Strasbourg in Germany, several European universities established departments of pharmacology.

Major breakthroughs in medical care came with the discovery of several important drugs. In 1847, Ignaz Semmelweis helped reduce deaths from puerperal fever by requiring those entering maternity wards to scrub their hands first in chlorinated limewater. In the 1860s, Joseph Lister introduced antiseptics into surgery with his use of carbolic acid for cleansing instruments and suture materials.

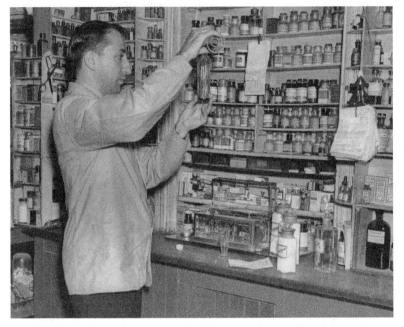

By the 1940s, pharmacies in the United States were employing many modern techniques and medications that are still in use today.

In 1907, Paul Ehrlich, a German bacteriologist, introduced arsphenamine, or Salvarsan, to treat syphilis. This rudimentary antimicrobial was the first chemical agent used to treat an infectious disease. In 1923, Sir Frederick Banting, a Canadian physiologist, and his assistant Charles Best successfully extracted the hormone insulin from the pancreas to create the first effective treatment for diabetes.

In the 1920s and 1930s, bacterial infections from *staphylococci* and *streptococci* claimed the lives of many. In 1935, the first sulfa drug, Prontosil, was introduced by German physician Gerhardt Domagk. Sulfa drugs were used to treat conditions such as meningitis, pneumonia, and gonorrhea. The introduction and use of penicillin, however, shifted use away from sulfa drugs. The first penicillin was discovered by bacteriologist Sir Alexander Fleming in 1928, but it wasn't until 1940 when Ernst Chain and Howard Florey, two fellow scientists, became interested in Fleming's work that penicillin was able to be mass produced and used during World War II.

2.2 Contemporary Pharmacy Practice

Today's pharmacy practice continues to build on past knowledge. Scientists research new, innovative drug treatments for the disorders and diseases that affect the human body. **Contemporary pharmacy** is a science based on systematic research to determine the origin, nature, chemistry, effects, and uses of drugs. Medications can affect certain mechanisms or functions in the body. For example, some medications can cause low blood sugar levels (hypoglycemia). Laboratory values may be used to assess a disease or the effect of a medication on a body, so it is important for pharmacy technicians to know what normal values are for certain tests. Basic laboratory values are presented in Table 2.2.

TABLE 2.2 Normal Laboratory Values*

Serum Plasma	Liver Enzymes
Albumin 3.2–5 g/dL	ALT (SGPT) <35 IU/L
Bicarbonate 19–25 mEq/L	AST (SGOT) <35 IU/L
Blood urea nitrogen (BUN) 7–20 mg/dL	GGT
Calcium 8.6–10.3 mg/dL	Male 11–63 IU/L
Chloride 98–108 mEq/L	Female 8–35 IU/L
Creatinine 0.5–1.4 mg/dL	
Glucose 80–120 mg/dL	**CBC**
Hemoglobin, glycosylated 4–8%	Hematocrit
Magnesium 1.6–2.5 mg/dL	Male 41–50 mL/dL
Potassium 3.5–5.2 mEq/L	Female 36–44 mL/dL
Sodium 134–149 mEq/L	Hemoglobin
	Male 13.5–16.5 g/dL
Cholesterol	Female 12.0–15.0 g/dL
Total <200 mg/dL	WBC with differential 4,500–11,000
LDL 65–170 mg/dL	per microliter
HDL 40–60 mg/dL	
Triglycerides 45–150 mg/dL	

ALT=alanine aminotransferase; AST=aspartate aminotransferase; CBC=complete blood count; GGT=gamma-glutamyl transferase; HDL=high-density lipoprotein; IU=International Unit; LDL=low-density lipoprotein; WBC=white blood cell count

*Values may vary slightly based on laboratory.

Though early drugs came from natural sources, many modern drugs are synthesized in the laboratory, and some have been developed through bioengineering advances. Hence, the growth of present-day pharmacologic knowledge has been greatly stimulated by the development of synthetic organic chemistry, which has provided new tools and led to the development of many new therapeutic agents. As new drugs are introduced, it is essential that those who prescribe and dispense them also thoroughly understand them and the process required for a medication to be approved for use.

Practice Tip

The roles of pharmacy personnel are evolving. Currently, pharmacists can administer vaccinations in all 50 states, but only some states allow pharmacy technicians to administer vaccines.

The Pharmacist and Pharmacy Technician

A **pharmacist** is licensed to prepare, sell, and dispense drugs and compounds; fill prescriptions; and advise patients and customers on proper usage. The primary responsibility of a pharmacist is to make sure that drugs are dispensed properly and used appropriately. The pharmacist is an integral professional on the healthcare team. Furthermore, as pharmacists are being asked increasingly to focus their expertise and judgment on direct patient care and counseling, responsibilities related to dispensing have shifted to the pharmacy technician.

The **pharmacy technician** is an important member of the healthcare team who works under the supervision of a licensed pharmacist to assist with activities not requiring the professional judgment of a pharmacist. Although pharmacy technicians legally cannot counsel patients, because doing so requires the judgment of a pharmacist, technicians are involved in all aspects of drug distribution. Depending on state law, a pharmacy technician's responsibilities could include the following:

- receiving written prescriptions or requests for prescription refills from patients or their caregivers
- verifying that the information on the prescription is complete and accurate
- counting, weighing, measuring, and mixing medication

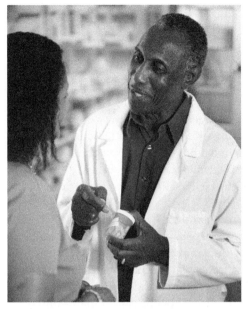

In addition to dispensing medications, the pharmacist plays an important role in instructing patients about side effects of medications, food and drug interactions, and dosing schedules.

- preparing sterile intravenous (IV) and chemotherapy compounds
- preparing prescription labels and selecting appropriate containers
- establishing and maintaining patient profiles
- ordering and stocking prescription and over-the-counter (OTC) medications
- assisting with drug studies
- transcribing prescriptions over the telephone
- transferring prescriptions
- tracking and reporting medication errors
- checking another technician's work in the preparation of medicine carts
- educating healthcare professionals about pharmacy-related issues
- obtaining laboratory results for pharmacists
- helping patients with OTC drugs
- making sure patients are counseled by the pharmacist (the technician should always ask whether there are any questions for the pharmacist)
- overseeing and maintaining automated dispensing systems
- maintaining pharmacy records
- cleaning the pharmacy (because the pharmacy is a restricted area, this responsibility is always completed by pharmacy personnel)

Pharm Fact

A unit dose cart is a movable cart that houses medications specifically dosed for patients within a hospital. It is filled by the pharmacy technician.

Technician responsibilities vary tremendously from state to state. In many states, a certified pharmacy technician can legally take a prescription over the phone. Some states allow "tech-check-tech." This describes when a technician checks the work of another technician. Although this may be allowed in community pharmacies, it is more common in hospital pharmacies. Most often, tech-check-tech is used to double-check unit dose medications that will be put into a unit dose cart or in an automated dispensing cabinet. Studies have shown that technicians who check each other's work are as accurate, or more accurate, as a pharmacist who checks the technician's work.

One of the most efficient measures to prevent medication errors is patient counseling. Even though the technician cannot counsel, it is the technician's duty to make sure the patient understands that the pharmacist is available for counseling. A patient should never leave the facility without being asked whether they have any questions regarding the drugs. Sometimes the technician can respond to these questions by reading information to the patient, but often the technician will need the pharmacist to talk to the patient. One drug-related problem in the United States is medication **nonadherence**, or not following the prescription instructions. Patients who understand their medications and know why and how to take them are more likely to take them appropriately.

One responsibility that technicians are claiming across the country is overseeing the **automated dispensing process**, which is a computerized drug storage device that automatically tracks drug distribution. As the pharmacy becomes more and more automated, someone must assume the responsibility of monitoring and refilling those machines. Technicians are now involved with complicated computer programs that ensure that safe and effective systems are in place to dispense drugs automatically.

Pharmacy Technician Certification

In 1995, five organizations—the American Pharmacists Association, the American Society of Health-System Pharmacists (ASHP), the Illinois Council of Health-System Pharmacists, the Michigan Pharmacists Association, and the National Association of Boards of Pharmacy—joined to form the **Pharmacy Technician Certification Board (PTCB)** to maintain a national certification program. The PTCB develops standards and acts as the nationally recognized credentialing agency. To become a credentialed pharmacy technician, one must pass a certification exam. The exam tests an individual's knowledge and skills required to perform as a technician and covers both hospital and retail pharmacy settings. Exams also cover pharmacy law, drug classes, dosage forms, common side effects, interactions, and indications. Practice tests are available from various sources.

Many states require certification by national examination. All states recognize the PTCB certification; other certifications are state specific. Several states recognize the Exam for the Certification of Pharmacy Technicians certification, which is offered by the National Healthcareer Association. Most states require that technicians register with their state board of pharmacy to do background checks and track pharmacy personnel. Each state has different requirements, but all are raising standards and maintaining a system to track pharmacy technicians. Most states require pharmacy technicians to have a high school diploma or GED, be at least 18 years of age, and have no felony convictions. Each state has different standards regarding what a technician may and may not do, so technicians must be knowledgeable of the laws in the state in which they practice. Renewal requirements also differ in each state.

Since 1983, ASHP has assumed the responsibility of accrediting technician-training programs. In 2014 the Pharmacy Technician Accreditation Commission was formed as a collaborative of ASHP and the Accreditation Counsel of Pharmacy Education (ACPE).

The two largest national pharmacy technician organizations are the American Association of Pharmacy Technicians (AAPT) and the National Pharmacy Technician Association (NPTA). AAPT was organized in 1979 to promote safe and cost-effective ways to dispense and distribute medications. It presents the pharmacy technician as an integral part of the healthcare team and provides leadership in representing the interests of its members and the healthcare community.

NPTA is an association dedicated to advancing the value of pharmacy technicians and the vital roles they play in pharmaceutical care. Founded in 1999, the organization is composed of pharmacy technicians practicing in a variety of practice settings, such as retail, independent, hospital, mail order, home care, long-term care, nuclear, military, correctional facility, formal education, training, management, sales, and many more. NPTA publishes the magazine *Today's Technician*.

The Pharmacy Technician Educators Council (PTEC) was organized in 1989 by Don Ballington. The purpose of this organization is to share information among those who are teaching in pharmacy technician programs across the country. PTEC's efforts focus on curriculums, educational materials, and instructional techniques. In July 1998, at the national meeting in Aspen, Colorado, the first pharmacology text written especially for technicians was introduced by Paradigm Education Solutions.

2.3 Drug Regulation

People have been concerned about the quality and safety of medicines throughout history. The manufacture, sale, and use of drugs are regulated by the US legal system. State and federal laws govern the development, prescription, and dispensation of drugs, providing a rational system of checks and balances to ensure everyone's safety. These laws have been developed and refined over the past century.

The Food and Drug Administration

The **Food and Drug Administration (FDA)** is the oldest consumer protection agency in the US federal government. The FDA's mission as it pertains to drugs is to protect public health by ensuring the safety, efficacy, and security of human and veterinary drugs, biologic products, and medical devices. The FDA is also responsible for ensuring the safety of the United States' food supply, cosmetics, and products that emit radiation. The regulation of drugs and food has evolved over time. In 1906, the Federal Food and Drug Act, often referred to as the Pure Food and Drug Act, was passed as the first attempt by the US government to regulate the sale of drugs or substances that affect the body. In 1927, the Food, Drug, and Insecticide Administration was formed. In 1930, its name was changed to the Food and Drug Administration. Recall that this agency is responsible for ensuring that any drug or food product approved for marketing is safe when used as directed on the label. The FDA controls purity, labeling accuracy, and product safety.

The passage of the Food, Drug, and Cosmetic Act of 1938 initiated the current system of drug regulation in the United States. The act required all new drugs to be proven safe before being marketed. The basic definition of "safe" under this act is "nontoxic" when used in accordance with the conditions set forth on the label. This act also specifies that every new drug must have been the subject of an approved **New Drug Application (NDA)** before US commercialization. The NDA is the vehicle through which a **drug sponsor**, usually a pharmaceutical company, formally proposes that the FDA approve a new legacy drug for sale and marketing in the United States.

In 1951, the **Durham-Humphrey Amendment** established two classes of drugs. A **legend drug** is sold only by prescription and is labeled "Rx only." An **over-the-counter (OTC) drug** may be sold without a prescription.

The FDA has the responsibility of regulating both legend and OTC drugs as well as medical and radiological devices, food, cosmetics, biologics, and veterinary drugs. In Canada, the corresponding federal agency is Health Canada. The FDA does not test drugs itself, although it does conduct limited research in the areas of drug quality, safety, and effectiveness. A company seeking to market a drug is responsible for testing it and submitting evidence that it is safe and clinically effective.

Drug Approval Process

The FDA requires that the manufacturer of any new drug provide evidence of its safety and effectiveness before the drug will be allowed to enter the US market. The drug must be shown to be safe through an intensive testing process that is undertaken by a drug sponsor, which is usually a pharmaceutical company.

The drug approval process can be broken into four main phases: preclinical, clinical, New Drug Application (NDA) Review, and postmarketing. The first stage is the preclinical phase, when the drug sponsor is developing a new compound and testing the drug on animals for toxicity. If major risks or early toxicity markers are not seen, the sponsor then submits an investigational drug application (IND) to the

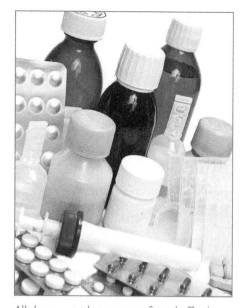

All drugs must be proven safe and effective through the FDA approval process to be used in the United States.

FDA. The IND includes information about the composition and manufacturing of the drug and a proposal for testing in humans (**clinical trial**).

Once the FDA reviews and approves the IND, the drug then moves to the second phase of development. This is also known as the clinical phase, when clinical trials are conducted on human volunteers. The third phase, or the NDA review, occurs once the clinical trials (described next) are complete and the sponsor officially files for approval.

All test results are made available to the FDA through the NDA, which also specifies proposed labeling (indications for use, dosing, safety information, and more) for the new drug. The NDA contains details on the entire history of the development and testing of the drug. It documents results of the animal studies and clinical trials; describes components and composition of the drug; explains how the drug behaves in the body; and provides the details of manufacturing, processing, and packaging, with a special emphasis on quality control. The FDA also requires that the NDA include samples of the drug and its labels. A team of FDA physicians, statisticians, chemists, pharmacologists, and other scientists then reviews the contents of the NDA. If the drug is shown to be safe and effective, the team will likely recommend that the FDA approve it. Drugs sometimes may be used for purposes other than the ones approved by the FDA. This is called **off-label use**, and insurance companies may not pay for drugs used for these purposes.

Clinical Trials

If initial laboratory and animal model research on a particular drug is sufficiently promising, the developer will submit an application to the FDA requesting permission to begin testing the drug on humans. An **investigational drug**, also known as an experimental drug, is a chemical or biological substance that the FDA has approved for testing on people during clinical trials. During clinical trials, scientists try to prove whether the drug is safe and effective, how the drug might be used to treat a disease, how much and what dose of the drug is needed, and the benefits and risks of taking the drug. Human testing, referred to as a clinical trial, is used to determine whether new drugs or treatments are both safe and effective. Protocols for testing are typically developed by researchers and are subject to the approval of an FDA review board. These protocols describe what type of people may participate in the trial, the schedule of tests and procedures, medications and their dosages, and the length of the study. Throughout the trial phases, participants are monitored to determine the safety and efficacy of the drug. Only about 20% of the drugs that enter clinical trials are ultimately approved for marketing.

During clinical trials, patients are typically separated into two groups. The experimental group receives the drug to be tested, while the control group receives either a standard treatment for the illness or a placebo. A **placebo** is an inactive substance that the patient believes is a medication but that has no pharmacologic effect. In general, neither trial participants nor the study investigators know whether a particular participant is in the experimental or the control group. This type of study, which allows for greater objectivity on the part of the investigators, is referred to as a **double-blind study**. It is considered the gold standard of clinical trials.

Pharm Fact

The US National Library of Medicine at the National Institutes of Health provides information to the public about clinical studies that are ongoing or completed. Currently, the database offers information on the thousands of clinical trials conducted in the United States and around the world. To access the website, go to https://Pharmacology7e.ParadigmEducation.com/trials.

Clinical trials of new drugs proceed through four phases:

- **Phase I** The drug is administered to a small group of healthy people (20 to 100) to evaluate its safety, determine a safe dosage range, and identify side effects. Phase I studies assess the most common acute adverse effects and clarify what happens to a drug in the human body.

- **Phase II** The drug is studied in patients who have the condition the drug is intended to treat. At this point, it is determined whether the drug has a favorable effect on the disease state. Short-term placebo-to-drug comparisons are made in double-blind trials to determine the range and response of various doses.

- **Phase III** The drug treatment is compared to commonly used treatments. During this phase, study investigators collect information that will allow the drug to be used safely. This phase continues the double-blind, placebo-to-drug comparisons begun in Phase II or the comparison of the new drug to the standard of care. Dose escalations are used to determine the efficacy of the drug in treating the target disease.

- **Phase IV** After completion of the Phase III trials, a drug may be approved for use by the FDA. After receiving FDA approval, Phase IV studies begin. The purpose of Phase IV studies is to evaluate how well the drug works in the real world and to monitor its safety.

In the past, the entire FDA approval process for a drug took approximately 7 to 10 years. Recently, however, the FDA has taken steps to make urgently needed drugs available sooner. The Prescription Drug User Fee Act of 1992 instituted reforms that shortened the review process for new drugs. This act required that drug companies pay fees upon the submission of NDAs; these funds are used to hire an adequate number of reviewers. Now the FDA must act on standard applications for new drugs within 10 months and act on priority applications for drugs used to treat serious diseases within 6 months. Figure 2.1 illustrates the FDA review process.

FIGURE 2.1
The Drug Review Process

After the government approves a manufacturer's IND application, a drug must pass through three phases of testing on human subjects before it is ready for final review by the FDA.

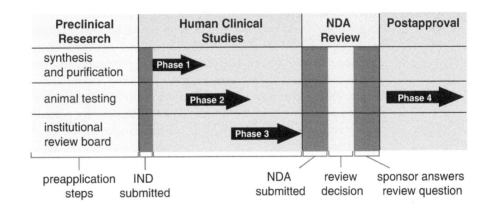

A classification system helps to determine the order in which applications are reviewed. Priority is given to drugs with the greatest potential benefit. Drugs that offer a significant medical advantage over existing therapies for any given disease state are assigned priority status. Drugs for life-threatening diseases are considered first.

It is important to remember that no drug is absolutely safe. The FDA's approval is based on a judgment about whether the benefits of a new drug to users will outweigh its risks (also known as risk-benefit analysis). The FDA will allow a product to present more of a risk when its potential benefit is great, especially if the product is used to treat a serious, life-threatening condition.

For example, drugs are not traditionally tested on pregnant individuals. Instead, the FDA uses all available information (mainly from animal studies) to assess the risks each drug marketed in the United States poses to pregnant and lactating individuals. The old FDA pregnancy categories (from safest to unsafe: A, B, C, D, and X) have been replaced with new labeling requirements. In the packaging information for each drug, the manufacturer must include the following three sections covering topics related to pregnancy: (1) pregnancy, (2) lactation, and (3) females and males of reproductive potential.

The new labeling system provides more helpful information about a medication's risks to the expectant mother, the developing fetus, and the breast-fed infant. Within each of these sections, more detailed information is included. For example, in the pregnancy section, information about a pregnancy exposure registry, a risk summary, clinical considerations, and data are included to help inform the healthcare provider and consumer.

Postmarketing Surveillance

The consumer's well-being is the FDA's most important concern. Public health cannot be protected without procedures to monitor the quality of drugs once they are marketed. The FDA's Office of Compliance oversees the drug manufacturing process, ensuring that manufacturers follow Current Good Manufacturing Practices as spelled out in FDA regulations.

In addition to demonstrating that a drug is safe and effective, a manufacturer must adhere to standards set by the US Pharmacopoeia–National Formulary (USP-NF). The USP-NF is a combination of two compendia, the US Pharmacopeia (USP) and the National Formulary (NF). The purpose of the USP-NF is to ensure the strength, quality, and purity of medicinal ingredients.

Some adverse reactions do not become known until after a drug has been approved and has been used by a larger number of people outside the clinical trial setting. Therefore, postmarketing surveillance (Phase IV trials) is important in identifying unexpected adverse effects so that appropriate action can be taken, if needed. Sometimes these actions could mean removal of a drug from the market or a change in the label of a medication. Professionals and consumers can report serious adverse reactions to **MedWatch**, the FDA's medical products reporting program. The purpose of this program is to improve the postmarketing surveillance of medical products and to ensure that new safety information pertaining to drug use is rapidly communicated to the medical community, thereby improving patient care. If a drug poses a health risk, the FDA will remove it from the market even though it has already been approved.

Medication Guides

Pharm Fact

Medication guides focus on a specific risk or on adherence to the medication.

At times, the FDA may require that a medication guide be provided with a filled prescription. **Medication guides**, a part of the Risk Evaluation and Mitigation Strategy program, are paper handouts that contain specific risk information and are dispensed to patients with certain medications. It is important to know that a medication guide is different from the consumer medication information printouts that are generated and dispensed with all medications that contain broad information on how to take a medication, store a medication, etc. Medication guides include FDA-approved information designed to help patients avoid serious adverse events, and they must be provided each time a medication is dispensed to a patient. Some medication guides are prepared for entire classes of drugs. Examples of such classes of drugs are nonsteroidal anti-inflammatory drugs and antidepressants. Other medication guides are prepared for specific drugs. Many retail computer systems are set up to print the medication guide automatically when the drug label is printed. Medication guides may also be obtained from the FDA. The pharmacy technician plays a vital role in making sure that the patient receives the proper medication guide. The technician can put the guide together with the drug for the pharmacist when the pharmacist verifies the drug.

FDA Recalls

A drug is considered safe if the FDA determines that the benefits of the drug outweigh the risks when the drug is used by patients for its approved indications. If a medication is used for indications not included in its FDA label, it is considered an unapproved or off-label use.

It is important to recognize that safe does not mean harmless and every drug has risks. When the FDA obtains information regarding safety concerns about a medication, the agency may issue a drug recall. A drug recall is an action taken by the drug manufacturer to remove a defective medication from the market. Drug recalls may happen by a company's own initiative or by FDA request.

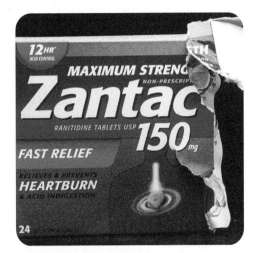

In 2020, the FDA requested manufacturers withdraw all products containing ranitidine. Certain products containing this common heartburn relief agent exposed consumers to unacceptable levels of impurities.

Practice Tip

Boxed warnings are the sternest warnings put on drug labels. As you are learning pharmacology, you should make special note of these warnings.

Boxed or Black Box Warnings

For drugs that are on the market and have been found to be problematic but still provide therapy for specific conditions, a **boxed** (or **black box**) **warning** is placed on the package insert (see Figure 2.2). This warning alerts prescribers to the known problems associated with the use of the drug. The prescriber must then weigh the advantages of using this drug against the associated risks. Thousands of drugs on the market have boxed warnings. They are deemed safe enough to continue using, but they have known problems. Within the boxed warning, each bullet is followed by a parenthetical. For example, in Figure 2.2, *(5.1)* can be found. This number reflects the section of the prescribing information where more detailed information is located.

FIGURE 2.2
Boxed Warning

The FDA requires a specific format for a boxed warning: the text must be in boldfaced type and have bullets or subheads that highlight the serious adverse effects of the drug.

> **WARNING: SUICIDAL THOUGHTS AND BEHAVIORS**
> *See full prescribing information for complete boxed warning.*
> - **Increased risk of suicidal thinking and behavior in children, adolescents, and young adults taking antidepressants (5.1).**
> - **Monitor for worsening and emergence of suicidal thoughts and behaviors (5.1).**
>
> *When using PROZAC and olanzapine in combination, also refer to Boxed Warning section of the package insert for Symbyax.*

Controlled Substances

The Comprehensive Drug Abuse Prevention and Control Act of 1970 (better known as the Controlled Substances Act) was designed to combat escalating drug abuse. It promoted drug education and research into the prevention and treatment of drug dependence; strengthened enforcement authority; and designated schedules, or categories, for drugs with a high potential for abuse, according to their probability of abuse. A drug listed on one of these schedules is known as a **controlled substance**.

The **Drug Enforcement Administration (DEA)** was established in 1973 as a branch of the US Department of Justice. The DEA is responsible for regulating the sale and use of specified drugs. It works at the national, state, and local levels. Individuals and institutions that handle or prescribe any controlled substances must be registered by the DEA. The prescriber's DEA registry number must be associated with the prescription when it is filled.

Controlled substances are divided among five categories, or schedules (CI–CV), each with its own set of restrictions imposed on the prescribing of such substances. For example, schedule I drugs have the highest potential for abuse and have no accepted medical use. They may be used solely for research purposes. Table 2.3 summarizes the five categories of controlled substance schedules and includes corresponding abuse potential, accepted medicinal uses, and examples of each category. Controlled substance product labels must indicate the schedule of the drug (see Figure 2.3).

The DEA mandates that C-III and IV drugs may be refilled only five times, for a total of six fillings per prescription, within a six-month period. Of the controlled substances, C-V drugs have the lowest potential for abuse and dependency. C-V drugs may be available in certain states without a prescription. In most states, prescriptions for C-V drugs have the same restrictions for refills as legend drugs, but some states are more restrictive and hold C-V drugs to the same requirements as C-III and C-IV medications. C-IIs are not allowed refills, but the length of time for which the prescription is good depends on the state. Of the available controlled substances, C-IIs have the greatest potential for abuse and may be stored separately from other drugs in a locked location. C-IIs are also high-alert medications because if they are involved in errors, they are more likely to result in patient harm. The pharmacy must have the original signed prescription for a C-II drug. An exception is an e-prescription, which must be sent from a secure location and requires two identifiers from the sender before it will transmit.

Federal laws determine how medications are handled and scheduled. However, some states have stricter laws. The strictest law always takes precedence. States also vary on who may write prescriptions for controlled substances.

Inventory control is critical when dealing with C-IIs. There are two ways to order C-II drugs: the Controlled Substance Ordering System (CSOS) or DEA Form 222. The CSOS allows for secure electronic ordering without requiring a DEA Form 222. When the CSOS is not used to order C-IIs, they must be ordered using **DEA Form 222**. The paper form is filled out in triplicate: the first and second copies are sent to the supplier, and the third is kept in the pharmacy. When the drugs arrive in the pharmacy, the pharmacy must document on the 222 exactly which and how many drugs were received—and this form must be kept for two years. When C-IIs have expired, DEA Form 106 must be completed to document the destruction of the supply, and there must be a witness to the destruction. The pharmacist usually receives (checks in) and destroys controlled substances.

TABLE 2.3 Schedules for Controlled Substances*

Manufacturer's Label	Abuse Potential	Physical and Psychological Dependence	Medical Use	DEA Dispensing Instructions	Examples
C-I	Highest potential for abuse	Severe physical or psychological dependence	No accepted medical use in the United States	For research only. Must have license to obtain.	Heroin, lysergic acid diethylamide (LSD), marijuana
C-II	High possibility of abuse, which can lead to severe psychological or physical dependence	Severe physical or psychological dependence	Currently accepted medical use	Dispensing is severely restricted. Cannot be prescribed by phone except in an emergency. No refills on prescriptions.	Oxycodone, meperidine, hydromorphone, fentanyl, morphine, hydrocodone
C-III	Moderate potential for abuse and addiction	Moderate to low physical or high psychological dependence	Currently accepted medical use	Prescriptions can be refilled up to five times within six months if authorized by a physician.	Codeine with aspirin, codeine with acetaminophen, anabolic steroids
C-IV	Low abuse potential	Limited physical or psychological dependence	Currently accepted medical use	Prescriptions can be refilled up to five times within six months if authorized by a physician.	Benzodiazepines, meprobamate, phenobarbital
C-V	Lowest abuse potential	Limited physical or psychological dependence	Currently accepted medical use	Some sold without a prescription depending on state law; purchaser must be over 18 years and is required to sign a log and show a driver's license.	Liquid codeine preparations, pregabalin

* This table represents federal law. Each state may have laws that differ from federal law. Marijuana is considered a C-I substance by the DEA. However, there is growing support for marijuana's medical use. Many states now have laws that allow its use for medical purposes, and some states have legalized marijuana's recreational use.

FIGURE 2.3
Prescription Drug Label

Schedule II controlled substances, such as narcotics and amphetamines, have the highest potential for abuse, drug tolerance, and psychological or physical dependence among drugs with accepted medical use.

NDC number (a unique 10- or 11-digit code specific to each FDA-approved medication)

controlled drug schedule

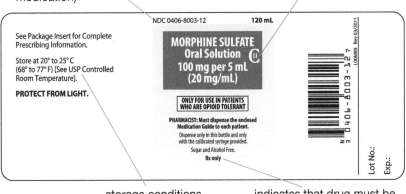

storage conditions

indicates that drug must be dispensed by prescription only

Generic Drugs

At some stage in the drug development process, a drug sponsor will apply for patent protection. A **patent** protects the drug sponsor's investment in developing the drug by granting the sponsor the sole right to manufacture the drug while the patent is in effect. Under patent protection, the generic and brand names of a drug both belong to the drug sponsor. The manufacturer's proprietary right to the drug expires as soon as the patent expires, leaving other companies free to produce the drug as a nonproprietary or generic drug, possibly under their own brand name as well as the generic name. When this occurs, the price differential between the brand-name drug and the generic preparation is frequently substantial.

The substitution of generic drugs for more expensive brands is an important means of reducing healthcare costs, and many insurance companies require the use of generics before they will reimburse patients for drug costs. Some insurance companies provide a list of brand-name drugs that they will reimburse.

Drug companies must submit an **abbreviated new drug application** to the FDA to obtain approval to market a generic product. In approving a generic drug, the FDA requires many rigorous tests and procedures to ensure that the drug is interchangeable with the innovator drug (the original brand-name, FDA-approved drug) under all approved indications and conditions of use. The generic drug must meet the following requirements:

- It must contain the same active ingredients as the original brand-name drug.
- It must be identical in strength, dosage form, and route of administration.
- It must have the same use indications.
- It must meet the same batch requirements for identity, strength, purity, and quality.
- It must yield similar blood absorption and urinary excretion curves for the active ingredient.

When the above criteria are met, the generic drug should produce pharmacologic effects similar to the innovator drug.

The FDA has devised an A/B rating system to establish the therapeutic equivalence of generic drugs. An A rating indicates that the agency has determined a drug to be therapeutically equivalent to the innovator drug by meeting the criteria of pharmaceutical equivalence, bioequivalence (the biological equivalence of two proprietary preparations of a drug), labeling, and Current Good Manufacturing Practices. The FDA has also identified generics that are not therapeutically equivalent. (This information is published in an FDA book referred to as the Orange Book.) Drugs given an A rating have been deemed therapeutically equivalent to the reference drug product. Medications designated a B rating have not shown equivalence to the reference drug product based on the FDA standards. Although few drugs fall into this latter category, be aware that such drugs do exist.

Biosimilar Medications

Some medications are categorized as biologic drugs. **Biologic drugs** are complex, large molecules that are created in a laboratory and derived from various living organisms such as bacteria, mammals, plants, insects, and birds. Because these biologic products are derived from living organisms, manufacturing them is much more complex and difficult to replicate. In contrast, small-molecule drugs are simpler, smaller, and more stable, so they are more easily replicated through predictable chemical reactions. This means that an exact copy of the active ingredient can be made, and a generic product can be produced.

In 2014, the FDA released the Purple Book. The Purple Book is a reference guide that lists biological products and the date each biologic was licensed, whether the FDA has evaluated that biological product for reference product exclusivity (meaning it was the originator product), and whether the medication has been determined to be biosimilar or interchangeable to a reference product. A **biosimilar drug** is highly similar to the reference or originator drug. There can be no clinically meaningful differences between that product and the reference product regarding safety, purity, and potency (safety and effectiveness). A manufacturer who is developing a proposed biosimilar product must submit comparative information from tests that demonstrate the product is highly similar to the reference product. Tests may include information on the structural and functional characteristics, animal study data, human pharmacokinetic and pharmacodynamic data, and other data showing its similarity. Differences in clinically inactive substances (e.g., stabilizers and buffers) are acceptable. Unlike generic medications, biosimilar products cannot automatically be substituted for the reference product. A prescriber must specifically write for the biosimilar medication to be used.

Interchangeable products are biosimilar products that meet additional requirements from more evaluations and tests. These requirements include showing that the interchangeable product is expected to produce the same clinical results as the reference drug. Furthermore, tests must also demonstrate there is no loss of efficacy or increased safety if a patient switches back and forth between the interchangeable product and the reference product versus if that patient were to remain on the reference product without any switching. If a drug has been determined to be an interchangeable product, it may be substituted for the reference product without consultation by the prescriber. At present, the FDA has not designated any biosimilar products as interchangeable. Part of the responsibility of the healthcare practitioner is to lower costs without compromising the health of the patient. Healthcare costs have risen at an alarming rate in the United States, and money can be saved when generics or biosimilar products are used.

Over-the-Counter Drugs

Many drugs used in the treatment of illnesses are OTC drugs. These drugs do not require a prescription. Drug companies recognize that consumers' instant recognition of OTC brand names has marketing value and sales potential. Consequently, companies are reluctant to change OTC brand names, even when the ingredients of the drugs change. Thus, drug companies commonly reuse brand names for products with different ingredients. Healthcare professionals are concerned about this practice, but a loophole in the federal regulations allows it. The confusion created by this practice is potentially dangerous. For example, Gaviscon, an OTC drug used for alleviating heartburn, previously contained alginic acid. Now it consists of aluminum hydroxide and a magnesium compound. Taking aluminum hydroxide can be dangerous for a patient with renal impairment, because it could lead to aluminum toxicity. Patients taking this OTC medication may not know it contains aluminum.

This is one area where the pharmacy technician has tremendous responsibility and can play an important role. Reading the ingredients when helping patients select OTC products is essential. It is also important to report product problems to the FDA's MedWatch or the Institute for Safe Medication Practices (ISMP). Both can be found online.

Whether ideal or not, the reality is that the pharmacy technician is often the individual who ultimately guides patients to these drugs. Although pharmacy technicians cannot counsel or recommend drugs, they certainly need to be able to inform patients what conditions these drugs treat. In most pharmacies, OTC drugs are shelved in sections according to broad categories of ailments. For example, drugs for constipation and drugs for diarrhea are in the same section. Although the labels contain information, patients might be easily confused and often do not understand the medical terms or cannot read the small print on the box. The technician can be a great resource to patients in helping them find the OTC medications they need and describe the various uses for drugs. In no way could this be construed as counseling. Often it is as simple as reading the label to an older patient who cannot read the small print. It is important that the pharmacy technician is familiar with these drugs.

Review and Assessment

History of Medicinal Drugs

- Historically, humans have sought to find relief for their ailments.

- Pharmacology is a broad term that includes the study of drugs and their interactions with the systems of living animals.

- The 20th century brought major breakthroughs in medical care.

Contemporary Pharmacy Practice

- Five organizations—the American Pharmacists Association, the American Society of Health-System Pharmacists (ASHP), the Illinois Council of Health-System Pharmacists, the Michigan Pharmacists Association, and the National Association of Boards of Pharmacy—joined to form the Pharmacy Technician Certification Board (PTCB) to maintain a national certification program.

- The American Association of Pharmacy Technicians (AAPT) is composed of pharmacy technicians. This organization provides leadership, promotes the interests of its members, and represents them as members of healthcare teams.

- The Pharmacy Technician Educators Council (PTEC) is an organization of educators that focuses on pharmacy technician training curriculums and networking to share ideas.

- PTCB maintains a national certification program for technicians.

- The National Pharmacy Technician Association (NPTA) is a technician organization that is dedicated to advancing the value and roles of pharmacy technicians.

- The National Healthcareer Association is an organization that provides pharmacy technician certification and preparation resources to assist students in earning a CPhT certification.

- Drugs are derived from sources such as plants, animals, minerals, synthetic materials, and bioengineering advances.

Drug Regulation

- Laws govern the drug industry and protect patients' rights.

- The FDA may require medication guides be dispensed with certain medications as another layer of communication about serious adverse events.

- A boxed or black box warning makes the prescriber aware of any serious problems that have occurred with a drug since it has been on the market.

- The FDA requires that all new drugs be proved effective and safe before they can be approved for marketing.

- Clinical trials, in which results observed in

patients receiving the drugs are compared to the results of patients receiving a different treatment or placebo, are the best way to determine the effects of a new drug.

- When the benefits outweigh the risks, the FDA considers a drug safe enough to be approved.

- Drugs are not tested on pregnant individuals, but, based on all available information, drugs are labeled to identify the risks each drug marketed in the United States poses to pregnant and lactating individuals.

- Federal law divides controlled substances into five schedules according to their potential for abuse and clinical usefulness: C-I (research only), C-II (dispensing is severely restricted), C-III (can be refilled up to five times in six months if authorized by the physician), C-IV (same restrictions as C-III), and C-V (may, depending on state law, be sold without a prescription).

- Generic drugs must be equivalent to the brand-name drugs and are given an A/B rating by the FDA.

- Pharmacy technicians can play an important role in helping patients identify ingredients in OTC medications, especially when it is possible that the ingredients of a previously purchased OTC medication have changed.

✓ CHECK YOUR UNDERSTANDING

Take a moment to review what you have learned in this chapter and answer the following questions.

1. The word *pharmakon* means
   a. "dosing methods."
   b. "remedy."
   c. "pharmacist" in Greek.
   d. a list of remedies found in Greek literature.

2. Claude Bernard
   a. was a French physiologist who demonstrated that certain drugs have specific sites of action within the body.
   b. grew herbs of medicinal value.
   c. is the father of American pharmacology.
   d. discovered penicillin.

3. A pharmacy technician should never
   a. take prescriptions over the telephone.
   b. advise patients about the use of their medicine.
   c. mix IV solutions.
   d. maintain patient profiles.

4. The FDA is required to
   a. ensure that a drug is safe and effective.
   b. monitor drug safety after a drug has been approved for sale.
   c. approve drugs in a timely manner.
   d. All of these are correct.

5. Which drug testing phase(s) involves human participants?
   a. Phase I
   b. Phase II
   c. Phase III
   d. All of these are correct.

6. A generic drug must
   a. contain the same active ingredients as the original brand-name drug.
   b. be identical in strength, dosage form, and route of administration.
   c. have the same use indications.
   d. All of these are correct.

7. Which of the following schedules includes drugs that have no accepted medical use in the United States?
   a. schedule I / C-I
   b. schedule II / C-II
   c. schedule III / C-III
   d. schedule IV / C-IV

8. Which of the following federal laws was designed to prevent drug abuse?
   a. Federal Food and Drug Act
   b. Durham-Humphrey Amendment
   c. Controlled Substances Act
   d. Prescription Drug User Fee Act

9. MedWatch is
   a. a program to shorten the review process for new drugs.
   b. an organization that sets standards for clinical trials.
   c. a system through which healthcare professionals can report adverse drug events.
   d. an organization that registers pharmacists.

10. The FDA's approval of a new drug is based on
    a. the completion of the first three phases of clinical trials.
    b. evidence that a drug is effective in treating the condition for which it was intended.
    c. a judgment that the benefits of a new drug to users will outweigh its risks.
    d. All of these are correct.

MAKE CONNECTIONS

Take a moment to consider what you have learned in this chapter and respond thoughtfully to the following prompts. Note that some of these activities will require internet access.

1. This chapter introduced the responsibilities most pharmacy technicians face in their jobs. Do any of your prior experiences relate to these skills? If so, how will you apply those experiences to this profession? If not, how might you pursue developing some of these skills outside of class?

2. How might you become more familiar with the work of a pharmacy technician outside of class?

 The online course includes additional review and assessment resources.

Pharmacology Study for the Pharmacy Technician

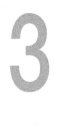

Learning Objectives

1 Paraphrase study strategies, such as spacing, interleaving, testing, and the contiguity principle. (Section 3.1)

2 Describe how eliminating distractions and adopting a growth mindset improve studying. (Section 3.1)

3 Explain how learning medications by drug class can assist with efficient pharmacology learning. (Section 3.2)

4 List common generic drug name endings and their associated drug classes. (Section 3.2)

5 Define *mnemonic device* and describe two pharmacy mnemonics. (Section 3.2)

6 Identify information included in a package insert. (Section 3.3)

7 Describe the subject matter of the FDA's Orange, Purple, and Green books. (Section 3.3)

8 Compare and contrast various electronic and smartphone-based drug resources. (Section 3.3)

9 Paraphrase the general health information available from the Centers for Disease Control, the National Institute of Health, MedlinePlus, and the FDA. (Section 3.4)

ASHP/ACPE Accreditation Standards
To view the *ASHP/ACPE Accreditation Standards* addressed in this chapter, refer to Appendix C.

Pharmacology may seem like an intimidating subject at first. It contains a vast amount of information to learn coupled with new terms and concepts. However, with a strategic approach, dedication, and a productive mindset, it is possible to master pharmacology. This chapter will highlight evidence-based study methods and offer pharmacology-specific study aids to assist learning. Furthermore, the chapter will offer resources to deepen medication and health knowledge that can be applied to all areas of the pharmacy technician profession.

3.1 Evidence-Based Study Methods

The previous chapter introduced the history of medicinal drugs and how the study and application of drugs improved and evolved over time. Most pharmacy personnel are aware of scientific research and how it applies to health care. The drug approval process discussed in Chapter 2 requires such research. Furthermore, the drugs presented in this book are the direct result of scientific research. Fewer pharmacy personnel may be aware of the existence of **educational research**, the scientific field of study that examines learning and education. Educational research can be used to a pharmacy technician student's advantage. Using proven and evidence-based study strategies may help learners more efficiently use their time and recall greater amounts of information for longer durations.

Educational research is constantly evolving. New studies and best practices continue to be uncovered. This section covers several examples of evidence-based strategies for studying and learning, including spacing, interleaving, testing, and the contiguity principle. Consider using these techniques to help you study wisely.

Spacing as a Study Method

Spacing is the method of having multiple small study sessions spread across a long period of time. Spacing can be contrasted with **massing** (sometimes referred to as cramming), which is studying just one or two times over a short period of time. Repeated experiments show that spacing results in better long-term retention of information compared to massing.

A calendar is helpful when attempting the spacing method of studying. Instead of studying for a larger block of time once a week (e.g., on Sunday) or the evening before an exam, multiple (and shorter) study times are identified and added to the calendar. This may include daily study sessions or sessions on an every-other-day basis.

Individuals who will take a certification exam in the future benefit from the spacing method since it improves long-term retention.

Interleaving versus Blocking as a Study Method

A common approach to studying is called blocking. **Blocking** involves practicing one skill at a time before moving on to the next. Although blocking is the more common approach, growing evidence suggests interleaving is a more effective way to study. **Interleaving** is the method of mixing (interleaving) practice of several related skills together.

Flash cards can be an easy way to incorporate the interleaving method in your studies.

Consider learning to play soccer. A learner using the blocking method would first learn to dribble a ball in a straight line before moving on to dribbling in a zigzag pattern. After learning to dribble in a zigzag pattern, the learner would move on to special moves to throw off a defender. Meanwhile, a learner using the interleaving method would alternate between dribbling in a straight line, dribbling in a zigzag pattern, and practicing special moves to throw off defenders.

Several studies show interleaving is superior to blocking in category learning. Since learners are working with a variety of concepts and categories at the same time, this method allows learners to quickly identify and compare the distinguishing features of each. It is hypothesized that interleaving benefits learning because it encourages greater attention and promotes retrieval skills and may promote higher-level thinking.

Interleaving can be easily applied to pharmacology using flash cards or other category-identification exercises. For example, if you are studying the musculoskeletal system, make a point to study a mixture of flash cards. Instead of studying only anatomy and physiology and then moving on to drugs related to this system, combine the flash cards and study them together. Consider combining flash cards from previous chapters and body systems as well.

Self-Testing as a Study Method

Students are familiar with tests administered by teachers as a means to assess a student's understanding of specific topics. A less familiar concept is **self-testing**, or self-assessment, as a means to study. Self-testing as a means of studying is the method of testing oneself on newly learned information. Another word for self-testing is *retrieval practice*. Testing as a study method has been shown to provide superior retention compared to providing more time and exposure to a subject (restudying).

Integrating this strategy requires the learner to give themselves a practice test during study time. This could be as simple as putting away study materials and trying to recall information. Taking advantage of practice tests or quizzes, writing information down, saying information aloud, or even sketching diagrams are other ways to use this method of study. Another way to self-test is by using flash cards or asking others to quiz you. After a self-testing activity, answers should be checked using course materials. Ideally one should self-test several times to prepare for an exam.

Contiguity Principle Study Method

Educational literature has identified and described various styles of learning. Visual learning (where the learner prefers seeing), auditory learning (where the learner prefers hearing), and kinesthetic learning (where the learner prefers doing) are three of the most common learning styles.

Although many instructors try to address the learning style preferences found within their classrooms, studies show using multiple styles at once can help increase information retention. The contiguity principle uses this approach. The **contiguity principle** is a method of study that aligns words to corresponding graphics. Research shows studying information as text together with diagrams or pictures improves retention.

To apply this method to pharmacology, consider summarizing information in a chapter using words and pictures together. When studying the side effects of a drug class, draw and write the most common effects (see Figure 3.1). If a drug has multiple boxed warnings, write the warnings in a box you draw.

FIGURE 3.1
Side Effects of Aspirin

The contiguity principle study method recommends that students use multiple learning styles to retain information. For example, to study a drug's side effects one might draw and label these impacts on the body.

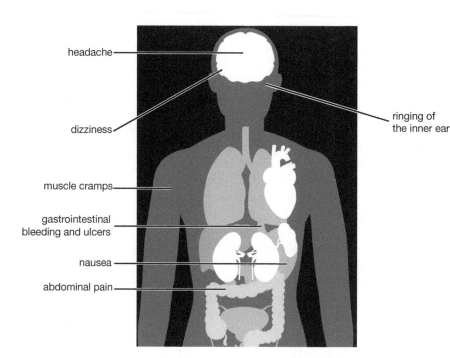

Work Wise

You may be multitasking while studying without even realizing it. Responding to text messages, checking your email, browsing social media, and answering or responding to alerts on your cell phone while studying all constitute multitasking.

Eliminating Distractions

Eliminating distractions may include studying in a location with minimal distractions (such as a library). It can also be a matter of minimizing the distractions technology presents, such as avoiding using a computer or phone. If a computer is not required for studying, consider not using it. Computer alerts and the internet can be distracting while studying. Other ways to minimize technology include turning off cell phones or using the do not disturb or airplane modes while studying. Another type of distraction to avoid is multitasking. **Multitasking** is the act of trying to complete multiple tasks at the same time. Educational research shows that multitasking can negatively affect study quality and increase the amount of time needed to learn materials.

Adopting a Growth Mindset

Research shows that beliefs about intelligence and academic ability can affect success and trajectory. The concept of mindset falls into two basic categories: fixed and growth.

Someone with a **fixed mindset** assumes that intelligence, character, and drive are static and will never change. As a result, they may not attempt to grow or learn new things. Those with fixed mindsets tend to have difficulty recovering from stumbles or challenges. They may give up after meeting adversity.

Contrast this with a growth mindset. A **growth mindset** views intelligence, character, and drive as evolving characteristics that can be changed. Those with growth mindsets tend to thrive on challenges and see failures as learning opportunities. Growth mindset individuals react to adversity by working harder and trying new strategies.

Mindsets can be applied to learning pharmacology. For example, if a technician approaches learning pharmacology with a fixed mindset, they may become quickly discouraged with this challenging topic. Discouragement may lead to giving up because they feel they will never master the information. However, if the same technician approaches pharmacology with a growth mindset, their reaction to a challenging topic may be completely different. Instead of wanting to quit, they may find the challenge exciting and see a complicated topic as an obstacle that they can and will overcome.

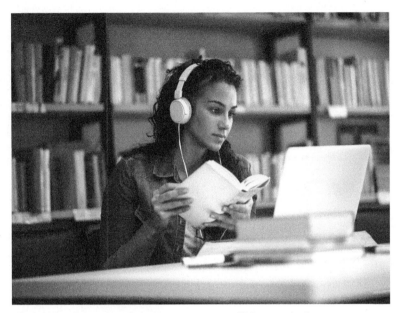

Eliminating distractions is one way to ensure efficient study time.

3.2 Pharmacy-Specific Study Aids

Up to this point, the chapter has focused on general methods to assist with studying. Although these techniques can be universally useful, there are methods that are *specific* to pharmacology. The following pharmacy-specific study aids include learning by drug class, generic name endings, and pharmacology-specific mnemonics.

Learning by Drug Class

Many learners find it best to break up pharmacology material into categories. Organizing medications by **drug classes**—categories of drugs having similar characteristics—is one way to break up study materials. Drugs in the same class share common features such as mechanism of action, therapeutic use, certain side effects, and contraindications. These commonalities can be used to help more efficiently learn pharmacology.

Consider drugs in the angiotensin converting enzyme (ACE) inhibitors class. ACE inhibitors share the same mechanism of action. These drugs are also used for similar therapeutic uses (lowering blood pressure and protecting kidneys) and share many common side effects such as cough and increased potassium. While studying this class of drugs, it may be helpful to first focus on the commonalities of the drug class (such as mechanism of action and therapeutic use). Next, it would be useful to focus on the unique features of specific drugs within the class. For example, learn the ACE inhibitors that are available in injectable forms, such as enalaprilat. Approaching the learning of drug classes in this way will help to quickly identify what a particular drug does and how it works by simply seeing or hearing its name. Although pharmacy personnel will also need to remember the few exceptions to each drug class rule, these typically exist only within the side effects and dosage forms.

Work Wise

If you are currently employed in the pharmacy practice setting, you can quiz yourself while you work. Every time you see a medication order or prescription for a drug, ask yourself what class the drug belongs to. Then name side effects, common doses, and contraindications of that drug class.

After learning the commonalities and differences of a drug class, one can focus on learning the drug names associated with that class. This will help consolidate the amount of information that needs to be memorized. See Figures 3.2 and 3.3.

FIGURE 3.2
Learning Drugs by Class Overview

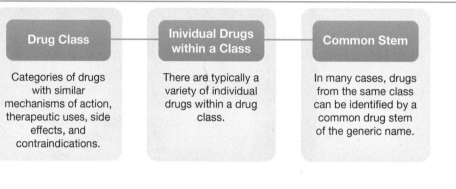

Drug Class	Inividual Drugs within a Class	Common Stem
Categories of drugs with similar mechanisms of action, therapeutic uses, side effects, and contraindications.	There are typically a variety of individual drugs within a drug class.	In many cases, drugs from the same class can be identified by a common drug stem of the generic name.

FIGURE 3.3
Learning by Drug Class

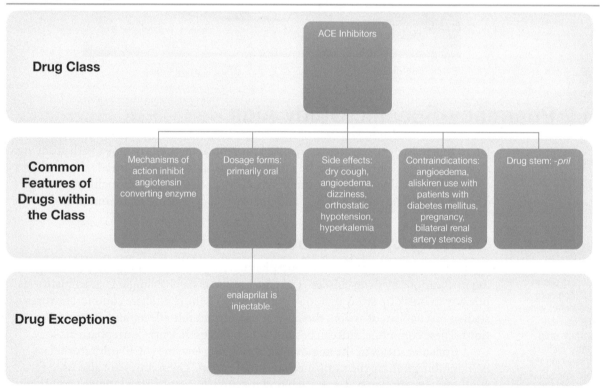

Identifying Drugs Using Generic Drug Stems

Once the common features of a drug class are learned, the next step is to identify which drugs belong to each class. Pharmacy technicians can usually identify a drug's class by looking at the generic name. Generic drugs of the same class often share a common drug stem. **Drug stems** are defined as a group of letters in a drug's generic name that can help identify the drug class. They are most often a **suffix** (a group of letters at the end of the drug name), but they can also be a **prefix** (found at the beginning of the drug name) or an **infix** (found in the middle of the drug name). Consider drugs in the ACE inhibitor class. Each contain the infix or suffix -*pril* (such as enalaprilat and lisinopril).

Older generic drug names were derived by shortening the name of the chemical compound. Consider the generic name *isoniazid* (an antibiotic). The name of the antibiotic's chemical compound is *isonicotinic acid hydrazide*—shortened to *isoniazid*. Although logical, this naming system led to complex names and overuse of common chemically derived syllables, both of which posed medication safety concerns. Today, generic names are assigned to reduce the risk of medical errors while also communicating important information about the drug to prescribers and pharmacy personnel. Generic drugs now have drug stems that denote chemical structure, indication, or mechanism of action.

Studying and memorizing common drug stems can be helpful in studying pharmacology. Once the common drug stem of a drug class is known, focus can shift to learning the features of the entire class instead of the individual drugs. Furthermore, knowing drug stems can help determine the class of a drug quickly, without necessarily memorizing the specific brand and generic name. Table 3.1 provides a list of common drug stems of drug classes. Pharmacy technicians may find it useful to memorize the generic drug stems and associated drug classes.

Practice Tip

Suffixes can help you learn which drugs belong to a certain class. Make flash cards with common drug class suffixes and quiz yourself or classmates, even if you have only a few minutes.

TABLE 3.1 Stems of Common Drug Classes

Stem	Drug Class	Therapeutic Use	Generic Examples
-afil	phosphodiesterase inhibitors	erectile dysfunction, pulmonary hypertension	sildenafil
-ane	inhaled anesthetics	anesthesia	halothane
-artan	angiotensin receptor blockers	hypertension	losartan
-azepam, -zolam	benzodiazepines	anxiety	lorazepam, midazolam
-azine	phenothiazines	antipsychotic	chlorpromazine
-azole	azole antifungals	antifungal	ketoconazole
-barbital	barbiturates	anxiety	phenobarbital
-caine	local anesthetics	anesthesia	lidocaine
-cillin	penicillin antibiotics	antibiotic	ticarcillin
-cycline	tetracyclines	antibiotic	doxycycline
-etine	selective serotonin reuptake inhibitors	depression	fluoxetine
-fene	selective estrogen response modifiers	osteoporosis, breast cancer	tamoxifen, clomifene
-floxacin	fluoroquinolones	antibiotic	levofloxacin
-fungin	echinocandins	antifungal	caspofungin
-gramostim, grastim	colony stimulating factors	blood dyscrasias	filgrastim, sargramostim
-ipine	dihydropyridine calcium channel blockers	high blood pressure	nifedipine
-ipramine	tricyclic antidepressants	depression	desipramine

continues

TABLE 3.1 Stems of Common Drug Classes—*Continued*

Stem	Drug Class	Therapeutic Use	Generic Examples
-lukast	LTD4 receptor antagonist	asthma	montelukast
-navir	protease inhibitor	antiviral	saquinavir
-olol	beta blocker	high blood pressure	propranolol
-oxin	cardiac glycoside	arrhythmias	digoxin
-phylline	methylxanthine	bronchodilator	theophylline
-pril	ace inhibitor	high blood pressure	lisinopril
-quine	quinolone derivatives	antimalarial	chloroquine
-statin	HMG-CoA reductase inhibitors	hyperlipidemia	simvastatin
-tecan	topoisomerase I inhibitor	chemotherapy	topotecan
-terol	β_2 agonist	bronchodilator	albuterol
-tidine	second-generation antihistamine	acid reflux	famotidine
-fine	allylamine antifungals	antifungal	terbinafine
-toposide	topoisomerase II inhibitor	chemotherapy	etoposide
-triptan	$5\text{-HT}_{1B}/_{1D}$ agonist	migraines	sumatriptan
-tropin	pituitary hormone	hormone deficiency	somatotropin
-vaptan	vasopressin receptor antagonist	hyponatremia	tolvaptan
-zosin	alpha-adrenergic blockers	high blood pressure, benign prostatic hypertrophy	terazosin

Using Mnemonic Devices

Mnemonic devices can be useful when learning side effects or other difficult-to-memorize pharmacology facts. A **mnemonic device** is a learning technique that uses a pattern of letters, ideas, or associations to assist in information retention or retrieval. Educational research demonstrates the efficacy of mnemonic devices in recalling lists of information. There are a variety of different types of mnemonics.

Pharm Fact

Mnemonics are not a new learning strategy. In fact, the ancient Greeks developed mnemonics more than 1,000 years ago.

Acronym Mnemonic

The acronym mnemonic method uses the first letters of a list of words to create a new or memorable word. A common example is the acronym ROYGBIV to recall the colors of the rainbow from low to high frequency. The acronym is made using the first letters of *red, orange, yellow, green, blue, indigo,* and *violet.*

Acrostic Mnemonic

The acrostic mnemonic method is similar to but varies from the acronym method. In the acrostic mnemonic method, the first letters in a list of words serve as the first letters in a new sentence or phrase. For example, to remember the colors of the rainbow from low to high frequency, one would use a sentence such as, Richard Of York Gave Battle In Vain. The first letters of each word in the sentence should remind you of *red, orange, yellow, green, blue, indigo,* and *violet.*

Songs, Stories, and Rhyming Mnemonics

Songs, stories, and rhymes are another way to use mnemonics. In this method, information to memorize is joined together in a song, story, or rhyme. A common rhyming mnemonic is "30 days hath September, April, June, and November."

Mnemonics in Pharmacology

Mnemonics can be used to remember side effects, cautions, and contraindications for drug classes. Consider the ACE inhibitor drug class and the acronym mnemonic CAPTOPRIL shown in Table 3.2. The information provided by the mnemonic applies to all ACE inhibitors. Captopril is also conveniently the generic name of an ACE inhibitor. Another mnemonic that may help recall drugs that increase potassium (K+) is K-BANK. Table 3.3 shows the K-BANK mnemonic.

TABLE 3.2 The CAPTOPRIL Mnemonic

Letter	Meaning
C	Cough (side effect)
A	Angioedema (side effect)
P	Proteinuria (side effect)
T	Taste changes (side effect)
O	Orthostatic hypotension (side effect)
P	Pregnancy contraindication
R	Renal failure (contraindication)
I	Increased potassium (side effect)
L	Leukopenia (side effect)

TABLE 3.3 The K-BANK Mnemonic

Letter	Meaning
K	K+ sparing diuretics
B	Beta-blockers
A	ACE inhibitors
N	Nonsteroidal anti-inflammatory drugs
K	K+ supplements

3.3 Drug Information Resources

In addition to study strategies and aids, a pharmacy technician and/or student will need to access multiple drug information resources. Pharmacy is an evolving field with new drugs being discovered and approved by the FDA every year. Furthermore, drugs currently on the market may have information updates such as newly discovered cautions and drug interactions. For these reasons, technicians will want to have a variety of drug information resources available, such as package inserts; Orange, Purple, and Green books; and electronic-based resources.

Practice Tip

The audience of the PI is the pharmacist and pharmacy technician, not the patient. Pharmacy technicians should expand their knowledge of new drugs by reading the PI documents when an opportunity arises in their workdays.

Package Inserts

Since technicians and pharmacists cannot be expected to remember everything about every drug, the FDA requires that manufacturers provide scientific information for pharmacy personnel with each drug. This information is contained in the FDA label information, otherwise known as the **package insert** (PI) or patient package insert, which accompanies the stock sent from the wholesaler. PIs are attached to or placed inside stock bottles. Alternately, PIs can be found online through their official provider, DailyMed, which is published by the US National Library of Medicine. The information on the insert is provided in a specific order (see Table 3.4). These inserts detail indications, contraindications, warnings, side effects, and dosages, along with how to handle and store the medications. They also include the date of the most recent labeling revision.

TABLE 3.4 Organization of a Package Insert (PI)

- Description
- Clinical studies
- Indications and usage
- Contraindications
- Warnings and precautions
- Adverse reactions
- Drug abuse and overdosage
- Dosage and administration
- How supplied/preparation
- Stability/storage and handling

FDA Orange, Purple, and Green Books

The FDA publishes three online reference books that catalog a variety of information about approved drugs and their uses. The first is called the *Approved Drug Products with Therapeutic Equivalence Evaluations*, commonly called the Orange Book. The Orange Book identifies all drugs that are approved for both their safety and efficacy. This reference is used by drug wholesalers and in pharmacies primarily to make sure that generic products can be safely substituted for brand-name products. Pharmacy technicians may use information contained in the Orange Book on a daily basis. However, many prescription order entry programs automatically integrate information from the Orange Book, decreasing the need to access the actual reference text.

The second FDA reference book is called the *Lists of Licensed Biological Products with Reference Product Exclusivity and Biosimilarity or Interchangeability Evaluations*. This publication is referred to as the Purple Book. The Purple Book provides information on interchangeable biologic-based drugs. The third FDA reference book is called *Approved Animal Drug Products* and is known as the Green Book. The Green Book focuses on veterinary medicine.

Electronic and Drug Resource Apps

Many drug information resources that were once available only in print are now available electronically and through smartphone-based apps. Electronic and smartphone-based drug references typically require a subscription or fee for use. However, many workplaces have institutional licenses that allow employees or students free access. A school's librarian (or pharmacy employer) may be able to assist pharmacy technicians with access. Common examples include the *Prescribers' Digital Reference* (PDR), Epocrates, Lexicomp, Micromedex, and RxList.

The PDR, formerly the *Physicians' Desk Reference*, is a publication with reprints of drug PIs from pharmaceutical manufacturers of most drugs. This digital resource is useful for identifying unknown drugs by color, shape, and coding and for alerting pharmacists and pharmacy technicians to boxed warnings. Pharmacy technicians can learn more about the drugs that they are dispensing by studying the PDR and reading PIs during any free or slow times in the pharmacy. This resource can be accessed as an ebook at pdr.net and via PDR smartphone applications.

Epocrates is a drug information app that provides prescribing and safety information for thousands of medications. Dosing guidelines, side effects, contraindications, cautions and considerations, pregnancy and lactation ratings, pharmacokinetics, and general pricing are included.

Lexicomp is a drug information resource available in print, online, and via smartphone apps. Dosing guidelines, side effects, contraindications, cautions and considerations, pregnancy and lactation ratings, and pharmacokinetics are included in the various Lexicomp products. Online and app versions also include an electronic drug interaction tool and intravenous drug compatability checker.

Micromedex is an online and app-based product that provides information on more than 1,400 drugs. Dosing guidelines, side effects, contraindications, cautions and considerations, pregnancy and lactation ratings, and pharmacokinetics are included in the online and app products. A drug interaction tool and an intravenous drug compatibility checker are also available.

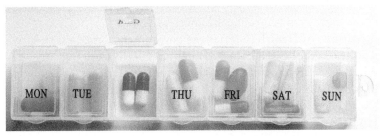

Patients may bring pills into your practice setting in pillboxes instead of the packaging that accompanied the medication at the time of dispensing. Online resources may help you identify the pills based on shape, color, and markings.

RxList is an online resource that includes general drug information. A unique feature is the Pill Identification Tool. This free tool allows the user to input information about a pill (such as color, shape, or imprint) to find out what the pill is. This may be helpful to a pharmacy technician if they need to identify a pill based on appearance. For example, a patient may bring a pillbox into a community pharmacy and ask to refill a specific medication without knowing the name. An institutional pharmacy technician may need to identify pills from a pillbox during the medication reconciliation process.

In addition to being a resource while practicing, drug resource apps may be helpful to pharmacy technician students for study purposes. For example, students could quiz themselves about boxed warnings for a certain drug and check their answers using these resources. Alternately, they could look up drugs by brand name and self-test on the associated generic name.

3.4 Health Information Resources

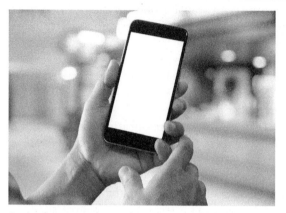

Smartphones can be used to access health information resources that previously were available only in print or on desktop computers.

In the digital age, people have more access to health information than ever before. A simple internet search for the word *acetaminophen* offers over 1 million results within seconds. Although there is no scarcity of information when searching online, not all information found online is accurate and to be trusted. One may be asked to research health information during pharmacy technician studies and will want to access trusted sources. Furthermore, when practicing as a pharmacy technician, it is important to access reputable health information resources for continuing education and be able to refer patients to these same reputable resources.

Always assess internet sources for validity. If the website is published by the government or a university, health organization, or hospital, it is more likely to be reputable. Check the "About" or "Contact" pages to identify who (or what entity) runs the website.

 Safety Alert

The US National Library of Medicine created a free tutorial and checklist that teaches consumers how to evaluate health information found on the internet. Both the tutorial and checklist can be found at https://medlineplus.gov/webeval/webeval.html.

Government Healthcare Websites

The **Centers for Disease Control and Prevention** (CDC) is a governmental organization aimed to protect Americans from health, safety, and security threats. The CDC has a regularly updated website that provides health alerts, communicates current outbreaks and breaking health news, provides fact sheets about common disease states and their treatments, and offers suggestions on healthy living. Travel-related health concerns and emergency preparedness information is also published on the CDC website. The pharmacy technician could benefit from regularly using the CDC as an information source to stay current on health matters.

The **National Institutes of Health** (NIH) is the governmental medical research agency of the United States. Like the CDC, the NIH has a regularly updated website that provides science-based health information on symptoms, diagnoses, treatments, research, and clinical trials. The NIH website also has a free alert subscription that provides email alerts when new health information is published.

MedlinePlus is a health information website published by the US National Library of Medicine. MedlinePlus provides information on health topics, drugs and supplements, and medical tests. A medical encyclopedia is also available as a resource. The website has a section devoted to videos that illustrate the anatomy of body parts and organ systems and how certain disease states affect them.

Health care is a constantly evolving field. Those in healthcare fields, such as pharmacy technicians, need to stay informed on health-related information. One way to keep informed is to regularly check health information resources, including the websites mentioned in this chapter. Verified social media accounts are another option to help you stay abreast of new and noteworthy health developments. Consider following the CDC and NIH on social media. Both organizations have Facebook, Instagram, and Twitter accounts. The FDA and MedlinePlus have Twitter accounts. If you prefer to watch videos, you can follow the CDC and the NIH on YouTube.

The FDA maintains a website that provides information on products under its jurisdiction, including food, drugs, medical devices, radiation-emitting products, vaccines, blood, biologics, animal and veterinary products, cosmetics, and tobacco products. Drug recalls and market withdrawals information can also be found on the website.

Safety Alert

The FDA's website publishes safety information regarding recent recalls of drugs, supplements, and food.

Medical Dictionaries and Encyclopedias

The medical field has a reputation for unique terminology, multiple abbreviations, and use of jargon. Many terms commonly used in the pharmacy practice setting may seem unusual at first. **Medical dictionaries**—resources that define commonly used terms in the healthcare field—may be helpful for pharmacy technicians as they become more familiar with the particular terminology of the healthcare setting.

Merriam-Webster, a publisher of dictionaries since the 1800s, has a specific dictionary dedicated to medical terms. Both medical terms and abbreviations are contained in the resource. The *Merriam-Webster Medical Dictionary* can be accessed online and is free for users.

Stedman's Medical Dictionary is a resource that contains over 38,000 terms. Definitions, images, and appendices are included. Tools such as term pronunciation and word origin are provided. *Stedman's Medical Dictionary* is currently available in both electronic book and online versions. The online version requires a subscription for user access.

MedlinePlus, the online health information resource published by the US National Library of Medicine offers medical definitions and a medical encyclopedia. The medical encyclopedia provides definitions, potential causes, symptoms, and test and examination basics of disease states. Treatment options and preventive steps are also included. MedlinePlus is available online and can be accessed for free.

Review and Assessment

CHAPTER SUMMARY

Evidence-Based Study Techniques

- Educational research is the scientific field of study that examines learning and education.

- Spacing is a study method that uses multiple study sessions spread across a long period of time. Spacing can be contrasted with massing (studying just once or twice over a short period of time). Spacing is shown to improve learning outcomes compared to massing.

- Interleaving is the process of mixing the study of several related skills together. Interleaving is superior compared to blocking (practicing one item before moving to the next) in category learning.

- Self-testing is the study method of testing oneself on newly learned information. Using practice tests or flash cards, writing information down, or saying information aloud are ways to self-test.

- The contiguity principle of study is a method that aligns words to corresponding graphics. Research shows this method improves information retention.

- Eliminating distractions may help the pharmacy technician use study time more efficiently.

- Research supports a growth mindset (seeing intelligence, character, and drive as evolving characteristics) over a fixed mindset (seeing intelligence, character, and drive as unchanging) for academic success.

Pharmacy-Specific Study Aids

- Medications are organized by drug class—groups of drugs with common features such as mechanism of action, therapeutic use, side effects, and contraindications.

- Pharmacy technicians may find it advantageous to learn commonalities and differences of a drug class before learning the names of individual drugs within a class.

- Drugs within the same class often share a common drug stem (a group of letters that are part of a word or name). Learning generic drug stems may be helpful in pharmacology study.

- A mnemonic device is a learning technique that uses a pattern of letters, ideas, or associations to assist in information retention or retrieval. Types of mnemonic devices include acronyms, acrostics, or songs, stories, and rhyming. Mnemonic devices can help recall lists of information.

Drug Information Resources

- A pharmacy technician will need to access current drug information resources while in training and practicing.

- Package inserts accompany drug stock sent from the wholesaler and include key information about the medication.

- The FDA publishes several drug references. The *Approved Drug Products with Therapeutic Equivalence Evaluations* (the Orange Book) identifies all drugs that are approved for both their safety and efficacy. Another publication, *Lists of Licensed Biological Products with Reference Product Exclusivity and Biosimilarity or Interchangeability Evaluations* (the Purple Book), contains information on biological products. The *Approved Animal Drug Products* (the Green Book) is for veterinary medicine.

- There are multiple electronic and smartphone-based based drug resources that may be used by the pharmacy technician. Examples include the Prescribers' Digital Reference (PDR), Epocrates, Lexicomp, Micromedex, and RxList.

Health Information Resources

- Accessing reputable health information resources is important for the pharmacy technician during their studies and while in practice.

- Government healthcare websites that may be useful to the pharmacy technician include the Centers for Disease Control and Prevention, National Institutes of Health, MedlinePlus, and the US Food and Drug Administration.

- The medical field is full of unique terms, and the pharmacy technician may need to access medical dictionaries and encyclopedias. The *Merriam-Webster Medical Dictionary*, *Stedman's Medical Dictionary*, and MedlinePlus are resources available to the pharmacy technician.

✔ CHECK YOUR UNDERSTANDING

Take a moment to review what you have learned in this chapter and answer the following questions.

1. Which of the following best describes spacing as a study method?
   a. mixing practice on several related skills together
   b. practicing one skill at a time before moving on to the next
   c. spreading out study sessions across a long period of time
   d. studying one or two times over a short period of time

2. Which of the following best describes interleaving as a study method?
   a. mixing practice on several related skills together
   b. practicing one skill at a time before moving on to the next
   c. spreading out study sessions across a long period of time
   d. studying one or two times over a short period of time

3. Which of the following is an example of using testing as a study method?
   a. adopting a growth mindset
   b. studying for a large block of the night before an exam
   c. taking practice tests and quizzes during study time
   d. using smaller blocks for study time on a daily basis

4. The contiguity principle of studying is best defined as
   a. aligning words to corresponding graphics to improve information retention.
   b. eliminating distractions so study time is used most efficiently.
   c. practicing one skill at a time prior to learning a new skill.
   d. studying at the same time each day to improve memory.

5. Which of the following is an example of eliminating distractions while studying?
   a. having multiple windows open on your computer so you can take a practice test and respond to email at the same time
   b. keeping your cell phone on a loud setting so calls and messages can be easily heard
   c. responding to computer alerts during study time
   d. studying in a location with minimal distractions, such as a library

6. A growth mindset views intelligence, character, and drive as
   a. characteristics unimportant to success.
   b. evolving characteristics that can be changed.
   c. static and unchangeable characteristics.
   d. ways to help others study more efficiently.

7. Drugs in the same class typically have which of the following common characteristics?
   a. common doses, generic name drug stems, mechanisms of action, and side effects
   b. contraindications, common doses, therapeutic uses, and side effects

   c. dosage forms, mechanisms of action, side effects, and contraindications
   d. mechanisms of action, therapeutic uses, side effects, and contraindications

8. The generic name suffix *-floxacin* indicates which of the following drug classes?
   a. ACE inhibitors
   b. fluoroquinolones
   c. loop diuretics
   d. tetracyclines

9. The generic names of beta-blockers end in which drug stem?
   a. *-pril*
   b. *-lukast*
   c. *-olol*
   d. *-phylline*

10. The FDA reference titled *Approved Drug Products with Therapeutic Equivalence Evaluations* is commonly known as the
   a. Blue Book.
   b. Green Book.
   c. Orange Book.
   d. Purple Book.

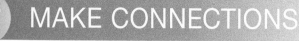

MAKE CONNECTIONS

Take a moment to consider what you have learned in this chapter and respond thoughtfully to the following prompts. Note that some of these activities will require internet access.

1. Using the evidence-based education research in this chapter, create an ideal weekly pharmacology study schedule. Your schedule should include study times, days, and locations. Make sure to include what you plan to do to study during each scheduled time.

2. Mnemonics can be useful when learning side effects or other difficult-to-memorize pharmacology facts. Create two different mnemonics (not listed in this chapter) to help you learn pharmacology information from any chapter in this book.

The online course includes additional review and assessment resources.

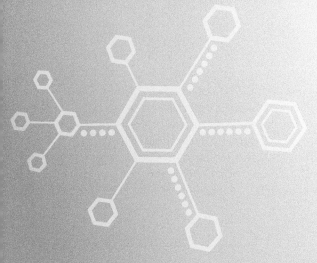

Prescription Orders and Medication Safety

4

Learning Objectives

1 Describe the components of a prescription. (Section 4.1)

2 State commonly used prescription abbreviations. (Section 4.1)

3 Explain the "rights" of correct drug administration. (Section 4.2)

4 Recognize common dosage forms. (Section 4.3)

5 Describe the routes of administration and dosage forms. (Section 4.3)

6 Recognize factors that influence the effects of drugs, particularly in older adults and pediatric populations. (Section 4.4)

7 Explain the importance of and the components of teaching patients medication management. (Section 4.5)

8 Describe the role of the pharmacy technician in medication safety. (Section 4.6)

ASHP/ACPE Accreditation Standards

To view the *ASHP/ACPE Accreditation Standards* addressed in this chapter, refer to Appendix C.

Pharmacy technicians play a key role in the dispensing of medications. This role requires a thorough understanding of the components of the prescription and the responsibilities of pharmacy personnel. The prescription includes all the information necessary for the pharmacist to fill the prescription with the correct dosage form and for the patient to take the medication correctly. Two age groups of patients—older adults and children—have special needs that must be considered in dispensing drugs.

4.1 The Prescription

A **prescription** is a written or oral direction for medication to be dispensed to a patient. A physician or other licensed practitioner issues a prescription, and it is filled by a pharmacist. When a prescription is issued and dispensed in an **institutional setting** (or facilities that assume total care of patients such as hospitals or long-term care facilities), it is called an **order** or a *medication order*. The term *prescription* is used in noninstitutional settings. The term **noninstitutional setting** describes facilities such as clinics or community pharmacies that offer same-day patient care.

There are two types of prescriptions being issued today: those that are handwritten and those that are transmitted electronically. A handwritten prescription is typically a piece of paper a patient receives from a prescriber that the patient then presents to a pharmacy for fulfillment. Or, more commonly, an e-prescription will be used. An **e-prescription** is transmitted electronically through secure systems directly from the prescriber to the pharmacy. Components of a valid prescription vary by state but typically should contain all of the information described in Table 4.1.

TABLE 4.1 Parts of a Prescription

Part	Description
prescriber's information	name, address, telephone number, and other information identifying the prescriber; NPI and DEA numbers; and, sometimes, the state license number
date	date on which the prescription was written; this date may differ from the date on which the prescription was received
patient's information	full name, address, telephone number, and date of birth of the patient
℞	symbol ℞, from the Latin verb *recipere* meaning "to take"
inscription	medication prescribed, including generic or brand name, strength, and amount to be dispensed
subscription	instructions to the pharmacist on dispensing the medication
signa	directions for the patient to follow (commonly called the *sig*)
additional instructions	any additional instructions that the prescriber deems necessary
signature	signature of the prescriber

If the prescription is for a controlled substance, as discussed in Chapter 1, the Drug Enforcement Agency (DEA) number of the prescriber must be on the prescription.

Figure 4.1 is an example of a prescription with the essential elements labeled. Figure 4.2 is an example of an e-prescription. The symbol at the top of the form, ℞ or Rx, is the symbol for prescription. If a medication has this symbol on the container, the medication may not be dispensed unless a prescriber writes an order or prescription for it. It cannot be sold over the counter (OTC).

Pharmacy technicians should always double-check a prescription for accuracy and to ensure that all of the legal requirements have been met. Depending on state laws, the label on the medication container given to the patient must include the patient's name, the date the prescription was filled, the inscription, the signa, the number of refills, the expiration or beyond use date, the prescriber's name, the Rx number, and the phone number and address of the pharmacy.

FIGURE 4.1
The Essential Elements of a Prescription

The pharmacy technician should always double-check these elements.

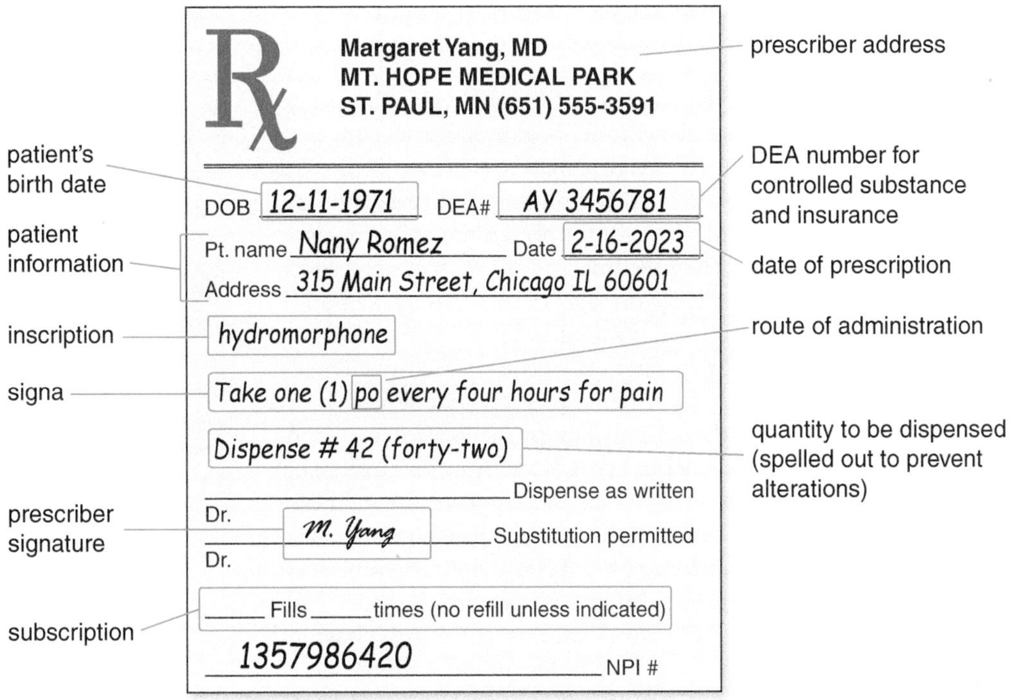

Margaret Yang, MD
MT. HOPE MEDICAL PARK
ST. PAUL, MN (651) 555-3591
prescriber address
patient's birth date
DOB 12-11-1971
DEA# AY 3456781
DEA number for controlled substance and insurance
patient information
Pt. name Nany Romez
Date 2-16-2023
date of prescription
Address 315 Main Street, Chicago IL 60601
inscription
hydromorphone
route of administration
signa
Take one (1) po every four hours for pain
Dispense # 42 (forty-two)
quantity to be dispensed (spelled out to prevent alterations)
Dispense as written
prescriber signature
Dr.
M. Yang
Substitution permitted
Dr.
subscription
Fills times (no refill unless indicated)
1357986420
NPI #

FIGURE 4.2
E-prescription

E-prescriptions contain the essential elements of a prescription in an electronic format.

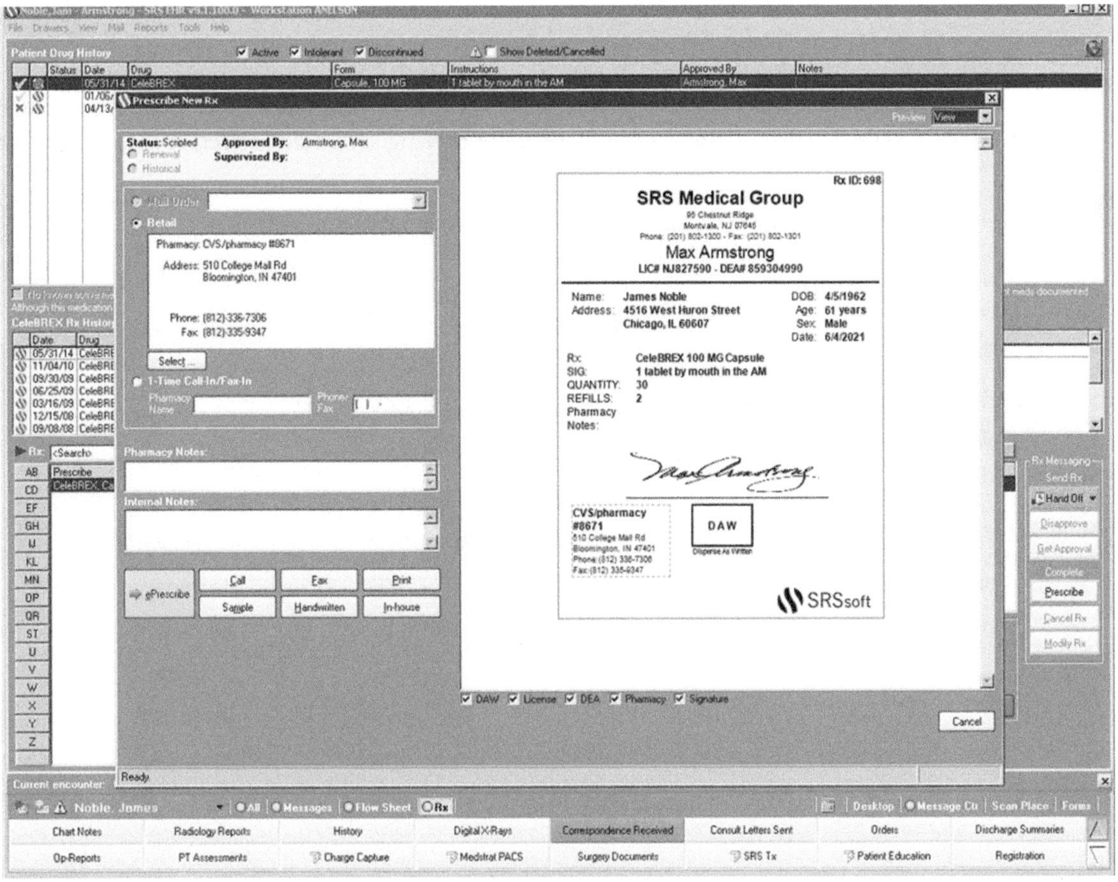

Patient Drug History
Prescribe New Rx
SRS Medical Group
Max Armstrong
Name: James Noble
Address: 4516 West Huron Street
Chicago, IL 60607
DOB: 4/5/1962
Age: 61 years
Sex: Male
Date: 6/4/2021
Rx: CeleBREX 100 MG Capsule
SIG: 1 tablet by mouth in the AM
QUANTITY: 30
REFILLS: 2
DAW
SRSsoft
Cancel

Abbreviations in the Pharmacy

To fill the prescription safely, the pharmacy technician should be familiar with common abbreviations used in prescriptions (see Table 4.2). Although these abbreviations are standard usage for prescribers, pharmacists, and their technicians, the instructions to the patient are not abbreviated but spelled out in full and phrased as simply as possible to ensure proper use of the medication. There is strong evidence to show that abbreviations are the source of many medication errors. A **medication error** is a preventable event that may cause or lead to inappropriate medication use or patient harm. When taking a verbal order or prescription, it is recommended that abbreviations *not* be used.

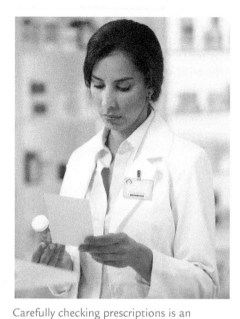

Carefully checking prescriptions is an important responsibility of the pharmacy technician.

The abbreviations in Table 4.3 have been identified by The Joint Commission as the cause of many errors and should never be used. Additional dangerous abbreviations are listed at the Institute for Safe Medication Practices (ISMP) website. Although many abbreviations are unapproved, the technician will frequently see them and will need to be able to interpret them to fill a prescription.

Most pharmacies give the patient an information sheet with additional details regarding the proper way to take the medication (especially in regard to food intake), possible side effects, and situations in which the prescribing physician should be consulted. Limiting the number of refills allowed without another physician consultation is a way to prevent the patient from encountering severe side effects from the medication.

℞ Put Down Roots

Many of the abbreviations used in writing prescriptions come from Latin. For example, the abbreviation *ac* is from the Latin words *ante cibum* and translates to "before meals."

Per os is Latin for "by mouth," hence the abbreviation *po*.

TABLE 4.2 Abbreviations Used in Writing Prescriptions

Abbreviation	Translation	Abbreviation	Translation
ac	before meals	IV	intravenous
am	morning	L	liter
bid	twice a day	mcg	microgram
c	with	mEq	milliequivalent
cap	capsule	mL	milliliter
DAW	dispense as written	NKA	no known allergy
d/C	discontinue	nKDA	no known drug allergy
g	gram*	npo	nothing by mouth
gr	grain	pc	after meals
gtt	drop	po	by mouth
h or hr	hour	prn	as needed
iM	intramuscular	q	every

continues

TABLE 4.2 Abbreviations Used in Writing Prescriptions—*Continued*

Abbreviation	Translation	Abbreviation	Translation
qh	every hour	tab	tablet
q2h	every two hours	tid	three times a day
qid	four times a day	ud	as directed
qs or qsad	a sufficient quantity	wk	week
stat	immediately		

* The abbreviation gm is sometimes used for gram.

Note: Some prescribers may write abbreviations using capital letters or periods. However, periods should not be used with metrics or medical abbreviations, because they can be a source of medication errors.

Work Wise

Many drugs look alike in spelling or packaging, such as azaTHIOprine and azaCITIDine. Other drugs sound alike, such as Celexa and Zyprexa. To help prevent errors, the ISMP publishes a list of Confused Drug Names. Many of these are also discussed in Appendix A.

TABLE 4.3 Official "Do Not Use" List of Abbreviations

Do Not Use	Potential Problem	Use Instead
U, u (unit)	mistaken for 0 (zero), the numeral 4, or cc	write "unit"
IU (International Unit)	mistaken for IV (intravenous) or the numeral 10	write "International Unit"
Q.D., QD, q.d., qd (daily)	mistaken for qod (every other day)	write "daily"
Q.O.D., QOD, q.o.d, qod (every other day)	mistaken for qd (daily), period after the Q mistaken for "I" and the "O" mistaken for "I" (four times daily)	write "every other day"
Trailing zero (X.0 mg)*	decimal point is missed, wrong amount administered	write "X mg" write "0.X mg"
Lack of leading zero (.X mg)	decimal point is missed, wrong amount administered	
MS	can mean morphine sulfate or magnesium sulfate	write "morphine sulfate" or "magnesium sulfate"
MSO4 and MgSO4	confused for one another	write "morphine sulfate" or "magnesium sulfate"

*A "trailing zero" may be used only where required to demonstrate the level of precision of the value being reported, such as for laboratory results, imaging studies that report size of lesions, or catheter/tube sizes. It may not be used in medication orders or other medication-related documentation.

Medication Orders in the Institutional Setting

Institutions and hospitals have organizational policies on the prescribing, dispensing, administration, and documentation of medication administration. These policies were created to ensure safe medication use within the facility. It is important that each organization's policies and procedures address the following topics:

- **Medication Orders** Defines which practitioners may prescribe medications per state and federal regulations. These policies and practices may also identify the format that must be used and if certain abbreviations may not be used. Generally, a complete medication order includes the patient name, the medication name, route of administration, and rate of administration (if applicable). Some institutions may require that an indication also be listed on the medication order.

- **Verbal Orders** Defines who may accept a verbal order and the process of transcribing the verbal order.
- **Stop Orders** Defines which medication orders have an automatic stop. This may be used for medications that have a specific duration limit on how long they should be used.
- **Controlled Substances** Defines the process and procedure on how controlled substances should be prescribed; who can prescribe them; and how they are stored, tracked, distributed, and documented.

4.2 Correct Drug Administration Rights

The "rights" of medication administration, illustrated in Figure 4.3, offer useful guidelines when filling prescriptions for patient medications. The healthcare professionals who are involved in the process from prescribing through administration use these concepts to prevent medication errors. A medication error can occur whenever the rights are not followed correctly. Seven of these rights are overviewed below. Hospitals or other institutional settings may include additional rights (e.g., reason) into their medication administration procedures.

- **Right Patient** Always verify the patient's name before dispensing medication. Always use at least two patient identifiers (name plus room number, address, birth date, phone number, or other data).
- **Right Drug** Always check the medication against the original prescription and the patient's disease state. The medication label contains important information about the drug that will be dispensed to the patient. Figure 4.4 provides an example of a medication label.
- **Right Strength** Check the original prescription for this information, and pay attention to the age of the patient.
- **Right Dose Form** Check the medication against the original label to make sure the dosage form being dispensed is appropriate.
- **Right Route** Check that the physician's order agrees with the drug's specified route of administration. Many medications can be given by a variety of routes, and the route of administration can affect the medication's absorption.
- **Right Time** Check the prescription to determine the appropriate time for the medication to be administered. Some medications must be taken on an empty stomach (one hour before or two hours after a meal), while others should be taken with food. Sometimes, a certain time span is needed between doses to maintain a therapeutically effective blood level.
- **Right Documentation** You must accurately record that the correct patient has been given the correct medication with the right strength, route, and time.

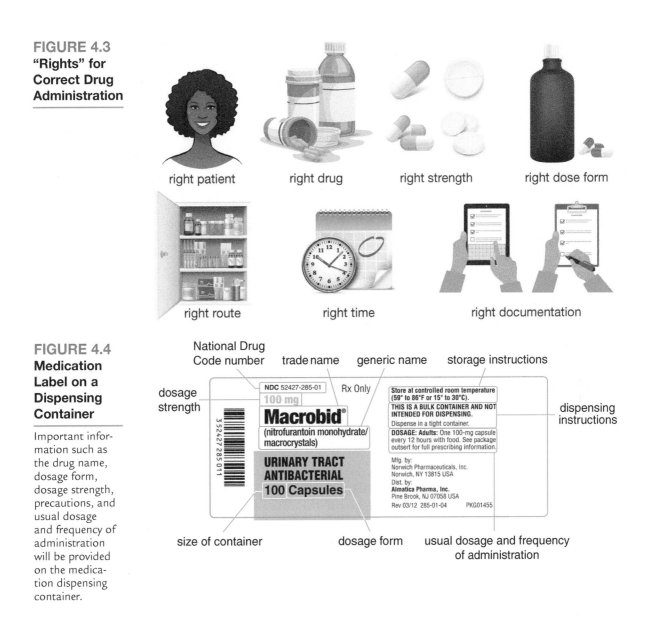

FIGURE 4.3
"Rights" for Correct Drug Administration

right patient   right drug   right strength   right dose form

right route   right time   right documentation

FIGURE 4.4
Medication Label on a Dispensing Container

Important information such as the drug name, dosage form, dosage strength, precautions, and usual dosage and frequency of administration will be provided on the medication dispensing container.

National Drug Code number   trade name   generic name   storage instructions

dosage strength

NDC 52427-285-01   Rx Only

100 mg

Macrobid®

(nitrofurantoin monohydrate/macrocrystals)

URINARY TRACT ANTIBACTERIAL

100 Capsules

Store at controlled room temperature (59° to 86°F or 15° to 30°C).

THIS IS A BULK CONTAINER AND NOT INTENDED FOR DISPENSING.

Dispense in a tight container.

DOSAGE: Adults: One 100-mg capsule every 12 hours with food. See package outsert for full prescribing information.

Mfg. by:
Norwich Pharmaceuticals, Inc.
Norwich, NY 13815 USA
Dist. by:
Almatica Pharma, Inc.
Pine Brook, NJ 07058 USA
Rev 03/12   285-01-04   PKG01455

dispensing instructions

size of container   dosage form   usual dosage and frequency of administration

4.3 Dosage Forms and Routes of Administration

A medication may be administered in many different forms for convenient and efficacious treatment of disease. The route and dosage form are determined by many factors, including the disease being treated, the area of the body that the drug needs to reach, and the chemical composition of the drug itself. Each drug has its own characteristics related to absorption, distribution, metabolism, and elimination (ADME). Drugs are prepared for administration by many conceivable routes, but the primary routes are oral, parenteral, and topical. Table 4.4 lists a few of these common routes and their common dosage forms.

The age and condition of the patient often determine the dosage form that will be used. Pediatric and older adult populations frequently have special needs. These two groups often need liquid dosage forms. Convenience may also play a role in the selection of the appropriate dosage form. Drugs with distinctive sizes, shapes, and colors are inherently easier to identify. Dosage forms that reduce the frequency of administration without sacrificing efficacy are often advantageous and improve patient **adherence** (taking a medication correctly or as prescribed).

TABLE 4.4 Common Routes of Administration and Dosage Forms

Route	Example	Primary Dosage Forms
oral (po, by mouth)	buccal (dissolves in the cheek) oral (swallowed) sublingual (under the tongue)	capsules elixirs gels powders solutions suspensions syrups tablets troches/lozenges
parenteral (not through the alimentary canal, but by injection through some other route)	epidural (fibrous membrane of spinal cord) intra-arterial (artery) intracardiac (heart) intramuscular (muscle) intraspinal/intrathecal (spinal fluid) intrasynovial (joint-fluid area) intravenous (vein) subcutaneous (beneath the skin)	solutions suspensions
topical (applied to surface of skin or mucous membranes)	inhalation (lung) intranasal (nose) ophthalmic (eye) otic (ear) rectal (rectum) transdermal (skin surface) urethral (urethra) vaginal (vagina)	aerosols creams emulsions enemas gels inhalants lotions ointments pastes powders sponges sprays suppositories transdermal patches

Oral Routes

The **oral** (po) route is the most economical and most convenient way to give medications. The term *po* comes from the Latin *per os*, meaning "by opening." This route was once referred to as the **peroral** route. The term *oral* means that the medication is given by mouth either in solid form (such as a tablet or capsule) or in liquid form (such as a solution or syrup). Once the medication enters the mouth, it must be swallowed to reach the stomach. Then it must pass to the area of absorption, most commonly the small intestine, although some medications are absorbed in the stomach.

The absorption process takes time and is affected by several factors, including the presence of food (which slows the process) or digestive disorders. It is important to refer to a reliable drug reference guide to determine whether the medication should be given with or without food and whether any specific assessments should be done before dispensing it.

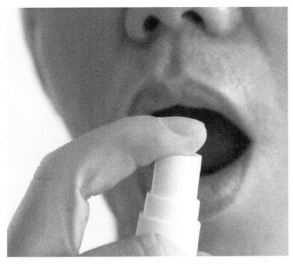

Nitroglycerin, a medication commonly used in patients with chest pain, is administered sublingually.

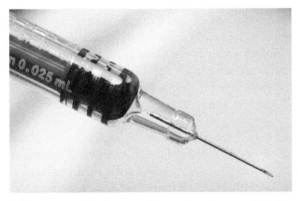

Subcutaneous injections require needles that are relatively short, as pictured above. Intramuscular injections require longer needles.

Sublingual (under the tongue) and **buccal** (between the cheek and gum) routes of administration are used when a rapid action is desired or when a drug is specifically designed to be easily absorbed into blood vessels. The medication enters the bloodstream directly from the richly vascularized mucous membrane of the mouth and produces its effects more quickly than drugs that are swallowed. This dosage form cannot obtain the same effect if swallowed.

When taking medication by the sublingual route, the patient should hold the tablet under the tongue until it dissolves completely. For buccal administration, the patient should place the tablet between the cheek and gums, close the mouth, and hold the tablet there until it is dissolved. It is important to remind the patient not to drink water or swallow excessively until the tablet is completely absorbed.

Parenteral Routes

Administration of drugs by injection is referred to as the **parenteral** route (meaning "outside the intestines"). Injections can be painful, and there is a risk of infection at the site of puncture, but parenteral administration may be necessary for several reasons. Some drugs, such as insulin, are inactivated in digestive juices, so swallowing them would be ineffective. Other medications would be inactivated by first-pass metabolism, described in Chapter 1, if they had to pass through the liver before entering the bloodstream, so they are injected directly into the tissues of the body. Parenteral routes also offer the potential for quick absorption of injected medication into the bloodstream and a rapid effect (especially for the intravenous route). Parenteral products also offer an alternative during times when the patient cannot tolerate oral medications, such as during severe vomiting.

Sometimes the prescriber forgets to write a prescription for the needle to inject these drugs. You may need to call the prescriber to clarify which needle is needed, because different medications need different size needles. For example, it can be dangerous to inject heparin intramuscularly (IM), so the prescription should indicate a subcutaneous (SQ, SC, or subcut) needle. If the prescription for the appropriate needle is in the patient profile, a lot of pain and confusion can be prevented. Drugs may be injected into the following locations:

- muscle: **intramuscular (IM)**
- vein: **intravenous (IV)**
- skin: **intradermal**
- tissue beneath the skin: **subcutaneous (SC, SQ, or subcut)**
- spinal column: **intraspinal** or **intrathecal**

Topical Routes

Topical medications are applied to the surface of the skin or mucous membranes (such as eyes and nose). The desired effect can be **local** (affecting only a small area of the body) or **systemic** (affecting the body as a whole). Other topical routes are inhalation, ophthalmic, otic, nasal, rectal, and vaginal.

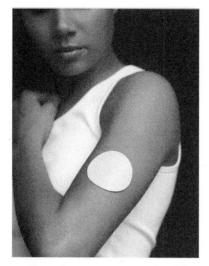

A nicotine patch is a topical medication that a patient can use to quit smoking. The effect of a nicotine patch is systemic in that it delivers nicotine to the entire body.

The **inhalation route** delivers medications to the respiratory system. These medications are usually intended for one or more of the following purposes: to alter the condition of the mucous membranes, to alter the character of the secretions in the respiratory system, to treat diseases and infections of the respiratory tract, or to produce general anesthesia.

Another route is the **ophthalmic route**, which describes administering medicine via drops of liquid preparation into the conjunctival sac of the eye or by application of a cream or ointment. Using drops is also known as **instillation**, or the administration of a medication drop by drop.

Drugs administered by the **otic route**, into the ear, are used locally to treat inflammation or infection of the external ear canal or to remove excess cerumen (wax) or foreign objects from the canal. Eardrops come in **solutions** (where the active drug is dissolved in liquid) and **suspensions** (where the active drug particles are mixed, but not dissolved, in liquid). If the patient has a tube in the ear, a suspension rather than a solution should be used. When a prescription for eardrops is dispensed, the technician should always ask whether the patient has an ear tube.

Medications can be administered via the **nasal route**, or through the nose. Nasal administration can result in local and/or systemic drug effects. Examples of intranasal drugs that are used for local effect include corticosteroids (used for rhinitis) and decongestants (used for congestion). Nasal drugs that are used for systemic effect include hormone products, migraine medications, and nicotine replacement. Nasal products are typically available as a spray or drops for instillation.

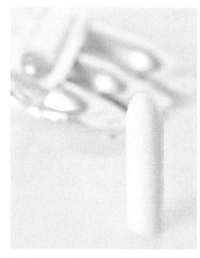

Rectal suppositories are usually packaged in foil and require refrigeration.

Medications that are administered by the **rectal route** are most commonly in the form of suppositories or enemas. A **suppository** is a soft, rounded piece of cocoa butter, glycerin, or a synthetic base containing medication. When inserted into the rectum, it melts at body temperature and releases the medication to be absorbed through the walls of the large intestine. An **enema** is a liquid or gas that is inserted into the rectum. The primary advantage of rectal administration is that the medication does not depend on the digestive system to be absorbed into the bloodstream. Therefore, this route is frequently used to treat nausea and vomiting. Suppositories can also be used for local effect to treat constipation. Additionally, the rectal route is ideal for treating fever in infants and young children.

Medications given by the **vaginal route** can be used to treat a **local infection** (restricted to or pertaining to one area of the body) caused by either bacteria or fungi. There can also be some **systemic absorption** (absorption into the bloodstream) through this route, enabling the medication to circulate and affect other parts of the body.

4.4 Factors That Influence Drug Action

Ensuring that patients receive the correct medication at the correct dosage and that a newly prescribed medication does not adversely interact with other drugs that a patient is taking is of paramount importance. A variety of factors can influence the effects of drugs and may require dosage adjustment.

Children and older adults may require a reduced dose because of alterations in metabolism of drugs and reductions in excretion or elimination from the body. In these instances, if the dosage is not decreased, it may have toxic effects on the patient. The prescriber can use a variety of formulas when prescribing medications for pediatric or older adult patients.

Patients with specific diseases may be unable to absorb, metabolize, or excrete certain medications. Impaired gastrointestinal (GI) function may affect absorption, impaired liver function may affect metabolism, and impaired kidney function may affect elimination. Inadequate nutritional intake may also adversely affect the metabolism of drugs. Therefore, the patient's disease state must be evaluated before medications can be prescribed.

Physicians also consider psychological and genetic factors when prescribing medications. The mental state of a patient can influence the body's ability to release chemical substances needed to absorb or metabolize a drug properly. Genes can also control the release of chemicals and the way the body absorbs or metabolizes various medications. Unfortunately, these factors are less predictable than age, gender, and disease state.

Before prescribing medications, healthcare practitioners must evaluate all patients for immune responses and document any allergic responses to foods or medications in the patient chart. Each time a new medication is dispensed, the pharmacy technician should ask whether the patient has had any additional allergic responses so that the records can be kept up to date.

Special Considerations in Older Adults

Older adults have special needs in relation to their medications. Aging affects both the chemical reactions that administered drugs undergo in the body (pharmacokinetics) as well as how the body reacts to the drugs (pharmacodynamics). In addition, older adults have more chronic diseases than the young and also tend to use more drugs—both prescription and nonprescription. Four out of five older individuals have at least one chronic disease, and many in this age group take numerous medications, three to four times daily. For some older adults, medications can support their self-reliance and help them lead independent lifestyles. As a result, geriatric medicine has emerged as a new and important medical specialty of the healthcare system.

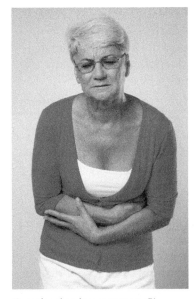

Constipation is a common GI change in older adults.

Changes in Physiologic Function

Aging can involve declines in both mental function (ability to continue to meet the demands of daily life) and physiologic well-being (normal functioning of the body). Physiologic changes do not occur at the same rate for all individuals, and many changes are not always predictable. Successful aging is characterized by losses in physiologic function that are **nonpathologic** (not related to disease). Impaired aging represents **pathologic** (manifestations of disease) changes with greater physiologic loss than in average persons of the same age group.

The following is a list of some of the changes that body systems may undergo with aging:

- **Visual Changes** As the lenses of the eye become less elastic, more dense, and yellow, visual acuity is compromised; this can often be improved with corrective lenses.

- **Auditory Changes** Hearing loss occurs in all sound frequencies, but especially in the high ranges. Impairment of sound localization and loudness perception is a problem for many older adults. A delay in central processing of auditory messages results in an increase in the time it takes for the person to respond to a question.

- **Gastrointestinal Changes** These changes create many problems, including decreases in saliva production, esophageal motility, hydrochloric acid secretion, absorptive surface, and rate of gastric emptying. Constipation may be a complaint.

- **Pulmonary Changes** Many older adults have chronic obstructive pulmonary disease (COPD). Aging brings on increased rigidity of the chest wall, decreased vital capacity (maximum intake and exhalation), decreased response to **hypoxia** (reduced oxygen in the blood), and **hypercapnia** (increased carbon dioxide in the blood). If an older adult patient also has cardiac disease, these functions are further compromised.

- **Cardiovascular Changes** Hypertension and coronary artery disease are major issues to address. Age-related cardiovascular changes are less appreciable at rest. Decreased cardiac response to exertion, however, is more noticeable. Cardiac output often decreases in older adults.

- **Renal Changes** Changes pertaining to the fluid excreted by the kidneys can result from a decrease in the number of functioning **nephrons** (structural and functional units of the kidney) and in renal blood flow. Older adults have a higher incidence of renal insufficiency (reduced capacity to filter blood). **Incontinence** (inability to retain urine in the bladder) is often a problem; with these individuals, adult diapers or pads become a necessity. Instability of the bladder muscle, overflow, and sphincter weakness are common causes. Diuretics, often necessary medications to treat an existing illness, may aggravate this condition. **Urinary retention**, which is the inability to partially or completely empty the bladder, may result from prostate hypertrophy, malignancies, kidney stones, anticholinergic drug (e.g., certain antidepressants, antihistamines) intake, or urinary tract infections.

- **Hormonal Changes** Functional changes pertaining to the endocrine system are a natural consequence of aging. Some hormone levels increase, some decrease, and some stay the same. Aldosterone release decreases, which can lead to light-headedness and orthostatic hypotension—when a drop in blood pressure occurs with a sudden position change. In women, estrogen and prolactin levels may decrease.

- **Body Composition Changes** The proportion of total body weight composed of fat increases with age, while lean body mass and total body mass decrease. Albumin (the main blood plasma protein) production decreases with aging, possibly because of poor nutrition, hepatic disorders, or other disease states. Loss in bone density (osteoporosis) causes some loss of height. Arthritis also takes its toll on the skeletal system.

Altered Drug Responses

Age-related changes in organ function and body composition can alter the response to medication. The following factors play an important part in selecting a drug and its dosage:

- **Absorption Changes** Changes in GI function with aging may affect the rate of drug dissolution, breakdown of enzymes, and drug ionization. Reduction in the rate of gastric emptying may delay intestinal absorption of some drugs. For most patients, the rate and extent of absorption are determined by passive diffusion during contact with the surface area of the gut. Reduction in absorptive surface decreases absorption. GI fluid secretion also decreases.

- **Distribution Changes** Alterations in body composition, such as protein binding (less protein means more free drug in plasma), affect the distribution of drugs. If a drug is highly protein bound, it may have enhanced pharmacologic or toxic effects in older adults. Other factors that affect distribution are decreases in total body water, lean body mass, and cardiac output.

- **Metabolism Changes** During metabolism, a drug is transformed biochemically to a more water-soluble compound. Older adults may have impaired metabolism, which decreases clearance and allows the drug to accumulate, sometimes to toxic levels. Decline in liver metabolism results from reductions in both enzyme activity and blood flow.

- **Elimination Changes** Elimination by the kidneys decreases because of reduced filtration rate, blood flow, and tubular secretion. The result of decreased kidney elimination of drug products is an increased half-life that may require a reduction in dose of a drug.

As mentioned, older patients are more likely than younger patients to have chronic diseases requiring long-term treatment. Many take from 3 to 12 or more medications, and they tend to have a disproportionate number of **adverse drug reactions** (**ADRs**; see Table 4.5), which are unintended, harmful responses to a drug. Maintaining accurate medication profiles is important in these cases. Many ADRs are attributable to antithrombotic, diuretic, and nonsteroidal anti-inflammatory drugs. The pharmacy technician must take special care when dispensing these drugs and double-check the dose and compare it to the patient profile.

TABLE 4.5 Common Adverse Reactions Potentiated in Older Adults

• central nervous system changes (often misdiagnosed as disease manifestations)	• GI upset
	• incontinence
• constipation	• insomnia
• dermatitis	• rheumatoid symptoms
• diarrhea	• sexual dysfunction
• drowsiness	• urinary retention
• falls	• xerostomia (dry mouth)

A group of drugs that is especially important to monitor for older adult patients is included in the **Beers Criteria** (commonly called the Beers List). This list, which was originally published to provide information on potentially problematic drugs for patients in long-term care facilities, is now useful for older adult patients in other settings. The Beers Criteria continues to grow and is periodically revised. Computer databases commonly contain warnings attached to these drugs. A warning does not mean that the patient should not take the drug but rather that drugs on this list should be closely monitored in the older adult population. There is a corresponding Canadian list of drugs that require careful monitoring when used in older adults. Drugs on both lists are identified in Table 4.6.

TABLE 4.6 Common Drugs Requiring Monitoring in Older Adults

- amitriptyline (Elavil)
- chlorpromazine (Thorazine)
- clorazepate (Tranxene)
- chlordiazepoxide (Librium)
- diazepam (Valium)
- dipyridamole (Persantine)
- indomethacin (Indocin)
- reserpine
- thioridazine (Mellaril)

Polypharmacy is the term often used to describe concurrent use of multiple medications (usually five or more). ADRs often result from overprescribing. When many drugs are prescribed for a patient, especially when the patient sees more than one physician, the potential for drug interactions or other problems is high. Owing to the slowing of drug metabolism with aging, older adults can often obtain the desired pharmacologic effect with a much lower dose than is normally prescribed, but this can be difficult to identify if the patient uses different pharmacies or does not disclose all of their conditions and medications.

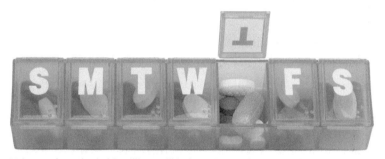

Using tools such as this pillbox will help patients who must take medications daily to remember to take them. The pharmacy technician can help inform patients about such medication management strategies.

Aging can also affect cognitive abilities. An inadequate understanding of the need for the medication and the dosage directions for the medication (e.g., whether it is to be taken with or without food) can lead to failure to take the drug, unintentional over dosing, taking the medication for the wrong reason, or taking drugs prescribed for another person. This failure to take a medication as prescribed is referred to as **nonadherence** and is especially prevalent among older adults. Pharmacy technicians can provide invaluable services in this area. They can make sure the patient gets written information and provide aids to dosing and ways to remember to take medication.

The older adult population presents a special challenge for the pharmacy technician and will constitute much of the pharmacy practice. As people age, they may need more drugs to maintain a healthy lifestyle. Patients usually visit a pharmacy not because they feel well but rather because they have health problems. Older patients may become frustrated because they can no longer function as they once did, and pharmacy technicians will encounter situations where older individuals may be irritated or upset. Technicians must develop skills that enable them to empathize and effectively communicate with older adults. Successful pharmacy technicians treat older adult patients with respect and understanding.

Special Considerations in Children

Providing drug therapy to children presents a unique set of challenges. As they grow, children undergo profound physiologic changes that affect drug absorption, distribution, metabolism, and elimination. Failure to understand these changes and their effects can lead to underestimating or overestimating drug dosage, with the resultant potential for failure of therapy, severe adverse reactions, or perhaps fatal toxicity.

Age may be the least reliable guide to drug administration in children because of the wide variation in the relationship between age and degree of organ-system development. Height correlates better with lean body mass than does weight. Body surface area may be the best measure because it correlates with all body parameters; however, it is not easily determined. Body weight is most commonly used because of its ease of calculation. Children who are small for their age should receive conservative doses, but larger children may require a dose recommended for the next higher age bracket.

Pediatricians often prescribe an OTC medication for a child without telling the parent how to dose the drug, or they think the dosing instructions will be on the package. A caretaker may purchase the medication only to find that the drug is intended for use in an older child and that appropriate dosage information for a younger or smaller child is not provided with the medication. The pharmacist may have to determine the child's dose for the caretaker. The pharmacy technician should always refer these questions to the pharmacist.

The following considerations are important when dosing children:

- The dosage should be appropriate for the child's age. A dose appropriate for a full-term infant may not be appropriate for a premature infant or a toddler.
- Calculations should be double-checked by the pharmacist and possibly by another pharmacy technician.
- All dosages should be reevaluated at regular intervals.

Allergic Response

An **allergy** is a state of hypersensitivity of the immune system induced by exposure to a particular substance. Many of these substances, called **allergens**, occur naturally in the environment; some are seasonal, some are found in food, whereas others occur in pharmaceutical products. In response to an allergy, the body releases chemicals such as **histamine**, which produces symptoms commonly known as the *allergic reaction*—red, watery eyes; sneezing; urticaria; rash; and bronchiolar constriction—when exposed to these substances. A histamine that causes such symptoms is designated as H_1 and is treated with antihistamines (see Chapter 11). Gastric mucosal cells release a different type of histamine, known as H_2, which is treated with the H_2 blockers (see Chapter 12). Both antihistamines and H_2 blockers are sold over the counter. Some allergic reactions are not as serious as others (e.g., seasonal allergies), and these antihistamines can be self-prescribed and administered. However, some allergic reactions can be life threatening.

Life-threatening allergies (e.g., food allergies, bee sting allergies) may result in anaphylaxis and require patients to carry an epinephrine auto-injector with them to reverse life-threatening symptoms in the event of an exposure to the allergen. In these types of allergies, antihistamines are not adequate substitutes to reverse the reaction.

The pharmacy technician must be keenly aware that dangerous allergic reactions are a possibility for some medications. One of the most important tasks for the technician is to screen patients for allergies. Allergies must be a part of the patient's medical record, and the technician must always make sure this issue has been addressed before any drugs are dispensed. If the patient has no allergies, the technician enters "NKA" (no known allergies) or "NKDA" (no known drug allergies) into the record. Under no circumstances should this field be left blank either in the computer or on the patient chart.

4.5 Teaching Patients Medication Management

The pharmacy technician can play an important role in helping patients learn how to manage medications. If the drug does not enter the body or enters it incorrectly, it will not work as desired. The pharmacy technician can positively affect patient adherence by providing clearly written instructions and aids to implement the process.

Federal law requires that the pharmacy collect the patient's history regarding drugs prescribed as well as side effects and adverse reactions experienced by the patient. The pharmacy technician can positively affect patient drug therapy by accurately collecting and recording the patient's medication history in the patient's profile. The pharmacist filling the prescription is responsible for providing information about the prescription drugs ordered and their proper administration to the patient. The pharmacist can help the patient understand the administration instructions as well as any precautions. The following are specific instructions to emphasize:

- methods for administering the drug
- how to make swallowing easier
- times and time intervals for administration and what to do if a dose is missed
- whether a medication can or should be taken with or without food
- possible side effects and which ones should be reported to the physician
- how long the medication should be taken

It is important that the pharmacy technician explain to patients that the pharmacist is available to answer questions or provide instructions. The technician is allowed to read to the patient the label, medication guide, or educational materials dispensed with the drug—this is *not* counseling and can be very helpful to the patient. However, technicians should read the exact wording of the written information and should bear in mind that they must not offer advice to patients.

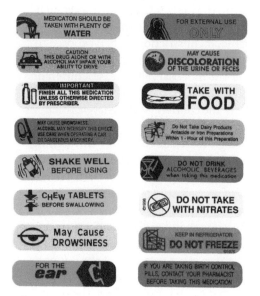

When a patient receives a prescription, it will sometimes include labels that provide instructions for how to self-administer the medication properly. These labels, referred to as *auxiliary labels*, use color and symbols to communicate their message.

Technicians can ensure that patients understand how to read medication labels. Important items to look for include the trade name and/or generic name, the dosage strength, frequency and route of administration, precautions and warnings, and potential interactions. It is important to remember, however, that technicians cannot—by law—counsel patients. Figure 4.5 provides an example of a doctor's prescription and the corresponding medication label that should be affixed to the drug container. The label provides directions that the patient needs to understand and follow. By federal law, many prescriptions require a medication guide, which is an explanation of how the drug works and its potential side effects. Pharmacists must dispense the guide with the drug.

Many drugs that are now available over the counter previously required a prescription. This change occurred because the drugs were found to help with common, uncomplicated problems and carry a relatively low risk of adverse effects. However, it is important that patients read the information provided with these drugs to understand their action, interactions, cautions, and possible side effects. OTC drugs can also interfere with the desired effects of prescription drugs ordered by the prescriber. That is why it is important to obtain information about the patient's OTC drug use as well as information about prescription medications.

A medication regimen can be effective only if the patient or caregiver follows the directions for administration. A care plan may include modifying the patient's lifestyle and keeping medical appointments for follow-up care.

When a patient does not adhere to instructions, there may be a relapse or aggravation of the disease. Hospitalization may then be required, causing healthcare costs to rise. The end result may even be the death of the patient.

FIGURE 4.5
Medication Label Information

The information on a prescription, as shown in (a), is translated for the patient as instructions on the medication label, as shown in (b). This label also includes the physician's name and the date the prescription was filled, the drug name, the number of refills, and the pharmacy's address and phone number.

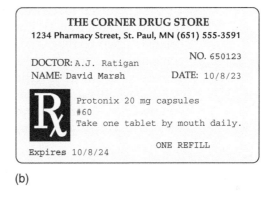

(a)

(b)

Reasons why a patient does not adhere to a care plan can be varied and often complex. They include side effects that cause discomfort, failure to understand the disease, confusion caused by cognitive impairment or the complexity of the regimen, and simple forgetfulness. In general, teenagers and older adults have the highest rates of nonadherence.

Side effects are a common reason for nonadherence. If a medication produces discomfort, the patient may discontinue its use. Although side effects of some medications subside as the drugs are continuously used, others may persist. It is important to educate patients about the importance and benefits of medication and potential side effects to promote adherence. Patients may be willing to tolerate some side effects if they are aware of them and understand that they will experience relief over the long term. For this reason, side effects should be addressed initially. The pharmacist should inform patients of potential side effects, the importance of correct dosing, what to do if an adverse effect occurs, and how to monitor treatment.

Lack of reliable information regarding disease states or medication treatments can be another barrier to adherence. Patients who do not understand how a drug may improve their disease state will be at a higher risk of nonadherence than patients who have some understanding of drug action and can see how the treatment will affect their disease. Patients lacking sufficient knowledge of their disease and the drug therapy for the disease may not understand the importance of consistent use. Thus, healthcare professionals should educate patients about their disease so that they will understand the drug therapy required. This education should include information about the assumed benefits of the drug regimen, side effects, and the consequences of failing to follow the drug regimen.

Adherence decreases as the number of daily medications and the complexity of the regimen increase. Multiple medications, multiple instructions regarding medications, and drugs that have to be taken at a certain time of the day or several different times of the day and with (or without) food may all confuse the patient, resulting in poor adherence. The result may be missed doses and a less-than-desired therapeutic response or an increased risk of ADRs and hospitalization. With a simpler regimen, there is a greater chance of patient adherence. Consequently, pharmacists and prescribers should evaluate therapeutic alternatives that ensure patient adherence. Patients with cognitive impairment that affects their ability to understand and follow directions concerning their drugs will be at a higher risk of nonadherence.

Forgetfulness is another reason for lack of adherence. Pharmacy technicians can encourage patients to use various kinds of reminders to aid their memory. Reminders may include taking medications at the time certain daily tasks are performed, placing colored stickers on the calendar after the medication is taken, using pillboxes with daily compartments, setting watches with alarms, using pill bottle cap alarms or other electronic devices, and using technology such as mobile device reminders and applications.

Above all, patients need to monitor their own medication regimens. Pharmacists and pharmacy technicians are in a position to build a trusting relationship in which the patient is generally willing to accept recommendations to promote adherence.

4.6 Medication Safety

Medications are used to help manage conditions, relieve symptoms, and treat diseases. As described earlier, adverse drug events (harm from using a medication) may occur. In addition to the known risks of using a medication (side effects, etc.), the complexity of the medication use process can lead to medication errors. The **medication use process** is an outline of the steps needed to provide medications to patients. At a high level, it includes the manufacturing, procurement, prescribing, filling or dispensing, administering, and monitoring of medications. Recall that a medication error is any preventable event that may cause or lead to inappropriate medication use or patient harm. Medication errors are preventable, and pharmacy technicians are an important layer of protection in helping prevent such errors.

All steps in the medication use process have potential for errors to occur. A list of potential errors appears in Table 4.7. This list is not comprehensive, but it provides examples of what errors may be encountered. Pharmacy technicians are most involved in the dispensing step of the medication use process. Errors can occur due to a number of different reasons, but rushing and miscommunication are common reasons. It is important for pharmacy technicians to follow processes and procedures and to inform the pharmacist when they have a concern or if a question arises. Many organizations have medication error reporting systems where the person who identifies the error can submit information regarding the incident. The reporting systems allow each institution or pharmacy to monitor and respond to errors. These error reporting systems are meant to improve patient care and are not meant to punish those involved in the original error. It is important to report errors or potential errors so that system changes can be made to prevent the error from happening again.

TABLE 4.7 Potential Errors in the Medication Use Process

Drug Relationship	Description
manufacturing	contamination of the medication
	incorrect or misleading labeling or packaging
prescribing	prescribing a medication to which a patient has an allergy
	illegible handwriting on the prescription order
	incorrect data entry (e.g., selecting a wrong medication in a computerized order entry system)
filling/dispensing	dispensing the incorrect medication from stock
	affixing the wrong label to a product
	dispensing the wrong medication to a patient
	incorrectly preparing the medication for dispensing
	delivering a medication to the wrong hospital unit
	filling a medication dispensing cabinet with the wrong medication
administration	administering an incorrect medication, dose, or dosage form
	administering a medication at the wrong time or with an incorrect technique
	omitting a dose

Technician Role

Technicians are an integral part of the medication dispensing process, and pharmacists rely heavily on them to help catch and prevent errors. Properly trained and educated technicians can make a tremendous difference in the quality of care a patient receives. Technicians must verify the patient's address, date of birth, phone numbers, allergies, and conditions such as pregnancy. Another role of the technician is to make sure the patient gets proper counseling from the pharmacist. This counseling process is very important in minimizing errors.

E-Prescribing

Pharm Fact

Examples of medication safety initiatives include e-prescribing, prescriber order entry, dispensing cautions, tamper-resistant pads, and medication reconciliation.

Recall that *e-prescribing* is a method of prescribing medications electronically. A prescriber enters a prescription into a computer program that communicates directly with a computer program at a designated pharmacy. E-prescribing eliminates the need for a written prescription and can potentially reduce errors and improve patient safety by eliminating illegible prescriptions and automatically checking for allergies, interactions, dosing errors, and therapeutic duplications. Accidental selection of the wrong drug, dose, or dosage form in the computer program by the prescriber could, however, create a new source of errors. E-prescribing is also costly because of the expense of installing appropriate computer programs.

Physician Order Entry

In hospitals, where physicians enter prescriptions into a database or electronic health record, a decrease in errors has been documented. This is called **computerized physician order entry (CPOE)** or prescriber order entry and is different from e-prescribing. In physician order entry, the prescriber (physician or other qualified prescriber) personally enters drug orders (as opposed to pharmacists or other professionals) that are then verified and dispensed by pharmacy personnel.

Dispensing Cautions

For safety reasons, some medications must be dispensed in their original containers. Most of these drugs are affected by light or moisture or can be stored only in glass containers. Patients cannot receive a partial prescription of any of these medications, because this would require them to be repackaged—and doing so might affect the drug. In some cases, the pharmacist or pharmacy technician should not handle the drugs. Table 4.8 lists examples of these medications.

TABLE 4.8 Examples of Drugs That Should Be Dispensed in Original Containers

Brand Name	Generic Name
Accolate	zafirlukast
Afinitor	everolimus
Aggrenox	dipyridamole, aspirin
Atripla	efavirenz, emtricitabine, tenofovir
Augmentin—chewable and oral suspension	amoxicillin-clavulanate
Creon, Pancrease, Zenpep, Viokase	pancrelipase
Crixivan	indinavir
Edarbi	azilsartan—and any combination of this drug
Effient	prasugrel
Ella	ulipristal
Hepsera	adefovir
Horizant	gabapentin
Intelence	etravirine
Kuvan	sapropterin
Mephyton	phytonadione
Nitrostat	nitroglycerin
Norvir	ritonavir
Pradaxa	dabigatran
Procardia	nifedipine
Sandimmune, Neoral, Gengraf	cyclosporine—capsules and oral solution
Tekturna	aliskiren—and any combination of this drug
Treximet	sumatriptan and naproxen
Trileptal	oxcarbazepine
Truvada	emtricitabine, tenofovir
Tyzeka	telbivudine
Viread	tenofovir

Note: Drugs that come in blister packs, drugs packaged in 30- or 90-day supplies, and powdered drugs to which water must be added are not included in this list.

Tamper-Resistant Prescription Pads

Prescribers who file for Medicaid reimbursement must use tamper-resistant paper for written prescriptions. Tamper-resistant prescription pads describe prescription paper with at least one tamper-resistant feature that is meant to prevent unauthorized copying of blank forms, modifying the form, and the use of counterfeit forms. If a tamper-resistant prescription pad has not been used, the technician must call and verify the prescription. The technician then documents the date and time of the call, the name of the person who verified it, and the technician's initials on the prescription. E-prescribing is commonly being used as an alternative to paper prescriptions.

Medication Reconciliation

One critical goal for community and hospital pharmacies is to share information from patient profiles—a process known as **medication reconciliation**. Such sharing of health information is allowed under the privacy provisions in Title II of the Health Insurance Portability and Accountability Act (HIPAA) and is part of the continuum of care and the effort to improve patient safety as patients move from one level of care to another. Studies show that patients are most vulnerable during transitions of care from one level of care to another when many medication errors occur. This applies to transitions that occur between hospitals; between hospital and community; and within a hospital, a rehabilitation center, an assisted living facility, or other healthcare facility. Hospitals should communicate drug regimen information to the patient's next care setting. In the future, retail pharmacies will receive greater numbers of calls from providers who need this information. Pharmacy technicians play a major role in making these transitions safer.

Medication Error Reporting Systems

Each organization will have its own process for reporting medication errors, so it is important to understand and follow this process. These systems are not designed to punish those involved in the error but rather to understand what mistakes have happened and where in the process the error occurred so that changes can be made to prevent another from happening. When completing an error report, it is important to report the facts and describe who, what, why, when, where, and how of the situation.

REMS Programs

The FDA is authorized to require drug manufacturers to have **Risk Evaluation and Mitigation Strategy (REMS)** programs for certain medications. The goal of REMS programs is to ensure that the benefits of a drug outweigh its risks. These REMS programs may be as simple as dispensing a medication guide to a patient, or they may involve special dispensing and/or prescribing requirements. REMS programs may require prescribers and dispensing pharmacists to complete training regarding certain drugs, and technicians may need to take special steps when dispensing the drug. REMS programs may vary from state to state, but the technician needs to be aware of REMS programs and the purpose behind them.

4.7 Understanding the Profession

The remainder of this book and course will introduce you to the various body systems and the diseases and conditions that can negatively affect a person, as well as the medications that can cure or lessen the severity of those conditions.

Along the way, you will also be presented with opportunities to stretch your understanding of medical topics and to realize what it means to be a member of the pharmacy profession. You will also be given opportunities to explore ethical decisions, the demands of effective communication, cultural differences, interpersonal relationships, and more.

As you pursue your studies, keep in mind your ultimate goals, one of which is obtaining certification as a pharmacy technician. Another is securing employment in your profession. This book and its accompanying online content are designed to help you reach those goals as well as understand your potential for career advancement. Be sure to check with your instructor about the variety of materials available with this textbook that are related to career preparation and professionalism as a pharmacy technician. It will be beneficial to familiarize yourself with the Pharmacy Technician Certification Board (PTCB), the American Association of Pharmacy Technicians (AAPT), and the National Pharmacy Technician Association (NPTA). These organizations offer highly informative websites for the pharmacy technician as well as other resources you will likely find helpful as you advance in your chosen career.

Review and Assessment

CHAPTER SUMMARY

The Prescription

- A request for the dispensing of medication to a patient is called an **order** in a hospital setting; outside the hospital setting it is called a **prescription**.

- To fill a prescription or order, the pharmacy technician must understand the meanings of abbreviations.

- Certain abbreviations should not be used on prescriptions or instructions because there is extensive evidence to document them as the source of medication errors.

Correct Drug Administration Rights

- The "rights" for correct drug administration are the right patient, the right drug, the right strength, the right route, the right dose form, the right time, and the right documentation.

Dosage Forms and Routes of Administration

- The three primary routes of administration are oral, parenteral, and topical. The pharmacy technician must be familiar with each dosage form.

- The most common dosage forms are:

oral (po)	parenteral	topical
capsules	epidural injections	creams
solutions		gels
suspensions	intramuscular (IM) injections	inhalants
syrups		lotions
tablets	intravenous (IV) injections	ointments
	subcutaneous injections	patches
		suppositories

Factors That Influence Drug Action

- Altered drug responses in older adults are due to age-related changes in organ function and body composition. These physiologic changes include visual, auditory, gastrointestinal, pulmonary, cardiovascular, renal, hormonal, and body composition alterations.

- Some special problems of older adults are poor nutrition, adverse drug reactions, and poor adherence with drug regimens.

- Body surface area is the best measure to use in determining dosage for children, but it is difficult to ascertain; consequently, weight is most frequently used.

- Allergic reactions are a dangerous possibility for some medications and are thus a vital piece of information in the patient's record.

- An important role for the pharmacy technician is recording patient allergies.

Teaching Patients Medication Management

- Patient adherence with the dose schedule and the specific requirements of a drug regimen is important.

- A pharmacy technician can positively influence patient drug therapy by accurately collecting and recording the patient's medication history in the patient profile.

- Pharmacy technicians can help patients understand how to read medication labels.

- Pharmacy technicians should encourage patients to read the information provided with OTC drugs to understand their action, interactions, cautions, and possible side effects.

- Pharmacy technicians cannot counsel patients about their medications and regimens, but they can recommend pharmacist counseling and explain the materials that accompany a medication.

Medication Safety

- E-prescribing helps eliminate errors related to poorly written prescriptions.

- Hospitals that use physician order entry have documented a decrease in errors.

- Medication reconciliation, a national patient safety goal, will prevent many errors by increasing accuracy of medication history as patients transition between care settings.

✓ CHECK YOUR UNDERSTANDING

Take a moment to reflect on what you have learned in this chapter and answer the following questions.

1. A prescription typically must contain the following parts except the
   a. patient's name.
   b. drug and dose.
   c. signa.
   d. drug expiration date.

2. All of the following are "rights" for correct drug administration except the right
   a. patient.
   b. drug.
   c. strength.
   d. doctor.

3. Which route of medication administration is usually the most economical and convenient?
   a. oral
   b. topical
   c. parenteral
   e. subcutaneous

4. How often should information on drug allergies be collected prior to drug dispensing?
   a. each time a new prescription is filled
   b. only when a patient has a documented drug allergy
   c. only when a prescriber writes the allergy on the prescription
   d. only when the patient requests the information

5. Federal law requires that pharmacies collect
   a. donations for hospitals.
   b. a patient history regarding the drug prescribed.
   c. pharmacokinetic data on animal models.
   d. a list of all the physicians in their state.

6. All of the following are administered via the oral route *except*
   a. tablets.
   b. syrups.
   c. capsules.
   d. ointments.

7. Factors that determine the best route of administration include all of the following *except* the
   a. patient's condition.
   b. type of container to be used.
   c. site of desired action.
   d. rapidity of the desired response.

8. A prescription label must have all of the following *except*
   a. the patient's and prescriber's names.
   b. the dosage and how to take the drug.
   c. the address of the pharmacy and date of fill.
   d. the date the patient saw the provider.

9. Parenteral forms
   a. do not pass through the liver before entering the bloodstream.
   b. are inactivated in digestive juices.
   c. are the most common drug forms.
   d. are the most painless way to administer medications.

10. Of the following, which is not a way a pharmacy technician can help to improve safety?
    a. create time-saving work-arounds
    b. inform someone of a concern
    c. verify a patient's address, date of birth, phone number, allergies, and conditions such as pregnancy
    d. report errors

MAKE CONNECTIONS

Take a moment to consider what you have learned in this chapter and respond thoughtfully to the following prompts. Note that some of these activities will require internet access.

1. Why are pharmacy technicians restricted from counseling patients? Do you think this is a good policy? Why or why not?

2. Visit the websites for PTCB, AAPT, ISMP, and NPTA. What resources do you see that already seem useful?

 The online course includes additional review and assessment resources.

UNIT
2 Body Systems and Corresponding Drug Therapies

Chapter 5	The Integumentary System and Drug Therapy	87
Chapter 6	The Musculoskeletal System and Drug Therapy	119
Chapter 7	The Nervous System and Drug Therapy	161
Chapter 8	The Nervous System, Mental Health, and Drug Therapy	211
Chapter 9	The Sensory System and Drug Therapy	263
Chapter 10	The Cardiovascular System and Drug Therapy	283
Chapter 11	The Respiratory System and Drug Therapy	343
Chapter 12	The Gastrointestinal System and Drug Therapy	405
Chapter 13	The Endocrine System and Drug Therapy	463
Chapter 14	The Reproductive System and Drug Therapy	497
Chapter 15	The Renal System and Drug Therapy	537

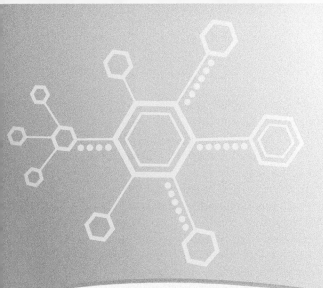

The Integumentary System and Drug Therapy

5

Learning Objectives

1. Describe the skin as an organ. (Section 5.1)

2. Describe the physiology of the skin. (Section 5.1)

3. Describe the classes of topical drugs and the skin conditions they treat. (Section 5.2 to 5.7)

4. Explain the action of topical treatments and their application. (Section 5.2 to 5.7)

5. Recognize the actions of antiseptics and disinfectants. (Section 5.7)

ASHP/ACPE Accreditation Standards
To view the *ASHP/ACPE Accreditation Standards* addressed in this chapter, refer to Appendix C.

Topical medications are used to treat a variety of skin conditions, such as acne, allergic and inflammatory reactions, infections, infestations, and autoimmune disorders that manifest on the skin. These classes of drugs range from mild agents to stronger forms of antibiotics, antiseptics, disinfectants, and corticosteroids.

5.1 Anatomy and Physiology of the Integumentary System

The **integumentary system** describes the tissue that covers the body, including skin, nails, and hair. This system protects the body from exposure to harmful pathogens and harsh substances and helps to regulate body temperature. Accounting for 16% of body weight, the skin is the largest organ of the body. It deals with microbial, chemical, and physical assaults on the body. It is also an important source of sensory input and is the main organ involved in temperature regulation. Healthcare practitioners may need to correct a skin defect, even when it does not pose a hazard to health, to aid the psychological well-being of the affected person.

Figure 5.1 illustrates the anatomy of the skin. The **epidermis** is the top layer of the skin and is derived from embryonic ectoderm. It continually forms new cells in the basal layer; sheds old, dead cells; and produces nails, hair, and glands. Pressure or friction on any part of the body stimulates skin growth, resulting in an area of thickened cells called a *callus*. Melanocytes, cells that produce the pigment melanin, exist throughout the basal layer of the epidermis.

The **dermis**, which is below the epidermis, includes connective tissue with upward projections into the epidermis. It is supplied with capillaries and sensory nerve terminals that do not penetrate the epidermis. The dermis contains smooth muscle at hair follicles (arrector pili), in sheets in the areola of the nipple, and in the scrotum, where the muscle action causes wrinkled skin.

Two types of glands are widely distributed in the dermis: sebaceous glands and sudoriferous glands, also known as *sweat glands*. A **sebaceous gland** secretes sebum, a substance that oils the skin and hair, preventing them from drying, and is also toxic to certain types of bacteria. Most sebaceous glands develop from hair follicles and empty their secretions into the follicles. The other sebaceous glands empty their secretions directly onto the surface of the epidermis. A **sweat gland**, also known as an *eccrine sweat gland*, produces sweat, which is made up of mostly water and salts. The larger, deeper sweat glands of the axillary, perineal, and genital regions (called *apocrine sweat glands*) produce sweat containing various organic materials that can produce an offensive odor when broken down by bacteria on the skin. The apocrine sweat glands in the skin of the external ear canal produce cerumen (earwax), which has antibacterial and antifungal activity; it also contains squamous cells and dust.

The **subcutaneous tissue** is the innermost layer of the skin and connects the dermis to underlying organs and tissues. This layer is composed of elastic fibers, also called *fascia*, and a layer of fat cells, called **adipose tissue**. The thickness of the subcutaneous tissue varies depending on the region of the body. Breast tissue arises from the subcutaneous tissue.

FIGURE 5.1
Anatomy of the Skin

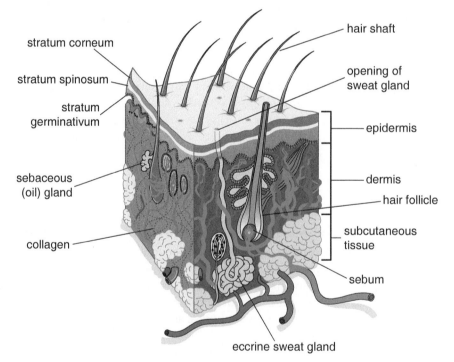

stratum corneum

stratum spinosum

stratum germinativum

sebaceous (oil) gland

collagen

hair shaft

opening of sweat gland

epidermis

dermis

hair follicle

subcutaneous tissue

sebum

eccrine sweat gland

5.2 Sun Exposure and Drug Treatments

Energy from the sun reaches the earth as electromagnetic radiation. Familiar examples of electromagnetic radiation are radio waves, microwaves, visible light, ultraviolet light, and x-rays. The energy from the sun warms the planet, provides energy as food (beginning with photosynthesis), and plays a critical role in climate and weather patterns. The energy also interacts with our skin.

With prolonged exposure, skin undergoes hypermelanization (heavily pigmented) and hyperkeratosis (abnormal thickening of the skin). The best way to prevent sun-damaged skin is to avoid excessive exposure to the sun and, while spending time outdoors, to protect the skin with sunscreen. To be effective, sunscreen should have a rating of at least **sun protection factor (SPF)** 30.

The rays responsible for suntans and sunburns are ultraviolet (UV) radiation. Ultraviolet radiation is higher in energy than visible light. Humans cannot see UV radiation, but this energy does interact with the atoms in the cells of our epidermis. Ultraviolet A (UVA) radiation is divided into two types, UVA-1 and UVA-2, and is informally referred to as the *suntan region*. UVB is referred to as the *sunburn region*. Both UVA and UVB radiation can cause skin cancer, so to be effective, sunscreen must protect against both. See Table 5.1 for a listing of available sunscreen active ingredients and their UV coverage.

TABLE 5.1 Commonly Used Active Ingredients in Sunscreens

Sunscreen Active Ingredient	UV Coverage
avobenzone	UVA-1, UVA-2
homosalate	UVB
octinoxate	UVB
oxybenzone	UVA-2, UVB
para-aminobenzoic acid (PABA)	UVB
titanium dioxide	UVA-2, UVB
zinc oxide	UVA-1, UVA-2, UVB

Individuals with fair skin are more likely to have atrophy and scaling of the epidermis than individuals with darker skin. In addition to irritated skin, overexposure to sunlight can also cause skin cancer. Although cancer treatments are covered in Chapter 20, it is necessary to understand the relationship between sun exposure and skin cancer. For all people with skin cancer, tumor growth is more common in areas of the body that are regularly exposed to the sun than in areas that are normally covered or shaded.

The following are several categories of skin cancer:

- **actinic keratosis:** a precancerous condition resulting from overexposure to sunlight
- **basal cell carcinoma:** a slow-growing tumor that rarely metastasizes
- **malignant melanoma:** a highly malignant cancer that forms from melanocytes; sunburn greatly increases the risk of this skin disorder
- **squamous cell carcinoma:** a type of cancer that grows more rapidly than basal cell carcinoma; cells tend to keratinize; metastasis is uncommon

Photosensitivity is an abnormal sensitivity to light, which can be caused by some drug therapies. In such cases, the skin can be extrasensitive to sunlight. Photosensitivity can increase the patient's susceptibility to phototoxicity. Patients taking these medications may find that they sunburn or experience second-degree burns (blistering) more easily with exposure to sunlight. Drugs in certain classes cause photosensitivity through biochemical interactions in the body, so it is important to alert the patient to this side effect when dispensing such a drug. The following classes have drugs that may cause photosensitivity: analgesics, angiotensin-converting enzyme (ACE) inhibitors, antibiotics, anticonvulsants, antidepressants, antifungals, antihistamines, antimalarials, antiplatelets, antipsychotics, antiretrovirals, antivirals, cardiovascular agents, chemotherapeutic agents, diabetes agents, diuretics, hormones, hypnotics, nonsteroidal anti-inflammatory drugs (NSAIDs), sedatives, statins, topicals, and vitamins. Table 5.2 lists some drugs that cause photosensitivity.

Technicians must watch for computer prompts on their pharmacy's computer system to know whether a particular drug needs a sticker warning the patient to avoid exposure to sunlight while taking the medication.

TABLE 5.2 Some Drugs That Cause Photosensitivity

Drug Class	Drug Example	Drug Class	Drug Example
ACE inhibitors	All agents	chemotherapeutic agents	dacarbazine
antibiotics	griseofulvin		fluorouracil (5-FU)
	quinolones		methotrexate
	sulfas		procarbazine
	tetracyclines		vinblastine
antidepressants	clomipramine	diuretics	acetazolamide
	maprotiline		furosemide
	sertraline		metolazone
	tricyclic antidepressants		thiazides
antihistamines	cyproheptadine	diabetes agents	sulfonylureas
	diphenhydramine	NSAIDs	all agents
antipsychotics	haloperidol		
	phenothiazines		
cardiovascular agents	amiodarone		
	diltiazem		
	quinidine		
	simvastatin		
	sotalol		

Drug Therapies for Sun Exposure

Pharmacologic treatment can help improve the condition of skin overexposed to the sun (see Table 5.3). For severe sunburn, corticosteroids are usually used. Aspirin can reduce irritation, pain, and edema.

TABLE 5.3 Commonly Used Agents for Sun-Damaged Skin

Generic (Brand)	Pronunciation	Dosage Form	Dispensing Status
benzocaine (Anacaine, Dermoplast, HurriCaine, Lanacane)	BEN-zoe-kayn	aerosol, gel, liquid, lozenge, ointment, swab	OTC
hydrocortisone (Cortaid, Cortizone)	hye-droe-KOR-ti-sone	cream, gel, lotion, ointment, topical solution	OTC, Rx
lidocaine (Lidoderm, Lidopin, Topicaine, Xolido, Xylocaine)	LYE-doe-kayn	cream, gel, ointment, patch	OTC, Rx
silver sulfadiazine (Silvadene, SSD)	SIL-ver sul-fa-DYE-a-zeen	cream	Rx

Benzocaine (Anacaine, Dermoplast, HurriCaine, Lanacane) and **lidocaine (Lidoderm, Lidopin, Topicaine, Xolido, Xylocaine)** are topical anesthetics that provide temporary relief from sunburn pain. These should be used only on intact skin for short periods.

Hydrocortisone (Cortaid, Cortizone) can be used on intact skin to decrease inflammation and accelerate healing. It also helps with pain relief.

Silver sulfadiazine (Silvadene, SSD) is a topical antiseptic product that can be used to prevent infection in serious burns. Silver sulfadiazine works on the bacterial cell wall and cell membrane. Silver sulfadiazine frequently darkens in its container or after being applied to the skin, but this color change does not interfere with its antimicrobial properties. Hypersensitivity to this drug is rare, and it is painless upon application.

Dosage Forms and Administration Benzocaine, lidocaine, and hydrocortisone should only be used on intact skin and should not be used in the eyes.

Side Effects Topical hydrocortisone may cause local sensitization.

Contraindications Benzocaine is contraindicated in patients with hypersensitivity to similar (ester-type classification) local anesthetics and in patients with secondary bacterial infections in the area of use. It should not be used in the eyes.

Topical lidocaine is contraindicated for the treatment of dermatitis associated with diaper use (diaper rash).

Pregnant patients and infants in the first two months of life should not use silver sulfadiazine products.

Cautions and Considerations Benzocaine is associated with **methemoglobinemia**, a disorder in which an abnormal form of hemoglobin is produced. Methemoglobinemia can be a medical emergency. For this reason, benzocaine use is not recommended in patients younger than two.

Topical corticosteroids should be applied sparingly so that systemic absorption does not happen.

Topical hydrocortisone may result in allergic contact dermatitis and local sensitization.

Patients who are allergic to sulfonamides can have an allergic reaction to silver sulfadiazine, so careful consideration must be given before its use. Because tissue necrosis (death) in the area of application has occurred in some patients, careful wound care and monitoring are necessary. Silver sulfadiazine does not protect against fungal organisms, so wounds treated with it should be monitored for development of a fungal infection.

Drug Interactions In general, drugs that are applied topically have few drug interactions.

5.3 Acne, Wrinkles, Rosacea, and Drug Treatments

In the United States, acne is the most common skin condition for which treatment, either over-the-counter (OTC) or prescription, is sought. Acne is initiated by the overproduction of **sebum**, which is produced by sebaceous glands around hair follicles. Such overproduction is most often stimulated by the hormonal changes encountered during puberty. Pimples, such as blackheads and whiteheads, appear as pores and follicles become clogged with oily material, dead skin cells, and dirt from the skin's surface. A **pimple** describes any type of clogged pore and can either be an open clogged pore, known as a *blackhead,* or a closed clogged pore, known as a *whitehead.* Mild forms of acne can be treated with OTC products. However, acne in its most

Safety Alert

Stickers warning patients to apply drugs appropriately should be placed on all topical drugs, especially liquids. It is not uncommon for someone to ingest a topical. This can be very dangerous.

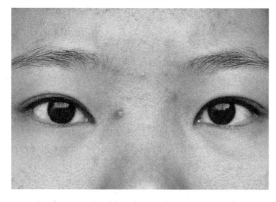

Acne is characterized by clogged pores and follicles.

severe forms, such as **nodular acne** and **acne vulgaris**, can cause deep cysts that permanently damage the dermal layer. Visible scars and pockmarks can form. Prescription drug therapy is needed to treat moderate to severe acne.

Wrinkles are another skin concern that affects many patients. A **wrinkle** is a line or crease in the skin. Wrinkles usually occur on parts of the body that receive the most sun exposure, such as the face, hands, and neck. Other factors such as smoking, lighter skin, and genetics can promote wrinkling as well.

Rosacea, a chronic inflammatory disorder seen in adults, is characterized by redness, visible blood vessels at the skin's surface, and raised bumps or pustules on the face and cheeks. Triggers of rosacea include stress, temperature, hot drinks, exercise, spicy food, alcohol, and any topical products that irritate the skin. Sunlight exposure is a major exacerbating factor for rosacea.

First-line treatment for mild to moderate acne is to cleanse the affected area twice a day. Although this cleansing will not eliminate acne, it can help prevent new blackheads and pimples from forming. Mild soap or cleanser is used twice a day to remove excess oil, dirt, and dead skin cells that clog pores.

Treatment of repeated acne lesions starts with OTC products, such as benzoyl peroxide. Moderate to severe acne requires the use of prescription products, starting with topical agents and progressing to oral agents when needed. Oral agents include antibiotics such as erythromycin, tetracycline, doxycycline, minocycline, and clindamycin (see Chapter 16). Some people may use oral contraceptives to decrease acne (see Chapter 14). The use of oral agents is associated with more side effects, so these medications are reserved for patients who do not gain adequate control with topical treatments.

Wrinkles are typically treated with retinoids.

When rosacea drug therapy is initiated, the specific triggers should be identified and then avoided. Because rosacea is not curable, antibiotics treat only its symptoms. Topical agent treatment options include azelaic acid, brimonidine, and metronidazole. Systemic tetracycline antibiotics (covered in Chapter 16) are oral treatments for rosacea.

Topical Antibiotics

Name Exchange

In practice, the drugs noted in this section will often include "topical" after the brand name to indicate the topical application—for example, Azelex topical and Finacea topical.

Topical antibiotics (see Table 5.4) are used alone to treat mild acne and may be used in combination with oral agents to treat moderate to severe acne. Benzoyl peroxide is a mainstay of treatment for mild acne.

Azelaic acid (Azelex, Finacea) is a topical treatment for mild to moderate inflammatory acne vulgaris. Hands should be washed after each application. Improvement usually occurs within four weeks.

Benzoyl peroxide (Benzac, Brevoxyl, Clearasil, Desquam, Oxy 10, PanOxyl) is another drug used to treat acne. It has antibacterial and mild drying effects, which help remove excess oils. Benzoyl peroxide produces oxygen, which is toxic to the bacteria that cause pimples.

Clindamycin (Cleocin-T, Clindagel, Clindets, Clindesse, Evoclin, Veltin, Ziana) is a topical drug product used to treat acne.

Dapsone (Aczone) is a topical antibiotic gel used for acne. The oral form of the drug (tablet) can be used to treat leprosy, spider bites, and other skin infections.

Erythromycin (Ery, Erygel) is a topical antibiotic used to treat acne.

Metronidazole (MetroCream, MetroGel, MetroLotion, Noritate, Rosadan) is a topical antibiotic used for rosacea.

TABLE 5.4 Commonly Used Agents for Acne, Wrinkles, and Rosacea

Generic (Brand)	Pronunciation	Dosage Form	Dispensing Status
Topical Antibiotics			
azelaic acid (Azelex, Finacea)	ay-ze-LAY-ik AS-id	cream, foam, gel	Rx
benzoyl peroxide (Benzac, Brevoxyl, Clearasil, Desquam, Oxy 10, PanOxyl)	BEN-zoe-il per-OX-ide	bar and liquid cleanser, cream, foam, gel, lotion, pad, soap, solution	OTC, Rx
clindamycin (Cleocin-T, Clindagel, Clindets, Clindesse, Evoclin, Veltin, Ziana)	klin-da-MYE-sin	foam, gel, lotion, topical solution	Rx
dapsone (Aczone)	DAP-sone	gel	Rx
erythromycin (Ery, Erygel)	eh-rith-roe-MYE-sin	gel, ointment, pads, solution	Rx
metronidazole (MetroCream, MetroGel, MetroLotion, Noritate, Rosadan)	me-troe-NI-da-zole	cream, gel, lotion	Rx
Retinoids			
adapalene (Differin)	a-DAP-a-leen	cream, gel, lotion, topical solution	Rx
isotretinoin (Absorica, Amnesteem, Claravis, Myorisan, Zenatane)	eye-soe-tret-i-NOE-in	capsule	Rx
tazarotene (Avage, Fabior, Tazorac)	ta-ZAR-oh-teen	cream, foam, gel	Rx
tretinoin (Altreno, Atralin, Avita, Refissa, Renova, Retin-A, Tretin-X)	tret-i-NOE-in	cream, gel, lotion	Rx
Miscellaneous			
brimonidine (Mirvaso)	bri-MOE-ni-deen	gel	Rx
salicylic acid (Clearasil, Fostex, Neutrogena products, Oxy, PROPA pH, Stri-Dex products)	sal-ah-SIL-ic AS-id	cleansing pad or wipe, cream, gel, liquid, lotion, ointment, pads, patch, shampoo, wipes	OTC
sodium sulfacetamide / sulfur (Avar Cleanser, Avar-E Emollient, Plexion, Plexion Cleanser, Sulfacleanse, Sulfamez Wash, Sumadan, Sumadan Wash, Sumaxin, Sumaxin CP)	sul-fa-SEE-ta-mide SUL-fur	cream, emulsion, foam, gel, liquid, lotion, pad, suspension	Rx

Dosage Form and Administration Topical treatments should be administered on skin that has been washed and patted dry. Azelaic acid is administered by gently applying a thin film to the affected area twice daily. Clindamycin is available as a foam, gel, lotion, and topical solution. When administered, a pea-sized amount of dapsone gel should be applied to clean skin of the affected area. Hands should be washed after each application of azelaic acid and dapsone. Erythromycin is available as a gel, ointment, pads, and solution. It should be applied sparingly as a thin layer to affected areas once or twice daily. Metronidazole is available as a cream, gel, and ointment and should be applied to clean, dry skin.

Side Effects Common side effects of topical acne products include dryness, redness, burning, and flaking or peeling skin. Moisturizer can be applied to control these side effects. If side effects are bothersome, less frequent use of these products is recommended. The oral form of dapsone has serious side effects, but the topical form is free of many of these side effects because it is not absorbed systemically. Dapsone should not be used by anyone younger than 12 years old.

Contraindications Acne products should not be used on moles, warts, or areas of skin that are infected, red, or irritated. In addition, prescribers should not prescribe topical acne products for infants or patients with impaired circulation, because their skin is more fragile.

Topical metronidazole is contraindicated in patients with hypersensitivity to parabens. It should not be used in patients who have taken disulfiram within the last two weeks or who have recently used or ingested alcohol or propylene glycol.

Cautions and Considerations These products are for external use only. Some topical antibiotic products are flammable. Products should be kept away from intense heat.

Drug Interactions Topical antibiotics are generally not associated with serious drug interactions.

Topical metronidazole may increase the adverse effects of alcohol, disulfiram, and lopinavir.

Retinoids

A **retinoid** is a vitamin A derivative. It works by increasing cell turnover in follicles, which pushes clogged material out of the pores. In acne, retinoids alter cell development and inflammatory processes to reduce swelling and redness.

Prescribers use retinoids to treat moderate to severe acne and to reduce the appearance of fine lines and wrinkles that accompany aging. Because of severe side effects and toxicities, prescribers reserve oral retinoid agents for the most severe forms of acne and psoriasis. Refer to Table 5.4 for more information on retinoids.

Adapalene (Differin) is a retinoid for acne treatment. It is less likely to cause skin irritation than tretinoin because it is water based, whereas tretinoin contains alcohol.

Isotretinoin (Absorica, Amnesteem, Claravis, Myorisan, Zenatane), a retinoid, is a treatment of last resort for severe acne. Isotretinoin is a known teratogen, which means it causes birth defects and comes with a boxed warning. The FDA mandates that patients may only use isotretinoin if they participate in a special program called iPLEDGE. Patients of all genders must sign an agreement to use birth control, and patients who have or might have the ability to become pregnant must undergo pregnancy testing while receiving isotretinoin. The prescriber must initiate enrollment of the patient in the iPLEDGE program, and then the patient must go online and register. Finally, the dispensing pharmacy must re-register the patient online. Failure of any of the parties to follow protocol will halt the dispensing of the drug by the pharmacist. In the pharmacy, a pharmacy technician is responsible for setting up the iPLEDGE program. A patient must have their iPLEDGE card to receive a prescription. Furthermore, if a patient has any form of mental illness, the program is unlikely to accept them. A depressed mood is a major side effect of this drug.

Tazarotene (Avage, Fabior, Tazorac), a synthetic retinoid, is approved for acne and psoriasis treatment. It modulates epithelial tissue and has some anti-inflammatory and immunological effects. Tazarotene is converted to its active form, tazarotenic acid. Some systemic absorption occurs with tazarotene, and because of the prolonged retention of the drug within the body, the therapeutic effects can last up to three months after discontinuation.

Pharm Fact

iPLEDGE is the name for the Risk Evaluation Mitigation Strategy (REMS) drug safety program that the FDA requires for drugs with safety concerns. This system restricts dispensing of drugs that pose significant risk of harm. Other drugs with REMS dispensing restrictions can be found at https://www.accessdata.fda.gov/scripts/cder/rems/index.cfm.

Work Wise

Pharmacy technicians should be aware that many insurance companies consider the use of retinoids to minimize the signs of aging to be a cosmetic rather than a therapeutic indication. Consequently, these companies deny insurance coverage for the cost of these medications. It can be helpful to warn patients that these products can be costly before they have their prescriptions filled.

Tretinoin (Altreno, Atralin, Avita, Refissa, Renova, Retin-A, Tretin-X), a retinoid, is a topical medication approved for the treatment of acne. It is also used to treat photodamaged skin and some skin cancers. Tretinoin makes epidermal cells in hair follicles become less adherent, then works by removing these cells (keratinocytes) and loosening the keratic (thickening) cells at the mouth of the follicle, causing easy sloughing and sebum discharge. Thus, the drug helps the skin to renew itself more quickly, improving its texture and appearance.

Dosage Forms and Administration Adapalene is applied once daily, usually at night. In addition to enrolling in the iPLEDGE program, patients using isotretinoin must take the medication with a full glass of water to prevent the capsule from dissolving in the esophagus. Tazarotene is administered by applying a thin layer to very dry skin in the evening, since this drug makes the skin highly sensitive to sunlight. Patients using tretinoin should also avoid direct sunlight.

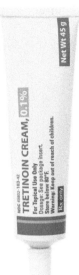

Tretinoin is a topical product for acne treatment.

Side Effects Common side effects of topical retinoid agents include burning, dry skin, itching, peeling, and redness. Sensitive skin may be especially prone to these effects. If these effects are severe or bothersome, the patient should stop using the product. In addition, retinoids should not be used along with topical antibiotics such as tetracyclines because the antibiotics can increase these side effects.

Oral agents such as isotretinoin have systemic side effects that can include depression, psychosis, pancreatitis, high triglyceride levels, and hepatotoxicity. Patients who already have any of these conditions should not take isotretinoin. Patients must be monitored closely for mental status changes, and regular laboratory blood tests must be performed to watch for pancreas and liver problems.

Contraindications Retinoids should not be used by patients with liver or kidney impairment. Because of their side effects, they should be used with caution in patients with depression or hypertriglyceridemia. Isotretinoin cannot be used by patients who are or might become pregnant. Severe birth defects are highly likely if a patient becomes pregnant while taking isotretinoin.

Cautions and Considerations As with all acne products, retinoids should not be used on areas of skin that are infected, red, or irritated. Care should also be taken to avoid applying these products close to the eyes or around the mouth.

Drug Interactions Topical products are generally not associated with serious drug interactions.

Alcohol, multivitamins, tetracyclines, and vitamin A may enhance the adverse effects of isotretinoin. Isotretinoin may decrease the effectiveness of oral contraceptives.

Miscellaneous Agents

Brimonidine (Mirvaso) is a topical alpha agonist used for rosacea. It decreases redness by causing constriction of blood vessels.

Salicylic acid (CeraVe, Clean and Clear, Clearasil, Fostex, Neutrogena products, Oxy, Stri-Dex products) is a **keratolytic** agent: an agent that breaks down and peels off dead skin cells, thereby preventing them from clogging pores. Salicylic acid is a mainstay of treatment for mild acne.

Sodium sulfacetamide / sulfur (Avar Cleanser, Avar-E Emollient, Plexion, Plexion Cleanser, Sulfacleanse, Sulfamez Wash, Sumadan, Sumadan Wash, Sumaxin, Sumaxin CP) is an acne treatment available by prescription as a cream, emulsion, foam, gel, liquid, lotion, pad, and suspension.

Dosage Forms and Administration A pea-sized amount of brimonidine gel should be applied to the face. Salicylic acid is available in various dosage forms and is commonly used.

Side Effects Side effects for these products are rare other than irritation to the skin at the site of application.

Contraindications Brimonidine and sodium sulfacetamide / sulfur do not have contraindications.

Salicylic acid should not be used on moles, warts, or areas of skin that are infected, red, or irritated. Salicylic acid also is not appropriate for infants and patients with impaired circulation because their skin is more fragile.

Sodium sulfacetamide / sulfur should not be used by patients with hypersensitivity to sulfa drugs.

Cautions and Considerations Worsening of erythema (abnormal redness of the skin or mucous membranes due to capillary congestion or inflammation) may occur with use of brimonidine. Serious adverse effects (such as cardiac and respiratory problems) may occur with ingestion of topical brimonidine.

Drug Interactions Topical brimonidine may increase the antihypertensive effects of other drugs that reduce blood pressure. The central nervous system (CNS) depressant side effects of other drugs may be enhanced by brimonidine.

5.4 Dermatitis, Eczema, Psoriasis, Dandruff, and Drug Treatments

Dermatitis is a **pruritic** (itchy) skin inflammation that can be caused by a variety of factors. The most severe cases can result in blisters and oozing erosions on the skin, but typical symptoms include areas of redness; dry, flaky skin; raised or bumpy skin; and pruritus (itching). Types of dermatitis include contact dermatitis, seborrheic dermatitis, diaper rash, and atopic dermatitis.

Contact dermatitis occurs in response to exposure to an irritant or allergenic substance. A rash appears wherever the skin has come into contact with the offending substance, such as a soap or detergent. Poison ivy, poison oak, and other plants can cause redness, itching, rashes, and blisters when their oils come into contact with the skin.

Seborrheic dermatitis, also called **cradle cap**, is a greasy, scaly area on the skin that sometimes appears red, brown, or yellow. It usually occurs in infants and in areas where hair follicles are concentrated, such as the scalp, ears, upper trunk, eyebrows, and around the nose. In adults who can grow facial hair, it can occur in the beard area.

Another skin rash common in infants is **diaper rash**. This acute and easily treated condition occurs most frequently in children who are not yet toilet trained, but it can

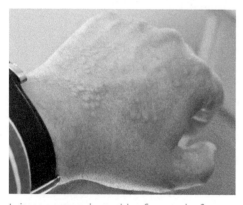

Irritant contact dermatitis often results from these common substances: soaps, cosmetics, rubbing alcohol, bleach, and solvents.

also occur in adults who must wear incontinence pads. When skin remains wet for long periods, tissue breakdown allows bacteria on the surface to enter deeper tissues. Diaper rash products treat irritation and redness when skin frequently contacts urine, feces, or both. These products contain a variety of ingredients that combine to promote healing, protect skin from further insult, and prevent infection. Common ingredients in diaper rash products include:

- balsam of Peru for wound healing and tissue repair
- camphor or menthol to provide local anesthetic action to relieve pain and itching
- eucalyptol (eucalyptus oil) for antimicrobial activity
- talc or kaolin for moisture absorption
- zinc oxide, a barrier with drying properties

These agents should be used as soon as redness appears in order to protect the skin from further damage and prevent infection from bacteria or fungi.

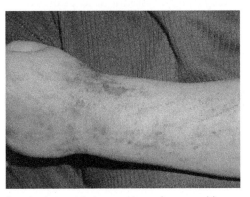

Atopic dermatitis (eczema) can be caused by allergies and a variety of other conditions.

Atopic dermatitis, also called **eczema**, is a chronic condition that usually first occurs in childhood and can continue into adulthood. Atopic dermatitis is not well understood but has an immunologic component, in that patients tend to have elevated levels of immunoglobulin E (IgE) in their blood. Patients with atopic dermatitis have an elevated risk of developing asthma or hay fever sometime in life. Eczema appears as dry, flaky, red skin that is very itchy. Patients sometimes scratch enough to cause secondary skin infections. Unlike other types of dermatitis, which are usually curable, atopic dermatitis is a chronic condition. Periods of severe symptoms (exacerbation) can cycle with periods of remission. Common triggers for exacerbations include stress, exposure to skin irritants, and food allergies.

Psoriasis is an immunologic condition affecting T-cell activity in the skin. It manifests on the skin as well-defined plaques (patches) that are raised, silvery or white, flaky, and pruritic. The plaques can appear anywhere on the body and may be very small or quite large and painful. Like eczema, psoriasis is characterized by periods of exacerbation that cycle with periods of remission. Stress and exposure to environmental factors that dry out skin can trigger exacerbation.

Dandruff is a malfunction of the oil-producing glands around hair follicles on the scalp, accompanied by accelerated cell proliferation in the scalp. Overproduction of sebum and cells results in layers of epidermis sticking together and flaking off as they dry. Specks of skin become visible in the hair and on the scalp. Although unsightly, dandruff is not harmful.

Table 5.5 identifies agents commonly used to treat dermatitis, eczema, psoriasis, and dandruff. Topical corticosteroids and calcineurin inhibitors are commonly used to treat dermatitis, eczema, and psoriasis.

Corticosteroids are usually first-line therapy for dermatitis and eczema. Therapy starts with topical medications but may include oral corticosteroids if severe. Seborrheic dermatitis can be treated with attention to good hygiene and topical antihistamines, anti-inflammatory agents, and moisturizing creams. Eczema treatment involves constant maintenance of skin with moisturizers to prevent exacerbations, along with topical corticosteroids for flare-ups. If the affected skin becomes infected, topical antibiotics may be used.

Psoriasis can be difficult to treat and does not always respond well to drug therapy. As they are for dermatitis and eczema, corticosteroids are the first-line treatment for psoriasis. Immunosuppressants and immunomodulators are sometimes required.

Immunosuppressants used to treat psoriasis include azathioprine, cyclosporine, and methotrexate. Immunomodulators for psoriasis treatment include biologic therapies such as adalimumab (Humira) and etanercept (Enbrel). Biologic agents such as tumor necrosis factor-alpha (TNF-alpha) inhibitors are costly but effective treatments for severe psoriasis. See Chapters 6 and 20 for more information on immunosuppressants and immunomodulators.

Topical Corticosteroids

Topical corticosteroids are anti-inflammatory agents that work by inhibiting redness, swelling, itching, and pain in the dermal layer of the skin. They can treat contact dermatitis, eczema, psoriasis, and allergic reactions. A thin layer of medication is applied to affected skin for a limited period. Because corticosteroids can penetrate the skin and can be absorbed systemically, they should be used sparingly. Systemic absorption can cause **hypothalamic-pituitary-adrenal (HPA) axis suppression**, which is associated with appetite changes, weight gain, fat redistribution, fluid retention, and insomnia.

Dosage Forms and Administration Treatment with topical corticosteroids starts with OTC-strength products, such as 0.5% and 1% hydrocortisone. Both strengths are usually effective for treatment of poison ivy and diaper rash (the lower strength should be used for infants and children). Combination products that contain an antifungal along with a corticosteroid can be useful for treating severe diaper rash.

Safety Alert

Hydrocortisone acetate is a low-potency corticosteroid, whereas hydrocortisone valerate is a high-potency corticosteroid. Be careful not to confuse these two different products. High-potency corticosteroids should be used for only a limited period because they can be systemically absorbed and can cause thinning of skin and other unwanted side effects.

TABLE 5.5 Commonly Used Agents for the Treatment of Dermatitis, Eczema, Psoriasis, and Dandruff

Generic (Brand)	Pronunciation	Dosage Form	Dispensing Status
Calcineurin Inhibitors and Calamine			
calamine	KAL-ah-mine	lotion	OTC
pimecrolimus (Elidel)	pim-e-KROE-li-mus	cream	Rx
tacrolimus (Protopic)	ta-KROE-li-mus	ointment	Rx
Vitamin D Analog			
calcipotriene (Calcitrene, Dovonex, Sorilux)	kal-si-poe-TRY-een	cream, ointment, topical solution	Rx
Topical Corticosteroids			
Low Potency			
alclometasone (Aclovate)	al-kloe-MET-a-sone	cream, ointment	Rx
hydrocortisone (Dermarest, Instacort, Lanacort)	hye-droe-KOR-ti-sone	cream, gel, liquid, lotion, ointment, spray	OTC
hydrocortisone (Ala-Cort, Aquanil, Cortaid, Instacort, Kericort, Lanacort, NuCort, Texacort)	hye-droe-KOR-ti-sone	cream, liquid, lotion, ointment, topical solution	Rx
hydrocortisone acetate (Cortaid, Cortef, Gynecort, Lanacort, Tucks)	hye-droe-KOR-ti-sone AE-seh-tate	cream, ointment	OTC, Rx

continues

TABLE 5.5 Commonly Used Agents for the Treatment of Dermatitis, Eczema, Psoriasis, and Dandruff—*Continued*

Generic (Brand)	Pronunciation	Dosage Form	Dispensing Status
hydrocortisone butyrate (Locoid)	hye-droe-KOR-ti-sone BYU-ty-rate	cream, lotion, ointment, topical solution	Rx
hydrocortisone probutate (Pandel)	hye-droe-KOR-ti-sone proe-BUE-tate	cream	Rx
prednicarbate (Dermatop)	pred-ni-KAR-bate	cream, ointment	Rx
High Potency			
betamethasone dipropionate (AlphaTrex, Diprolene, Sernivo)	bay-ta-METH-a-sone dye-PRO-pee-on-ate	aerosol, cream, lotion, ointment	Rx
betamethasone valerate (Apexicon, Luxiq, Psorcon)	bay-ta-METH-a-sone VAL-ur-rate	cream, foam, lotion, ointment	Rx
clocortolone (Cloderm)	kloe-KOR-toe-lone	cream	Rx
desoximetasone (Topicort)	des-ox-i-MET-a-sone	cream, gel, ointment spray	Rx
fluocinolone (Capex, Synalar)	floo-oh-SIN-oh-lone	cream, gel, ointment, shampoo, topical solution	Rx
fluocinonide (Lidex, Vanos)	floo-oh-SIN-oh-nide	cream, gel, ointment, topical solution	Rx
fluticasone (Cutivate)	floo-TIK-a-sone	cream, lotion, ointment	Rx
halcinonide (Halog)	hal-SIN-oh-nide	cream, ointment, topical solution	Rx
hydrocortisone valerate (Instacort, Locoid, Pandel)	hye-droe-KOR-ti-sone va-LAIR-ate	cream, ointment	Rx
mometasone furoate (Elocon)	moe-MET-a-sone FYUR-o-ate	cream, lotion, ointment, topical solution	Rx
triamcinolone (Kenalog, Triderm)	trye-am-SIN-oe-lone	aerosol, cream, lotion, ointment	Rx
Very High Potency or Superpotency			
amcinonide	am-SIN-oh-nide	cream, lotion, ointment	Rx
betamethasone dipropionate, augmented (Diprolene)	bay-ta-METH-a-sone dye-PRO-pee-on-ate	cream, gel, lotion, ointment	Rx
clobetasol propionate (Clobex, Clodan, Olux, Temovate, Tovet)	kloe-BAY-ta-sawl PRO-pee-on-ate	cream, foam, gel, lotion, ointment, shampoo, topical solution, spray	Rx
desonide (DesOwen, Tridesilon, Verdeso)	DESS-oh-nide	cream, foam, gel, lotion, ointment	Rx
halobetasol propionate (Lexette, Ultravate)	hal-oh-BAY-ta-sawl PRO-pee-on-ate	cream, foam, ointment	Rx
Selenium Sulfide and Pyrithione Zinc			
selenium sulfide (Head & Shoulders Intensive Treatment, Selsun Blue, SelRex)	suh-LEE-nee-um SUL-fide	shampoo	OTC, Rx
pyrithione zinc (Denorex Everyday Dandruff Shampoo, T/Gel Daily Control)	peer-i-THYE-own ZINK	shampoo	OTC

Practice Tip

Make your own flash cards for studying the topical corticosteroids. Use color coding to differentiate potency levels: for example, green for low potency, yellow for high potency, and red for very high potency (superpotency).

Corticosteroid products vary in potency depending on the formulation. Ointments are typically more potent than creams. (See Table 5.5 for topical corticosteroid potency information.) Ointments are most appropriate for treating dry, scaly lesions, whereas creams are most effective for treating moist or oozing lesions. When using gels, patients should follow package and prescription instructions. Creams, gels, and ointments are not interchangeable and should not be substituted for each other.

Side Effects Common side effects of topical corticosteroids include burning, itching, dryness, excessive hair growth, dermatitis, acne, hypopigmentation, and thinning of the skin. Use of the least amount over the smallest area for the shortest period possible is recommended to minimize these effects.

Contraindications Topical corticosteroids have no contraindications.

Cautions and Considerations Occlusive wound dressings should not be applied over topical corticosteroid products, especially the high-potency ones. To reduce the potential for systemic absorption and HPA axis suppression, superpotent (very high potency) corticosteroid products are restricted in the length of treatment and/or total amount of product that may be used. These agents should not be used for longer than two consecutive weeks. The total amount used in one week should not exceed 50 g, and these products should not be applied close to the eyes or mucous membranes.

Drug Interactions In general, topical corticosteroids do not have drug interactions.

Calcineurin Inhibitors

These medications are immunomodulators that work by inhibiting T-cell activation, which prevents release of chemical mediators that promote inflammation. **Calcineurin inhibitors** are treatments for severe eczema, especially when topical corticosteroids have not been effective.

Pimecrolimus (Elidel) and tacrolimus (Protopic) are topical immunomodulators used in the treatment of eczema. They are immunosuppressant agents that reduce itching and inflammation by suppressing the releasse of cytokines from T-cells. The advantage of these products over a steroid is they do not result in thinning of the skin or other side effects of long-term steroid use.

Dosage Forms and Administration Calcineurin inhibitors are available in the following forms: capsule, cream, ointment, and solution. Oral calcineurin inhibitors are available, but they are used to prevent rejection after an organ transplant. Pimecrolimus should be applied as a thin layer to all areas of the skin diagnosed as having eczema (and not to areas without eczema). Tacrolimus may be used anywhere on the body, even the face. Products with a concentration of 0.03% tacrolimus are approved for use in children between 2 and 15 years old, and products containing 0.1% tacrolimus can be used by adults. The areas with eczema should remain free of other skin products.

Side Effects Common side effects of calcineurin inhibitors include burning, itching, tingling, acne, and redness at the site of application. Other effects include headache, muscle aches and pains, sinusitis, and flu-like symptoms. To minimize these effects, these agents should be used sparingly for a short treatment period.

Contraindications No contraindications exist for topical calcineurin inhibitors.

Cautions and Considerations Calcineurin inhibitors have been associated with increased occurrences of cancer (skin cancer and lymphoma). Topical application is less likely to cause malignancy, but patients must be informed of this risk. Use of calcineurin inhibitors, even topical application, can cause alcohol intolerance. Facial flushing can occur when drinking alcohol and using these medications. Prolonged use of pimecrolimus and tacrolimus is usually avoided because it has been associated with rare cases of malignancy.

Drug Interactions Topical tacrolimus may increase the adverse effects of alcohol. Antidepressants, antifungals, calcium channel blockers, cyclosporine, and danazol may increase tacrolimus levels.

Immunosuppressant side effects may be enhanced by tacrolimus use. Topical tacrolimus may enhance the kidney-damaging effects of cyclosporine and sirolimus.

Pimecrolimus may enhance the adverse effects of immunosuppressants.

Vitamin D Analogs

Calcipotriene (Calcitrene, Dovonex, Sorilux) is a synthetic form of Vitamin D, also known as a Vitamin D analog, that regulates the growth and development of skin cells. In psoriasis, skin cells reproduce abnormally and rapidly to form plaques. Vitamin D and Vitamin D analogs regulate this cell process.

Dosage Forms and Administration **Vitamin D analogs** are available in several forms, including creams, foam, ointment, and solution. Some dosage forms can effectively treat psoriatic lesions on the scalp when other creams and ointments are too greasy and thick to use where hair is dense.

Side Effects Common side effects of Vitamin D analogs, such as calcipotriene, include burning, itching, and redness at the site of application. Less common effects include inflamed hair follicles (folliculitis), skin irritation, change in skin color at the site of application, and thinning of the skin. Patients who experience these problems should stop using calcipotriene and contact their healthcare practitioners.

Contraindications Patients who have hypercalcemia, vitamin D toxicity, or acute psoriasis should not use calcipotriene.

Cautions and Considerations Vitamin D analogs can cause alterations in calcium metabolism, so patients who have had problems with too much calcium in the blood (such as a history of kidney stones) should not use them without medical supervision. Periodic blood tests may be performed to monitor calcium levels.

Drug Interactions Calcipotriene may increase concentrations of aluminum hydroxide. It may decrease concentrations of sucralfate.

Multivitamins and other vitamin D analogs may enhance the toxic effects of calcipotriene.

Calamine

Mild itching from insect bites, rashes, hives, poison ivy or poison oak, or other allergic reactions can be relieved with **calamine** (see Table 5.5). Calamine works through a counterirritant action that involves evaporation and cooling, which soothe the itchy sensation. Many calamine products also contain zinc oxide, an ingredient with antiseptic properties that protects against infection from repeated scratching.

Dosage Forms and Administration Calamine is a lotion that can be applied as needed.

Side Effects Patients may use calamine frequently, and it has few side effects.

Contraindications Patients should not use calamine on broken or blistered skin. The drug is not recommended for children younger than two years.

Cautions and Considerations If the itching and rash are not relieved within a few days of using calamine, the patient should see their healthcare practitioner. Stronger prescription products may be needed, or the patient may have an underlying problem that requires medical treatment.

Drug Interactions Calamine has no known drug interactions.

Selenium Sulfide and Pyrithione Zinc

The most common active ingredients in OTC dandruff products are **selenium sulfide (Head & Shoulders Intensive Treatment, Selsun Blue)** and **pyrithione zinc**

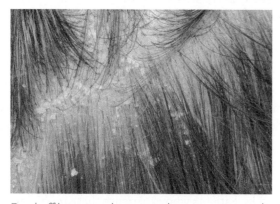

Dandruff is a cosmetic concern that appears as specks of skin in the hair and on the scalp.

(Denorex Everyday Dandruff Shampoo, T/Gel Daily Control). Selenium sulfide can also be found in prescription strength (SelRex). Patients should use these products once a day or on a regular basis to control dandruff. Coal tar shampoos, including Neutrogena T/Gel, are also available over the counter, but only patients with severe cases tend to use them. Coal tar is safe, but it can be messy and odorous, and most patients find long-term use unpleasant.

All of these active ingredients work by slowing cell and oil production, which results in reduced skin flaking. In addition, these products have antipruritic properties that reduce the itching associated with dry, flaking skin.

Dosage Forms and Administration The products identified here are mainly shampoos or cleansers that are applied and then washed out of the hair.

Side Effects Side effects of dandruff products are rare and mild. However, possible effects include contact dermatitis, photosensitivity, and aggravation of preexisting skin conditions such as acne or psoriasis. If such effects occur, the patient should stop using the product, and the effects will subside.

Contraindications No contraindications exist for these products.

Cautions and Considerations If dandruff and scalp itching continue with repeated use of these products, patients should seek medical advice to determine whether the issue has an alternative cause.

Drug Interactions Topical products generally do not have serious drug interactions.

5.5 Skin Infections and Drug Treatments

Skin infections are common. Although patients can manage most with nonprescription topical antimicrobial products, some do not respond to ordinary products, necessitating treatment with a prescription drug. The severity of a skin infection depends on the extent to which the skin and its structures are affected. Patients can experience drainage, swelling, fever, and malaise.

Skin infections can be caused by a bacteria, fungus, or a virus. In many cases, skin infections can be treated topically. Topical antibiotics and antivirals work quickly, but topical antifungals require longer treatment times to be effective. In rare circumstances and severe infection, oral drugs may be needed. Table 5.6 identifies common topical agents used to treat skin infections.

TABLE 5.6 Commonly Used Topical Products for Infections

Generic (Brand)	Pronunciation	Dosage Form	Dispensing Status
Topical Antibacterials			
bacitracin	bas-i-TRAY-sin	ointment	OTC
bacitracin / neomycin / polymyxin B (Mycitracin Triple Antibiotic, Neosporin, Triple Antibiotic Ointment)	bas-i-TRAY-sin nee-oh-MYE-sin pol-ee-MIX-in BEE	ointment	OTC
mupirocin (Centany)	myoo-PEER-oe-sin	cream, ointment	Rx
retapamulin (Altabax)	ret-a-PAM-yoo-lin	ointment	Rx
Topical Antifungals			
butenafine (Lotrimin Ultra, Mentax)	byoo-ten-a-feen	cream	OTC, Rx
ciclopirox (Ciclodan, Loprox, Penlac)	sye-kloe-PEER-ox	cream, gel, shampoo, topical solution, topical suspension	Rx
clotrimazole (Alevazol, Desenex, Gyne-Lotrimin, Lotrimin AF, Pro-Ex)	kloe-TRIM-a-zole	cream, ointment, suppository, topical solution	OTC, Rx
ketoconazole (Extina, Ketodan Kit, Nizoral, Xolegel)	kee-toe-KOE-na-zole	cream, foam, gel, shampoo	OTC, Rx
miconazole (DermaFungal, Desenex, Lotrimin AF, Micaderm, Micatin, Neosporin AF, Zeosorb)	mi-KON-a-zole	cream, ointment, powder, spray, suppository	OTC, Rx
sertaconazole (Ertaczo)	ser-ta-KON-a-zole	cream	Rx
terbinafine (Lamisil, Lamisil AT)	ter-BI-na-feen	cream, gel, spray	OTC, Rx
tolnaftate (Fungi-Guard, Lamisil AF Defense, Podactin, Tinactin)	tol-NAFF-tate	aerosol, cream, powder, topical solution	OTC
Topical Antivirals			
acyclovir (Sitavig, Zovirax)	ay-SYE-kloe-veer	buccal tablet, cream, ointment	Rx
docosanol (Abreva)	doe-KOE-sa-nole	cream	OTC

Topical Antibacterials

Bacterial skin infections most frequently involve *Staphylococcus aureus*, which is considered normal flora and is not generally harmful, unless overgrowth occurs or it is introduced internally through a cut or sore. Methicillin-resistant *Staphylococcus aureus* (MRSA), an organism that is particularly difficult to treat when introduced internally, is common to have on the skin. Therefore, patients take systemic antibiotics prior to surgery to prevent infection from an incision through the skin.

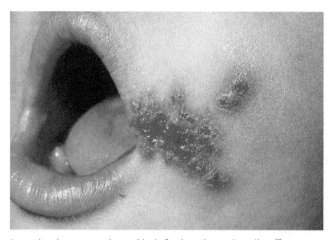

Impetigo is a contagious skin infection that primarily affects young children.

Impetigo is a skin infection caused by *S. aureus* or *Streptococcus*. It is a superficial but highly contagious skin infection that is common in early childhood, particularly in warm, humid climates and where hygiene is poor. It is uncommon in adults but does occur, particularly in older adults and immunocompromised patients.

Erysipelas, a form of cellulitis, is characterized by redness and warmth, local pain, swollen plaques with sharply established borders, chills, malaise, and fever. The infection spreads progressively and rapidly through the superficial layers of the skin. On the face, erysipelas may assume a butterfly distribution. Erysipelas usually responds well to oral antibiotics. However, if systemic toxicity (high fever with elevated white blood cell count) results, parenteral antibiotics should be administered.

Folliculitis is an inflammation of a hair follicle that is characterized by a minute, red, pustulated nodule without involvement of the surrounding tissues. Patients experience little pain. Folliculitis commonly occurs on the bearded part of the face in patients who can grow beards.

A **furuncle** (boil) is a staphylococcal infection beginning in a sebaceous gland and the associated hair follicle. The follicular infection is more extensive and deeper than in folliculitis. It begins with itching, local tenderness, and erythema, followed by swelling, marked local pain, and pus formation within the lesion. A **carbuncle** is a coalescent mass of infected follicles with deeper penetration than a furuncle. Pain, erythema, swelling, purulent (containing pus) drainage, and fever can occur. The infection causing carbuncles can spread through the blood or with contact to other parts of the body.

Bacterial skin infections can be treated with topical products and systemic therapies. Systemic antibiotics are covered in Chapter 16. Generic names for topical antibiotic agents differ from names of oral antibiotics, so familiarity with oral antibiotics does not automatically confer knowledge of topical products. Topical antibiotics are used to treat local skin infections such as impetigo, diaper rash, and infections in cuts and scrapes.

Certain antibiotic combinations are available over the counter (OTC). Bacitracin and **bacitracin-neomycin-polymyxin B (Mycitracin Triple Antibiotic, Neosporin, Triple Antibiotic Ointment)** are used to prevent or treat minor skin infections.

Mupirocin (Centany) is a common topical treatment for impetigo caused by *Staphylococcus aureus* or *Streptococcus pyogenes*. It should not be applied to the eye; patients should discontinue use if rash, itching, or irritation occurs or if they experience no improvement within 5 days.

Retapamulin (Altabax) is an ointment approved for the topical treatment of impetigo in both adults and children. The active ingredient is derived from an edible mushroom. Retapamulin should be used twice a day for 5 days. Retapamulin is slower acting than mupirocin, the other topical agent used for impetigo.

Erythromycin and metronidazole, discussed previously in this chapter, may be used for bacterial skin infections.

Dosage Forms and Administration See Table 5.6 for dosage forms of these topical antibacterials. Mupirocin is applied three times a day for 12 days. Retapamulin should be used twice a day for 5 days.

Side Effects Side effects of topical antibacterials include burning, itching, dryness, tenderness, or swelling of the treated area.

Contraindications Patients with a known allergy to an antibiotic should not use a topical product with that same drug in it. Pharmacy personnel must remember that when a patient is allergic to one antibiotic, they are allergic to all antibiotics in the same drug class. Patients can check with their pharmacist if they are not sure whether an allergy should prevent them from using one of these medications.

Cautions and Considerations These products are for external use only and should be kept away from the eyes and other mucous membranes during application. Patients should not apply these products over large areas of skin, because systemic absorption can occur.

Drug Interactions Topical antibiotics are generally not associated with serious drug interactions.

Topical Antifungals

Skin, mucous membranes, and nails are susceptible to various fungal infections. Candidiasis (see also Chapter 16) is an infection caused by *Candida albicans*, a fungus that usually gives rise to lesions in the vagina (where it is called a *yeast infection*) or the mouth (where it is called *thrush*). Candidiasis may be treated with antifungal agents such as clotrimazole and miconazole. Nystatin suspension is used to treat thrush. Table 5.6 lists common products used for skin and nail fungal infections.

Tinea infections are caused by a microscopic fungus that infects the horny (scaly) layer of the skin or the nails. Tinea causes ringworm (tinea corporis), athlete's foot (tinea pedis), and jock itch (tinea cruris). In **ringworm**, the infection spreads outward as the center heals, leaving a ring. Tinea infections respond well to topical antifungal agents such as **butenafine (Lotrimin Ultra, Mentax)** and **terbinafine (Lamisil, Lamisil AT)**. Because they are fungicidal (they kill the fungus), butenafine and terbinafine are more effective than other antifungal agents that are fungistatic (they only slow or stop fungal growth).

Lotrimin Ultra is available OTC and is identical to Mentax, the prescription form of butenafine. Only Lotrimin Ultra is butenafine; Lotrimin AF cream is clotrimazole, and Lotrimin AF sprays and powder are miconazole. It is important to know the generic and brand names of these drugs.

Ciclopirox (Ciclodan, Loprox, Penlac) is probably the most effective topical medication for onychomycosis, which is extremely difficult to treat. The aging population in the United States is very prone to this infection, which causes the nail to thicken and can lead to foot problems. Nail fungus infections are difficult to treat topically because topical treatments have difficulty penetrating the nail and/or are difficult to place under the nail so that they can attack the fungus directly. Because

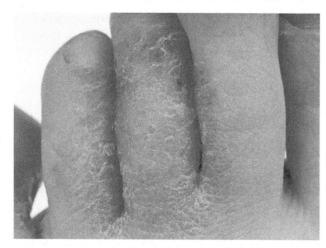

Athlete's foot causes scaling, flaking, and itching of the skin.

of this, these infections are commonly treated with oral medications.

Clotrimazole (Alevazol, Desenex, Gyne-Lotrimin, Lotrimin AF, Pro-Ex) can treat ringworm, athlete's foot, jock itch, and vaginal yeast infections. It is in a class of antifungal medications called imidazoles. The imidazole class, sometimes referred to as *-azole antifungals*, is fungistatic in low doses but fungicidal at higher dosages. It inhibits the synthesis of ergosterol, a key component in the cell membrane of a fungi.

Sertaconazole (Ertaczo) is also an imidazole. It is available by prescription, and it is used to treat athlete's foot. Sertaconazole can treat ringworm that affects the scalp, feet, hands, groin, or toenails. It also treats athlete's foot. These infections generally spread through close human contact or through indirect contact. Because the infections are superficial, topical therapy is generally sufficient to halt the growth of the fungi.

Antifungal products used for vaginal yeast infections include butoconazole, clotrimazole, miconazole, terconazole, and tioconazole. These products come in creams, ointments, and vaginal suppositories. Depending on the product, they are used for three to seven days for symptoms of vaginal yeast infections, which include itching, pain, irritation, swelling, and white-colored discharge. These products are availble over the counter.

Dosage Forms and Administration Butenafine is applied once daily for four weeks. After the last application, the drug may maintain its effect for an additional four weeks, making it a popular treatment for athlete's foot and ringworm. Ciclopirox is available as a cream but is also available as a topical solution (Penlac Nail Lacquer).

Ketoconazole (Extina, Ketodan Kit, Xolegel) is a 2% gel indicated for seborrheic dermatitis for persons 12 years and older. **Ketoconazole (Nizoral)** is available as a shampoo for patients with fungal infections of the scalp. It is used daily for two weeks. Patients should wait 20 minutes after application before using sunscreen or makeup on the affected areas.

Miconazole (DermaFungal, Desenex, Lotrimin AF, Micaderm, Micatin, Neosporin AF, Zeosorb) is available as a powder or liquid spray.

Sertaconazole is applied to the affected area two times a day for four weeks. The most common side effect is contact dermatitis.

Terbinafine is a topical cream, gel, and spray that can treat fungi. It inhibits the biosynthesis of fungal membranes. For athlete's foot, it should be applied twice daily, and four times daily for ringworm and jock itch. The treatment course takes only one week, as opposed to four weeks for other antifungal agents. Further, systemic absorption of the topical medication is low. Terbinafine remains active for one week or longer after the patient stops using it.

Tolnaftate (Fungi-Guard, Lamisil AF Defense, Podactin, Tinactin) is an OTC drug recommended for treatment of jock itch. It is not recommended for nail infections and should not be used around the eyes.

Side Effects Side effects of topical antifungals include irritation and stinging. Side effects of tolnaftate include pruritus, contact dermatitis, irritation, and stinging. If skin irritation develops, infection worsens, or there is no improvement within 10 days, the patient should consult a physician.

Pharm Fact

Note that Lotrimin AF spray and powder are miconazole, whereas Lotrimin AF cream is clotrimazole.

Contraindications The topical antifungals presented do not have contraindications.

Cautions and Considerations Discontinue use of these products if sensitivity or skin irritation occurs. Ciclopirox may cause a burning sensation upon application.

Ketoconazole is for external use only and should not be used on mucous membranes. Ketoconazole cream contains sulfites and should be avoided in patients with sulfite sensitivity.

Drug Interactions Antifungal agents can reduce the effectiveness of progesterone, especially vaginal dosage forms.

Topical Antivirals

Viral infections can cause several skin disorders, including herpes labialis (cold sores) and warts. Herpes simplex virus (HSV) is associated with painful dermatitis and blisters. HSV type 1 is usually associated with orofacial disease (herpes labialis), and HSV type 2 is usually associated with genital infection.

A **wart** is a virally caused epidermal tumor. Remission is due to developing immunity, but the virus may lie dormant and later cause reinfection. Genital warts are transmitted by sexual contact.

Topical treatment of HSV is palliative; it affords relief but does not cure, although antivirals such as oral acyclovir (see Chapter 17), if initiated early enough, may prevent recurrent outbreaks. Warts can be removed by surgery or destroyed by local freezing. Some OTC products may be effective if the wart is small. Most agents contain salicylic acid (discussed previously) as an active ingredient.

Refer to Table 5.6 for a list of topical products commonly used for viral infections.

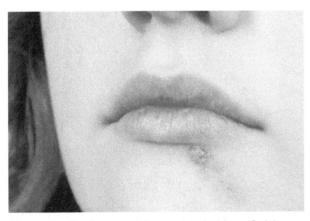

Herpes simplex virus type 1 is associated with orofacial lesions, as shown.

Acyclovir (Zovirax) is a prescription topical antiviral medication. It is used for genital herpes simplex virus, herpes labialis, and mucocutaneous (areas around the lips, nostrils, eyes, urethra, vagina, foreskin, and anus) HSV. Acyclovir is also available as a buccal tablet (**Sitavig**) for oral herpes simplex (cold sores).

Docosanol (Abreva) is another OTC topical medication that treats cold sores. Acyclovir and docosanol block the virus from invading the cells and are most effective when administered at the first sign of an outbreak.

Dosage Forms and Administration Acyclovir is available as both a topical cream and ointment and as a tablet. Docosanol is available as a cream and must be applied five times a day to be effective.

Side Effects Side effects of topical antivirals include dryness and flaking skin, burning, stinging, and itching.

Contraindications Topical acyclovir is contraindicated in patients with hypersensitivity to valacyclovir. Docosanol has no contraindications.

Cautions and Considerations Docosanol may contain benzyl alcohol, which is associated with potentially fatal neonatal gasping syndrome.

Drug Interactions Topical acyclovir and docosanol have no known significant interactions.

5.6 External Parasites and Drug Treatments

Two common types of external parasites use the human body as a host: scabies mites and lice. The mites that cause scabies may spend part of their life cycle on the skin surface and the remainder burrowed in the host's skin. In contrast, lice spend their entire life cycle on the skin surface, body, hair, and clothing and bedding fibers of their host. An infestation of lice is called **pediculosis**. Agents used to treat external parasites are listed in Table 5.7.

TABLE 5.7 Commonly Used Topical Agents for External Parasites

Generic (Brand)	Pronunciation	Dosage Form	Dispensing Status
ivermectin (Sklice, Soolantra)	eye-ver-MEK-tin	cream, lotion	Rx
permethrin (Elimite, Nix)	per-METH-rin	cream, lotion	OTC
pyrethrin (Licide, RID)	pye-REE-thrin	shampoo, topical liquid	OTC

Mites called *Sarcoptes scabiei*, or itch mites, cause **scabies** (the intense itching and threadlike lesions caused by these mites). These tiny mites (0.2–0.4 mm long) are white, flat, and oval. Along with spiders and ticks, mites belong to the class of animals called arachnids (similar to insects, but having eight legs rather than six).

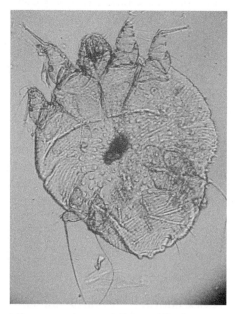

Mites cause intense itching while they are living on the skin.

The female mite burrows into the epidermis and secretes substances that disintegrate the skin. It digests the skin and sucks in the intracellular fluid but does not consume any blood because the capillaries are below the epidermis.

An infected patient experiences an intense itching that worsens at night after their bed is warmed by body heat. This heightened itching may be due to the mites' increased activity, feeding, and excretion of feces.

Scabies lesions appear as light-gray, threadlike burrows that are thin, wavy, and slightly elevated. They occur most often in the webs between the fingers. Burrows usually range from 1 to 10 mm long. Figure 5.2 shows the common sites of scabies infestation. Drug treatment for scabies usually involves permethrin. Permethrin (discussed with lice) should be massaged thoroughly into the skin from the neck to the soles of the feet in adults. The hairline, neck, temples, and forehead may be infested in infants and older adults; in these patients, permethrin should also be applied to the scalp and face, avoiding the eyes. Permethrin should be washed off 8 to 12 hours later.

Patients rarely need further repeated treatment. Persistent inflammation and itching may be due to scratching, contact dermatitis, or a secondary infection rather than the mite infestation. Additional applications could cause dermatitis.

FIGURE 5.2
Sites of Scabies Infestation

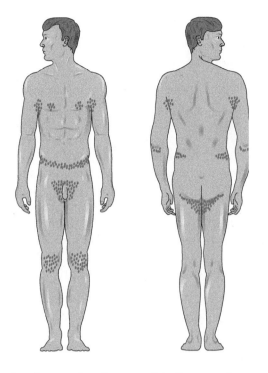

Pharm Fact

Lice, like other pathogens, can develop resistance to medications. In the past, most lice were susceptible to medications containing permethrin or pyrethrin. Now lice are developing resistance to these OTC products. A prescription agent may be required to eliminate them.

Lice are wingless insects that live parasitically on various animals, including most mammals. The lice that only live on humans exist in all climate zones, from polar to tropical, and may infest persons from any walk of life. Human blood is the only source of nourishment for these lice. They live up to 30 days, but they may die prematurely due to scratching, combing, or disease. Injured or weak lice fall off the host. Lice spread through direct contact with the infested person's head, body, or personal items such as hats, hairbrushes, combs, or bedding. The symptom of a lice infestation is itching.

Three types of lice can infest humans: body lice, head lice, and pubic lice. DNA studies suggest that body lice evolved from head lice, possibly when *Homo sapiens* first began to wear clothing (possibly 70,000 years ago). In contrast, pubic lice are more closely related to lice that live on nonhuman primates, such as gorillas, than to human head or body lice.

Body lice are 2 to 4 mm long and live in clothing and moist areas of the body, such as the waistline and armpits. Body lice do not always require treatment with drugs. Instead, they can often be treated by removing clothing, bathing, changing bedding, and putting on clean clothing. Body lice are sensitive to heat, so washing clothing and bedding in hot water or using a clothes dryer can eliminate both adult lice and eggs.

The head louse, *Pediculus humanus capitis*, is 1 to 2 mm long and lives on the scalp and hair, but not on eyebrows or eyelashes. Head lice are not generally believed to transmit any viral or bacterial diseases. They feed on blood from the scalp, which produces the intense pruritus in patients with an infestation. A female head louse has a life span of 30 days, during which it lays approximately 10 eggs (nits) per day. The louse cements its nits to hair shafts close to the scalp, where they can take advantage of body heat, which allows them to hatch in approximately 8 days. Some OTC medications only treat adult lice and cannot kill the nits. This is why the treatment must be repeated. Shining a bright light on the scalp is the best way to see nits. They appear white and look like dandruff. They cannot be shaken off but can be removed using a delousing comb.

Pubic lice, or crab lice, are 0.8 to 1.2 mm long and live in the pubic area. An infestation may resemble dermatitis and may be very itchy; corticosteroids worsen this condition. Sexual contact can transmit pubic lice. To eliminate pubic lice, patients

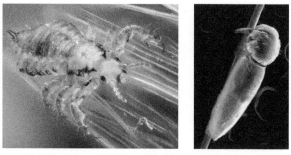

An adult head louse (left) can live for up to 30 days on the scalp. The heat from the scalp allows nits (right) to hatch in 8 days.

must apply a topical treatment. In rare cases, pubic lice may inhabit the scalp.

Ivermectin (Sklice, Soolantra) is a topical product used for head lice. It may also be used for inflammatory lesions of rosacea in adults. This drug requires a prescription.

Permethrin (Elimite, Nix) produces virtually no effects on the CNS. A 1% concentration is the drug of choice for treating head lice. It has residual action lasting up to 14 days that continues to kill any lice hatched after the initial application.

Pyrethrin (Licide, RID) is an OTC drug usually used for head lice. The mechanism of action involves disruption of neuronal transmission in lice and is similar to the action of the now-banned insecticide DDT. Pyrethrin must be applied to premoistened hair and scalp for 10 minutes and then rinsed off; treatment is repeated in one week.

Dosage Forms and Administration Products used to treat lice and scabies are available as cream, lotion, shampoo, and topical liquid.

Side Effects Common side effects of ivermectin include skin irritation, rash, dry skin, dandruff, and eye irritation. The most common side effects of permethrin are related to skin irritation: itching, burning redness, or rash. Rarely, permethrin has caused headache, diarrhea, dizziness, nausea or vomiting. Pyrethrin is usually well tolerated, but it can cause skin or eye irritation.

Contraindications Permethrin use is contraindicated in patients with hypersensitivity to pyrethroids or pyrethrin. OTC pyrethrin should not be used near eyes; inside the nose, mouth, or vagina; or on infestations in eyebrows or eyelashes.

Cautions and Considerations Patients should only use topical ivermectin on the scalp and hair.

Permethrin may cause difficulty breathing in patients with asthma.

Patients sensitive to ragweed may be sensitive to impurities in pyrethrin. Allergic reactions to pyrethrin can be serious. Patients experiencing any of the following

WORKPLACE WISDOM

Table 5.7 lists agents most commonly used to treat lice. Instructions to the patient vary with the type of lice infestation:

- Body lice: Shower or bathe and apply 20–30 g of cream or lotion to the whole body from the neck down; then wash off in 24 hours. Repeat in one week.

- Head lice: Massage 2 ounces or less of cream or lotion into premoistened hair for four minutes, and rinse out. Repeat after one week. The repetition is important to eliminate eggs.

- Pubic lice: Apply a thin layer of cream or lotion that extends to the thighs, trunk, pubic region, and armpits; wash off within 24 hours. Repeat in one week.

For both head and pubic lice, it is important to comb the hair with a clean, fine-tooth comb for at least eight days (the life cycle of a common louse) to ensure that all nits and adult lice are removed.

should seek medical care: hives; swelling of the mouth, face, lips, or tongue; blisters; peeling skin; wheezing; or trouble swallowing or breathing.

Drug Interactions The products listed for the treatment of lice do not have drug interactions.

5.7 Antiseptics and Disinfectants

Safety Alert

Antiseptics and disinfectants should only be used topically and never swallowed. The nearest poison control center should be consulted if a patient has ingested one of these products.

Chemicals have long been used to control **suppuration** (formation or discharge of pus), prevent the spread of disease, and preserve food. In the mid-19th century, scientists including Robert Koch and Louis Pasteur showed that microorganisms are what cause infection and putrefaction. Still, it took until the 1860s and 1870s for physicians to begin to appreciate the importance of disinfection. This was the period when Joseph Lister developed techniques for antiseptic surgery and the control of postoperative sepsis. These techniques, still in use today, included disinfecting the surgical patient's skin, the surgeon's hands, the instruments, and the operating theater.

Antiseptics and disinfectants have two uses. Healthcare practitioners and patients use them to disinfect instruments and to treat accessible infections in the oral cavity and on body surfaces. The ideal antiseptic must possess the ability to inhibit all forms of infectious organisms without being toxic to the patient or inducing sensitization of human tissues. It should be capable of penetrating tissues and of acting in the presence of body fluids such as serum, pus, and mucus. It should be soluble in water, stable, noncorrosive, and inexpensive. No agent meets all these requirements. As a result, it is always best to use two separate agents with different mechanisms of action to clean instruments or to maintain sterility in a cleanroom. Table 5.8 lists the most commonly used antiseptics and disinfectants.

TABLE 5.8 Commonly Used Antiseptics and Disinfectants

Generic (Brand)	Pronunciation	Dosage Form	Dispensing Status
Topical Products			
benzalkonium chloride (Viroxyn)	benz-al-KOE-nee-um KLOR-ide	topical solution	OTC
hydrogen peroxide (various brands)	HYE-droe-jen per-OX-ide	topical solution	OTC
isopropyl alcohol (various brands)	eye-so-PROE-pil AL-koe-hawl	liquid disinfectant	OTC
povidone / iodine (Aplicare, Betadine, NuPrep)	POE-vi-done EYE-oh-dyne	aerosol, gel, ointment, topical solution	OTC
sodium hypochlorite (Clorox)	SOE-dee-um hye-poe-KLOR-ite	liquid disinfectant	OTC
zinc oxide (Desitin Maximum Strength Original)	ZINK OX-ide	ointment	OTC
Miscellaneous Products			
benzocaine (Anacaine, Dermoplast, HurriCaine, Lanacane)	BEN-zoe-kayn	gel, topical liquid, lozenge, ointment, spray	OTC, Rx
carbamide peroxide (Gly-Oxide Oral)	KAR-ba-mide per-OX-ide	topical solution	OTC
chlorhexidine gluconate (Biopatch, Dyna-Hex, Hibiclens)	klor-HEX-i-deen GLOO-koe-nate	external liquid, oral liquid antiseptic, pad	OTC

Topical Antiseptics and Disinfectants

A variety of agents, listed in Table 5.8, serve as antiseptics and disinfectants. Disinfectants kill bacteria, while antiseptics prevent bacterial growth. These chemicals each have specific actions (see Table 5.9). The most desirable property of a disinfectant is its ability to destroy microorganisms rapidly and completely. No single disinfectant is equally effective against all types of organisms. Furthermore, many agents that rapidly destroy organisms may be too toxic to apply to human or animal tissue cells.

Aesthetic factors, such as odor, taste, and staining quality, may also influence disinfectant selection. If a disinfectant is used in or around the mouth, bad odor or taste may reduce patient adherence. Patients also may object to materials that stain the oral mucosa, skin, or clothing.

Benzalkonium chloride (Viroxyn) is used as a preoperative skin disinfectant. Instruments and hospital utensils are also often stored in a solution of benzalkonium chloride.

Hydrogen peroxide is a strongly disinfecting, cleansing, and bleaching agent. It is used to prepare dental surfaces before filling and to clean wounds. The release of oxygen provides the antiseptic action.

TABLE 5.9 Actions of Antiseptics and Disinfectants

Agent	Action
antiseptic	a substance that inhibits growth and development of microorganisms but does not necessarily kill them
disinfectant	a chemical applied to objects to free them from pathogenic organisms or render such organisms inert
fungicide	a substance that destroys fungi
germicide	a substance that destroys bacteria but not necessarily spores
preservative	an agent that prevents decomposition by either chemical or physical means
sanitizer	an agent that reduces the number of bacterial contaminants to a safe level
sporicide	a substance that destroys spores

Isopropyl alcohol is supplied in 70%–90% concentrations. This alcohol is inexpensive, spreads well, and dries slowly. It primarily removes bacteria but can also kill some bacteria. Isopropyl alcohol denatures proteins and produces a marked stinging reaction when applied to cuts or abrasions. To be effective, alcohol must dry and be left on the wound for at least two minutes.

Povidone-iodine (Aplicare, Betadine, NuPrep) is an aqueous solution that does not stain and causes little discomfort when applied to an open wound. It is among the most effective disinfectants available. It has a broad spectrum of activity against bacteria, fungi, viruses, protozoa, and yeasts.

Sodium hypochlorite (Clorox) disinfects and deodorizes by killing most germs and their odors. It is a common laundry and household product (chlorine bleach) that is used in cleaning and stain removal.

Zinc oxide (Desitin Maximum Strength Original) is a mild antiseptic and astringent used for some conjunctival (relating to the mucous membrane lining the eyelids' inner surface) and skin diseases. It is an ingredient in some brands of calamine lotion. The oxide salt, a zinc salt, is combined with a petroleum jelly and a waxy lanolin base for use in treating diaper rash and other minor skin irritations.

Miscellaneous Products

Unlike the disinfectants used on the skin outlined so far, the following antiseptics can be used in the mouth. The oral cavity is very difficult to disinfect. Very few drugs adhere to the mucosal lining long enough to overcome bacteria or ease pain.

Benzocaine (Anacaine, Dermoplast, HurriCaine, Lanacane) is a local anesthetic, but it also forms a protective barrier over the mucous membrane in the mouth. The patient should not eat for an hour after applying an oral mucosa. Benzocaine should not be applied to broken skin.

Carbamide peroxide (Gly-Oxide Oral) releases oxygen on contact with oral tissues and reduces inflammation; inhibits odor-forming bacteria; and relieves pain in periodontal pockets, oral ulcers, and dental sores. It is also used to **emulsify** (enable mixing with water) and disperse earwax.

Chlorhexidine gluconate (Biopatch, Dyna-Hex, Hibiclens) is a skin cleanser for surgical scrubbing, skin wounds, germicidal hand rinsing, and antibacterial dental rinsing. It is active against gram-positive and gram-negative organisms and yeast. Studies show that patients on ventilators who have scheduled mouth cleansings throughout the day with chlorhexidine gluconate have significantly decreased incidences of pneumonia.

5.8 Complementary and Alternative Therapies

Aloe gel has soothing and wound-healing properties. It inhibits bradykinin, a pain-inducing agent, and slows the synthesis of thromboxane, which may speed the healing of burns and sun overexposure. Aloe gel also has antibacterial and antifungal properties. When combined with lidocaine, aloe gel is especially soothing.

Clove oil is an antiseptic used on exposed dentin (dense material that composes the principal mass of a tooth). Mixed with zinc oxide or zinc acetate, it is used as a dental application in temporary fillings and cements and in periodontal and intra-alveolar packs.

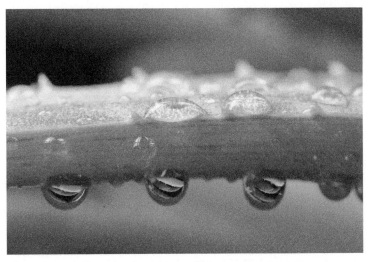

Aloe gel comes from the aloe plant and has soothing properties.

Review and Assessment

📖 CHAPTER SUMMARY

Anatomy and Physiology of the Integumentary System

- The skin is a major organ in the human body and accounts for 16% of body weight. It is the main organ involved in temperature regulation.

- The dermis is composed of connective tissue with upward projections into the epidermis.

- Two types of glands receive widespread distribution in the skin: sebaceous glands and sweat glands.

Sun Exposure and Drug Treatments

- A suntan may look good but can permanently damage the skin.

- A sunscreen should protect against both UVA and UVB rays.

- Sun-damaged skin can be a precursor to skin cancer.

Acne, Wrinkles, Rosacea, and Drug Treatments

- Acne is treated with cleansers, antibiotics, retinoids, and salicylic acid.

- Retinoids also treat wrinkles.

- Isotretinoin cannot be used by patients who are or may become pregnant.

- Rosacea is treated with azelaic acid, brimonidine, and metronidazole.

Dermatitis, Eczema, Psoriasis, Dandruff, and Drug Treatments

- Dermatitis is itchy, inflamed skin.

- Topical corticosteroids are commonly used for dermatitis, eczema, and psoriasis.

- Creams, gels, and ointments are not interchangeable.

- Topical corticosteroids should be applied sparingly as a very thin film. Significant quantities may be absorbed systemically because these drugs can penetrate the skin.

- Eczema may be treated with the calcineurin inhibitors pimecrolimus (Elidel) and tacrolimus (Protopic).

- Dandruff results from a malfunction of oil-producing glands on the scalp and overproliferation of cells.

- Dandruff is treated with selenium sulfide.

Skin Infections and Drug Treatments

- Skin infections are common, and many can be managed with topical antimicrobial products.

- Impetigo is a highly contagious skin infection common in early childhood.

- Fungal infections include thrush and other yeast infections, ringworm, and nail fungus.

- Ringworm is caused by a fungus. It may be treated with butenafine and terbinafine.

- Viral infections may cause skin disorders such as warts and herpes simplex virus types 1 and 2.

- Acyclovir treats genital herpes simplex virus, herpes labialis, and mucocutaneous HSV.

External Parasites and Drug Treatments

- Scabies results from mites that burrow into the epidermis.

- Lice are insects that live on mammals. They can live on the scalp, skin, and pubic area.

- Treatment for lice infestations includes both OTC and prescription products.

- Head lice treatment must be repeated after one week to eliminate eggs.

Antiseptics and Disinfectants

- When an antiseptic is used to disinfect instruments or to maintain sterility in a cleanroom, it is always best to use two separate cleansers with different mechanisms of action.

Complementary and Alternative Therapies

- Aloe gel has soothing and wound healing properties.

- Clove oil is an antiseptic used on exposed dentin.

DRUG LIST

Sun-Damaged Skin
aloe gel
benzocaine (Anacaine, Dermoplast, HurriCaine, Lanacane)
hydrocortisone (Cortaid, Cortizone)
lidocaine (Lidoderm, Lidopin, Topicaine, Xolido, Xylocaine)
silver sulfadiazene (Silvadene, SSD)

Skin Diseases and Disorders

Acne—Topical Antibiotics
azelaic acid (Azelex, Finacea)
benzoyl peroxide (Benzac, Brevoxyl, Clearasil, Desquam, Oxy 10, PanOxyl)
Clindamycin (Cleocin T, Clindagel, Clindets, Evoclin, Veltin, Ziana)
dapsone (Aczone)
erythromycin (Ery, Erygel)

Acne—Retinoids
adapalene (Differin)
isotretinoin (Absorica, Amnesteem, Claravis, Myorisan, Zenatane)
tazarotene (Avage, Fabior, Tazorac)

tretinoin (Altreno, Atralin, Avita, Refissa, Renova, Retin-A, Tretin-X)

Acne—Miscellaneous
salicylic acid (Clearasil, Fostex, Neutrogena products, Oxy, PROPA pH, Stridex products)

Bacterial Skin Infections
bacitracin
bacitracin-neomycin-polymyxin B (Triple Antibiotic Ointment, Neosporin)
mupirocin (Centany)
retapamulin (Altabax)

Dandruff
ketoconazole (Nizoral)
pyrithione zinc
selenium sulfide (Head & Shoulders Intensive Treatment, Selsun Blue)

Dermatitis, Eczema, and Psoriasis
calamine
calcipotriene (Calcitrene, Dovonex, Sorilux)
pimecrolimus (Elidel)
tacrolimus (Protopic)
topical corticosteroids (see following page)

Fungal Skin Infections

butenafine (Lotrimin Ultra, Mentax)
ciclopirox (Ciclodan, Loprox, Penlac)
clotrimazole (Alevazol, Desenex, Gyne-Lotrimin, Lotrimin AF, Pro-Ex)
ketoconazole (Extina, Ketodan Kit, Nizoral, Xolegel)
miconazole (DermaFungal, Desenex, Lotrimin AF, Micaderm, Micatin, Neosporin AF, Zeosorb)
sertaconazole (Ertaczo)
terbinafine (Lamisil, Lamisil AT)
tolnaftate (Fungi-Guard, Lamisil AF Defense, Podactin, Tinactin)

Rosacea

brimonidine (Mirvaso)
metronidazole (MetroCream, MetroGel, MetroLotion, Noritate, Rosadan)

Wrinkles

tretinoin (Altreno, Atralin, Avita, Refissa, Renova, Retin-A, Tretin-X)

Topical Corticosteroids

Low Potency

alclometasone (Aclovate)
hydrocortisone (Cortaid, Cortizone-10, Dermarest, Instacort, Lanacort)
hydrocortisone (Ala-Cort, Aquanil, Cortaid, Instacort, Kericort, Lanacort, NuCort, Texacort)
hydrocortisone acetate (Cortaid, Cortef, Gynecort, Lanacort, Tucks)
hydrocortisone butyrate (Locoid)
hydrocortisone probutate (Pandel)
prednicarbate (Dermatop)

High Potency

betamethasone dipropionate (AlphaTrex, Diprolene, Sernivo)
betamethasone valerate (Apexicon, Luxiq, Psorcon)
clocortolone (Cloderm)
desoximetasone (Topicort)
fluocinolone (Capex, Synalar)
fluocinonide (Lidex, Vanos)
fluticasone (Cutivate)
halcinonide (Halog)

hydrocortisone valerate (Instacort, Locoid, Pandel)
mometasone furoate (Elocon)
triamcinolone (Kenalog, Triderm)

Very High Potency or Superpotency

amcinonide
betamethasone dipropionate, augmented (Diprolene)
clobetasol propionate (Clobex, Clodan, Olux, Temovate, Tovet)
desonide (DesOwen, Tridesilon, Verdeso)
halobetasol propionate (Lexette, Ultravate)

Topical Antivirals

acyclovir (Sitavig, Zovirax)
docosanol (Abreva)

Treatments for Lice

ivermectin (Sklice, Soolantra)
permethrin (Elimite, Nix)
pyrethrin (Licide, RID)

Antiseptics and Disinfectants

Topical

benzalkonium chloride (Viroxyn)
hydrogen peroxide
isopropyl alcohol
povidone-iodine (Aplicare, Betadine, NuPrep)
sodium hypochlorite (Clorox)
zinc oxide (Desitin Maximum Strength Original)

Other

benzocaine (Anacaine, Dermoplast, HurriCaine, Lanacane)
carbamide peroxide (Gly-Oxide Oral)
chlorhexidine gluconate (Biopatch, Dyna-Hex, Hibiclens)

Boxed Warnings

isotretinoin (Claravis)
pimecrolimus (Elidel)
tacrolimus (Protopic)
tretinoin (Altreno, Atralin, Avita, Refissa, Renova, Retin-A, Tretin-X)

Medication Guides

isotretinoin (Claravis)
tacrolimus (Protopic)

Take a moment to review what you have learned in this chapter and answer the following questions.

1. Which of the following tissues makes up the outermost layer of the skin?
   a. dermis
   b. epidermis
   c. subcutaneous
   d. sebum

2. Which of the following treatments is *not* used for acne?
   a. adapalene
   b. erythromycin
   c. fluticasone
   d. tretinoin

3. Which of the following is a product used to treat psoriasis?
   a. bacitracin
   b. sertaconazole
   c. retapamulin
   d. tazarotene

4. Which drug is used to treat dandruff?
   a. Dovonex
   b. Azelex
   c. selenium sulfide
   d. Retin-A

5. Which oral agent should *not* be used in patients who are or may become pregnant?
   a. mupirocin
   b. isotretinoin
   c. selenium sulfide
   d. tretinoin

6. Which of the following is used to treat head lice?
   a. salicylic acid
   b. tacrolimus
   c. mupirocin
   d. pyrethrin

7. Which class of drug does *not* cause photosensitivity?
   a. ACE inhibitors
   b. diuretics
   c. macrolide antibiotics
   d. NSAIDs

8. Which of the following drugs is a high potency corticosteroid?
   a. hydrocortisone
   b. triamcinolone
   c. clobetasol
   d. calcipotriene

9. Which of the following antifungal agents would be most likely to be used for nail fungus?
   a. clotrimazole
   b. docosanol
   c. ketoconazole
   d. ciclopirox

10. The main organ involved in temperature regulation is the
    a. skin.
    b. liver.
    c. heart.
    d. spleen.

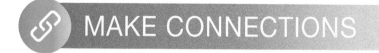

MAKE CONNECTIONS

Take a moment to consider what you have learned in this chapter and respond thoughtfully to the following prompts. Note that some of these activities will require internet access.

1. Consider the distinction between helping a customer select an OTC medication and counseling that person. Explain the difference and what is acceptable for a pharmacy technician.

2. A patient brings in a prescription for isotretinoin. The patient says they forgot to enroll in the iPLEDGE program and is asking you to make an exception and fill the prescription. Explain what you would do and why.

The online course includes additional review and assessment resources.

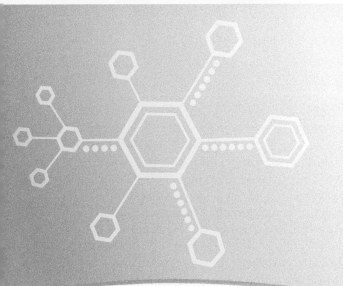

The Musculoskeletal System and Drug Therapy

6

Learning Objectives

1 Describe the anatomy and physiology of the musculoskeletal system. (Section 6.1, Section 6.2)

2 List drug classes used to treat osteoarthritis and describe their usage, side effects, contraindications, and cautions/considerations. (Section 6.3)

3 State the antidote for acetaminophen overdose. (Section 6.3)

4 Compare and contrast traditional NSAIDs with COX-2 inhibitors. (Section 6.3)

5 Identify agents commonly used to treat rheumatoid arthritis and discuss their usage, side effects, contraindications, and cautions/considerations. (Section 6.4)

6 List agents used to treat gout and describe their usage, side effects, contraindications, and cautions/considerations. (Section 6.5)

7 Identify drug classes commonly used to treat osteoporosis and discuss their usage, side effects, contraindications, and cautions/considerations. (Section 6.6)

8 Describe special administration instructions for bisphosphonate drugs. (Section 6.6)

9 State commonly used muscle relaxants. (Section 6.7)

10 Summarize drug class options for the treatment of inflammation and swelling. (Section 6.8)

11 List complementary and alternative therapies for disorders of the musculoskeletal system. (Section 6.9)

ASHP/ACPE Accreditation Standards
To view the *ASHP/ACPE Accreditation Standards* addressed in this chapter, refer to Appendix C.

The musculoskeletal system encompasses a large portion of the body. Bones, cartilage, ligaments, joints, muscles, and tendons are all components of the musculoskeletal system. Together these components create the supporting framework of the body, allow for movement, and protect internal organs. Disorders related to the musculoskeletal system include arthritis, osteoporosis, muscle spasms, and inflammation. Drug therapies for the musculoskeletal system vary. Some drugs, such as acetaminophen and nonsteroidal anti-inflammatory drugs (NSAIDs), are also used for other indications. Other drugs—such as agents used for osteoporosis—are more specific to the musculoskeletal system.

6.1 Anatomy of the Musculoskeletal System

The framework of the human body is made of bones and muscles (see Figure 6.1). The human skeleton is made of 206 bones. Each bone is formed by compact and cancellous (spongy) tissue. The outside of bone is formed from compact tissue, which is relatively solid. The interior of bone is formed from cancellous tissue and is less solid. In addition to this tissue, long bones (such as the femur) contain a substance called marrow. Bone marrow is a spongy substance found in the center of these bones and is responsible for creating blood cells.

Bones are connected by cartilage, ligaments, and other connective tissue. The place of union or junction between two or more bones of the skeleton is called a **joint**. The human body contains a wide variety of joints. The anatomy of a typical joint where two bones meet is shown in Figure 6.2.

FIGURE 6.1
Skeletal and Muscular Systems

Bones, pictured on the left, and muscles, seen on the right, create the framework of the human body.

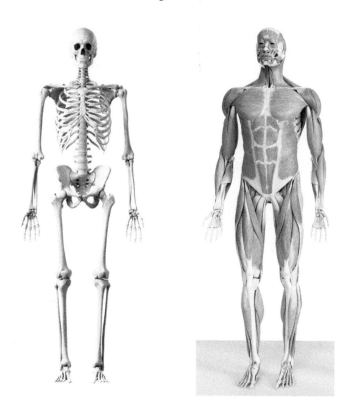

Another component of a joint is ligaments. Ligaments are noncontractile connective tissue (tissue that does not contract or relax) that ties one bone to another bone. They keep bones aligned and form the fibrous capsule that encloses the moving parts. One method of classifying joints is according to the surfaces of the articulating bones.

For example, a cartilaginous joint is a joint whose surfaces are covered with cartilage, a fibrous joint is a joint whose surfaces are attached by fibrous connective tissue, and a synovial joint is a joint whose surfaces are covered by a fluid-filled, fibrous sac.

Joints can also be classified based on the degree of movement they permit. This may be no movement, a slight degree of movement, or a variety of types of movement.

A **muscle** is an organ that produces movement by contracting (shortening itself). Muscles are connected to bones by tough, cordlike tissues called tendons. Muscles are typically grouped into three types: skeletal, smooth, and cardiac (see Figure 6.3).

FIGURE 6.2
Anatomy of a Joint

A typical joint is made up of the bones and the joint capsule.

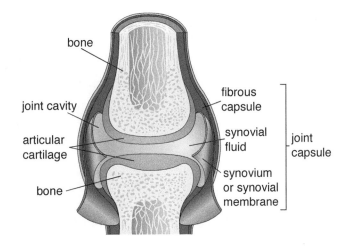

Skeletal muscle is **striated** (or striped) muscle in which contraction is voluntary; this contraction is used for locomotion and maintaining posture.

Smooth muscle is muscle in which contraction is involuntary. For example, the smooth muscles in the esophagus move food down to the stomach without the individual's direct control. Smooth muscle occurs in the lining of various organs, including the stomach, esophagus, uterus, and bladder.

Cardiac muscle is found only in the heart and is also known as heart muscle. This muscle works involuntarily and pumps blood throughout the body, but the texture of the muscle is striated like skeletal muscle.

FIGURE 6.3
Types of Muscle Tissue

Muscle comes in several types, including skeletal, smooth, and cardiac muscle.

6.2 Physiology of the Musculoskeletal System

Bones do more than provide structural support for the body and protect organs. They also allow movement and store essential nutrients. Without bones to attach to and pull on, muscles would have a difficult time moving parts of the body effectively. Figure 6.4 shows some of the bones, muscles, and tendons involved in producing movement at the elbow joint. In addition to creating skeletal movement, muscle contraction pumps blood, facilitates movement in the gastrointestinal tract, and produces uterine contractions during childbirth, among other involuntary movements.

FIGURE 6.4
**Bones,
Muscles, and
Tendons**

In this figure, the
involvement of
bones, muscles,
and tendons
produce move-
ment at the elbow
joint.

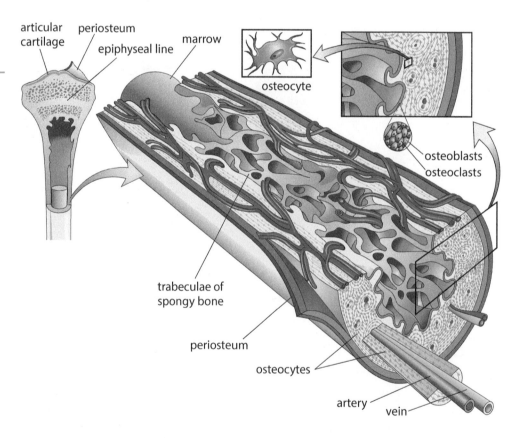

Bones also store minerals, such as calcium and phosphorus, and lipids. A
constant process of buildup and breakdown of bone, called **bone remodeling**, occurs
to maintain appropriate mineral balance in the body. An **osteoclast** is a cell that
breaks down bone and releases calcium into the bloodstream. Conversely, an **osteoblast** is a cell that takes this calcium from the blood and uses it to build bone tissue
(see Figure 6.5). Long bones such as the femur are also responsible for the production
of blood cells, including red blood cells and white blood cells.

FIGURE 6.5
**Microscopic
View of Bone**

Osteoclasts and
osteoblasts break
down, build up,
and repair bone,
a continual
process called
bone remodeling.

Skeletal muscles are controlled by impulses originating in the central nervous
system (CNS). Electrical impulses are conducted through the spinal cord by somatic
neurons (sensory and motor nerve cells) that communicate with the muscle at the
neuromuscular junction (the area of connection between a neuron and muscle fiber).

The somatic neurons release the neurotransmitter **acetylcholine (ACh)**. When the neurotransmitter binds to the receptor, the muscle cell releases calcium, causing a contraction in the muscle fibers. Skeletal muscles relax when ACh is broken down by acetylcholinesterase. Skeletal muscle contractions can be either voluntary (causing movement) or involuntary (maintaining posture and muscle tone).

Joints and muscles work together to allow the body to maintain posture and to produce movement. Any injury or illness that affects a joint or muscle can impede movement of that part of the body and may have a negative effect on the individual's quality of life. Even relatively minor injuries or stiffness can be problematic. Muscles commonly injured or strained tend to be those of the lower back, head and neck, and legs.

The most common disorders of the musculoskeletal system are arthritis (a condition affecting the joints) and osteoporosis (a condition affecting the bones). Although less common, muscle disorders can also be problematic for patients. An understanding of common prescriptions and over-the-counter treatments for musculoskeletal disorders will serve the pharmacy technician well.

6.3 Osteoarthritis and Drug Treatments

The word *arthritis* is derived from the Greek word for joint, *arthron*. **Arthritis** means "joint inflammation" and is a disorder characterized by joint pain. Although arthritis can take many forms, the most common complaint of arthritis patients is persistent pain. This pain is caused by functional problems of the joints such as inflammation, damage to joint tissues from wear and tear, and muscle strain caused by overworked muscles attempting to protect the joint.

Osteoarthritis (OA) is a degenerative joint disease in which cartilage in joints becomes thinner and less elastic, eventually causing bone to wear and become deformed (see Figure 6.6). It is a common age-related condition of synovial joints. The most commonly affected joints are the sternoclavicular joint (where the clavicle meets the sternum, or breastbone), and the joints of the spine, hips, knees, fingers, and big toes. Joints carrying large loads (knees) and those under repetitive stress (fingers) are especially likely to be affected. Osteoarthritis generally appears after age 40. The disease is characterized by progressive pain, stiffness, limitation of motion, and deformed joints. Stiffness in the morning or after inactivity (such as sitting) is the most prevalent complaint. Drug therapy for OA is aimed at the reduction of symptoms and the prevention of disability. If OA is severe enough, surgery or joint replacement is performed.

Drug treatment for osteoarthritis is unique in that several over-the-counter drugs are used as standards of therapy. Acetaminophen, for example, is commonly used by itself or in combination with other drugs. Nonsteroidal anti-inflammatory drugs are used in both oral and topical formulations. Duloxetine, which is typically used for depression, anxiety, and pain, may also be prescribed. See Table 6.1 for a list of agents used to treat osteoarthritis.

Analgesics

One of the most commonly used analgesics is acetaminophen. **Acetaminophen (Tylenol)** decreases pain and can reduce fever. These effects are known as **analgesic** (pain reducing) and **antipyretic** (fever reducing). The exact way acetaminophen works to decrease pain and fever is not fully understood. Acetaminophen may decrease the production of prostaglandins (PGs), chemicals that cause inflammation and swelling. It also elevates the pain threshold.

FIGURE 6.6
Osteoarthritis

Compared to a healthy joint, a joint with osteo-arthritis may have exposed bone, erosion, and bone spurs. Pain is a common charac-teristic of osteo-arthritis. Pain may be caused by inflammation and damage to joint tissues, as pictured. Muscle strain is another cause of osteoar-thritis pain.

Healthy Joint

Osteoarthritis

cartilage

exposed bone

cartilage beginning to break down

eroding meniscus

bone spurs

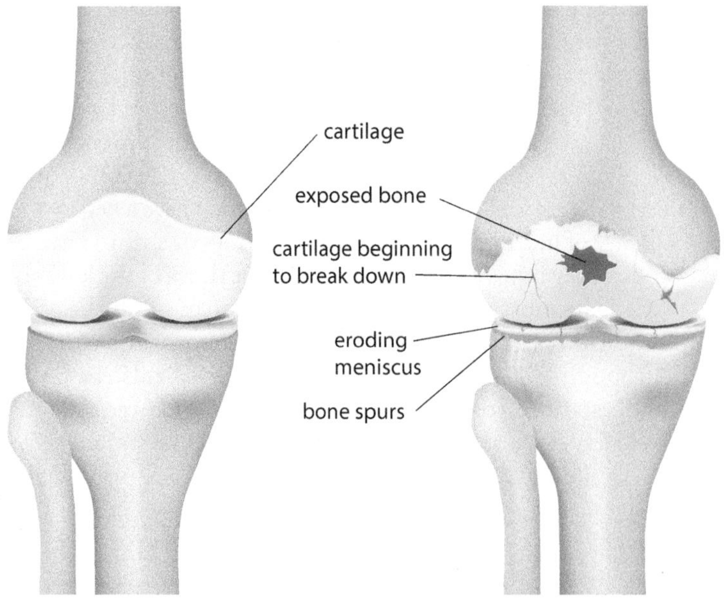

TABLE 6.1 Commonly Used Agents to Treat Osteoarthritis

Generic (Brand)	Pronunciation	Dosage Form	Common Dosage	Dispensing Status
Analgesics				
acetaminophen (Tylenol)	a-seet-a-MIN-oh-fen	caplet, capsule, chewable tablet, injection, oral elixir, oral gel, oral packet, oral solution, oral suspension, oral syrup, rectal suppository, tablet	IV/PO/PR: 325–650 mg every 4–6 hr, but not to exceed 4 g in 24 hr	Rx, OTC
Antidote for Acetaminophen				
acetylcysteine (Acetadote, Mucomyst)	uh-see-til-SIS-teen	oral solution, inhalation solution, injection	varies	Rx
Conventional NSAIDs				
diclofenac (Cambia, Zipsor, Zorvolex, Pennsaid, Voltaren Gel)	dye-KLOE-fen-ak	capsule, oral packet, ophthalmic solution, transdermal patch, tablet, transdermal gel, transdermal solution, topical solution	PO: 100–200 mg a day Topical: 2–4 g every 6 hr	Rx, OTC
etodolac (Lodine)	ee-TOE-doe-lak	capsule, tablet	600–1,000 mg a day	Rx
ibuprofen (Advil, Motrin)	eye-byoo-PROE-fen	capsule, caplet, chewable tablet, cream, injection, oral drops, oral suspension, tablet	OTC: 200 mg every 6–8 hr Rx: 400–800 mg every 6–8 hr	OTC, Rx
indomethacin (Indocin, Tivorbex)	in-doe-METH-a-sin	capsule, injection, oral suspension, suppository	PO: 50–200 mg a day (taken 1–3 times a day) Rectal: 50–200 mg a day (divided into 2–3 doses) IV (pediatric use): 0.1–0.2 mg/kg every 12–24 hr for 3 doses	Rx

continues

TABLE 6.1 **Commonly Used Agents to Treat Osteoarthritis—*Continued***

Generic (Brand)	Pronunciation	Dosage Form	Common Dosage	Dispensing Status
ketoprofen	kee-toe-PROE-fen	capsule, cream	200–300 mg a day	Rx
ketorolac (Toradol)	kee-toe-ROLE-ak	injection, nasal spray, ophthalmic solution, tablet	IM/IV: 30–60 mg every 4–6 hr PO: 10–20 mg every 4–6 hr, but not to exceed 40 mg in 24 hr	Rx
meloxicam (Mobic)	mel-OX-i-kam	capsule, oral disintegrating tablet, oral suspension, tablet	7.5–15 mg a day	Rx
nabumetone (Relafen)	na-BYOO-met-tone	tablet	1,000–2,000 mg a day	Rx
naproxen (Aleve, Anaprox, Anaprox DS, EC-Naprosyn, Flanax, Naprelan, Naprosyn)	na-PROX-en	capsule, cream, oral suspension, tablet	7.5–15 mg a day	OTC, Rx
piroxicam (Feldene)	peer-OX-i-kam	capsule	20 mg a day	Rx
Combination NSAIDs				
diclofenac / misoprostol (Arthrotec)	dye-KLOE-fen-ak mye-soe-PROST-awl	tablet	diclofenac 50 mg and misoprostol 200 mcg 3 times a day	Rx
ibuprofen / famotidine (Duexis)	eye-byoo-PROE-fen fa-MOE-ti-deen	tablet	ibuprofen 800 mg and famotidine 26.6 mg 3 times a day	Rx
naproxen / esomeprazole (Vimovo)	na-PROX-en ee-soe-MEP-ra-zole	tablet	naproxen 375–500 mg and esomeprazole 20 mg 2 times a day	Rx
COX-2 Inhibitor				
celecoxib (Celebrex)	sel-a-KOX-ib	capsule	200 mg a day	Rx

Safety Alert

Doses of acetaminophen above recommended levels may cause serious liver damage. Acetaminophen poisoning has become the most common cause of acute liver failure in the United States.

Acetaminophen was once the most popular treatment for OA, particularly the noninflammatory type. However, recent studies have suggested that other options are more effective.

Acetaminophen is used for mild to moderate pain, including pain caused by sources unrelated to osteoarthritis. When used appropriately, acetaminophen has relatively few side effects. It can be especially useful in patients who

- have a peptic ulcer,
- take a uricosuric agent for gout,
- take an oral anticoagulant,
- have a clotting disorder,
- are at risk for Reye's syndrome,
- are intolerant to aspirin (there is still a 6% chance of cross reactivity), or
- have postsurgical pain.

Acetaminophen is available over the counter and does not require a prescription. However, acetaminophen is available in several combination products that do require a prescription.

Dosage Forms and Administration Acetaminophen is most commonly used via the oral route. Oral routes of administration include tablets, caplets, and oral liquids. Other dosage forms include rectal suppositories, which may be helpful for pediatric patients or those who are vomiting and cannot tolerate oral medication. Intravenous acetaminophen is commercially available and may be used in the hospital setting.

Regardless of the route of administration, acetaminophen is dosed every four to six hours. Frequent dosing to maintain pain control can be inconvenient, and many patients choose other treatments for arthritis for this reason. Additionally, arthritis may become so severe that acetaminophen no longer manages the pain.

Side Effects Acetaminophen is generally well tolerated. Unlike other drugs for osteoarthritis, acetaminophen does not cause gastrointestinal (GI) irritation, bleeding, alteration of platelet adhesiveness, or potentiation (increase in strength) of oral anti-coagulants. The most common side effect of acetaminophen is nausea.

Acetaminophen is found in many pain prescription medications as well as OTC products. Due to this, an overdose can occur without the patient or the prescriber realizing it. Overdoses can be lethal, and pharmacy technicians need to be aware of the maximum acetaminophen dose when dispensing combination pain medications (such as hydrocodone with acetaminophen, also known as Vicodin). If the prescription allows the patient to take more than 4,000 mg (4 g) per day, the prescriber must be notified.

Contraindications Patients who have severe liver impairment or severe active liver disease should avoid acetaminophen use.

Cautions and Considerations Acetaminophen should be used cautiously and monitored in patients with alcoholic liver disease or who consume three or more alcoholic drinks each day.

An acute overdose of acetaminophen or doses greater than 4,000 mg (4 g) a day may cause liver toxicity. Long-term daily use of this medication may lead to liver damage in some patients. Use caution with **concomitant** (accompanying) acetaminophen and alcohol use.

Acetylcysteine (Acetadote, Mucomyst) is the only antidote for an acetaminophen overdose; it is also approved for some bronchial diseases. Acetylcysteine works by detoxifying the active (and harmful) metabolite of acetaminophen.

Acetylcysteine has a strong, rotten egg–like smell, which limits its use. The IV form is primarily used because of the convenience. For bronchial conditions, it comes in an inhaled, vaporized, or oral dosage form. When used for acetaminophen poisoning, acetylcysteine can be administered orally or intravenously. Each has a different dosing regimen: 72 hours when administered orally and 21 hours when intravenously, varying based on patient-specific factors. Both regimens include a loading dose and are followed by maintenance doses. Administration may vary depending on acetaminophen levels. Acetylcysteine should be administered as soon as possible, preferably within 4 hours of ingestion of the medication, but it can be effective in patients treated up to 10 hours after ingestion.

Drug Interactions Probenecid may increase the blood concentration of acetaminophen.

Conventional Nonsteroidal Anti-Inflammatory Drugs

Nonsteroidal anti-inflammatory drugs (NSAIDs) are often used as first-line therapy in patients with inflammatory OA. In noninflammatory OA, NSAIDs are used when patients experience inadequate pain reduction with acetaminophen. Other indications for the use of NSAIDs include inflammation associated with injury, dysmenorrhea (painful menstrual cycle), and fever. NSAIDs relieve inflammation, swelling, and pain. They may take longer to reduce fever than other agents, but the effects last longer, and they do not cause euphoria.

Work Wise

Acetaminophen is often abbreviated as APAP (pronounced eh-pap). This is an abbreviation of acetaminophen's chemical name, acetyl-para-aminophenol.

Safety Alert

Acetaminophen is a component within hundreds of medications and should be monitored to reduce chances of overdose.

NSAIDs work by inhibiting PG synthesis in tissues, thereby preventing pain receptors from becoming even more sensitive to other elements of inflammation. Thus, they generally act in the affected tissues, rather than centrally as opioids do. Any central actions that NSAIDs exhibit are usually unwanted side effects, except for lowered body temperature. It is unlikely, though, that all NSAIDs act only on PGs and by only one mechanism.

Various NSAIDs are available, most of which work similarly. Commonly used NSAIDs include diclofenac (Cambia, Pennsaid, Voltaren Gel, Zipsor, Zorvolex), etodolac (Lodine), ibuprofen (Advil, Motrin), indomethacin (Indocin, Tivorbex), ketoprofen, ketorolac (Toradol), meloxicam (Mobic), nabumetone (Relafen), naproxen (Aleve, Anaprox, Anaprox DS, EC-Naprosyn, Flanax, Naprelan, Naprosyn), and piroxicam (Feldene) (see Table 6.1).

Dosage Forms and Administration Several NSAIDs are OTC, or their manufacturer has requested OTC status. This means they will be used to self-medicate. It is important to realize that, although all NSAIDs have similar mechanisms of action, patient response to these drugs varies widely. Clinical trials have not shown any of these agents to be superior to the others for managing osteoarthritis. Given the wide variation in patients' reactions, inadequate response or loss of response to one NSAID does not imply inefficacy of others. If one drug does not achieve the desired results, treatment with another NSAID is appropriate before considering adding other agents. Rotating these agents is common, and patients seem to get better results when this is done, although it is important to allow two to three weeks with one agent before switching to another.

The only NSAIDs with parenteral forms are ibuprofen, indomethacin, and ketorolac, and these are for short-term use only. **Ketorolac (Toradol)** is indicated for short-term use (less than five days) in moderate to severe pain. It acts peripherally to inhibit PG synthesis. It is useful in patients who cannot tolerate narcotics. When injected, a dose of 30 mg provides pain relief comparable to 12 mg of morphine.

Topical NSAIDs are desirable due to their localized effect and decreased side effect profile. NSAIDs with topical formulations include diclofenac, ibuprofen, and ketoprofen. **Prescription topical diclofenac (Solaraze, Pennsaid, Voltaren Gel)** should be dispensed with dosing cards. Patients should squeeze an even line of medication onto the card, using the marks on it to measure the prescribed dose. OTC diclofenac is sold with an enclosed dispensing card. The prescribed amount should be massaged into the area that is painful, and the area where the drug is applied should not be washed for at least an hour.

Diclofenac (Flector Patch) is available as a transdermal patch. It should be applied to the most painful area and changed every 12 hours. The patch should be kept dry and away from heat.

Indomethacin (Indocin, Tivorbex) is the only NSAID available as a rectal suppository.

Ibuprofen (Advil, Motrin) comes in oral liquid and other dosage forms and is the first OTC analgesic for children since acetaminophen was approved. Ibuprofen has a slower onset of action than acetaminophen but a longer duration. Consequently, alternating ibuprofen and acetaminophen works well. The adult formulations are also available OTC in strengths of 200 mg per tablet, caplet, or capsule. However, the

Practice Tip

Tips for safe NSAID use include the following:

- Take with food.
- Take sufficient fluids.
- Use antacids.
- Avoid gastric irritants such as alcohol.
- Use the lowest possible dose.
- Know the side effects.

1 mL single-dose vial
15 mg/mL

Ketorolac tromethamine ®

IM or IV

Ketorolac injection is an NSAID commonly used to treat the moderate to severe pain associated with OA. Labels for injectable products and oral products often look different.

patient can easily take more than one tablet at a time and attain the 400 mg, 600 mg, or 800 mg prescription doses. Unless recommended by a prescriber, this could be very dangerous. If the patient is taking OTC agents, the physician should be notified if a fever lasts more than 3 days or pain lasts longer than 10 days.

Etodolac (Lodine) tablets should not be crushed.

Piroxicam (Feldene) has the advantage of once-a-day dosing. It is for acute or long-term therapy for arthritis.

Certain NSAIDs come in combination products. These products combine NSAIDs with products aimed to decrease GI side effects. **Arthrotec** is diclofenac combined with misoprostol; it protects the stomach from NSAID-induced ulcers. **Ibuprofen / famotidine (Duexis)** has been shown to reduce NSAID-induced ulcers. It is dosed three times daily and is often used in patients who cannot tolerate a proton pump inhibitor. It is meant for patients with low cardiovascular risk who need GI protection. **Naproxen / esomeprazole (Vimovo)** is an NSAID and a proton pump inhibitor. The proton pump inhibitor portion of the drug decreases the risk of NSAID-associated gastric ulcers. This drug is approved to treat osteoarthritis, rheumatoid arthritis, and ankylosing spondylitis and to decrease the risk of gastric ulcers in patients at risk of developing them from treatment with NSAIDs. This drug is enteric coated, so it should not be halved or crushed. The tablet should be taken 30 minutes before a meal. The drug should be used at the lowest effective dose for the shortest amount of time, and it should not be used for a period longer than six months.

Side Effects The action of NSAIDs in inhibiting PG synthesis explains their primary side effect: GI upset. PGs perform three protective functions in the GI tract: increasing mucosal blood flow, increasing mucus production, and decreasing free acid production. Thus, by inhibiting PG synthesis, NSAIDs also inhibit the protective effect of PGs on the gastric mucosa, so it is no surprise that one in five chronic NSAID users develops some type of GI gastropathy (stomach disease). Patients should be told to report abdominal pain and dark or tarry stools to a healthcare provider immediately, as these may indicate a GI bleed. This drug class should always be taken with food, be administered at the lowest dose for the shortest period of time possible, and be dispensed with a Medication Guide.

The next most common side effect of NSAID use is kidney damage. Acute renal failure, fluid retention, hypertension, increased potassium, and kidney damage can all be attributed to NSAID use. Other side effects include liver abnormalities, blood clotting irregularities, bone marrow depression (decreased number of hematopoietic cells in the bone marrow), tinnitus (ringing in the ears), jaundice, dizziness, drowsiness, rash, and dry mouth.

Diclofenac can induce signs and symptoms of hepatotoxicity (toxic damage to liver): nausea, fatigue, pruritus, jaundice, upper-right-quadrant tenderness, and flu-like symptoms. Therefore, regular liver function tests are necessary.

Indomethacin (Indocin, Tivorbex) is a potent NSAID; however, it has more adverse effects than the newer agents. Because of its side effect profile, indomethacin is not used as frequently as the other NSAIDs for arthritis.

Contraindications All NSAIDs that appear in Table 6.1 are contraindicated for perioperative pain (pain related to or occurring around the time of a surgical operation) during coronary artery bypass graft (CABG) surgery. NSAID use is also contraindicated if an individual has asthma, hives, or other allergic reactions after taking aspirin or other NSAIDs. For example, if an individual experienced hives and an asthma exacerbation with ibuprofen use, all other NSAIDs would also be contraindicated due to concerns about cross reactivity.

Ketorolac has additional contraindications. It should not be used in patients with peptic ulcer disease, a history of GI bleeding or perforation, advanced kidney disease or risk of kidney failure, suspected or confirmed cerebral bleeding, or a high risk of bleeding.

Indomethacin suppositories should not be used in people with inflammation of the rectal lining or recent rectal bleeding.

Diclofenac/misoprostol is contraindicated in pregnancy. Misoprostol can cause abortion, premature birth, or birth defects.

Safety Alert

Pharmacy technicians who are pregnant should be aware of which drugs, such as misoprostol, require special handling.

Cautions and Considerations The following cautions and considerations apply to all the drugs listed in Table 6.1 unless otherwise stated.

Technicians should be aware that NSAIDs carry boxed warnings for an increased risk of serious (and potentially fatal) heart attack and stroke as well as an increased risk of GI inflammation, ulceration, and bleeding.

A Medication Guide describing an increased risk of heart attack and stroke (which may lead to death), an increased risk of bleeding, and the need to avoid celecoxib before and after coronary artery bypass surgery must be dispensed with NSAID prescriptions. The combination diclofenac/misoprostol product carries a boxed warning for women of childbearing potential because it can cause abortion, premature birth, or birth defects.

Practice Tip

NSAIDs must be dispensed with a Medication Guide.

Drug Interactions NSAIDs can interact with the following drugs:

- other NSAIDs, including aspirin
- beta-blockers
- cyclosporine
- digoxin
- diuretics
- methotrexate
- oral hypoglycemics
- warfarin

Because NSAIDs are protein bound, concentrations can be altered by other drugs, including aspirin. Consequently, concurrent use of the two should be discouraged, as the combination may lead to additive or synergistic toxicity (toxicity equal to or greater than the sum of the toxicity of each agent) rather than increased efficacy. Also, NSAIDs may interfere with the cardioprotective effects of low-dose (81–325 mg) aspirin.

Additionally, ketorolac should not be used with probenecid or pentoxifylline.

COX-2 Inhibitor

Celecoxib (Celebrex), a type of NSAID, works slightly differently from the aforementioned NSAIDs. The other NSAIDs discussed (such as ibuprofen and naproxen) inhibit **cyclooxygenase-1 (COX-1)** and **cyclooxygenase-2 (COX-2)**. COX-1 and COX-2 are enzymes that promote the production of PGs and cause pain and inflammation. COX-1 also produces PGs that protect the stomach lining.

Celecoxib works by selectively inhibiting COX-2. This means celecoxib decreases pain and inflammation without the unwanted effect of reducing GI protection. In other words, celecoxib has anti-inflammatory and pain-relieving properties without dramatically increasing the risk of GI side effects.

Celecoxib is the only selective COX-2 inhibitor available in the United States. Celecoxib is taken for arthritis pain and other pain in patients with a history of ulcers or GI bleeding. Other indications for use include rheumatoid arthritis and primary dysmenorrhea.

Dosage Forms and Administration Celecoxib is only available in oral dosage forms. It is available as a capsule in a variety of strengths. Celecoxib can be taken on a short-term or long-term basis. A label should be attached when dispensing this drug to instruct patients to take it with food

Side Effects Celecoxib has a slightly different side effect profile than other NSAIDs. Although GI upset is reduced compared to other NSAIDs, it remains the primary side effect. Fluid retention is another significant side effect with this drug.

Contraindications As with the NSAIDs discussed previously, celecoxib should not be used for treatment of perioperative pain related to CABG surgery. Allergy to sulfonamides, aspirin, or other NSAIDs contraindicates celecoxib use.

Cautions and Considerations Technicians should be aware that celecoxib, like other NSAIDs, carries boxed warnings for an increased risk of serious (and potentially fatal) heart attack and stroke as well as an increased risk of GI inflammation, ulceration, and bleeding.

A Medication Guide describing an increased risk of heart attack and stroke (which may lead to death), an increased risk of bleeding, and the need to avoid celecoxib before and after coronary artery bypass surgery must be dispensed with celecoxib prescriptions.

Practice Tip

Celecoxib must be dispensed with an FDA Medication Guide.

Drug Interactions Celecoxib has the potential for cross reactivity in patients who are allergic to sulfonamides.

Nephrotoxic agents (agents toxic to the kidneys, such as other NSAIDs and angiotensin-converting enzyme [ACE] inhibitors) increase the nephrotoxic effects of celecoxib. Anticoagulants may increase bleeding risk.

6.4 Rheumatoid Arthritis and Drug Treatments

Work Wise

A diagnosis of RA can be emotionally taxing for patients. As a pharmacy technician, you have the opportunity to make a positive and lasting impact by smiling when appropriate and showing respect and empathy.

Rheumatoid arthritis (RA) is an autoimmune disorder in which the immune system destroys the synovial membrane of the joint, producing inflammation. The synovial membrane, also called the synovium (see Figure 6.2), swells and thickens. Fingerlike projections grow from the synovial membrane into cartilage, bone, tendon, and joint spaces, causing reabsorption of bone and cartilage. As the disease progresses, bone-to-bone contact occurs, eventually causing joint fusion. Most destruction occurs close to the inflamed synovial membrane. Because cartilage has no nerves,

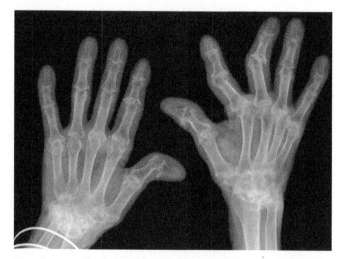

X-ray images of wrists and hands affected by rheumatoid arthritis.

pain originates from the surrounding joint structures, such as bones, tendons, ligaments, and muscles. The same joints on both sides are affected approximately 70% of the time. The small joints of the hand are usually affected first, followed by the feet, ankles, knees, wrists, elbows, shoulders, temporomandibular joints (joints connecting the jawbone to the skull), and vertebral column.

Symptoms of RA include morning pain and stiffness. These symptoms are usually symmetrical, last longer than an hour, and are not relieved by activity. Patients may feel their symptoms aggravated by cold temperatures and can feel changes in barometric pressure. Four main laboratory tests are used to help diagnose RA: rheumatoid factor (RF), anticyclic citrullinated peptide (anti-CCP) antibodies, erythrocyte sedimentation rate (ESR), and C-reactive protein (CRP). The disease is not curable but can be slowed with medication.

The goal of drug therapy in RA is to maintain mobility and delay disability for as long as possible. Medication cannot cure RA, but it can improve pain symptoms, increase function, and slow the progression of the disease, which eventually erodes and distorts joints.

To treat rheumatoid arthritis, drugs that turn off the immune system must be administered. This makes the body very susceptible to infections, cancer, and other diseases. That is why infection and malignancies are the primary side effects of the drugs.

The existing treatments for rheumatoid arthritis are divided into two categories:

1. agents that provide only symptomatic relief
2. agents that can potentially modify the course and progression of the disease

The former category includes NSAIDs, discussed earlier, and corticosteroids, discussed in Chapter 11. The latter category includes a variety of agents that are collectively referred to as disease-modifying antirheumatic drugs (DMARDs).

Disease-Modifying Antirheumatic Drugs (DMARDs)

The latest evidence shows that early, mild RA should be treated with more than NSAIDs, because joint damage occurs earlier than previously thought. The newer therapeutic approaches to the treatment of RA focus on the use of new **biologic response modifiers** that target the part of the immune system responsible for inflammation and joint damage. These drugs are collectively referred to as DMARDs. **Disease-modifying antirheumatic drugs (DMARDs)** are defined as agents that can potentially modify the disease progression of rheumatoid arthritis. Table 6.2 gives an overview of the most commonly used DMARDs.

FIELD NOTES

Never assume a patient has a specific disease state just because they are using a particular drug. Some drugs may be used for multiple indications. For example, methotrexate can be used as a DMARD for rheumatoid arthritis. The medication is also indicated to treat leukemia, breast cancer, head and neck cancer, lung cancer, lymphoma, psoriasis, and juvenile idiopathic arthritis. Furthermore, methotrexate may have more FDA-approved indications in the future. A research article published in 2019 suggested methotrexate may be an effective treatment for cancers that cause overproduction of red blood cells. Technicians should always ask patients what they are using medications for instead of assuming.

TABLE 6.2 Commonly Used DMARDs

Generic (Brand)	Pronunciation	Dosage Form	Common Dosage	Dispensing Status
auranofin (Ridaura)	aw-RAN-noh-fin	capsule	6–9 mg/kg/day, divided 2–3 times a day	Rx
azathioprine (Azasan, Imuran)	az-a-THYE-oh-preen	tablet	3–5 mg/kg/day initially, then 1–3 mg/kg/day	Rx
hydroxychloroquine (Plaquenil)	hye-drox-ee-KLOR-oh-kwin	tablet	200–300 mg a day	Rx
leflunomide (Arava)	le-FLOO-noe-mide	tablet	100 mg a day for 3 days, then 10–20 mg once a week	Rx
methotrexate (Rheumatrex, Xatmep)	meth-oh-TREX-ate	injection, oral solution, tablet	7.5–15 mg a week	Rx
sulfasalazine (Azulfidine, Azulfidine EN-tabs)	sul-fa-SAL-a-zeen	tablet	500 mg twice a day, then increase to 1 g twice a day	Rx
Biologic Response Modifiers				
adalimumab (Humira)	a-da-LIM-yoo-mab	injection	40 mg every 2 weeks	Rx
anakinra (Kineret)	an-a-KIN-ra	injection	100 mg a day	Rx
etanercept (Enbrel)	ee-TAN-er-sept	injection	25 mg twice a week or 50 mg once a week	Rx
golimumab (Simponi, Simponi Aria)	goe-LIM-ue-mab	injection	50 mg once a month	Rx
infliximab (Remicade)	in-FLIX-i-mab	injection	3 mg/kg at 0, 2, and 6 weeks, then every 8 weeks	Rx
upadacitinib (Rinvoq)	ue-PAD-a-SYE-ti-nib	tablet	15 mg a day	Rx

℞ Put Down Roots

It may be helpful to remember that some of the generic names of the biologic DMARDs end with *-mab*. This ending is an abbreviation for *monoclonal antibody,* a laboratory-produced molecule designed to mimic the antibodies in humans.

Pharm Fact

Methotrexate is often prescribed as an off-label treatment for ectopic pregnancies.

DMARDs are taken regularly to slow the progression of disease—they maintain disease control and symptom control. If one agent does not generate a response or causes intolerable adverse effects, others are tried, or combinations of multiple DMARDs are prescribed. DMARDs work best when started within the first three months after RA diagnosis. Disease remission can sometimes be achieved. At a minimum, early therapy slows the joint destruction that creates disability.

Auranofin (Ridaura) is a DMARD that is indicated for the treatment of RA. Auranofin is unique in that it is formulated with gold.

When used for RA, **azathioprine (Azasan, Imuran)** may not show therapeutic response for up to three months. Azathioprine depresses bone marrow function, thereby increasing the potential for infection.

Hydroxychloroquine (Plaquenil) is an antimalarial drug also used to treat RA and lupus.

Methotrexate (Rheumatrex, Xatmep) is an antineoplastic (chemotherapeutic) agent used to treat cancers, arthritic conditions, and psoriasis.

Sulfasalazine (Azulfidine, Azulfidine EN-Tabs) is used to treat ulcerative colitis and rheumatoid arthritis. Sulfasalazine helps to reduce joint pain, swelling, and stiffness.

The injectable biologic response modifiers, including **adalimumab (Humira), anakinra (Kineret), etanercept (Enbrel), golimumbab (Simponi Simponi Aria), and infliximab (Remicade)**, are made through recombinant DNA technology and work by inhibiting tumor necrosis factors (TNFs) or interleukin-1 (IL-1), two substances that cause inflammation and joint damage.

Adalimumab is approved for RA but also for ankylosing spondylitis, Crohn's disease, juvenile idiopathic arthritis, plaque psoriasis, psoriatic arthritis, rheumatoid arthritis, and ulcerative colitis.

Etanercept is a biologically engineered protein that inhibits the action of tumor necrosis factor (TNF), a protein that induces the destruction of some tumor cells and the activation of white blood cells. Growing evidence suggests that TNF plays a key role in the pathogenesis (origination and development of a disease) of RA. Etanercept was the first biologically engineered product approved for the treatment of RA. This drug is indicated in the treatment of moderate to severe RA in patients who have experienced an inadequate response to one or more of the other arthritis drugs.

Golimumab is a TNF inhibitor used to treat RA, psoriatic arthritis, and ankylosing spondylitis.

Infliximab was initially approved for Crohn's disease, but it is now approved for RA, ankylosing spondylitis, plaque psoriasis, psoriatic arthritis, and ulcerative colitis.

Leflunomide (Arava) is a pyrimidine synthesis inhibitor that interferes with the proliferation of lymphocytes. Leflunomide slows the progression of rheumatoid arthritis, reduces pain and joint swelling, and improves functional ability. Evidence suggests that this drug exhibits an additive effect when combined with methotrexate.

Upadacitinib (Rinvoq) is a newer drug indicated for moderately to severely active rheumatoid arthritis. The mechanism of action is unique from other DMARDs. Upadacitinib is a janus kinase (JAK) inhibitor. Upadacitinib is indicated for the treatment of adults with moderately to severely active rheumatoid arthritis who have had an inadequate response or intolerance to methotrexate.

Dosage Forms and Administration DMARDs are available in oral and injectable dosage forms. The various dosage forms of DMARDs are presented in Table 6.2.

Adalimumab is available as a prefilled syringe or a pen injector. It is administered every other week as a subcutaneous injection. Adalimumab is stored in the refrigerator.

Anakinra is available as an injection.

Auranofin comes as a capsule and is taken once or twice a day initially. After six months of therapy, it may be taken three times daily.

Etanercept is available as an injection and must be stored in the refrigerator.

Golimumab is injected subcutaneously once a month. Golimumab should be used with methotrexate for RA, with or without methotrexate for psoriatic arthritis, and alone for ankylosing spondylitis.

Infliximab is given intravenously with an induction regimen of 3 mg/kg at weeks 0, 2, and 6, followed by a maintenance regimen every 8 weeks.

In the event of leflunomide overdose or toxicity, cholestyramine should be administered. Leflunomide tablets should be protected from light.

Methotrexate is available in oral and injectable dosage forms. The oral form should be taken on an empty stomach. Exposure to sunlight should be avoided.

Sulfasalazine tablets should be administered in evenly divided doses, preferably after meals. Enteric-coated tablets should be swallowed whole.

Side Effects Side effects of individual DMARDs are presented in Table 6.3.

Contraindications Contraindications to DMARD use are presented in Table 6.3.

Cautions and Considerations DMARDs are unique in that most of them have special cautions and considerations. Please see Table 6.4 for a review of cautions, considerations, and drug interactions of DMARDs.

Drug Interactions Drug interactions associated with DMARDs are listed in Table 6.4.

Pharm Fact

One way to remember the boxed warnings for the DMARD auranofin is to dissect the generic name. The drug name starts with "au," which is the elemental abbreviation for gold. The boxed warnings for auranofin all relate to gold toxicity.

TABLE 6.3 Side Effects and Contraindications of DMARDs

Generic (Brand)	Side Effects	Contraindications
auranofin (Ridaura)	diarrhea, nausea, vomiting, abdominal pain, anorexia, indigestion, gas, constipation, itching, rash, hair loss, photosensitivity, blood disorders, kidney and liver damage, lung problems (serious but rare)	severe toxicity to gold
azathioprine (Azasan, muran)	malaise, nausea, vomiting, leukopenia, neoplasia, thrombocytopenia, liver toxicity, myalgia, fever	in patients with RA: pregnancy and history of use of alkylating agents
hydroxychloroquine (Plaquenil)	corneal deposits, retinal changes, GI upset, skin rash	hypersensitivity to 4-aminoquinoline derivatives or retinal or visual changes attributable to 4-aminoquinoline derivatives long-term use in children
leflunomide (Arava)	headache, dizziness, diarrhea, abdominal pain, indigestion, weight loss, liver problems, peripheral neuropathy (nerve pain), hair loss, high blood pressure, anemia, blood disorders, lung disease	pregnancy
methotrexate (Rheumatrex)	mouth sores, nausea, vomiting, abdominal distress, anemia and blood disorders, liver and kidney damage, Stevens-Johnson syndrome, eye irritation, heart problems	breast-feeding, pregnancy, alcoholism, alcoholic liver disease or other chronic liver disease, immunosuppressed states, and preexisting blood diseases
sulfasalazine (Azulfidine, Azulfidine EN-tabs)	anorexia, diarrhea, abdominal pain, indigestion, headache, nausea, vomiting, colitis, blood disorders, rash, Stevens-Johnson syndrome, liver and kidney problems, hair loss, male infertility	hypersensitivity to sulfa drugs or salicylates intestinal or urinary obstruction porphyria
Biologic Response Modifiers		
adalimumab (Humira)	headache, nausea, vomiting, flu-like symptoms, rash, itching, heart problems, anemia and blood disorders, secondary malignancy, nephrotic syndrome, confusion, tremor, reactivation of hepatitis B	no known contraindications
anakinra (Kineret)	headache, nausea, vomiting, diarrhea, redness and pain at injection site, flu-like symptoms, blood disorders	hypersensitivity to proteins derived from Escherichia coli
etanercept (Enbrel)	injection site reactions, headache, nausea, vomiting, hair loss, cough, dizziness, abdominal pain, rash, indigestion, swelling, mouth sores, blood disorders, secondary lymphoma, Stevens-Johnson syndrome, seizures, heart problems, pancreatitis, difficulty breathing	sepsis
golimumab (Simponi, Simponi Aria)	upper respiratory tract infections, runny nose, fever/chills, dizziness, redness at injection site	no known contraindications
infliximab (Remicade)	nausea, vomiting, headache, diarrhea, abdominal pain, cough, indigestion, fatigue, back pain, fever, chills, chest pain, flushing, dizziness, heart failure, nerve problems, seizures, Stevens-Johnson syndrome	hypersensitivity to murine (mouse) proteins
upadacitinib (Rinvoq)	upper respiratory infections, nausea, cough, and fever	no known contraindications

TABLE 6.4 Cautions, Considerations, and Drug Interactions of Commonly Used DMARDs

Generic (Brand)	Cautions and Considerations	Drug Interactions
auranofin (Ridaura)	Contains gold. Auranofin's boxed warnings include: warnings related to gold toxicity (rash, stomatitis, pruritis); gastrointestinal effects such as persistent diarrhea, nausea, vomiting, or ulcerative colitis; hematologic effects such as decreased hemoglobin, white blood cells, and platelets; proteinuria and hematuria.	Auranofin has no known drug interactions.
azathioprine (Azasan, Imuran)	Boxed warning includes: increased risk of development of malignancy (such as lymphoma); only experienced prescribers should prescribe azathioprine; severe gastrointestinal toxicity may occur with use (nausea, vomiting, diarrhea, myalgia, hypotension, and liver enzyme abnormalities).	Adverse effects of other immuno-suppressants may be enhanced. Febuxostat may increase serum concentrations of azathioprine. Azathioprine may increase the risk of infection with live vaccines. Concurrent use should be avoided.
hydroxychloroquine (Plaquenil)	Hydroxychloroquine's boxed warning advises that only an experienced prescriber should be prescribing.	Artemether may enhance the adverse effects of hydroxychloroquine. Hydroxychloroquine may enhance the toxicities of lumefantrine and mefloquine.
leflunomide (Arava)	Boxed warnings include: patients' liver function should be monitored, and they should be monitored for hepatotoxicity; patients who are or plan to become pregnant should not take leflunomide. May increase risk of serious infection; considered a hazardous agent (special handling precautions should be taken).	Bile acid sequestrants may decrease serum concentrations of the active metabolite. Cholestyramine (a bile acid sequestrant) can be used for an overdose. Activated charcoal may also decrease serum concentrations. Adverse effects of natalizumab, teriflunomide, and tofacitinib may be enhanced by leflunomide. Pimecrolimus and tacrolimus may enhance the adverse effects of leflunomide. Live vaccines may cause infection; avoid concurrent use.
methotrexate (Rheumatrex)	Boxed warnings include: may cause kidney damage; bone marrow suppression (that may be fatal); severe and potentially fatal dermatologic reactions; gastrointestinal toxicity; liver damage (acute and fatal); immune suppression (leading to potentially fatal infections); pneumonitis; malignant lymphomas; tumor lysis syndrome; decreased elimination in patients with ascites or kidney impairment; or severe bone marrow suppression with concurrent NSAID use. May cause fetal death or congenital abnormalities in pregnant patients. Concurrent use with radiotherapy may increase the risk of soft tissue necrosis and osteonecrosis. Products that contain preservatives should not be used for intrathecal administration.	Acitretin, foscarnet, pimecrolimus, and tacrolimus may enhance the toxic effects of methotrexate. May increase the toxic effects of clozapine, dipyrone, and natalizumab. Live vaccines may cause infection; avoid concurrent use.

continues

TABLE 6.4 Cautions, Considerations, and Drug Interactions of Commonly Used DMARDs—*Continued*

Generic (Brand)	Cautions and Considerations	Drug Interactions
sulfasalazine (Azulfidine, Azulfidine EN-tabs)	May have cross-reactivity in patients with sulfa allergy. Blood diseases have occurred with use. Severe skin reactions, including fatal ones, have occurred. Enteric-coated tablets may not be fully absorbed in some patients. If tablets pass in stool, discontinue this formulation.	Sulfasalazine interacts with ketorolac and methotrexate. Live vaccines may cause infection; avoid concurrent use.
Biologic Response Modifiers		
adalimumab (Humira)	Boxed warnings include: increased risk of serious infection that may result in hospitalization and death; lymphoma risk and other malignancies in children; risk of hepatosplenic T-cell lymphoma (a rare disease reported primarily in patients using adalimumab for Crohn's disease or ulcerative colitis); risk of tuberculosis (TB) reactivation with use (patients should be evaluated for latent TB prior to therapy initiation).	Adalimumab may increase the adverse effects of abatacept, anakinra, belimumab, canakinumab, certolizumab, infliximab, natalizumab, pimecrolimus, rilonacept, tacrolimus, tocilizumab, tofacitinib, and vedolizumab. Adalimumab may decrease serum concentration of warfarin. Live vaccines may cause infection; avoid concurrent use.
anakinra (Kineret)	Hypersensitivity reactions may occur (including anaphylaxis). Use with caution in asthma because of an increased risk of infection. Needle cover of anakinra contains latex (avoid in latex sensitivity). Contains polysorbate 80.	Live vaccines may cause infection; avoid concurrent use.
etanercept (Enbrel)	Boxed warnings include: increased risk of serious infection that may lead to hospitalization or even death; lymphoma and other malignancies in children; risk of tuberculosis (TB) reactivation with use (patients should be evaluated for latent TB prior to therapy initiation).	Etanercept may increase the adverse effects of abatacept, anakinra, belimumab, canakinumab, certolizumab, cyclophosphamide, infliximab, natalizumab, rilonacept, tacrolimus, tofacitinib, and vedolizumab. Pimecrolimus and tocilizumab may enhance the adverse effects of etanercept. Live vaccines may cause infection; avoid concurrent use.
golimumab (Simponi, Simponi Aria)	Boxed warnings include: increased risk of serious infection that may lead to hospitalization or even death; lymphoma and other malignancies in children; risk of tuberculosis (TB) reactivation with use (patients should be evaluated for latent TB prior to therapy initiation).	Golimumab may increase the adverse effects of abatacept, anakinra, belimumab, canakinumab, certolizumab, cyclophosphamide, infliximab, natalizumab, rilonacept, tacrolimus, tofacitinib, and vedolizumab. Pimecrolimus and tocilizumab may enhance the adverse effects of golimumab. Live vaccines may cause infection; avoid concurrent use.

continues

TABLE 6.4 Cautions, Considerations, and Drug Interactions of Commonly Used DMARDs—*Continued*

Generic (Brand)	Cautions and Considerations	Drug Interactions
infliximab (Remicade)	Boxed warnings include: increased risk of serious infection that may lead to hospitalization or even death; lymphoma and other malignancies in children; risk of tuberculosis (TB) reactivation with use (patients should be evaluated for latent TB prior to therapy initiation).	Infliximab may increase the adverse effects of abatacept, anakinra, belimumab, canakinumab, certolizumab, natalizumab, pimecrolimus, rilonacept, tacrolimus, tofacitinib, and vedolizumab. Adalimumab, etanercept, golimumab, tocilizumab, and ustekinumab may enhance infliximab's toxicities. Live vaccines may cause infection; avoid concurrent use.
upadacitinib (Rinvoq)	Boxed warnings include: increased risk of serious infection that may result in hospitalization or death; lymphoma and other malignancy risk; risk of blood clots.	Drugs that inhibit CYP3A4 may increase levels (such as ketoconazole). Drugs that induce CYP3A4 (such as rifampin) more decrease levels. Upadacitinib should be used with caution in patients using drugs that strongly inhibit (such as ketoconazole) or induce (such as rifampin) CYP3A4. Avoid concurrent use. Live vaccines may cause infection; avoid concurrent use.

6.5 Gouty Arthritis and Drug Treatments

Pharm Fact

Gout was once known as the "disease of kings." This moniker came from the disease's association with rich food and alcohol consumption—goods accessible only to the wealthy.

Gouty arthritis is a form of arthritis resulting from the body's improper excretion of uric acid. Often referred to merely as *gout*, the disease usually affects single joints, causing a **tophus** (a deposit of sodium urate) to form around the joint. Tophi may form in tissues, joint cartilage, earlobes, and metatarsals. Typically, the first joint affected is the joint in the big toe, which becomes painful, swollen, and red.

The disease is related to the patient's metabolism of uric acid, which is normally excreted by the kidneys. The affected patient overproduces or has improper excretion of uric acid, so aspirin is contraindicated because it competes with uric acid for kidney excretion. The condition is usually inherited. Persons prone to gout should avoid the following drugs, which could cause an attack:

- cytotoxic agents
- diuretics
- ethanol
- nicotinic acid
- salicylates

Uricosuric Agents, Xanthine Oxidase Inhibitors, and Antigout Agents

Treatment for gout can be used for an acute attack or for prevention purposes. A gout attack is a severe and debilitating pain episode, with the worst pain occurring in the first 24 hours. Most attacks usually resolve in 3 to 10 days with proper medication. Potent and fast-acting NSAIDs (such as indomethacin and naproxen) are often used. NSAIDs may help with pain and swelling. Colchicine may also be used. Cortico–steroids such as triamcinolone and prednisone (discussed in Chapter 11) are also used for acute gout attacks.

Preventive therapy for chronic gout is indicated in certain patients. Allopurinol, colchicine (also used for acute gout attacks), febuxostat, and probenecid are all common preventive gout options.

An overview of the medicines used to treat both acute gout attacks and preventive gout therapy is presented in Table 6.5.

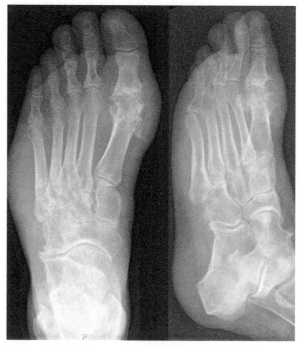

X-rays of the left foot of a person with gout show the characteristic swelling of the joint of the big toe.

TABLE 6.5 Common Drugs Used to Treat Gout

Generic (Brand)	Pronunciation	Dosage Form	Common Dosage	Dispensing Status
Acute Gout Attack Therapy				
colchicine (Colcrys, Gloperba, Mitigare)	KOL-chi-seen	oral solution, injection, tablet	1.2 mg initially, followed in 1 hr with 0.6 mg; maximum dose of 1.8 mg within 1 hr	Rx
Preventive Gout Therapy				
allopurinol (Aloprim, Zyloprim)	al-oh-PURE-i-nawl	IV solution, tablet	200–600 mg a day	Rx
colchicine (Colcrys, Gloperba, Mitigare)	KOL-chi-seen	oral solution, tablet	0.6 mg 1 or 2 times a day	Rx
febuxostat (Uloric)	feb-UX-oh-stat	tablet	80–120 mg a day	Rx
probenecid	proe-BEN-e-sid	tablet	250 mg twice a day for 1 week, then 500 mg twice a day for 2 weeks; may increase up to 2,000 mg a day if needed	Rx

Colchicine

Colchicine (Colcrys, Gloperba, Mitigare) can be used to treat an acute gout attack and to reduce the frequency of recurrent episodes of gouty arthritis. When used for preventive gout treatment, therapy is often short-term because of its potentially toxic side effects. Colchicine's exact mechanism of action is not completely known, but the drug is thought to work as an anti-inflammatory and may decrease uric acid accumulation.

Dosage Forms and Administration Colchicine is available in an oral tablet and an injectable form. Therapy may be short-term when used for an acute gout attack. Long-term therapy is used to prevent gout attacks.

Side Effects Side effects of colchicine include diarrhea, nausea, and vomiting. Neutropenia (abnormally low neutrophils, a type of white blood cell, in the blood) may also occur with colchicine use and may be worsened by other drugs (such as HMG-CoA reductase inhibitors [statins]).

Contraindications Colchicine use is contraindicated in patients with kidney or liver impairment. Colchicine should not be used in combination with drugs that may slow the drug's clearance from the body.

Cautions and Considerations Colchicine should be used with caution in older adults, and dosage adjustments should be considered. Clearance of colchicine is decreased in patients with liver or kidney impairment.

Grapefruit juice may increase serum concentrations of colchicine. The effect may be heightened with associated hepatic or renal impairment.

Drug Interactions Colchicine-associated neutropenia may be worsened when taken with statin drugs. Increased colchicine concentrations may occur when used with clarithromycin, cyclosporine, or erythromycin.

Allopurinol

Allopurinol (Aloprim, Zyloprim) is often used for preventive gout treatment and is usually one of the top 200 drugs dispensed in pharmacies. Allopurinol works by inhibiting the production of uric acid. It is classified as a xanthine oxidase inhibitor.

Safety Alert

Allopurinol can be mistaken for Apresoline (hydralazine, a vasodilator), especially if an error is made in dosing. Allopurinol comes in 100 mg, 300 mg, and 500 mg forms. Hydralazine comes in 10 mg, 25 mg, 50 mg, and 100 mg forms.

Dosage Forms and Administration Allopurinol is available as a tablet and a reconstituted solution for injection.

Allopurinol should be taken after meals. Patients using allopurinol should be instructed to drink plenty of fluid.

Side Effects Side effects include skin rash, nausea, and diarrhea.

Contraindications Allopurinol does not have any reported contraindications.

Cautions and Considerations Allopurinol use has been associated with severe hypersensitivity reactions and should be discontinued if signs of allergic reaction are present. Allopurinol should be used with caution in patients with kidney impairment because of the increased risk of hypersensitivity reactions.

Drug Interactions Diuretics may increase the toxic effects of allopurinol. ACE inhibitors may increase the risk of allergic reactions to allopurinol. Allopurinol may increase the risk of hypersensitivity to certain antibiotics. The anticoagulant effects of warfarin may be enhanced by allopurinol use.

Febuxostat

Febuxostat (Uloric) works by inhibiting uric acid production. Like allopurinol, it is classified as a xanthine oxidase inhibitor. Febuxostat is used for chronic management of high uric acid levels in patients with gout.

Dosage Forms and Administration Febuxostat is available as a tablet for oral ingestion.

Side Effects Side effects include diarrhea, headache, and angioedema (swelling that resembles hives but is under the skin instead of on the surface). Liver dysfunction may also occur.

Contraindications Febuxostat should not be used concurrently with azathioprine or mercaptopurine.

Cautions and Considerations Technicians should be aware that febuxostat carries a boxed warning for increased risk of cardiovascular disease. Febuxostat should be dispensed with an FDA Medication Guide.

Febuxostat use has been associated with severe hypersensitivity reactions and should be discontinued if signs of allergic reaction are present. Liver failure has been reported with febuxostat use. Febuxostat should also be used with caution in patients with severe hypersensitivity reactions to allopurinol.

Drug Interactions Febuxostat may increase the serum concentrations of azathioprine, didanosine, mercaptopurine, pegloticase, and active metabolites of theophylline derivatives.

Probenecid

Probenecid is used for preventive gout treatment in patients with relatively low kidney uric acid excretion. This treatment works by inhibiting the renal reabsorption of uric acid and therefore promotes uric acid excretion.

Dosage Forms and Administration Probenecid is used orally only in tablet form. The dose is typically increased over several weeks.

Probenecid may be taken with food or antacids if GI upset occurs. Patients using probenecid should drink 6 to 8 glasses of water each day to prevent the development of kidney stones.

Side Effects Side effects include nausea, vomiting, and anorexia.

Contraindications Probenecid should not be used in children less than two years of age, and therapy should not be initiated during an acute gout attack.

Cautions and Considerations Probenecid use has been associated with severe hypersensitivity reactions and should be discontinued if signs of allergic reaction are present.

Drug Interactions Probenecid may increase the concentrations of doripenem, ketorolac, meropenem, methotrexate, and penicillins. Salicylates (such as aspirin) may also interact with probenecid.

6.6 Osteoporosis and Drug Treatments

Bone is a living tissue that is continuously being replaced as a result of the balance between osteoclast (a cell that resorbs—breaks down and assimilates the components of—bone) and osteoblast (a cell that forms bone) activity. In normal, healthy bone, the opposing activities of osteoclasts and osteoblasts are balanced. As adults age, however, resorption of bone tissue exceeds the deposit of new bone. Furthermore, newly formed bone is less dense and more fragile than original bone. Reduction or weakening of bone mass increases the risk of bone fracture. For adults over 50 years old, these processes usually occur at a faster rate for women (cis- and transgender) compared to men (cis- and transgender). The condition of reduced bone mineral density, disrupted microarchitecture of bone structure, and increased likelihood of fracture is known as **osteoporosis**. Osteoporosis occurs as a result of deficiency in estrogen, calcium, and vitamin D. The reduction in bone mass is accelerated and more severe in patients who have had an early hysterectomy, because the body of a person who has had their uterus removed produces less estrogen. With less estrogen, lower amounts of calcium are used by bony tissue. Daily calcium intake with vitamin D is essential to the prevention of bone loss.

Osteoporosis can cause fractures in the hips, spine, and wrists that are painful and debilitating. A **hip fracture** can be life-threatening because the subsequent hip replacement surgery, recovery, and potential complications are often stressful. Older patients may never return to normal function after a hip fracture.

Individuals at risk for developing osteoporosis typically have one or more of these characteristics:

- cis- or transgender woman
- Caucasian or Asian descent
- family history of osteoporosis
- small body frame
- history of smoking
- heavy caffeine intake
- suboptimal nutrition (e.g., low calcium intake)

The risk for osteoporosis can be assessed using a **bone mineral density (BMD)** machine. This machine uses x-ray and ultrasound technology to determine bone density measurements. Typically, the heel bone is measured because it is a good estimate of hip and spine bone density. The result of a BMD screening yields a **T-score**, which compares a measured BMD with that of a healthy young adult. BMD screening may occur at a provider office, hospital, or even community pharmacy. Armed with BMD information, patients can make changes in their lives, such as performing weight-bearing exercises, eating foods high in calcium, quitting smoking, and decreasing caffeine intake, which are all ways to increase bone density. If a diagnosis of osteoporosis is made by a healthcare practitioner, drug therapy may be prescribed.

It makes sense that supplementing estrogen in women whose estrogen levels are declining would stave off drastic drops in bone mineral density. However, the increased risk of heart disease, cancer, and stroke associated with estrogen replacement products has been found to outweigh this benefit. Consequently, hormone replacement therapy (HRT) with estrogen has fallen out of favor as a treatment for osteoporosis. When taken, it is at the lowest dose for the shortest time possible with the sole goal of alleviating menopausal symptoms. The most common drugs to treat osteoporosis include the bisphosphonates. These drugs work by inhibiting bone resorption (breakdown and assimilation of bone). Other treatments aim to mimic the beneficial effects of estrogen without the deleterious effects. Some osteoporosis therapies suppress osteoclasts or regulate calcium and phosphate metabolism. Table 6.6 lists the most commonly used agents for the prevention and treatment of osteoporosis.

TABLE 6.6 Common Drugs Used to Treat Osteoporosis

Generic (Brand)	Pronunciation	Dosage Form	Common Dosage	Dispensing Status
Bisphosphonates				
alendronate (Binostro, Fosamax)	a-LEN-droe-nate	effervescent tablet, oral solution, tablet	5–10 mg a day; 35–70 mg 1 time a week	Rx
ibandronate (Boniva)	eye-BAN-droh-nate	tablet, injection	PO: 150 mg 1 time a month IV: 3 mg every 3 months	Rx
risedronate (Actonel, Atelvia)	ris-ED-roe-nate	tablet	Delayed release: 35 mg 1 time a week Immediate release: 5 mg a day, 35 mg a week, or 150 mg a month	Rx
zoledronic acid (Reclast)	zo-le-DROE-nik AS-id	injection	5 mg 1 time a year	Rx
Selective Estrogen Receptor Modulator (SERM)				
raloxifene (Evista)	ra-LOX-i-feen	tablet	60 mg a day	Rx
Other Drugs for Osteoporosis				
denosumab (Prolia, Xgeva)	den-OH-sue-mab	injection	60 mg every 6 months	Rx
romosozumab (Evenity)	ROE-moe-SOZ-ue-mab	injection	210 mg 1 time a month	Rx
teriparatide (Forteo)	ter-i-PAR-a-tide	injection	20 mcg a day	Rx

Pharm Fact

Pamidronate (Aredia) is a bisphosphonate that is not FDA approved for osteoporosis. It is approved for hypercalcemia of malignancy, osteolytic bone metastases and lesions, and Paget's disease. It is available only as an injection and is administered at varying intervals based on use.

Bisphosphonates

Bisphosphonates inhibit osteoclasts from removing calcium from bone tissue. These medications prevent bone breakdown so that stronger bones are maintained. Over time, bone density can be maintained, and hopefully, fractures can be prevented. Bisphosphonates are used primarily for osteoporosis but can be used to treat Paget's disease (a chronic disorder that results in weakened bones, fractures, and arthritis). Sometimes, bisphosphonates are used in bone and spinal injury cases to promote bone regrowth and strengthening.

Dosage Forms and Administration Depending on the product chosen, bisphosphonates can be taken orally on a daily, weekly, or monthly basis. They can even be administered intravenously (IV) every month, every three months, or annually. The variety of dosage regimens allows prescribers to individualize drug therapy.

Alendronate (Binostro, Fosamax) is dosed once daily or once weekly, depending on the dosage. **Ibandronate (Boniva)** is manufactured in a once-a-month tablet or an IV formulation that is administered every three months.

Risedronate (Actonel, Atelvia) is an oral bisphosphonate that is taken daily, weekly, or monthly. **Zoledronic acid (Reclast)** is a bisphosphonate for IV infusion.

Oral bisphosphonates are poorly absorbed from the GI tract and are adversely affected by food. Therefore, they must be taken on an empty stomach (preferably first thing in the morning) with water. After taking a bisphosphonate, patients should wait at least 30 minutes before eating. Bisphosphonates are also highly irritating to the GI tract, so they must be taken with a full glass of water to ensure that they do not become lodged in the esophagus. Patients must remain upright for at least 30 minutes after medication administration to prevent reflux. In most cases, bisphosphonate infusions are administered in a physician's office or clinic.

Side Effects Side effects of bisphosphonates can include headache, nausea, vomiting, diarrhea, constipation, abdominal pain, indigestion, and esophagitis (inflammation of the esophagus). Taking oral dosage forms with a full glass of water and remaining upright afterward can reduce side effects such as reflux and esophageal issues. Other side effects include insomnia and anemia, for which patients must seek medical advice to manage. A less common yet severe side effect is osteonecrosis (bone tissue death) of the jaw. The IV dosage forms can cause fever, so acetaminophen is given simultaneously.

Contraindications Bisphosphonates are contraindicated in the case of hypersensitivity to other bisphosphonates. For example, if a patient has a hypersensitivity to alendronate, the use of all other bisphosphonates is contraindicated.

Specific bisphosphonates have unique contraindications. Alendronate, ibandronate, and risedronate are contraindicated in patients with hypocalcemia (deficiency of calcium in the blood), abnormalities of the esophagus, or an inability to stand or sit upright for at least 30 minutes. The effervescent tablets and oral solution of alendronate are contraindicated in patients at increased risk for aspiration (breathing foreign matter into the lungs). Zoledronic acid should not be used in patients with hypocalcemia and kidney dysfunction.

Put Down Roots

The generic names of the drugs in the bisphosphonate class have a common stem. They all end in *-dronate*.

Cautions and Considerations Oral bisphosphonates can cause irritation to the upper GI system. Serious damage to the esophagus (such as erosion or strictures) can occur. For these reasons, oral bisphosphonates should always be taken as instructed (first thing in the morning, on an empty stomach, without food, and with water). Food should be avoided for at least 30 minutes after bisphosphonate ingestion. Bisphosphonates should be used with caution in patients with GI issues (such as ulcers or gastritis) or difficulty swallowing.

Severe bone, joint, and muscle pain are associated with bisphosphonate use. Specifically, osteonecrosis of the jaw has been reported. It appears that risk increases with bisphosphonate use extending longer than four years. Bone fractures have also been reported in bisphosphonate users.

Oral bisphosphonates should be avoided after certain types of bariatric surgery.

Drug Interactions Antacids, calcium, iron, magnesium, and multivitamins may decrease the concentration of oral bisphosphonates. Antacids should be taken two hours before or one hour after bisphosphonates. Proton pump inhibitors may decrease the effectiveness of bisphosphonates.

Put Down Roots

Note that the drugs in the SERM class end in *-ifene*.

Selective Estrogen Receptor Modulators

Selective estrogen receptor modulators (SERMs) work as estrogen receptors by mimicking the beneficial effects of estrogen on bone mineral density. However, they do not increase the risk of breast or uterine cancer the way regular estrogen can. In fact, SERMs may even decrease the risk of breast cancer and improve cholesterol levels, although they are not used for hyperlipidemia (excess fat or lipids in the blood).

While multiple SERMs are on the market, **raloxifene (Evista)** is the one indicated to treat osteoporosis (see Table 6.6).

Dosage Forms and Administration Raloxifene is available exclusively as a tablet for oral ingestion.

Side Effects Common side effects of SERMs are hot flashes, headache, diarrhea, joint pain, leg cramps, and flu-like symptoms. The most serious side effects are deep vein thrombosis and other blood clots.

Contraindications Raloxifene is contraindicated in patients who have a history of or currently have venous thromboembolic disorders (including deep vein thrombosis and pulmonary embolism). This medication should not be taken by patients who are pregnant or could become pregnant or by patients who are breast-feeding.

Practice Tip

Raloxifene, a SERM indicated for the treatment of osteoporosis, must be dispensed with an FDA Medication Guide.

Cautions and Considerations Raloxifene carries a boxed warning for increased risk of blood clots and stroke. Patients with active blood clots or a past history of blood clots should not use raloxifene. Raloxifene should be dispensed with a Medication Guide outlining the increased risk of blood clots and stroke with raloxifene use.

Raloxifene should not be taken if prolonged immobility is anticipated due to the increased risk of blood clots or stroke. If patients using SERMs experience pain, swelling, or bruising in one leg or difficulty breathing, they should seek medical care immediately.

Drug Interactions Cholestyramine may decrease absorption of raloxifene, and concurrent use should be avoided. Raloxifene may decrease the effectiveness of warfarin.

Other Osteoporosis Medications

Several other medications are used for osteoporosis in addition to those previously mentioned. These medications include denosumab, teripartide, and romosozumab.

Denosumab (Prolia, Xgeva) inhibits osteoclast formation, which decreases bone resorption and increases bone mass strength. Denosumab is indicated for patients who have failed other osteoporosis therapy and are at high risk for fracture.

Teriparatide (Forteo) is a human parathyroid hormone used for treating osteoporosis. It stimulates bone formation and resorption by regulating calcium and phosphate metabolism with bony tissue. Whereas other drugs only slow osteoporosis, teriparatide actually stimulates new bone growth. Teriparatide is indicated to increase bone mass in patients with primary or hypogonadal osteoporosis at high risk for fracture, for the treatment of postmenopausal patients at high risk for fracture, and in those with osteoporosis associated with chronic glucocorticoid therapy at high risk for fracture.

Romosozumab (Evenity) works rapidly to increase bone mineral density. It builds more high-density, strong bone. It is indicated in postmenopausal patients at high risk for fracture and in patients who have failed or are intolerant to other available osteoporosis therapies.

Pharm Fact

Recall that a REMS program is a drug safety program required by the FDA.

Dosage Forms and Administration Denosumab comes as a prefilled syringe or solution for injection and is administered by a healthcare professional subcutaneously every six months. Patients should take calcium and vitamin D with this drug (typically 1,000 mg of calcium daily and at least 400 international units, or IUs, of vitamin D daily). The solution may appear clear and colorless, or it may look pale yellow. Denosumab must be stored in a refrigerator and should be removed 15 to 30 minutes before administration. No other method should be used to warm the drug.

The Prolia formulation of denosumab is part of a REMS program, and special prescribing, counseling, and dispensing precautions must be taken. See the Cautions and Considerations section for more information.

Teriparatide is administered via pen injection device (a device that appears similar to a writing pen). It is injected subcutaneously and must be stored in a refrigerator.

Romosozumab is available as an injection (subcutaneous) only. The drug comes in single-use prefilled syringes. The full dose requires two syringes and should be administered by a healthcare professional in the abdomen, thigh, or upper arm. Use should be limited to 12 monthly doses. Patients should supplement romosozumab with calcium and vitamin D.

Side Effects Side effects such as dermatitis, eczema, and skin rash are reported with denosumab use.

Teriparatide use is associated with hypercalcemia (an excess of calcium in the blood) and dizziness.

The most common side effects of romosozumab are arthralgia (joint pain) and headache.

Contraindications Denosumab is contraindicated in pregnancy and preexisting hypocalcemia.

Teriparatide use has no contraindications.

Hypocalcemia contraindicates use of romosozumab.

Practice Tip

The Prolia form of denosumab is used for individuals at high risk for fracture. Prolia is part of the FDA's REMS program and has special counseling requirements. In addition, Prolia must be dispensed with an FDA Medication Guide.

Cautions and Considerations Prolia, one of the brand names for denosumab, is part of the FDA's REMS program. The purpose of the REMS program is to inform healthcare providers and patients about Prolia's serious risks of hypocalcemia, osteonecrosis of the jaw, atypical femoral fractures, serious infections, and dermatologic reactions. A Medication Guide must also accompany any Prolia dispensed.

Use teriparatide with caution in patients who have an increased risk for dizziness or falling. Teriparatide has been associated with osteosarcoma, so patients with Paget's disease or with an increased risk for bone cancer should not use teriparatide. Teriparatide has a boxed warning for this.

Romosozumab has a boxed warning for the risk of heart attack, stroke, and cardiovascular disease. Therefore, the medication should not be initiated in patients who experienced a heart attack or stroke in the preceding year. If a patient experiences a heart attack or stroke while on therapy, romosozumab should be discontinued. Hypocalcemia may occur with romosozumab use. Hypocalcemia should be corrected prior to using romosozumab. Patients should supplement with calcium and vitamin D during therapy, and calcium levels should be monitored. Osteonecrosis of the jaw and bone fractures may occur with use. Hypersensitivity reactions have occurred with romosozumab use. Patients may experience angioedema, itching, and rash. Use should be discontinued in patients with serious reactions such as anaphylaxis.

Drug Interactions Denosumab may enhance the adverse effects of immunosuppressants. Teriparatide and romosozumab have no known drug interactions.

6.7 Muscle Spasms and Drug Treatments

A **muscle spasm**, also known as a cramp, is a sudden and involuntary contraction of one or more muscles. Muscle spasms are often the result of muscle overexertion, pain, or fatigue. Spasms may present the patient with a spectrum of discomfort ranging from annoyance to severe pain. Skeletal muscles of the limbs and spine (see Figure 6.4) and the smooth muscles lining the internal organs of the body are the muscles that are most often involved in muscle spasms.

Muscle spasms can be either acute or chronic. Acute muscle spasms are often the result of muscle injury or overuse. In fact, spasms from back injuries are one of the most common types of muscle spasms experienced in the United States. Another common cause of spasms is completing vigorous exercise without proper warm-up. Chronic muscle spasms may result from prolonged injury or underlying medical conditions. Hormonal, nutritional, and vascular conditions may all manifest in muscle cramps or spasms.

Drug therapy for muscle spasms includes a variety of options. NSAIDs and acetaminophen (discussed previously) are often used as first-line therapies. However, in many cases, additional medication is needed, and muscle relaxants are used. If pain from muscle spasms is severe, medication such as tramadol and opioids may be used (covered in Chapter 18).

Skeletal Muscle Relaxants

A **muscle relaxant** is a drug that reduces or prevents skeletal muscle contraction and spasms and provides pain relief. Muscle relaxants act on motor neurons (nerve cells that conduct nerve impulses that cause movement) or at the neuromuscular junction. These substances block normal muscle function through one of the following mechanisms:

- blocking release of acetylcholine (ACh)
- preventing destruction of ACh
- preventing ACh from reaching specific receptors

Agents that continuously bind to ACh nicotinic receptors can also block normal muscle function and may cause paralysis by fatigue, an unwanted outcome. Table 6.7 presents the most commonly used muscle relaxants.

Muscle relaxants are also used to reduce spasticity in multiple sclerosis, cerebral palsy, skeletal muscle injuries, orthopedic surgery, postoperative recovery, and spinal cord injury (see Figure 6.7).

FIGURE 6.7
Muscle Control and Relaxation

Muscle relaxants work by (1) slowing CNS signal conduction, (2) preventing intracellular calcium release, or (3) inhibiting ACh at the neuromuscular junction.

Three Potential Ways to Block Muscle Contraction

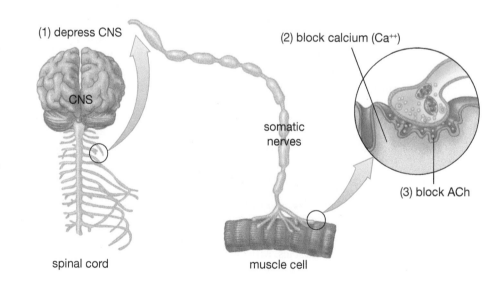

(1) depress CNS

CNS

spinal cord

somatic nerves

muscle cell

(2) block calcium (Ca^{++})

(3) block ACh

TABLE 6.7 Commonly Used Muscle Relaxants

Generic (Brand)	Pronunciation	Dosage Form	Common Dosage	Dispensing Status
baclofen (EnovaRX-Baclofen, First-Baclofen, Gablofen, Lioresal)	BAK-loe-fen	cream, intrathecal injection, oral solution, oral suspension, tablet	5–20 mg 3 times a day	Rx
carisoprodol (Soma)	kar-eye-soe-PROE-dawl	tablet	250–350 mg 4 times a day	Rx, C-IV in some states
chlorzoxazone (Lorzone)	klor-ZOX-a-zone	tablet	250–500 mg 3–4 times a day	Rx
cyclobenzaprine (Amrix, EnovaRx, Fexmid, Tobradol FusePaq, Tobradol RapidPaq)	sye-kloe-BEN-za-preen	cream, oral suspension, tablet	IR: 5 mg 3 times a day ER: 15 mg a day	Rx
dantrolene (Dantrium, Revonto, Ryanodex)	DAN-troe-leen	capsule, reconstituted solution for injection	varies	Rx
diazepam (Diastat, Valium)	dye-AZ-e-pam	auto-injector, injection, nasal liquid, oral concentrate, oral solution, rectal gel, tablet	varies	Rx, C-IV
metaxalone (Metaxall, Skelaxin)	me-TAX-a-lone	tablet	800 mg 3–4 times a day	Rx
methocarbamol (Robaxin)	meth-oh-KAR-ba-mawl	injection, tablet	1,000 mg 4 times a day or 750 mg every 4 hr, or 1,500 mg 3 times a day	Rx
orphenadrine	or-FEN-a-dreen	injection, tablet	100 mg 2 times a day	Rx
tizanidine (Zanaflex)	tye-ZAN-i-deen	capsule, tablet	varies	Rx

Pharm Fact

The term *intrathecal* means introduced into the space under the arachnoid membrane of the brain or spinal cord.

Safety Alert

The Institute for Safe Medication Practices (ISMP) includes baclofen on its list of drugs that have a heightened risk of causing significant patient harm when used in error.

Some dispensing issues are common among the muscle relaxants. To prevent possible drug interactions, a drug history should be completed for a patient before administering any of these drugs. The pharmacy technician often obtains this history from the healthcare practitioner and updates it as necessary. Once the patient takes the muscle relaxant, its sedative properties cause the patient to relax. Side effects of muscle relaxants include sedation, reduced mental alertness, reduced motor abilities, and gastrointestinal (GI) upset. Patients taking these drugs should avoid alcohol.

Dosage Forms and Administration Dosage considerations for individual muscle relaxants are presented in Table 6.8.

Side Effects Muscle relaxants cause drowsiness and dizziness. Side effects unique to specific muscle relaxants are listed in Table 6.8.

Contraindications Topical and oral baclofen do not have contraindications. The intrathecal formula should not be given intravenously, intramuscularly, subcutaneously, or via epidural.

Hypersensitivity to carbamates (such as meprobamate) or acute intermittent porphyria contraindicates carisoprodol use.

Chlorzoxazone has no contraindications.

TABLE 6.8 Dosage Considerations and Side Effects of Common Muscle Relaxants

Generic (Brand)	Dosage Considerations	Side Effects
baclofen (EnovaRX-Baclofen, First-Baclofen, Gablofen, Lioresal)	Take with food or milk. Avoid alcohol consumption while taking this medication.	Baclofen may cause drowsiness, and it may impair coordination and judgment. Concurrent alcohol use may enhance these effects.
carisoprodol (Soma)	Use only for short durations (two to three weeks). Avoid alcohol consumption. Do not operate heavy machinery or engage in tasks that require mental alertness.	Carisoprodol may cause drowsiness and dizziness.
chlorzoxazone (Lorzone)	Avoid alcohol consumption.	Chlorzoxazone may cause drowsiness and dizziness. Liver toxicity may occur.
cyclobenzaprine (Amrix, EnovaRx, Fexmid, Tobradol FusePaq, Tobradol RapidPaq)	Onset of action usually occurs within one hour. Do not use for more than three weeks. Administer at the same time each day. Swallow tablets or capsules whole, or sprinkle contents onto a tablespoon of applesauce and consume immediately without chewing; rinse mouth to ensure all contents have been swallowed.	Cyclobenzaprine may cause drowsiness, dizziness, dry mouth, and acne.
dantrolene (Dantrium, Revonto, Ryanodex)	Avoid sun exposure. Avoid alcohol consumption.	Dantrolene may cause malaise, weakness, fatigue, liver toxicity, and photosensitivity.
diazepam (Diastat, Valium)	Administer with food or water. Measure liquid dose only with calibrated dropper provided. Dilute or mix oral concentrate with water, juice, applesauce, or pudding before use. If used long-term, dose tapering may be required prior to discontinuation.	Diazepam may cause drowsiness, fatigue, and loss of body control.
metaxalone (Metaxall, Skelaxin)	Administer with or without food. Serum concentrations may be increased when administered with food (especially in older adults), heightening general CNS depression.	Metaxalone may cause dizziness, drowsiness, skin rash, or yellowish discoloration of the skin or eyes.
methocarbamol (Robaxin)	Protect from light and moisture.	Methocarbamol may cause drowsiness, vertigo, skin rash, jaundice, blurred vision, nasal congestion, and discoloration of urine (blue, black, or green).
orphenadrine	The tablet should be swallowed whole, not crushed or chewed. Avoid alcohol consumption. Do not operate heavy machinery or engage in tasks that require mental alertness.	Orphenadrine may cause lightheadedness, dizziness, syncope, and dryness of the mouth.
tizanidine (Zanaflex)	Capsules may be opened and contents sprinkled on food.	Tizanidine may cause hypotension, drowsiness, dizziness, dry mouth, and lack of energy.

Contraindications of cyclobenzaprine include use with or within 14 days of MAOI use, hyperthyroidism, heart failure, heart block, and use during the acute recovery phase of heart attacks.

Dantrolene use is contraindicated in patients with active hepatic disease, such as hepatitis and cirrhosis; where spasticity is used to sustain upright posture and balance in locomotion; and whenever spasticity is used to obtain or maintain increased function.

Children less than six months of age and patients with acute narrow-angle glaucoma should not use diazepam.

Metaxalone use is contraindicated in patients with significantly impaired hepatic or renal function or a history of drug-induced hemolytic anemias or other anemias.

The injectable form of methocarbamol is contraindicated in renal impairment.

Orphenadrine is contraindicated in patients with glaucoma, GI obstruction, peptic ulcers, prostatic hypertrophy, neck obstruction, cardiospasm, or myasthenia gravis.

Tizanidine use is contraindicated with concurrent use of ciprofloxacin or fluvoxamine.

Cautions and Considerations Cautions and considerations for muscle relaxants are covered in Table 6.9.

Drug Interactions Drug interactions for muscle relaxants are covered in Table 6.9.

Pharm Fact

Many drugs are prescribed for unlabeled uses. Baclofen, for example, is sometimes used to control hiccups.

TABLE 6.9 Cautions and Considerations and Drug Interactions for Common Muscle Relaxants

Generic (Brand)	Cautions and Considerations	Drug Interactions
baclofen (EnovaRX-Baclofen, First-Baclofen, Gablofen, Lioresal)	Abrupt withdrawal after prolonged use may cause hallucinations, tachycardia, or spasticity. Intrathecal baclofen carries a boxed warning against abrupt discontinuation. Abrupt withdrawal has resulted in severe reactions that led to organ failure and death in some cases. Use with caution in older adults, as they may be more sensitive to CNS side effects.	The use of CNS depressants may exacerbate the CNS side effects of baclofen.
carisoprodol (Soma)	Carisoprodol is converted to an active metabolite in the body called meprobamate (which is a Schedule IV controlled substance). Because of the abuse potential, carisoprodol is a scheduled substance in many states. Carisoprodol is on the AGS Beers Criteria as a drug that may be inappropriate for use in older adults. Use with alcohol and other CNS depressants increases the risk of toxicity.	Carisoprodol interacts with clindamycin, phenothiazines, and monoamine oxidase inhibitors (MAOIs). The use of CNS depressants may exacerbate the CNS side effects of carisoprodol.
chlorzoxazone (Lorzone)	Chlorzoxazone is on the AGS Beers Criteria as a drug that may be inappropriate for use in older adults. Liver toxicity has occurred with use. Liver enzymes should be monitored. Discontinue if elevated liver enzymes develop.	The use of CNS depressants may exacerbate the CNS side effects of chlorzoxazone.
cyclobenzaprine (Amrix, EnovaRx, Fexmid, Tobradol FusePaq, Tobradol RapidPaq)	Cyclobenzaprine is on the AGS Beers Criteria as a drug that may be inappropriate for use in older adults. Cyclobenzaprine may impair the ability to perform hazardous activities requiring physical coordination. Cyclobenzaprine may cause serotonin syndrome when used with other serotonergic drugs. Anticholinergic effects may present with use.	The use of CNS depressants may exacerbate the CNS side effects of cyclobenzaprine. Anticholinergic medications may decrease the therapeutic effects of cyclobenzaprine.

continues

TABLE 6.9 **Cautions and Considerations and Drug Interactions for Common Muscle Relaxants—***Continued*

Generic (Brand)	Cautions and Considerations	Drug Interactions
dantrolene (Dantrium, Revonto, Ryanodex)	Dantrolene has a boxed warning for hepatotoxicity. Patients using dantrolene should have their liver function monitored.	Estrogen may increase the risk of liver toxicity. The use of CNS depressants may exacerbate the CNS side effects of dantrolene.
diazepam (Diastat, Valium)	Diazepam carries a boxed warning for profound sedation, respiratory depression, coma, and death when used with opioids. Diazepam is a controlled substance. The potential for dependence and abuse exists. Patients with hypersensitivity to other benzodiazepines may also react to diazepam. Diazepam should be used with caution in these patients. Benzodiazepines are on the AGS Beers Criteria as being potentially inappropriate for use in older adults.	Cimetidine and protease inhibitors may decrease clearance of benzodiazepines. Coadministration with disulfiram may produce alcohol intolerance. The use of CNS depressants may exacerbate the CNS side effects of diazepam.
metaxalone (Metaxall, Skelaxin)	Metaxalone may cause CNS depression, and patients should be warned about decreased ability to perform tasks that require mental alertness. Metaxalone should be used with caution in patients with liver or kidney impairment. Caution must be exercised when used by older adults because of the increased risk of CNS and anticholinergic side effects. Metaxalone may cause serotonin syndrome when used with other serotonergic drugs. Anticholinergic effects may present with use.	Metaxalone may enhance the effects of alcohol, barbiturates, and other CNS depressants.
methocarbamol (Robaxin)	Methocarbamol may cause CNS depression, and patients should be warned about decreased ability to perform tasks that require mental alertness. Methocarbamol is on the AGS Beers Criteria as a drug that may be inappropriate for use in older adults.	Methocarbamol may enhance the effects of alcohol and other CNS depressants.
orphenadrine	Orphenadrine may cause CNS depression, and patients should be warned about decreased ability to perform tasks that require mental alertness. The injectable form of orphenadrine contains sulfites, which may cause allergic reaction in certain patients. Orphenadrine is on the AGS Beers Criteria as a drug that may be inappropriate for use in older adults.	Anticholinergic medications may enhance the anticholinergic side effects of orphenadrine. The use of CNS depressants may exacerbate the CNS side effects of orphenadrine.
tizanidine (Zanaflex)	Tizanidine may induce hypersensitivity reactions (such as anaphylaxis). Liver toxicity is a concern. Patients with liver impairment should avoid use of tizanidine. Use with caution in patients with kidney impairment. Low blood pressure may result from use. Visual hallucinations and delusions may occur. Abrupt withdrawal may result in rebound hypertension and tachycardia. Doses should be tapered prior to discontinuation.	The use of CNS depressants may exacerbate the CNS side effects of tizanidine. Ciprofloxacin may increase tizanidine levels.

6.8 Inflammation and Swelling and Drug Treatments

When the body experiences injury or infection, a cascade of events occurs, including the release of various chemical messengers. The chemical messengers arachidonic acid, cyclooxygenase (discussed previously), and PGs are released and ultimately lead to vasodilation (widening of blood vessels) and increased vascular permeability (permeability of blood vessels) near the site of injury or infection. Both vasodilation and increased vascular permeability allow more blood and fluid to flow to the area of injury or infection. This allows white blood cells to arrive and help the body heal. However, vasodilation and increased vascular permeability can lead to **inflammation**, the body's response to tissue injury or infection. Common characteristics of inflammation include heat, redness, and swelling. Inflammation may also result in pain. Figure 6.8 provides a graphic representation of the inflammatory response to injury.

Reduction of inflammation, pain, or both is the primary target for drug therapy. NSAIDs, discussed with osteoarthritis, are commonly used for inflammation. NSAIDs work by inhibiting PG synthesis in tissues, thereby preventing the sensitization of pain receptors to other chemical messengers of inflammation. Salicylates are another drug class commonly used to treat inflammation. Salicylates can also be classified as nonsteroidal anti-inflammatory agents. However, their mechanism and side effects make them unique from other NSAIDs and are discussed separately in this text. Acetaminophen, discussed with osteoarthritis, is also used for inflammation and pain.

FIGURE 6.8
The Inflammatory Response to Injury

Tissue injury leads to the release of various chemical messengers and ultimately to inflammation.

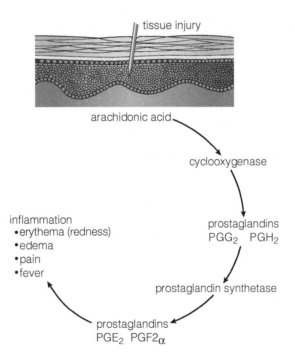

Salicylates

Salicylates were initially discovered and isolated from the bark of the white willow tree and were first used for rheumatic fever. Table 6.10 lists commonly used salicylates. These drugs have analgesic, antipyretic, and anti-inflammatory properties. The primary analgesic action is peripheral rather than central. In contrast, the primary antipyretic action is central, presumably in the hypothalamus. Salicylates reduce fever by increasing blood flow to the skin and inhibiting PG synthesis.

TABLE 6.10 Commonly Used Salicylates

Generic (Brand)	Pronunciation	Dosage Form	Common Dosage	Dispensing Status
aspirin (Durlaza)	AS-pir-in	capsule, chewable tablet, gum, suppository	325–650 mg every 4–6 hr, not to exceed 4 g per day	OTC, Rx
buffered aspirin (Ascriptin, Bufferin)	BUF-erd AS-pir-in	tablet	325–650 mg every 4–6 hr, not to exceed 4 g per day	OTC
choline magnesium trisalicylate (Trilisate)	KOE-leen mag-NEE-zhum trye-sa-LIS-il-ate	oral liquid	individualize based on patient response	Rx
salsalate (Disalcid)	SAL-sa-late	tablet	3 g per day in 2–3 divided doses	Rx

Salicylates are indicated for the following symptoms and conditions:

- inflammation of arthritis and rheumatism
- menstrual cramps
- muscular aches and pains
- pain and fever for influenza or other infections
- simple headache (headache other than migraine)

Work Wise

Aspirin is sometimes abbreviated as ASA. This stands for its chemical name, acetylsalicylic acid.

Aspirin, also known as acetylsalicylic acid, is a commonly used OTC salicylate. Low-dose (81–325 mg) aspirin taken daily has been shown to reduce the risk of heart attacks and strokes in patients with a prior history of cardiovascular disease (heart attack, stroke, bypass surgery). At low doses, aspirin appears to irreversibly inhibit the formation of thromboxane A2, a prostaglandin molecule that facilitates platelet adhesion aggregation in blood vessels.

Choline magnesium trisalicylate (Trilisate) is a salicylate approved for the treatment of arthritis. It acts on the hypothalamus to reduce fever and block pain impulses. A much lower dose of choline magnesium trisalicylate is necessary to have an antipyretic effect than is needed to inhibit pain.

Salsalate (Disalcid), another salicylate, is approved for the treatment of signs and symptoms of osteoarthritis, rheumatoid arthritis, and related rheumatic disorders. Salsalate is unique in that it does not inhibit platelet aggregation as much as other salicylates. This potentially decreases the risk of bleeding. Salsalate should be taken with food. The fact that it will not "thin" the blood makes it a very important member of this drug class.

Dosage Forms and Administration As a class, salicylates must be taken with food.

Low dosages (300–900 mg per day) of a salicylate can usually be taken safely. More than 4 g per day may cause problems; 10 g per day can be lethal. It is not uncommon, however, for a patient with rheumatoid arthritis to take 3–6 g per day under a prescriber's supervision.

The liquid form of choline magnesium trisalicylate may be mixed with fruit juices, but one needs to remain in an upright position for 30 minutes after ingestion.

Side Effects The side effects of salicylates include GI upset, tinnitus (ringing in the ears), and platelet changes. The nonionized portion of acetylsalicylic acid is lipid soluble and is easily absorbed into the gastric mucosal cells, which in turn causes further damage that can disrupt the integrity of the gastric mucosal barrier. This is why pharmacy databases provide the pharmacy technician with warnings when these drugs are dispensed and also why the FDA stipulates that they be accompanied by a Medication Guide.

Contraindications Aspirin use is contraindicated for viral infections in children and teenagers. Aspirin is also contraindicated in patients with hypersensitivity to NSAIDs. Patients with asthma, rhinitis, or nasal polyps should not use aspirin.

Hypersensitivity to other salicylates contraindicates use of choline magnesium trisalicylate.

Contraindications to salsalate include asthma, urticaria (hives), and allergic reaction.

Safety Alert

Aspirin, which is OTC, may increase the risk of bleeding in patients who use the blood thinner warfarin.

Practice Tip

Prescription salicylates must be dispensed with an FDA Medication Guide.

Safety Alert

The advent of childproof caps for medicine has reduced the incidence of pediatric intoxication.

Cautions and Considerations The following cautions and considerations apply to all salicylates discussed. Cautions and considerations unique to specific salicylates are presented in Table 6.11.

NSAIDs, including salicylates, may increase the risk of cardiovascular events (serious and potentially fatal) as well as GI inflammation, ulceration, and bleeding. Salicylates carry boxed warnings for these potentially serious complications. Prescription salicylates must be dispensed with an FDA Medication Guide.

Patients should be on alert for signs or symptoms of salicylate toxicity. Salicylism, mild salicylate intoxication, is characterized by tinnitus, dizziness, headache, and mental confusion. Severe intoxication is characterized by **hyperpnea** (abnormal increase in the depth of breathing), nausea, vomiting, acid-base disturbances, petechial hemorrhages, hyperthermia, delirium, convulsions, and coma.

Salicylates should be avoided after surgery or tooth extraction in patients with hemophilia (because they can interfere with normal clotting); in patients with asthma, nasal polyps, or chronic sinusitis (because salicylates may trigger an allergic-like hypersensitivity reaction); and in patients with bleeding ulcers (due to bleeding risk).

If used during pregnancy, salicylates may result in anemia; prolonged pregnancy and labor; and excessive bleeding before, during, and after delivery. They can also contribute to birth defects. Use of salicylates in the last trimester may result in prematurity, stillbirth, newborn death, low birth weight, and bleeding into the fetal brain. Salicylates can also cause closure of the ductus arteriosus (a fetal blood vessel that connects the pulmonary artery to the aorta), causing premature distribution of blood to the lungs. Moreover, the gastric irritation caused by salicylates and other NSAIDs must not be treated with misoprostol (Cytotec), a PG analog, in pregnant patients, because PGs stimulate uterine contraction. Pharmacy technicians who are pregnant should wear gloves when dispensing misoprostol.

Drug Interactions Some drug interactions apply to all discussed salicylates. Patients taking probenecid should not take a salicylate, which can prevent the excretion of uric acid and precipitate an attack of gout. Salicylates should not be taken with methotrexate, because they can increase methotrexate levels to a life-threatening toxic range. If a patient taking warfarin (Coumadin) is also taking aspirin, the pharmacy technician should alert the pharmacist. Some prescribers use the two drugs in combination, but this increases bleeding times. Drug interactions specific to certain salicylates are presented in Table 6.10.

Aspirin is avoided when treating children due to the possibility that the child will develop Reye's syndrome. Reye's syndrome is a rare condition that can develop in children who have been given aspirin after having been exposed to chicken pox or other viral infections. This syndrome includes a range of mental changes (mild amnesia, lethargy, disorientation, and agitation) that can culminate in coma and progressive unresponsiveness, seizures, relaxed muscles, dilated pupils, and respiratory failure.

TABLE 6.11 Unique Cautions, Considerations, and Drug Interactions of Commonly Used Salicylates

Generic (Brand)	Cautions and Considerations	Drug Interactions
aspirin (Durlaza)	Beware of aspirin toxicity and the risk of overdose. The lethal dose for aspirin is usually over 10 g for an adult. Aspirin should not be given to children. Pharmacy technicians must be mindful of combination preparations (e.g., Alka-Seltzer) that contain aspirin, if these preparations are intended for pediatric use. Use caution in patients with fluid retention or heart failure.	Use with other salicylates increases risk of toxicity. Aspirin increases the risk of bleeding when taken with anticoagulants. Concurrent administration of salsalate, and potentially other nonselective NSAIDs, may interfere with aspirin's cardioprotective effect.
choline magnesium trisalicylate (Trilisate)	Choline magnesium trisalicylate should be used with caution in patients with asthma or with liver or kidney dysfunction. Because of the increased risk of salicylate-related toxicities, older adults should use the lowest possible effective dose.	This drug may enhance adverse reactions of corticosteroids. Other salicylates may enhance side effects. Warfarin's anticoagulant effect may increase with concurrent use.
salsalate (Disalcid)	There are no unique cautions and considerations for salsalate.	Salsalate may enhance the adverse effects of corticosteroids. NSAIDs may increase the toxic side effects of salsalate.

6.9 Complementary and Alternative Therapies for Disorders of the Musculoskeletal System

Acupuncture, a method that involves penetrating the skin with thin needles in specific areas, is used for pain. Acupuncture has been used for thousands of years in Chinese medicine. Several studies show acupuncture to be beneficial for acute and chronic pain. In fact, some insurance plans cover acupuncture as a benefit.

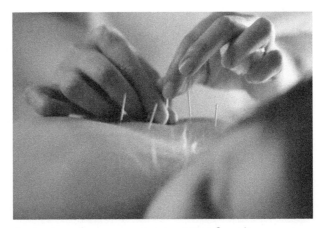
A person receives acupuncture treatment for pain.

Chiropractic care involves the physical manipulation of the spine based on the theory that proper alignment of the body's musculoskeletal structure will enable the body to heal. Chiropractors, practitioners of chiropractic care, often use hands-on approaches to spinal manipulation (sometimes in concert with other alternative therapies). Chiropractic care is primarily used to relieve pain associated with muscles, joints, bones, and connective tissue. Insurance plans may provide chiropractic care benefits.

The dietary supplement **chondroitin** is taken by some individuals in combination with glucosamine for hip and knee osteoarthritis (OA). However, studies do not clearly show that chondroitin taken with glucosamine is effective for OA. Chondroitin is derived from shark cartilage and bovine (cow) sources and is thought to work by inhibiting an enzyme that promotes inflammation. If patients want to take chondroitin, typical dosing is 200–400 mg two or three times a day. Common side effects tend to be mild and include nausea, heartburn, diarrhea, and constipation. Rare side effects include eyelid swelling, lower limb swelling, hair loss, and allergic reaction. If patients experience any of these effects, they should stop taking chondroitin.

Glucosamine is a drug supplement used by some individuals to improve pain and stiffness from OA. This supplement is derived from the exoskeleton of shellfish and is thought to slow joint degeneration. If patients want to take glucosamine, typical dosing is 1,500 mg a day (given in divided doses, 500 mg 3 times a day). Side effects are usually mild and include nausea, heartburn, diarrhea, and constipation. Taking glucosamine with food can decrease these effects. Although studies have not proven glucosamine to be harmful, it is recommended that patients with shellfish allergies avoid taking it.

Willow bark (*Salix alba*), a bark that contains salicin, has been used to treat many kinds of pain. Willow bark is a traditional analgesic therapy for osteoarthritis. Several studies have confirmed this finding. Additional studies comparing willow bark to conventional medicinal agents for safety and effectiveness are warranted.

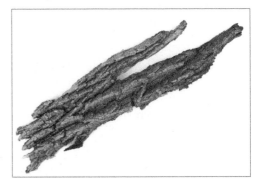
Willow bark contains salicin and is used for pain.

Review and Assessment

CHAPTER SUMMARY

Anatomy of the Musculoskeletal System

- The musculoskeletal system comprises the bones of the skeleton as well as cartilage, ligaments, joints, muscles, and tendons.

- Bones provide structural support for the body, protect organs, and allow muscle movement.

Physiology of the Musculoskeletal System

- Bones provide storage for lipids and minerals.

- The most common disorders of the musculoskeletal system are arthritis (a condition impacting the joints) and osteoporosis (a condition affecting the bones).

Osteoarthritis and Drug Treatments

- The most common complaint from arthritis patients is persistent pain.

- Acetaminophen is a common OTC drug used to treat OA. It is available orally, rectally, and intravenously. Acetaminophen is an analgesic and antipyretic. Patients with severe liver disease or who consume three or more drinks per day should not take acetaminophen.

- Acetaminophen is generally well tolerated when used appropriately.

- At a dose of more than 4 g of acetaminophen per day, liver toxicity can occur. Acetylcysteine is the antidote for acetaminophen overdose.

- Alcohol can cause a problem with OTC analgesics. For acetaminophen, the problem is liver toxicity; for NSAIDs, gastric irritation.

- NSAIDs are used for OA, inflammation associated with injury, painful menstrual cycles, and fever.

- NSAIDs take longer to reduce fever than other products, but the effect may last longer.

- NSAIDs inhibit PG synthesis in inflamed tissues, thereby preventing the sensitization of pain receptors to mediators of inflammation. Thus, they generally act peripherally rather than centrally as other pain relievers do.

- NSAIDs are available OTC and by prescription.

- PGs perform three protective functions in the GI tract: increasing mucosal blood flow, increasing mucus production, and decreasing free acid production.

- All NSAIDs should be administered with food and dispensed with an FDA Medication Guide.

- Side effects of NSAIDs are GI upset, nausea, kidney damage, fluid retention, hypertension, hyperkalemia, liver abnormalities, blood clotting irregularities, bone marrow depression, ringing in the ears, jaundice, dizziness, drowsiness, rash, and dry mouth.

- All NSAIDs carry boxed warnings for an increased risk of heart attack, stroke, and death, as well as GI complications (such as inflammation or bleeding).

- Some patients will need to take a proton pump inhibitor with NSAIDs.

- Concurrent use of multiple NSAIDs (including aspirin) should be discouraged, because the combination may lead to additive or synergistic toxicity rather than increased efficacy.

- Celecoxib (Celebrex) is a COX-2 inhibitor that works differently from other NSAIDs. Celecoxib provides pain and inflammation relief without the unwanted effect of reducing GI protection.

- Celecoxib should be dispensed with an FDA Medication Guide.

Rheumatoid Arthritis and Drug Treatments

- Rheumatoid arthritis is an autoimmune disorder with symptoms that include morning pain and stiffness.

- Treatment for rheumatoid arthritis includes agents that provide symptomatic relief and agents that potentially modify disease progression called disease-modifying antirheumatic drugs (DMARDs).

- NSAIDs and corticosteroids may be used to treat discomfort and other symptoms of RA.

- DMARDs are disease-modifying antirheumatic drugs that may slow the progression of the disease.

- Methotrexate (Rheumatrex, Trexall) is an antineoplastic agent commonly used to treat RA. It should be taken on an empty stomach, and exposure to the sun should be avoided.

Gouty Arthritis and Drug Treatments

- Aspirin should not be given to a patient with gout; it competes with uric acid for kidney excretion.

- Cytotoxic agents, diuretics, ethanol, nicotinic acid, and salicylates can precipitate a gout attack.

- Colchicine and NSAIDs are used for acute gout attacks.

- Allopurinol, colchicine, febuxostat, and probenecid are all used as preventative therapies for gout.

Osteoporosis and Drug Treatments

- Osteoporosis is a condition marked by reduced bone mineral density, disrupted microarchitecture of bone structure, and increased likelihood of fracture.

- Lifestyle changes to decrease bone loss include increasing calcium intake, ceasing cigarette smoking and heavy caffeine use, and engaging in weight-bearing exercise.

- Bisphosphonates are the drug class most commonly used to treat osteoporosis.

- Bisphosphonates may be oral or injectable. Special attention must be given to patients regarding oral bisphosphonate administration. These drugs must be taken on an empty stomach with a full glass of water. Patients must wait at least 30 minutes after bisphosphonate ingestion before eating.

- SERMs, denosumab (Prolia, Xgeva), romosozumab (Evenity), and teriparatide (Forteo) are other drugs used to treat osteoporosis.

Muscle Spasms and Drug Treatments

- Muscle spasms are treated with NSAIDs, acetaminophen, and muscle relaxants.

- The side effects of muscle relaxants include sedation, reduced mental alertness, reduced motor abilities, and GI upset. Patients taking these drugs should avoid alcohol.

- Muscle relaxants are available in oral, topical, and injectable dosage forms.

Inflammation and Swelling and Drug Treatments

- Inflammation is treated with a variety of drugs, including NSAIDs, acetaminophen, and salicylates.

- Salicylates have analgesic (pain-relieving), anti-inflammatory, and antipyretic (fever-reducing) properties.

- The primary analgesic actions of salicylates are peripheral rather than central. Their primary antipyretic action is central and presumed to be in the hypothalamus.

- Salicylates are indicated for simple headache, inflammation of arthritis and rheumatism, pain and fever with influenza, muscular aches and pains, menstrual cramps, and inflammation.

- More than 4 g of aspirin per day can cause problems; 10 g can be lethal.

- Mild salicylate intoxication is characterized by ringing in the ears (tinnitus), dizziness, headache, and mental confusion.

- Salicylates cause gastrointestinal ulceration. They should be avoided by patients with asthma, nasal polyps, chronic sinusitis, or bleeding ulcers. Patients with hemophilia should not take salicylates after surgery or tooth extraction.

Complementary and Alternative Therapies

- Acupuncture and chiropractic care may be used to treat pain.

- Glucosamine and chondroitin may be used to treat symptoms associated with osteoarthritis.

- Willow bark contains salicin and may be used for pain.

DRUG LIST

Conventional NSAIDs
diclofenac (Cambia, Pennsaid, Voltaren Gel, Zipsor, Zorvolex)
etodolac (Lodine)
ibuprofen (Advil, Motrin)
indomethacin (Indocin, Tivorbex)
ketoprofen (Orudis, Oruvail)
ketorolac (Toradol)
meloxicam (Mobic)
nabumetone (Relafen)
naproxen (Aleve, Anaprox, Anaprox DS, EC-Naprosyn, Flanax, Naprelan, Naprosyn)
piroxicam (Feldene)

Combination NSAIDs
diclofenac / misoprostol (Arthrotec)
ibuprofen / famotidine (Duexis)
naproxen / esomeprazole (Vimovo)

COX-2 Inhibitor
celecoxib (Celebrex)

DMARDs
adalimumab (Humira)
anakinra (Kineret)
auranofin (Ridaura)
azathioprine (Azasan, Imuran)
etanercept (Enbrel)
golimumab (Simponi, Simponi Aria)

hydroxychloroquine (Plaquenil)
infliximab (Remicade)
leflunomide (Arava)
methotrexate (Rheumatrex, Xatmep)
sulfasalazine (Azulfidine, Azulfidine EN-tabs)

Gout Therapies
allopurinol (Aloprim, Zyloprim)
colchicine (Colcrys, Gloperba, Mitigare)
febuxostat (Uloric)
probenecid

Bisphosphonates
alendronate (Binostro, Fosamax)
ibandronate (Boniva)
pamidronate (Aredia)
risedronate (Actonel, Atelvia)
zoledronic acid (Reclast)

Selective Estrogen Receptor Modulators (SERMs)
raloxifene (Evista)

Other Agents for Osteoporosis
denosumab (Prolia, Xgeva)
romosozumab (Evenity)
teriparatide (Forteo)

Muscle Relaxants
baclofen (EnovaRX-Baclofen, First-Baclofen, Gablofen, Lioresal)
carisoprodol (Soma)
chlorzoxazone (Lorzone)
cyclobenzaprine (Amrix, EnovaRx, Fexmid, Tobradol FusePaq, Tobradol RapidPaq)
dantrolene (Dantrium, Revonto, Ryanodex)
diazepam (Diastat, Valium)
metaxalone (Metaxall, Skelaxin)
methocarbamol (Robaxin)
orphenadrine
tizanidine (Zanaflex)

Salicylates
aspirin (Durlaza)
buffered aspirin (Ascriptin, Bufferin)
choline magnesium trisalicylate (Trilisate)
salsalate (Disalcid)

✓ CHECK YOUR UNDERSTANDING

Take a moment to review what you have learned in this chapter and answer the following questions.

1. A joint is best described as
   a. an organ that produces movement by contracting.
   b. noncontractile connective tissue that ties one bone to another bone.
   c. the breakdown of bone and release of calcium into the bloodstream.
   d. the junction between two or more bones of the skeleton.

2. Which of the following is an approved medication to treat acetaminophen overdose?
   a. acetylcysteine
   b. flumazenil
   c. naloxone
   d. zoledronic acid

3. Acetaminophen doses greater than 4 g (4,000 mg) a day are associated with which of the following?
   a. breathing abnormalities
   b. gastrointestinal bleeding
   c. kidney failure
   d. liver toxicity

4. All the following nonsteroidal anti-inflammatory drugs are available in topical formulations *except*
   a. diclofenac.
   b. ibuprofen.
   c. nabumetone.
   d. ketoprofen.

5. NSAIDs carry boxed warnings for all the following adverse effects *except*
   a. increased risk of GI inflammation, ulceration, and bleeding.
   b. increased risk of liver toxicity.
   c. increased risk of serious heart attack.
   d. increased risk of serious stroke.

6. Celecoxib has the potential for cross-reactivity in patients who are allergic to which of the following drug classes?
   a. aminoglycosides
   b. fluoroquinolones
   c. penicillins
   d. sulfonamides

7. Which of the following is a drug used to treat gout that is available in oral and injectable dosage forms?
   a. colchicine
   b. febuxostat
   c. probenecid
   d. sulfasalazine

8. Which of the following is a common side effect of allopurinol?
   a. changes in skin color
   b. discoloration of urine
   c. neutropenia
   d. skin rash

9. Oral bisphosphonates should be administered
   a. on an empty stomach.
   b. while lying down.
   c. with meals.
   d. without regard to meals.

10. Salicylate toxicity is characterized by all the following *except*
    a. acid-base disturbances.
    b. hypothermia.
    c. mental confusion.
    d. tinnitus.

MAKE CONNECTIONS

Take a moment to consider what you have learned in this chapter and respond thoughtfully to the following prompts. Note that some of these activities will require internet access.

1. Use online resources to find the most recent list of the top 200 prescribed drugs. Cross-reference this list with the drug list provided at the end of Chapter 6. Which drugs in Chapter 6 are considered top 200 drugs?

2. Nonsteroidal anti-inflammatory drugs may be prescribed in combination with proton pump inhibitors or histamine receptor blockers. Describe the rationale behind this practice (include a description of the mechanism of action of NSAIDs).

The online course includes additional review and assessment resources.

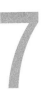

The Nervous System and Drug Therapy

Learning Objectives

1 List the divisions of the nervous system and their functions. (Section 7.1)

2 Discuss the classes of drug therapy that are used to treat conditions affecting the nervous system. (Section 7.1)

3 Describe the physiologic processes that occur in epilepsy. (Section 7.2)

4 Classify seizures and the goals of antiseizure therapy. (Section 7.2)

5 Describe the specific drugs used in the treatment of different classes of seizures. (Section 7.2)

6 Describe the pathophysiology and manifestations of Parkinson's disease. (Section 7.3)

7 Explain drug treatments for Parkinson's disease. (Section 7.3)

8 Recognize drugs used for multiple sclerosis. (Section 7.4)

9 Recognize drugs used to manage Alzheimer's disease. (Section 7.5)

10 Identify drugs used to treat attention deficit hyperactivity disorders. (Section 7.6)

ASHP/ACPE Accreditation Standards
To view the *ASHP/ACPE Accreditation Standards* addressed in this chapter, refer to Appendix C.

The nervous system is the main coordinator and controller for all the systems in the body. It also acts to interpret, integrate, and respond to the environment around us and our body's internal environment. The nervous system does this through electrical and chemical signals that transmit rapidly through the body. In general, the nervous system works continuously to maintain a state of homeostasis. Most drugs commonly used to anesthetize patients and relieve pain and migraine headache interact with the body by influencing the electrical and chemical signaling of the nervous system or its target tissues. This chapter concentrates on disorders related to the central nervous system and their corresponding drug therapies.

7.1 Anatomy and Physiology of the Nervous System

The nervous system can be organized into anatomical and functional divisions. Understanding these divisions can aid in understanding the site of action, mechanism of action, and effects of a drug in the body.

Anatomical Divisions

The nervous system has two anatomical divisions, the **central nervous system (CNS)** and the **peripheral nervous system (PNS)**. The CNS consists of the brain and spinal cord, the two organs that process and evaluate incoming information and determine responses. The CNS coordinates and controls the activity of the other body systems as well. The PNS consists of nerves and sensory receptors, which are located outside of the CNS. The PNS carries neural signals between the body and the CNS.

Functional Divisions

Functionally, the peripheral nervous system consists of sensory and motor divisions, as shown in Figure 7.1. The sensory division carries information to the CNS from sensory receptors that detect heat, cold, pain, and the presence of chemicals. This division is called the **afferent system**. The afferent system is further divided into the somatic sensory and visceral sensory systems. The **somatic sensory system** includes nerves that sense touch, pressure, temperature, and painful stimuli on the surface of the body such as muscles and joints. The **visceral sensory system** includes nerves that sense pain or reflex signals in the internal organs and blood vessels. The motor division carries information from the CNS to parts of the body such as muscles and glands to produce a response. This division is called the **efferent system**. The motor division can be further subdivided into the **autonomic nervous system** and the **somatic nervous system**. The autonomic nervous system regulates motor activity that is involuntary or not consciously controlled (e.g., motor activity of cardiac muscle, smooth muscle, and glands). The somatic nervous system regulates motor activity that is voluntary or conscious (e.g., motor activity of skeletal muscles).

FIGURE 7.1 Functional Organization of the Nervous System

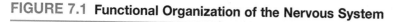

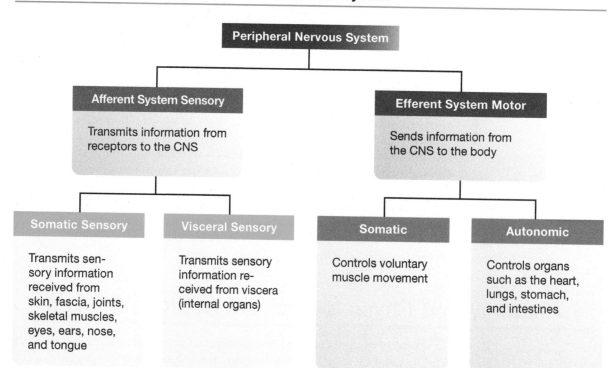

The autonomic nervous system can be further subdivided into the **sympathetic nervous system** and the **parasympathetic nervous system**, which control specific autonomic functions. As shown in Figure 7.2, the sympathetic nervous system transmits information to the body from the sympathetic ganglion chain in the thoracic and lumbar regions of the spinal cord. The parasympathetic nervous system transmits information to the body from the brain and from the cervical and sacral regions of the spinal cord.

FIGURE 7.2
The Autonomic Nervous System

The autonomic nervous system is divided into the sympathetic and parasympathetic nervous systems. The sympathetic controls the fight-or-flight functions, and the parasympathetic controls rest, digestion, and homeostasis.

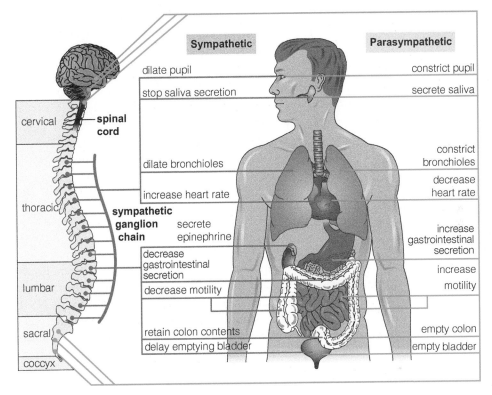

Neurons and Neurotransmitters

The nervous system is responsible for transmitting information over a vast network throughout the body. This network is primarily made up of a specific type of cell, called a **neuron**, as well as supporting cells. A neuron transmits information through electrical and chemical signals. For neurons to transmit their signal, or impulse, they must be connected to one another, and this connection is called a **synapse**. The nerve impulse reaches the synaptic vesicle (which stores neurotramitters) and causes the release of neurotransmitters. **Neurotransmitters** are chemical messengers that carry the signal across the synapse to the next neuron.

These chemical signals are then received by receptors on the cell body or by dendrites. A **dendrite** is a branchlike extension from a neuron's cell body. The receptors or dendrites convert the chemical signals into electrical signals, also called *impulses*, which travel down the neuron's axon away from the cell body until it ends at the axon terminal. Schwann cells assist the nerve signal to travel along axons of nerves smoothly and efficiently.

The neuron's axon terminal bulbs contain neurotransmitters that can then be released onto subsequent cells, as shown in Figure 7.3, to stimulate or inhibit the activity of that cell or target tissue.

FIGURE 7.3 Release of Neurotransmitters from a Neuron

Neurotransmitters are released from one neuron's axon and received by the receptors on the dendrites of the next neuron.

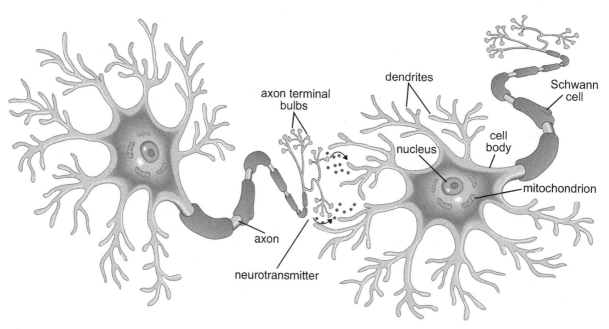

The process of transmitting signals in the nervous system involves the release of neurotransmitters at each neuron junction. Some of these neurotransmitters are excitatory (also called *stimulatory*), and others are inhibitory. The primary CNS transmitters are acetylcholine (ACh), gamma-aminobutyric acid (GABA), dopamine, epinephrine (adrenaline), norepinephrine (noradrenaline), serotonin (also known as *5-hydroxytryptamine*, or *5-HT*), and glutamate. Glutamate is the most common neurotransmitter in the brain, and it is always excitatory. The primary PNS neurotransmitters are ACh and norepinephrine. In the autonomic nervous system, ACh and norepinephrine can be excitatory or inhibitory; however, ACh is the only neurotransmitter of the somatic nervous system, where it is excitatory. Most neurons voluntarily or involuntarily communicate with motor neurons in the spinal cord, which then stimulate muscle fibers to contract for movement.

Every neuron is in one of three states: resting, firing, or returning to rest. The balance between excitatory and inhibitory impulses determines whether a neuron fires. Neurons operate through the movement of ions across the cell membrane. When negatively charged ions, such as chloride, enter a neuron, they inhibit firing; conversely, when positively charged ions, such as sodium and calcium, enter the cell, they excite it and make it more likely to fire.

The flow of ions is controlled by ion channels, a type of molecule in the cell membrane. A neurotransmitter is a chemical that controls these channels. Some neurotransmitters bind to receptors in the cell membrane that let positive ions in and excite the cell, whereas others bind to receptors that let negative ions in and inhibit firing. Table 7.1 identifies the various type of neurotransmitters, their anatomical divisions, and their effects.

TABLE 7.1 Neurotransmitters

Neurotransmitter	Anatomical Division	Roles and Effects
acetylcholine (ACh)	CNS and PNS	PNS-ACh stimulates skeletal muscle, inhibits cardiac muscle, and both inhibits and excites smooth muscle and glands CNS-ACh is involved in signals that control memories, sleep, and perception of pain
gamma-aminobutyric acid (GABA)	CNS	primary inhibitory neurotransmitter in the brain; can impact muscle tone
dopamine	CNS	inhibitory neurotransmitter in the brain; has important roles in cognition (the ability to perceive, think, and remember), motivation, behavior, and mood
epinephrine (adrenaline)	CNS	affects thalamus, hypothalamus, and spinal cord
norepinephrine (noradrenaline)	CNS and PNS	PNS-norepinephrine modulates the sympathetic nervous system CNS-norepinephrine increases arousal, alertness, retrieval of memories, and focused attention
serotonin (5-hydroxytryptamine)	CNS	has various functions in the brain related to sleep, appetite, cognition, and mood
glutamate	CNS	stimulatory neurotransmitter that increases activity in the nervous system to promote cognitive function in the brain (the ability to perceive, think, and remember); most common neurotransmitter in the brain

Safety Alert

The anticholinergic drugs can have important side effects. Some reactions include decreased GI motility (constipation), decreased sweating, decreased urination (urinary retention), dilated pupils (mydriasis) and blurred vision, dry eyes, and dry mouth.

Neurotransmitter Mechanism of Action

When a neurotransmitter binds to a receptor on a cell membrane, it causes downstream changes. For many receptors, neurotransmitter binding increases cell membrane permeability to various ions, which then directly stimulate or inhibit an electrical signal in the receiving cell. Other receptors activate enzymatic systems that promote chemical reactions within the cell.

The effect of a neurotransmitter on a cell can depend on the type of receptor it binds to. In the nervous system, adrenergic receptors are sensitive to both epinephrine and norepinephrine. The three types of adrenergic receptors are alpha, beta-1, and beta-2. The binding of epinephrine and norepinephrine to these receptors facilitates the following responses:

- **Alpha receptor:** causes blood vessels to constrict (vasoconstriction, raising blood pressure), but also causes decongestion
- **Beta-1 receptor (ß1):** increases the heart rate and contractile force of the heart
- **Beta-2 receptor (ß2):** influences dilation of both bronchial tubes (bronchodilation) and blood vessels (vasodilation)

In general, the most important action of adrenergic receptors are bronchodilation and heart stimulation. Notice, though, that alpha and beta-2 receptors have opposite effects on blood vessels. The overall action of an adrenergic neurotransmitter depends on its concentration. Beta-2 receptors widen blood vessels in response to moderate neurotransmitter levels, whereas higher levels stimulate the alpha receptors to narrow blood vessels.

A receptor's response to a neurotransmitter can be affected by the tissue where the cell is located. For example, a specific type of acetylcholine receptor called a muscarinic receptor has a very different effect when found in smooth muscle than when found in cardiac muscle. In smooth muscle, activation of muscarinic receptors leads to muscle contraction. In cardiac muscle, activation of muscarinic receptors slows heart contractions and reduces their force.

Many drugs facilitate an effect in the body by mimicking or influencing the action of neurotransmitters. The action of a neurotransmitter can be affected by influencing neurotransmitter release, enzyme degradation, and neurotransmitter reabsorption.

Drugs may also act by blocking receptors, thereby preventing neurotransmitters from binding to them. This can facilitate a physiologic response that is the opposite of the normal effect when those neurotransmitters bind to the receptors. For example, anticholinergic drugs block acetylcholine receptors. As described previously, when ACh binds to cardiac muscle, their heart rate and force of contractions decrease. When a patient takes an anticholinergic drug, their heart rate and force of contractions increase.

Central nervous system (CNS) disorders cause a range of complex, distressing, and life-threatening symptoms, some of which are nonresponsive to treatment. These disorders often leave patients unable to function normally. The chemicals involved in thought processes and motor activity cause some of these diseases and provide rationales for their treatments. These diseases include epilepsy in its various forms, Parkinson's disease, myasthenia gravis, attention deficit disorders, amyotrophic lateral sclerosis, multiple sclerosis, Alzheimer's disease, restless legs syndrome, fibromyalgia, and Huntington's disease. For some of these diseases, medical researchers are still searching for definitive treatments.

7.2 Seizure Disorders and Drug Treatments

A **seizure** is a change in behavior or function caused by abnormal electrical discharges in the cerebral cortex (the main portion of the brain). Seizures result from the sudden excessive firing of a small number of neurons, often without an exogenous (outside the organism) trigger and the spread of the electrical activity to adjacent neurons.

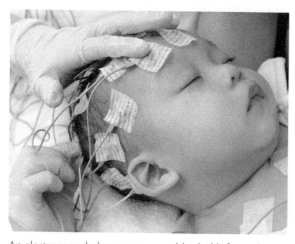

An electroencephalogram can provide vital information on the cause of seizures, helping the physician to select the best option for treatment.

These firings can result in a **convulsion**, an involuntary contraction or series of contractions, of the voluntary muscles. Conscious periods may or may not be accompanied by loss of control over movements or distortion of the senses. When body movement is lost, it may be in only one area of the body or in the entire body.

Epilepsy is a fairly common neurologic disorder characterized by **paroxysmal** (sudden and recurring) seizures. It involves disturbances of neuronal electrical activity that interfere with normal brain function. These abnormal discharges may occur only in a specific area of the brain or may spread extensively throughout the brain. Though seizures may not provoke obvious clinical symptoms, seriously imbalanced electrical discharges may still occur.

Epilepsy is a symptom of brain dysfunction. All epilepsy patients have seizures, but not all patients with seizures have epilepsy. Some patients with seizures have a single unprovoked seizure in their lifetime; 1%–2% have chronic epilepsy.

Healthy individuals have a balance between neuronal excitation and inhibition, but individuals diagnosed with epilepsy have an imbalance. When excitation is excessive relative to inhibition, neurons can fire uncontrollably, leading to a seizure. Glutamate, an excitatory neurotransmitter, and gamma-aminobutyric acid (GABA), an inhibitory neurotransmitter, play the greatest role in seizures. Other contributors are CNS chemicals involved in thought processes and motor activity, such as the following:

- acetylcholine (ACh)
- aspartate
- dopamine
- glycine
- norepinephrine
- serotonin

Neurotransmitter levels are determined in part by the levels of the enzymes that produce them. An **enzyme** is a biological molecule that catalyzes chemical reactions in the body. Upsetting those enzymes disrupts the balance between excitation and inhibition in neurons and leads to seizures, especially if the disruption results in a high ratio of glutamate to GABA. The majority of seizures are caused by the following events or conditions:

- illegal or recreational drug use
- alcohol withdrawal or extreme intoxication
- epilepsy
- high fever
- hypoglycemia (low blood glucose) or hyperglycemia (high blood glucose)
- meningitis infection
- neoplasm (tumor) in the brain
- head trauma or injury

The two major types of seizures are focal and generalized (see Figure 7.4). Each type is further subdivided according to its manifestations.

Focal Seizures

A **focal seizure** is localized in a specific hemisphere or area of the brain. Focal seizures, formerly known as *partial seizures*, generally result from injury to the cerebral cortex. They occur in two distinct types, each of which can progress to a generalized seizure.

In a **simple focal seizure**, the patient does not lose consciousness and may have:

- some muscular activity manifested as twitching
- sensory hallucinations (visual or auditory phenomena)

In a **complex focal seizure**, the patient experiences:

- impaired consciousness, often with confusion
- a blank stare
- postseizure amnesia

FIGURE 7.4
Focal and Generalized Seizure Activity

A focal seizure and a generalized seizure affect brain activity differently, as shown on the simulated electro-encephalograms (EEGs).

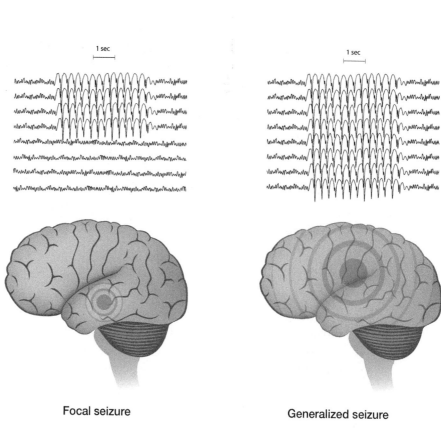

Focal seizure   Generalized seizure

Generalized Seizures

A **generalized seizure** involves simultaneous malfunction in both hemispheres of the brain and has no local origin. This type of seizure sometimes occurs in the absence of injury or known structural abnormality. Generalized seizures are classified by type and include tonic-clonic, status epilepticus, absence, myoclonic, and atonic seizures.

- A **tonic-clonic seizure** (formerly called a **grand mal seizure**) occurs in two general phases. The tonic portion of the seizure begins with the patient's body becoming rigid, which may result in a fall. This phase lasts for a minute or less. The clonic portion usually is initiated with muscle jerks and may be accompanied by shallow breathing, loss of bladder control, and excess saliva- tion (foaming at the mouth). Jerking continues for a few minutes. After the attack, the patient is drowsy and confused for moments or hours.

- **Status epilepticus** is a serious disorder involving continuous tonic-clonic convulsions, with or without a return to consciousness, that last at least 30 minutes. It is characterized by a high fever and lack of oxygen severe enough to cause brain damage or death. Of the patients who have convulsive status epilepticus, 10% die regardless of treatment, often as a complication of sudden drug withdrawal.

- An **absence seizure** (formerly called a **petit mal seizure**) begins with inter- ruption of the patient's activities by some or all of the following signs: blank stare, rotating eyes, momentary break in consciousness, uncontrolled facial movements, chewing, rapid eye blinking, and twitching or jerking of an arm or a leg. However, this includes no generalized convulsions. Absence seizures can last from 10 seconds to 2 minutes but are rarely longer than 30 seconds. The patient may experience up to 100 attacks a day. Often, the person has a premonition of the attack through unusual sensations of light, sound, and taste, known as an **aura**. After the attack, the patient continues normal activities. Absence seizures are most prevalent during the first 10 years of life; 50% of children with absence seizures have tonic-clonic activity as they grow older.

- A **myoclonic seizure** occurs with sudden, massive, brief muscle jerks, which may throw the patient down, or smaller, quick jerks of the arms, hands, legs, or feet. Consciousness is not lost, and this seizure type can occur during sleep.

- An **atonic seizure** begins with sudden loss of both muscle tone and consciousness. The patient may collapse, the head may drop, and the jaw may slacken. An arm or a leg may go limp. The seizure lasts a few seconds to a minute, and then the patient can stand and walk again.

Antiepileptic Therapy

Epilepsy can have profound effects on an individual's health, quality of life, and ability to function. The optimum antiepileptic therapy would be complete seizure control without compromising the patient's quality of life. Thus, therapy with anticonvulsant drugs has two goals: (1) to control seizures or reduce their frequency so that the patient can live an essentially normal life, and (2) to prevent emotional and behavioral changes that may result from the seizures.

Seizures occur when the effect of excitatory neurotransmitters is excessive relative to the effect of inhibitory neurotransmitters. Drugs to control seizures work by reducing the excitation or increasing the inhibition so that neurons do not fire out of control. Not surprisingly, many drugs used to control seizures are used, or have been used, to treat other conditions characterized by excessive excitation, such as mania, anxiety, and panic.

Monotherapy, use of a single drug, is tried first, and other agents may be added to control seizures. Except in life-threatening situations, single-drug therapy, or monotherapy, should be initiated at one-fourth to one-third of the usual daily dosage. The dosage is then increased gradually over three to four weeks until seizures are controlled or adverse side effects occur. Once an optimal dosage has been determined, it is essential that the plasma concentration (amount of drug found in the blood) of the drug remains stable to ensure seizure control and minimize the risk of side effects. **Combination therapy**, or polytherapy, is using two or more drugs from different classes. Polytherapy is common among patients with severe forms of epilepsy. It can take up to a month to see the full benefit from these drugs. Monotherapy is preferred to combination therapy because it costs less and patients may have fewer adverse effects, drug interactions, and compliance problems.

One possible reason for nonresponsiveness to antiepileptic drug therapy is that the agent is inappropriate for the seizure type. In the past, most patients with epilepsy were treated with phenytoin, phenobarbital, or both drugs. Clinicians now recognize that different seizure types respond better to specific antiepileptic agents. A drug that controls one seizure type may exacerbate another type. The newer drugs are seizure specific; that is, their pharmacologic action is directed toward controlling a certain type of seizure activity.

The need for therapy should be evaluated periodically. Some patients can discontinue therapy if they have been seizure free for several years. To discontinue an antiepileptic drug, the dosage should be decreased gradually over two to six months. Abrupt discontinuation should be avoided because of the risk of triggering status epilepticus or other withdrawal seizures.

The potential for drug interactions during antiepileptic therapy is high. Antiepileptic drugs interact with each other and with other drugs through two major mechanisms. They can induce or inhibit the liver enzymes responsible for drug metabolism. They can also displace drugs from their binding sites on plasma proteins.

Table 7.2 presents the most commonly used anticonvulsant drugs. An **anticonvulsant** is a drug used to control seizures. Anticonvulsants have a relatively narrow therapeutic index, meaning that small differences in dose can lead to overdose or serious adverse reactions. The amount of drug that must be given to reach the desired effect is not much lower than the point where serious side effects or toxicity can occur. In some patients, even minor changes in bioavailability can compromise control or result in toxicity. Factors that affect bioavailability include storage conditions, the drug's physical and chemical characteristics, the dosage form, and the patient's physical condition. In some cases, blood levels are used to monitor therapy closely.

TABLE 7.2 Commonly Used Anticonvulsants

Generic (Brand)	Pronunciation	Dosage Form	Dispensing Status	Controlled Substance Schedule
Sodium Channel Blockers				
carbamazepine (Carbatrol, Epitol, Equetro, Tegretol)	kar-ba-MAZ-e-peen	capsule, oral suspension, tablet	Rx	
eslicarbazepine (Aptiom)	es-li-kar-BAZ-e-peen	tablet	Rx	
fosphenytoin (Cerebyx)	fos-FEN-i-toyn	injection	Rx	
lacosamide (Vimpat, Vimpat IV)	la-KOE-sa-mide	injection, oral solution, tablet	Rx	C-V
oxcarbazepine (Oxtellar XR, Trileptal)	ox-kar-BAZ-e-peen	oral suspension, tablet	Rx	
phenytoin (Dilantin, Phenytek)	FEN-i-toyn	capsule, injection, oral suspension, tablet	Rx	
rufinamide (Banzel)	roo-FIN-a-mide	tablet	Rx	
vigabatrin (Sabril)	vye-GA-ba-trin	oral powder, tablet	Rx	
Calcium Channel Blockers				
divalproex sodium (Depakote, Depakote ER)	dye-vall-PRO-ex SO-dee-um	tablet	Rx	
ethosuximide (Zarontin)	eth-oh-SUX-i-mide	capsule, syrup	Rx	
zonisamide (Zonegran)	zoh-NIS-a-mide	capsule	Rx	
GABA Enhancers				
gabapentin (Neurontin)	gab-a-PEN-tin	capsule, oral solution, tablet	Rx	
phenobarbital	fee-noe-BAR-bi-tal	elixir, injection, tablet	Rx	C-IV
pregabalin (Lyrica)	pree-GAB-a-lin	capsule, oral solution, tablet	Rx	C-V
primidone (Mysoline)	PRYE-mih-done	tablet	Rx	
tiagabine (Gabitril)	ty-AG-a-been	tablet	Rx	
Glutamate Inhibitors				
felbamate (Felbatol)	FEL-ba-mate	oral suspension, tablet	Rx	

continues

TABLE 7.2 Commonly Used Anticonvulsants—*Continued*

Generic (Brand)	Pronunciation	Dosage Form	Dispensing Status	Controlled Substance Schedule
lamotrigine (Lamictal Lamictal CD, Lamictal ODT, Lamictal XR)	la-MOE-tri-jeen	tablet	Rx	
perampanel (Fycompa)	per-AM-pa-nel	oral suspension, tablet	Rx	C-III
Glutamate Inhibitors				
topiramate (Qudexy XR, Topamax, Trokendi XR)	toe-PYRE-a-mate	capsule, tablet	Rx	
Synaptic Vesicle Protein Binders				
brivaracetam (Briviact)	briv-a-RA-se-tam	injection, oral solution, tablet	Rx	C-V
levetiracetam (Elepsia XR, Keppra, Keppra XR, Roweepra, Spritam)	lev-a-tur-AS-a-tam	injection, oral solution, tablet	Rx	

Safety Alert

Medication Guides must be given to patients upon dispensing anticonvulsant drugs. Technicians should remember to include these materials when patients pick up their medications from the pharmacy.

Work Wise

Carbamazepine has a narrow therapeutic index, and maintaining therapeutic drug concentrations is important. Patients may need to use carbamazepine produced by only one manufacturer, which may require the pharmacy to dispense the brand-name drug, not a generic drug.

Anticonvulsants have many drug interactions, which can also impact therapeutic ranges (see Table 7.3). Because of the narrow therapeutic index of this class of drugs, even the very small allowable differences in manufacturing can affect the ability of the drug to control episodes. For this reason, prescribers may not allow generic drugs to be used, so pharmacy technicians should double-check these drugs' prescriptions for the instructions "DAW" (dispense as written) or "brand only." If the computer automatically changes the brand name of one of these drugs to its generic name, the technician may have to change it back to the brand name. Medication Guides are required when dispensing all antiepileptics.

Sodium Channel Blockers

A **sodium channel blocker** works on sodium channels (ion channels for sodium ions). Blocking sodium (a positive ion) makes neurons less likely to fire. Alteration of sodium currents is the most common mechanism of action of existing anticonvulsants. Sodium channel blockers include carbamazepine, eslicarbazepine, fosphenytoin, lacosamide, oxcarbazepine, phenytoin, rufinamide, and vigabatrin. See Table 7.2 for the various dosage forms of sodium channel blockers. Side effects and drug interactions of each are listed in Table 7.3.

Carbamazepine, Eslicarbazepine, and Oxcarbazepine

Carbamazepine (Carbatrol, Epitol, Equetro, Tegretol) is a sodium channel blocker used to treat tonic-clonic seizures and certain focal seizures, mixed seizures (both generalized and focal), and other generalized seizures. It is also used to treat bipolar disorders, as described in Chapter 8. Its antiepileptic effect may be related to its effects on sodium channels to limit sustained, repetitive firing and alter synaptic transmission. Blood monitoring is important to assure the dose of carbamazepine is appropriate for the patient. **Eslicarbazepine (Aptiom)** is used for focal seizures. **Oxcarbazepine (Oxtellar XR, Trileptal)** blocks voltage-sensitive sodium channels and thereby stabilizes hyperexcited neurons. This drug is most frequently used as an adjunct to other therapies, but it can be used as monotherapy for focal seizures.

TABLE 7.3 Common Uses, Side Effects, and Drug Interactions for Sodium Channel Blockers

Generic (Brand)	Common Uses	Side Effects	Selected Drug Interactions
carbamazepine (Carbatrol, Epitol, Equetro, Tegretol)	tonic-clonic seizure, focal seizure (no effect on absence seizure)	dizziness, drowsiness, nausea, rash, unsteadiness, vomiting, abnormal vision, hyponatremia, hepatotoxicity, arrhythmias, bleeding, bruising, jaundice, abdominal pain, pale stools, mental disturbances, fever, chills, sore throat, mouth ulcers	Cimetidine, diltiazem, erythromycin, isoniazid, itraconazole, nefazodone, theophylline, and troleandomycin increase concentrations. Phenobarbital, phenytoin, theophylline, and valproic acid decrease concentrations.
eslicarbazepine (Aptiom)	focal seizure	dizziness, drowsiness, headache, nausea/vomiting, hypertension, rash, hyponatremia, urinary tract infection, tremor, weakness, blurred vision, cough difficultly concentrating, stomach pain	abemaciclib, avapritinib, bedaquiline, bosutinib, carbamazepine, clarithromycin, clozapine, cobimetinib, codeine, dasabuvir, deflazacort, encorafenib, estrogens, fedratinib, flibanserin, grazoprevenir, guanfacine, lemborexant, lumateperone, neratinib, opiates and other CNS depressants, oxcarbazepine, pimavanserin, pretomanib, ranolazine, sonidegib, velpatasvir, venetoclax, zanubrutinib
fosphenytoin (Cerebyx)	status epilepticus (short-term use until phenytoin can be given)	dizziness, itching, numbness, headache, tiredness, decreased movement, hypotension, cardiovascular collapse (rare but serious)	Anticoagulants, chloramphenicol, cimetidine, diltiazem, disulfiram, isoniazid, phenylbutazone, sulfonamides, and trimethoprim may increase phenytoin concentrations. Fosphenytoin may increase anticoagulant effects and chloramphenicol concentrations. Antineoplastic drugs, diazoxide, folic acid, and rifampin may decrease the effect of fosphenytoin.
lacosamide (Vimpat, Vimpat IV)	focal seizure	dizziness, fatigue, headache, nausea, tremors, slurred speech, blurred or double vision	Nicardipine may increase concentrations.
oxcarbazepine (Oxtellar XR, Trileptal)	focal seizure (alternative uses: bipolar disorder, diabetic neuropathy, neuralgia)	abdominal pain, headache, trouble walking, abnormal or double vision, difficulty moving, dizziness, fatigue, nausea, tremors, vomiting, hyponatremia, rapid eye movement, shaking or slowed movements, muscle weakness, sweating	Carbamazepine, phenobarbital, phenytoin, valproic acid, and verapamil may decrease levels. Oxcarbazepine may decrease the effects of oral contraceptives, felodipine, and lamotrigine. Oxcarbazepine may increase levels of phenobarbital and phenytoin.
phenytoin (Dilantin, Phenytek)	tonic-clonic seizure, focal seizure, status epilepticus	decreased coordination, decreased movement, mental confusion, slurred speech, dizziness, headache, insomnia, twitches, nervousness, hepatotoxicity, gingival hyperplasia, hair growth	Anticoagulants, chloramphenicol, cimetidine, diltiazem, disulfiram, isoniazid, phenylbutazone, sulfonamides, and trimethoprim may increase phenytoin concentrations. Phenytoin may increase anticoagulant effects and chloramphenicol concentrations. Antineoplastic drugs, folic acid, and rifampin may decrease the effect of phenytoin.

continues

TABLE 7.3 Common Uses, Side Effects, and Drug Interactions for Sodium Channel Blockers—*Continued*

Generic (Brand)	Common Uses	Side Effects	Selected Drug Interactions
rufinamide (Banzel)	adjunctive treatment of Lennox-Gastaut syndrome	dizziness, drowsiness, headache, nausea, vomiting, aggressive behavior, hyperactivity, anxiety, suicidal ideation, rash, constipation, anemia	ethinyl estradiol, norethindrone, ubrogepant, valproate
vigabatrin (Sabril)	focal seizure	fatigue, headache, confusion, poor coordination, memory loss, tremors, weight gain, blurred vision, depression	Vigabatrin may decrease fosphenytoin and phenytoin levels. Vigabatrin enhances the effects of other CNS depressants.

Dosage Forms and Administration Carbamazepine comes as an oral capsule (that should not be chewed) and an oral suspension that are taken every 12 hours. Carbamazepine is also available in tablet form, some of which can be chewed and some which cannot. Close attention should be paid to providing the correct instructions to patients. Eslicarbazepine is a tablet taken by mouth, and it can be swallowed whole or crushed. Oxcarbazepine comes as a tablet and a suspension usually taken every 12 hours with or without food, and as an extended-release tablet usually taken once a day on an empty stomach.

Side Effects The most common side effect of carbamazepine is a rash that occurs after several weeks of use. The drug should be taken with food to offset gastrointestinal (GI) disturbances. See Table 7.3 for a list of common side effects for these three agents.

Contraindications Carbamazepine use is contraindicated in bone marrow depression, with monoamine oxidase inhibitors (MAOIs) or within 14 days of MAOI use, and with nefazodone. Use of delavirdine or other nonnucleoside reverse transcriptase inhibitors (NNRTIs) is contraindicated with carbamazepine drug therapy. There are no contraindications for eslicarbazepine or oxcarbazepine except in patients with allergies to carbamazepine, oxcarbazepine, or eslicarbazepine. If someone is allergic to one of these drugs, it is likely they are allergic to the others as well.

Cautions and Considerations Carbamazepine has two boxed warnings. One warning is for potentially fatal dermatologic reactions that certain patient populations are more likely to experience. For this reason, genotype testing is recommended for Asian patients who are at a higher risk than patients of other ethnicities. The other boxed warning is for aplastic anemia and agranulocytosis. Hyponatremia is a concern with carbamazepine and oxcarbazepine, and sodium levels should be monitored. Blood monitoring is necessary for patients using these agents, because they can cause anemia and a rare but potentially life-threatening side effect called *drug reaction with eosinophilia and systemic symptoms (DRESS)*.

Drug Interactions As with many other anticonvulsants, carbamazepine, eslicarbazepine, and oxcarbazepine have numerous drug interactions. Patients must work closely with their prescriber and pharmacist to monitor for interactions. Patients who may become pregnant who are taking carbamazepine, eslicarbazepine, and oxcarbazepine must be warned that this drug decreases the effectiveness of oral contraceptives. Patients should also be warned about the potentially debilitating drowsiness associated with oxcarbazepine therapy.

Carbamazepine will not be as effective when taken with these other medications. Because carbamazepine can slow the heartbeat, it should not be taken with antiarrhythmics or other medications that can have this same effect.

Lacosamide and Rufinamide

Lacosamide (Vimpat, Vimpat IV) and **Rufinamide (Banzel)** both work by decreasing abnormal activity in the brain. The mechanism of action for rufinamide is unknown, but in vitro studies suggest that it works by inhibiting sodium channels, making neurons less likely to fire. Lacosamide has few interactions and is a Schedule V drug because it promotes a sensation of euphoria.

Dosage Forms and Administration Lacosamide comes as a tablet, injection, and oral solution. Rufinamide is only available in tablet form.

Side Effects Side effects of lacosamide include dizziness, fatigue, headache, nausea, tremors, slurred speech, and blurred or double vision. Common side effects of rufinamide are similar in that it can cause dizziness, headache, and nausea. Rufinamide can also cause aggressive behavior, anxiety, suicidal ideation, rash, constipation, and anemia.

Contraindications Use of lacosamide is contraindicated in patients with liver abnormalities and blood disorders. There are no contraindications for rufinamide.

Cautions and Considerations Lacosamide has cardiac side effects. Cardiac function should be monitored in patients using it. Rufinamide is used in addition to other anticonvulsants to treat seizures associated with Lennox-Gastaut syndrome. It has a rare but serious, and potentially fatal, side effect called DRESS. Like some other anticonvulsants, rufinamide can also cause Stevens-Johnson syndrome. Patients experiencing rash or fever should be evaluated by their provider right away for more serious effects.

Drug Interactions Lacosamide interacts with lidocaine, mefloquine, mexiletine, and orlistat. Rufinamide can interact with other anticonvulsants such as carbamazepine, phenytoin, and divalproate sodium. In addition, it can interact with clozapine, birth control pills, and alcohol (or other substances that cause drowsiness such as pain medication).

Phenytoin

Safety Alert

When diluting phenytoin for a safe infusion, normal saline is the only suitable vehicle. Phenytoin is one of the few drugs that might be mixed by a nurse outside the pharmacy because it precipitates so quickly.

Phenytoin (Dilantin, Phenytek) is used to manage tonic-clonic and absence seizures and to prevent seizures after head trauma or neurosurgery. It works by promoting sodium ion outflow from cells, thus stabilizing the cell. In some patients, small changes in dosage result in large changes in how much of the drug is present in the blood.

Phenytoin is a drug for which pharmacy technicians may receive requests to dispense the brand-name product. Requests to use the same manufacturer for all phenytoin dispenses for a

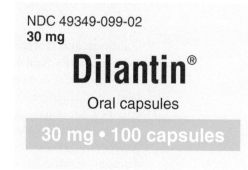

NDC 49349-099-02
30 mg

Dilantin®
Oral capsules

30 mg • 100 capsules

Phenytoin (Dilantin) is most often administered orally. For intravenous administration, fosphenytoin is more frequently used.

particular patient may also occur. The rationale behind these requests is based on the drug's narrow therapeutic index, which is so small that legally allowable differences in drug formulations may pose problems for patients. For most drugs, changes

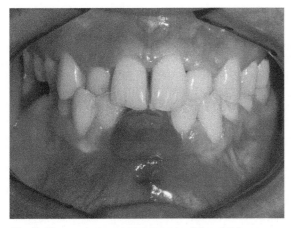

Gingival hyperplasia, or overgrowth of the gingiva (gum), is a side effect of phenytoin use.

this small are negligible, but for antiepileptic drugs, these changes can result in significant variations in efficacy.

Dosage Forms and Administration IV phenytoin should be mixed or prepared using only normal saline. Oral suspensions of phenytoin must be shaken well—as should any medication in suspension form.

Side Effects Phenytoin should be discontinued if a rash appears. A phenytoin rash, even a mild one, can progress to life-threatening Stevens-Johnson syndrome and should prompt concern. Side effects may or may not be related to dosage and may be reversible when the dosage is reduced. Table 7.4 lists phenytoin's side effects related and unrelated to dose.

Contraindications Phenytoin has a particularly large number of drug interactions, so it is important for technicians to obtain accurate drug lists for patients using phenytoin. Use of delavirdine or other nonnucleoside reverse transcriptase inhibitors (NNRTIs) is contraindicated with carbamazepine, phenytoin, and fosphenytoin drug therapy. Due to absorption problems, phenytoin and antacids should be administered several hours apart.

TABLE 7.4 **Phenytoin's and Fosphenytoin's Side Effects**

Dose Related	ataxia (irregularity of muscular action)
	diplopia (the perception of two images of a single object)
	dizziness
	drowsiness
	encephalopathy (degenerative brain disease)
	involuntary movements when concentration is greater than 30 mcg/mL
Nondose Related	gingival hyperplasia (abnormal tissue growth that increases the volume of the tissue covering the tooth-bearing border of the jaw)
	peripheral neuropathy (noninflammatory pathologic disturbance or pathologic change in peripheral nerves, commonly in the arms or legs; pain in the extremities)
	vitamin deficiencies

Cautions and Considerations Intravenous (IV) phenytoin is considered a "high alert" drug due to safety concerns with use. This drug is considered a vesicant (agent that induces blistering), and injection can cause **phlebitis** (inflammation of the vein). Extravasation (when a drug administered intravenously leaks into the tissue surrounding the vein in which it is being given) should be avoided. Additionally, IV phenytoin may cause hypotension and should be infused no faster than 50 mg/min.

Phenytoin should be avoided in patients who have certain cardiac issues (including sinus bradycardia, sinoatrial block, second- or third-degree atrioventricular [AV] block, and Stokes-Adams syndrome), who experience a rash during treatment, or who are being treated for absence seizures. Phenytoin should be avoided in patients with a hypersensitivity to hydantoins.

Drug Interactions Phenytoin is highly bound to protein in the bloodstream, and it interacts with many other medications that are also bound to protein. All alerts for drug interactions should be taken seriously, and the pharmacist must evaluate each one carefully. Phenytoin can adhere to nasogastric (nasal passage to stomach) tubing. If it is given through a tube into the stomach, it must be mixed well with normal saline and separated by two hours from feedings given through the same tube.

Fosphenytoin

Safety Alert

Fosphenytoin is dosed differently from other drugs. Instead of being based on weight (such as milligrams), fosphenytoin is dosed as milligrams of phenytoin equivalents: 1 mg of phenytoin = 1 mg phenytoin equivalent = 1.5 mg fosphenytoin. Pharmacy technicians should be aware that milligrams of fosphenytoin are not the same as milligrams of phenytoin equivalents.

Fosphenytoin (Cerebyx) can be used instead of IV phenytoin. It is a prodrug (precursor or inactive form) that is rapidly converted to phenytoin after administration. It has the advantage of being water soluble and, therefore, better tolerated.

Dosage Forms and Administration Fosphenytoin is available as an injection. Being water soluble means fosphenytoin has fewer infusion reactions (pain, burning, or tissue damage) and is a more reliable treatment than phenytoin.

Side Effects Fosphenytoin does have an unusual side effect of brief, intense itching, usually in the groin, which might be a reaction to the phosphate in the injection, but this reaction is not an allergic response. Other side effects of fosphenytoin can include dizziness, headache, tiredness, and decreased movement. Fosphenytoin can lower blood pressure and must be monitored as it can potentially contribute to cardiovascular collapse.

Fosphenytoin should be discontinued if a rash appears. A fosphenytoin rash, even a mild one, can progress to life-threatening Stevens-Johnson syndrome and should prompt concern.

Contraindications Use of delavirdine or other nonnucleoside reverse transcriptase inhibitors is contraindicated with phenytoin and fosphenytoin drug therapy. Fosphenytoin is not a vesicant like phenytoin is; thus, it can be safer to administer.

Cautions and Considerations Fosphenytoin has a boxed warning regarding the rate of infusion. Fosphenytoin is always dosed in phenytoin equivalents (PE) per kilogram. The rate of administration of fosphenytoin (PE/min) should not exceed 150 PE/min due to risk of severe hypotension and cardiac arrythmias. Fosphenytoin should be avoided in patients who have certain cardiac issues (including sinus bradycardia, sinoatrial block, second- or third-degree atrioventricular [AV] block, or Stokes-Adams syndrome), who experience a rash during treatment, or who are being treated for absence seizures. Fosphenytoin should be avoided in patients with a hypersensitivity to hydantoins.

Drug Interactions Like phenytoin, fosphenytoin is highly bound to protein in the bloodstream, and it interacts with many other medications that are also bound to protein. All alerts for drug interactions should be taken seriously, and the pharmacist must evaluate each one carefully. Fosphenytoin can adhere to nasogastric tubing. If it is given through a tube into the stomach, it must be mixed well with normal saline and separated by two hours from feedings given through the same tube.

Vigabatrin

Vigabatrin (Sabril) is used only as an adjunct drug for seizures that do not respond to other drugs, because it can cause permanent loss of vision. Only qualified prescribers (those who have undergone required training) can order this drug, and it is shipped directly to the patient.

Dosage Forms and Administration Vigabatrin is available as an oral powder and tablet. Patients using the drug receive baseline vision testing as well as follow-up visits every three months. These visits continue for up to six months after the patient has stopped taking the drug.

Side Effects Side effects of vigabatrin include fatigue, headache, confusion, poor coordination, memory loss, tremors, weight gain, blurred vision, and depression.

Contraindications There are no contraindications for vigabatrin.

Cautions and Considerations Serious vision problems may occur in patients who take vigabatrin, so frequent eye examinations are necessary.

Calcium Channel Blockers

Calcium channel blockers are anticonvulsants that work to stabilize the neuronal membrane. Calcium is a positively charged ion, which excites neuronal cells and makes them more likely to fire. Blocking calcium channels makes neurons less likely to inappropriately fire. Calcium channel blockers include ethosuximide, valproate, and zonisamide.

Ethosuximide (Zarontin) is used for absence seizures and increases the seizure threshold. A **seizure threshold** is a person's likelihood to have a seizure. The higher the threshold, the less likely it is that a seizure will occur. Patients should have a complete blood count (CBC) every four months during therapy.

Zonisamide (Zonegran) is a sulfonamide with anticonvulsant activity. Patients must be warned about potentially serious sulfonamide reactions, and pharmacy technicians should check for sulfa allergies when dispensing this drug. Patients should also be instructed to report any skin rashes and to drink six to eight glasses of water a day to reduce the risk of developing kidney stones.

Valproate is a drug available as **divalproex sodium (Depakote, Depakote ER, Depakote Sprinkle)**. Valproate blocks sodium channels, and it increases GABA levels. It is also indicated for treating manic episodes in bipolar disorder (see Chapter 8) and for managing absence seizures, mixed seizure types, and tonic-clonic seizures. Valproate may also be effective for focal seizures and infantile (early childhood) spasms.

Dosage Forms and Administration Patients should take oral divalproex sodium with water (not with a carbonated beverage) and should pay close attention to intructions about whether they can chew, break, or crush the tablets or capsules. Some of the products can be chewed, but others cannot. Some capsules can be opened and the contents sprinkled on food. Patients should be warned not to use aspirin or aspirin products, because these products could lead to serious valproate toxicity. Routine hepatic and hematologic tests are indicated during therapy. Patients should report severe or persistent sore throat, fever, fatigue, bleeding, or bruising. Because of its long half-life, ethosuximide can usually be given once daily to achieve therapeutic plasma concentrations, but it is often divided between two daily doses to reduce GI side effects. Patients should be told to take the dose with food and not to discontinue it abruptly. See Table 7.3 for additional dosage information for calcium channel blockers.

Side Effects Calcium channel blockers may cause headaches, drowsiness, dizziness, nausea, vomiting, and impaired judgment and coordination.

Contraindications Ethosuximide is contraindicated in patients with a history of sensitivity to succinimides. Divalproex sodium should not be used in patients who have a hypersensitivity to divalproex or divalproex derivatives, liver disease, urea cycle disorders, and mitochondrial disorders. Zonisamide use should be avoided in patients with a sulfonamide hypersensitivity.

Cautions and Considerations Divalproex sodium has several boxed warnings. One warning is for liver failure, which usually occurs within the first six months of therapy. The risk is increased in patients with inherited deoxyribonucleic acid (DNA) mutations. Liver function tests should be performed in patients using valproic acid. Other boxed warnings are for pancreatitis and for the risk of fetal malformations when used during pregnancy. Divalproex sodium should not be taken with aspirin or carbonated beverages. Ethosuximide, however, works best when taken with food. Zonisamide has been associated with glaucoma; metabolic acidosis; elevated ammonia in the bloodstream; signficiant psychiatric, including suicidal ideation; and serious allergic reactions. Patients will be monitored closely for any of these effects.

Drug Interactions Selected drug interactions are listed in Table 7.5.

TABLE 7.5 Common Uses, Side Effects, and Drug Interactions for Calcium Channel Blockers

Generic (Brand)	Common Uses	Side Effects	Selected Drug Interactions
ethosuximide (Zarontin)	absence seizure	drowsiness, headache, dizziness, hiccups, aggression, fatigue, difficulty moving, loss of appetite, stomach upset, diarrhea, nightmares	Carbamazepine, nevirapine, phenytoin, phenobarbital, primidone, ritonavir, and valproic acid decrease levels.
divalproex sodium (Depakote)	focal, absence, and tonic-clonic seizures	dizziness, headache, nausea, vomiting, tremors, diarrhea, drowsiness, hair loss, hepatotoxicity	estrogen-containing oral contraceptives, meropenem, rifampin concentrations Salicylates increase effects.
zonisamide (Zonegran)	focal seizure (alternative uses: binge-eating disorder, obesity)	drowsiness, dizziness, loss of appetite, headache, nausea, irritability, difficulty thinking, sulfa allergy, kidney stones	Carbamazepine, phenobarbital, and phenytoin may decrease levels.

GABA Enhancers

Gamma-aminobutyric acid (GABA) is a neurotransmitter that is present throughout the CNS. GABA is capable of inhibiting neuron firing. Reducing GABA can be proconvulsant; increasing GABA can be anticonvulsant.

Gabapentin (Neurontin) is used as an adjunct for drug-refractory (not responsive to treatment) focal seizures. It is not effective for absence seizures. Gabapentin was designed to mimic the neurotransmitter GABA, but studies have shown that it must have another mechanism of action.

Gabapentin is a well-accepted treatment option for patients with diabetic neuropathy, a stinging and burning pain that results from nerve damage due to complications of diabetes. Because it is generally well tolerated and easy to use, gabapentin is a very popular drug.

Pregabalin (Lyrica) reduces the release of several neurotransmitters, including glutamate, norepinephrine, and substance P (a sensory neurotransmitter mediating pain, touch, and temperature). Pregabalin is thought to bind to calcium channels and modulate calcium influx. Pregabalin is structurally similar to gabapentin. Pregabalin produces fewer side effects than gabapentin and other anticonvulsant drugs, probably because it is efficacious at lower doses. Pregabalin can be titrated (dose adjusted) more readily and may have a faster onset. It is approved as an adjunct only for focal seizures. It is important to remember that pregabalin is classified as a controlled substance (Schedule V) because it can cause euphoria and withdrawal. It is also approved to treat diabetic neuropathy and nerve pain that continues after shingles. It must not be stopped abruptly.

Phenobarbital is used for tonic-clonic and focal seizures because it interferes with the transmission of impulses from the thalamus to the cortex of the brain.

Primidone (Mysoline) is indicated in tonic-clonic and complex focal seizures. Metabolic reactions in the liver transform primidone into phenobarbital, so the therapeutic and side effect profiles are similar to those of phenobarbital. Because megaloblastic anemia is a rare and serious side effect of primidone, annual CBCs are recommended.

Tiagabine (Gabitril) blocks the reabsorption of GABA, which allows GABA to bind to nerve cells that may enhance normal brain activity. Tiagabine should be taken with food and must be tapered if stopped. Tiagabine can cause seizures, which has occurred in patients who do not have epilepsy but take tiagabine for other uses.

Dosage Forms and Administration All GABA enhancers are available in oral dosage formulations. The various dosage forms are listed in Table 7.3. Tiagabine should be taken with food and must be tapered if stopped.

Side Effects Side effects of gabapention include fatigue, headache, confusion, poor coordination, memory loss, and blurred vision. These effects can subside after a few weeks of therapy. Other side effects can include tremors, weight gain, and depression.

Contraindications Gabapentin and pregabalin do not have contraindications. Phenobarbital should not be used in patients with liver impairment, shortness of breath or airway obstruction, porphyria, or sedative addiction. Primidone use is contraindicated in porphyria. Tiagabine has no contraindications.

Cautions and Considerations Tiagabine has a boxed warning for an increased risk of seizures when used to treat conditions other than epilepsy. Phenobarbital and pregabalin are controlled substances. With the use of these drugs, patients can develop tolerance. Use of alcohol and other CNS depressants should be avoided when taking phenobarbital. The drug should not be stopped abruptly. Phenobarbital is a Schedule IV agent because it has abuse potential. It can cause drowsiness and paradoxical hyperexcitability in children and older adults. Periodic blood tests are required. If the patient has a rash or exhibits excessive drowsiness, ataxia, dysphagia (difficulty swallowing), slurred speech, or confusion while taking this drug, the prescriber should be notified immediately.

Drug Interactions When filling a prescription for phenobarbital, the pharmacy technician should always check the patient's profile in the computer for other drugs being prescribed because phenobarbital has several interactions. Patients taking primidone must be warned that this drug decreases the effectiveness of oral contraceptives. Other selected drug interactions are listed in Table 7.6.

TABLE 7.6 Common Uses, Side Effects, and Drug Interactions for GABA Enhancers

Generic (Brand)	Common Uses	Side Effects	Selected Drug Interactions
gabapentin (Neurontin)	focal seizure (alternative uses: diabetic neuropathy, neuralgia, shingles, fibromyalgia, hot flashes, hiccups, restless legs syndrome, others)	dizziness, drowsiness, fatigue, nausea, vomiting, diarrhea, dry mouth, swelling in legs/arms, abnormal thinking, difficulty moving, weight gain	Gabapentin enhances the effects of other CNS depressants.
phenobarbital	tonic-clonic seizure, status epilepticus (alternative use: sedative for anxiety and insomnia)	fatigue, drowsiness, hepatotoxicity, aggression or mood changes, hypotension	Oxcarbazepine, phenytoin, rufinamide, and valproic acid increase levels. Alcohol ingestion may enhance CNS depression.
pregabalin (Lyrica)	focal seizure, neuropathic pain, fibromyalgia	dizziness, drowsiness, dry mouth, blurred vision, fluid retention, weight gain	Pregabalin enhances the effects of other CNS depressants.
primidone (Mysoline)	tonic-clonic seizure (alternative use: tremors)	difficulty moving, dizziness, nausea, vomiting, loss of appetite, fatigue, mood changes, impotence, double vision	Carbamazepine and phenytoin decrease levels of primidone and its metabolite, phenobarbital. Primidone deceases levels of carbamazepine, dronedarone, protease inhibitors, ticagrelor, and tolvaptan. Levels and the effects of estrogen-based oral contraceptives are decreased. Alcohol ingestion may enhance CNS depression.
tiagabine (Gabitril)	focal seizure (alternative use: bipolar disorder)	dizziness, drowsiness, nausea, nervousness, tremors, abdominal pain, abnormal thinking, depression	Barbiturates, carbamazepine, and phenytoin decrease levels. Tiagabine enhances the effects of other CNS depressants.

Glutamate Inhibitors

Glutamate is an excitatory neurotransmitter. Blocking glutamate decreases neuronal activity and has anticonvulsant action.

Lamotrigine (Lamictal, Lamictal CD, Lamictal ODT, Lamictal XR) provides **adjunct therapy** (used in combination with another drug for improved effect) for adults with focal seizures, with or without generalized secondary seizures. (A secondary seizure is a seizure that occurs from something other than epilepsy, such as a fever.) Lamotrigine can also be used to treat bipolar disorder. Lamotrigine works by blocking sodium channels, thereby reducing neuron excitation.

Perampanel (Fycompa) is prescribed for tonic-clonic and focal seizures in children and adults. Perampanel should be used with caution in patients with psychiatric conditions or prior history of aggressive behavior, because it can worsen these conditions.

Topiramate (Qudexy XR, Topamax, Trokendi XR) is prescribed for treating focal seizures in adults. Although its mechanism of action is not well understood, the most common theories propose that topiramate blocks sodium channels, enhancing the activity of GABA and antagonizing glutamate receptors. It is used as an adjunct therapy to carbamazepine and phenytoin. It works well but causes significant cognitive effects (including slowed thinking, slowed speech, and difficulty concentrating). Therapy should start with a low dose and be titrated slowly over eight weeks.

Felbamate (Felbatol) is used for tonic-clonic and focal seizures.

Dosage Forms and Administration Topiramate therapy should start with a low dose that is slowly adjusted over eight weeks. See Table 7.2 for dosage forms and routes of administration for glutamate inhibitors.

Side Effects Common side effects of glutamate inhibitors include dizziness and nausea. For a more detailed list of side effects and drug interactions for each drug, see Table 7.7.

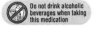

Contraindications Felbamate use should be avoided in patients with carbamate sensitivity, a history of blood dyscrasia, or liver impairment. Topiramate in the extended-release formula is contraindicated in patients with recent alcohol use and in those with metabolic acidosis who are also taking metformin. Lamotrigine, perampanel, and immediate-release topiramate have no contraindications.

Cautions and Considerations Glutamate inhibitors can increase suicidal ideation. Patients should be monitored in the first few weeks of therapy for this effect. Felbamate has boxed warnings for aplastic anemia and liver failure. Felbamate should not be used in patients with liver dysfunction or hematologic problems. Both conditions may be exacerbated by felbamate. Lamotrigine has a boxed warning for potentially fatal rashes. In fact, lamotrigine doses must be adjusted slowly because of the risk of rash. Slow titration decreases the incidence of rash. Topiramate may cause metabolic acidosis. Blood chemistries should be monitored in patients using topiramate. Parampanel must be used with caution in patients with psychiatric disorders, especially depression. Because parampanel can cause dizziness, it can pose a fall risk for older patients.

Lamotrigine does not affect serum concentrations of phenobarbital, phenytoin, or primidone, but it may affect the pharmacokinetics or pharmacodynamics of carbamazepine and valproate. The drug has a boxed warning about fatal rashes. Patients should be advised to call their physician immediately if a rash appears, but the drug should not be discontinued abruptly. Life-threatening rashes with this drug are much more common in children, and lamotrigine is not to be used in patients less than 16 years old.

Use of alcohol while taking perampanel should be avoided. This drug should be used with caution in patients with kidney or liver impairment.

Patients should drink plenty of water during use of topiramate.

Felbamate poses the risk of developing aplastic anemia, liver failure, or both (it has both boxed warnings). Patients must be fully advised of these risks and sign a waiver consenting to the use of felbamate.

Drug Interactions Patients who may become pregnant and are taking topiramate must be warned that this drug may decrease the effectiveness of oral contraceptives. As with many other anticonvulsants, perampanel has numerous drug interactions. Patients must work closely with their prescriber and pharmacist to monitor for interactions.

Topiramate can increase phenytoin levels. It is a weak carbonic anhydrase inhibitor, so it increases the risk of kidney stones. Other drug interactions are listed in Table 7.7.

TABLE 7.7 Common Uses, Side Effects, and Drug Interactions for Glutamate Inhibitors

Generic (Brand)	Common Uses	Side Effects	Selected Drug Interactions
felbamate (Felbatol)	tonic-clonic seizure, focal seizure	insomnia, loss of appetite, weight loss, nausea, vomiting, headache, dizziness, fatigue, acne, rash, constipation, diarrhea	Carbamazepine and phenytoin decrease levels. Felbamate enhances the effects of drugs that increase the QT interval.
lamotrigine (Lamictal, Lamictal CD, Lamictal ODT, Lamictal XR)	tonic-clonic seizure, focal seizure (alternative use: bipolar disorder)	rash, decreased coordination/movement, dizziness, headache, insomnia, fatigue, rash, nausea, vomiting, blurred or double vision	Acetaminophen, carbamazepine, estrogen-containing oral contraceptives, phenobarbital, phenytoin, and rifampin decrease concentrations. Valproic acid increases levels.
perampanel (Fycompa)	tonic-clonic seizure, focal seizure	dizziness, vertigo, hostility, aggressive behavior, drowsiness, headache, rash, nausea, vomiting, urinary tract infection, bruising, back pain, blurred or double vision, cough	azelastine, buprenorphine, carbamazepine, CNS depressants, dabrafenib, droperidol, enzalutamide, lemborexant, mefloquine, mitotane, opiates, oxomemazine, thalidomide, zolpidem
topiramate (Qudexy XR, Topamax, Trokendi XR)	tonic-clonic seizure, focal seizure (alternative use: migraine)	dizziness, numbness, memory problems, depression, kidney stones, insomnia, nausea, fatigue, loss of appetite, weight loss	Carbamazepine, phenytoin, and valproic acid decrease levels. Hydrochlorothiazide increases concentrations. Topiramate may decrease the effectiveness of digoxin, oral contraceptives, and valproic acid.

Synaptic Vesicle Protein Binders

Synaptic vesicle protein binder anticonvulsants include brivaracetam and levetiracetam. **Brivaracetam (Briviact)** is used for focal seizures in patients at least 4 years old (oral dosage form) and in patients at least 16 years old (injectible dosage form). Brivaracetam can cause decreased white blood cell count and DRESS, so it must be monitored with blood testing.

Levetiracetam (Elepsia XR, Keppra, Keppra XR, Roweepra, Spritam) is an adjunct therapy for focal seizures. Its mechanism of action is unknown, and it is structurally unrelated to other anticonvulsants. It was initially developed to improve cognition (learning, memory). The pharmacokinetics of this drug are predictable. There is little potential for drug interactions, and no serum monitoring is required, so dispensing this drug is fairly easy. However, there is no evidence that dosages greater than 3,000 mg a day are effective, so pharmacy technicians should watch the dosage and alert the pharmacist if a prescriber orders a higher dosage.

Dosage Forms and Administration Brivaracetam and levetiracetam can be taken with or without food. Brivaracetam should be swallowed whole (not chewed or crushed). Brivaracetam must be monitored with blood testing. See Table 7.2 for additional dosage information for synaptic vesicle protein binders.

Side Effects Levetiracetam and brivaracetam both cause drowziness. See Table 7.8 for additional details and selected drug interactions.

Contraindications Brivaracetam and levetiracetam have no contraindications.

Cautions and Considerations Levetiracetam and brivaracetam may cause CNS depression. It should be used with caution in patients using other CNS depressants.

Psychiatric symptoms such as psychosis, paranoia, and hallucinations may occur with levetiracetam use. Suicidal ideation may also occur. Patients should be monitored for changes in behavior that suggest suicidal thoughts and depression. Selected drug interactions are listed in Table 7.8.

Drug Interactions Levetiracetam and brivaracetam have numerous drug interactions. Prescribers and pharmacists should be informed of a patient's medications to ensure interactions are avoided.

TABLE 7.8 Common Uses, Side Effects, and Drug Interactions for Synaptic Vesicle Protein Binders

Generic (Brand)	Common Uses	Side Effects	Selected Drug Interactions
brivaracetam (Briviact)	focal seizure	drowsiness, fatigue, abnormal gait, vertigo, psychiatric disturbances, weakness, vision disturbances, nausea, vomiting, constipation, blood abnormalities, suicidal ideation	azelastine, droperidol, CNS depressants, flunitrazepam, lemborexant, levetiracetam, opiates, orphenadrine, oxomemazine, suvorexant, thalidomide, zolpidem
levetiracetam (Elepsia XR, Keppra, Keppra XR, Roweepra, Spritam)	focal seizure	dizziness, drowsiness, lack of energy, depression, behavioral changes, psychosis	Levetiracetam enhances the effects of other CNS depressants.

7.3 Parkinson's Disease and Drug Treatments

Parkinson's disease (PD) is characterized by muscular difficulties and postural abnormalities. It usually affects individuals over age 60. Three characteristic signs of PD are tremors while resting, rigidity, and akinesia (absence of movement). These signs may manifest as poor posture control, shuffling gait, and loss of overall muscle control (e.g., flexed stance, difficulty turning, and hurried gait). With the population of older adults increasing in number, this debilitating disease may become more prevalent in the coming years.

PD occurs as a result of pathologic alterations in the extrapyramidal system, a complex functional unit of the CNS involved in controlling motor activities. The extrapyramidal system is composed of the **basal ganglia** (also known as *basal nuclei*); these are symmetric masses of gray matter (a type of neural tissue in the CNS) embedded in the lower portions of the brain. PD is the most common of the extrapyramidal diseases. No definitive test exists for this disease, so it is diagnosed almost exclusively by its symptoms.

Voluntary movement requires complex neurochemical messaging in the brain. Electrical currents and neurotransmitters carry nerve impulses from the cerebral cortex to the basal nuclei and back to the cerebral cortex via the thalamus (see Figure 7.5 for the features of the brain). Transmission of information about the initiation of movement, muscle tone, and posture is affected by the balance of neurotransmitters in the basal nuclei. Normal movement requires that two neurotransmitters—dopamine, an inhibitor, and ACh, an excitatory—be in balance.

In a healthy person, dopaminergic neurons (neurons that release dopamine when they fire) in the **substantia nigra** (a dark-gray structure in two parts found deep within the midbrain and illustrated in Figure 7.6) release an amount of dopamine sufficient to control the stimulating effect of ACh on muscle movements. In PD, however, there is progressive destruction of dopaminergic neurons in the nigrostriatal pathway (pathway joining the substantia nigra and the corpus striatum; see Figures 7.5 and 7.6), so an insufficient amount of dopamine is produced to counterbalance ACh production. This dopamine deficiency results in a predominance of cholinergic neuronal activity, which produces excessive motor nerve stimulation.

Currently, there is no cure for PD, so the goals of treatment are to minimize disability and help patients maintain the highest possible quality of life. Drug therapy for PD has greatly improved the functional ability and clinical status of patients, and temporary remission from the disease can allow patients to live productive lives. Nevertheless, drug therapy is aimed only at symptomatic relief; it cannot alter the underlying disease process. Levodopa / carbidopa is the most commonly used drug therapy for PD, but the search continues for new agents to prolong the length of effective treatment or reverse the disease. Table 7.9 presents the most commonly used agents for patients who have PD.

The side effects of the drugs can be a problem in the treatment of PD, which may necessitate constant changes in medication. Often, the patient needs emotional and psychological support as well.

FIGURE 7.5
Cutaway View of the Brain

Major features of the brain.

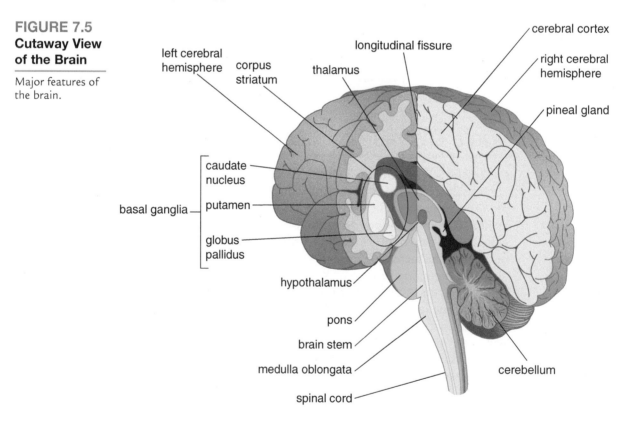

FIGURE 7.6
Substantia Nigra

In PD, damaged or destroyed cells in the substantia nigra result in an interruption of nerve impulses to the part of the brain that controls movement.

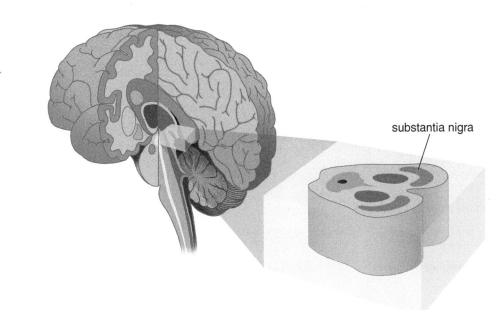

substantia nigra

TABLE 7.9 Commonly Used Agents for Parkinson's Disease

Generic (Brand)	Pronunciation	Dosage Form	Common Dosage	Dispensing Status
levodopa / carbidopa (Duopa, Rytary, Sinemet)	lee-voe-DOE-pa kar-bi-DOE-pa	capsule, oral suspension, tablet	individualized to patient	Rx
levodopa / carbidopa / entacapone (Stalevo)	lee-voe-DOE-pa kar-bi-DOE-pa en-TAK-a-pone	tablet	individualized to patient	Rx
Dopamine Agonists				
apomorphine (Apokyn)	a-poe-MOR-feen	sublingual tablet, injection	0–30 mg per dose up to 5 times a day	Rx
bromocriptine (Cycloset, Parlodel)	broe-moe-KRIP-teen	capsule, tablet	individualized to patient	Rx
pramipexole (Mirapex, Mirapex ER)	pra-mi-PEX-ole	tablet	0.375 mg–4.5 mg a day	Rx
ropinirole (Requip, Requip XL)	ro-PIN-a-role	tablet	12–24 mg a day	Rx
rotigotine (Neupro)	roe-TIG-oh-teen	transdermal patch	2–6 mg a day	Rx
Anticholinergics				
benztropine (Cogentin)	BENZ-troe-peen	tablet	3–6 mg a day	Rx
trihexyphenidyl	trye-hex-ee-FEN-i-dill	oral solution, tablet	5–15 mg per day	Rx
Catechol-O-Methyltransferase (COMT) Inhibitors				
entacapone (Comtan)	en-TAK-a-pone	tablet	200 mg with each levodopa / carbidopa dose	Rx
tolcapone (Tasmar)	TOLE-ka-pone	tablet	100 mg with each levodopa / carbidopa dose	Rx

continues

TABLE 7.9 Commonly Used Agents for Parkinson's Disease—*Continued*

Generic (Brand)	Pronunciation	Dosage Form	Common Dosage	Dispensing Status
Monoamine Oxidase Inhibitors (MAOIs)				
rasagiline (Azilect)	ra-SAJ-i-leen	tablet	0.5–1 mg a day	Rx
safinamide (Xadago)	sa-FIN-a-mide	tablet	50 mg a day	Rx
selegiline (Eldepryl, Emsam, Zelapar)	seh-LEDGE-ah-leen	capsule, tablet, transdermal patch	1.25–5 mg a day	Rx
Other Agents				
amantadine (Gocovri, Osmolex ER, Symmetrel)	a-MAN-ta-deen	capsule, oral syrup, tablet	100 mg	Rx
istradefylline (Nourianz)	IS-tra-DEF-i-lin	tablet	20–40 mg a day	Rx

Levodopa / Carbidopa and Dopamine Agonists

Dopamine agonists are the mainstay of treatment for PD. This group of drugs either replaces dopamine or mimics its action in the brain. Levodopa is widely recognized as the most effective treatment for PD because it significantly improves movement and restores normal function. Unfortunately, the effects of this drug (especially its ability to restore control of movement, or "on" time, to patients) wear off over time.

Levodopa crosses the blood-brain barrier (a barrier that prevents many substances from crossing capillary walls into brain tissues) and is metabolized in the brain into dopamine, which does not itself cross the blood-brain barrier. Levodopa is also converted into dopamine by the peripheral tissues, so the brain does not receive the full dose. On its own, levodopa has very undesirable effects, so it is usually taken in a combination product that includes carbidopa.

The addition of carbidopa prevents loss of levodopa from the CNS by conversion to dopamine in the peripheral nervous system, resulting in fewer dopaminergic side effects. Carbidopa does not affect the CNS's metabolism of levodopa, and lower doses of levodopa can be used as brain concentrations of dopamine increase. Levodopa / carbidopa provides a smoother, more rapid induction into therapy than levodopa alone. Consequently, **levodopa / carbidopa (Duopa, Rytary, Sinemet)** is the most commonly used drug combination for PD.

Another problem with levodopa is the **on-off phenomenon**, which occurs in as many as two-thirds of patients after about five years of therapy. This phenomenon is a wide fluctuation of functional states, ranging from hyperkinetic to hypokinetic, potentially occurring several times a day. The hyperkinetic (abnormally increased motor function) state is characterized by **dyskinesia** (impairment of the power of voluntary movement) and good functional status; the hypokinetic (abnormally diminished motor activity) state is characterized by akinesia or "freezing" episodes and painful dystonic (characterized by disordered muscle tone) spasms. These fluctuations are associated primarily with the availability of levodopa at dopamine receptors in the CNS. The dosage of levodopa / carbidopa must be limited because of the potential for nausea, vomiting, and cardiac arrhythmia.

Patients may be well controlled on levodopa for several years and then suddenly assume a state of akinesia, masked facies (a relentless, unblinking stare without emotional expressiveness), and stooped posture. The drug may just as suddenly start working again. It also causes neuropsychiatric disorders, dementia (organic loss of intellectual function), loss of memory, hallucinations, and orthostatic hypotension (reduced blood pressure in certain positions, due to inhibition of neurons responsible for vasoconstriction). Levodopa should be carefully titrated to provide optimal control at minimal doses so that the on-off phenomenon is delayed as long as possible.

Apomorphine (Apokyn) is a self-injected agent used for acute treatment of intermittent "off" time (the inability to move). Despite its name, apomorphine is not an opioid drug. It should not be used regularly; instead, it is saved for when levodopa wears off more quickly than anticipated. Apomorphine boosts the effects of levodopa until the next dose can be taken. If repeated doses of apomorphine are needed, adjustments in other therapies should be made to prevent frequent "off" times. Apomorphine is only available through specialty pharmacies.

Bromocriptine (Cycloset, Parlodel) is an ergot alkaloid with dopaminergic properties. It improves symptoms of PD by directly stimulating dopamine receptors in the corpus striatum (see Figure 7.5). It is typically used with levodopa or levodopa / carbidopa.

Dopamine agonists offer an alternative without some of the movement effects that levodopa causes, but they are not always as effective as levodopa. The average period for which a dopaminergic drug will work without significant side effects is about five years. **Pramipexole (Mirapex, Mirapex ER)** is a dopamine agonist. This drug works as well as other antiparkinsonian drugs but has fewer side effects. Unlike bromocriptine, pramipexole is not an ergot derivative. Pramipexole should be prescribed early in the disease, either as a monotherapy or in combination with levodopa / carbidopa. It should be taken with food to reduce nausea. Pramipexole is approved for restless legs syndrome (see the section on restless legs syndrome later in this chapter). It may help with the pain of fibromyalgia and with bipolar disorder but is not yet approved for these uses.

Ropinirole (Requip, Requip XL), like pramipexole, is a dopamine agonist. The precise mechanism of action is unknown. Ropinirole can be taken without regard to food. Hypotension, especially at the beginning of therapy or dose escalation, can cause severe dizziness, especially with a change in position. Ropinirole is also approved for restless legs syndrome.

Rotigotine (Neupro) is a dopamine agonist used for treatment of PD and restless syndrome in adults. The benefit of rotigotine is that it comes as a patch and thus can help patients avoid having to take multiple doses a day. It is applied once daily. Rotigotine is generally well tolerated but can cause stomach upset, drowsiness, headache, and irritation at the site of application.

Dosage Forms and Administration Bromocriptine should be taken with food or milk. The patient should limit use of alcohol and avoid exposure to cold. Blood pressure should be closely monitored when taking bromocriptine. Pramipexole should be taken with food. Apomorphine and levodopa / carbidopa can be taken without regard to food. Levodopa / carbidopa capsules should not be chewed or crushed.

Side Effects In addition to the on-off phenomenon and the dyskinesia that levodopa / carbidopa can cause, common side effects can include dizziness, headache, nausea, constipation, and low blood pressure. Some patients experience insomnia, anxiety, and abnormal dreams. It can also cause changes in kidney function that should be monitored. Drowsiness, nausea, and hypotension are the most common side effects of bromocriptine. Bromocriptine also inhibits prolactin secretion and has been used to stop milk production in patients who are breast-feeding.

Contraindications Use of levodopa / carbidopa is contraindicated in patients with narrow-angle glaucoma, recent MAOI use, melanoma, or undiagnosed skin lesions. Apomorphine should not be administered intravenously, and its use is contraindicated in patients taking a serotonin (5-HT) antagonist. Bromocriptine should be avoided in patients with a hypersensitivity to ergot alkaloids. Pramipexole, ropinirole, and rotigotine do not have contraindications.

Cautions and Considerations Apomorphine should not be taken along with antiemetic agents such as ondansetron, granisetron, or alosetron. If a patient complains of nausea and drug treatment is needed, other antiemetic medications should be used.

Apomorphine comes in a self-injector pen. The pharmacist should teach the patient how to use the pen if that patient has not been instructed already. Ampules and cartridges for the injector can be stored at room temperature. If syringes are prefilled with apomorphine, they can be stored in the refrigerator for one day.

Drug Interactions Antipsychotics and anticholinergics may diminish the antiparkinsonian effects of these drugs. The adverse effects of bupropion may be enhanced by levodopa and dopamine agonists. These agents may enhance the hypotensive effects of MAOIs.

Apomorphine's hypotensive effects may be enhanced by antiemetics such as ondansetron, alesotron, and granisetron. Apomorphine may enhance the effects of agents that prolong the QT interval. (See Chapter 10.) Apomorphine may also increase the serum concentration of pimozide.

Pramipexole and ropinirole may diminish the therapeutic effect of sulpiride. Sulpiride may diminish the therapeutic effect of pramipexole and ropinirole.

Rotigotine can cause hallucinations in patients with preexisting psychotic disorders. It can also affect or increase impulse control disorders, such as gambling, shopping, and binge eating. Because interactions are numerous for these drugs, patients should inform their prescriber and pharmacist about all medications that they take.

Anticholinergics

Anticholinergic agents are used early in PD to treat mild symptoms (primarily tremors). They are used later in the disease progression as adjunct therapy for the movement side effects caused by levodopa. By blocking muscarinic receptors in the brain, anticholinergics help balance cholinergic activity and reduce tremors. (See Table 7.9 for information on these drugs.)

Benztropine (Cogentin) blocks central cholinergic receptors, helping to balance cholinergic activity in the basal ganglia. Indications for the use of this drug are acute dystonic reactions, PD, and drug-induced extrapyramidal reactions (such as those caused by antipsychotics). Benztropine may also prolong dopamine's effects by blocking dopamine reuptake.

Trihexyphenidyl is a widely used, centrally acting anticholinergic agent. It appears to be useful for relieving tremors in PD.

Dosage Forms and Administration Trihexyphenidyl should be administered after meals to prevent GI irritation. Trihexyphenidyl should not be discontinued abruptly. The starting dosage of trihexyphenidyl is 0.5 to 1 mg twice a day, with a gradual increase to 2 mg three times a day.

Side Effects Constipation is the primary side effect of benztropine.

Contraindications Benztropine should not be prescribed for children younger than three years old. Trihexyphenidyl does not have contraindications.

Cautions and Considerations Because these agents can cause drowsiness and confusion, patients should avoid alcohol, which can intensify these effects. Patients may also be advised to drink plenty of fluids and eat foods high in fiber to counteract the constipation these agents can cause.

Drug Interactions These agents increase the anticholinergic effects of other anti-cholinergics, including ipratropium, oxybutynin, solifenacin, and tiotropium.

Catechol-O-Methyltransferase Inhibitors

Catechol-O-methyltransferase (COMT) inhibitors are drugs that inhibit the action of catechol-O-methyltransferase. As an adjunct therapy, COMT inhibitors, such as entacapone and tolcapone, help when levodopa starts to wear off at the end of each dosing interval. Typically, one of these agents (see Table 7.9) is given with each dose of levodopa to increase the amount of "on" time by one to two hours each day. Usually, the levodopa dosage is decreased by approximately 100 mg a day when one of these drugs is added. This class of drug works by blocking an enzyme that metabolizes dopamine. COMT inhibitors boost the effects of levodopa and dopamine by allowing dopamine to remain active longer.

Tolcapone (Tasmar) was the first COMT inhibitor to be discovered. The inhibition of COMT allows greater amounts of levodopa to reach the brain, thereby extending the drug's beneficial life. The COMT inhibitors have no clinical effect unless they are combined with levodopa. Tolcapone was approved by the FDA in 1998, but it has since been linked to three fatal liver injuries. As a result, the medication now carries a boxed warning recommending that its use be limited to people who do not respond to or are not appropriate candidates for other available treatments. Tolcapone has been shown to increase patient "on" time by an average of two to three hours per day. The drug should be discontinued if the patient does not demonstrate any improvement within three weeks.

Entacapone (Comtan) is the second COMT inhibitor to be approved by the FDA. Whereas tolcapone penetrates the CNS, entacapone acts peripherally. Thus, entacapone is expected to be less toxic than tolcapone. Entacapone is indicated for patients who are experiencing a deteriorating response to levodopa in the earlier stages of motor fluctuations.

Dosage Forms and Administration Entacapone and tolcapone can be taken without regard to food.

Side Effects A common side effect of entacapone is urine discoloration.

Contraindications Entacapone does not have contraindications. Tolcapone is contraindicated in patients with liver disease.

Cautions and Considerations Entacapone can cause urine discoloration (urine may appear red, brown, or black), so patients should be warned about this sometimes alarming but harmless effect. Tolcapone has a boxed warning for liver damage, so this medication should be used only when other drug therapies for PD fail.

Drug Interactions Entacapone and tolcapone should not be taken with azelastine, orphenadrine, or thalidomide. COMT inhibitors can enhance the side effects of CNS depressants, such as alcohol, sedatives, and pain medications.

Monoamine Oxidase Inhibitors

Mild dopamine-boosting drugs that are used early on in disease progression or as adjunct therapy in advanced PD are known as monoamine oxidase inhibitors (MAOIs). These agents block monoamine oxidase (MAO), an enzyme that breaks down dopamine in neurons. Rasagiline is often used for mild PD symptoms. Selegiline is usually used as an adjunct therapy when levodopa begins wearing off. (See Table 7.9 for information on these drugs.)

Rasagiline (Azilect) is an MAOI, so it blocks the breakdown of dopamine. It is similar to selegiline. Rasagiline is used as initial therapy in early stages of PD to improve symptoms. It can also be added to levodopa to prolong the effects of levodopa. Rasagiline should not be taken for two weeks prior to surgery. Like other MAOIs, rasagiline can cause a hypertensive crisis, as described in Chapter 8, if the patient ingests foods that contain tyramine. Examples of tyramine-containing foods include aged cheese, concentrated yeast extracts, pickled fish, sauerkraut, soy sauce, beer, and broad beans.

Selegiline (Eldepryl, Emsam, Zelapar) is a potent MAOI that plays a major role in the metabolism of dopamine and may increase dopaminergic activity by interfering with dopamine breakdown. Emsam is the transdermal form of selegiline and is approved only for depression, not for the treatment of PD; therefore, Emsam is discussed in Chapter 8.

Safinamide (Xadago) is a monoamine oxidase inhibitor added to levodopa / carbidopa treatment for "off" times in which that drug therapy stops working intermittently.

Dosage Forms and Administration The daily dose of selegiline should not exceed 10 mg. Zelapar is a form that dissolves in the mouth. Because absorption is higher with Zelapar, doses are lower than for related drugs. Safinamide doses start at 50 mg a day but can be increased to 100 mg a day after two weeks. Safinamide is long acting, so it can be taken only once a day, whereas other MAOIs have to be taken multiple times a day.

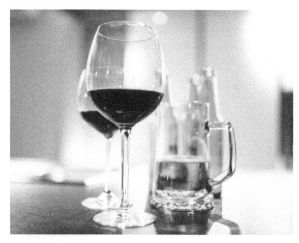

Red wine and beer are among beverages that contain tyramine. Tyramine-containing foods and beverages should be avoided in patients using MAOIs.

Side Effects Common side effects related to MAOIs include nausea and abdominal pain. Side effects of safinamide include difficulty moving, nausea, and insomnia.

Contraindications Rasagiline should be avoided with concurrent use of other MAOIs, meperidine, methadone, tramadol, cyclobenzaprine, dextromethorphan, or St. John's wort. Selegiline should not be used with meperidine. Patients using the oral disintegrating tablet form of selegiline should not concurrently use dextromethorphan, methadone, tramadol, or other MAOIs. The transdermal form of selegiline is contraindicated in patients with a pheochromocytoma; with concomitant use of bupropion, selective serotonin reuptake inhibitors, tricyclic antidepressants, tramadol, propoxyphene, methadone, dextromethorphan, St. John's wort, mirtazapine, cyclobenzaprine, oral selegiline and other MAOIs, carbamazepine, and oxcarbazepine; in patients undergoing elective surgery requiring general anesthesia; with use of sympathomimetics; with foods high in tyramine (see Cautions and Considerations section below); and with supplements containing tyrosine, phenylalanine, tryptophan, or caffeine.

Cautions and Considerations MAOIs block the metabolism of tyramine, a substance in many aged and pickled foods. If tyramine concentrations rise high enough in the blood, blood pressure may increase to dangerous levels. Therefore, patients should be instructed to limit their intake of the following tyramine-rich foods and beverages:

- aged cheese
- beef
- beer
- peppers
- red wine
- sauerkraut
- sausage

Drug Interactions MAOIs have many serious drug interactions. In particular, they should never be administered with tramadol, methadone, dextromethorphan, sympathomimetics, fluoxetine, or fluvoxamine.

Other Agents for Parkinson's Disease

Other agents used to treat Parkinson's disease include amantadine and istradefylline. See Table 7.9 for information on these drugs.

Amantadine (Gocovri, Osmolex ER, Symmetrel), an antiviral drug used for influenza and to treat PD, inhibits the reuptake of dopamine into nerve endings. This inhibition allows dopamine to accumulate in the synapse and stimulate dopamine receptors.

Istradefylline (Nourianz) is used in addition to levodopa / carbidopa for "off" times in which that drug therapy stops working intermittently. The mechanism of action is not known.

Dosage Forms and Administration Amantadine is taken once or twice a day, and the second dose of the day should be taken in the early afternoon to decrease the incidence of insomnia. Abrupt discontinuation of therapy should be avoided. Smoking can stimulate the metabolism of istradefylline. Patients who smoke more than 20 cigarettes a day may have to take a higher dose of istradefylline to get sufficient effect.

Side Effects Common side effects of amantadine include nausea, dizziness, and insomnia. Common side effects related to istradefylline include involuntary movement, constipation, and nausea.

Contraindications Amantadine and istradefylline do not have contraindications.

Cautions and Considerations Istradefylline has been associated with compulsive behaviors such as pathological gambling, hypersexuality, and binge eating. This drug can also cause mental status change and psychotic-like behavior. Patients who develop these behaviors should have their dose reduced or stop taking istradefylline.

Drug Interactions Istradefylline has numerous drug interactions, including lemborexant, lomitapide, lorlatinib, triazolam, and ubrogepant. Close monitoring must be performed if taken with phenobarbital, phenytoin, rifampin, St. John's wort, or corticosteroids. Istradefylline may not work as well when taken with these drugs.

7.4 Multiple Sclerosis and Drug Treatments

Multiple sclerosis (MS) is an autoimmune disease in which the myelin sheaths around nerves, which serve as electrical insulation, degenerate. This degeneration causes patients to lose skeletal muscle control, making it difficult to use their muscles. MS can also affect eyesight. In the later stages of the disease, patients experience severe trembling. Some drugs can slow the progression of the disease, but it has no cure. MS is treated with beta interferons and other disease-modifying therapies. Table 7.10 lists the agents most commonly used to treat MS.

Beta Interferons

Interferons are used for a variety of conditions affecting the immune system, including MS. Beta interferons closely resemble interferons (a type of cytokine) naturally produced by the body. The exact way that beta interferons help in the treatment of MS

TABLE 7.10 Commonly Used Agents for Multiple Sclerosis

Generic (Brand)	Pronunciation	Dosage Form	Common Dosage	Dispensing Status
Beta Interferons				
interferon beta-1a (Avonex)	in-ter-FEER-on BAY-ta won-aye	injection	IM and SC: 30 mcg 1 time a week	Rx
interferon beta-1a (Rebif)	in-ter-FEER-on BAY-ta won-aye	injection	SC: 22–44 mcg 3 times a week	Rx
interferon beta-1b (Betaseron, Extavia)	in-ter-FEER-on BAY-ta won-bee	injection	0.25 mg every other day	Rx
Other Disease-Modifying Therapies (Noninterferons)				
cladribine (Leustatin, Mavenclad)	KLA-dri-been	injection, tablet	1.75–3.5 mg/kg given in multiday cycle over two years	Rx
dimethyl fumarate (Tecfidera)	dye-METH-il FYOO-ma-rate	capsule	240 mg 2 times a day	Rx
diroximel fumarate (Vumerity)	dye-ROX-i-mel FYOO-ma-rate	capsule	231–462 mg 2 times a day	Rx
fingolimod (Gilenya)	fin-GO-li-mod	capsule	0.5 mg 1 time a day	Rx
glatiramer acetate (Copaxone, Glatopa)	gla-TIR-a-mer a-SET-tate	injection	20 mg 1 time a day	Rx
mitoxantrone (Novantron)	mye-toe-ZAN-trone	injection	12 mg/m^2 1 time a day	Rx
natalizumab (Tysabri)	na-ta-LIZ-yoo-mab	injection	300 mg every 4 weeks	Rx
siponimod (Mayzent)	si-PON-i-mod	tablet	0.25–2 mg 1 time a day	Rx
teriflunomide (Aubagio)	ter-i-FLOO-noe-mide	tablet	7–14 mg 1 time a day	Rx

is not fully understood. However, they can prevent CNS inflammation and demyelination (loss of myelin). Interferon therapy is costly (tens of thousands of dollars a year) and often dispensed only in specialty pharmacies or hospitals.

Interferon beta-1a (Avonex, Rebif) is used for ambulatory patients with relapsing-remitting MS (MS with periods of new or increasing symptoms followed by periods of partial or complete recovery). It reduces the frequency of attacks in patients with this form of MS and delays disability. This drug should not be exposed to high temperatures or freezing.

Interferon beta-1b (Betaseron, Extavia) is approved to reduce the frequency of episodes and for patients with a single episode plus consistent magnetic resonance imaging (MRI) findings.

Interferon beta-1b differs from a naturally occurring protein by a single amino acid and a lack of carbohydrate side chains. Its mechanism of action in MS is unknown, but it does suppress T-cell activity, thereby reducing MRI lesions, decreasing relapses, and lessening the severity of these relapses.

Dosage Forms and Administration Interferon beta-1a is dosed every other day. Most patients report flu-like symptoms with interferon beta-1a; to avoid these symptoms, prophylaxis with acetaminophen is indicated. It is also recommended that interferon beta-1a be taken in the evening. A photosensitivity reaction may occur. Interferon beta-1b is injected subcutaneously every other day.

Side Effects The most common side effects of interferon betas are flu-like symptoms and injection site reactions. Injection site reactions are common and can include skin necrosis. Other side effects include anemia (Avonex), leukopenia and increased liver enzymes (Rebif), and asthenia and menstrual disorders (interferon beta-1b).

Contraindications Interferons are contraindicated in patients with a hypersensitivity to human albumin.

Cautions and Considerations Hypersensitivity reactions are a concern with interferon betas. Anaphylaxis is associated with interferon use and may occur immediately after initiation of therapy or after prolonged use.

The interferon betas are associated with asymptomatic liver dysfunction. Caution should be exercised in patients using other potentially hepatotoxic drugs.

Hematologic abnormalities including leukemia and anemia have been reported with use of interferon betas. Routine monitoring of CBCs is recommended.

Drug Interactions Interferons should not be used with deferipone, pexidartinib, or pretomanid, as these agents increase the toxicities of one another.

Other Disease-Modifying Therapies

There are several disease-modifying therapies for MS in addition to the interferon betas. Unlike interferon betas, which are injectable products, these medications are available in various dosage forms.

Cladribine (Leustatin, Mavenclad) is a potent immunosuppressant (drug that suppresses immune response) used to treat relapsing forms of MS and secondary progressive MS, a severe form of MS that occurs in later stages of the disease. Cladribine has a boxed warning about its increased risk of cancer and birth defects, and it is associated with an increased risk of infections. Periodic blood tests must be performed to monitor for changes in blood cells and severe anemia.

Dimethyl fumarate (Tecfidera) is an oral drug used to reduce relapse rates and the development of new brain lesions in patients who have MS. The starting dose is titrated after approximately a week.

Diroximel fumarate (Vumerity) is used to treat relapsing forms of MS and secondary progressive MS. Its mechanism of action is similar to that of dimethyl fumarate. Patients taking diroximel fumarate are monitored closely due to increased risk of infection. Rare but serious side effects include reduced lymphocytes in the blood.

Fingolimod (Gilenya) is an immunomodulator (a drug that helps activate, amplify, or otherwise modify immune system function) taken orally that prevents lymphocyte cells from migrating to the CNS. It reduces the frequency of exacerbations and delays disability. Patients should be tested for immunity to chicken pox and varicella zoster, and these immunizations should not be administered until at least one month after the patient has completed treatment with this drug. The primary side effects are cardiac.

Glatiramer acetate (Copaxone, Glatopa) is an injectable that seems to block the autoimmune reaction against myelin that leads to nerve damage. It decreases the frequency of relapses, but it has not been shown to slow disease progression.

Mitoxantrone (Novantrone) is a medication given by intravenous infusion, which is used for relapsing-remitting MS.

Pharm Fact

Severe chicken pox has occurred in patients on fingolimod. Although administration would not be delayed if a patient was not immune, knowing they would be susceptible means they could take precautions to avoid infection. A vaccine could be administered a month after fingolimod treatment ends.

REFRIGERATE

Natalizumab (Tysabri) is an intravenous infusion that is used for relapsing forms of MS.

Siponimod (Mayzent) is used to treat relapsing forms of MS as well as secondary progressive MS. Its mechanism of action is similar to that of fingolimod. Siponimod is associated with risk of PML like natalizumab.

Teriflunomide (Aubagio) is an oral drug used for relapsing forms of MS. Oral dosing is a main advantage of teriflunomide. Hepatotoxicity may occur with use. A rare side effect is hair thinning. More information on side effects can be found in Table 7.11.

TABLE 7.11 Common Side Effects of Other Disease-Modifying Therapies

Generic (Brand)	Side Effect
cladribine (Leustatin, Mavenclad)	fatigue, headache, fever, rash, nausea, respiratory tract infection, coughing, hypertension, dizziness, insomnia, depression, hair loss, itching, nausea, vomiting, diarrhea, abdominal pain, constipation, back or joint pain, rash
dimethyl fumarate (Tecfidera)	flushing, abdominal pain, diarrhea
diroximel fumarate (Vumerity)	flushing, abdominal pain, diarrhea, nausea, rash
fingolimod (Gilenya)	increased liver enzymes, infections, diarrhea
glatiramer acetate (Copaxone, Glatopa)	injection-site reactions, chest pain, flushing, dyspnea
mitoxantrone (Novatrone)	nausea, alopecia, menstrual disorders
natalizumab (Tysabri)	headache, fatigue, arthralgia
siponimod (Mayzent)	hypertension, headache, falls, liver dysfunction, swelling, slowed heart rate, dizziness, nausea, diarrhea, tremor, limb pain, macular edema, reduced lung function, increased risk of infections
teriflunomide (Aubagio)	diarrhea, nausea, hair thinning

Dosage Forms and Administration As an oral, once-a-day dose, fingolimod is more likely to have better patient compliance. Glatiramer acetate is given every day by subcutaneous injection. The injection must be refrigerated when stored but brought to room temperature before injection. It may cause local injection-site reactions and brief flushing, chest pain, and shortness of breath; these side effects are bothersome but benign. Patients must be enrolled in a REMS program to receive natalizumab. Natalizumab is given as an IV infusion every four weeks.

Side Effects Common side effects for these disease-modifying therapies are noted in Table 7.11.

Contraindications Fingolimod is contraindicated in heart disease, stroke, heart failure, atrioventricular (AV) block, and sick sinus syndrome. It should not be used concurrently with class Ia antiarrhythmics (disopyramide, procainamide, quinidine) or class III antiarrhythmics. Contraindications to glatiramer acetate include mannitol hypersensitivity. Natalizumab should not be used by patients with a history of progressive multifocal leukoencephalopathy. Teriflunomide is contraindicated in patients with severe liver impairment, patients who may have the ability to become pregnant and who do not use contraception reliably, and patients who are pregnant. Dimethyl fumarate and mitoxantrone do not have contraindications.

Cautions and Considerations Dimethyl fumarate may decrease lymphocyte counts; consequently, these counts should be monitored while patients are undergoing therapy. Fingolimod is associated with the risk of varicella-zoster virus infections and tumor development. Mitoxantrone therapy may lead to bone marrow suppression and typically should not be used in patients with neutropenia. Myocardial toxicity may occur with mitoxantrone use, and the risk increases with cumulative dosing. Severe local tissue damage can occur with mitoxantrone extravasation. Natalizumab has a boxed warning about its association with progressive multifocal leukoencephalopathy (PML), a disease affecting the brain's white matter, which can be fatal. For this reason, natalizumab is part of a Risk Evaluation and Mitigation Strategy (REMS) program. REMS programs are risk management plans that use risk minimization strategies beyond professional labeling to ensure that the benefits of certain drugs outweigh the risks. Monitoring of signs and symptoms of PML is required. Teriflunomide use is associated with a risk of liver toxicity; therefore, patients with liver disease should be cautious when taking this drug. This agent is not recommended during pregnancy, so patients who may become pregnant should also be cautious.

Drug Interactions These drugs increase the adverse effects of live vaccines:

- Fingolimod and siponimod have an additive effect with other drugs that prolong the QT interval. These drugs may enhance the effects of antiarrhythmic agents.
- Glatiramer acetate, cladribine, natalizumab, and teriflunomide may enhance the adverse effects of immunosuppressants.
- Mitoxantrone may decrease levels of digoxin and hydantoins.

7.5 Alzheimer's Disease and Drug Treatments

Alzheimer's disease was first described by Alois Alzheimer, a German psychiatrist, in 1906. It is a degenerative disorder of the brain that leads to progressive dementia (loss of memory, intellect, judgment, orientation, and speech) and changes in personality and behavior. In the early stages of the disease, the patient complains of memory deficit, forgetfulness, misplacement of ordinary items, or a combination of these. Depression is a part of the disease profile. As the disease progresses, complex tasks become impossible (for example, managing personal finances), and concentration becomes poor. In the final stages, the patient suffers complete incapacitation, disorientation, and failure to thrive.

Two neurochemical mechanisms for cognitive impairment have been identified. One underlying cause is that not enough of the neurotransmitter ACh is produced to transmit reliable signals. The other underlying cause is that some of the receptors for the neurotransmitter glutamate are hyperactive and cause the neuron to fire even when there is no glutamate present.

Table 7.12 lists the drugs most commonly used to manage Alzheimer's disease. These drugs slow the disease but do not cure or reverse it. There are no agents that will reverse the cognitive abnormalities. The depression associated with the disease is often treated with antidepressants, as determined by existing symptoms and adverse drug reaction profiles. Amitriptyline should be avoided in patients with Alzheimer's disease because it blocks ACh receptors. Agitation and sleep disturbances should be treated with short-acting benzodiazepines.

TABLE 7.12 Commonly Used Agents for Alzheimer's Disease

Generic (Brand)	Pronunciation	Dosage Form	Common Dosage	Dispensing Status
Acetylcholinesterase Inhibitors				
donepezil (Aricept, Aricept ODT, Namzaric)	doe-NEP-a-zil	tablet	5–23 mg a day	Rx
galantamine (Razadyne, Razadyne ER)	ga-LAN-ta-meen	capsule, oral liquid, tablet	8–24 mg a day	Rx
rivastigmine (Exelon)	riv-a-STIG-meen	capsule, oral liquid, transdermal patch	3–12 mg a day	Rx
NMDA Antagonist				
memantine (Namenda)	MEM-an-teen	capsule, oral solution, tablet	5–20 mg a day	Rx

Safety Alert

The labels for Aricept and AcipHex (rabeprazole, a drug for gastroesophageal reflux disease) are nearly identical.

Acetylcholinesterase Inhibitors

Acetylcholinesterase inhibitors are used to treat mild symptoms early in disease progression and will not work once severe memory and functional loss have occurred. These agents work by inhibiting enzymes that break down ACh, a neurotransmitter thought to be deficient in the early stages of Alzheimer's disease.

Donepezil (Aricept, Aricept ODT, Namzaric) is an acetylcholinesterase inhibitor that improves memory and alertness.

Galantamine (Razadyne, Razadyne ER) is an acetylcholinesterase inhibitor derived from daffodil bulbs. It may be better tolerated than rivastigmine, but it is not as well tolerated as donepezil. This drug is not used as much as the other acetylcholinesterase inhibitors.

Rivastigmine (Exelon) is similar to donepezil, but it may be more difficult to dose and administer. The patch form, which uses a matrix design, was specifically designed for patients with Alzheimer's disease. This drug is thought to increase brain ACh levels through inhibition of acetylcholinesterase. It is approved to treat mild to moderate dementia associated with PD or Alzheimer's disease.

TAKE WITH FOOD

Dosage Forms and Administration Donepezil is taken orally, once a day at bedtime. The oral forms of galantamine should be taken with meals. Rivastigmine is taken daily. If side effects occur, it can be stopped and then restarted at a lower dose.

Side Effects Common side effects of acetylcholinesterase inhibitors include nausea, vomiting, agitation, rash, loss of appetite, weight loss, and confusion. These effects can be significant, so doses must be started low and increased slowly. If these effects do not ease with time or are particularly bothersome, the drug should be discontinued.

Contraindications Donepezil is contraindicated in patients with piperidine hypersensitivity. Contraindications to rivastigmine include a hypersensitivity to related compounds and a history of an application-site reaction to a rivastigmine patch. Galantamine does not have contraindications.

Cautions and Considerations Patients with cardiac disease, liver problems, or PD should not take donepezil.

Drug Interactions Donepezil can interact with nonsteroidal anti-inflammatory drugs (NSAIDs), theophylline, and nicotine (through smoking). These substances should be avoided while taking donepezil. Galantamine may increase the adverse effects of other agents that prolong the QT interval. Rivastigmine may decrease the effects of anticholinergic agents.

NMDA Antagonist

Work Wise

The brand name for memantine is Namenda. It works as an NMDA receptor inhibitor. You can remember this mechanism of action by making the connection between the brand name and the abbreviation that gave rise to this name: Namenda (NMDA).

NMDA antagonists work by blocking the glutamate receptors known as *NMDA receptors* (named this because they also respond to the chemical *N*-methyl-D-aspartate). These receptors are excessively excitable in Alzheimer's disease and can cause neurons to fire even without the neurotransmitter.

Memantine (Namenda) is an NMDA antagonist that is used to treat Alzheimer's disease. Memantine may have less severe side effects and may be better tolerated than other drugs used to treat this disease.

Dosage Forms and Administration The prescriber will provide starter doses to titrate the patient to the optimal dose. After the patient is stabilized and the optimal dose is established, the pharmacy will receive a prescription. The results of clinical trials suggest that memantine slows the advancement of Alzheimer's disease.

Side Effects Common side effects of memantine include dizziness, headache, drowsiness, constipation, vomiting, confusion, high blood pressure, and rash. Patients who experience difficulty breathing should seek medical care immediately.

Contraindications Memantine does not have contraindications.

Cautions and Considerations Memantine should be used with caution in patients with seizure disorder, heart disease, kidney disease, or liver disease. Trimethoprim may enhance the adverse effects of memantine.

Drug Interactions Memantine has very few interactions that necessitate changes to therapy.

7.6 Attention Deficit Hyperactivity Disorder and Drug Treatments

Attention deficit hyperactivity disorder (ADHD) has received significant media attention and carries with it many misconceptions about diagnosis and treatment. The condition is characterized by inattention, impulsivity, and hyperactivity. To be diagnosed with ADHD, an individual must exhibit six or more symptoms of inattention and six or more symptoms of hyperactivity/impulsivity that impair daily life in at least two settings for at least six months. Although many people think environment and stressors cause an individual to have ADHD, research has shown that these factors merely exacerbate the condition rather than cause it.

According to some estimates, 4%–11% of school-aged children have some aspect of the disorder, whereas 5% of adults have ADHD. Onset occurs by 12 years of age. Although hyperactivity symptoms decline with age, the inattention and impulsivity can persist into adulthood for half of those individuals who have this condition. Usually, symptoms improve after puberty when the frontal lobe of the brain is closer to maturity. Several other disorders can coexist with ADHD. Learning disabilities are the most common of these; depression and anxiety are less frequent. Proper diagnosis

Safety Alert

All stimulant drugs used for the treatment of ADHD are contraindicated with MAOIs or within 14 days of MAOI use.

of and assistance with learning disabilities are important steps in helping children with ADHD perform well in school. Counseling and behavioral strategies can help with the development of good coping mechanisms. Without adequate treatment and effective coping mechanisms, adults with ADHD can sometimes have problems with substance abuse. Therefore, ADHD and its coexisting conditions can be a difficult mix to treat effectively. Table 7.13 identifies agents commonly used to treat ADHD.

TABLE 7.13 Commonly Used Agents for Attention Deficit Hyperactivity Disorders

Generic (Brand)	Pronunciation	Dosage Form	Dispensing Status	Controlled Substance Schedule
Central Nervous System Stimulants				
amphetamine (Adzenys, Dyanavel, Evekeo)	am-FET-a-meen	capsule, tablet, chewable tablet, oral disintegrating tablet (ODT), suspension	Rx	C-II
dexmethylphenidate (Focalin, Focalin XR)	dex-meth-il-FEN-i-date	capsule, tablet	Rx	C-II
dextroamphetamine / amphetamine (Adderall, Mydayis)	dex-troe-am-FET-a-meen am-FET-a-meen	capsule, tablet	Rx	C-II
lisdexamfetamine (Vyvanse)	liss-dex-am-FET-a-meen	capsule, tablet	Rx	C-II
methylphenidate extended release (Adhansia XR, Aptensio XR, Concerta, Cotempla XR, Daytrana, Jornay PM, Metadate CD, Quillichew ER, Quillivant XR, Ritalin LA)	meth-il-FEN-i-date	capsule, chewable tablet, tablet, transdermal patch	Rx	C-II
methylphenidate immediate release (Ritalin, Methylin)	meth-il-FEN-i-date	oral solution, chewable tablet, tablet	Rx	C-II
Nonstimulant Drugs				
atomoxetine (Strattera)	at-oh-MOX-e-teen	capsule	Rx	

Note: All these drugs require a Medication Guide.

Central Nervous System Stimulants

Common therapy for children and adults with ADHD includes the use of CNS stimulants. A **CNS stimulant** is a drug that affects the levels of certain chemicals in the brain, temporarily boosting mental and physical processes. These agents work best when used with behavioral therapy. CNS stimulants include methylphenidate, dexmethylphenidate, amphetamine, dextroamphetamine / amphetamine, and lisdexamfetamine.

Methylphenidate (immediate and extended release; see Table 7.13 for brand names), a Schedule II controlled substance, is commonly used to treat ADHD. Methylphenidate improves concentration for many patients by increasing levels of neurotransmitters in the brain. It should be used as an adjunct to psychosocial measures.

Dexmethylphenidate (Focalin, Focalin XR) consists of the dextrorotatory isomer of methylphenidate. An **isomer** is one of two (or more) compounds that

Safety Alert

A Medication Guide must be distributed for the medications used to treat ADHD.

contain the same number and type of atoms but have different molecular structures. Many biologically active substances have isomers whose molecules are mirror images of each other, like a pair of gloves. Such isomers are often distinguished using the terms *dextrorotatory* (right) and *levorotatory* (left). Methylphenidate is such a compound, with D (dextrorotatory) and L (levorotatory) isomers. Dexmethylphenidate contains only the more active dextrorotatory isomer of methylphenidate. Because dexmethylphenidate only contains one isomer, it is expected to have fewer side effects than methylphenidate. Like methylphenidate, it is a Schedule II controlled substance.

Amphetamine (Adzenys, Dyanavel, Evekeo) and **dextroamphetamine / amphetamine (Adderall, Mydayis)** are Schedule II controlled substances. They are alternatives to other stimulants. Depending on the dosage form, the effects can last about six to twelve hours, long enough to get some children through the school day.

Lisdexamfetamine (Vyvanse) is dextroamphetamine chemically bonded to the amino acid lysine. Enzymes in the GI tract cleave the lysine, leaving dextroamphetamine, an active drug. The attachment to lysine is intended to reduce the abuse potential of the drug, which is a problem with dextroamphetamine. Once the lysine is cleaved, the dextroamphetamine is absorbed rapidly, so this drug is still a Schedule II controlled substance. A Medication Guide must be distributed with this drug.

Safety Alert

Adderall can look like *Inderal* (propranolol, a beta-blocker used as an anti-anxiety agent).

Dosage Forms and Administration Dosing starts low and is increased until optimal improvement in symptoms is seen without side effects. Immediate-release products are usually tried first. Children starting therapy are often given the first dose before school; if a second dose is needed, it is usually given after school. (See Table 7.13 for more information.) When longer effects are needed, extended-release products may be used. Transdermal patches are applied in the morning, worn for nine hours, and then removed. To help prevent the development of tolerance, the patient can skip methylphenidate doses, especially during times of low stress, such as during weekends and vacations. Most adults taking methylphenidate take it daily without skipping days or doses. A patient resuming medication after skipping doses may be able to decrease the necessary dosage. The patient should get plenty of rest.

Many dosage forms of methylphenidate are taken once per day, which allows them to be given only in the morning. In some cases, the outer layer of the tablet dissolves to release part of the dose immediately. The rest of the tablet is an osmotic-controlled release oral delivery system (OROS) tablet, which releases the drug slowly through pores in the tablet, leaving a ghost tablet that passes through the stool. Daytrana is the patch form of methylphenidate. It is worn for nine hours and then removed. Caution should be used with administration of the patch, as the drug is contained in the adhesive. The patches should be disposed of carefully, as they will continue to contain active drug and pose a risk of abuse.

Side Effects Common side effects of stimulants include headache, loss of appetite, and insomnia. The primary side effect of dextroamphetamine / amphetamine is depression and insomnia.

Contraindications All stimulant drugs that are mentioned in this chapter for the treatment of ADHD are contraindicated with MAOIs and within 14 days of the use of MAOIs. Amphetamine salts, dextroamphetamine, and methylphenidate are contraindicated in patients with cardiovascular disease, high blood pressure, hyperthyroidism, glaucoma, or agitated states and in patients with a history of drug abuse. Contraindications to dexmethylphenidate include high levels of anxiety, tension, and agitation; glaucoma; and motor tics or a diagnosis of Tourette's syndrome.

Cautions and Considerations The CNS stimulants for ADHD have boxed warnings for potential drug dependence. Dextroamphetamine / amphetamine also carries a boxed warning for associated cardiovascular events. Rare but serious (even fatal) cardiac abnormalities have occurred with the use of all CNS stimulants. All CNS stimulants are controlled substances (Schedule II) and have abuse and addiction potential. Therefore, no refills are allowed, and only a limited supply can be dispensed at each pickup. Many of the medications for ADHD (such as amphetamine, atommoxetine, and dexmethylphenidate) have Medication Guides that must be given to patients when dispensing them.

The patient's CBC with differential (number of types of cells) and platelet counts should be monitored during long-term therapy with methylphenidate. This drug does have abuse potential.

Drug Interactions These drugs may enhance the desired effects of analgesics. Stimulants may decrease the desired effects of sedatives. Antipsychotic agents may decrease the desired effects of stimulants. Atomoxetine and MAOIs may increase the hypertensive effects of stimulants. Caffeine may decrease methylphenidate's efficacy, so the patient should avoid coffee, tea, and other caffeinated beverages.

NDC 49999-636-30
25 mg

Strattera®

Oral capsules

25 mg • 30 capsules

Atomoxetine (Strattera) is a drug for ADHD.

Pharm Facts

Other nonstimulant agents can be used to control some of the impulsive behaviors associated with ADHD, such as anxiety, tics, and insomnia. These drugs include clonidine (Catapres, Kapvay) and guanfacine (Intuniv, Tenex), which were originally developed as antihypertensive medications.

Nonstimulant Drugs

Nonstimulant drugs are also used to treat ADHD. These include atomoxetine, bupropion, desipramine, nortriptyline, venlafaxine, clonidine, and guanfacine. The most common of these is atomoxetine.

Atomoxetine (Strattera) may be a good choice for a patient who also has substance abuse problems, because it does not have the potential for abuse and, therefore, is not a controlled substance.

Atomoxetine is a nonstimulant medication that selectively inhibits reuptake of norepinephrine, which controls impulsivity and activity. It is the only nonstimulant indicated for the treatment of ADHD in patients as young as six years old. Atomoxetine has been shown to be as effective as psychostimulants and therefore can be a reasonable alternative with a lower risk for abuse. It is not a controlled substance, so prescriptions can be refilled and called in as a verbal order. Atomoxetine should be used as a first-line agent. Like other drugs for attention deficit hyperactivity disorders, atomoxetine can cause weight loss and slow growth.

Dosage Forms and Administration Atomoxetine is available as a capsule and does not have potential for abuse.

Side Effects Common side effects of atomoxetine are nausea, heartburn, fatigue, and decreased appetite.

Contraindications Atomoxetine should be avoided in patients with narrow-angle glaucoma, pheochromocytoma, or heart disorders.

Cautions and Considerations Atomoxetine can cause severe liver injury; therefore, laboratory tests should be conducted and results monitored for patients taking this medication. Patients with preexisting liver problems should avoid atomoxetine if possible. Finally, atomoxetine has been associated with increased suicidal ideation and has a boxed warning regarding increased risk of suicide. Children and adolescents who are prescribed atomoxetine should be monitored closely. Patients with depression may not be good candidates for this drug therapy.

Drug Interaction Atomoxetine may prolong the QT interval or enhance the effects of other medications used for heart arrhythmias.

7.7 Other Central Nervous System Disorders and Drug Treatments

Several other neurologic disorders share signs and symptoms with the seizure disorders, PD, MS, Alzheimer's disease, and ADHD. They include myasthenia gravis, amyotrophic lateral sclerosis (ALS), and Huntington's disease. Restless legs syndrome and fibromyalgia are treated with many of the same drugs, so they are also discussed in this section of the text.

Myasthenia Gravis

Myasthenia gravis is a disorder of the interface between nerves and muscles, resulting from autoimmune damage to ACh receptors at the **motor end plate** (connection between a neuron and muscle fiber; see Figure 7.7). As a result, the muscles cannot respond to the nerve signal to contract. The disorder is characterized by weakness and increased fatigability, especially of the skeletal muscles. For some individuals, weakness is relatively constant; for others, weakness is typically caused by exercise and diminishes with rest. The first symptoms may be **ptosis** (paralytic drooping of the upper eyelid), **diplopia** (double vision), or blurred vision; these symptoms may be accompanied or followed by **dysarthria** (imperfect articulation of speech), **dysphagia** (difficulty in swallowing), extremity weakness, or respiratory difficulty. The clinical course is variable and includes spontaneous remissions and exacerbations.

FIGURE 7.7
Neuro-muscular Junction

The interface between the nervous system and the muscular system is called the *neuromuscular junction*.

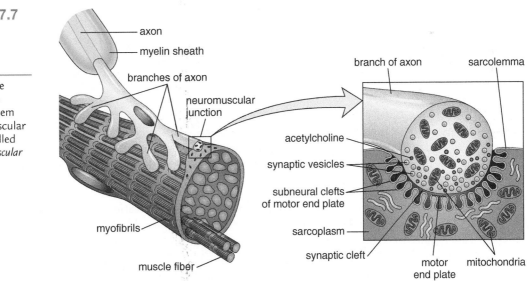

Symptomatic treatment of myasthenia gravis includes several different agents. Among these are acetylcholinesterase inhibitors, alkylating agents, disease-modifying antirheumatic drugs (DMARDs), and immunomodulators. The class of drugs known as *acetylcholinesterase inhibitors* (commonly pyridostigmine) can be used to treat symptoms. Acetylcholinesterase inhibitors can produce clinical improvement in all forms of myasthenia gravis. They allow ACh to remain in the neuromuscular junction longer and may be used with corticosteroids. Although drug therapy does not inhibit or reverse the basic immunologic flaw, it does enable the ACh remaining in the junctions to interact with ACh receptors for longer periods. In addition, many patients require the use of immunotherapy (such as azathioprine and cyclophosphamide). Table 7.14 lists the most commonly used drugs for the treatment of myasthenia gravis.

TABLE 7.14 Commonly Used Agents for Myasthenia Gravis

Generic (Brand)	Pronunciation	Dosage Form	Common Dosage	Dispensing Status
azathioprine (Azasan, Imuran)	ay-za-THYE-oh-preen	injection, tablet	1–5 mg/kg a day	Rx
cyclophosphamide (Cytoxan)	sye-kloe-FOS-fa-mide	injection, tablet	1–5 mg/kg a day	Rx
pyridostigmine (Mestinon)	peer-id-oh-STIG-meen	injection, oral syrup, tablet	600 mg a day in 5–6 doses	Rx

Pyridostigmine (Mestinon) is used to treat myasthenia gravis or to reverse the effects of nondepolarizing muscle relaxants. Pyridostigmine is an acetylcholinestrase inhibitor. It blocks ACh breakdown by acetylcholinesterase, resulting in ACh accumulation at cholinergic synapses and thereby increasing stimulation of cholinergic receptors at the neuromuscular junction.

Azathioprine (Azasan, Imuran) is classified as both a DMARD and an immunosuppressant. It suppresses cell-mediated hypersensitivity and alters antibody production.

Cyclophosphamide (Cytoxan), an alkylating agent, prevents cell division by cross-linking DNA strands. Cyclophosphamide is covered in depth in Chapter 20. Guidelines for preparing and disposing of chemotherapeutic agents should be followed when handling this drug.

Dosage Forms and Administration Pyridostigmine should be taken with food or milk. It is equally important to take it exactly as directed and at the same time each day. Azathioprine should be taken with food to prevent nausea. Fluids should be taken liberally (3 L a day) when taking cyclophosphamide.

Side Effects Side effects of pyridostigmine are generally due to exaggerated pharmacologic effects. The most common side effects are salivation and **muscle fasciculation** (a small, local, involuntary muscular contraction visible under the skin). The prescriber should be notified of any nausea, vomiting, muscle weakness, severe abdominal pain, or difficulty in breathing.

The side effects of immunosuppressive drugs such as azathioprine are pancytopenia (abnormal depression of leukocytes, erythrocytes, and platelets), infection, GI irritation, and abnormal liver function tests.

Cystitis (inflammation of the urinary bladder) is a frequent side effect of cyclophosphamide use, even months after therapy has been discontinued. Other urinary tract effects may include urinary bladder fibrosis, hematuria (blood or blood cells in urine), and renal tubular necrosis. Alopecia (hair loss) is also a side effect of cyclophosphamide, as are nausea, vomiting, and bone marrow depression.

Contraindications Pyridostigmine has no contraindications other than when a patient is allergic to it.

Cautions and Considerations When using cyclophosphamide, uric acid, CBCs, and renal and hepatic functions should be monitored. Use caution when using these agents and beta blockers.

Drug Interactions Pyridostigmine interacts with procainamide, quinidine, corticosteroids, succinylcholine, and magnesium.

Amyotrophic Lateral Sclerosis

Amyotrophic lateral sclerosis (ALS), also known as *Lou Gehrig's disease*, is a progressive, degenerative disease of the motor nerves that leads to muscle weakness, paralysis, and eventually, death. It is thought to be caused by excessive levels of glutamate, an excitatory neurotransmitter, which causes nerve damage. A glutamate inhibitor, such as riluzole, is commonly prescribed for ALS.

The only glutamate inhibitor on the market is riluzole and its brand-name counterparts. **Riluzole (Rilutek, Tiglutik)** inhibits the release of glutamate, inactivates sodium channels, and interferes with intracellular events following neurotransmitter binding at excitatory receptors. Riluzole is the only drug that prolongs ALS patient survival. Riluzole is generally well tolerated. Weakness, dizziness, GI effects, and liver enzyme elevation are the most common side effects.

Dosage Forms and Administration Riluzole is taken orally twice a day.

Side Effects Riluzole is generally well tolerated. Common side effects can include nausea, diarrhea, drowsiness, dizziness, weakness, stomach pain, headache, and runny nose.

Contraindications Patients who are pregnant should not take riluzole.

Cautions and Considerations Patients with liver disease will need to be monitored closely while taking riluzole.

Drug Interactions Riluzole can interact with acetaminophen, amitriptyline, allopurinol, methyldopa, omeprazole, methotrexate, ACE inhibitors, antibiotics, cholesterol medications, and seizure medications. Riluzole can make oral contraceptives less effective so patients should know that other forms of birth control are needed to prevent pregnancy.

Huntington's Disease

Huntington's disease (also known as *Huntington's chorea*) is a neurodegenerative disorder characterized by brief, repetitive, jerky, involuntary movements (known as *chorea*). It is also characterized by emotional disturbances and other problems with brain function, such as memory and reasoning skills.

Tetrabenazine (Xenazine) is approved to treat this condition. This drug works by reducing the activity of chemicals (especially dopamine) in the brain, thereby reducing the involuntary movements associated with the disease. Tetrabenazine must be dose-titrated to the optimal dose. It has serious side effects, including neurologic side effects, which should be carefully monitored. This drug is dispensed from a specialty pharmacy.

Dosage and Administration The dosing of tetrabenazine is slowly adjusted up to the effective dose to reduce side effects. It is available as an oral tablet.

Side Effects Common side effects of tetrabenazine include slowed heartbeat, fainting, aggressive behavior, confusion, dizziness, suicidal ideation, skin rash, and tremor. The dose is increased slowly to avoid these effects.

Contraindications Tetrabenazine is contraindicated in patients with liver disease and with active suicidal ideation.

Cautions and Considerations Tetrabenazine must be used with caution in patients with depression, heart arrythmias, or PD. Tetrabenazine has a boxed warning about use in patients with depression because it can increase risk of suicide.

Drug Interactions Tetrabenazine has a number of known drug interactions. Some agents increase the effects of tetrabenazine (and vice versa) through synergism. These include deutetrabenazine, selegiline, and valbenazine. Administration with certain drugs runs a risk of acute hypertensive disorder. These agents include isocarboxazid, linezolid, phenelzine, procarbazine, rasagiline, selegiline, and tranylcypromine.

Restless Legs Syndrome and Fibromyalgia

Restless legs syndrome (RLS) causes pain or unpleasant sensations in the legs, especially between the knees and ankles. These sensations can be uncomfortable and overwhelming. The cause is generally unknown, although stress can worsen the condition. This syndrome occurs most often in middle-aged or older adults, usually at bedtime, which can create serious sleep disturbances. RLS may be linked to kidney disease, diabetes, PD, peripheral neuropathy, and iron deficiency. Pregnancy or withdrawal from sedatives may also cause these symptoms, as well as the use of lithium, calcium channel blockers, or caffeine. The cause of RLS is thought to be genetic, although the responsible abnormality has not yet been identified.

A person with **fibromyalgia** suffers from long-term pain across the entire body as well as tenderness in the joints, muscles, and tendons. This syndrome has been linked to sleep problems, fatigue, headaches, anxiety, and depression. There is no known cause, but the disorder may be triggered by trauma, sleep disturbances, or infection. Fibromyalgia is most common in women between ages 20 and 50.

There is no cure for RLS or fibromyalgia, so treatment is focused on relieving pain and stress. For RLS, a healthcare practitioner may recommend stretching exercises, massage, or warm baths. **Gabapentin (Neurontin)** (see Table 7.2) is approved to treat RLS. Antiparkinsonian medications, such as **pramipexole (Mirapex, Mirapex ER), ropinirole (Requip, Requip XL)**, and **rotigotine (Neupro)**, are also used to treat this ailment (see Table 7.9).

In treating fibromyalgia, a physician may start by recommending physical therapy, an exercise and fitness regimen, light massage, and relaxation techniques. Again, there is no consensus on proper treatment, but prescribers may try an antidepressant such as duloxetine (Cymbalta) discussed in Chapter 8 or an anticonvulsant such as pregabalin (Lyrica, Lyrica CR).

7.8 Complementary and Alternative Therapies

Yoga, an ancient practice, is used to help patients cope with the effects of many CNS disorders, including epilepsy and ADHD. It is generally considered safe for most individuals. Of note, certain yoga breathing techniques should be avoided in patients with lung or heart disease.

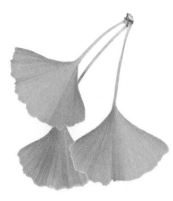

Ginkgo biloba may be used to improve memory.

Certain complementary and alternative therapies are used in patients with PD. One, **5-hydroxytryptophan**, is the chemical precursor to serotonin and improves motor symptoms in patients with PD. It should be used with caution in patients taking antidepressants or other medications for PD. Music therapy may improve motor symptoms, speech, and bradykinesia (slowness of movement).

Although patients in the early stage of Alzheimer's disease may benefit from the use of ginkgo biloba, serious side effects have occurred with its use. These include bleeding, seizures, and even coma. Results of studies are inconclusive and do not necessarily show dramatic improvement in memory or thinking. The benefits of taking ginkgo biloba to prevent Alzheimer's disease are questionable, although many patients take it for this purpose. If patients choose to take ginkgo biloba, they should clearly and fully understand the risks and benefits. Typical doses are 120 to 720 mg ginkgo extract, and commercially available products vary in their content. Ginkgo biloba has antiplatelet effects that affect bleeding. Patients taking warfarin or aspirin for coagulation effects should not use ginkgo biloba without medical supervision. This supplement also interacts with several other prescription medications, particularly anticonvulsants. Therefore, patients who take other prescription medications should discuss taking ginkgo biloba with their prescribers and pharmacists before doing so.

Review and Assessment

CHAPTER SUMMARY

Anatomy of the Nervous System

- The nervous system has two anatomical divisions: the central nervous system (CNS) and the peripheral nervous system (PNS).

- The nervous system is responsible for transmitting information over a vast network throughout the body.

- The autonomic nervous system regulates motor activity that is involuntary or not consciously controlled.

- The somatic nervous system regulates motor activity that is voluntary or conscious.

- Parts of nerve cells, also called *neurons*, include the body, axon, axon terminals, and dendrites.

Physiology of the Nervous System

- The neurons respond to chemical neurotransmitters to send messages through the nervous system.

- Many drugs facilitate an effect in the body by mimicking or influencing the action of neurotransmitters.

Seizure Disorders

- Epilepsy is a common neurologic disorder characterized by recurring seizures. It involves disturbances of neuronal electrical activity that interfere with normal brain function.

- Two major classifications of seizures are focal seizures and generalized seizures.

- The objective of antiepileptic drug therapy is to eliminate seizures without compromising the patient's quality of life because of adverse effects.

- Different seizure types require different drugs.

- All anticonvulsants have very narrow dose/therapeutic ranges. A slight dosage change can result in a loss of seizure control or an increase in toxicity; therefore, prescribers often specify the brand-name drug.

Parkinson's Disease (PD)

- For normal movements to be performed, two neurotransmitters—dopamine (an inhibitor) and acetylcholine (an excitatory)—must be in balance. In PD, these transmitters are not in balance.

- Dopamine does not cross the blood-brain barrier.

- Levodopa / carbidopa is the drug that is most often prescribed to treat PD.

- Bromocriptine (Cycloset, Parlodel) is a dopamine agonist used to treat PD.

- Selegiline (Eldepryl, Emsam, Zelapar) is an MAOI used to treat PD.

Multiple Sclerosis (MS)

- MS is an autoimmune disease in which the myelin sheaths around nerves degenerate.

- Beta interferons are one class of drugs used to treat MS.

- Glatiramer acetate (Copaxone, Glatopa), a drug used to treat MS, must be kept refrigerated.

Alzheimer's Disease

- Alzheimer's disease is a progressive form of dementia.

- Data from clinical trials suggests that memantine (Namenda) slows the progression of Alzheimer's disease.

Attention Deficit Hyperactivity Disorder (ADHD)

- ADHD is a condition characterized by inattention, impulsivity, and hyperactivity.

- Methylphenidate is a CNS stimulant and Schedule II controlled substance used for attention deficit disorders. Many dosage forms allow the drug to be taken only in the morning, and one form is administered through a patch.

- Atomoxetine (Strattera) is for treatment of ADHD in patients as young as six years old.

Other Central Nervous System Disorders

- Acetylcholinesterase inhibitors can produce clinical improvement in all forms of myasthenia gravis.

- Other CNS disorders include amyotrophic lateral sclerosis (ALS), Huntington's disease, restless legs syndrome, and fibromyalgia.

DRUG LIST

Anticonvulsants

brivaracetam (Briviact)
carbamazepine (Epitol, Equetro, Tegretol)
divalproex sodium (Depakote, Depakote ER, Depakote Sprinkle)
eslicarbazepine (Aptiom)
ethosuximide (Zarontin)
felbamate (Felbatol)
fosphenytoin (Cerebyx)
gabapentin (Neurontin)
lacosamide (Vimpat, Vimpat IV)
lamotrigine (Lamictal, Lamictal CD, Lamictal ODT, Lamictal XR)
levetiracetam (Elepsia XR, Keppra, Keppra XR, Roweepra, Spritam)
oxcarbazepine (Oxtellar XR, Trileptal)
parampanel (Fycompa)
phenobarbital
phenytoin (Dilantin, Phenytek)
pregabalin (Lyrica)
primidone (Mysoline)
rufinamide (Banzel)
tiagabine (Gabitril)
topiramate (Qudexy XR, Topamax, Trokendi XR)
vigabatrin (Sabril)
zonisamide (Zonegran)

Antiparkinsonian Agents

amantadine (Gocovri, Osmolex ER, Symmetrel)
apomorphine (Apokyn)
benztropine (Cogentin)
bromocriptine (Cycloset, Parlodel)
entacapone (Comtan)
istradefylline (Nourianz)
levodopa / carbidopa (Duopa, Rytary, Sinemet)
levodopa / carbidopa / entacapone (Stalevo)

pramipexole (Mirapex, Mirapex ER)
rasagiline (Azilect)
ropinirole (Requip, Requip XL)
rotigotine (Neupro)
safinamide (Xadago)
selegiline (Eldepryl, Emsam, Zelapar)
tolcapone (Tasmar)
trihexyphenidyl

Multiple Sclerosis (MS)
cladribine (Leustatin, Mavenclad)
dimethyl fumarate (Tecfidera)
diroximel fumarate (Vumerity)
fingolimod (Gilenya)
glatiramer acetate (Copaxone, Glatopa)
interferon beta-1a (Avonex, Rebif)
interferon beta-1b (Betaseron, Extavia)
mitoxantrone (Novantron)
natalizumab (Tysabri)
siponimod (Mayzent)
teriflunomide (Aubagio)

Alzheimer's Disease
donepezil (Aricept, Aricept ODT, Namzaric)
galantamine (Razadyne, Razadyne ER)
memantine (Namenda)
rivastigmine (Exelon)

Attention Deficit Hyperactivity Disorder (ADHD)
amphetamine (Adzenys, Dyanavel, Evekeo)
atomoxetine (Strattera)
dexmethylphenidate (Focalin, Focalin XR)
dextroamphetamine (Dexedrine)
dextroamphetamine / amphetamine (Adderall, Mydayis)
lisdexamfetamine (Vyvanse)
methylphenidate (Adhansia XR, Aptensio XR, Concerta, Cotempla XR, Daytrana, Jornay PM, Metadate CD, Quillichew ER, Quillivant XR, Ritalin LA)
methylphenidate immediate release (Ritalin, Methylin)

Myasthenia Gravis
azathioprine (Azasan, Imuran)
cyclophosphamide (Cytoxan)
pyridostigmine (Mestinon)

Amyotrophic Lateral Sclerosis (ALS)
riluzole (Rilutek, Tiglutik)

Huntington's Disease
tetrabenazine (Xenazine)

Restless Legs Syndrome (RLS)
gabapentin (Horizant, Neurontin)
pramipexole (Mirapex, Mirapex ER)
ropinirole (Requip, Requip XL)
rotigotine (Neupro)

Fibromyalgia
duloxetine (Cymbalta)
pregabalin (Lyrica, Lyrica CR)

Complementary and Alternative Therapies
ginkgo biloba

Boxed Warnings
amphetamine (Adzenys, Dyanavel, Evekeo)
atomoxetine (Strattera)
azathioprine (Azasan, Imuran)
carbamazepine (Epitol, Equetro, Tegretol)
cladribine (Leustatin, Mavenclad)
dexmethylphenidate (Focalin, Focalin XR)
dextroamphetamine / amphetamine (Adderall)
felbamate (Felbatol)
fosphenytoin (Cerebyx)
lamotrigine (Lamictal, Lamictal CD, Lamictal ODT, Lamictal XR)
lisdexamfetamine (Vyvanse)
methylphenidate (Concerta, Daytrana, Metadate, Methylin, Ritalin)
mitoxantrone (Novantrone)
natalizumab (Tysabri)
tetrabenazine (Xenazine)
tiagabine (Gabitril)
tolcapone (Tasmar)
valproic acid (Depakene)

Medication Guides
amphetamine (Adzenys, Dyanavel, Evekeo)
atomoxetine (Strattera)
dexmethylphenidate (Focalin, Focalin XR)
dextroamphetamine (Dexedrine)
dextroamphetamine / amphetamine (Adderall, Mydayis)
divalproex sodium (Depakote)
ethosuximide (Zarontin)
fosphenytoin (Cerebyx)
gabapentin (Neurontin)
interferon beta-1a (Avonex, Rebif)

interferon beta-1b (Betaseron, Extavia)
lamotrigine (Lamictal, Lamictal CD, Lamictal ODT, Lamictal XR)
levetiracetam (Elepsia XR, Keppra, Keppra XR, Roweepra, Spritam)
lisdexamfetamine (Vyvanse)
methylphenidate (Adhansia, Aptensio, Concerta, Cotempla, Daytrana, Jornay, Metadate, Methylin, Quillichew, Quillivant, Ritalin)

mitoxantrone (Novantrone)
oxcarbazepine (Oxtellar XR, Trileptal)
phenytoin (Dilantin, Phenytek)
pregabalin (Lyrica)
primidone (Mysoline)
topiramate (Qudexy XR, Topamax, Trokendi XR)
valproic acid (Depakene)
zonisamide (Zonegran)

✔ CHECK YOUR UNDERSTANDING

Take a moment to review what you have learned in this chapter and respond thoughtfully to the following prompts. Note that some of these activities will require internet access.

1. Which of the following generalized seizure types would be most consistent with symptoms of a blank stare followed by rapid eye blinking and uncontrolled facial movements?
   a. absence
   b. atonic
   c. status epilepticus
   d. tonic-clonic

2. Which of the following would be *least* likely to cause a seizure?
   a. alcohol withdrawal
   b. Alzheimer's disease
   c. head injury
   d. high fever

3. Which of the following drugs prevents seizure by inhibiting the neurotransmitter glutamate in the brain?
   a. lamotrigine
   b. tiagabine
   c. vigabatrin
   d. zonisamide

4. Which of the following drugs is used to treat neuropathic pain and fibromyalgia in addition to focal seizures?
   a. carbamazepine
   b. lacosamide
   c. pregabalin
   d. primidone

5. Parkinson's disease results from the destruction of neurons in the substantia nigra that transmit which of the following neurotransmitters?
   a. dopamine
   b. glutamate
   c. norepinephrine
   d. serotonin

6. Which of the following is the most commonly used drug for treatment of Parkinson's disease?
   a. Azilect
   b. Focalin XR
   c. Sinemet
   d. Zelapar

7. Which of the following drug products contains methylphenidate in a long-acting dosage form?
   a. Adderall
   b. Aptensio XR
   c. Focalin XR
   d. Vyvanse

8. Which of the following drugs would be a good choice to treat ADHD in a patient who also has a substance abuse disorder?
   a. atomoxetine
   b. clonidine
   c. dexmethylphenidate
   d. dextroamphetamine

9. Which of the following drugs should *not* be used to treat Alzheimer's disease in patients who smoke?
   a. donepezil
   b. galantamine
   c. memantine
   d. rivastigmine

10. Which of the following drugs is used for multiple sclerosis and comes in an oral dosage form?
    a. Avonex
    b. Betaseron
    c. Gilenya
    d. Novantrone

🔗 MAKE CONNECTIONS

Take a moment to consider what you have learned in this chapter and respond thoughtfully to the following prompts. Note that some of these activities will require internet access.

1. What limitations do patients with ADHD and their families face when they are prescribed methylphenidate but their insurance limits them to getting only a 30-day supply at a time?

2. The medications used to treat seizures have many drug interactions, and many of them cause drowsiness. Identify the drugs that have a recognized drug interaction with other CNS depressant medications.

The online course includes additional review and assessment resources.

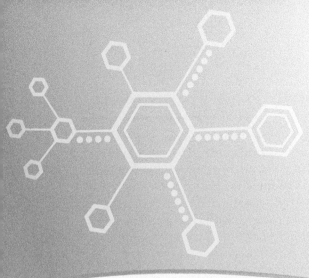

8

The Nervous System, Mental Health, and Drug Therapy

Learning Objectives

1 Differentiate antidepressant, antipsychotic, and antianxiety agents. (Sections 8.1, 8.3, 8.4)

2 Discuss the antidepressant classes, their uses, and their side effects. (Section 8.1)

3 Describe the mechanism of lithium and other drugs used in treating bipolar disorders. (Section 8.2)

4 Discuss the antipsychotic agents, their uses, and their side effects. (Section 8.3)

5 Define anxiety, state its symptoms, and describe the drugs used in its treatment. (Section 8.4)

6 Recognize the course and treatment of panic disorder, insomnia, and alcoholism. (Sections 8.4 through 8.6)

ASHP/ACPE Accreditation Standards

To view the *ASHP/ACPE Accreditation Standards* addressed in this chapter, refer to Appendix C.

Mental health disorders can be debilitating for patients living with them and challenging for the healthcare professionals caring for them. Many of these disorders have their cause in the interaction of central nervous system (CNS) chemicals. (Refer to the previous chapter for information on the anatomy and physiology of the nervous system.) Often, control of symptoms is the only treatment that can be offered. Psychiatric disorders include depression, posttraumatic stress disorder, seasonal affective disorder, bipolar disorder, schizophrenia, psychosis, anxiety, and panic attacks. While sleep disorders and alcohol abuse are not considered psychiatric disorders, this chapter will also cover these topics.

The anatomy and physiology of the nervous system are covered in the Anatomy and Physiology of the Nervous System section in Chapter 7. Refer to Chapter 7 for a review of neurons, neurotransmitters, and the function of the central nervous system.

8.1 Depression, Mood Disorders, and Drug Treatments

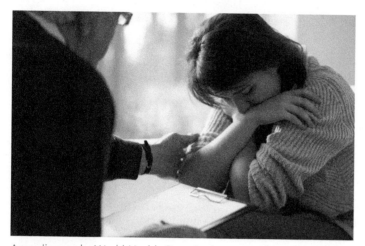

According to the World Health Organization, more than 350 million individuals worldwide have depression.

Depression is the most common severe psychiatric disorder. **Depression** is characterized by feelings of pessimism, worry, intense sadness, loss of concentration, slowing of mental processes, and problems with eating and sleeping. Its key symptoms include dysphoric mood (feelings of being unwell or unhappy) and loss of interest in usual activities. Other symptoms include low self-esteem, self-pity, weight loss or gain, insomnia or hypersomnia, extreme restlessness, loss of energy, feelings of worthlessness, diminished ability to think, feelings of guilt, recurrent thoughts of death, and suicide attempts.

In addition to depression, other recognized types of mood disorders include mania, bipolar disorder, posttraumatic stress disorder, and seasonal affective disorder. **Mania** is characterized by mental and physical hyperactivity, disorganized behavior, and elevated mood. Individuals with bipolar disorder experience alternating episodes of depression and mania. Major depressive disorder (MDD) is depression with no previous occurrence of mania. **Posttraumatic stress disorder (PTSD)**, is a mental health condition triggered by a traumatic event that leaves a person with intense, disturbing thoughts and feelings long after the event. Although the majority of individuals involved in a traumatic event experience a brief period of difficulty, if persistent anxiety or recurrent fear lasts more than a month or disturbs work or personal life, the disorder should be treated. Finally, **seasonal affective disorder (SAD)** is a form of major depression that occurs in the fall and winter and remits (goes into remission) in the spring and summer.

Recall that a neurotransmitter is a chemical produced by a nerve cell and is involved in transmitting information in the body. Neurotransmitters are important in mood disorders and other mental health disorders. Drug therapy for depression is aimed at changing the levels of neurotransmitters, specifically serotonin, norepinephrine, and dopamine. Antidepressants are classified based on which neurotransmitter they affect and how.

Unlike most other drugs, antidepressants generally have a delay of onset of 10 to 21 days. These medications should never be used on an as needed basis to treat depression. Pharmacy personnel are required by the FDA to include a Medication Guide with each antidepressant dispensed. These guides address concerns regarding the drug class. It is also important to remember that antidepressants are *not* controlled substances. Types of antidepressants include selective serotonin reuptake inhibitors (SSRI), serotonin-norepinephrine reuptake inhibitors (SNRI), cyclic antidepressant (TCA), (tricyclic and tetracyclic antidepressants), and monoamine oxidase inhibitors (MAOI). Table 8.1 lists the most common agents used to treat depression and mood disorders.

Practice Tip

Patients who have been prescribed antidepressants should be aware that it may take four weeks for these drugs to achieve full effect. However, antidepressants should help with sleep problems within a week or so.

Pharm Fact

PTSD was first recognized in World War I combat veterans. At that time, this disorder was called *shell shock*. PTSD became more recognized as a major civilian illness after the Iraq War and Hurricane Katrina.

TABLE 8.1 Commonly Used Agents for Depression and Mood Disorders

Generic (Brand)	Pronunciation	Dosage Form	Common Dosage	Dispensing Status
Selective Serotonin Reuptake Inhibitors (SSRI)				
citalopram (Celexa)	sye-TAL-oh-pram	oral solution, tablet	10–40 mg a day	Rx
escitalopram (Lexapro)	es-sye-TAL-oh-pram	oral solution, tablet	5–20 mg a day	Rx
fluoxetine (Prozac Prozac Weekly, Sarafem)	floo-OX-e-teen	capsule, oral solution, tablet	10–80 mg a day	Rx
fluvoxamine (Luvox)	floo-VOX-a-meen	capsule, tablet	25–150 mg a day	Rx
paroxetine (Brisdelle, Paxil, Paxil CR, Pexeva)	pa-ROX-e-teen	capsule, oral solution, tablet	10–60 mg a day	Rx
sertraline (Zoloft)	SER-tra-leen	oral concentrate, tablet	50–200 mg a day	Rx
Serotonin-Norepinephrine Reuptake Inhibitors (SNRIs)				
desvenlafaxine (Pristiq)	des-ven-la-FAX-een	tablet	50 mg a day	Rx
duloxetine (Cymbalta)	doo-LOX-a-teen	capsule	20–60 mg a day	Rx
levomilnacipran (Fetzima)	lee-voe-mil-NAY-ci-pran	capsule	20–120 mg a day	Rx
Serotonin-Norepinephrine Reuptake Inhibitors (SNRIs)				
milnacipran (Savella)	mil-NAY-ci-pran	tablet	12.5–50 mg 1 or 2 times a day	Rx
venlafaxine (Effexor, Effexor XR)	ven-la-FAX-een	capsule, tablet	75–375 mg a day	Rx
Tricyclic Antidepressants (TCAs)				
amitriptyline	a-mee-TRIP-ti-leen	tablet	30–300 mg a day	Rx
clomipramine (Anafranil)	cloe-MIP-ra-meen	capsule	25–75 mg a day	Rx
desipramine (Norpramin)	des-IP-ra-meen	tablet	75–200 mg a day	Rx
doxepin (Silenor Zonalon)	DOX-e-pin	capsule, oral concentrate, topical cream	25–150 mg a day	Rx
imipramine (Tofranil)	im-IP-ra-meen	capsule, tablet	75–200 mg a day	Rx
nortriptyline (Aventyl, Pamelor)	nor-TRIP-ti-leen	capsule, oral liquid	25–100 mg a day	Rx
Tetracyclic Antidepressant				
mirtazapine (Remeron, Remeron SolTab)	meer-TAZ-a-peen	tablet	15–45 mg a day	Rx
Monoamine Oxidase Inhibitors (MAOIs)				
phenelzine (Nardil)	FEN-el-zeen	tablet	45–90 mg a day	Rx
selegiline (Eldepryl, Emsam, Zelapar)	seh-LEDGE-i-leen	capsule, oral disintegrating tablet, transdermal patch	6–12 mg a day	Rx
tranylcypromine (Parnate)	tran-il-SIP-roe-meen	tablet	30–60 mg a day	Rx

continues

Generic (Brand)	Pronunciation	Dosage Form	Common Dosage	Dispensing Status
Miscellaneous Antidepressants				
bupropion (Aplenzin, Forfivo XL, Wellbutrin, Wellbutrin SR, Wellbutrin XL, Zyban)	byoo-PROE-pee-on	tablet	100–450 mg a day	Rx
trazodone	TRAZ-oh-done	tablet	150–600 mg a day	Rx

Selective Serotonin Reuptake Inhibitors

A **selective serotonin reuptake inhibitor (SSRI)** blocks the reuptake (reabsorption) of serotonin, thus increasing the concentration of that neurotransmitter in the synapses between nerve cells with little effect on another important neurotransmitter, norepinephrine. SSRIs have the benefit of producing fewer side effects than historically older antidepressants.

A **serotonin-norepinephrine reuptake inhibitor (SNRI)** blocks the reuptake of both serotonin and norepinephrine. SSRIs and SNRIs are generally safer than tricyclic antidepressants (TCAs) or tetracyclic antidepressants. However, if combined with certain other drugs, they can be fatal. This effect, known as **serotonin syndrome**. Serotonin syndrome occurs when drugs that increase serotonin levels are combined with drugs that stimulate serotonin receptors, causing the receptors to be overstimulated. Although serotonin syndrome is rare, it can be fatal, partly because it is difficult to diagnose. It causes mental state changes and neuromuscular abnormalities as well as other symptoms. Because prescribers may not have a complete medication history for a patient, they may be unaware of these dangerous interactions. Pharmacy personnel will receive warnings on their computer screens (from pharmacy database information) and from insurance companies. If a patient is prescribed drugs that could cause such an interaction, the pharmacy technician should notify the pharmacist.

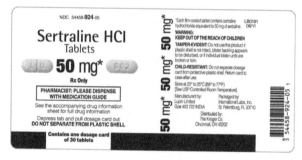

Sertraline is a commonly used SSRI.

The most commonly used SSRIs for the treatment of depression are listed in Table 8.1. SSRIs share many common side effects, contraindications, cautions, and considerations.

Side Effects The most common side effects of SSRIs are usually tolerable and typically last one to two weeks from the start of therapy. These side effects include nausea, vomiting, diarrhea, anxiety, and headache. Either insomnia or drowsiness can occur with all SSRIs, depending on the patient. Side effects can subside over time, but if they are bothersome, a different agent may be prescribed. Most of these medications can also cause sexual dysfunction, including decreased libido, inability to achieve orgasm, or impaired ejaculation. In fact, sexual dysfunction is a frequent reason why patients stop SSRI therapy.

Contraindications SSRIs are contraindicated with the use of monoamine oxidase inhibitors (MAOIs). SSRIs should not be started in patients who are receiving line-zolid or intravenous (IV) methylene blue. Pimozide use is contraindicated with SSRIs.

Cautions and Considerations SSRIs have been associated with an increased risk of suicide in the first few weeks of therapy, especially in pediatric and adolescent patients. Because of this potentially fatal hazard, SSRIs have a boxed warning for children, adolescents, and young adults. Patients should be monitored until the drug's full effects are experienced. Patients should be offered counseling and psychotherapy in addition to medication. The FDA has a warning that discusses the dangers of combining 5HT-3 agonists (triptans; serotonin receptor agonists used to treat migraines, discussed in Chapter 18) with antidepressants, a combination that can occur frequently because many people who suffer from migraine headaches are also depressed. All SSRIs must be dispensed with a Medication Guide.

When discontinued abruptly, SSRIs can be associated with withdrawal syndrome. Depression can suddenly worsen if an SSRI is stopped abruptly. Doses should be slowly decreased to avoid this effect.

Drug Interactions The sedating side effects of alcohol and benzodiazepines may be increased by SSRIs. The anticoagulant effect of warfarin may be enhanced with SSRI use. SSRIs may lower the seizure threshold and should be used cautiously in patients taking antiepileptic drugs. The risk of gastrointestinal (GI) bleeding increases when nonsteroidal anti-inflammatory drugs (NSAIDs) are used with SSRIs. MAOIs when combined with SSRIs may lead to an increased risk of hypertensive crisis. SSRIs can increase the risk of serotonin syndrome when combined with other serotonergic drugs (such as 5HT-3 agonists, TCAs, lithium, tramadol, tryptophan, and buspirone).

SSRIs increase the concentration of IV methylene blue. SSRIs may decrease the effects of tamoxifen. SSRIs decrease the patients' metabolism of mexiletine. Tryptophan may enhance the serotonergic effects of SSRIs.

Citalopram and Escitalopram

Safety Alert

Celexa is often confused with Cerebyx (fos-phenytoin, an anticonvulsant) and Celebrex (celecoxib, for treating arthritis pain). Technicians should be careful in dispensing these medications.

Citalopram (Celexa) is considered to be an SSRI, although it is structurally different from the other drugs in this class. Citalopram has relatively few drug interactions because it is metabolized through an alternative pathway. It is ideal for patients who are required to take a number of different prescriptions concurrently. In addition to depression, citalopram is approved to treat OCD. **Escitalopram (Lexapro)** is the S-isomer of citalopram. An isomer is one of two or more chemical compounds of identical composition but with a different arrangement of atoms. Escitalopram is more potent than citalopram, and patients who take it generally experience fewer side effects than with citalopram. Escitalopram is used to treat both depression and generalized anxiety disorder.

Dosage Forms and Administration Citalopram and escitalopram are available in tablet and oral solution dosage forms.

Side Effects In addition to the common SSRI side effects noted earlier, some of the most common adverse effects of citalopram include insomnia, headache, drowsiness, anxiety, nervousness, and yawning. These side effects are less pronounced with escitalopram.

Contraindications See the most common SSRI contraindications noted earlier.

Cautions and Considerations In addition to the common SSRI cautions and considerations noted earlier, conivaptan, fusidic acid, and idelalisib may increase concentrations of escitalopram. Citalopram and escitalopram can prolong the **QT interval** (the time between depolarization and repolarization of the ventricles of the heart during a heartbeat, as shown on an electrocardiogram). They should be used with caution in patients with prexisiting cardiac arrhythmias. This medication must be dispensed with a Medication Guide.

Drug Interactions See the common SSRI drug interactions noted earlier.

Fluoxetine

Fluoxetine (Prozac, Prozac Weekly, Sarafem) is indicated for major depression and **obsessive-compulsive disorder (OCD)**, which is characterized by recurrent, persistent thoughts (obsessions) or behaviors (compulsions), such as urges to perform repetitive acts like handwashing. Adverse effects include nervousness, insomnia, drowsiness, **anorexia** (loss of appetite for food), nausea, and diarrhea. Most patients lose weight with fluoxetine use, but some may gain weight. Patients should avoid alcohol. They should also take the drug in the morning to prevent insomnia. Fluoxetine plus light therapy (exposure to white light for a specific time period early in the morning, upon awakening) may be effective for treating SAD.

Sarafem is a brand of fluoxetine specifically targeted for patients suffering from **premenstrual dysphoric disorder (PMDD)**, a severe form of premenstrual syndrome (PMS). Serotonin levels are thought to influence the hormonal fluctuation that occurs just prior to the onset of menstruation.

Safety Alert

The drug names Prozac and Proscar (finasteride, used to treat prostate enlargement) are LASA (look-alike, sound-alike) drugs. Caution needs to be taken to ensure the technician dispenses the correct medication. Finasteride (Proscar) is pregnancy category X, and should not be handled by women who are pregnant.

Dosage Forms and Administration Fluoxetine is taken most often on a daily basis. For patients with PMDD, fluoxetine may be taken only during the week before menses. For this purpose, it comes as a seven-day pack containing 10 mg or 20 mg capsules.

Side Effects See the common SSRI side effects noted earlier.

Contraindications In addition to the SSRI contraindications noted earlier, fluoxetine should not be used with thioridazine.

Cautions and Considerations See the common SSRI cautions and considerations noted earlier. This medication must be dispensed with a Medication Guide.

Drug Interactions In addition to the SSRI drug interactions noted earlier, fluoxetine may increase the effects of metoprolol and propranolol. It may also increase the levels of the antiepileptics carbamazepine and phenytoin and the antipsychotics clozapine, haloperidol, and risperidone. Fluoxetine and paroxetine may increase each other's concentrations.

Fluoxetine may enhance the effects of other medications that prolong the QT interval, such as haloperidol, ivabradine, mifepristone, ondansetron, pimozide, propafenone, thioridazine, and ziprasidone. Pharmacists and technicians should be alert for possible interaction with phenytoin (Dilantin). This interaction can raise the serum phenytoin to toxic levels.

Fluvoxamine

Fluvoxamine (Luvox) is effective for the treatment of major depression and may be useful in managing anxiety; it is also approved for treatment of OCD. The primary side effect is nausea.

Dosage Forms and Administration Fluvoxamine is available as a capsule and tablet.

Side Effects The primary side effect is nausea. Hard candy can relieve the side effect of dry mouth.

Contraindications In addition to the SSRIs contraindications noted earlier, fluvoxamine should not be used with thioridazine, alosetron, rameloten, and tizanidine. SSRIs are contraindicated with the use of MAOIs. SSRIs should not be started in patients who are receiving linezolid or IV methylene blue. Pimozide use is contraindicated with SSRIs.

Cautions and Considerations See the most common SSRI cautions and considerations noted earlier. This medication must be dispensed with a Medication Guide.

Drug Interactions In addition to the SSRI drug interactions noted earlier, fluvoxamine has many drug interactions. Fluvoxamine may decrease the patients' metabolism of rameloten and increase the serum concentration of pirfenidone, pomalidomide, and thioridazine. Combining fluvoxamine with these medications should be avoided. Alcohol should be avoided, as should administration of phenytoin (Dilantin).

Paroxetine

Paroxetine (Brisdelle, Paxil, Paxil CR, Pexeva) is indicated for treatment of depression, OCD, social anxiety disorder, generalized anxiety disorder, posttraumatic stress disorder, premenstrual dysphoric disorder, hot flashes, and panic disorder.

Dosage Forms and Administration Paroxetine is available in oral solution, capsule, and tablet dosage forms.

Side Effects Side effects include nausea, headache, ejaculatory disturbances, and sweating.

Contraindications See the most common SSRI contraindications noted earlier.

Cautions and Considerations See the most common SSRI cautions and considerations noted earlier. This medication must be dispensed with a Medication Guide.

Drug Interactions In addition to the SSRI drug interactions noted earlier, paroxetine may increase the effects of metoprolol, propranolol, and rivaroxaban. Paroxetine may increase the levels of the antiepileptics carbamazepine and phenytoin and the antipsychotics clozapine, haloperidol, and risperidone. Fluoxetine and paroxetine may increase each other's concentrations. Paroxetine may decrease the effects of tamoxifen.

Sertraline

Sertraline (Zoloft) is used to treat depression, obsessive-compulsive disorder, panic attacks (sudden, unexpected attacks of extreme fear and worry about these attacks), posttraumatic stress disorder, and social anxiety disorder (extreme fear of interacting with others or performing in front of others). It is also used to relieve the symptoms of premenstrual dysphoric disorder, including mood swings, irritability, bloating, and breast tenderness.

Dosage Forms and Administration Sertraline is available in oral solution and tablet form. It should be taken once a day without regard for food. Patients should show improvement in the first eight weeks of therapy.

Side Effects The primary side effect of sertraline reported by patients is nausea when they first begin to take the drug; sertraline may also cause drowsiness.

Contraindications See the most common SSRI contraindications noted earlier.

Name Exchange

Fluvox, the first brand name of fluvoxamine, has been voluntarily removed from the market. However, many prescribers still write "Fluvox" on prescriptions and medication orders. In those situations, Luvox should be dispensed instead.

Safety Alert

Paxil can be easily confused with Pepcid (famotidine, a gastric acid reducer) because the strengths are the same and the two words sound very similar.

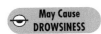

May Cause DROWSINESS

Safety Alert

Zoloft and Zocor (simvastatin, a blood cholesterol reducer) have been mistakenly dispensed for each other.

Cautions and Considerations See the most common SSRI cautions and considerations noted earlier. This medication must be dispensed with a Medication Guide.

Drug Interactions See the most common SSRI drug interactions noted earlier.

Serotonin-Norepinephrine Reuptake Inhibitors

When SSRIs are not effective, SNRIs offer potential relief. SNRIs affect both serotonin and norepinephrine reuptake, increasing the levels of these neurotransmitters in the synapses between nerve cells. This may make them more effective for treating pain than drugs that affect only one neurotransmitter. These drugs may be prescribed for pain alone. The most commonly used SNRIs in the treatment of depression are listed in Table 8.1.

Side Effects SNRIs are commonly associated with nausea, vomiting, insomnia, agitation, and drowsiness. SNRIs, like SSRIs, may cause sexual dysfunction.

Contraindications SNRIs are contraindicated with the use of MAOIs intended to treat psychiatric disorders. SNRIs should not be started in patients who are receiving linezolid or IV methylene blue.

Cautions and Considerations SNRIs have been associated with an increased risk of suicide in the first few weeks of therapy, especially in pediatric and adolescent patients. Because of this potentially fatal hazard, SNRIs have a boxed warning for children, adolescents, and young adults. Patients should be monitored until the drug's full effects are experienced. Patients should be offered counseling and psychotherapy in addition to medication. All SNRIs must be dispensed with a Medication Guide.

Drug Interactions Linezolid, MAOIs, and IV methylene blue may enhance the serotonergic effects of SNRIs.

SNRIs should not be used with MAOIs due to an increased risk of serotonin syndrome. SNRIs should be used cautiously with other serotonergic drugs such as SSRIs, 5HT-3 agonists, TCAs, lithium, tramadol, tryptophan, and buspirone. SSRIs can cause QT prolongation, so they should be used with caution in patients taking other medications that also have this potential.

Desvenlafaxine and Venlafaxine

Venlafaxine (Effexor, Effexor XR) is prescribed for depression. A sustained increase in blood pressure may result from its use, and it may produce manic episodes. At lower doses, venlafaxine primarily affects serotonin, whereas at higher doses, it also affects norepinephrine.

Desvenlafaxine (Pristiq), is approved to treat depression and hot flashes. Pharmacokinetically, it works in the same way as venlafaxine, but it does not produce all the unpleasant side effects. Additionally, desvenlafaxine is a nonestrogenic drug available for hot flashes. This distinction is significant because many of the estrogens previously used for hot flashes have been taken off the market. It is anticipated that patients who cannot tolerate estrogen will be prescribed desvenlafaxine. Desvenlafaxine is also used for fibromyalgia and neuropathic pain.

Dosage Forms and Administration Desvenlafaxine is available as a tablet. Venlafaxine is available as both a capsule and a tablet.

Side Effects In addition to the SNRI side effects noted earlier, venlafaxine may cause sweating, headache, drowsiness, nausea, vomiting, dry mouth, blurred vision, and abnormal ejaculation or orgasm.

Contraindications In addition to the SNRI contraindications noted earlier, desvenlafaxine is contraindicated in patients with a hypersensitivity to venlafaxine.

Cautions and Considerations In addition to the SNRI cautions and considerations noted earlier, desvenlafaxine should not be used in pediatric patients. These medications must be dispensed with a Medication Guide.

Drug Interactions In addition to the SNRI drug interactions noted earlier, patients using venlafaxine should avoid the concurrent use of agents that prolong the QT interval.

Duloxetine

Duloxetine (Cymbalta) is approved for the treatment of major depression and the management of pain associated with diabetic neuropathy. It is a potent inhibitor of serotonin and norepinephrine reuptake and a weak inhibitor of dopamine reuptake.

Dosage Forms and Administration Duloxetine is available as a capsule. It cannot be discontinued abruptly; instead, its dosage must be tapered.

Side Effects See the most common SNRI side effects noted earlier.

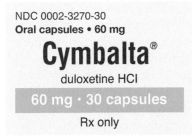

NDC 0002-3270-30
Oral capsules • 60 mg

Cymbalta®
duloxetine HCl
60 mg • 30 capsules
Rx only

Duloxetine (Cymbalta), an SNRI, was recently approved by the FDA for the treatment of major depression.

Contraindications See the most common SNRI contraindications noted earlier.

Cautions and Considerations See the most common SNRI cautions and considerations noted earlier.

Drug Interactions In addition to the SNRI drug interactions noted earlier, duloxetine affects metabolism of many drugs, which can increase levels of drugs (such as TCAs, carvedilol, diphenhydramine, fluoxetine, metoclopramide, metoprolol, tamoxifen, and venlafaxine). Concurrent use of anticoagulant drugs should be avoided when possible. Duloxetine has more interactions than the other drugs in this class.

Levomilnacipran

TAKE WITH FOOD

Levomilnacipran (Fetzima) is approved for the treatment of MDD. It is a more potent inhibitor of norepinephrine reuptake than the other SNRIs.

Dosage Forms and Administration Levomilnacipran is available in capsule form. Food may improve the ability to tolerate this medication. The drug must be adjusted. If the drug is discontinued, the dosage must be tapered.

Side Effects See the most common SNRI side effects noted earlier.

Contraindications In addition to the SNRI contraindications noted earlier, levomilnacipran is contraindicated in patients with a hypersensitivity to milnacipran or with narrow-angle glaucoma.

Cautions and Considerations In addition to the SNRI cautions and considerations noted earlier, levomilnacipran should be used with caution in older adults and in individuals with kidney dysfunction. This medication must be dispensed with a Medication Guide.

Drug Interactions See the most common SNRI drug interactions noted earlier.

Milnacipran

Milnacipran (Savella) is approved for treatment of depression and fibromyalgia.

Dosage Forms and Administration Milnacipran is available in tablet form and must be adjusted up or down in dose so as not to cause undue side effects.

Side Effects In addition to the SNRI side effects noted earlier, side effects of milnacipran can include decreased urine output, prostatitis, and testicular swelling. Rarer side effects include fever, urinary tract infection, and swelling in legs and feet.

Contraindications See the most common SNRI contraindications noted earlier.

Cautions and Considerations In addition to the SNRI cautions and considerations noted earlier, older adults and individuals with kidney dysfunction should use caution when using milnacipran. This medication must be dispensed with a Medication Guide.

Drug Interactions See the SNRI drug interaction noted earlier.

Cyclic Antidepressants

The cyclic antidepressants include varieties that contain three fused rings (tricyclic) and four fused rings (tetracyclic) of carbon atoms. A **tricyclic antidepressant (TCA)** is a member of a class of antidepressant drugs that were developed earlier than the SSRIs and SNRIs. Like SSRIs and SNRIs, TCAs prevent neuron reuptake of norepinephrine, serotonin, or both. TCAs produce a response in greater than 50% of patients. Usually, a therapeutic course of 10 to 20 days is needed before improvements are apparent. Once the acute phase has subsided, the patient should continue to take the drug for 6 to 12 months to reduce the risk of relapse. TCAs have anticholinergic effects (blocking the neurotransmitter acetylcholine), which can decrease urinary urgency; therefore, TCAs may be used in children with bed-wetting problems. Table 8.1 includes the most commonly used cyclic antidepressants. Sedation may occur with multiple antidepressants but is most common with cyclic antidepressants.

Tricyclic Antidepressants

Name Exchange

Although amitriptyline is currently only available as a generic medication, some prescribers or pharmacists may still refer to it by its former brand name, Elavil.

Amitriptyline, clomipramine, desipramine, doxepin, imipramine, and nortriptyline are all TCAs. As a class, they behave similarly. However, they do have some differences. For example, **imipramine (Tofranil)** is used primarily for nocturnal enuresis (bed-wetting) in children.

Dosage Forms and Administration TCAs come in oral capsules or tablets and are usually taken at bedtime, since they frequently cause drowsiness. Oral forms should not be taken with carbonated beverages or grape juice because these drinks can reduce their effectiveness.

In addition to a capsule form, **doxepin (Silenor)** comes in a cream form which is used for pruritis (itching) in adults. The cream form is applied three to form times a day and should not be used for more than eight days. An oral liquid dosage form of doxepin is used by dentists as a topical for "burning mouth syndrome."

Side Effects Sedation is a common side effect, especially in the first few days of treatment. This effect may last several weeks; however, most patients become tolerant to this effect. It is usually prudent to advise the patient to take these drugs at bedtime. Dry mouth, blurred vision, constipation, and urinary retention (an anticholinergic effect) may all resolve within a few weeks. Patients also need to avoid prolonged sun exposure.

Contraindications TCAs should not be used with MAOIs because serotonin syndrome could develop. If a TCA is not working and an MAOI must be tried, the TCA must be discontinued for two weeks prior to initiation of an MAOI. This time in between therapies is called a **washout period**.

Amitriptyline, clomipramine, desipramine, and imipramine are contraindicated in the days to weeks after a heart attack. Clomipramine, desipramine, and imipramine are contraindicated in patients using linezolid or IV methylene blue.

Cautions and Considerations TCAs have a boxed warning for an increased risk of suicidal thoughts and behavior in children, adolescents, and young adults. However, patients of all ages should be closely monitored for the emergence of suicidal thoughts and behaviors. All TCAs must be dispensed with a Medication Guide.

TCAs can cause cardiotoxicity and heart arrhythmias. Patients with preexisting heart conditions or who have recently had a heart attack should not take TCAs. These drugs can also cause **orthostatic hypotension** (a drop in blood pressure upon sitting or standing up). An overdose of TCAs may result in CNS toxicity and potentially fatal cardiac arrhythmias. Treatment should begin with a low dose and should be increased as needed to attain a response. Due to the potential for orthostatic hypotension, patients should be advised to change positions slowly—that is, from a supine (lying down) position to a seated position, or from a seated position to a standing position.

TCAs can lower the seizure threshold, so most patients with seizure disorders should not take these drugs. Because these agents can also cause liver toxicity, patients with liver problems should not take TCAs. Periodic blood tests are required to monitor liver function.

An overdose of TCAs can be fatal, so prescriptions written for a large supply of medication all at once can be dangerous. Pharmacists may be resistant to filling such prescriptions for patients at risk for suicide. Technicians should be aware that many prescribers are also wary of warning patients that an overdose could be lethal, because that message could suggest a pathway to suicide. It is important for healthcare prescribers to assess a patient's risk for suicide when prescribing TCAs.

Drug Interactions Aclidinium, ipratropium, and umeclidinium may enhance the anticholinergic effects of TCAs. TCAs may enhance the CNS depressant effects of azelastine, thalidomide, and tiotropium. TCAs may increase the adverse effects of glucagon.

Linezolid, MAOIs, and IV methylene blue may enhance the serotonergic effects of TCAs.

Amitriptyline may enhance the effects of cisapride, which can cause cardiac arrhythmias.

Despiramine may increase concentrations of bosutinib, ibrutinib, ivabradine, lomitapide, naloxegol, olaparib, simeprevir, thioridazine, tolvaptan, trabectedin, and ulipristal.

Clomipramine and imipramine may increase the concentration of thioridazine.

Tetracyclic Antidepressants

Mirtazapine (Remeron) is a tetracyclic antidepressant used to treat mild to severe depression. It may be useful for patients who suffer from nausea. Like other antidepressants, mirtazepine increases levels of serotonin and norepinephrine. But rather than blocking the reuptake of these neurotransmitters, it is thought to work by blocking receptors that normally inhibit the release of the neurotransmitters.

Dosage Forms and Administration Mirtazepine should be taken at bedtime because it can cause drowsiness.

Side Effects Common side effects of mirtazapine are similar to those of TCAs. As mirtazapine can cause significant drowsiness, it should be taken at bedtime.

Contraindications Mirtazapine is contraindicated in patients using MAOIs. Mirtazapine should not be initiated in patients receiving linezolid or IV methylene blue.

Cautions and Considerations Mirtazapine has a boxed warning for an increased risk of suicidal thoughts and behavior in children, adolescents, and young adults. However, patients of all ages should be closely monitored for the emergence of suicidal thoughts and behaviors. Mertazepine must be dispensed with a Medication Guide.

Drug Interactions Alcohol, azelastine, orphenadrine, and thalidomide may enhance the CNS side effects of mirtazapine.

Linezolid, MAOIs, and IV methylene blue may enhance the serotonergic effects of mirtazapine.

Pimozide concentrations may be increased by mirtazapine.

Conivaptan, fusidic acid, and idelalisib may increase the concentration of mirtazapine.

Monoamine Oxidase Inhibitors

Monoamine oxidase inhibitors (MAOIs) are antidepressants that inhibit the activity of the enzymes that break down serotonin and catecholamines (a group of neurotransmitters used by the sympathetic nervous system, including epinephrine, dopamine, and norepinephrine), thus allowing these transmitters to build up in the nerve synapse. Because of their many interactions with other drugs and foods, MAOIs are not first-line treatments for depression, but they may be effective for certain patients. These drugs may be beneficial in atypical depression. They are similar in efficacy and adverse effects to TCAs, but they are not as cardiotoxic and may offer some advantages to patients with angina or cardiac conduction defects. At present, they are primarily used to treat conditions other than depression. Table 8.1 lists the most commonly used MAOIs.

When dispensing any of these drugs, the pharmacist should check the patient profile for interactions with other drugs. If a patient is taking an MAOI and the physician changes to another class of antidepressant, the patient must wait at least two weeks for the MAOI to clear their system (sometimes referred to as a *washout period*) before starting the second drug. MAOIs generally cause weight gain and edema. Severe interactions may also occur when someone taking an MAOI takes amphetamine, ephedrine, levodopa, meperidine, or methylphenidate. MAOIs impact serotonin and may increase the risk of serotonin syndrome, especially when used with other drugs that effect serotonin.

Severe hypertensive reactions have occurred when an MAOI is taken with food containing a high level of tyramine, a compound

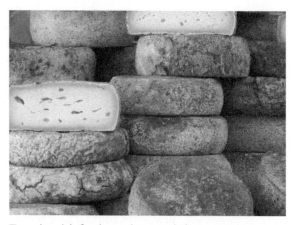

Tyramine-rich foods—such as aged cheese, concentrated yeast extracts, pickled fish, sauerkraut, and broad beans—should be avoided in patients taking MAOIs.

that occurs in aged cheese and many meats and vegetables. The clinical result is a sudden onset of a painful, throbbing, occipital headache; if severe, the condition may progress to severe hypertension; profuse sweating; pallor; palpitations; and, occasionally, death. Patients taking these drugs should never ingest aged cheeses, concentrated yeast extracts, pickled fish, sauerkraut, or broad bean pods (fava beans) because of the high levels of tyramine in these foods.

Although **phenelzine (Nardil)** and **tranylcypromine (Parnate)** are available, selegiline is the MAOI that is most often prescribed. **Selegiline (Eldepryl, Emsam, Zelapar)** may be used to treat depression but is primarily used in Parkinson's disease as an adjunct in the management of patients in whom levodopa / carbidopa therapy is becoming ineffective. Selegiline may also be used in the management of Alzheimer's disease.

Dosage Forms and Administration Selegiline can be administered either orally or via a transdermal patch. The patch has some distinct advantages over the oral forms. For one, the patch allows selegiline to bypass the first-pass effect, an effect through which the concentration of a drug administered orally is reduced before reaching systemic circulation. Bypassing the first-pass effect lets selegiline reach higher levels in the CNS than can be achieved with oral administration. Patch administration also carries less potential for food interactions, although patients still need to be mindful of their diets. A patch should be used immediately upon removal from the sealed packet; applied to dry, intact skin on the upper body; and worn for 24 hours. The patch usually increases patient adherence. Because of the potential for serotonin syndrome, selegiline should not be taken with other antidepressants.

Side Effects Weight gain is a common side effect of all MAOIs.

Contraindications MAOIs should not be used in patients with cardiovascular disease, a cerebrovascular defect, a history of headache or liver disease, pheochromocytoma, or severe kidney impairment. MAOIs are also contraindicated with the use of antihistamines, blood pressure medications, bupropion, buspirone, caffeine (excessive use), depressants (such as alcohol), dextromethorphan, diuretics, general anesthetics, meperidine, other MAOIs or TCAs, carbamazepine, SNRIs, SSRIs, spinal anesthesia, sympathomimetics, and foods high in tyramine content.

Cautions and Considerations MAOIs have boxed warnings. MAOIs interact with tyramine, a substance found in aged and pickled foods. This interaction causes serotonin syndrome, a life-threatening condition involving a rapid heart rate, high blood pressure, headache, and fever. Patients who take MAOIs should avoid consuming foods and beverages containing tyramine, such as aged cheeses, beer, wine, sauerkraut, and other pickled foods. All MAOIs must be dispensed with a Medication Guide.

Drug Interactions These agents interact with numerous other drugs. When patients are taking an MAOI, they should work closely with their physicians and pharmacists to manage any additional prescription or over-the-counter (OTC) medications they want to take.

Other Antidepressant Drugs

Some antidepressant medications do not fit into the aforementioned classes. Two of these medications, also listed in Table 8.1, are bupropion and trazodone.

Bupropion

Bupropion (Aplenzin, Forfivo XL, Wellbutrin, Wellbutrin SR, Wellbutrin XL, Zyban) is a dopamine-norepinephrine reuptake inhibitor (DNRI) that has no direct effect on serotonin or monoamine oxidases, and it does not present anticholinergic, antihistaminic, or adrenergic effects. Bupropion has been approved to treat depression and SAD and aid smoking cessation. It may take three to four weeks for the full effects to be realized. Bupropion should not be discontinued abruptly.

Dosage Forms and Administration Bupropion is manufactured in several forms, which can cause confusion for the pharmacy technician. At times it is difficult to determine which dosage form the prescriber intended. Forms of bupropion, together with daily dosing rates, include the following:

- Wellbutrin, three times a day
- Wellbutrin SR, two times a day
- Wellbutrin XL, one time a day

Prescriptions for bupropion may be written in any of these forms. The dosing indicates which drug to dispense. When in doubt, always clarify the form and dosage with the prescriber. The buproprion brand Zyban, which is for smoking cessation, is initiated at 1 time a day for 3 days, then 2 times a day for 7 to 12 weeks. Aplenzin is a once-daily dose that allows the patient to take one dose of 300 mg or greater.

Side Effects Bupropion has negligible anticholinergic and adrenergic effects. It does not cause sedation, blood pressure effects, or electrocardiographic changes. Effects that may occur include headache, impairment of cognitive skills, nausea and vomiting, dry mouth, constipation, seizures, and impotence. Bupropion may cause less erectile dysfunction than other antidepressants.

Contraindications Contraindications to bupropion include seizure disorder; history of anorexia or bulimia; abrupt discontinuation of ethanol or sedatives, including benzodiazepines, barbiturates, and antiepileptic drugs; use of MAOIs concurrently or within 14 days of discontinuing the MAOI; and concurrent use of other dosage forms of bupropion. Initiating administration of bupropion in a patient receiving linezolid or IV methylene blue is also contraindicated.

Aplenzin and Wellbutrin XL should not be used in patients with other conditions that increase seizure risk, including arteriovenous malformation, severe head injury, severe stroke, CNS tumor, and CNS infection.

Cautions and Considerations Bupropion has two boxed warnings. The first warning is for a risk of suicidal thoughts and behavior in children, adolescents, and young adults. However, patients of all ages should be closely monitored for the emergence of suicidal thoughts and behaviors. The second warning describes serious neuropsychiatric events that can occur in patients taking bupropion for smoking cessation. This medication must be dispensed with a Medication Guide.

Drug Interactions MAOIs may enhance the hypertensive effects of bupropion. Bupropion may increase concentrations of pimozide and thioridazine. Bupropion may decrease concentrations of tamoxifen.

Trazodone

Trazodone exerts its effect by preventing the reuptake of serotonin and norepinephrine. It is a serotonin inhibitor/antagonist, which means its mechanism of action is slightly different from that of the SNRIs.

Dosage Forms and Administration Trazodone is available as a tablet and should be taken at bedtime because it can cause drowsiness. Patients should avoid alcohol and sun exposure.

Side Effects Trazodone has fewer side effects than the TCAs. It has no anticholinergic effects and no effects on cardiac conduction. It may cause orthostatic hypotension, which can be offset by changing positions gradually.

Contraindications Trazodone is contraindicated in patients using MAOIs. In addition, trazodone should not be given to a patient receiving linezolid or IV methylene blue.

Cautions and Considerations Trazodone has a boxed warning for risk of suicidal thoughts and behavior in children, adolescents, and young adults. However, patients of all ages should be closely monitored for the emergence of suicidal thoughts and behaviors. This medication must be dispensed with a Medication Guide.

If trazodone is to be used in combination with other antidepressants, such as SNRIs, SSRIs, TCAs, or MAOIs, the patient should be monitored closely for symptoms of serotonin syndrome. Therapy should be stopped immediately if any of the following symptoms occur, especially if in combination: fever, agitation, hallucinations, racing heart rate, flushing, tremors, diarrhea, or nausea and vomiting.

Trazodone has been associated with a serious and potentially fatal cardiac arrhythmia called *torsades de pointes*. Patients with a history of heart disease should not take trazodone. Trazodone has also been associated with lowering of blood pressure and subsequent fainting. Therefore, it should be used with caution in combination with antihypertensive medications.

Cases of **priapism** (prolonged penile erection) have been reported with trazodone use; some patients have even required surgical intervention. This drug should not be prescribed for younger individuals who have a penis.

Drug Interactions Trazodone may increase the CNS side effects of CNS depressants. Taking trazodone with other serotonergic drugs may increase the risk of serotonin syndrome.

Trazodone may increase digoxin blood levels and the risk of bleeding with anticoagulants. There is also concern that it might have a serious interaction with ginkgo biloba.

8.2 Bipolar Disorder and Drug Treatments

Bipolar disorder is related to the dysfunction of neurotransmitters such as gamma-aminobutyric acid (GABA), serotonin, and norepinephrine. This disorder is characterized by periods of depression alternating with periods of mania, a state of overly high energy, excitement, hyperactivity, optimism, and increased psychomotor activity, during which the patient exhibits irritability, excessive involvement in work or other activities, grandiose ideas, racing thoughts, and a decreased need for sleep. Patients vary in how much they experience mania versus depression.

Patients with bipolar disorder can struggle with other symptoms of psychosis, such as thought disorders, hallucinations, or delusions. Half of patients with bipolar disorder will have at least one psychotic episode in their lifetime. Frequently, other psychiatric disorders coexist with bipolar disorder. If a patient is experiencing signs of increased mood or activity or three or more of the following symptoms, the diagnosis could be mania:

- decreased need for sleep
- increased distractibility
- elevated or irritable mood
- excessive involvement in pleasurable activities with a large potential for painful consequences (e.g., financial irresponsibility, sexual indiscretions, alcohol or drug abuse, or reckless driving)
- grandiose ideas
- increase in activity (socially, at work, or sexually)
- emotional lability (frequently or easily changing emotions)
- racing thoughts

Depressive episodes are characterized by the following symptoms:

- sadness or excessive crying
- low energy
- loss of pleasure
- difficulty concentrating
- irritability
- thoughts of death or suicide

The first episode of bipolar disorder typically occurs at about age 30, may last several months, and usually remits spontaneously. Without treatment, however, many patients experience one or more subsequent episodes. The objective of therapy is to treat acute episodes and prevent subsequent attacks.

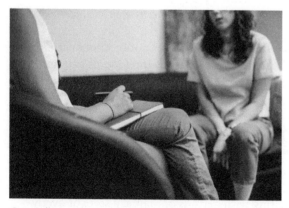

Counseling and cognitive behavioral therapy are key components in the treatment of bipolar disorder.

Lithium is a commonly prescribed drug in the treatment of bipolar disorder to manage the manic episodes. It works best when combined with psychotherapy, counseling, or cognitive behavioral therapy. An antipsychotic agent may be added initially to the regimen to control the hostility and agitation that sometimes accompany mania. Valproic acid and lamotrigine, traditionally thought of as anticonvulsants, are also commonly used (see Chapter 7 for more details on these medications). Antidepressants and some antipsychotic medications can also be used in the treatment of bipolar disorder, but close monitoring is required. Antidepressants are used very carefully when a patient is in depression, because they can trigger a manic episode. Table 8.3 presents the drugs most often used to treat bipolar disorder.

TABLE 8.3 Commonly Used Agents for Treating Bipolar Disorder

Generic (Brand)	Pronunciation	Dosage Form	Common Dosage	Dispensing Status
carbamazepine (Carbatrol, Epitol, Equetro, Tegretol)	kar-ba-MAZ-e-peen	capsule, oral liquid, tablet	1,200–1,600 mg a day	Rx
divalproex (Depakote)	dye-VAL-pro-ex	capsule, tablet	60 mg/kg a day	Rx
lithium (Lithobid)	LITH-ee-um	capsule, oral liquid, tablet	600–900 mg a day in 2 to 3 doses	Rx
valproate (Depakote, Depakote ER, Depakote Sprinkles)	val-PRO-ate	capsule, injection, oral liquid	varies by dosage form	Rx

Lithium

Safety Alert

Lithobid tablets expire after six months. Technicians should be sure to highlight expiration dates on containers.

Lithium (Lithobid) compounds are the most commonly prescribed drugs for bipolar mood disorders; these compounds are generally referred to simply as *lithium*.

Lithium's specific mechanism of action is unknown, but it is believed it affects the synthesis and storage of neurotransmitters. Lithium promotes norepinephrine reuptake and increases sensitivity of serotonin receptors. Lithium may indirectly interfere with sodium transport in nerve and muscle cells.

When the blood level of lithium reaches therapeutic levels, other antipsychotic agents can then be discontinued. Lithium is the only mood stabilizer that has consistently been shown to decrease the risk of suicide for patients with bipolar disorder.

Dosage Forms and Administration Lithium is available as a capsule, tablet, or oral liquid. A common dosage of lithium is 300 mg two to three times a day. Therapeutic blood levels are usually attained 5 to 10 days after the start of therapy. Lithium has a narrow therapeutic index, so periodic lab tests are used to check blood levels. Levels of 0.6 to 0.8 mEq/L are effective for most patients. To prevent toxicity, the patient must have regular blood tests and take the medication at specific times each day. Even if the patient is taking a therapeutic dosage, slight tremors, especially of the hands, may occur. Lithium may also cause liver damage. Salt intake should remain constant during treatment because it can affect lithium blood levels. Alcohol intake increases the potential for toxicity.

Side Effects Common side effects that can occur in a patient initiating lithium therapy include dry mouth, thirst, fine hand tremors, and mild nausea. These effects usually subside with continued treatment. Lithium can affect thyroid function and can cause hypogonadism. Patients taking lithium sometimes complain of fatigue, mental dullness, somnolence, and impotence. These side effects do not go away with continued use of lithium. Should these effects become bothersome, patients should discuss these side effects with their prescriber before stopping therapy on their own. Symptoms associated with elevated levels of lithium in the blood include diarrhea, vomiting, muscular weakness, slowed heart rate, low blood pressure (which can result in fainting), blackouts, incontinence, frequent urination, confusion, and hallucinations. If any of these effects occur, patients should seek medical attention right away.

Contraindications Contraindications to lithium include severe cardiovascular or kidney disease, dehydration, and sodium depletion.

Cautions and Considerations Lithium can become toxic, even in doses at the upper end of the normal dosing range; therefore, regular laboratory tests to check blood concentration are needed to appropriately dose and monitor therapy. Lithium should be used with caution in patients with kidney disease, cardiovascular disease, or dehydration, as these conditions could increase the risk of lithium toxicity. Lithium should be dispensed with a Medication Guide.

Drug Interactions Patients taking diuretics or angiotensin-converting enzyme inhibitors should not take lithium, as these medications can increase the risk of lithium toxicity. Patients taking NSAIDs or thyroid hormone with lithium should be monitored closely.

Carbamazepine

Carbamazepine (Carbatrol, Epitol, Equetro, Tegretol) affects the sodium channels that regulate nerve cells. This drug is indicated in bipolar disorder and is also used as an anticonvulsant. It is considered a second-line treatment to lithium and is used for patients who do not respond to lithium or cannot tolerate its side effects. Carbamazepine produces a response within 10 days in many patients experiencing a manic episode. Side effects, which may be alleviated by briefly decreasing the dose to slow the rate of accumulation in the blood, include dizziness, ataxia (inability to coordinate voluntary muscular movements), clumsiness, slurred speech, double vision, and drowsiness. More information on carbamazepine can be found in Chapter 7.

Divalproex and Valproic Acid

Divalproex (Depakote) and **valproic acid (Depakene)**, referred to as *valproates*, are particularly effective in older adults and in patients with rapid changes of mood (rapid cyclers). These medications also work well as an adjunct to lithium and may replace lithium for some patients. They should be taken with food or milk but not with carbonated beverages. Bleeding or bruising symptoms of thrombocytopenia (a decrease in the number of platelets) should be reported to the physician. Valproates may also cause drowsiness and impair judgment or coordination. See Chapter 7 for more information on these medications.

8.3 Schizophrenia, Psychosis, and Drug Treatments

The primary indication for using an **antipsychotic drug** (or **neuroleptic drug**, as these drugs are sometimes called) is schizophrenia. **Schizophrenia** is a chronic mental health disorder characterized by delusions, disorganized speech and behavior, decrease in emotional range, and neurocognitive deficits. In general, schizophrenia comprises positive symptoms (including hallucinations and delusions) and negative symptoms (including withdrawal, ambivalence, behavior changes, memory loss, and confusion). Schizophrenia is associated with thought disorders in which the patient displays language and communication that is illogical, contradictory, irregular, distracting, and tangential. The onset of symptoms usually occurs in the teenage or early adult years.

Dopamine and, to a lesser degree, serotonin are the major neurotransmitters implicated in schizophrenia. Dopamine receptors are present in four pathways: the limbic system (nerve fibers surrounding the upper brain stem), which controls emotions; the frontal cortex, which controls thought, learning, and memory; the basal ganglia, which affect control of voluntary muscle movement; and the pathway for the release of the hormone prolactin, which can cause sexual dysfunction. The first of these four pathways, involving the limbic system, is the one responsible for psychotic experiences when dopamine levels are excessive. The "older" or "typical" antipsychotic drugs antagonize dopamine receptors in all four of the dopamine pathways, leading to unfavorable side effects. In particular, drug action in the pathway involving the basal ganglia causes muscle control problems. This type of problem is referred to as an **extrapyramidal symptom (EPS)**, or *EPS effect*.

At the beginning of the 21st century, antipsychotic agents with improved efficacy and fewer negative side effects were developed. The "new" or "atypical" antipsychotic medications are designed to limit their dopamine-blocking ability to the limbic system pathway rather than functioning in all four pathways. The atypical agents are now considered first-line agents in the treatment of schizophrenia. Table 8.4 identifies common agents used to treat schizophrenia and other psychoses.

TABLE 8.4 Commonly Used Antipsychotic Agents

Generic (Brand)	Pronunciation	Dosage Form	Common Dosage	Dispensing Status
Typical Antipsychotics				
fluphenazine	floo-FEN-a-zeen	injection, oral liquid, tablet	IM: 12.5–25 mg every 2–4 weeks PO: 2.5–20 mg a day	Rx
haloperidol (Haldol, Haldol Decanoate)	hal-oe-PAIR-i-dawl	injection, oral liquid, tablet	IM: 50–200 mg every 4 weeks PO: 0.5–30 mg a day	Rx
loxapine (Adasuve)	LOKS-a-peen	capsule, aerosol (MDI)	10–100 mg a day	Rx
molindone	moe-LIN-done	tablet	30–100 mg a day	Rx
perphenazine	per-FEN-a-zeen	tablet	4–64 mg a day	Rx
pimozide (Orap)	PI-moe-zide	tablet	0.2–10 mg a day	Rx
prochlorperazine (Compro)	proe-klor-PAIR-a-zeen	suppository, tablet	PO: 15–40 mg a day suppository: 40 mg a day	Rx
thioridazine	thye-oh-RID-a-zeen	tablet	100–800 mg a day	Rx
trifluoperazine	trye-floo-oh-PAIR-a-zeen	tablet	2–20 mg a day	Rx
Atypical Antipsychotics				
aripiprazole (Abilify)	air-i-PIP-ra-zole	injection, oral disintegrating tablet, oral solution, tablet	IM: 5.25–15 mg every 2 hr (daily maximum = 30 mg) PO: 10–30 mg a day	Rx
aripiprazole lauroxil (Aristada)	ay-ri-PIP-ray-zole lawr-OX-il	injection	IM: 41 mg every 4–6 weeks	Rx
asenapine (Saphris)	a-SEN-a-peen	transdermal patch, sublingual tablet	PO: 5–10 mg 2 times a day patch: apply 3.8–5.7 mg patch every 24 hr	Rx
brexpiprazole (Rexulti)	breks-PIP-ra-zole	tablet	2–4 mg a day	Rx
cariprazine (Vraylar)	kar-IP-ra-zeen	capsule	1.5–6 mg a day	Rx

continues

TABLE 8.4 Commonly Used Antipsychotic Agents—*Continued*

Generic (Brand)	Pronunciation	Dosage Form	Common Dosage	Dispensing Status
clozapine (Clozaril, FazaClo ODT, Versacloz)	KLOE-za-peen	oral disintegrating tablet, oral suspension, tablet	25–500 mg a day	Rx
iloperidone (Fanapt)	eye-loe-PER-i-done	tablet	1–12 mg twice a day	Rx
lumateperone (Caplyta)	loo-ma-TE-per-one	capsule	42 mg a day	Rx
lurasidone (Latuda)	loo-RAS-i-done	tablet	80–120 mg a day	Rx
olanzapine (Zyprexa, Zyprexa Relprevv)	oh-LAN-za-peen	injection, oral disintegrating tablet, tablet	IM: 150–300 mg every 2 weeks or 300–405 mg every 4 weeks PO: 5–20 mg a day	Rx
paliperidone (Invega, Invega Sustenna, Invega Trinza)	pal-ee-PAIR-i-doan	injection, tablet	IM: 39–234 mg every 4 weeks PO: 6–12 mg a day	Rx
pimavanserin (Nuplazid)	pim-a-VAN-ser-in	capsule, tablet	10–34 mg a day	Rx
quetiapine (Seroquel, Seroquel XR)	kwe-TYE-a-peen	tablet	300–800 mg a day	Rx
risperidone (Perseris, RisperDAL, RisperDAL Consta, RisperDAL M-TAB)	ris-PAIR-i-doan	injection, oral disintegrating tablet, oral solution, tablet	IM: 25–50 mg every 2 weeks PO: 1–8 mg a day	Rx
ziprasidone (Geodon)	zi-PRAS-i-doan	capsule, injection	IM: 10 mg every 2 hr or 20 mg every 4 hr (daily maximum = 40 mg) PO: 40–160 mg a day	Rx

Antipsychotic drugs are chosen on the basis of cost, intensity of adverse effects, and the patient's response history. Drugs do not alter the natural course of schizophrenia. They do reduce symptoms such as thought disorders, hallucinations, and delusions, but medications rarely eliminate them. Symptoms such as emotional and social withdrawal, ambivalence (conflicting emotional attitudes), and poor self-care usually do not respond to drug treatment. Most therapeutic gains occur in the first 6 weeks, but maximum response may take 12 to 18 weeks. Discontinuation of these drugs leads to recurrence of symptoms. Evidence shows that drug therapy does not reverse memory impairment, confusion, or intellectual deterioration.

Typical Antipsychotics

"Typical" or "first-generation" antipsychotics may be effective, but serious long-term side effects limit their use. As a result, prescribers are moving toward the newer "atypical" antipsychotics, described in the following section. Typical antipsychotics are used rarely and only when multiple atypical antipsychotics have been tried first.

Side effects of antipsychotic drugs run the gamut from minor annoyances to serious irreversible problems. Sedation that lasts as long as two weeks is a common side effect, which is minimized by administering the total daily dose at bedtime. The patient may also experience the following side effects:

- **Anticholinergic** Dryness of the mouth, eyes, and throat; blurred vision; and constipation. Problems occur at the beginning of treatment, but the patient develops tolerance.

- **Cardiovascular** Postural hypotension and an increase in pulse rate of about 20 beats per minute (bpm) with a change in position. These events may cause fainting or falling, most often in older adults.

- **Dermatologic** Excessive tanning or burning and a steely-gray appearance to the skin after years of therapy, due to drug accumulation in melanocytes. With increased usage of the newer drugs, this effect is becoming rare.

- **Endocrine** Hyperglycemia (high blood glucose), lack of menses, lactation in nonpregnant patients, breast enlargement in patients who would not otherwise develop breasts, change in sexual function and drive (increased in females, decreased in males). Patients taking antipsychotics should be monitored closely for weight gain, development of diabetes, and increase in cholesterol levels.

- **Hematologic** Reversible or irreversible bone marrow depression.

- **Neurologic** EPS effects due to an imbalance of cholinergic and dopaminergic transmitters. Dopaminergic blockade can result in excessive cholinergic effects. The coadministration of anticholinergic drugs can balance some of these effects. These side effects develop in 40%–60% of patients, with early-onset symptoms developing within the first four weeks.

The following muscle coordination conditions may develop as early-onset side effects from the cholinergic and dopaminergic imbalance:

- ~ **Akathisia** Motor restlessness. Patients may complain that they are unable to sit or stand still and that they feel a compulsion to pace. Feelings of apprehension, irritability, and uneasiness may also appear. While standing, the patient may rock to and fro or shift weight from one leg to the other. This symptom occurs most frequently in middle-aged patients.

- ~ **Dystonia** Involuntary tonic contraction of skeletal muscles, mostly of the head, face, and shoulders. The tongue may protrude, and the patient experiences difficulty talking and swallowing.

- ~ **Pseudoparkinsonism** Tremors, rigidity, and slow movement; apathy with little facial expression; difficulty walking or a shuffling gait; and drooling. The treatment is reducing the dose, changing to an agent less likely to produce EPS effects, or prescribing anticholinergics.

- **Ophthalmologic** Deposits of melanin-drug complex in lens and retina, potentially resulting in blindness.

- **Withdrawal** Relapse (when symptoms return or get worse) may occur.

Late-onset neurologic side effects occur after six months of treatment. **Tardive dyskinesia** involves involuntary movements of the mouth, lips, and tongue that are sometimes accompanied by involuntary movements of the limbs or trunk. These actions are worsened by emotional distress and disappear during sleep. Onset of these side effects can be insidious (develop so gradually that it is not noticed until well established). The condition is potentially irreversible, even if the drug is discontinued. Once tardive dyskinesia appears, it is rarely progressive and usually either becomes static or slows, improving gradually over weeks or months. Currently, there is no satisfactory treatment for this condition. Anticholinergics make the condition worse.

Table 8.5 lists drugs that are commonly used to minimize the side effects of antipsychotic medications. **Benztropine** is an anticholinergic that may produce an immediate but not necessarily complete response to excessive muscle activity resulting from antipsychotic administration. **Diphenhydramine (Benadryl)** is an antihistamine.

TABLE 8.5 Commonly Used Drugs to Minimize the Side Effects of Antipsychotic Drugs

Generic (Brand)	Pronunciation	Dosage Form	Common Dosage	Dispensing Status
benztropine	BENZ-troe-peen	injection, tablet	1–6 mg a day	Rx
diphenhydramine (Benadryl, various brands)	dye-fen-HYE-dra-meen	capsule, injection, oral liquid, tablet	25–50 mg a day	OTC, Rx

Atypical Antipsychotics

The mechanisms of action for **atypical antipsychotics** are not fully understood and vary among agents. Some block dopamine and others enhance it. Atypical antipsychotics are first-line therapy for schizophrenia and other psychoses. Each agent varies in its effectiveness for individual patients. If one agent does not work, others are tried until a medication and dose are found that control symptoms. Unlike typical antipsychotics, atypical antipsychotics may be effective for the negative symptoms of schizophrenia.

Although atypical antipsychotic agents are much better tolerated than the older agents, they are associated with metabolic side effects, such as weight gain, hyperglycemia, diabetes, and dyslipidemia. The most commonly prescribed atypical antipsychotic medications are listed in Table 8.4 and briefly discussed below.

Dosage Forms and Administration See Table 8.4 for a list of dosage forms and common dosages for both typical and atypical antipsychotic agents.

Side Effects The side effects of atypical antipsychotics are similar to those of typical antipsychotics, but their incidence is lower. Common side effects of atypical antipsychotics include drowsiness, headache, constipation, dry mouth, urinary incontinence or retention, rash, excitation, and, occasionally, frequent hiccups. Taking these medications at bedtime can help with drowsiness, an effect that decreases with time. Atypical antipsychotic agents can cause EPS effects, but to a much lesser extent than do typical antipsychotic agents.

Contraindications See the individual drug entries that follow for contraindications.

Cautions and Considerations Atypical antipsychotics have boxed warnings. The first is for increased mortality in older adults with dementia-related psychosis. Another warning is for a risk of suicidal thoughts and behavior in children, adolescents, and young adults. However, patients of all ages should be closely monitored for the emergence of suicidal thoughts and behaviors. Many antipsychotics must be dispensed with a Medication Guide.

Atypical antipsychotics can lower the seizure threshold, so patients with seizure disorders must be monitored closely when taking these medications. Patients with liver or kidney problems should avoid taking atypical antipsychotics if possible. Some atypical antipsychotics can cause bone marrow suppression, a rare but serious side effect. Regular laboratory tests are necessary to check for this condition. Atypical antipsychotics should be used with caution in older adults because excessive dizziness, drops in blood pressure, and sedation can cause falls. Patients must be monitored closely. Because kidney and liver functions are often reduced in older adult patients, these patients cannot effectively eliminate atypical antipsychotics. Therefore, reduced doses are necessary.

Because patients at any age who have schizophrenia or psychosis can have thought disorders, it is important for patients to be monitored closely and offered counseling or psychotherapy in addition to drug treatment.

Patients should not drink alcohol while taking atypical antipsychotic medications, because excessive sedation and hallucinations can occur. Pharmacy technicians should affix an auxiliary label warning against alcohol use when dispensing these medications.

Drug Interactions Both typical and atypical antipsychotics may increase the CNS effects of azelastine and thalidomide. Metoclopramide may increase the adverse effects of all antipsychotics. Atypical antipsychotics can enhance the CNS depressant effects of other drugs. Atypical antipsychotics can affect many other drugs and be affected by many other drugs. Close attention to drug interactions is needed to evaluate appropriate use in individual patients. Metoclopramide may increase the adverse effects of antipsychotics.

Aripiprazole and Aripiprazole Lauroxil

Aripiprazole (Abilify) and **aripiprazole lauroxil (Aristada)** are dopamine system stabilizers. Unlike typical antipsychotic agents, their actions may vary throughout the brain, depending on endogenous dopamine activity. Also, unlike some atypical antipsychotics, aripiprazole does not prolong the QT interval, and it may cause less weight gain than typical antipsychotic drugs. These drug characteristics can make aripiprazole a favorable option for the treatment of schizophrenia. It is thought that this drug improves dopamine activity and modulates motor function and prolactin secretion. It is used primarily for bipolar disorder but has also received approval for major depressive disorder.

Dosage Forms and Administration Aripiprazole is available as an injection, oral disintegrating tablet, tablet, and oral solution.

Side Effects Aripiprazole has a low risk of motor and other side effects.

Contraindications See the most common typical antipsychotic contraindications noted earlier.

Cautions and Considerations See the most common typical antipsychotic cautions and considerations noted earlier. This medication must be dispensed with a Medication Guide.

Drug Interactions Refer to the list of atypical antipsychotic drug interactions noted earlier.

Asenapine

Asenapine (Saphris) is a mixed serotonin-dopamine antagonist. This mechanism of action is thought to improve the negative symptoms of psychosis and reduce EPS effects. It is used to treat bipolar disorder and schizophrenia.

Dosage Forms and Administration Asenapine is available as a transdermal patch (applied one time a day) and a sublingual tablet.

Side Effects Side effects include dizziness, drowsiness, agitation, constipation, dry mouth, weight gain, and joint pain. Liver function must be monitored regularly.

Contraindications In addition to the contraindications noted earlier, asenapine cannot be used in patients with liver disease.

Cautions and Considerations In addition to the cautions and considerations noted earlier, liver function must be monitored regularly when using asenapine.

Drug Interactions In addition to the atypical antipsychotic drug interactions noted earlier, asenapine may enhance the effects of other medications that prolong the QT interval (such as quinolones and ivabradine). Asenapine may enhance anticholinergic side effects of other drugs (such as ipratropium and umeclidinium), and it may enhance the CNS depressant effects of other drugs (such as alcohol, azelastine, and thalidomide).

Brexpiprazole

Brexpiprazole (Rexulti) is a mixed serotonin-dopamine agonist and antagonist. It is used to treat major depressive disorder and schizophrenia.

Dosage Forms and Administration Brexpiprazole is available in tablet form.

Side Effects Side effects include headache, EPS effects, drowsiness, dizziness, anxiety, restlessness, heartburn, increased appetite, tremor, and sinus infection.

Contraindication Brexpiprazole is contraindicated in individuals with brexpiprazole hypersensitivity.

Cautions and Considerations In addition to the cautions and considerations noted earlier, brexpiprazole can cause a reduction in white blood cells. Sometimes this effect is serious and life threatening. Regular laboratory tests are necessary to check for this condition. This medication must be dispensed with a Medication Guide.

Drug Interactions In addition to the antipsychotic drug interactions noted earlier, brexpiprazole may enhance anticholinergic side effects of other drugs (such as ipratropium and umeclidinium) and the CNS depressant effects of other drugs (such as alcohol, azelastine, and thalidomide). It can also enhance the effects of antidepressants and many other drugs. Close attention to drug interactions is needed to evaluate appropriate use in individual patients.

Cariprazine

Cariprazine (Vraylar) causes partial stimulation and partial inhibition of dopamine and serotonin receptors. It is used for the acute management of manic episodes in bipolar disorder as well as for treatment of schizophrenia. It is also sometimes used for major depressive disorder and psychosis associated with dementia.

Dosage Forms and Administration Cariprazine is available in capsule form.

Side Effects Side effects include dizziness, drowsiness, agitation, anxiety, constipation, vomiting, stomach pain, weight gain, and tooth pain. Liver function must be monitored regularly.

Contraindications Cariprazine is contraindicated in patients with cariprazine hypersensitivity.

Cautions and Considerations In addition to the cautions and considerations noted earlier, cariprazine can cause a reduction in white blood cells. Sometimes this effect is serious and life threatening. Regular laboratory tests are necessary to check for this condition. This medication must be dispensed with a Medication Guide.

Drug Interactions In addition to the antipsychotic drug interactions noted earlier, cariprazine may enhance anticholinergic side effects of other drugs (such as ipratropium and umeclidinium) and the CNS depressant effects of other drugs (such as alcohol, azelastine, and thalidomide). It can also enhance the effects of antidepressants and many other drugs. Close attention to drug interactions is needed to evaluate appropriate use in individual patients.

Clozapine

Safety Alert

Clozapine can cause agranulocytosis, a serious decrease in white blood cells. Patients, physicians, and the pharmacy must be enrolled in the clozapine REMS program.

Clozapine (Clozaril, FazaClo ODT, Versacloz), a blocker of dopamine and serotonin receptors, is indicated for managing patients who have schizophrenia. It also blocks other dopaminergic, alpha-adrenergic, and histamine CNS receptors. Its most serious side effect is a reduction in white blood cells (WBCs); leukocyte counts should be obtained weekly for the duration of therapy.

Dosage Forms and Administration Clozapine is available as a tablet, oral disintegrating tablet, and oral suspension. Frequent blood samples *must* be taken and the results documented by the pharmacy. Before the drug is dispensed, the pharmacy must receive blood-work reports, and the technician must document that the WBC count is greater than $3,500/mm^3$ and that the absolute neutrophil count (ANC) is greater than $2,000/mm^3$.

Side Effects The patient should report any lethargy, fever, throat soreness, flulike symptoms, or symptoms of infection. However, the medication should not be stopped abruptly.

Cautions and Considerations In addition to the cautions and considerations noted earlier, clozapine's most serious side effect is **agranulocytosis**, a reduction in WBCs, for which it carries a boxed warning. Patients showing hematologic changes should be monitored. Another boxed warning is for orthostatic hypotension, bradycardia, and cardiac arrest. Seizure risk, which is thought to be dose related, is another warning. Clozapine also carries a warning for potentially fatal myocarditis and cardiomyopathy.

Clozapine may cause QT prolongation, which can lead to serious and life-threatening arrhythmias.

Drug Interactions Clozapine may enhance the effects of other medications that prolong the QT interval (such as quinolones and ivabradine). Clozapine may enhance anticholinergic side effects of other drugs (such as ipratropium and umeclidinium) and the CNS depressant effects of other drugs (such as alcohol, azelastine, and thalidomide). Carbamazepine and other myelosuppressive drugs may increase the hematologic adverse effects of clozapine.

Iloperidone

Iloperidone (Fanapt) has mixed activity in blocking dopamine and serotonin receptors. This mechanism of action is thought to improve the negative symptoms of psychosis and reduce EPS effects. Iloperidone is used to treat schizophrenia and psychosis.

Dosage Forms and Administration Iloperidone is available in tablet form.

Side Effects Side effects include dizziness, drowsiness, agitation, constipation, nausea, dry mouth, diarrhea, skin rash, sexual dysfunction, weight gain, joint pain, and nasal congestion. Rare cases of priapism have been reported.

Contraindications Iloperidone is contraindicated in patients with iloperidone hypersensitivity.

Cautions and Considerations In addition to the atypical antipsychotic cautions and considerations noted earlier, iloperidone can cause QT prolongation. It must be used with caution in patients with recent acute myocardial infarction or uncompensated heart failure and with concurrent use of other drugs that prolong the QT interval (such as arsenic trioxide, chlorpromazine, dofetilide, dolasetron, droperidol, gatifloxacin, mefloquine, moxifloxacin, other class Ia and III antiarrhythmics, pentamidine, pimozide, quinidine, sotalol, tacrolimus, or thioridazine).

   Iloperidone must be adjusted slowly when withdrawing therapy to avoid symptoms of withdrawal.

Drug Interactions In addition to the atypical antipsychotic drug interactions noted earlier, iloperidone may enhance anticholinergic side effects of other drugs and the CNS depressant effects of other drugs (such as alcohol, azelastine, and thalidomide). It can also enhance the effects of antidepressants and many other drugs. Close attention to drug interactions is needed to evaluate appropriate use in individual patients.

Lumateperone

Lumateperone (Caplyta) has strong inhibition of serotonin receptors and mild activity on dopamine receptors. It is used for schizophrenia in adults.

Dosage Forms and Administration Lumateperone is available as a capsule taken one time a day.

Side Effects Side effects include dizziness, drowsiness, nausea, dry mouth, and decreased appetite. Liver function must be monitored regularly.

Contraindications Lumateperone is contraindicated in patients with lumateperone hypersensitivity.

Cautions and Considerations In addition to the atypical antipsychotic cautions and considerations noted earlier, lumateperone can cause a reduction in white blood cells. Sometimes this effect is serious and life threatening. Regular laboratory tests are necessary to check for this condition.

   Lumateperone must be adjusted slowly when withdrawing therapy to avoid symptoms of withdrawal.

Drug Interactions See the atypical antipsychotic drug interactions noted earlier. In addition, other drugs can alter the effectiveness of lumateperone. Close attention to drug interactions is needed to evaluate appropriate use in individual patients.

Lurasidone

Lurasidone (Latuda) has mixed activity on serotonin and dopamine receptors. This mechanism of action is thought to improve the negative symptoms of psychosis and reduce EPS effects. It is used to treat bipolar disorder and schizophrenia.

Dosage Forms and Administration Lurasidone is available as a tablet.

Side Effects Side effects include dizziness, drowsiness, agitation, anxiety, nausea, vomiting, dry mouth, weight gain, and increased incidence of infection.

Contraindications Lurasidone is contraindicated in patients also taking ketoconazole, clarithromycin, ritonavir, voriconazole, rifampin, St. Johns' wort, phenytoin, and carbamazepine.

Cautions and Considerations See the atypical antipsychotic cautions and considerations noted earlier. In addition, lurasidone can cause a reduction in white blood cells. Sometimes this effect is serious and life threatening. Regular laboratory tests are necessary to check for this condition. This medication must be dispensed with a Medication Guide.

Drug Interactions Lurasidone can enhance the CNS depressant effects of other drugs (such as alcohol, azelastine, and thalidomide). Lurasidone can affect and be affected by many other drugs. Close attention to drug interactions is needed to evaluate appropriate use in individual patients.

Olanzapine

Olanzapine (Zyprexa, Zyprexa Relprevv) is used to treat schizophrenia. Like clozapine and risperidone, olanzapine blocks dopamine and serotonin receptors, but it causes fewer movement disorders. It does not affect WBCs as clozapine does, so frequent blood monitoring is not necessary. Patients *must* avoid alcohol. Olanzapine appears to help patients by decreasing distorted thinking and compulsive behavior concerning

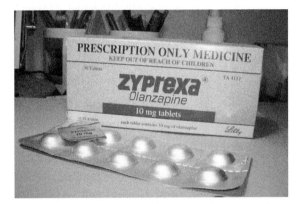

Atypical antipsychotics, such as olanzapine (Zyprexa), can be used to treat schizophrenia.

food. It helps patients respond better to behavioral therapy. In addition to treating schizophrenia, it can be used to treat anorexia nervosa or to promote weight gain.

Dosage Forms and Administration Olanzapine has a once-monthly injectable dosage form, which may improve patient adherence. Patients must be enrolled in a REMS program to receive the injectible form.

Side Effects Common side effects include dizziness, drowsiness, constipation, dry mouth, and weight gain.

Contraindications Olanzapine does not have any contraindications.

Cautions and Considerations See the cautions and considerations of atypical antipsychotics noted earlier. This medication must be dispensed with a Medication Guide.

Drug Interactions See the atypical antipsychotic drug interactions noted earlier. In addition, olanzapine may enhance the adverse effects of benzodiazepines. It may also increase the anticholinergic side effects of other anticholinergic drugs (such as diphenhydramine and umeclidinium).

Pimavanserin

Pimavanserin (Nuplazid) works to inhibit serotonin receptors. Pimavanserin is used primarily for hallucinations and delusions associated with Parkinson's disease.

Dosage Forms and Administration Pimavanserin is available as a capsule and a tablet.

Side Effects Side effects include fluid retention, confusion, nausea, and constipation.

Contraindications Pimavanserin is contraindicated in patients with pimavanserin hypersensitivity.

Cautions and Considerations See the atypical antipsychotic cautions and considerations noted earlier. In addition, pimavanserin can cause QT prolongation. It must be used with caution in patients with recent acute myocardial infarction or uncompensated heart failure and with concurrent use of other drugs that prolong the QT interval (such as arsenic trioxide, chlorpromazine, dofetilide, dolasetron, droperidol, gatifloxacin, mefloquine, moxifloxacin, other class Ia and III antiarrhythmics, pentamidine, pimozide, quinidine, sotalol, tacrolimus, or thioridazine).

Lurasidone can cause a reduction in white blood cells. Sometimes this effect is serious and life threatening. Regular laboratory tests are necessary to check for this condition.

Drug Interactions In addition to the atypical antipsychotic drug interactions noted earlier, pimavanserin can be affected by many other drugs. Close attention to drug interactions is needed to evaluate appropriate use in individual patients.

Drug Interactions Refer to the previously identified common atypical antipsychotic drug interactions.

Quetiapine

Quetiapine (Seroquel, Seroquel XR) is structurally related to clozapine but has a lower incidence of the hematologic toxicities associated with clozapine.

Dosage Forms and Administration Quetiapine is available in tablet form.

Side Effects Side effects may include blurred vision, constipation, drowsiness, dry mouth, upset stomach, tiredness, and weight gain.

Contraindications Quetiapine does not have contraindications.

Cautions and Considerations See the cautions and considerations noted earlier. In addition, quetiapine can increase a patient's risk for cataracts, so regular eye examinations are necessary. This medication must be dispensed with a Medication Guide.

Drug Interactions See the atypical antipsychotic drug interactions noted earlier.

Risperidone and Paliperidone

Risperidone (Perseris, RisperDAL, RisperDAL Consta, RisperDAL M-TAB) is a mixed antagonist of serotonin and dopamine receptors. It binds to serotonin receptors in the CNS and the peripheral nervous system with high affinity, and it binds to dopamine receptors with less affinity. Its binding to serotonin receptors and dopamine receptors is thought to improve negative symptoms of psychosis and reduce the incidence of EPS effects. Risperidone is indicated for the management of psychotic disorders (such as schizophrenia) and dementia in older adults.

Paliperidone (Invega, Invega Sustenna, Invega Trinza) is an active metabolite of risperidone. It is used in the treatment of schizophrenia. Paliperidone works as well as risperidone, but it causes fewer side effects. The sustained-release tablet dosage form is used most often. It is taken once a day. It has few interactions with other drugs because it is not extensively metabolized in the liver. Advantages of paliperidone include low weight gain, fewer EPS effects than risperidone, and significant efficacy in the treatment of schizophrenia.

Dosage Forms and Administration Risperidone is available as an injection, tablet, oral disintegrating tablet, and oral solution. Paliperidone is available as an injection and a tablet. The tablets must not be crushed or broken. Invega uses an extended-release technology called osmotic controlled-release oral delivery system (OROS), in which the drug dissolves through pores in the tablet shell. When the tablet is empty, the tablet shell, known as a **ghost tablet**, is excreted in the stool. It is recommended that the drug be taken in the morning.

Paliperidone comes in extended-release tablets only. Consequently, these tablets should not be chewed or crushed.

Side Effects The primary side effects of risperidone are hypotension, sedation, and anxiety. Patients taking paliperidone should be monitored for the development of orthostatic hypotension.

Contraindications Risperidone does not have contraindications. Paliperidone is contraindicated in patients with risperidone hypersensitivity.

Cautions and Considerations See the cautions and considerations for atypical antipsychotics noted earlier. Risperidone and paliperidone have boxed warnings for an increased mortality in older adults with dementia-related psychosis.

Drug Interactions See the atypical antipsychotic drug interactions noted earlier. In addition, risperidone has a significant drug interaction with the SSRI paroxetine. Risperidone levels may increase with concurrent use.

The effects of agents that prolong the QT interval may be enhanced when used with risperidone or paliperidone.

Ziprasidone

Ziprasidone (Geodon), which is used to treat schizophrenia, may cause less weight gain than other antipsychotic agents. This drug characteristic is an important advantage, because weight gain is often the reason patients quit taking their antipsychotic medication. The major problem with ziprasidone is that it prolongs the QT interval, which may lead to arrhythmia and death.

Dosage Forms and Administration Ziprasidone can be given intramuscularly.

Side Effects See the most common atypical antipsychotic side effects noted earlier.

Contraindications Contraindications to ziprasidone include a known history of QT prolongation, recent acute myocardial infarction, uncompensated heart failure, and concurrent use of other drugs that prolong the QT interval (such as arsenic trioxide, chlorpromazine, dofetilide, dolasetron, droperidol, gatifloxacin, mefloquine, moxifloxacin, other class Ia and III antiarrhythmics, pentamidine, pimozide, quinidine, sotalol, tacrolimus, or thioridazine).

Cautions and Considerations See the cautions and considerations for atypical antipsychotics noted earlier.

Drug Interactions See the atypical antipsychotic drug interactions noted earlier.

8.4 Anxiety and Drug Treatments

Anxiety is a state of uneasiness characterized by apprehension and worry about possible events. Anxiety is a common complaint made to physicians. It is a collection of unpleasant feelings similar to the fearful feelings experienced under conditions of actual danger. The patient feels generalized tension and apprehension and startles easily. Other symptoms include uneasiness and nervousness at work or with people or vague, nagging uncertainty about the future. These feelings may lead to chronic fatigue, headaches, and insomnia. Uncontrolled anxiety can lead to self-treatment with alcohol or other substances. As such, individuals suffering from anxiety are at increased risk for substance abuse.

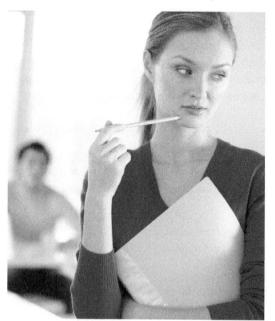

Anxiety and emotional disorders can separate people from their friends and loved ones. Medications can relieve the symptoms so that patients may lead productive, positive lives.

Exogenous anxiety (anxiety caused by factors outside the person) develops in response to external stresses. The response may be appropriate if conditions warrant apprehension and fear.

Endogenous anxiety (anxiety caused by factors within the person) is not related to any identifiable external factors but occurs spontaneously as a result of a defined abnormality in cellular function in the CNS.

Antianxiety drugs include drugs from multiple classes including benzodiazepines (controlled-substances), antidepressants, antihistamines, and anxiolytics (see Table 8.6). SSRIs and SNRIs are key therapies used short term to treat anxiety. Benzodiazepines, which are effective in the treatment of insomnia, panic disorders, alcohol withdrawal syndrome, convulsive disorders, and muscle spasms, are also used short term to treat anxiety. Benzodiazepines are used in the lowest possible doses that control symptoms while minimizing side effects.

TABLE 8.6 Commonly Used Antianxiety Agents

Generic (Brand)	Pronunciation	Dosage Form	Common Dosage	Dispensing Status	Control Schedule
SSRIs and SNRIs					
citalopram (Celexa)	sye-TAL-oh-pram	oral solution, tablet	20–40 mg a day	Rx	
duloxetine (Cymbalta)	doo-LOX-a-teen	capsule	30–120 mg a day	Rx	
escitalopram (Lexapro)	es-sye-TAL-oh-pram	oral liquid, tablet	5–20 mg a day	Rx	
paroxetine (Brisdelle, Paxil, Paxil CR, Pexeva)	pa-ROX-e-teen	oral liquid, tablet	10–80 mg a day	Rx	
sertraline (Zoloft)	SER-tra-leen	oral liquid, tablet	37.5–60 mg a day	Rx	
venlafaxine (Effexor, Effexor XR)	ven-la-FAX-een	capsule, tablet	50–200 mg a day	Rx	

continues

TABLE 8.6 Commonly Used Antianxiety Agents—*Continued*

Generic (Brand)	Pronunciation	Dosage Form	Common Dosage	Dispensing Status	Control Schedule
Benzodiazepines					
alprazolam (Xanax, Xanax XR)	al-PRAZ-oh-lam	oral disintegrating tablet, oral liquid, tablet	0.5–10 mg a day	Rx	C-IV
chlordiazepoxide (Librium)	klor-dye-az-e-POX-ide	capsule	50–300 mg a day	Rx	C-IV
Benzodiazepines					
clonazepam (Klonopin)	kloe-NA-ze-pam	oral disintegrating tablet, tablet	0.25–4 mg a day	Rx	C-IV
clorazepate (Tranxene)	klor-AZ-e-pate	tablet	15–60 mg a day	Rx	C-IV
diazepam (Diastat, Valium, Valtoco)	dye-AZ-e-pam	injection, oral solution, rectal gel, tablet	2–40 mg a day	Rx	C-IV
lorazepam (Ativan, Lorazepam Intensol)	lor-AZ-e-pam	injection, oral liquid, tablet	0.5–10 mg a day	Rx	C-IV
oxazepam	ox-AZ-e-pam	capsule	10–30 mg 3 or 4 times a day	Rx	C-IV
Other Antianxiety Agents					
buspirone	byoo-SPYE-rone	tablet	10–60 mg a day	Rx	
hydroxyzine (Vistaril)	hye-DROX-i-zeen	capsule, injection, oral solution, syrup, tablet	37.5–100 mg a day	Rx	

Safety Alert

Patients who consistently request refills of benzodiazepines a few days early could be exhibiting physical or psychological dependence. Technicians should alert the prescriber if they receive frequent refill authorization requests, as this could be a sign that dependence is developing. Some patients may need help to stop taking these drugs and may benefit from intervention.

Patients taking antianxiety drugs should be monitored closely for the onset of depression, which occurs in about one-third of cases. Patients who discontinue these medications have a high rate of relapse. Antianxiety drugs must be tapered (slowly decreased in dose over time) prior to discontinuation to avoid withdrawal reactions.

Panic disorder is characterized by a form of intense, overwhelming, and uncontrollable anxiety. This anxiety is not a voluntary, controllable emotion, nor is panic disorder a condition that can be avoided by ignoring it or wishing it away.

Panic attacks have a definite onset and end spontaneously. They occur in public or at home, sometimes interrupting sleep. They are characterized by intense fear or apprehension and may involve anticipation of a serious illness or life-threatening attack. The criteria for diagnosis are three attacks in a three-week period; not stimulated by physical exertion, life-threatening situations, or exposure to phobic stimulus; and at least four of the following symptoms: dyspnea (labored breathing), palpitations, chest pain or discomfort, a choking sensation, dizziness, feelings of unreality, tingling in the hands or feet, hot or cold flashes, sweating, numbness, and trembling.

Panic disorder appears to result from a neurochemical dysfunction in part of the brain stem. This disorder, often characterized by progressively heightened sensitivity to certain signals entering the brain, can develop at any age. It is believed that the neurochemical dysfunction occurs in the *locus coeruleus*, a group of synapses in the brain stem at the level of the pons and medulla. The locus coeruleus determines a person's level of responsiveness to stimuli, also called arousal. Sensory information that arrives from all parts of the body passes through this major neurologic junction before being distributed to other parts of the brain. If an abnormality occurs in the locus coeruleus, it affects the signals it receives in ways that depend on both the current state of the patient and the nature of the arriving messages. If it inappropriately amplifies these messages to signal a life-threatening stressor, the patient is aroused to defense or flight. Excessive amplification of these messages gives rise to a state of excessive arousal, excessive autonomic discharges, and increased respiratory drive. If incoming messages are calm and nonthreatening, the locus coeruleus does not overreact.

Patients who have panic disorder are unusually sensitive to the stimulant effects of low doses of caffeine and sodium lactate. When infused, these substances alter intracellular pH and increase impulse transmission through the brain, causing panic symptoms.

A panic attack is postulated to be of neurochemical origin and has both emotional and physical components. The most successful treatment combines medication and behavioral therapy.

Psychotherapy is the preferred treatment for panic disorders in patients whose symptoms cause significant discomfort or impairment. Panic disorder has a true biochemical basis and can be effectively treated. It should be viewed with the same objectivity as other chronic, incurable diseases that can be controlled with medications.

Short-term administration of an antianxiety agent may be indicated in patients with anxiety disorder. Drug therapy blocks the autonomic expression of the panic. SSRIs, benzodiazepines, buspirone, and, to a lesser extent, the beta-adrenergic blocking agents (i.e., beta-blockers [see Chapter 10]) are the most appropriate pharmacologic alternatives.

Benzodiazepines

Benzodiazepines are used to treat anxiety, panic disorder, and PTSD. They are regularly used as preanesthetic medications to calm patients prior to procedures such as a colonoscopy or surgery. Benzodiazepines are also part of the standard treatment for alcohol withdrawal symptoms and status epilepticus.

Benzodiazepines work by stimulating GABA receptors in the CNS, thereby causing drowsiness and relaxation. When used to treat anxiety, benzodiazepines have a calming and sometimes euphoric effect. When used for sleep, they reduce the time it takes to fall asleep, decrease early-morning waking, and generally improve sleep quality.

Dosage Forms and Administration Benzodiazepine agents are available in a variety of dosage forms. See Table 8.6 for details.

Side Effects Common side effects of benzodiazepines include muscle weakness, impaired reflexes, and constipation. Patients may also experience difficulty waking up in the morning and residual drowsiness the following day. Pharmacy technicians should affix an auxiliary label about drowsiness to each benzodiazepine prescription. Other concerning effects include oversedation and respiratory depression (slowed breathing). Patients should be informed of these effects and should notify their physician if they occur.

Contraindications **Alprazolam (Xanax)** is contraindicated in patients with narrow-angle glaucoma and in individuals taking ketoconazole or itraconazole. **Clonazepam (Klonopin)** should not be used in patients with acute narrow-angle glaucoma or liver disease. Clorazepate is contraindicated in patients with narrow-angle glaucoma. Contraindications to **diazepam (Valium)** include myasthenia gravis, respiratory insufficiency, liver disease, sleep apnea, and acute narrow-angle glaucoma. **Lorazepam (Ativan)** is contraindicated in patients with acute narrow-angle glaucoma, sleep apnea, and respiratory insufficiency. **Chlordiazepoxide (Librium)** and **oxazepram** do not have contraindications.

Cautions and Considerations All benzodiazepines have dependence and abuse potential. Consequently, they are considered Schedule IV controlled substances. Patients can become both physically and psychologically dependent on benzodiazepines, making it difficult to stop therapy. Patients should be made aware of this potential and understand that benzodiazepines should be used only for a short time. If a benzodiazepine is used for longer than two weeks, doses must be slowly tapered to avoid withdrawal symptoms. All benzodiazepines must be dispensed with a Medication Guide.

Because these drugs are controlled substances, benzodiazepine prescriptions have a limited number of refills and may have specific storage requirements. Technicians should be familiar with regulations and follow their facility's policies and procedures for dispensing benzodiazepines. Patients with heart conditions may not be able to take benzodiazepines and should be monitored closely. These medications can increase heart rate.

In settings where patients taking benzodiazepines can be observed, such as in inpatient or long-term care facilities, caregivers should monitor them for slowed breathing and excessive sleepiness. Patients should not drink alcohol or take other medications that cause sedation (e.g., opiate pain medications) because excessive sedation and drastically slowed breathing can occur. Breathing can slow to the point of causing death.

Drug Interactions The effects of CNS depressants may be enhanced by benzodiazepines. Azole antifungals may decrease the patients' metabolism of benzodiazepines. Digoxin and phenytoin concentrations may be increased by benzodiazepines. TCA levels may increase when used with benzodiazepines. Benzodiazepines may cause physical or psychological dependence, or both.

Other Antianxiety Agents

Additional antianxiety medications are available. Diphenhydramine, hydroxyzine, and other antihistamines are sometimes prescribed, especially for older adults. TCAs have also proven to be effective. Two noteworthy medications are buspirone and hydroxyzine.

Buspirone

TAKE WITH FOOD

Buspirone acts by selectively antagonizing serotonin receptors without affecting the receptors for benzodiazepine and GABA. Buspirone is not a controlled substance. It has shown little potential for abuse. Buspirone is also used for depression.

Dosage Forms and Administration Buspirone is available as a tablet and should be taken with food. The patient should report any changes in the senses (hearing, smell, or taste). It takes about two weeks to see the full effect of this drug.

Side Effects Buspirone has few side effects; nausea and headache are the most common.

Contraindications Buspirone does not have contraindications.

Cautions and Considerations Buspirone has been associated with depression and increased suicidal tendencies. Patients taking this medication should be monitored closely. Counseling should accompany buspirone therapy when warranted.

Drug Interactions Buspirone, when combined with MAOIs, may elevate blood pressure. It should not be used with sedative hypnotic drugs because it may increase CNS depression. Buspirone may worsen OCD in patients using fluoxetine.

Hydroxyzine

Hydroxyzine (Vistaril), used for some anxious patients, is a sedative and is widely used as a preoperative sedative and sleeping pill. This drug is thought to depress subcortical areas of the CNS. Hydroxyzine chloride (Atarax) is used for itching.

8.5 Sleep Disorders and Drug Treatments

Sleep is fundamental to human health as well as to the health of all mammals and many other vertebrates. Sleep research has recognized four stages of sleep:

- Stage I involves nonrapid eye movements (NREMs). The subject is somewhat aware of their surroundings and is relaxed (4%–5% of sleep time).
- Stage II also involves NREMs. The subject is unaware of surroundings but can be easily awakened (50% of sleep time).
- Stages III and IV involve rapid eye movements (REMs). The subject's sleep is characterized by increased autonomic activity and by episodes of REM sleep with dreaming, if possible. This deep sleep (20%–25% of sleep time), which occurs four to five times per night (for a total of more than 90 minutes), is important for physical rest.

The two most common sleep disorders are insomnia (the inability to fall asleep) and narcolepsy (the inability to stay awake). Table 8.7 identifies the common agents used to treat these sleep disorders. These include hypnotics (such as ramelteon and Z-drugs) to induce sleep and stimulants to treat narcolepsy.

TABLE 8.7 Common Agents Used to Treat Sleep Disorders

Generic (Brand)	Pronunciation	Dosage Form	Common Dosage	Dispensing Status	Control Schedule
Benzodiazepines for Insomnia					
estazolam	es-TAZ-oe-lam	tablet	1–2 mg	Rx	C-IV
flurazepam	floo-RAZ-e-pam	capsule	15–30 mg	Rx	C-IV
quazepam (Doral)	KWA-ze-pam	tablet	7.5–15 mg	Rx	C-IV
temazepam (Restoril)	tem-AZ-e-pam	capsule	7.5–30 mg	Rx	C-IV
triazolam (Halcion)	trye-AY-zoe-lam	tablet	0.25–0.5 mg	Rx	C-IV
Non-Benzodiazepine Hypnotics (Z-Drugs)					
eszopiclone (Lunesta)	es-zo-PIK-lone	tablet	1–3 mg immediately before bedtime	Rx	C-IV
zaleplon (Sonata)	ZAL-e-plon	capsule	5–20 mg immediately before bedtime	Rx	C-IV
zolpidem (Ambien, Ambien CR, Edluar, Intermezzo, Zolpimist)	ZOLE-pi-dem	oral spray, sublingual tablet, tablet	5–12.5 mg immediately before bedtime	Rx	C-IV

continues

TABLE 8.7 Common Agents Used to Treat Sleep Disorders—*Continued*

Generic (Brand)	Pronunciation	Dosage Form	Common Dosage	Dispensing Status	Control Schedule
Miscellaneous Hypnotic					
ramelteon (Rozerem)	ra-MEL-tee-on	tablet	8 mg within 30 min of bedtime	Rx	
Stimulants for Narcolepsy					
armodafinil (Nuvigil)	ar-moe-DAF-i-nil	tablet	150–250 mg 1 time a day	Rx	C-IV
modafinil (Provigil)	moe-DAF-i-nil	tablet	200 mg 1 time a day	Rx	C-IV
pitolisant (Wakix)	pi-TOL-i-sant	tablet	17.8–35.6 mg 1 time a day	Rx	
solriamfetol (Sunosi)	sol-ri-AM-fe-tol	tablet	37.5–150 mg 1 time a day	Rx	C-IV

Many adults have trouble sleeping. Approximately 6% of these individuals seek a physician's help. **Insomnia** is characterized by difficulty falling or staying asleep and by not feeling refreshed upon awakening. The symptoms of insomnia are indications for using a **hypnotic** (a drug that induces sleep).

Therapeutic approaches for narcolepsy include drug and nondrug therapy. Nondrug therapy includes lifestyle changes to establish a consistent sleep schedule, avoidance of shift work, and avoidance of alcohol. Stimulants such as methylphenidate and dextroamphetamine have been the drug therapy mainstay for sleepiness. (These drugs are discussed in Chapter 7.) TCAs and SSRIs work well in the treatment of cataplexy. Drugs specifically approved for narcolepsy include armodafinil, modafinil, pitolisant, and solriamfetol.

Insomnia may be a chronic condition or an occasional or short-term problem. Transient insomnia is not really a sleep disorder. It is usually a response to an acute stressful event and can typically be expected to improve with time as the person adapts to the stress. Chronic insomnia often has multifaceted origins. The first evaluation of a patient should include sleep, drug, medical, and psychiatric histories.

Insomnia can be caused by various events or conditions. The causes can be:

- **situational:** job stress, hospitalization, or travel
- **medical:** pain, respiratory problems, or GI problems
- **psychiatric:** schizophrenia, depression, or mania
- **drug induced:** alcohol, caffeine, or sympathomimetic agents

In these cases, diagnosis and effective treatment of the cause can usually eliminate the need for using hypnotic drugs. Treating only the symptoms of insomnia can make it difficult to recognize and treat the underlying illness. Furthermore, it can subject patients to psychological or physical dependence on hypnotic drugs.

Effective treatment of sleep disorders necessitates both pharmacologic and nonpharmacologic measures. For patients with clearly defined insomnia, pharmacologic treatment consists primarily of the adjunctive use of hypnotics. Therapy with hypnotic agents decreases the time it takes to fall asleep, reduces early-morning awakenings, increases total sleep, and improves quality of sleep. Three specific criteria guide the choice when prescribing a hypnotic drug:

- The agent must have low addiction and suicide potential.
- The agent must minimally alter electroencephalographic patterns (brain activity) and must not depress REM sleep.
- The agent must have minimal interaction with other drugs.

Hypnotics are associated with behavior changes and abnormal thinking. Aggression, bizarre behavior, agitation, and hallucinations have all occurred in patients using hypnotics. Drug classes that are considered hypnotic drugs include benzodiazepines, non-benzodiazepine hypnotics (Z-drugs), and melatonin receptor agonists.

Table 8.7 lists the most commonly used agents for sleep disorders, several of which are among the antianxiety medications listed in Table 8.6. Nonpharmacologic treatment includes supportive counseling and behavioral treatment. The components of this therapy include:

- normalizing the sleep schedule for bedtime and waking time
- increasing physical exercise during the daytime
- discontinuing use of alcohol as a sedative
- sleeping a total of only 7–8 hours in a 24-hour period
- reducing caffeine and nicotine intake
- eliminating any drug (e.g., decongestant) that could lead to insomnia.

A person facing a clearly identified external stress (such as a grief reaction) may become anxious and have difficulty sleeping. A one- to three-week course of treatment with a hypnotic agent may be justified in such instances. Hypnotic drugs should be used only as an adjunct to medical therapeutic measures.

Patients should be informed of the limitations of drugs used to induce sleep. To reduce the risk of habituation and increase the duration of effectiveness, these drugs should be taken as needed, rather than every night. It is easy to slip into the habit of taking these drugs every night, and the patient may become unable to sleep without them. Therapy should be started with a small dose, to be increased only if the initial dose is ineffective. Some sleep agents work best if taken 30 minutes prior to bedtime, while some work best if taken right at bedtime.

The primary side effect of sleep medications (seen more often with high doses) is CNS depression, which results in dizziness, confusion, next-day drowsiness, and impaired reflexes. Some patients, particularly older adults, may exhibit paradoxical reactions (excitation, irritability, and, occasionally, aggressive behavior). Anterograde amnesia (impaired memory immediately following a precipitating event) may also occur after taking a hypnotic.

Non-Benzodiazepine Hypnotics (Z-Drugs)

The class of hypnotic drugs called non-benzodiazepine hypnotics (or Z-drugs) has become the mainstay for the treatment of sleep disorders. Z-drugs have relatively short half-lives and, unlike other hypnotics, do not significantly impact REM sleep. Consequently, the Z-drugs are the most commonly used sleep aids.

Eszopiclone (Lunesta) is similar to zolpidem; however, the FDA has approved it for chronic insomnia. It may cause an unpleasant taste in the mouth, which usually disappears after a couple of weeks. The medication should be taken immediately before bedtime.

Zaleplon (Sonata), the shortest-acting hypnotic, has a four-hour duration of action. It can be taken in the middle of the night. Depending on when the drug is taken, there should be little leftover morning grogginess. Use should be limited to 7–10 days. Zaleplon has the advantage of having the lowest risk of next-day impairment of cognitive function. Patients should be warned to take this drug right before going to bed and to allow enough time to sleep before the drug wears off.

Zolpidem (Ambien, Ambien CR, Edluar, Intermezzo, Zolpimist) has the hypnotic (and many of the anxiety-relieving) properties of the benzodiazepines, but it is structurally dissimilar. It has a high affinity for benzodiazepine receptors, but it

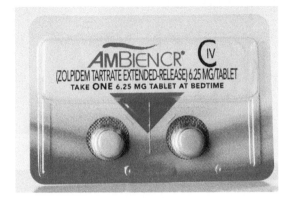

Zolpidem is available in a controlled-release formulation under the brand name Ambien CR.

has reduced effects on skeletal muscle and seizure threshold. Rarely is mechanical ventilation required for an overdose. Zolpidem is used for short-term treatment of insomnia. Its side effects are dizziness, headache, nausea, diarrhea, and next-day drowsiness. Like zaleplon, this drug should not be taken for more than 10 days. Pharmacy technicians should monitor the prescriptions and alert the pharmacist if it is prescribed for a longer period. Of course, there may be exceptions. Ambien CR is approved for long-term use. It is a controlled-release form that contains 12.5 mg, of which 10 mg is released immediately, then 2.5 mg later in the night to help maintain sleep. It prevents early awakening. Zolpimist is the spray form.

Dosage Forms and Administration See Table 8.7 for specific forms. Patients using a hypnotic should use it only a limited number of times each week, and that use should be restricted to a four- to six-week period. Drug-specific administration notes are included in the previous paragraphs.

Side Effects Side effects of the Z-drugs may include sleepwalking or eating, with no recall of the events. There have also been reports of people driving with no recall of the event. The FDA is investigating these reports and encouraging manufacturers to include these side effects in their labeling.

Contraindications Z-drugs do not have contraindications.

Cautions and Considerations Eszopiclone, zaleplon, and zolpidem are Schedule IV controlled substances. Pharmacy technicians should be aware of laws regarding controlled substances in the state in which they practice. Eszopiclone, zaleplon, and zolpidem must be dispensed with a Medication Guide.

CNS depression may result with Z-drug use, including impaired physical and mental capabilities. Patients should be warned about performing tasks that require mental alertness.

Hypnotics are associated with behavior changes and abnormal thinking. Aggression, bizarre behavior, agitation, and hallucinations have all occurred in patients using hypnotics.

Drug Interactions The Z-drugs cause CNS depression with and enhance the adverse effects of other CNS depressants (such as opioids, orphenadrine, paraldehyde, and thalidomide).

Conivaptan and fusidic acid may increase levels of Z-drugs.

Stimulants for Narcolepsy

Narcolepsy is a sleep disorder involving recurring inappropriate episodes of sleep during the daytime hours. It has no known cause. Onset usually occurs in adolescents or young adults, and this disorder continues throughout life. Narcolepsy exhibits four characteristic symptoms. First, the patient feels sleepy during the daytime, pro-ceeding almost immediately into REM sleep without first entering NREM. The patient can only briefly resist the desire to sleep. Second, the patient experiences **cataplexy**, or short periods of muscle weakness or loss of muscle tone, associated with sudden emotions such as joy, fear, or anger. Third, sleep paralysis occurs as the patient falls asleep or immediately upon awakening. The patient wishes to move but finds that, for a brief period, they cannot. Fourth, the patient has vivid hallucinations at the onset of sleep.

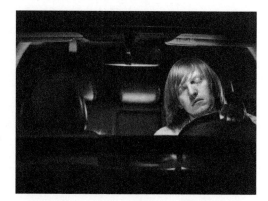

Narcolepsy may make driving or operating heavy machinery unsafe.

Modafinil

One drug approved for narcolepsy is **modafinil (Provigil)**. It is a nonamphetamine stimulant, but it is a Schedule IV controlled substance. Modafinil is also approved for shift-work sleep disorder, which is a disturbance in the circadian rhythm, the cycle of changes the body typically goes through each 24-hour period, and is a response to changes in exposure to light and dark. This problem affects people who work at night. The mechanism of action is unclear, but modafinil does increase mental alertness.

Dosage Forms and Administration Modafinil is available in tablet form.

Side Effects Side effects include nausea, headache, decreased appetite, and stomachache.

Contraindications Hypersensitivity to armodafinil contraindicates the use of modafinil.

Cautions and Considerations Modafinil may impair the ability to engage in hazardous activities, and patients should be warned about performing activities that require mental alertness, such as driving. This medication must be dispensed with a Medication Guide.

Modafinil may increase blood pressure and heart rate. It should be used with caution in patients with cardiac issues.

Patients should avoid alcohol when using modafinil.

Drug Interactions Modafinil may decrease concentrations of axitinib, bosutinib, enzalutamide, nisoldipine, olaparib, simeprevir, and sofosbuvir. Conivaptan may increase modafinil levels. Idelalisib and pimozide concentrations may increase with modafinil use.

Armodafinil

Armodafinil (Nuvigil) is structurally related to modafinil. It is approved for exces-sive sleepiness caused by sleep apnea, narcolepsy, or shift-work sleep disorder. The mechanism of action is unknown. Armodafinil is a Schedule IV controlled substance.

Dosage Forms and Administration Armodafinil should be taken in the morning or one hour before going to work if taken for shift-work sleep disorder. It will not cure sleep apnea, but it will help diminish the symptoms. Armodafinil should not be taken close to the time of sleep and should not be taken for longer than 12 weeks. When prescribed to treat sleep apnea, armodafinil is commonly combined with a continuous positive airway pressure (CPAP) machine. The CPAP machine consists of an air pump, connected to a mask, that blows pressurized air into the nose while its user is sleeping. It does not interrupt normal sleep patterns.

Side Effects The most serious side effect of armodafinil is a skin rash. If a rash appears, the patient should immediately stop taking armodafinil.

Contraindications Hypersensitivity to modafinil contraindicates its use.

Cautions and Considerations Armodafinil may impair the ability to engage in hazardous activities, and patients should be warned about performing activities that require mental alertness, such as driving. Because the drug works on the CNS, patients should avoid alcohol while taking this drug. This medication must be dispensed with a Medication Guide.

Armodafinil should never be used in place of getting enough sleep, and it may decrease the effectiveness of oral contraceptives.

Drug Interactions Conivaptan and fusidic acid may increase armodafinil levels. Idelalisib concentrations may increase with armodafinil use.

Pitolisant

Pitolisant (Wakix) has an unknown mechanism but is thought to work through activity on histamine receptors. Pitolisant is a noncontrolled substance that is used to improve wakefulness in adults with excessive daytime sleepiness. Pitolisant is not a controlled substance.

Dosage Forms and Administration Pitolisant is available as a tablet.

Side Effects Side effects include headache, insomnia, anxiety, irritability, nausea, stomach pain, muscle pain, and increased upper respiratory tract infections.

Contraindications Pitolisant should not be used in patients with severe liver disease.

Cautions and Considerations Pitolisant can cause QT prolongation. It must be used with caution in patients with cardiac arrhythmias or a history of heart disease. Pitolisant should not be taken with other drugs that also have this effect, which include some antibiotics and antidepressants. Pitolisant should be used with caution in patients with kidney or liver disease.

Drug Interactions Pitolisant may reduce the effectiveness of hormonal contraceptives. Patients should use alternative birth control during treatment with pilolisant and for 21 days after the last dose.

Antihistamines and some antidepressants (such as TCAs and mirtazapine) can reduce the effectiveness of pitolisant.

Solriamfetol

Solriamfetol (Sunosi) has an unknown mechanism but is thought to work through activity on dopamine and norepinephrine reuptake. Solriamfetol is used to treat excessive daytime sleepiness associated with narcolepsy and obstructive sleep apnea. Solriamfetol is a Schedule IV controlled substance.

Dosage Forms and Administration Solriamfetol is available as a tablet.

Side Effects Side effects include anxiety, insomnia, irritability, decreased appetite, nausea, diarrhea, dry mouth, and heart palpitations.

Contraindications Solriamfetol should not be used within 14 days of taking an MAOI.

Cautions and Considerations Solriamfetol can cause increases in blood pressure and heart rate. This effect must be monitored as therapy is started with solriamfetol. Patients with unstable heart disease or other serious cardiac disease may not be good candidates to take solriamfetol.

Because solriamfetol can cause anxiety, insomnia, and irritability, it should be used with caution in patients with a history of psychosis or bipolar disorder. It must either be avoided or closely monitored to avoid exacerbation of the underlying disease.

Drug Interactions Other drugs that have stimulant effects (such as bupropion, venlafaxine, and MAOIs) can enhance these side effects of solriamfetol. Antiparkinson drugs can also enhance the hypertensive effects of solriamfetol. Caution should be taken to avoid the additive effects of solriamfetol with these other drugs.

Miscellaneous Hypnotic Agent

Ramelteon (Rozerem) is a hypnotic drug approved for sleep-onset insomnia. It is a melatonin receptor agonist, so there is no potential for abuse, and it is not a controlled substance. It is more potent than melatonin. It has not been shown to be effective in sleep maintenance disorders, just for initiating sleep. It has a rapid onset and no next-day morning grogginess.

Dosage Forms and Administration Ramelteon is available in tablet form.

Side Effects As with most hypnotics, ramelteon's effects may include aggression and agitation.

Contraindications Contraindications include a history of angioedema with previous ramelteon therapy and concurrent use of fluvoxamine.

Cautions and Considerations CNS depression may result from the use of ramelteon, including impaired physical and mental capabilities. Patients should be warned about performing tasks that require mental alertness. This medication must be dispensed with a Medication Guide.

Ramelteon should not be taken with or immediately following a high-fat meal. Patients with liver problems should discuss use of ramelteon with their healthcare practitioners before taking it.

Drug Interactions Ramelteon is a CNS depressant and may enhance the effects of other CNS depressants (such as azelastine, orphenadrine, paraldehyde, and thalidomide). Fluvoxamine may decrease the patients' metabolism of ramelteon.

Benzodiazepines for Insomnia

May Cause **DROWSINESS**

Benzodiazepines, discussed earlier with antianxiety agents, are also used for insomnia. The FDA has approved five benzodiazepines specifically for hypnotic use: **estazolam**, **flurazepam**, **quazepam (Doral)**, **temazepam (Restoril)**, and **triazolam (Halcion)**.

Dosage Forms and Administration Benzodiazepines are available in tablet or capsule form, depending on the drug prescribed.

Side Effects Common side effects of benzodiazepines include muscle weakness, impaired reflexes, and constipation. Patients may also experience difficulty waking up in the morning and residual drowsiness the following day. Pharmacy technicians should affix an auxiliary label about drowsiness to each benzodiazepine prescription.

Contraindications Benzodiazepines are contraindicated in pregnant patients. They may cause fetal damage when administered during pregnancy. Allergy to one benzodiazepine contraindicates use of others.

Quazepam is contraindicated in patients with established or suspected sleep apnea and pulmonary insufficiency.

Triazolam is contraindicated in patients taking itraconazole, ketoconazole, or HIV protease inhibitors.

Safety Alert

All benzodiazepines must be dispensed with a Medication Guide.

Cautions and Considerations All benzodiazepines have dependence and abuse potential. Consequently, they are considered Schedule IV controlled substances. Patients can become both physically and psychologically dependent on benzodiazepines, making it difficult to stop therapy. Patients should be aware of this potential and should understand that benzodiazepines should be used only for a short time. If a benzodiazepine is used for longer than a couple of weeks, doses must be slowly tapered to prevent withdrawal symptoms. All benzodiazepines must be dispensed with a Medication Guide. Because these drugs are controlled substances, their prescriptions have a limited number of refills and may have specific storage requirements. Pharmacy technicians should be familiar with regulations and follow their facility's policies and procedures for dispensing benzodiazepines. Patients with heart conditions may not be able to take benzodiazepines and should be monitored closely. These medications can increase a patient's heart rate.

Do not drink alcoholic beverages when taking this medication

Drug Interactions The effects of CNS depressants may be enhanced by benzodiazepines. Azole antifungals may decrease the patients' metabolism of benzodiazepines. Digoxin and phenytoin concentrations may be increased by benzodiazepines. TCA levels may increase when used with benzodiazepines.

8.6 Alcohol Dependence and Drug Treatments

Alcohol dependence, sometimes referred to as *alcoholism*, is a pattern of alcohol use that involves problems controlling drinking, preoccupation with alcohol, use of alcohol even when it causes problems, drinking more to get the same effect, or experiencing withdrawal symptoms upon rapidly decreasing or stopping drinking. The World Health Organization estimates that 75 million people suffer from alcohol dependence globally. Genetic, psychological, social, and environmental factors all contribute to alcohol dependence. Theories suggest that, for certain people, drinking has a different and stronger impact that can lead to alcohol use disorder.

Alcohol dependence can impact health. Liver disease, digestive problems, cardiac complications, diabetes, sexual dysfunction, immune system weakening, and neurologic complications can all result. Furthermore, alcohol dependence can impact safety and can increase the risk of motor vehicle accidents, drowning, and legal problems.

Alcoholism is a complex genetic disease. The abuser has different levels of brain chemicals, different levels of enzymes, or altogether different enzymes that metabolize alcohol at different rates and quantities than someone without alcohol use disorder. Thus, genetic makeup may affect a person's likelihood of experiencing alcohol dependence.

Ethanol (alcohol), the intoxicating agent in liquors, is an anesthetic. As with any anesthetic, intake of a large quantity of ethanol causes loss of consciousness. However, the margin between loss of consciousness and medullary paralysis (loss of function of the brain's respiratory centers) is smaller than with general anesthetics. The **emetic** (vomit-inducing) action of ethanol usually prevents death by reducing absorption to less-than-lethal concentrations. Many deaths from alcohol are due to cirrhosis of (irreversible damage to) the liver or aspiration of vomitus during unconsciousness.

Habitual drinkers have an increased ability to metabolize ethanol rapidly, which increases tolerance. Neurons in the CNS adapt to the presence of ethanol, and habitual drinkers learn to compensate to some extent for the depressant action.

Alcohol use disorder takes a substantial toll on many aspects of health. Heavy drinking may lead to obesity coupled with vitamin deficiency. In the later stages of alcohol use disorder, gastritis and loss of appetite, organic brain damage, alcoholic psychosis, and dementia occur. Cirrhosis of the liver results from fatty synthesis and excessive buildup of lipid compounds.

Treatment for alcohol dependence involves multiple modalities, including counseling, behavior modification, and pharmacologic therapy. In the most severe form, alcohol dependence is likely to require drug therapy to treat withdrawal symptoms.

Dependence on and Withdrawal from Alcohol

Chemical dependence is a person's inability to control their use of some chemical substance; they are unable to stop their use or limit the amount they use. Dependence is often a physical condition that cannot be cured by willpower. A person can be chemically dependent without showing obvious signs. Table 8.8 lists symptoms of dependence. To resolve this health issue, people with alcohol dependence must take four steps toward recovery:

1. Acknowledge the problem.
2. Limit time spent with substance users.
3. Seek professional help.
4. Seek support from people recovering from alcohol dependence.

TABLE 8.8 Alcohol Dependence Symptoms

blackouts or lapses of memory

concerns of family, friends, and employers about drinking

doing things while under the influence of alcohol that cause regret afterward

financial or legal problems from drinking

loss of pleasure without alcohol

neglecting responsibilities

trying to cut down or quit drinking but failing

drinking alone; hiding evidence

drinking to forget about problems

willingness to do almost anything to get alcohol

Abrupt withdrawal of alcohol can precipitate a variety of symptoms, some of which are serious and even life threatening. Table 8.9 lists withdrawal symptoms. The first signs of withdrawal appear within a few hours. In mild withdrawal, symptoms may disappear in one to two days; in severe withdrawal, symptoms may last one to two weeks.

TABLE 8.9 Alcohol Withdrawal Symptoms

agitation	mental disturbances
circulatory disturbances	nausea and vomiting
convulsions	restlessness
delirium tremens	sweating
digestive disorders	temporary suppression of REM sleep
disorientation	tremors
extreme fear	weakness
hallucinations	

Benzodiazepines are frequently used during detoxification, the process of freeing a person from their dependence on a substance. Their dosage must be adjusted to the needs of individual patients. Benzodiazepines prevent detoxification-related seizures and **delirium tremens**, a condition caused by cessation of alcohol consumption in which coarse, irregular tremors are accompanied by vivid hallucinations.

Alcohol withdrawal may also necessitate administering a sedative, anticonvulsant, beta-blocker, or antipsychotic or a combination of these drugs. In addition, when a person with alcohol dependence enters a treatment program, arrives at an emergency department, or is admitted into a hospital, they are usually given folic acid, thiamine (vitamin B_1), and a multipurpose vitamin. This treatment is given because liver damage, imbalanced fluid intake, and imbalanced nutrition cause people with alcohol dependence to be deficient in vitamins, particularly the water-soluble ones.

Name Exchange
Although folic acid is only available in generic, the old brand name (Folvite) may still be referenced in the pharmacy.

Drugs Used for Alcohol Dependence

Three drugs are approved for treating alcohol dependence (see Table 8.10). They work in different ways and are prescribed taking into consideration individual circumstances. Any drug regimen for alcohol dependence must be accompanied by psychosocial support.

TABLE 8.10 Commonly Used Drugs for Alcohol Dependence

Generic (Brand)	Pronunciation	Dosage Form	Common Dosage	Dispensing Status
acamprosate (Campral)	a-kam-PROE-sate	tablet	666 mg 3 times a day	Rx
disulfiram (Antabuse)	dye-SUL-fi-ram	tablet	125–500 mg 1 time a day	Rx
naltrexone (ReVia, Vivitrol)	nal-TREX-one	injection, tablet	PO: 50 mg a day IM: 380 mg every 4 weeks	Rx

Acamprosate

TAKE WITH FOOD

Acamprosate (Campral) is thought to work by restoring balance between neuronal excitation and neuronal inhibition. This reestablishment of balance reduces the negative effects of abstinence from alcohol and may diminish the chance of relapse. A combination of disulfiram and acamprosate may work better than either drug alone.

Dosage Forms and Administration Drug therapy should be combined with a comprehensive management program that includes psychosocial support. Acamprosate is taken three times a day, with meals, because food increases absorption. This regimen may also improve patient adherence and help prevent alcohol cravings and relapses. Acamprosate, however, is not an effective treatment for delirium tremens.

Side Effects The most common adverse effects include headache, diarrhea, flatulence, and nausea.

Contraindications Acamprosate is contraindicated in patients with severe renal failure.

Cautions and Considerations Acamprosate use may cause CNS depression. Patients using acamprosate have attempted suicide. Patients should be monitored for depression and suicidal thinking. Dose adjustment is needed in patients with renal insufficiency.

Drug Interactions Acamprosate has no known drug interactions.

Disulfiram

Do not drink alcoholic beverages when taking this medication

Disulfiram (Antabuse) stops the patients' metabolism of alcohol, allowing acetaldehyde to accumulate in body tissues. When a patient taking disulfiram consumes alcohol, the acetaldehyde causes violent effects almost instantaneously. These effects include:

- blurred vision
- confusion
- difficulty breathing
- hot, flushed face
- intense throbbing in head and neck
- chest pain

- nausea
- severe headache
- severe vomiting
- thirst
- uneasiness

These effects are known as **disulfiram-like reactions**. The patient usually becomes exhausted and sleeps for several hours after symptoms have worn off. Patients who are taking disulfiram must examine food labels to be sure they do not inadvertently ingest alcohol in an everyday product (such as a cough medicine, mouthwash, salad dressing, or wine vinegar). Several other prescription drugs can produce a disulfiram-like reaction when combined with alcohol. These medications include metronidazole, some cephalosporins, and certain oral hypoglycemic drugs. Pharmacy technicians should place an auxiliary label about alcohol use on these medication containers during the dispensing process.

Dosage Forms and Administration Disulfiram is available as a tablet.

Side Effects The main effects of this drug are identified above.

Contraindications Contraindications to disulfiram include severe myocardial disease, coronary occlusion, psychosis, and known hypersensitivity to disulfiram or other thiuram derivatives. Disulfiram is generally avoided in individuals who are pregnant or nursing.

Cautions and Considerations Disulfiram has a boxed warning. It should never be administered to a patient during a state of ethanol intoxication, within 12 hours after they have consumed alcohol, or without their knowledge.

Liver dysfunction is associated with disulfiram use. Consequently, liver function should be monitored in patients taking this drug.

Drug Interactions The adverse effects of alcohol and products that contain alcohol (such as lopinavir / ritonavir and ritonavir oral solution) are potentiated (made active or made more active) with disulfiram use. Disulfiram may enhance the adverse effects of metronidazole. The levels of paraldehyde and phenytoin in the body may be increased by disulfiram. Tinidazole may enhance the adverse effects of disulfiram.

Naltrexone

Naltrexone (ReVia, Vivitrol) is a pure opiate antagonist that blocks the effects of endogenous opioids released as a result of alcohol consumption, making alcohol consumption less pleasurable. It is used to treat alcohol dependence. Patients should have reached a point of stability after alcohol withdrawal before starting this drug. In opiate-dependent patients, naltrexone can cause an acute withdrawal syndrome, including nausea, dizziness, headache, and weight loss. To prevent withdrawal symptoms, those individuals with a history of opiate intake must be opiate free before starting the drug. Vivitrol is the injectable extended-release form of this drug. It decreases the effectiveness of opiates for pain, cough, and diarrhea. Patients taking this drug should wear a medical alert pendant or bracelet so that if they are treated in an emergency department, the staff will know not to provide opiates.

REFRIGERATE

Dosage Forms and Administration Naltrexone is available as a tablet or injection. The injection, Vivitrol is administered intramuscularly, monthly, in alternating buttocks. It is packaged in a single-use carton that contains the drug in powdered form, the diluent, and a syringe. The entire carton should be stored under refrigeration, but can be stored at controlled room temperature for up to 7 days prior to administration.

Side Effects Side effects of naltrexone include headache, nausea, vomiting, dizziness, abdominal pain, and insomnia.

Contraindications Contraindications include opioid dependence, current use of opioid analgesics (including partial opioid agonists), acute opioid withdrawal, failure to pass the naloxone challenge (a test that assesses physical dependence), and a positive urine screen for opioids.

Cautions and Considerations Accidental opioid overdose may occur with naltrexone use. Patients using naltrexone may respond to lower opioid doses than previously used, leading to life-threatening opioid intoxication.

Use naltrexone with caution in patients with hepatic dysfunction.

Drug Interactions Naltrexone may enhance the adverse effects of methylnaltrexone and naloxegol.

8.7 Complementary and Alternative Therapies

Melatonin is used for sleep and insomnia disorders as well as for benzodiazepine and nicotine withdrawal. It is used occasionally for a variety of other disorders, including headache.

Melatonin is a naturally produced hormone that helps regulate circadian rhythms (sleep-wake cycles). People generally take 0.3 to 5 mg before bedtime to induce sleep. Common side effects include drowsiness, headache, and dizziness. Melatonin can also cause mild tremors, anxiety, abdominal cramps, irritability, confusion, nausea, and low blood pressure. Melatonin interacts with other medications; it should never be taken with CNS depressants because excessive sedation could occur.

Kava, an extract derived from a *Piper methysticum* plant, is used to treat anxiety and insomnia. It has been found to be effective but dangerous. Kava can induce hepatotoxicity and liver failure, so patient self-treatment is not recommended. Kava lactone is the active ingredient and is thought to work by affecting GABA and dopamine in the brain. Other side effects include stomach upset, headache, dizziness, drowsiness, dry mouth, and EPS effects. Patients should also realize that herbal, dietary, and other supplements are not subject to the standardization among manufacturers that is required for prescription and OTC drugs.

St. John's wort is taken orally for mild depression with some success. It has also been used to relieve the psychological symptoms of menopause when used with black cohosh (Remifemin). Patients should discuss St. John's wort with their healthcare practitioners before taking it and make sure it is documented in their medication history.

The active ingredient in St. John's wort is hypericin, which has activity similar to that of SSRIs. Common starting doses range from 300 to 400 mg three times a day. Maintenance doses are often lower and may range from 300 to 900 mg a day. Side effects include insomnia, vivid dreams, restlessness, anxiety, irritability, upset stomach, diarrhea, fatigue, dry mouth, dizziness, and headache. Usually these effects are mild. St. John's wort can cause photosensitivity, so proper skin protection should be used.

St. John's wort should not be taken with other antidepressants, because serotonin syndrome could develop. In addition, it should not be taken with CNS depressants, such as digoxin, phenytoin, or phenobarbital. St. John's wort can alter the effectiveness of these and other drugs, including warfarin and some drugs for HIV and acquired immune deficiency syndrome (AIDS).

TABLE 8.11 Agents and Drug Classes that Interact with St. John's Wort

Severe Interactions

alfentanil (Alfenta)	digoxin (Lanoxin)	(various contraceptives)
alprazolam (Xanax)	docetaxel (Taxotene)	omeprazole (Prilosec)
antifungals (ketoconazole, itraconazole)	fluoxetine (Prozac)	omeprazole (Prilosec)
	glucocorticoids	ondansetron (Zofran)
calcium channel blockers (diltiazem, nicardipine, verapamil)	Imatinib (Gleevec)	oxycodone (Oxycontin)
	ketamine (Ketalar)	pentobarbital (Nembutal)
	losartan (Cozaar)	phenobarbital
chemotherapeutic agents (etoposide, paclitaxel, vinblastine, vincristine, vindesine)	mephenytoin (Mesantoin)	propranolol (Inderal)
	midazolam (Versed)	protease inhibitors (PIs)
	non-nucleoside reverse transcriptase inhibitors (NNRTIs)	secobarbital (Seconal)
cisapride (Propulsid)		tacrolimus (Prograf)
cyclosporine (Neoral, Sandimmune)	norethindrone and ethinyl estradiol	warfarin (Coumadin)

Moderate Interactions

bupropion (Wellbutrin)	imipramine (Tofranil)	zolmitriptan (Zomig)
clopidogrel (Plavix)	mexiletine (Mexitil)	dexamethasone (Decadron)
clozapine (Clozaril)	olanzapine (Zyprexa)	amitriptyline (Elavil)
cyclobenzaprine (Flexeril)	propranolol (Inderal)	carisoprodol (Soma)
fluvoxamine (Luvox)	tacrine (Cognex)	citalopram (Celexa)
haloperidol (Haldol)	zileuton (Zyflo)	diazepam (Valium)
lansoprazole (Prevacid)		

Patients taking natural products for mood disorders or insomnia should discuss those therapies with their healthcare practitioners. Herbal and dietary supplements may not adequately treat symptoms of depression or insomnia. Patients who display symptoms of mental illness should be evaluated by a physician and should not be self-treated. Pharmacy technicians should encourage patients to communicate with their healthcare practitioners.

Review and Assessment

Depression, Mood Disorders, and Drug Treatments

- Antidepressants are not controlled substances.

- Antidepressant drug classes include SSRIs, SNRIs, tricyclic and tetracyclic antidepressants, and MAOIs.

- TCAs can be cardiotoxic in high doses.

- Because of their many interactions with other drugs and foods, MAOIs are not first-line therapy for depression.

- It may take at least two weeks for most antidepressants to be effective.

Bipolar Disorder and Drug Treatments

- Lithium is commonly used to treat bipolar (manic-depressive) disorder and acute mania and for prophylaxis of unipolar and bipolar disorders.

- A patient taking lithium must have frequent blood tests to assess lithium levels and maintain a therapeutic range.

- Carbamazepine Carbatrol, Epitol, Equetro, (Tegretol), divalproex (Depakote), or valproic acid (Depakene) may be used to treat bipolar disorder.

Schizophrenia, Psychosis, and Drug Treatments

- The older agents are identified as "typical" antipsychotics and are effective, but serious long-term side effects limit their use. Prescribers are moving away from these drugs and toward the newer "atypical" antipsychotics, such as aripiprazole (Abilify), clozapine (Clozaril, FazaClo ODT, Versacloz), olanzapine (Zyprexa, Zyprexa Relprevv), paliperidone (Invega, Invega Sustenna, Invega Trinza), quetiapine (Seroquel, Seroquel XR), risperidone (Perseris, RisperDAL, RisperDAL Consta, RisperDAL M-TAB), and ziprasidone (Geodon).

- Anticholinergics can minimize some of the side effects of typical antipsychotic drugs.

Anxiety and Drug Treatments

- Anxiety is a state of uneasiness characterized by apprehension and worry about possible events.

- Panic disorder is characterized by intense, overwhelming, and uncontrollable anxiety.

- SSRIs, SNRIs, benzodiazepines, buspirone, and hydroxyzine are used to treat anxiety.

Sleep Disorders and Drug Treatments

- Benzodiazepines that are FDA approved for hypnotic use are estazolam, flurazepam, quazepam (Doral), temazepam (Restoril), and triazolam (Halcion).

- Many sleep agents should be administered one hour before bedtime.

- The Z-drugs are the preferred treatment for sleep disorders.

- Zaleplon (Sonata) is the shortest-acting hypnotic, with a duration of action of four hours. Therefore, it may be taken in the middle of the night.

- Zolpidem (Ambien) has many of the same properties as the benzodiazepines, but it is structurally dissimilar.

- Eszopiclone (Lunesta) is approved for chronic insomnia.

- Rozerem is not a controlled substance because it works in a different way from other hypnotics.

Alcohol Dependence and Drug Treatments

- Alcohol dependence is a serious disorder that is treated nonpharmacologically as well as with medications.

- Three drugs have been approved for treatment of alcohol dependence: disulfiram (Antabuse), acamprosate (Campral), and naltrexone (Revia, Vivitrol).

Complementary and Alternative Therapies

- Melatonin, a naturally produced hormone, can be used for sleep and insomnia disorders.

- Kava, a plant extract, is used to treat anxiety and insomnia.

- St. John's wort is taken orally for mild depression with some success.

DRUG LIST

Selective Serotonin Reuptake Inhibitors (SSRIs)
citalopram (Celexa)
escitalopram (Lexapro)
fluoxetine (Prozac, Prozac Weekly, Sarafem)
fluvoxamine (Luvox)
paroxetine (Brisdelle, Paxil, Paxil CR, Pexeva)
sertraline (Zoloft)

Serotonin-Norepinephrine Reuptake Inhibitors (SNRIs)
desvenlafaxine (Pristiq)
duloxetine (Cymbalta)
levomilnacipran (Fetzima)
milnacipran (Savella)
venlafaxine (Effexor, Effexor CR)

Tricyclic Antidepressants (TCAs)
amitriptyline
clomipramine (Anafranil)
desipramine (Norpramin)
doxepin (Silenor, Zonalon)
imipramine (Tofranil)
nortriptyline (Aventyl, Pamelor)

Tetracyclic Antidepressant
mirtazapine (Remeron)

Monoamine Oxidase Inhibitors (MAOIs)
phenelzine (Nardil)
selegiline (Eldepryl, Emsam, Zelapar)
tranylcypromine (Parnate)

Miscellaneous Antidepressants
bupropion (Aplenzin, Forfivo XL, Wellbutrin, Wellbutrin SR, Wellbutrin XL, Zyban)
trazodone

Agents for Treating Bipolar Disorders
carbamazepine (Carbatrol, Epitol, Equetro, Tegretol)
divalproex (Depakote)
lithium (Lithobid)
valproic acid (Depakene)

Antipsychotics
aripiprazole (Abilify)
aripiprazole lauroxil (Aristada)
asenapine (Saphris)
brexpiprazole (Rexulti)
cariprazine (Vraylar)
clozapine (Clozaril, FazaClo ODT, Versacloz)
fluphenazine
haloperidol (Haldol, Haldol Decanoate)
iloperidone (Fanapt)
lumateperone (Caplyta)
lurasidone (Latuda)
loxapine (Adasuve)
olanzapine (Zyprexa, Zyprexa Relprevv)
molindone
paliperidone (Invega, Invega Sustenna, Invega Trinza)
pimavanserin (Nuplazid)
perphenazine
pimozide (Orap)
prochlorperazine (Compro)
quetiapine (Seroquel, Seroquel XR)
risperidone (Perseris, RisperDAL, RisperDAL Consta, RisperDAL M-TAB)
thioridazine
trifluoperazine
ziprasidone (Geodon)

Agents for Minimizing the Effects of Antipsychotics
benztropine
diphenhydramine (Benadryl)

Antianxiety Agents
buspirone
citalopram (Celexa)
duloxetine (Cymbalta)
escitalopram (Lexapro)
hydroxyzine (Vistaril)
paroxetine (Brisdelle, Paxil, Paxil CR, Pexeva)
sertraline (Zoloft)
venlafaxine (Effexor, Effexor XR)

Benzodiazepines
alprazolam (Xanax, Xanax XR)
chlordiazepoxide (Librium)
clonazepam (Klonopin)
clorazepate (Tranxene)
diazepam (Diastat, Valium, Valtoco)
estazolam
flurazepam
lorazepam (Ativan, Lorazepam Intensol)
oxazepam
quazepam (Doral)
temazepam (Restoril)
triazolam (Halcion)

Stimulants for Narcolepsy
armodafinil (Nuvigil)
modafinil (Provigil)
pitolisant (Wakix)
solriamfetol (Sunosi)

Agents for Insomnia
diphenhydramine (Benadryl)
eszopiclone (Lunesta)
ramelteon (Rozerem)
zaleplon (Sonata)
zolpidem (Ambien, Ambien CR, Edluar, Intermezzo, Zolpimist)

Agents for Alcohol Use Disorder
acamprosate (Campral)
disulfiram (Antabuse)
naltrexone (ReVia, Vivitrol)

Boxed Warnings
amitriptyline (Elavil)
aripiprazole (Abilify)
aripiprazole lauroxil (Aristada)
armodafinil (Nuvigil)
asenapine (Saphris)
brexpiprazole (Rexulti)
bupropion (Aplenzin, Forfivo XL, Wellbutrin, Wellbutrin SR, Wellbutrin XL, Zyban)
cariprazine (Vraylar)
citalopram (Celexa)
clomipramine (Anafranil)
clozapine (Clozaril, FazaClo ODT, Versacloz)
desipramine (Norpramin)
desvanlafaxine (Pristiq)
disulfiram (Antabuse)
doxepin (Silenor, Zonalon)

duloxetine (Cymbalta)
escitalopram (Lexapro)
fluoxetine (Prozac, Prozac Weekly, Sarafem)
fluvoxamine (Luvox)
iloperidone (Fanapt)
imipramine (Tofranil)
levomilnacipran (Fetzima)
lithium (Eskalith, Lithobid)
lumateperone (Caplyta)
lurasidone (Latuda)
milnacipran (Savella)
mirtazapine (Remeron)
nortriptyline (Aventyl, Pamelor)
olanzapine (Zyprexa, Zyprexa Relprevv)
paliperidone (Invega, Invega Sustenna,
    Invega Trinza)
paroxetine (Brisdelle, Paxil, Paxil CR, Pexeva)
phenelzine (Nardil)
pimavanserin (Nuplazid)
quetiapine (Seroquel, Seroquel XR)
risperidone (Perseris, RisperDAL, RisperDAL
    Consta, RisperDAL M-TAB)
selegiline (Eldepryl)
sertraline (Zoloft)
tranylcypromine (Parnate)
trazodone
venlafaxine (Effexor, Effexor XR)
ziprasidone (Geodon)

Medication Guides

Note that in addition to the agents listed below, all antidepressants and all agents for treating bipolar disorder (except for Lithobid) must be dispensed with a Medication Guide.

aripiprazole (Abilify)
aripiprazole lauroxil (Aristada)
armodafinil (Nuvigil)
brexpiprazole (Rexulti)
cariprazine (Vraylar)
clorazepate (Tranxene)
estazolam
eszopiclone (Lunesta)
flurazepam
levomilnacipran (Fetzima)
lurasidone (Latuda)
modafinil (Provigil)
olanzapine (Zyprexa, Zyprexa Relprevv)
paroxetine (Brisdelle, Paxil, Paxil CR, Pexeva)
quazepam (Doral)
quetiapine (Seroquel, Seroquel XR)
ramelteon (Rozerem)
triazolam (Halcion)
zaleplon (Sonata)
zolpidem (Ambien, Ambien CR, Edluar,
    Intermezzo, Zolpimist)

✓ CHECK YOUR UNDERSTANDING

Take a moment to review what you have learned in this chapter and answer the following questions.

1. Which of the following drugs is a selective serotonin reuptake inhibitor used for depression?
   a. aripiprazole
   b. escitalopram
   c. mirtazapine
   d. alprazolam

2. Which of the following drugs is a selective serotonin reuptake inhibitor that is sometimes used for anxiety?
   a. buspirone
   b. diazepam
   c. paroxetine
   d. trazodone

3. Which of the following is a typical (1st generation) antipsychotic?
   a. Abilify
   b. Clozaril
   c. Geodon
   d. Haldol

4. Which of the following is an atypical antipsychotic?
   a. Aristada
   b. Latuda
   c. Vraylar
   d. All answers are correct.

5. Which of the following is an antipsychotic drug that can cause significant weight gain associated with high cholesterol and onset of diabetes?
   a. estazolam
   b. sertraline
   c. lithium
   d. olanzapine

6. Which of the following antianxiety drugs is a controlled substance?
   a. Lexapro
   b. Librium
   c. Vistaril
   d. Zoloft

7. Which of the following drugs is used to discourage alcohol consumption by causing flushing, blurred vision, chest pain, and vomiting?
   a. acamprosate
   b. disulfuram
   c. naltrexone
   d. All answers are correct.

8. Which of the following is an injectable antipsychotic drug given just one time every four to six weeks?
   a. aripiprazole lauroxil
   b. haloperidol
   c. paliperidone
   d. All answers are correct.

9. Which of the following drugs used as sleep aids activates receptors for melatonin, a natural hormone that causes sleepiness?
   a. Doral
   b. Restoril
   c. Rozerem
   d. Sonata

10. Which of the following drugs is the drug used most often for treatment of bipolar disorder?
    a. nortriptyline
    b. selegiline
    c. lithium
    d. Wellbutrin

MAKE CONNECTIONS

Take a moment to consider what you have learned in this chapter and respond thoughtfully to the following prompts. Note that some of these activities will require internet access.

1. How long does it take for the full effect of antidepressants to be achieved? Describe how a patient starts taking antidepressants and what they can expect when starting therapy.

2. Charles is a patient with schizophrenia to whom you have been providing refills of olanzapine for the past six months. You notice that he has improved in his mood and appears more well groomed than he did a few months ago. Yet he has gained quite a bit of weight. Describe the effect olanzapine can have on body weight and metabolism. What other conditions is Charles at risk for developing with this effect?

 The online course includes additional review and assessment resources.

The Sensory
System and
Drug Therapy

Learning Objectives

1 Identify the anatomy and physiology of the eyes and ears. (Section 9.1 and 9.5)

2 Identify the classes of ophthalmic drugs and the conditions they treat. (Section 9.2 to 9.4)

3 Describe how to properly use eye drops and ointments. (Section 9.3 and 9.4)

4 Identify the classes of otic agents and their uses. (Section 9.6)

5 Explain how to properly use eardrops. (Section 9.6)

ASHP/ACPE Accreditation Standards
To view the *ASHP/ACPE Accreditation Standards* addressed in this chapter, refer to Appendix C.

Ophthalmic and otic (eye and ear) medications are used to treat a variety of conditions, including glaucoma, conjunctivitis, and otalgia (earache). These classes of drugs range from antibiotics and corticosteroids to prostaglandin analogs and beta-blockers for glaucoma.

9.1 Anatomy and Physiology of the Eyes

For the EYE
The eyes are sensory organs adapted to sense light and produce vision. Light enters the eye through the pupil and is focused by the lens (see Figure 9.1). The lens is located just behind the **pupil**, the black center of the eye. The **lens** of the eye acts like a lens in a camera, focusing light onto the back of the eye. The **iris**, which surrounds the pupil, determines eye color. The **sclera**, commonly referred to as the white of the eye, is the outer layer of the eyeball.

Sight begins with light that travels through the cornea and lens to the retina in the back of the eye. In the **retina**, photoreceptor cells detect light and color. These rod- and cone-shaped sensory cells send signals via the optic nerve to the brain, where sight is ultimately perceived and interpreted. **Rod cells** are sensitive to light in dimly lit conditions. They are responsible for night vision. Vitamin A deficiency can cause malfunctions in retinal rod cells, affecting night vision. Rod cells are also considered responsible for black-and-white vision. **Cone cells** sense color and are responsible for day vision. Color blindness, usually caused by a genetic trait that primarily affects men, is a condition in which cone cells do not differentiate certain colors. The most common form of color blindness is the inability to differentiate red from green. Inside the **macula**, a yellowish spot near the center of the retina, is the focal point (fovea centralis), where light is concentrated for vision (see Figure 9.1). The macula is rich in cone cells.

Other parts of the eye relevant to drug therapy include the cornea, anterior chamber, aqueous humor, vitreous humor, ciliary body and muscle, and conjunctiva. The **cornea**, which is transparent, is a protective cover over the anterior chamber, iris, and pupil. The **anterior chamber** is the container behind the cornea that holds **aqueous humor**, a fluid that lubricates and protects the lens. **Vitreous humor** is the fluid inside the eye, behind the lens. The **ciliary muscle** holds the lens in place. The **conjunctiva** is the mucous membrane that covers the sclera and inner eyelids.

Some eye disorders require chronic (recurring, long-term) treatment, whereas others need only acute (short-term) treatment. For example, glaucoma and chronic dry eye are managed primarily with repeated or chronic use of medications. Conversely, conjunctivitis requires acute treatment to resolve the eye infection. Most eye disorders are treated with topical opthalmic agents, either eye drops or eye ointment.

FIGURE 9.1
The Structures of the Eye

(a) The external eye

(b) Cross section of the internal eye

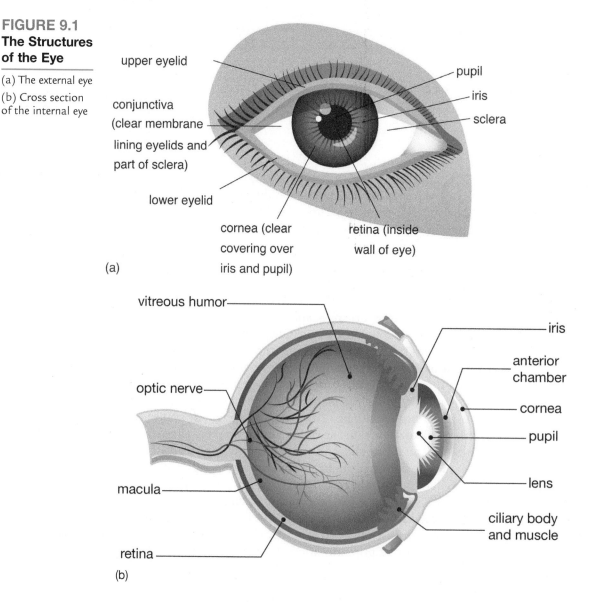

(a)

(b)

9.2 Glaucoma and Drug Treatments

Glaucoma is a condition in which abnormally high **intraocular pressure** (a buildup of force inside the eye) pushes on the optic nerve and damages it. The **optic nerve** is the nerve connecting the eye to the brain. Glaucoma can lead to blindness if it is not treated. The increased pressure comes from either overproduction of aqueous humor or blockage of its outflow from the anterior chamber. (See the parts of the eye in Figure 9.1.) As fluid builds up in the anterior chamber, intraocular pressure behind the anterior chamber increases, and pressure is applied to the optic nerve. **Open-angle glaucoma** is a slowly progressing, chronic condition managed with medication alone. **Narrow-angle glaucoma** is an acute condition that comes on quickly and is resolved with surgery followed by drugs. Table 9.1 lists common agents used to treat glaucoma.

Safety Alert

Betagan, Betoptic, and Betoptic S are easily confused.

Ophthalmic glaucoma agents come as eye drops and work by reducing the production of aqueous humor or by enhancing its drainage from the anterior chamber. Some agents constrict the pupil slightly by contracting the ciliary muscle, which enhances aqueous humor outflow. These agents include prostaglandin analogs, beta-blockers, alpha receptor agonists, and carbonic anhydrase inhibitors. See Table 9.1 for a list of common agents to treat glaucoma.

TABLE 9.1 Ophthalmic Agents for Glaucoma

Generic (Brand)	Pronunciation	Dosage Form	Common Dosages	Dispensing Status
Prostaglandin Analogs				
bimatoprost (Lumigan)	bye-MAT-oe-prost	ophthalmic solution	1 drop each night	Rx
latanoprost (Xalatan)	la-TAN-oe-prost	ophthalmic solution	1 drop each night	Rx
latanoprostene bunod (Vyzulta)	la-TAN-oe-PROS-teen buh-NOD	ophthalmic solution	1 drop each night	Rx
tafluprost (Zioptan)	TA-flu-prost	ophthalmic solution	1 drop each night	Rx
travoprost (Travatan Z)	TRAV-oe-prost	ophthalmic solution	1 drop each night	Rx
unoprostone (Rescula)	yoo-noe-PROS-tone	ophthalmic solution	1 drop each night	Rx
Beta-Blocker				
betaxolol (Betoptic S)	be-TAX-oe-lawl	ophthalmic solution, ophthalmic suspension	1 drop 2 times a day	Rx
carteolol (generic only)	KAR-tee-oh-lole	ophthalmic solution	1 drop 2 times a day	Rx
levobunolol (Betagan)	LEE-voe-BYOO-no-lahl	ophthalmic solution	1 drop 2 times a day	Rx
metipranolol (OptiPranolol)	MET-i-PRAN-oh-lol	ophthalmic solution	1 drop 2 times a day	Rx
timolol (Betimol, Timoptic, Timoptic GFS, Timoptic-XE)	TYE-moe-lawl	ophthalmic solution, ophthalmic gel (extended release)	1 drop 2 times a day	Rx
Alpha Receptor Agonists				
apraclonidine (Iopidine)	ap-pra-KLOE-ni-deen	ophthalmic solution	1 drop 3 times a day	Rx
brimonidine (Alphagan P, Lumify, Quoliana)	bri-MOE-ni-deen	ophthalmic solution	1 drop 3 times a day	OTC, Rx

continues

TABLE 9.1 Ophthalmic Agents for Glaucoma—*Continued*

Generic (Brand)	Pronunciation	Dosage Form	Common Dosages	Dispensing Status
Carbonic Anhydrase Inhibitors				
acetazolamide (Diamox)	ah-SET-ah-ZOE-la-mide	oral capsule, oral tablet	1 drop 2–3 times a day	Rx
brinzolamide (Azopt)	brin-ZOE-la-mide	ophthalmic solution	1 drop 2–3 times a day	Rx
dichlorphenamide (Keveyis)	die-KLOR-fen-a-mide	tablet	1 drop 2–3 times a day	Rx
dorzolamide (Trusopt, Trusopt Ocumeter Plus)	door-ZOE-la-mide	ophthalmic solution	1 drop 2–3 times a day	Rx
methazolamide	meth-a-ZOE-la-mide	tablet	1 drop 2–3 times a day	Rx

Prostaglandin analogs are first-line therapy for glaucoma because they are the most effective and need only be used once a day. Prostaglandin analogs work by increasing aqueous humor outflow from the anterior chamber.

Beta-blockers are also considered first-line therapy for glaucoma and usually cost less than prostaglandin analogs. However, beta-blockers must be used twice a day.

Other agents for glaucoma include carbonic anhydrase inhibitors and ophthalmic alpha receptor agonists. Both classes of drugs must be used three times a day, which many patients find challenging. Oral dosage forms of beta-blockers and alpha receptor agonists are available (see Chapter 10), but they are not usually used to treat glaucoma.

Dosage Forms and Administration Medications used to treat glaucoma are primarily available as eye drops. Local administration in the eye reduces the potential for systemic side effects. Some classes of medications are administered once a day, and others are administered two or three times a day. The once-a-day formulations are preferred because they are easiest for patients to remember to use as directed. Contacts must be removed before application of eye drops and must be left out for at least 15 minutes afterward. To instill eye drops, patients should lie down or tilt their head back, pull the lower eyelid downward, and gently squeeze the container to allow the required number of drops to fall into the eye without touching the tip of the applicator to the eye, eyelid, eyelashes, or fingers.

Side Effects Glaucoma agents are usually well tolerated. Side effects include mild stinging, tearing, itchiness, and dryness of the eyes. These effects generally improve with time. Many glaucoma agents have the potential to cause systemic effects if enough medication is absorbed into the bloodstream. These effects are primarily associated with beta-blockers and include slowed heart rate, heart problems, insomnia, dizziness, vertigo, headaches, tiredness, and difficulty breathing. If any of these effects occur, patients should contact their prescribers right away. A change in drug therapy will be needed.

Contraindications Prostaglandin analogs do not have contraindications.

Beta-blocker ophthalmic products are contraindicated in patients with heart problems, including sinus bradycardia, heart block greater than first degree, cardiogenic shock, and uncompensated heart failure. Carteolol and levobunolol should not be used in patients with respiratory problems such as chronic obstructive pulmonary disease (COPD), bronchial asthma, or pulmonary edema.

Put Down Roots

Note the following drug stems to identify each class.
-olol: beta blocker
-prost-: prostaglandin analog
-nidine: alpha agonists
-zolamide: carbonic anhydrase inhibitor

Practice Tip

Use color-coded flash cards to help you learn the generic and brand names of eye and ear products. Choose one color card for eye products and another for ear products. You may also want to use different-colored pens to represent the various drug classes.

Oral forms of carbonic anhydrase inhibitors are active systemically. They are contraindicated in patients with a sulfa allergy, a kidney impairment, a liver impairment, closed-angle glaucoma, or an electrolyte imbalance.

The alpha receptor agonist brimonidine should not be used in children younger than two years.

Cautions and Considerations Patients with heart or thyroid problems should discuss their choices for glaucoma treatment with their prescribers before selecting and using an ophthalmic glaucoma agent. In particular, the systemic effects of beta-blockers can affect heart and thyroid conditions and interfere with the drug therapies used to treat them.

Alpha receptor agonists should be used with caution in patients with cardiovascular disease, impaired kidney function, cerebrovascular disease, diabetes, or depression. Prostaglandin analogs have a unique effect in that they cause the iris of the eye to turn brown. Patients should be informed of this effect, because their eye color will likely change or darken permanently. Prostaglandin analogs also stimulate eyelash growth.

Drug Interactions NSAIDS may decrease the effectiveness of prostaglandin analogs. Beta agonists may decrease the effectiveness of beta-blockers.
Alpha receptor agonists may decrease the effectiveness of oral alpha-blockers. Alpha agonists can interact with some antidepressants, specifically tricyclic antidepressants and monoamine oxidase inhibitors. Alpha receptor agonists must be used with caution in patients taking these other medications. Ophthalmic beta-blockers can interact with many medications (see Chapter 10), but only when systemically absorbed. Administering the drops only at bedtime or pinching the tear duct closed during administration and holding it closed for a few minutes afterward can reduce such absorption.

9.3 Chronic Dry Eye and Drug Treatments

Anyone can experience dry eyes. This condition may occur periodically, usually due to temporary evaporation of the tear film from the surface of the eyes. Seasonal allergies, environmental factors, and stress can cause dry eyes, usually on a short-term basis, but sometimes can contribute to chronic dry eye. Although uncomfortable, this condition is temporary and easily treated. Chronic dry eye, in contrast, is a long-term condition. The chronic form of dry eye results from an inability to produce adequate tear film to properly lubricate the eyes. Not only is this condition uncomfortable, but it can cause vision impairment and can impact a patient's ability to engage in the tasks of daily living.

Old age, menopause hormonal changes, and autoimmune disorders like Sjögren's syndrome are associated with chronic dry eye. Many drug therapies contribute to dry eye as well (see Table 9.2). Patients who take one of these medications and experience dry eyes should be referred to their provider for evaluation.

TABLE 9.2 Some Drugs That Cause Dry Eye

Drug Class	Drug Example
antidepressants	selective serotonin reuptake inhibitors (see Chapter 8)
	tricyclic antidepressants (see Chapter 8)

continues

TABLE 9.2 Some Drugs That Cause Dry Eye—*Continued*

Drug Class	Drug Example
antihistamines	cetirizine
	chlorpheniramine
	diphenhydramine
	fexofenadine
	loratadine
antipsychotics	chlorpromazine
	fluphenazine
	haloperidol
	olanzapine
	risperidone
analgesics	aspirin
	ibuprofen
chemotherapeutic agents	(see Chapter 20)
beta-blockers	See Table 9.1
diuretics	furosemide
	hydrochlorothiazide
	metolazone
	triamterene
hormone therapy	estrogens (see Chapter 14)
narcotic (opiate and opioid) analgesics	codeine
	fentanyl
	hydromorphone
	meperidine
	morphine
	oxycodone
	oxymorphone
retinoids	isotretinoin

Treating dry eye most often addresses the symptoms but may not affect the underlying condition. Treatment usually begins with reducing environmental factors such as exposure to smoke or prolonged use of computer screens. Over-the-counter artificial tear products can be used to supplement tear production and may provide short-term relief (see Table 9.3). Treatments for dry eye include ophthalmic lubricants, topical corticosteroids, and certain disease-modifying agents.

To instill eye drops, patients should lie down or tilt their head back, pull the lower eyelid downward, and gently squeeze the container to allow the required number of drops to fall into the eye without touching the tip of the applicator to the eye, eyelid, eyelashes, or fingers (see Figure 9.2).

Propylene glycol (Refresh, Soothe, Systane, Tears) is an ophthalmic lubricant (artificial tears) that works by providing the eye with additional lubrication.

Topical corticosteroids work by reducing inflammation, including itching and redness. For dry eye, topical corticosteroids include **dexamethasone, fluorometholone (FML), lotepredninol (Lotamox),** and **prednisolone (Pred Forte).**

FIGURE 9.2
**Instilling Eye
Drops**

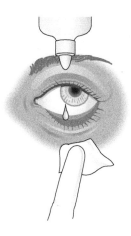

The lower eyelid
should be pulled
downward to
allow the drops to
fall into the eye.

TABLE 9.3 Commonly Used Ophthalmic Agents for Dry Eye

Generic (Brand)	Pronunciation	Dosage Form	Common Dosage	Dispensing Status
Ophthalmic Lubricant				
artificial tears (Refresh, Soothe, Systane, Tears)	AR-ti-fi-shul teers	ophthalmic solution	1–2 drops as needed	OTC, Rx
Topical Corticosteroids				
dexamethasone (generic only)	dex-a-METH-a-sone	ophthalmic solution, ophthalmic suspension	1–2 drops every 2 hr as needed	Rx
fluorometholone (Flarex, FML)	flor-oh-METH-oh-lone	ophthalmic solution, ophthalmic suspension	suspension: 1–2 drops 2–4 times a day ointment: apply small amount 1–3 times a day	Rx
loteprednol (Alrex, Inveltys, Lotemax, Lotemax SM, Zylet)	low-te-PRED-nol	ophthalmic ointment, ophthalmic suspension	suspension: 1 drop 3 times a day ointment: small amount 4 times a day	Rx
prednisolone (AK-Pred, Pred Forte, Pred Mild)	pred-NIS-oh-lone	ophthalmic suspension	1–2 drops 2–4 times a day	Rx
Other Agents				
cyclosporine (Restasis)	SYE-kloe-spor-reen	ophthalmic emulsion, ophthalmic solution	1 drop 2 times a day	Rx
lifitegrast (Xiidra)	lif-i-TEG-rast	ophthalmic solution	1 drop every 12 hr	Rx

Other disease-modifying agents can be used to treat dry eye. These include **cyclosporine (Restasis)** and **lifitegrast (Xiidra)**. These agents modify the underlying disease. Both of these agents affect the immune response which effectively reduces dry eye itself.

Opthlamic products are produced to be sterile, so special instructions for use and cleaning must be followed.

Dropper bottles should be stored in a clean place, and contact between the drop applicator and nonsterile surfaces (including eyes and fingers) should be avoided. Alcohol swabs can be used to clean the applicator, but patients should allow the alcohol to evaporate before dispensing drops into the eye.

Dosage Forms and Administration Contacts must be removed before application of eye drops and must be left out for at least 15 minutes afterward. To instill eye drops, patients should lie down or tilt their head back, pull the lower eyelid downward, and gently squeeze the container to allow the required number of drops to fall into the eye.

Side Effects Topical corticosteroids are usually well tolerated. Side effects may include stinging, blurred vision, eye pain, or headache. Cyclosporine taken systemically has chemotoxic effects (see Chapter 20). When used locally in the eye, these side effects can be avoided.

Contraindications Topical corticosteroids can increase intraocular pressure, which may cause glaucoma if used long term. Therefore, topical corticosteroids should be prescribed for no longer than four weeks for any patients, and they should not be used at all for patients with glaucoma.

Cautions and Considerations When used properly, cyclosporine is well tolerated. However, cyclosporine is an immunosuppressant and has a boxed warning for its potential to cause certain cancers. Patients need to be taught how to use and store this product safely, so that those around them are not exposed to these potentially harmful effects.

Topical corticosteroids do not usually interact with other medications, as they are not systemically absorbed. Patients may use dry-eye products in combination with other drugs, but they should not use other ophthalmic products at the same time as corticosteroids, cyclosporine, or lifitegrast without consulting their eye care specialist.

Drug Interactions Artificial tears, prostaglandin analogs, cyclosporine, and lifitegrast do not interact with other drugs. Use of NSAIDs can enhance the side effects of ophthalmic steroids. Patients will need to monitor for these effects and reduce use of NSAIDs, if possible, when necessary.

9.4 Conjunctivitis and Drug Treatments

Conjunctivitis (commonly called *pink eye*) is an inflammation caused by bacteria or viruses in the mucous membranes surrounding the eye. Symptoms include redness of the sclera and the insides of the eyelids, itching, pain, tearing, and the release of exudate (fluid that oozes out). This exudate can be white, yellow, or green. Being an infectious disease, conjunctivitis is usually treated with anti-infective agents. It is common to also be prescribed opthalmic corticosteroids to reduce inflammation. Conjunctivitis usually clears on its own, but bacterial conjunctivitis requires treatment with antibiotics.

If a person who gives birth to a newborn has untreated gonorrhea, the newborn is at high risk for gonococcal conjunctivitis. Treatment for newborns who might be infected includes topical ophthalmic anti-infectives for prevention and systemic antibiotics. Pregnant people should be tested for gonorrhea and treated before giving birth, if possible.

The number of ophthalmic anti-infective agents is large and can be intimidating to learn. However, this extensive number of products ensures that proper treatment of eye infections can be achieved easily (see Table 9.4).

TABLE 9.4 Commonly Used Ophthalmic Anti-Infectives to Treat Conjunctivitis

Generic (Brand)	Pronunciation	Dosage Form	Common Dosages	Dispensing Status
Aminoglycosides				
gentamicin (Garamycin Ophthalmic, Genoptic, Gentak, Gentasol)	jen-ta-MYE-sin	ophthalmic ointment and solution	1–2 drops every 4 hr	Rx
tobramycin (Tobrex)	toe-bra-MYE-sin	ophthalmic ointment and solution	1–2 drops every 4 hr	Rx
Macrolides				
azithromycin (AzaSite, Klarity-A)	az-ith-roe-MYE-sin	ophthalmic solution	1 drop 2 times a day	Rx
erythromycin (Romycin Ophthalmic)	eh-RITH-roe-MYE-sin	ophthalmic ointment	apply small amount 6 times a day	Rx
Quinolones				
besifloxacin (Besivance)	beh-see-FLOX-a-sin	ophthalmic suspension	1 drop 3 times a day	Rx
ciprofloxacin (Ciloxan)	sip-roe-FLOX-a-sin	ophthalmic ointment and solution	solution: 1–2 drops every 2 hr ointment: apply small amount 3 times a day	Rx
gatifloxacin (Zymaxid)	gat-i-FLOX-a-sin	ophthalmic solution	1 drop 2–4 times a day	Rx
levofloxacin (Iquix, Quixin)	le-voe-FLOX-a-sin	ophthalmic solution	1 drop 2–4 times a day	Rx
moxifloxacin (Moxeza, Vigamox)	mox-ee-FLOX-a-sin	ophthalmic solution	1 drop 2–3 times a day	Rx
ofloxacin (Ocuflox)	oh-FLOX-a-sin	ophthalmic solution	1–2 drops 2–4 times a day	Rx
Sulfonamide				
sulfacetamide (Bleph-10, Bleph-30, Cetamide, Sodium Sulamyd)	SUL-fa-SEE-a-mide	ophthalmic ointment and solution	1–2 drops every 3–4 hr	Rx
Miscellaneous Combinations				
gentamicin / prednisolone (Pred-G)	jen-ta-MYE-sin pred-NIS-oe-lone	ophthalmic ointment and suspension	suspension: 1 drop 2–4 times a day ointment: apply small amount 1–3 times a day	Rx
neomycin / polymyxin B / dexamethasone (Maxitrol)	nee-oh-MYE-sin pol-i-MIX-in dex-a-METH-a-sone	ophthalmic suspension	1–2 drops every 3–4 hr	Rx
sulfacetamide / fluorometholone	sul-fa-SEE-ta-mide flor-oh-METH-oe-lone	ophthalmic solution and suspension	2 drops every 4 hr	Rx

continues

Generic (Brand)	Pronunciation	Dosage Form	Common Dosages	Dispensing Status
Anti-infective/Corticosteroid Combinations				
sulfacetamide / prednisolone (Blephamide, Vasocidin)	sul-fa-SEE-ta-mide pred-NIS-oe-lone	ophthalmic ointment, solution, and suspension	solution: 2 drops every 4 hr ointment: apply small amount 3–4 times a day	Rx
tobramycin / dexamethasone (TobraDex)	toe-bra-MYE-sin dex-a-METH-a-sone	ophthalmic ointment and suspension	1–2 drops every 4–6 hr	Rx

Drug classes that are commonly used to treat conjunctivitis include aminoglycosides, macrolides, quinolones, sulfonamides, and anti-infective/corticosteroid combinations. Aminoglycosides used to treat conjunctivitis include **gentamicin (Gentak, Genoptic)** and **tobramycin (Tobrex)**.

Another drug class, macrolides, are also available for conjunctivitis. **Macrolides** include **azithromycin (AzaSite, Klarity-A)** and **erythromycin (Ilotycin)**. One sulfonamide, **sulfacetamide (Bleph-10)**, is appropriate to use to treat conjunctivitis. Quinolones include **besifloxacin (Besivance)**, **ciprofloxacin (Ciloxan)**, **gatifloxacin (Zymaxid)**, **levofloxacin (Iquix, Quixin)**, **moxifloxacin (Moxeza, Vigamox)**, and **ofloxacin (Ocuflox)**. Combination agents are also available.

Pharm Fact

Some eye medications are stored in the refrigerator. AzaSite is one of these medications. Other eye medications that are refrigerated include chloramphenicol, cyclopentolate, latanoprost, and timolol / latanoprost.

Dosage Forms and Administration Many of these medications are given as an **ophthalmic ointment** (eye ointment) and, therefore, require patients to learn a specific administration technique. This technique is similar to instilling eye drops and requires the same care in keeping the product sterile. Instead of a drop of liquid, the patient squeezes a continuous ribbon of ointment (roughly half an inch long) along the space between the eyeball and lower lid (see Figure 9.3). The patient then closes the eye for a few minutes to allow the ointment to liquefy and dissipate.

Side Effects Common side effects of topically administered anti-infectives are few, and, if present, they are usually mild and tolerable. Although systemic absorption is typically low with these dosage forms, systemic side effects are possible. To learn more about the systemic side effects of anti-infectives, see Chapters 16 and 17.

FIGURE 9.3 Applying Eye Ointment

Applying eye ointment is similar to applying eye drops, but the ointment is squeezed in a continuous ribbon along the space between the lower eyelid and the eye.

ointment

Contraindications Certain aminoglycosides, a type of anti-infective, have contraindications. Tobramycin should not be used in patients with hypersensitivities to other aminoglycosides. Gentamicin does not have contraindications.

Opthalmic erythromycin is contraindicated in patients who are allergic to macrolides.

Azithromycin is contraindicated in pregnancy patients with allergy to macrolides, and patients with myasthenia gravis or heart arrhythmia.

Sulfacetamide, a sulfonamide, is contraindicated in patients with a hypersensitivity to sulfonamides.

Trimethoprim-polymyxin B is contraindicated in patients who are allergic to sufonamides.

All the anti-infective and corticosteroid combination products in Table 9.4 that contain an aminoglycoside or steroid are contraindicated in patients with a hypersensitivity to aminoglycosides or corticosteroids. In addition, all the combination products are contraindicated in viral disease of the cornea or conjunctiva and in mycobacterial or fungal infections of the eye.

Cautions and Considerations Anti-infectives are drugs to which many patients have allergies. Therefore, technicians should ask each patient about their allergies and document them in the patient's record. Even topical anti-infective agents can cause serious allergic reactions, so updated allergy information is important for patient safety.

Drug Interactions In general, ophthalmic anti-infectives do not have significant drug interactions.

WORKPLACE WISDOM

To help ensure safety and accuracy when dispensing ophthalmic and otic products, pharmacy personnel should understand common obstacles related to dispensing these products. The technician should be aware of the packaging when dispensing ophthalmic and otic preparations. Often, the packaging is smaller than the pharmacy labeling. If so, the technican may have to "butterfly" or "flag" the label, making sure not to cover the National Drug Code (NDC). Another way to ensure that the label is visible is to place the drug, in its container, in a plastic bag and put the pharmacy label on the bag.

Determining the most appropriately sized bottle to select for an ophthalmic or otic medication can be challenging. The technician should assure accuracy using the following steps:

1. Determine the number of drops needed for an entire prescription
2. Convert the number of drops to milliliters. (Remember that 20 drops are approximately 1 milliliter.)
3. Select the smallest bottle that holds that number of milliliters or more

Ophthalmic and otic products may require auxiliary labels in addition to the main label. Most eye drops and eardrops are stored at room temperature, but some must be stored in the refrigerator and should receive auxiliary labels with that information. Technicians should pay close attention when dispensing ophthalmic and otic products to ensure that all necessary auxiliary labels are affixed to the packaging and are easy to read.

9.5 Anatomy and Physiology of the Ears

The ears are sensory organs that sense sound waves and produce hearing. As seen in Figure 9.4, the ear is divided into three parts: external, middle, and inner. The **external ear** (auricle or pinna) captures sound waves and directs them through the **ear canal** to the **tympanic membrane** (eardrum). **Cerumen** (earwax) is produced by follicles lining the auditory canal.

The eardrum separates the **middle ear** from the external ear. It vibrates in response to sound waves, causing the three bones in the ossicular chain (**malleus, incus,** and **stapes**) of the middle ear to move. The stapes taps on the **oval window,** the entrance to the inner ear. The **eustachian tube** connects the middle ear to the throat to allow fluid to drain and to allow equalization of the pressure in the middle ear when atmospheric air pressure changes. The **inner ear** includes the vestibule, semicircular canals, and the cochlea, which is spiral shaped. Fluid in the **cochlea** responds to the tapping on the oval window, producing pressure waves that flow through the cochlea (see Figure 9.4). Sensory hairs line the surface of the cochlea in what is called the **organ of Corti.** Sound is perceived and interpreted when corresponding vibrations in these tiny hairs send signals via nerves to the brain. Damage to sensory hairs in the inner ear occurs naturally with age and exposure to loud noise. This kind of hearing loss is called **presbycusis.** The first sounds lost to perception are those produced by high-pitched sound waves.

Fluid in the **semicircular canals** maintains the body's balance and orientation. Gravity pulls the fluid in these channels downward. The vestibular nerves detect this fluid movement and in turn send signals to the brain about body position. **Vertigo** is a malfunction of the semicircular canals, resulting in balance problems and dizziness.

Work Wise

The recognized medical abbreviations for both ears is AU and both eyes is OU. However, these abbreviations are easy to get confused and can lead to mistakes in dispensing. Pharmacy professionals are encouraged not to use these abbreviations so as to prevent errors.

FIGURE 9.4
The Structural Components of the Ear

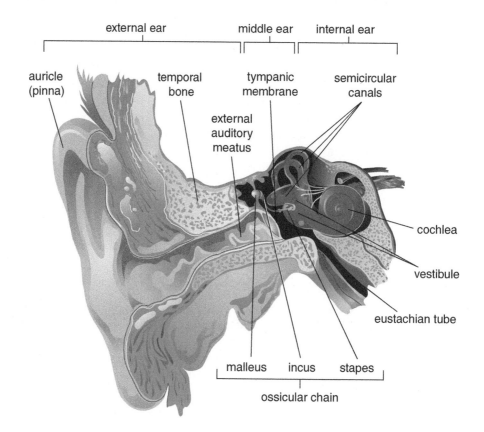

external ear   middle ear   internal ear

auricle (pinna)

temporal bone

tympanic membrane

semicircular canals

external auditory meatus

cochlea

vestibule

eustachian tube

malleus   incus   stapes

ossicular chain

The ear's structure can determine the appropriate route of administration for a drug affecting an ear condition. Infections make up the majority of ear disorders that require drug therapy. Oral drug therapy is usually necessary for middle ear infections (see Chapter 16). Antibiotic eardrops will not effectively treat an infection of the middle ear because medication applied to the external ear will not reach the intended site of action unless the tympanic membrane is ruptured.

9.6 Otitis (Media and Externa) and Drug Treatments

Pharm Fact

Although antibiotic eye drops are sometimes prescribed for the ear, eardrops must never be used in the eye. Note that it is extremely easy to mix up an ophthalmic and an otic, since the words are so similar.

Middle ear infection (otitis media) is most common in children. Because the eustachian tube is more horizontal in children than in adults, fluid from the middle ear does not drain well, allowing bacteria and viruses to flourish. Most middle ear infections are viral and clear on their own. However, some otitis media develops after a viral respiratory tract infection in which mucus and fluid build up and provide a growing medium for bacteria. Symptoms of an ear infection include ear pain (otalgia), jaw pain, sinus pain, itching, and fever. Pain is often intense enough to cause patients (or their parents) to seek medical attention. Sometimes, congestion in the ear can cause fluid pressure on the semicircular canals, resulting in dizziness (vertigo).

An **external ear infection (otitis externa)** is an inflammation of the ear canal usually caused by a bacterial or fungal infection. Bacteria and fungi thrive in moist environments such as that found in cerumen (earwax). When cerumen builds up, hearing can become impaired, and infection can follow. Regular swimmers have the highest propensity to develop external ear infections, because pool water and moisture may not fully evaporate from their ears. For that reason, otitis externa is commonly known as *swimmer's ear*.

Agents that are commonly used to treat otitis are identified in Table 9.5.

TABLE 9.5 Commonly Used Otic Agents

Generic (Brand)	Pronunciation	Dosage Form	Common Dosage	Dispensing Status
Analgesic				
benzocaine / benzethonium chloride / glycerin (Otocaine, Pinnacaine)	BEN-zoe-kayn BEN-ze-thoe-neeum KLOR-ide	otic solution	4–5 drops as needed	Rx
Antibiotics				
Quinolones				
ciprofloxacin (Cetraxal, Otiprio)	sip-roe-FLOX-a-sin	otic solution and suspension	0.2–0.25 mL 2 times a day	Rx
ofloxacin (Floxin Otic)	oh-FLOX-a-sin	otic solution	5–10 drops 1–2 times a day	Rx
Combinations				
ciprofloxacin / dexamethasone (Ciprodex)	sip-roe-FLOX-a-sin dex-a-METH-a-sone	otic suspension	4 drops 2 times a day	Rx
ciprofloxacin / hydrocortisone (Cipro HC)	sip-roe-FLOX-a-sin hye-droe-KOR-ti-sone	otic suspension	3 drops 2 times a day	Rx

continues

TABLE 9.5 **Commonly Used Otic Agents** —*Continued*

neomycin / polymyxin / hydrocortisone (Cortisporin Otic Solution, Casporyn HC Otic Suspension)	nee-oh-MYE-sin pol-i-MIX-in hye-droe-KOR-ti-sone	otic solution and suspension	3–4 drops 3–4 times a day	Rx
Drying Agents				
acetic acid	ah-SEE-tik	otic solution	3–5 drops every 4–6 hr	OTC
boric acid (AuroDri, EarDry)	BOR-ick	otic solution	3–5 drops every 4–6 hr	OTC
isopropyl alcohol / glycerin (Acetasol, Burrows, Cortane, Murine)	eye-soh-PRO-pill AL-coh-hall GLEH-ser-in	otic solution	3–5 drops every 4–6 hr	OTC
Earwax Dissolver				
carbamide peroxide (Debrox, Murine Ear Wax Removal)	KAR-ba-mide per-OX-ide	otic solution	3–5 drops every 4–6 hr	OTC

Oral and Otic Antibiotics

Practice Tip

Eardrops come in suspensions and solutions. Pharmacy technicians should place auxiliary labels on suspensions reminding patients to shake well. They should also instruct patients to avoid contaminating the dropper tip by touching it to surfaces, fingers, or ears.

To treat otitis media, healthcare practitioners prescribe oral antibiotics (see Chapter 16) to eradicate the infection and topical analgesics to relieve the pain. To reduce antibiotic resistance, practitioners attempt to be judicious when prescribing antibiotics for ear infections. Patients experiencing dizziness can use decongestants to reduce pressure in the middle ear.

Fewer otic antibiotics exist than oral antibiotics. Otic preparations usually serve as adjunct therapy to oral antibiotics for severe ear infections in patients who have a ruptured eardrum or tubes in their ears. Antibiotics in the form of eye drops are also sometimes used in the ear. Topical otic analgesics are used for patients with severe ear pain associated with infection. These products work by temporarily numbing the ear canal (see Table 9.6).

Dosage Forms and Administration Antibiotic otic agents are available as otic solutions and otic suspensions.

Side Effects The few side effects of otic agents are rarely experienced. Although systemic absorption is seldom seen with otic agents, allergic reactions are still possible. Technicans should be sure to update the patient's allergy profile each time new orders are written.

Contraindications Quinolone otic products are contraindicated in patients with a sensitivity to other quinolones. **Ciprofloxacin-dexamethasone (Ciprodex)** should not be used in patients with a quinolone or steroid hypersensitivity or a viral infection of the external ear canal. **Neomycin / polymyxin / hydrocortisone (Cortisporin Otic Solution, Casporyn HC Otic Suspension)** should not be used in patients with viral infections, fungal diseases, or mycobacterial infections.

Cautions and Considerations Few problems are encountered with otic antibiotics. In severe cases, children can have conjunctivitis along with an ear infection. If both eye drops and eardrops are prescribed, technicians should be sure to inform the patient about the difference between these medications.

Drug Interactions In general, otic antibiotics do not have significant drug interactions.

Topical Otic Preparations

Treating external ear infections calls for removing moisture, wax, and any bacteria or fungi present from the ear canal. Topical otic preparations are necessary, as oral administration would not reach the desired site of action. These preparations, commonly known as **eardrops**, are effective only for otitis externa. If an infection is in the middle ear or inner ear, medication applied to the external ear will not reach the intended site of action. Systemic absorption of otic preparations usually is not possible. When administering eardrops, the patient should lie down with the affected ear directed upward. In children younger than three years (whose ears are not fully grown), the caregiver should pull the earlobe gently down and back. In older children and adults, the earlobe should be pulled up and out. This manipulation of the earlobe creates the best angle for administration (see Figure 9.5).

FIGURE 9.5
Administering Otic Drops

(a) Children age three and older and adults should have the earlobe pulled up and out when otic medications are administered.

(b) Children under age three should have the earlobe pulled down and back.

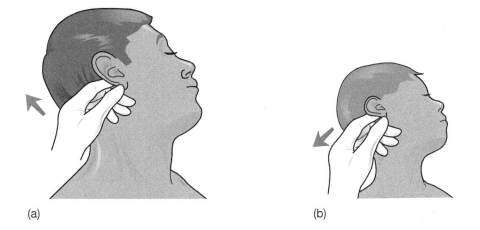

(a)   (b)

Practice Tip

Special instructions should be given to patients who have tubes in their ears. This patient population should only instill suspensions and should be extra careful to keep otic preparations sterile to prevent introducing infection in the ears.

A **drying agent** is used for the treatment or prevention of otitis externa. Treatment may be given on a short-term basis for active infection or on a regular (even daily) basis to help prevent infection. An **earwax dissolver** is used for patients with cerumen impaction. An earwax remover first loosens and dissolves cerumen, after which irrigation with warm water flushes it out. See Table 9.5 for drugs commonly used as drying agents and earwax removers.

Side Effects Side effects from the instillation of otic drying agents and earwax removers are rare.

Contraindications Drying agents are contraindicated in patients with a perforated tympanic membrane. Carbamide peroxide is also contraindicated in patients with a perforated tympanic membrane or with ear drainage, ear pain, or a rash in the ear. benzocaine / benzethonium chloride / glycerin should not be used in patients with a perforated tympanic membrane or with ear discharge.

Cautions and Considerations No other notable cautions or considerations are associated with the use of otic drying agents and earwax removers.

In general, otic drying agents and earwax removers do not have significant drug interactions.

9.7 Complementary and Alternative Therapies

Vitamin A, which the body manufactures from **beta-carotene**, is essential for photoreceptor cell growth and regeneration. Deficiency in vitamin A can cause night blindness. Vitamin A, vitamin C, vitamin E, copper, and zinc may slow the disease progression of age-related macular degeneration. Ocuvite is a brand-name product containing a combination of vitamins and minerals made especially for this use. Ocuvite is taken in doses of two tablets each morning and evening with food. This combination of vitamins does not cure or prevent macular degeneration. It can help to halt the progression of the disease. Patients who smoke or have a high risk of certain types of cancer may not be good candidates for therapy with this product. Patients should talk with their healthcare practitioners before starting to take any vitamin products to treat eye conditions.

Olive oil is an ingredient in some natural otic products used to soften earwax to help remove it from the ears. Docusate sodium, a common stool softener, is combined with olive oil as a base and applied in the ear to soften earwax.

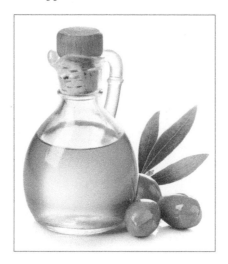

Review and Assessment

CHAPTER SUMMARY

Anatomy and Physiology of the Eyes

- The eyes are sensory organs specially designed to sense light and produce vision.

- The anterior chamber holds aqueous humor, a fluid that lubricates the lens.

- The conjunctiva forms the mucous membrane that covers the sclera and inner eyelids.

Glaucoma and Drug Treatments

- Glaucoma is a condition in which abnormally high intraocular pressure pushes on the optic nerve and damages it.

- Glaucoma can lead to blindness if left untreated.

- Topical prostaglandin analogs, beta-blockers, alpha receptor agonists, and carbonic anhydrase inhibitors are used to treat glaucoma.

- Eye drops can be used to treat glaucoma.

Chronic Dry Eye and Drug Treatments

- Many prescription and over-the-counter medications contribute to dry eye.

Conjunctivitis and Drug Treatments

- Conjunctivitis is a common eye disorder, and treatments include topical antibiotics and steroids.

Dispensing Ophthalmic Products

- Be aware of the packaging when dispensing ophthalmic and otic preparations. Often, the packaging is smaller than the pharmacy labeling.

- To dispense ophthalmic products safely, determine the number of drops needed in the prescription, convert those drops to milliliters, and then select the correct product volume.

- Ophthalmic and otic products may require auxiliary labels in addition to the main label.

Anatomy and Physiology of the Ears

- The tympanic membrane separates the external ear from the middle ear.

- The malleus, incus, and stapes are three bones inside the ear that transmit vibrations from sound by tapping on the oval window.

- The semicircular canals are involved in balance and sensing body position.

Otitis and Drug Treatments

- Otitis media (middle ear infection) is a common condition treated with antibiotics formulated as eardrops.

- Ophthalmics (eye drops and eye ointment) are often prescribed for use in the ear, but otics (eardrops) should never be used in the eye.

- Antibiotic eye drops are frequently dispensed for ear infections.

- External ear infections are often treated with drying agents and earwax dissolvers.

Complementary and Alternative Therapies

- Deficiency in vitamin A can cause night blindness.

- Olive oil is an ingredient in some natural otic products used to soften earwax to remove it from the ears. Ophthalmics

DRUG LIST

Topical Ophthalmic Agents

Corticosteroids Combinations

neomycin / polymyxin B-dexamethasone (Maxitrol)
sulfacetamide / prednisolone (Blephamide, Vasocidin)
tobramycin / dexamethasone (TobraDex)

Dry Eye Agents

artificial tears (Refresh, Soothe, Systane, Tears)
cyclosporine (Restasis)
dexamethasone
fluorometholone (Flarex, FML)
lifitegrast (Xiidra)
loteprednol (Alrex, Inveltys, Lotemax, Lotemax SM, Zylet)
prednisolone (AK-Pred, Pred Forte, Pred Mild)

Glaucoma Treatments

Ophthalmic Agents—Alpha Receptor Agonists

apraclonidine (Iopidine)
brimonidine (Alphagan P, Lumify, Quoliana)

Ophthalmic Agents—Beta-Blockers

betaxolol (Betoptic S)
carteolol
levobunolol (Betagan)
metipranolol (OptiPranolol)
timolol (Betimol, Timoptic, Timoptic GFS, Timoptic-XE)

Ophthalmic Agents—Carbonic Anhydrase Inhibitors

brinzolamide (Azopt)
dichlorphenamide (Keveyis)
dorzolamide (Trusopt)
methazolamide

Ophthalmic Agents—Prostaglandin Analogs

bimatoprost (Lumigan)
latanoprost (Xalatan)
latanoprostene bunod (Vyzulta)
tafluprost (Zioptan)
travoprost (Travatan-Z)
unoprostone (Rescula)

Ophthalmic Anti-Infectives

Aminoglycosides

gentamicin (Garamycin Ophthalmic, Genoptic, Gentak, Gentasol)
gentamicin-prednisolone (Pred-G)

Quinolones

besifloxacin (Besivance)
ciprofloxacin (Ciloxan)
gatifloxacin (Zymaxid)
levofloxacin (Iquix, Quixin)
moxifloxacin (Moxeza, Vigamox)
ofloxacin (Ocuflox)

Sulfonamides

sulfacetamide (Bleph-10, Bleph-30, Cetamide, Sodium Sulamyd)
sulfacetamide-fluorometholone

Otics

Analgesic

benzocaine / benzethonium chloride / glycerin (Otocaine, Pinnacaine)

Antibiotics

ciprofloxacin (Cetraxal, Otiprio)

ciprofloxacin-dexamethasone (Ciprodex)

ciprofloxacin-hydrocortisone (Cipro HC)

neomycin / polymyxin / hydrocortisone (Cortisporin Otic Solution, Casporyn HC Otic Suspension)

ofloxacin (Floxin Otic)

Earwax Dissolver

carbamide peroxide (Debrox, Murine Ear Wax Removal)

Drying Agents

acetic acid

boric acid (AuroDri, EarDry)

isopropyl alcohol / glycerin (Acetasol, Burrows, Cortane, Murine)

Boxed Warnings

None

Medication Guides

None

✓ CHECK YOUR UNDERSTANDING

Take a moment to review what you have learned in this chapter and answer the following questions.

1. Which of the following drugs is a topical analgesic used in otitis media for pain?
   a. Otocaine
   b. Ciprodex
   c. Cortisporin Otic
   d. Debrox

2. Which of the .following is an ophthalmic alpha receptor agonist?
   a. aspirin
   b. brimonidine
   c. latanoprost
   d. timolol

3. Which eye drop is a sulfonamide?
   a. Bleph-10
   b. Ciloxan
   c. Gentak
   d. Maxitrol

4. Which of the following statements is *not* true?
   a. Most middle ear infections are viral and clear on their own.
   b. Glaucoma may lead to blindness if untreated.
   c. Eardrops may be prescribed for use in the eye.
   d. Lifitegrast is used to treat dry eye.

5. Which of the following drugs can a patient with a perforated ear drum use?
   a. benzocaine / benzethonium chloride / glycerin
   b. carbamide peroxide
   c. isopropyl alcohol / glycerin
   d. ofloxacin

6. Which of the following drugs can cause a patient to have dry eyes?
   a. azithromycin
   b. bimatoprost
   c. ciprofloxacin
   d. loratadine

7. Which of the following drugs is contraindicated in patients with heart failure?
   a. Alphagan P
   b. Miostat
   c. Rescula
   d. Timoptic

8. Which of the following is a condition in which increased intraocular pressure damages the optic nerve?
   a. conjunctivitis
   b. glaucoma
   c. otitis externa
   d. otitis media

9. Which of the following drugs is used for chronic dry eye?
   a. fluorometholone
   b. levobunolol
   c. tafluprost
   d. tobramycin / dexamethasone

10. Which of the following drugs is likely to darken or change a patient's eye color to brown?
    a. Betagan
    b. Lumigan
    c. Vigamox
    d. Xiidra

MAKE CONNECTIONS

Take a moment to consider what you have learned in this chapter and respond thoughtfully to the following prompts. Note that some of these activities will require internet access.

1. You have a patient who brings in a prescription for Restasis. When you go to fill it, you discover that her insurance coverage will not pay for this product, and it is very expensive. The pharmacist offers to contact her provider and explains that other less expensive products can be used, depending on the severity of her condition. The pharmacist asks you to help the patient find the alternative in the OTC section while the pharmacist calls the provider. Research common prices of dry-eye drug products and list alternatives for this patient.

2. A pregnant patient with an eye infection comes to the pharmacy to fill a prescription for erythromycin eye ointment. When it is filled, she is surprised to see that it comes in a tube rather than as eye drops. The pharmacist explains that many of the antibiotic products that come as eye drops cannot be used during pregnancy. She will need to use an ophthalmic ointment. What are the differences in administration between an eye drop and an eye ointment?

The online course includes additional review and assessment resources.

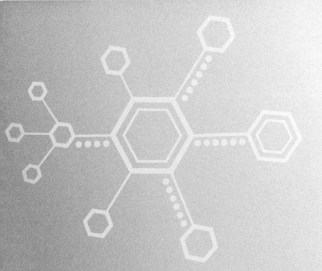

The Cardiovascular System and Drug Therapy

10

Learning Objectives

1 Describe the anatomy and physiology of the cardiovascular system. (Section 10.1)

2 List and describe drug classes used to treat hypertension. (Section 10.2)

3 Outline the multiple therapeutic indications for drugs used to treat hypertension. (Section 10.2)

4 Identify and describe agents commonly used to treat cardiac arrhythmia. (Section 10.3)

5 Compare and contrast the drug classes used to treat angina and myocardial infarction. (Section 10.4)

6 List and describe agents used to treat angina and myocardial infarction. (Section 10.4)

7 Identify drug classes commonly used to treat heart failure and discuss their usage and side effects. (Section 10.5)

8 Describe drug classes used to treat hyperlipidemia. (Section 10.6)

9 Summarize drug classes used to treat clotting disorders and stroke. (Section 10.7)

10 State the antidotes for dabigatran, heparin, oral factor Xa inhibitors, and warfarin. (Section 10.7)

11 List common complementary and alternative therapies used for disorders of the cardiovascular system. (Section 10.8)

10.1 Anatomy and Physiology of the Cardiovascular System

The **cardiovascular system** circulates blood throughout the body (see Figure 10.1) and is responsible for bringing oxygen and nutrients to tissues and for carrying away carbon dioxide and toxic by-products. The cardiovascular system, also known as the *circulatory system*, is composed of the heart and blood vessels (arteries, veins, and capillaries). Without a properly functioning cardiovascular system, human life is not sustainable. The heart pumps blood to the body through arteries and veins. An **artery** carries blood away from the heart to the body. A **vein** carries blood from tissues back to the heart.

FIGURE 10.1
**Overview
of the
Cardiovascular
System**

The cardiovascular system includes the heart, arteries, veins, and capillaries.

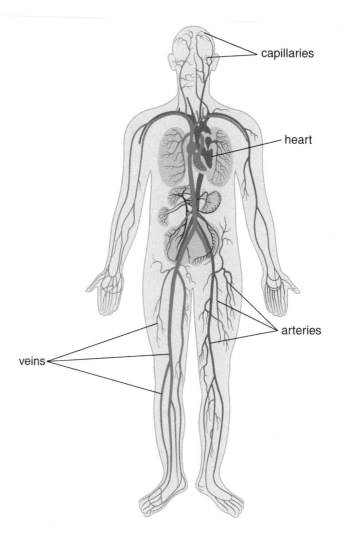

capillaries

heart

arteries

veins

The path that the blood takes through the body ensures that it carries deoxygenated blood to the lungs (for gas exchange) and then sends that reoxygenated blood to other tissues in the body (see Figure 10.2). A capillary is a tiny blood vessel. In the capillaries, critical fluids, gases, and nutrients are exchanged between the blood and body tissues. For additional information on gas exchange, see Chapter 11.

The heart is a hollow organ that has three functional parts: the cardiac muscle (also called the *myocardium* or *heart muscle*), which contracts to pump blood out of the heart and maintain blood flow through the body; the **conduction system**, which consists of cardiac muscle cells and conducting fibers that coordinate contraction; and blood supply, which is pumped in and out of each chamber.

The heart is made of specialized cardiac muscle fibers and is divided into four chambers. These chambers, each named for its location within the heart, are the right atrium, the left atrium, the right ventricle, and the left ventricle (see Figure 10.3). The atria *receive* the blood that is brought to the heart from the veins, and the ventricles pump the blood *out* through the arteries. The arteries direct blood either to the lungs or other body tissues.

The heart both contracts (effectively pumping blood) and relaxes (fills with blood). **Systole** refers to the period during which the heart is contracting and actively pumping blood. **Diastole** describes the period when the cardiac muscle relaxes, allowing blood to passively flow into the heart and fill the heart's chambers. Valves within the heart prevent blood from flowing in the wrong direction.

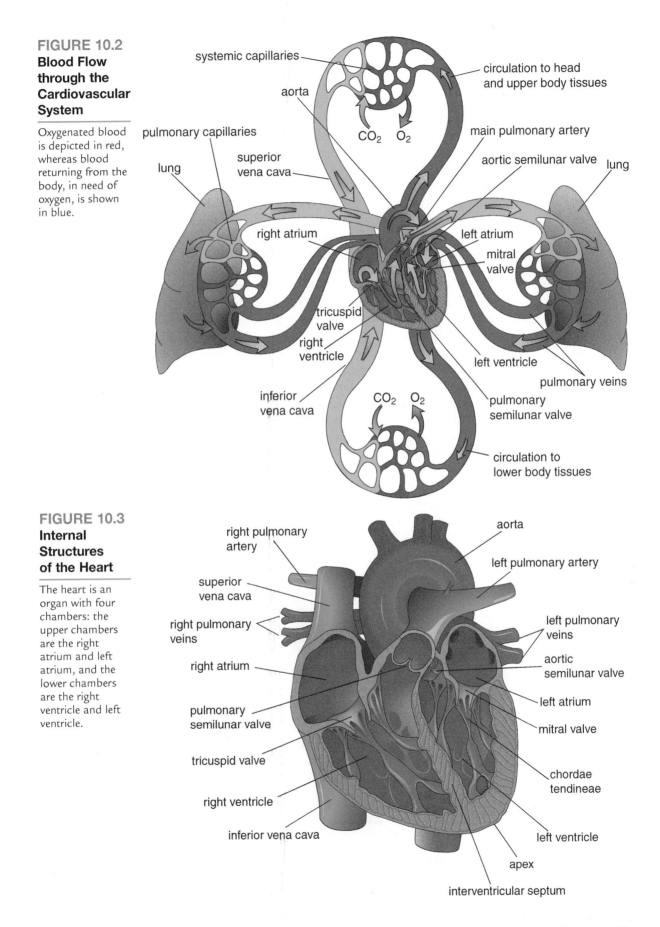

FIGURE 10.2
Blood Flow through the Cardiovascular System

Oxygenated blood is depicted in red, whereas blood returning from the body, in need of oxygen, is shown in blue.

systemic capillaries

aorta

pulmonary capillaries

superior vena cava

lung

right atrium

tricuspid valve

right ventricle

inferior vena cava

circulation to head and upper body tissues

CO_2 O_2

main pulmonary artery

aortic semilunar valve   lung

left atrium

mitral valve

left ventricle

pulmonary veins

pulmonary semilunar valve

CO_2 O_2

circulation to lower body tissues

FIGURE 10.3
Internal Structures of the Heart

The heart is an organ with four chambers: the upper chambers are the right atrium and left atrium, and the lower chambers are the right ventricle and left ventricle.

right pulmonary artery

superior vena cava

right pulmonary veins

right atrium

pulmonary semilunar valve

tricuspid valve

right ventricle

inferior vena cava

aorta

left pulmonary artery

left pulmonary veins

aortic semilunar valve

left atrium

mitral valve

chordae tendineae

left ventricle

apex

interventricular septum

Cardiac Contractility

A normal heartbeat is the result of a coordinated series of electrical events in the conduction system, a group of cardiac muscle cells that send signals to the heart muscle. It begins in the membranes of myocardial conducting cells in the **sinoatrial (SA) node**, often called the heart's natural pacemaker. Between beats, these cells are polarized; that is, the inside of each cell is at a negative voltage relative to the outside. The beat originates when ion channels in a cell membrane open to allow positively charged sodium and calcium ions to flow into the cell, making the voltage positive instead of negative (**depolarization**). Other channels then open to allow positively charged potassium ions to flow out of the cell, making the voltage negative again (**repolarization**). The resulting **action potential** (the electrical signal that causes a muscle to contract) spreads through the conduction system to the other muscle cells of the myocardium, called *myocardial contractile cells*. When the action potential arrives at a myocardial contractile cell, which is also polarized, the cell depolarizes with a rapid inflow of sodium and a slower inflow of calcium. Then the cell repolarizes with an outflow of potassium.

If the depolarizing and repolarizing flows were the only ion flows, the cell would run out of potassium and accumulate huge amounts of sodium and calcium. Other proteins in the cell membrane continually restore the balance by using energy to pump sodium and calcium out and potassium in simultaneously.

The electrical signal from the SA node is carried through the atria and at the same time down to the **atrioventricular (AV) node**. After a delay, the signal travels through the bundle of His (pronounced "hiss") and the bundle branches to the heart's apex. At this point, the electrical signal branches into the Purkinje fibers. A Purkinje fiber is one of the fibers that stretch from the apex up into the ventricles to contract the lower—and largest—part of the heart. This conduction system is shown in Figure 10.4.

The typical rate at which the SA node fires to initiate each heartbeat is 60 to 100 times per minute. This **heart rate (HR)** is typically reported in beats per minute (BPM) and is measured by taking a person's pulse. Common places to take a pulse include the carotid artery on the neck (this pulse is called a carotid pulse) and the thumb side of the wrist (this pulse is called a radial pulse).

FIGURE 10.4
Conduction System of the Heart

Heartbeat is regulated by the conduction system, which initiates impulses and conducts them throughout the heart. The numbers in this figure represent the order in which the electrical signals travel through the heart.

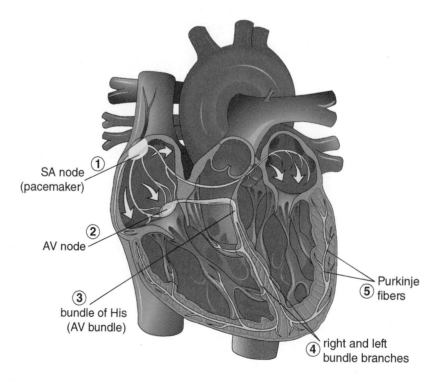

SA node (pacemaker) ①

AV node ②

bundle of His (AV bundle) ③

right and left bundle branches ④

Purkinje fibers ⑤

Blood Pressure

Blood pressure (BP) describes the force of blood in the circulatory system and is maintained by various feedback mechanisms. In simple terms, blood pressure is a function of capacitance, cardiac output, peripheral vascular resistance, and the renin-angiotensin system:

- **Capacitance:** the amount of blood held in the veins and venules (small veins that collect blood from capillaries)
- **Cardiac output (CO):** the force and volume of blood coming from the heart
- **Peripheral vascular resistance (PVR):** the degree to which the blood vessels, particularly small vessels called arterioles, are constricted or relaxed
- **Renin-angiotensin system:** the feedback mechanism that is regulated by the kidneys and balances fluid volume and vessel constriction

The sympathetic nervous system, part of the central nervous system, also plays a role in blood pressure regulation by influencing peripheral vascular resistance and the renin-angiotensin system. Figure 10.5 illustrates the complex feedback mechanisms that work together to balance blood pressure.

FIGURE 10.5
Maintaining Blood Pressure

Blood pressure is maintained by a variety of mechanisms.

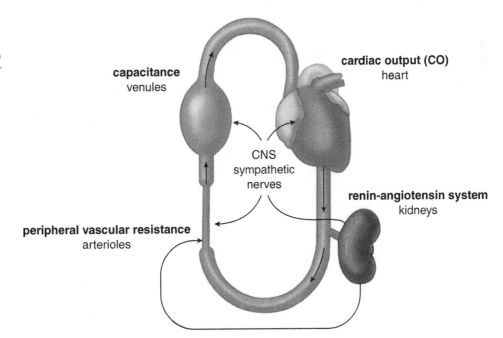

If blood vessels are constricted, causing increased PVR, the heart has to work harder to maintain the same cardiac output to keep blood pressure stable. Therefore, **constriction** (narrowing) or **dilation** (widening) of blood vessels raises or lowers blood pressure, respectively. High blood pressure is often caused by elevated PVR. Stress on the heart from high blood pressure may cause cardiac disease. High blood pressure also affects vital organs and can eventually result in kidney failure and stroke. Sympathetic nerves in the autonomic nervous system regulate that multifaceted system. Alterations in any one of the compensatory checks and balances in the feedback mechanisms that maintain blood pressure can cause hypertension. Losing large amounts of blood lowers blood pressure to dangerous levels. If blood pressure falls low enough, the patient may go into shock, a condition during which vital organs are not supplied with blood and begin to shut down.

Blood pressure is expressed as the **systolic blood pressure** reading, which measures the pressure when the heart contracts and ejects blood (systole), and the **diastolic blood pressure** reading, which measures the pressure when the heart relaxes and fills (diastole). Cardiac output is the major determinant of systolic pressure, which is the product of cardiac output and peripheral vascular resistance. Diastolic pressure is related to the volume of venous blood return. Both readings are in millimeters of mercury (abbreviated *mm Hg*)—that is, the height of a mercury column whose weight offsets the pressure. The reading is stated as systolic *over* diastolic pressure; measurements of 120 mm Hg systolic and 80 mm Hg diastolic are written *120/80* and read *120 over 80*. A blood pressure of 120/80 is often considered normal.

10.2 Hypertension and Drug Treatments

Hypertension, defined as elevated blood pressure, affects approximately 75 million people in the United States. While patients cannot immediately feel the effects of hypertension, damage is still being done to vital organs of the body, such as the heart, kidneys, eyes, and brain. Hypertension puts patients at risk for heart disease and stroke, which are the leading causes of death in the United States. Hypertension is also a risk factor for heart failure and kidney disease. This is why hypertension is referred to as the *silent killer*.

Practice Tip

Hypertension may be abbreviated on prescriptions and in medical records as *HTN*.

The underlying basis of most hypertension cases is unknown, although family history, cigarette smoking, and diet and lifestyle choices are definite factors. This type of hypertension, of unknown cause, is known as primary or essential hypertension. Other factors that may contribute to hypertension include kidney disease; obesity; adrenal tumor; decreased blood pressure or delayed pulse in the lower extremities; and use of drugs such as oral contraceptives, corticosteroids, nonsteroidal anti-inflammatory drugs (NSAIDs), decongestants, and appetite suppressants. When the source, or cause, of the hypertension is identified, it is known as secondary hypertension.

An elevation of systolic blood pressure, diastolic blood pressure, or both is considered hypertension. Blood pressure goals are determined by the patient and prescriber. The "2017 . . . Guideline for the Prevention, Detection, Evaluation, and Management of High Blood Pressure in Adults: A Report of the American College of Cardiology/American Heart Association Task Force on Clinical Practice Guidelines," published in the *Journal of the American College of Cardiology*, offers recommendations for the management of hypertension. It covers lifestyle interventions to decrease blood pressure, including weight loss for overweight or obese patients, a heart-healthy diet, physical activity, and alcohol consumption limits. The guideline also suggests criteria for treating high blood pressure in various patient populations. Treatment with medication is recommended in patients:

- with a history of cardiovascular events (such as myocardial infarction) when blood pressure is ≥ 130 / ≥ 80 mm Hg
- without a history of cardiovascular disease when their estimated 10-year risk of a cardiovascular event is ≥ 10% and their blood pressure is ≥ 130 / ≥ 80 mm Hg

Treatment of hypertension often requires more than one medication. Drug classes commonly used to treat hypertension include angiotensin-converting enzyme (ACE) inhibitors, angiotensin receptor blockers (ARBs), calcium channel blockers, and thiazide diuretics. Less commonly used are alpha-blockers, beta-blockers, and direct renin inhibitors. See Table 10.1 for a list of agents in each of these classes that are used to treat hypertension.

TABLE 10.1 Commonly Used Agents for the Treatment of Hypertension

Generic (Brand)	Pronunciation	Dosage Form	Common Dosage	Dispensing Status
Angiotensin-Converting Enzyme (ACE) Inhibitors				
benazepril (Lotensin)	ben-AZ-eh-pril	tablet	5–40 mg a day	Rx
captopril	KAP-toe-pril	tablet	25–100 mg a day	Rx
enalapril (Epaned, Vasotec)	e-NAL-a-pril	oral solution, tablet	5–20 mg a day	Rx
enalaprilat	e-NAL-a-pril-at	injection	1.25 mg every 6 hr	Rx
fosinopril	foe-SIN-oh-pril	tablet	10–40 mg a day	Rx
lisinopril (Prinivil, Qbrelis, Zestril)	lyse-IN-oh-pril	oral solution, tablet	5–40 mg a day	Rx
moexipril	moe-EX-i-pril	tablet	7.5–30 mg a day	Rx
perindopril (Aceon)	per-IN-doe-pril	tablet	4–16 mg a day	Rx
quinapril (Accupril)	KWIN-a-pril	tablet	10–80 mg a day	Rx
ramipril (Altace)	RA-mi-pril	capsule	2.5–20 mg a day	Rx
trandolapril (Mavik)	tran-DOE-la-pril	tablet	1–4 mg a day	Rx
Angiotensin Receptor Blockers (ARBs)				
azilsartan (Edarbi)	ay-zil-SAR-tan	tablet	40–80 mg a day	Rx
candesartan (Atacand)	kan-de-SAR-tan	tablet	8–32 mg 1–2 times a day	Rx
eprosartan (Teveten)	ep-roe-SAR-tan	tablet	400–800 mg a day	Rx
irbesartan (Avapro)	ir-be-SAR-tan	tablet	75–150 mg a day	Rx
losartan (Cozaar)	loe-SAR-tan	tablet	25–100 mg a day	Rx
olmesartan (Benicar)	ohl-me-SAR-tan	tablet	20–40 mg a day	Rx
telmisartan (Micardis)	tel-me-SAR-tan	tablet	20–80 mg a day	Rx
valsartan (Diovan)	val-SAR-tan	tablet	80–320 mg a day	Rx
Calcium Channel Blockers				
Dihydropyridine Agents				
amlodipine (Katerzia, Norvasc)	am-LOE-di-peen	oral suspension, tablet	5–10 mg a day	Rx
felodipine (Plendil)	fe-LOE-di-peen	tablet	2.5–10 mg a day	Rx
isradipine	iz-RAD-i-peen	capsule	5–20 mg a day	Rx
nicardipine (Cardene)	nye-KAR-di-peen	capsule, injection	IV: 0.5–2.2 mg/hr continuous infusion PO: 20–40 mg 3 times a day	Rx
nifedipine (Adalat CC, Afeditab, Afeditab CR, Nifediac, Procardia, Procardia XL)	nye-FED-i-peen	capsule, tablet	30–120 mg a day	Rx
nisoldipine (Sular)	nye-SOLE-di-peen	tablet	2 mg a day	Rx

continues

Generic (Brand)	Pronunciation	Dosage Form	Common Dosage	Dispensing Status
Nondihydropyridine Agents				
diltiazem (Cardizem, Cardizem CD, Cardizem LA, Cartia XT, Dilt-XR, Dilacor XR, Matzim LA, Tatzia XT, Tiadylt ER, Tiazac)	dil-TYE-a-zem	capsule, injection, tablet	IV: 20–25 mg infused over 2 min or 5–10 mg/hr continuous infusion for 24 hr PO: 180–240 mg a day	Rx
verapamil (Calan, Verelan)	ver-AP-a-mil	capsule, injection, tablet	IV: 5–10 mg infused over 2–3 min PO: 240–320 mg a day	Rx
Beta-Blockers				
Cardioselective Beta-Blockers				
acebutolol (Sectral)	a-se-BYOO-toe-lawl	capsule	400–800 mg a day	Rx
atenolol (Tenormin)	a-TEN-oh-lawl	tablet	50–100 mg a day	Rx
betaxolol	be-TAX-oh-lawl	tablet	10–20 mg a day	Rx
bisoprolol (Zebeta)	bis-OH-proe-lawl	tablet	5–20 mg a day	Rx
esmolol (Brevibloc)	ES-moe-lawl	injection	varies based on patient weight	Rx
metoprolol (Kaspargo, Lopressor, Toprol-XL)	me-TOE-proe-lawl	injection, oral solution, sprinkle, tablet	IV: 2.5–15 mg a day PO IR (tartrate): 100–450 mg a day PO XR (succinate): 50–100 mg a day	Rx
nebivolol (Bystolic)	neh-BIV-oh-lawl	tablet	5–20 mg a day	Rx
Nonselective Beta-Blockers				
carvedilol (Coreg, Coreg CR)	KAR-ve-dil-ole	capsule, tablet	6.25–80 mg a day	Rx
labetalol	la-BET-a-lawl	injection, tablet	IV: 50–200 mg a day PO: 100–400 mg 2 times a day	Rx
nadolol (Corgard)	naye-DOE-lawl	tablet	40–320 mg a day	Rx
propranolol (Inderal LA, Inderal XL, InnoPran XL)	proe-PRAN-oh-lawl	capsule, injection, oral solution, tablet	dose and frequency vary depending on indication and use	Rx
sotalol (Betapace, Sorine, Sotylize)	SOE-ta-lawl	oral solution, tablet	80–160 mg 2 times a day	Rx
timolol	TYE-moe-lawl	tablet	10–40 mg 2 times a day	Rx
Direct Renin Inhibitor				
aliskiren (Tekturna)	a-lis-KYE-ren	tablet	300 mg a day	Rx
Alpha-Blockers (discussed in Chapter 15)				
Thiazide Diuretics (discussed in Chapter 15)				
Vasodilators				
hydralazine	high-DRAL-uh-zeen	injection, tablet	PO: 100–200 mg a day divided in 3–4 doses IM/IV: 10–20 mg every 4 to 6 hr prn	Rx

Angiotensin-Converting Enzyme (ACE) Inhibitors

An **angiotensin-converting enzyme (ACE) inhibitor** is a drug class that regulates blood pressure through the renin-angiotensin system. Renin is an enzyme produced in the kidneys that is converted in the bloodstream to angiotensin I. Angiotensin I is further converted to angiotensin II by **angiotensin-converting enzyme**. Angiotensin II is a potent vasoconstrictor (agent that narrows blood vessels) in the body. By blocking the conversion of angiotensin I to angiotensin II, the use of ACE inhibitors results in blood vessel relaxation. This, in turn, lowers vascular resistance and overall blood pressure.

In addition to hypertension, ACE inhibitors are used for angina (sudden attacks of chest pain), myocardial infarction (heart attack), heart failure, and kidney disease.

Dosage Forms and Administration ACE inhibitors are typically used by patients on a long-term basis. ACE inhibitors come in oral tablets and capsules. The ACE inhibitor enalaprilat is available in an injectable form and is administered intravenously. Enalaprilat should be infused over five minutes.

Side Effects A persistent cough is one of the most common side effects of ACE inhibitors. It is believed that ACE inhibitors cause it by impeding the breakdown of bradykinin (a hormone that acts in the vasodilation of small arterioles). The resulting dry and unproductive cough can be extremely annoying. As a result, patient adherence with ACE inhibitors may be poor. The most dangerous side effect is angioedema. It most commonly presents as swelling of the face and tongue, which may begin a few hours after initiation of therapy or may not occur for several years into the treatment. ACE inhibitors may cause dizziness, especially during the first few days. The patient should be told to stand up slowly to prevent orthostatic hypotension (lowering of blood pressure upon standing). Increased potassium levels occur with ACE inhibitor use, and patients are usually instructed to avoid salt substitutes, which often contain potassium.

Contraindications ACE inhibitors should not be used in patients who have experienced angioedema with previous ACE inhibitor use. Other contraindications include idiopathic (of unknown origin) or hereditary angioedema and concomitant use with aliskiren in patients with diabetes mellitus.

Pregnant patients should not take ACE inhibitors, because these agents can cause severe birth defects. ACE inhibitors carry a boxed warning for this contraindication. Patients with a kidney condition called *bilateral renal artery stenosis* also should not take ACE inhibitors, because the kidneys could shut down.

Cautions and Considerations ACE inhibitors carry boxed warnings for injury and death to a developing fetus. ACE inhibitors should not be used by patients who are pregnant or who are trying to become pregnant. In rare instances, hypotension, or low blood pressure, can occur. With ACE inhibitors, hypotension can happen dramatically, sometimes on the first dose. Careful monitoring is necessary when a patient starts taking an ACE inhibitor. In some cases, the first dose may be given in the prescriber's office, so the patient's blood pressure can be monitored for drastic drops.

Hyperkalemia, or an elevated potassium level, is another rare but serious side effect. It tends to occur when patients are also taking potassium-sparing diuretics such as spironolactone. Periodic blood tests for potassium levels should be conducted.

Patients who take diuretics along with an ACE inhibitor should be warned against taking potassium supplements.

Patients who have kidney problems (other than bilateral renal artery stenosis) can take ACE inhibitors, but doses are adjusted downward.

Drug Interactions Drugs with hypotensive effects should be used cautiously in patients taking ACE inhibitors. Other drugs that have hyperkalemic side effects (such as spironolactone) may enhance similar side effects from ACE inhibitors. ACE inhibitors should not be used with angiotensin receptor blockers because of possible increased adverse effects. ACE inhibitors should be given with caution to patients taking lithium.

Angiotensin Receptor Blockers (ARBs)

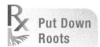

Put Down Roots

ARBs are identified by the drug stem *-sartan* in the generic name.

An **angiotensin receptor blocker (ARB)** is a type of agent used to treat hypertension and is an acceptable alternative for patients who cannot tolerate ACE inhibitors.

ARBs work by binding to the same receptors to which angiotensin II binds. Instead of stimulating vasoconstriction, as angiotensin II does, ARBs *block* these receptors, thereby preventing constriction and causing blood vessels to relax, which lowers blood pressure. ARBs do not cause bradykinin buildup, as ACE inhibitors do, so coughing is not a typical side effect.

ARBs are used for hypertension and other indications. However, not all ARBs have the same indications. Table 10.2 identifies indications for common ARBs.

TABLE 10.2 Commonly Used ARBs and Their Indications

Generic (Brand)	Indications
azilsartan (Edarbi)	hypertension
candesartan (Atacand)	hypertension, heart failure
eprosartan (Teveten)	hypertension
irbesartan (Avapro)	hypertension, diabetic nephropathy
losartan (Cozaar)	hypertension, diabetic nephropathy
olmesartan (Benicar)	hypertension
telmisartan (Micardis)	hypertension, cardiovascular risk reduction
valsartan (Diovan)	hypertension, heart failure, post–myocardial infarction

Dosage Forms and Administration ARBs are available in tablet dosage forms for oral consumption. ARBs with special dosing and administration needs are noted below.

Azilsartan (Edarbi) is sensitive to moisture and light and must be dispensed and stored in the original bottle. **Candesartan (Atacand)** is only available as a tablet. However, an oral suspension using tablets can be made for children or patients unable to swallow solids. **Olmesartan (Benicar)** is a selective ARB. It is a prodrug that is converted to its active form during absorption in the GI tract. **Telmisartan (Micardis)** has the longest half-life of all the ARBs. It is sensitive to moisture and is provided by the manufacturer in a foil blister pack. Because of this sensitivity to moisture, a telmisartan tablet cannot be cut in half. Pharmacy technicians should be aware that telmisartan will lose potency when the pack is opened.

Side Effects Common side effects of ARBs include headache, dizziness, fatigue, and mild diarrhea. Dizziness occurs most frequently in patients who also have heart failure. Patients using ARBs may have more respiratory tract infections, but the reason for this is unknown.

Contraindications ARBs are contraindicated in patients with diabetes mellitus who are taking aliskiren.

Cautions and Considerations ARBs should not be used during pregnancy. If pregnancy is detected, ARBs should be discontinued as soon as possible. ARBs have a boxed warning for causing injury or death to the developing fetus.

Patients taking diuretics along with ARBs may experience hypotension. Patients should be careful not to get up too quickly from a sitting or lying position until they know how these drugs affect them. Dizziness, fainting, and falling down may be signs of hypotension. Patients with kidney or liver impairment may need special dosing and monitoring if they are to take these medications.

Drug Interactions Drugs with hypotensive effects may enhance the hypotensive effects of ARBs. ARBs may enhance the adverse effects of ACE inhibitors. Pimozide concentrations may be increased by irbesartan and losartan. Telmisartan may enhance the adverse effects of ramipril.

Calcium Channel Blockers

The **calcium channel blocker** drug class is used to treat hypertension alone or in combination with other drugs and may also be used for other cardiac conditions such as heart failure and **arrhythmias** (any deviation from normal sinus rhythm).

A calcium channel blocker prevents calcium from entering the cells of the heart and arteries. Calcium causes the heart to contract more strongly. When calcium is kept from entering heart cells, the result is decreased heart contractility. Blocking the entrance of calcium to vasculature cells results in the relaxation of blood vessels. The relaxation increases blood flow, which increases oxygen delivery throughout the body. The combination of these effects decreases the oxygen demands of heart muscle tissue and increases the supply of oxygen.

Calcium channel blockers are categorized as dihydropyridine or nondihydropyridine. Dihydropyridine calcium channel blockers work by causing vasodilation while having less effect on pacemaking and conduction in the heart. Non-dihydropyridines typically vasodilate less but depress pacemaking and conduction more profoundly.

Dihydropyridine calcium channel blockers are first-line therapy for hypertension. A **dihydropyridine calcium channel blocker** reduces blood pressure by dilating the arterioles, which decreases energy consumption, oxygen requirements, and peripheral vascular resistance to blood flow.

Nondihydropyridine calcium channel blockers are commonly used to treat most supraventricular tachyarrhythmias (rapid, irregular beats). They slow conduction through the AV node, slow SA node action, and relax coronary artery smooth muscle. They are used to control fast ventricular rates in patients with atrial flutter or atrial fibrillation, two types of abnormal heart rhythms.

Dosage Forms and Administration Calcium channel blockers are available in oral and injectable dosage forms. Select calcium channel blockers come in extended-release dosage forms that need to be taken just once a day. These products should be swallowed whole, not crushed or chewed. Crushing or chewing the medication alters the release mechanism and could result in drastically lowered blood pressure because the entire large dose could be released at once.

Patients should be warned that some of the extended-release dosage forms (such as some oral forms of verapamil) work by releasing the drug from a capsule or tablet called a *ghost pill* while in the digestive system. The ghost pill casing then moves through the GI tract and appears in patients' stool. Patients should be assured that although they may see the casing in their stool, the medication was absorbed by the body.

Side Effects Side effects of calcium channel blockers include **bradycardia** (slowed heart rate), hypotension, heart block, cardiac failure, nausea, constipation, headache, dizziness, and fatigue, all of which lead to poor patient adherence. Patients sometimes do not understand that the drug is helping, because they may feel worse after taking it. The most common side effect is constipation. Some patients experience drowsiness when they begin taking a calcium channel blocker. Some of these drugs should be taken with food, and caffeine should be limited.

Contraindications Felodipine and nisoldipine should not be used in patients with a hypersensitivity to other calcium channel blockers. Nicardipine should not be used in patients with aortic stenosis. Nifedipine is contraindicated in patients with cardiogenic shock or acute myocardial infarction (MI).

Contraindications to diltiazem include sick sinus syndrome, second- or third-degree atrioventricular (AV) block, severe hypotension, acute MI, and pulmonary congestion. Contraindications to verapamil include severe left ventricular dysfunction, hypotension, cardiogenic shock, sick sinus syndrome, second- or third-degree AV block, Wolff-Parkinson-White syndrome, and Lown-Ganong-Levine syndrome. The IV form of verapamil is also contraindicated with concurrent use of beta-blockers and in patients with ventricular tachycardia. Amlodipine and isradipine do not have contraindications.

Safety Alert

Cardura (doxazosin, an alpha-blocker) and Cardene (nicardipine, a calcium channel blocker) can also be misread for each other.

Cautions and Considerations Some calcium channel blockers cause fluid retention (edema) and heart palpitations. To balance the positive and negative effects on the heart, healthcare practitioners closely monitor patients taking this class of drugs.

Drug Interactions Additive or increased adverse effects occur when calcium channel blockers are used concurrently with beta-blockers. Calcium channel blockers may increase digoxin levels.

Azole antifungals may increase concentrations of amlodipine, felodipine, isradipine, and nifedipine. Diltiazem and verapamil may result in altered drug levels and increased toxicity in lithium-using patients. Diltiazem, when used with amiodarone, may result in cardiotoxicity. Nafcillin decreases the effectiveness of nifedipine. Verapamil may increase tolvaptan concentrations.

Put Down Roots

Beta-blockers are identified by the drug stem *-olol* in the generic name.

Beta-Blockers

In response to increased anxiety, physical activity, or emotional stress, the sympathetic nervous system stimulates the release of catecholamines (the class of neurotransmitters that includes epinephrine and norepinephrine). The action of these neurotransmitters on the beta-1 receptors (see Chapter 7), in particular, increases heart rate and contractile force. A **beta-blocker** is a drug that is similar in molecular structure to a catecholamine and, therefore, competes for the same receptor sites. This action, in turn, inhibits neurotransmitter activity.

Beta-blockers are designed to exert action on two types of beta-receptors: beta-1 receptors and beta-2 receptors (see Chapter 7). Beta-1 receptors are found primarily in the heart and kidneys. Activation of beta-1 receptors in the heart ultimately lead to increased heart rate and contractility. Beta-1 receptor activation in the kidneys leads to the release of renin, which increases blood pressure. Beta-2 receptors are found primarily in the lungs. Activation on beta-2 receptors in the lungs leads to relaxation. In choosing a drug for the heart, a drug with more beta-1 blockage than beta-2 blockage may be preferred because beta-1 receptors are associated with cardiovascular function. Beta-blockers that are more selective for beta-1 receptors than beta-2 receptors are referred to as *cardioselective beta-blockers*. Drugs that block beta-2 receptors can adversely affect respiration in patients with asthma, chronic obstructive pulmonary disease (COPD), or other respiratory problems.

Beta-blockers may be used to treat hypertension, but they are also used to treat angina. Angina, atrial fibrillation, heart failure, tachycardia associated with operations, myocardial infarction, and arrhythmias are cardiac-related indications for specific beta-blockers. Noncardiac indications for beta-blockers include migraine prevention, glaucoma, hyperthyroidism, and essential tremors.

Dosage Forms and Administration Most beta-blockers are available in oral formulations. Injectable beta-blockers are typically reserved for emergent situations (such as arrhythmias and intraoperative tachycardia). **Esmolol (Brevibloc)** is a beta-1 selective beta-blocker available in an intravenous (IV) dosage form only. **Metoprolol (Kaspargo, Lopressor, Toprol-XL)**, **propranolol (Inderal LA, Inderal XL, InnoPran XL)**, and **labetalol** are available in oral and intravenous forms. Pharmacy technicians should be aware that an IV dose of metoprolol is much smaller than an oral dose.

Beta-blocker doses are typically titrated (meaning doses begin low and are slowly increased). Dose titration decreases the risk of adverse effects, especially **orthostatic hypotension** (a sudden decrease in blood pressure upon standing).

Atenolol (Tenormin), metoprolol, **nadolol (Corgard)**, propranolol, and **timolol** should not be discontinued abruptly. Doses should be decreased gradually to prevent the risk of worsening cardiac symptoms.

Oral metoprolol comes in immediate-release and extended-release forms. These tablets may be divided in half; however, they should not be crushed or chewed. Immediate-release tablets should be taken with meals.

Oral forms of propranolol include immediate-release and long-acting formulations. Immediate-release forms should be taken on an empty stomach; long-acting forms can be taken without regard to meals but should be taken consistently. Long-acting forms should not be crushed or chewed. As with metoprolol, the IV dose is much lower than the oral dose.

Side Effects Most adverse events related to beta-blockers are mild and transient and rarely require withdrawal of therapy. The most common adverse effect is fatigue. The primary side effect of beta-blockers is bradycardia.

Contraindications Beta-blockers are contraindicated in bradycardia, cardiogenic shock, and heart block. Specific beta-blockers may have additional contraindications. Atenolol should not be used in patients with pulmonary edema or in patients who are pregnant. **Carvedilol (Coreg)**, labetalol, pindolol, propranolol, **sotalol (Betapace, Sorine, Sotylize)**, and timolol are contraindicated in lung disorders such as asthma and COPD. Nebivolol should not be used in patients with liver impairment. Sotalol should be avoided in patients with long QT syndrome, kidney dysfunction, or low potassium levels.

Cautions and Considerations Atenolol, metoprolol, nadolol, propranolol, and timolol have boxed warnings for increased cardiac symptoms (including worsening of angina and MI) with abrupt discontinuation. Gradual dose reduction is recommended over several weeks, and physical activity should be limited during dose reduction. Sotalol has a boxed warning for increased risk of life-threatening arrhythmias.

Nonselective beta-blockers should be used with caution in patients with bronchospastic disease, because these drugs may inhibit the bronchodilating effects of endogenous catecholamines. Blocking of beta-2 receptors constricts airways in the lungs in addition to lowering blood pressure. This effect can be harmful to patients with impaired respiratory function. For these individuals, care must be taken to choose drugs that selectively block beta-1 receptors only. Beta-blockers that may be used by patients with asthma or COPD include **acebutolol (Sectral)**, atenolol, **betaxolol, bisoprolol (Zebeta), esmolol,** metoprolol, and **nebivolol (Bystolic)**.

Abrupt withdrawal from a beta-blocker can cause severe cardiac problems, such as an MI, angina, or arrhythmia. Thus, patients should not stop taking a beta-blocker suddenly. If a change in medication is made, the dose must be decreased slowly until it is discontinued.

Patients with diabetes should use beta-blockers with caution. These drugs can inhibit the usual signs and symptoms of low blood glucose. A patient taking a beta-blocker who experiences low blood sugar might only have sweating and hunger as symptoms. The pharmacist should counsel patients with diabetes who are taking beta-blockers.

Drug Interactions Beta-blockers may enhance the bradycrotic (inducing slowness of pulse) effects of other drugs. Concurrent use with another drug that causes bradycardia is generally not recommended.

Beta-blockers should not be used with beta-agonists.

Over-the-counter (OTC) decongestants are vasoconstrictors that can raise blood pressure. Patients taking beta-blockers to treat hypertension should avoid taking oral decongestants.

Sotalol should not be combined with other drugs that cause QT prolongation.

Direct Renin Inhibitors

Several drug classes used for the treatment of hypertension involve the renin-angiotensin system. Two such drug classes, ACE inhibitors and ARBs, were discussed previously in this chapter. A newer drug class, the direct renin inhibitors, also works on the renin-angiotensin system.

Renin is an enzyme produced in the kidneys. Renin is converted to angiotensin I, which is subsequently converted to angiotensin II. Angiotensin II is a potent vasoconstrictor in the body. Direct renin inhibitors decrease the activity of renin. This inhibition leads to a reduction in angiotensin I and II and results in blood vessel relaxation. This lowers vascular resistance and overall blood pressure. **Aliskiren (Tekturna)** is the only direct renin inhibitor available in the United States at the time of publication.

Dosage Forms and Administration Aliskiren is available exclusively in oral dosage forms. Aliskiren may be taken with or without meals; however, consistent administration is recommended. High-fat meals increase absorption of aliskiren.

Side Effects Common side effects of aliskiren include diarrhea, skin rash, increased serum creatinine, and cough.

Contraindications Contraindications include hypersensitivity to aliskiren or any component of the formulation and concomitant use with an ACE inhibitor or ARB in patients with diabetes. It is contraindicated in children younger than two years of age.

Cautions and Considerations Aliskiren has a boxed warning related to pregnancy. Injury and death to a developing fetus may occur with use during pregnancy.

Drug Interactions Aliskiren may increase the risk of hyperkalemia. The risk is higher in patients with kidney impairment or diabetes and in those using other medications that increase potassium (such as NSAIDs and potassium-sparing diuretics). Angioedema and anaphylaxis have occurred with aliskiren use. Use with caution in patients with a history of angioedema. Kidney function may worsen with aliskiren use. This risk is higher in patients with diabetes. Aliskiren should be used with caution in patients with renal impairment.

Aliskiren may enhance the hypotensive effects of drugs that lower blood pressure. Aliskiren may enhance the potassium-raising effects of other drugs (such as ACE inhibitors, ARBs, NSAIDs, and potassium supplements).

Aliskiren levels may be increased by atorvastatin, cyclosporine, and itraconazole.

Safety Alert

Beta-blockers should not be withdrawn abruptly. Dosage should be reduced gradually over one to two weeks.

Safety Alert

Aliskiren (Tekturna), a direct renin inhibitor, has a boxed warning for the risk of injury or death to a developing fetus.

Alpha-Blockers

Alpha-blockers are a class of drugs used to treat patients with hypertension by inhibiting the alpha-1 receptors in the body. This relaxes the blood vessels and decreases blood pressure. Blocking alpha-1 receptors also delays bladder emptying, which is why this class is used to treat benign prostatic hypertrophy, a condition in which the prostate enlarges with age. More information can be found in Chapter 15.

Thiazide Diuretics

Thiazide diuretics are commonly used in the treatment of hypertension. Thiazides work by eliminating sodium and water from the body. The loss of sodium and water contributes to a lowering of blood pressure. Chapter 15 addresses this drug class in detail.

Vasodilators

Hydralazine decreases blood pressure by directly causing vasodilation within the body. Hydralazine primarily acts as an arteriolar vasodilator with little effect on the venous circulation. Hydralazine is FDA indicated to treat hypertensive emergency.

Dosage Forms and Administration Oral hydralazine tablets may be administered with or without food, but consistent administration is recommended. Injected hydralazine may be administered undiluted.

Side Effects Side effects include headache, loss of appetite, dizziness, and anxiety.

Contraindications Coronary artery disease and mitral valve rheumatic heart disease contraindicate use of hydralazine.

Cautions and Considerations Hydralazine should be used with caution in patients with stroke and suspected heart disease due to the risk of angina and other cardiac abnormalities. Hydralazine may cause a lupus-like syndrome where patients exhibit symptoms of lupus. Reductions in red blood cells and white blood cells may occur with use. Some dosage forms contain propylene glycol or tartrazine.

Drug Interactions Hydralazine may enhance the blood pressure lowering effects of other antihypertensives.

10.3 Cardiac Arrhythmias and Drug Treatments

Normal heart rhythm is called *sinus rhythm* because it originates in the sinoatrial (SA) node, or pacemaker, which is located in the right atrium. Normal sinus rhythm is generated by the SA node at a rate of 70 to 80 beats per minute. Any deviation from normal sinus rhythm is considered an arrhythmia. Abnormalities of heart rate, rhythm, or both occur when the heart rate is too slow or too fast or when the contractions of the ventricles and atria are not synchronized.

An electrocardiogram (ECG or EKG) records and documents the signals sent through the conduction system of the heart, as shown in Figure 10.6. An ECG produces a graphical representation of the electrical activity of the heart. The spikes and dips on an ECG are referred to as waves. Different waves and segments correspond to electrical activity in various portions of the heart. The P wave illustrates activity in the atria. The PQ interval is when electrical activity moves from the atria, through the bundle of His, and to the ventricles. The interval called the QRS complex shows activity in the ventricles. The ST segment corresponds to when the ventricle is

FIGURE 10.6
**ECG
Recording
of Normal
Electrical
Heart Activity**

ECG's show spikes
and dips called
waves. The color
coded waves
correspond to
electrical activity
in various parts of
the heart.

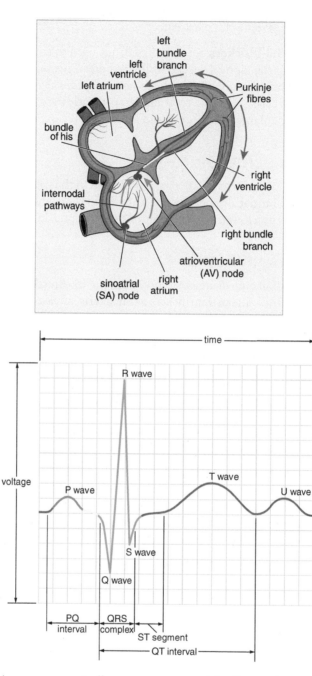

contracting. This segment typically appears as a straight line as there is no electrical conduction during this time. The T wave indicates the lower portion of the heart is repolarizing and preparing to contract again. ECG readings are used to observe heart function and diagnose arrhythmias.

Tachycardia refers to an increased heart rate, while bradycardia is a decreased heart rate. Other terms, such as *flutter* and *fibrillation*, refer to the ways certain parts of the heart beat out of sync with each other. **Flutter** occurs when select portions of the heart (the atria, for example) are slightly out of sync with the rest of the heart. It is not necessarily life threatening. **Fibrillation** occurs when large portions of the heart beat out of sequence. Atrial fibrillation is not necessarily life threatening. Ventricular fibrillation, however, is an emergency situation. In ventricular fibrillation, no blood flows through the heart; therefore, the use of an electronic defibrillator is necessary to shock the heart components back into sequence.

Table 10.3 shows abnormal heart rhythms and rates and their ECG tracings. These conditions may be caused by ischemia (deficient supply of blood to part of the body), myocardial infarction, or alteration of pacemaking cells. The symptoms of abnormal heart rhythms or rates include palpitations, syncope (loss of consciousness), lightheadedness, visual disturbances, pallor (paleness), cyanosis (bluish skin discoloration), weakness, sweating, chest pain, and hypotension.

TABLE 10.3 Abnormal Heart Rhythms

Arrhythmia	Beats per Minute	Electrocardiogram
tachycardia	>100	
bradycardia	<60	
atrial flutter	200–350	
atrial fibrillation	100–175	
premature atrial contraction	variable	
premature ventricular contraction	variable	
ventricular fibrillation	variable	

Pharmaceutical treatment for arrhythmias is directed at preventing these life-threatening conditions by restoring normal sinus rhythm. The various classes of antiarrhythmic drugs have characteristic electrophysiologic effects on the myocardium and the conduction system. Some drugs influence the heart rate directly or indirectly by affecting the movement of ions into or out of heart muscle cells. The excitability of the cells of the SA node is influenced by the permeability of the cell membranes to sodium and calcium ions. The sodium and calcium ions cross the cell membranes through openings called ion channels, which are actually protein molecules that are sensitive to specific electrical and chemical conditions. An ion channel acts as a gate or valve through which ions pass (see Figure 10.7). Drugs may act to tighten the valve, allowing fewer ions to penetrate the membrane, or to open the valve, allowing more ions to penetrate.

FIGURE 10.7
The Gatekeeper Role of Cardiovascular Drugs

Drugs may act to close ion channels, allowing fewer ions to penetrate cell membranes, or to open ion channels, allowing more ions to penetrate.

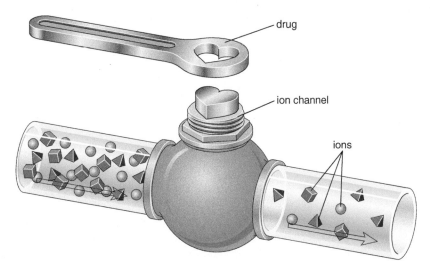

drug

ion channel

ions

Table 10.4 lists the most commonly used antiarrhythmic agents. Antiarrhythmics are organized into classes based on their mechanism of action. These classes include membrane-stabilizing agents or sodium channel blockers (class I antiarrhythmics) and potassium channel blockers (class III antiarrhythmics). Beta-blockers (class II antiarrhythmics) and calcium channel blockers (class IV antiarrhythmics) were discussed earlier in the Hypertension and Drug Treatments section.

TABLE 10.4 Commonly Used Antiarrhythmic Agents

Generic (Brand)	Pronunciation	Dosage Form	Common Dosages	Dispensing Status
Membrane-Stabilizing Agents/Sodium Channel Blockers (Class I)				
disopyramide (Norpace)	dye-soe-PEER-a-mide	capsule	varies	Rx
flecainide (Tambocor)	FLEK-a-nide	tablet	50–200 mg 2 times a day	Rx
lidocaine (Xylocaine)	LYE-doe-kane	injection	50–100 mg for 1 or 2 doses	Rx
mexiletine (Mexitil)	mex-IL-a-teen	capsule	150–300 mg every 8–12 hr	Rx
procainamide	proe-KANE-a-mide	injection	2–6 mg/min	Rx
propafenone (Rythmol)	proe-PAF-e-none	capsule, tablet	150–300 mg 3 times a day	Rx
quinidine	KWIN-i-deen	injection, tablet	varies	Rx
Beta-Blockers (Class II), see Table 10.1				
Potassium Channel Blockers (Class III)				
amiodarone (Cordarone, Nexterone, Pacerone)	am-ee-OH-da-rone	injection, tablet	varies	Rx
dofetilide (Tikosyn)	doe-FET-il-ide	capsule	500 mcg 2 times a day	Rx
dronedarone (Multaq)	droe-NE-da-rone	tablet	400 mg 2 times a day	Rx
Calcium Channel Blockers (Class IV), see Table 10.1				
Miscellaneous Antiarrhythmic Agents				
atropine	AT-roe-peen	injection, tablet	varies	Rx
digoxin (Digitek, Digox, Lanoxin)	di-JOX-in	injection, oral solution, tablet	varies	Rx
isoproterenol	eye-soe-proe-TER-e-nawl	injection	2–10 mcg/min	Rx
Antidote for Digoxin Toxicity				
digoxin immune Fab (DigiFab)	di-JOX-in i-MYUN fab	injection	varies	Rx

Membrane-Stabilizing Agents/Sodium Channel Blockers (Class I Antiarrhythmics)

A **membrane-stabilizing agent** slows the movement of sodium ions into myocardial cells, which is why this class of antiarrhythmics is also known as sodium channel blockers. As a result, the cells require a stronger signal to trigger an action potential. The reduced ability to generate an action potential dampens potential abnormal rhythms and heart rates. Common membrane-stabilizing agents used to treat life-threatening ventricular arrhythmias include **disopyramide (Norpace), flecainide (Tambocor), lidocaine, mexiletine**, and **propafenone (Rythmol)**. The agent procainamide is used for life-threatening atrial arrhythmias. See Tables 10.5 and 10.6 for additional information on these agents.

TABLE 10.5 Membrane-Stabilizing Agents (Class I Antiarrhythmics) Side Effects, Cautions and Considerations, and Drug Interactions

Generic (Brand)	Side Effects	Cautions and Considerations	Significant Drug Interactions
disopyramide (Norpace)	hypotension, anticholinergic effects, headache, gas, muscle aches and pains	Avoid use in heart failure due to heart rate reduction.	clarithromycin, erythromycin, fluoroquinolones
flecainide (Tambocor)	dizziness, shortness of breath, headache, nausea, fatigue, palpitations, tremor, angina	Avoid use in heart failure due to heart rate reduction.	cisapride, ritonavir
lidocaine	bradycardia, hypotension, dizziness, drowsiness, blurred vision, confusion	Often used to treat acute myocardial infarction.	anticonvulsants
mexiletine	palpitations, chest pain, dizziness, tremor, nervousness, insomnia, nausea, vomiting, blurred vision, headache, shortness of breath	Can cause leukopenia (low number of white blood cells) and agranulocytosis (a severe blood condition).	caffeine, cimetidine, rifampin, theophylline
procainamide	anorexia, nausea, vomiting, diarrhea, lupus-like syndrome	Can cause heart failure in patients with ventricular dysfunction. Can cause leukopenia (low number of white blood cells) and agranulocytosis (a severe blood condition).	amiodarone, antiarrhythmics, cimetidine, fluoroquinolones, ranitidine, thioridazine, ziprasidone
propafenone (Rythmol)	new arrhythmias, dizziness, nausea, vomiting	May worsen heart failure and interfere with pacemakers. Patients should be connected to a cardiac monitor at the beginning of therapy or with any increase in dosage.	cimetidine, digoxin, ritonavir, selective serotonin reuptake inhibitors, theophylline
quinidine	hypotension, anticholinergic effects, headache, tinnitus, confusion, nausea	Gluconate, polygluconate, and sulfate salts of quinidine contain varying amounts of active drug and are not interchangeable. Can cause thrombocytopenia (low platelets).	amiodarone, antacids, cimetidine

Dosage Forms and Administration Dosage form information for membrane-stabilizing medications can be found in Table 10.4.

Side Effects Common and life-threatening side effects of membrane-stabilizing agents can be found in Table 10.5.

Contraindications Disopyramide is contraindicated in patients with cardiogenic shock, preexisting second- or third-degree AV block, long QT syndrome, or sick sinus syndrome.

Contraindications to flecainide include preexisting second- or third-degree AV block, cardiogenic shock, coronary artery disease, or concurrent use of ritonavir or amprenavir.

Systemic lidocaine should be avoided in patients with Stokes-Adams syndrome; Wolff-Parkinson-White syndrome; or severe degrees of SA, AV, or intraventricular heart block. Some commercially available forms of premixed lidocaine for injection may include corn-derived products and, therefore, should be avoided in patients with corn hypersensitivity. Mexiletine is contraindicated in patients with cardiogenic shock or second- or third-degree AV block. Procainamide should not be used in patients with complete heart block, second-degree AV block, or an abnormal heart rhythm called *torsades de pointes*. Contraindications to propafenone include SA, AV, and intraventricular disorders; Brugada syndrome; sinus bradycardia; cardiogenic shock; uncompensated cardiac failure; marked hypotension; bronchospastic disorders; severe pulmonary disease; and uncorrected electrolyte abnormalities. Quinidine should not be used in patients with thrombocytopenia, thrombocytopenic purpura, myasthenia gravis, heart block greater than first degree, or idiopathic conduction delays, or with concurrent use of quinolone antibiotics, cisapride, amprenavir, or ritonavir.

Cautions and Considerations Disopyramide, flecainide, mexiletine, procainamide, propafenone, and quinidine carry boxed warnings stating they should be reserved for patients with life-threatening ventricular arrhythmias. Procainaide carries additional boxed warnings for the risk of drug-induced lupus-like syndrome and the risk of hematologic disorders. Other cautions and considerations unique to specific membrane-stabilizing agents are presented in Table 10.5. These agents should be used cautiously in patients with heart failure due to potential overreduction of heart rate.

Drug Interactions See Table 10.6 for a list of drug interactions.

Beta-Blockers (Class II Antiarrhythmics)

Beta-blockers are commonly used in the treatment of cardiac arrhythmias. Information on beta-blockers can be found in the Hypertension and Drug Treatments section of this chapter and in Table 10.1.

Potassium Channel Blockers (Class III Antiarrhythmics)

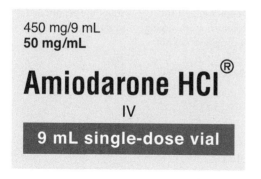

450 mg/9 mL
50 mg/mL

Amiodarone HCl®
IV

9 mL single-dose vial

As their name suggests, potassium channel blockers (class III antiarrhythmics) block potassium channels in cardiac muscle cells. Similar to class I antiarrhythmic drugs, potassium channel blockers slow the influx of a positively changed ion (potassium, in this case). This makes the cell membrane more stable and lowers its ability to depolarize. Consequently, the electrical charge must be stronger to make the heart beat. This effect regulates heart rhythm because it decreases the incidence of abnormal beats. See Table 10.6 for details on side effects, cautions and considerations, and drug interactions.

TABLE 10.6 Potassium Channel Blockers (Class III Antiarrhythmics) Side Effects, Cautions and Considerations, and Drug Interactions

Generic (Brand)	Side Effects	Cautions and Considerations	Significant Drug Interactions
amiodarone (Nexterone, Pacerone)	fatigue, tremor, photosensitivity, anorexia, constipation, nausea, vomiting, blurred vision	Takes days to months for full effects. Must use glass bottle for IV solution. Can cause fatal toxicities to lungs, liver, and heart—use with caution. Contains iodine.	azole antifungals, cimetidine, fentanyl, fluoroquinolones, loratadine, macrolide antibiotics, other antiarrhythmics, statins, warfarin
dofetilide (Tikosyn)	new arrhythmias, headache, chest pain, dizziness, shortness of breath, nausea	Used in cardioversion procedures to restore normal rhythm.	cimetidine, ketoconazole, trimethoprim, verapamil
dronedarone (Multaq)	dermatitis, fatigue, hypokalemia, kidney dysfunction, liver dysfunction, skin rash	Similar to amiodarone, but without the iodine. May increase risk of death in patients with symptomatic heart failure. May increase risk of death and stroke in patients with permanent atrial fibrillation.	azole antifungals, cimetidine, fentanyl, fluoroquinolones, loratadine, macrolide antibiotics, other antiarrhythmics, statins, warfarin

Dosage Forms and Administration **Amiodarone (Nexterone, Pacerone)** is a drug with an unusually long half-life. This means establishing control over the arrythmia may take several days to several weeks with the IV form and one to four weeks with the oral dose. **Dofetilide (Tikosyn)** must be initiated or reinitiated in a hospital setting. The patient must be placed in a facility that can provide monitoring and resuscitation for a period of three days. **Dronedarone (Multaq)** should be taken with the morning and evening meals. Grapefruit should be avoided.

Side Effects Potassium channel blockers are known to cause a variety of unique and sometimes serious and fatal side effects. Side effect information on these drugs can be found in Table 10.6.

Contraindications Amiodarone is contraindicated in patients with hypersensitivity to iodine, severe sinus node dysfunction, second- or third-degree AV block, bradycardia, or cardiogenic shock.

Dofetilide is contraindicated in patients with a long QT interval or severe kidney impairment. Concurrent use of cimetidine, dolutegravir, hydrochlorothiazide, itraconazole, ketoconazole, megestrol, prochlorperazine, trimethoprim, or verapamil contraindicates the administration of dofetilide.

Dronedarone should not be used in patients with permanent atrial fibrillation, symptomatic heart failure, liver or lung toxicity from amiodarone use, second- or third-degree AV block, bradycardia (heart rates below 60 beats per minute), or severe liver impairment or patients who are pregnant or breast-feeding. Agents that prolong the QT interval should not be used with dronedarone.

Safety Alert

The potassium channel blockers amiodarone, dofetilide, and dronedarone all carry boxed warnings.

Cautions and Considerations Amiodarone has several boxed warnings. One states that amiodarone should be used only in patients who have life-threatening arrhythmias. Another warns of the risk of severe liver toxicity. An additional warning advises that amiodarone has the potential to exacerbate arrhythmias. Amiodarone also carries a boxed warning that pulmonary toxicity may occur with use.

Dofetilide has a boxed warning stating that it must be initiated in a setting with clinical monitoring due to a risk of arrhythmias. Dofetilide should be used cautiously in patients with renal impairment.

Dronedarone also has boxed warnings. One warns that it should not be used in patients with symptomatic heart failure due to increased risk of death. When used in patients with permanent atrial fibrillation, dronedarone may also increase mortality.

Amiodarone, dofetilide, and dronedarone must all be dispensed with FDA-approved Medication Guides.

Other cautions and considerations for potassium channel blockers can be found in Table 10.6.

Drug Interactions Drug interactions associated with potassium channel blockers are listed in Table 10.6.

Calcium Channel Blockers (Class IV Antiarrhythmics)

The calcium channel blockers diltiazem and verapamil (nondihydropyridines) may be used in the treatment of cardiac arrhythmias. Information on these drugs can be found in the Hypertension and Drug Treatments section of this chapter and in Table 10.1.

Other Agents Used to Treat Arrhythmias

In addition to the class I–IV antiarrhythmics, other agents are used to treat cardiac arrhythmias. Atroprine, digoxin, and isoproterenol are three such agents. Each has a different mechanism of action, which is discussed below.

Atropine is an anticholinergic agent that increases heart rate and cardiac output. Atropine is used to treat bradycardia. Low doses of atropine may worsen bradycardia, whereas high doses may cause the heart rate to increase too much, which increases oxygen demand, which can result in ischemia and lead to arrhythmias. Atropine is also used as a preoperative medication to inhibit salivation and secretions during surgery.

Digoxin (Digitek, Digox, Lanoxin) may be used in the management of atrial flutter and fibrillation. Digoxin is also often used to treat symptoms of heart failure. Digoxin works by inhibiting sodium-potassium adenosine triphosphatase (ATPase), an enzyme that regulates the influx of ions into cardiac muscle cells. It also alters SA node conductivity, conduction velocity through the heart, and rest time between beats. Digoxin increases the force of velocity of muscle contraction, making the heart pump more efficiently.

Isoproterenol (Isuprel) dilates coronary vessels. It is used parenterally to treat ventricular arrhythmias due to AV block, and it is used in bradyarrhythmias (slow, irregular heartbeats). It may be used temporarily to treat third-degree AV block until pacemaker insertion is performed. It increases heart rate and contractility.

Safety Alert

Digoxin (Digitek, Digox, Lanoxin) is considered a narrow therapeutic index drug. This means there is a small difference between its therapeutic dose and toxic dose.

Dosage Forms and Administration Dosage form information for atropine, digoxin, and isoproterenol is listed in Table 10.4.

Side Effects Side effect information for atropine, digoxin, and isoproterenol is listed in Table 10.7.

Contraindications Atropine has no contraindications.

Patients who have hypersensitivity to digitalis or digoxin or a diagnosis of ventricular fibrillation should not use digoxin.

Isoproterenol is contraindicated in patients with angina, preexisting ventricular arrhythmias, tachyarrhythmias, or cardiac glycoside intoxication.

Pharm Fact

Digoxin was originally derived from the foxglove plant.

Cautions and Considerations General cautions and considerations for atropine, digoxin, and isoproterenol can be found in Table 10.7.

Digoxin should be used with caution because of the possibility of systemic accumulation of the drug. Patients who take digoxin commonly experience digitalis toxicity, commonly referred to as *dig* (pronounced "didge") *toxicity*. This effect is especially common among older adults. The three primary signs of digitalis toxicity are nausea, vomiting, and arrhythmias. Patients may also experience vertigo or general weakness, and they may see yellow-green halos around objects. If any of these signs or symptoms occur, the drug should be withdrawn immediately. **Digoxin immune Fab (DigiFab)** is an antidote for digitalis toxicity. It is an antibody fragment that binds to digoxin, inactivating the drug, which is then excreted by the kidneys.

Drug Interactions Significant drug interactions associated with antiarrhythmic agents are listed in Table 10.7.

TABLE 10.7 Miscellaneous Antiarrhythmic Agents Side Effects, Cautions and Considerations, and Drug Interactions

Generic (Brand)	Side Effects	Cautions and Considerations	Significant Drug Interactions
atropine	dry mouth, dry skin, blurred vision, urinary retention, tachycardia, constipation	Anaphylaxis may occur with use. Risk of hyperthermia in the presence of high environmental temperature. Psychosis can occur in sensitive individuals. Use with caution in patients with heart failure, tachyarrhythmia, or hypertension. Avoid use in patients at risk of gastrointestinal obstruction, obstructive uropathy, or other conditions resulting in urinary retention. Renal and hepatic impairment may prolong the effects of atropine.	other agents that increase heart rate, ipratropium, potassium citrate, tiotropium, umeclidinium
digoxin (Digitek, Digox, Lanoxin)	dizziness, confusion, nausea, gynecomastia (breast enlargement), anorexia, mental disturbances, heart block	Avoid switching between brand and generic versions. Digoxin has a narrow therapeutic index. Blood levels should be monitored. Patients should be monitored for signs and symptoms of toxicity. Use with caution in patients with renal impairment (dosage adjustment needed). Use with caution in patients with hypothyroidism.	amiodarone, atorvastatin, dronedarone, itraconazole, metronidazole, ombitasvir / paritaprevir / ritonavir, quinidine, ritonavir, siponimod, sucralfate, thyroid hormones
isoproterenol (Isuprel)	headache, nervousness, restlessness, hypokalemia, tremor, blurred vision, pulmonary edema	Use with caution in patients with diabetes (may increase glucose levels). Contains sulfites and may cause allergic reaction in susceptible patients. May cause ischemia. Use with caution in patients with hyperthyroidism.	inhaled anesthetics, linezolid, theophylline

10.4 Angina, Myocardial Infarction, and Corresponding Drug Treatments

Ischemia, inadequate blood supply to an organ, usually occurs as a result of blockage in the coronary arteries that supply the heart with blood. **Angina pectoris** (often referred to simply as *angina*) is chest pain caused by myocardial ischemia. In angina, tissue damage is not extensive enough to be considered a myocardial infarction but does cause recurring chest pain episodes.

Common types of angina include the following:

Stable angina is characterized by effort-induced pain from physical activity or emotional stress. This pain is relieved by rest and is usually predictable and reproducible. Stable angina is the most common form of angina.

Unstable angina is characterized by pain that occurs with increasing frequency, diminishes the patient's ability to work, and has a decreasing response to treatment. It may be a warning sign of an impending myocardial infarction.

Variant angina is characterized by pain due to a coronary artery spasm. This pain may occur at certain times of the day and is often induced by cold weather, stress, medications that constrict blood vessels, or smoking.

The characteristic symptom of angina is severe chest discomfort, which may be described as heaviness, pressure, tightness, choking, a squeezing sensation, or a combination of these sensations. Other symptoms may include sweating, dizziness, or dyspnea (shortness of breath). Diagnosis is made from physical examination, electrocardiograms, a coronary angiogram, and a radioisotope study. Risk factors for angina include:

- advanced age
- coronary artery disease
- hypertension
- increased serum glucose levels (diabetes)
- increased serum lipoprotein levels
- obesity
- smoking
- stress

Angina is typically treated with beta-blockers, calcium channel blockers, and nitrates. Ranolazine may also be used.

When one or more coronary arteries become significantly blocked (usually 70% or more), tissue damage in that area of the heart ensues. When cardiac muscle is deprived of oxygen long enough, cells die (infarct), causing a **myocardial infarction (MI)**, or heart attack. An MI is signaled by the following symptoms:

- tightness, heaviness, or a squeezing sensation in the chest
- chest, neck, or jaw pain
- chest pain that radiates down the left arm
- indigestion or nausea
- a sense of impending doom

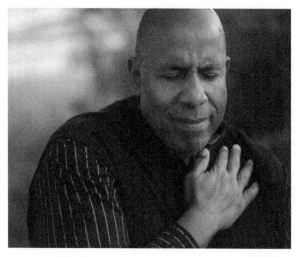

A myocardial infarction may cause pain in the chest that radiates down the left arm.

- weakness or fatigue
- sweating

Factors that increase the risk of an MI include a history of angina, alcohol consumption, reduced pulmonary vital capacity (amount of air a person can expel after a full inhalation), cigarette smoking, and atherosclerosis (buildup of fats and other substances on artery walls). Each year, approximately 1 million individuals in the United States have an MI, and roughly 50% of these individuals die from this event. For that reason, preventive measures are important.

Various lifestyle modifications may be recommended to reduce the risk of an MI, such as:

- eliminating smoking
- controlling blood pressure
- getting regular physical activity
- choosing healthy foods and beverages
- keeping a healthy weight
- using preventive medications when appropriate (such as aspirin and statins)
- managing diabetes

Acute MI is considered a medical emergency. Treatment of MI is initially aimed at opening blocked arteries, controlling blood pressure, and regulating heart rhythm. Oxygen, nitroglycerin, and aspirin may be used acutely. Chronic treatment of MI includes the use of other drugs. Anticoagulants, discussed later in this chapter, may be used. Beta-blockers, ACE inhibitors, and medications to treat cholesterol (antihyperlipidemics) are also considered standard of care. Calcium channel blockers and nitrates may be used in patients with ischemia. See Table 10.8 for common treatments for angina and MI.

TABLE 10.8 Commonly Used Agents for Angina and Myocardial Infarction

Generic (Brand)	Pronunciation	Dosage Form	Common Dosage	Dispensing Status
ACE Inhibitors, see Table 10.1				
Anticoagulants, see Table 10.11				
Antihyperlipidemics, see Table 10.10				
Beta-Blockers, see Table 10.1				
Calcium Channel Blockers, see Table 10.1				
Nitrates				
Short-Acting Nitrates				
nitroglycerin (GoNitro, Minitran, Nitro-Bid, Nitro-Dur, Nitro-Time, Nitrolingual, NitroMist, Nitrostat, Rectiv)	nye-troe-GLISS-er-in	capsule, injection, rectal ointment, sublingual tablet, transdermal ointment, transdermal patch, translingual solution, translingual spray	varies	Rx

continues

TABLE 10.8 Commonly Used Agents for Angina and Myocardial Infarction—*Continued*

Long-Acting Nitrates

isosorbide dinitrate (Dilatrate-SR, Isordil)	eye-soe-SOR-bide dye-NYE-trate	capsule, tablet	extended release: 40–160 mg a day immediate release: 10–40 mg 2 or 3 times a day	Rx
isosorbide mononitrate	eye-soe-SOR-bide mon-oh-NYE-trate	tablet	extended release: 60–120 mg 1 time a day immediate release: 20 mg 2 times a day	Rx

Metabolic Modifier

ranolazine (Ranexa)	ra-NOE-la-zeen	tablet	500–1,000 mg 2 times a day	Rx

℞ **Put Down Roots**

The drug stem *nitr-* in the generic name identifies a nitrate.

Nitrates

Vasodilators are drugs that relax smooth muscle and dilate blood vessels. The most frequently used vasodilators belong to a drug class called *nitrates*. A **nitrate** dilates coronary vessels, allowing more oxygen and nutrients to reach cardiac muscle cells. These actions relieve chest pain and ischemia.

Nitrates can be categorized as short acting or long acting. Short-acting nitrates are typically used for angina attacks and acute MI. Long-acting nitrates are used to prevent frequent angina attacks. See Table 10.9 for more details on nitrates.

Dosage Forms and Administration **Nitroglycerin (GoNitro, Minitran, Nitro-Bid, Nitro-Dur, Nitro-Time, Nitrolingual, NitroMist, Nitrostat)** is used for angina attacks and acute MI. The intravenous form is also indicated for the use of heart failure. **Nitroglycerin (Rectiv)** is an ointment that is applied rectally and is used for chronic anal fissures. Dosing instructions depend on the dosage form and the indication for which the drug is being used.

Only the sublingual and translingual (absorption through the tongue into systemic circulation) routes should be used for acute angina attacks. These include the sublingual tablet (Nitrostat), sublingual packet (GoNitro), translingual solution (Nitrolingual), and sublingual/translingual spray (Nitromist). The sublingual and translingual dosage forms are applied under the tongue. For an acute angina attack, a patient should place one tablet or apply one to two sprays every 3 to 5 minutes, with a maximum of three doses in a 15-minute period. If pain does not subside within 5 minutes after taking one dose, the patient should call 911. When nitroglycerin is used for angina prophylaxis, it should be taken a few minutes before the activity or stress that might cause an anginal attack.

Nitroglycerin patches (Nitro-Dur) should not be allowed to remain on the skin for 24 hours. There should be a drug-free time, usually when the patient is sleeping, or tolerance will develop. The label should instruct the patient in this procedure. Nitroglycerin topical ointment (Nitro-Bid) also requires a drug-free interval.

In capsule and sublingual tablet dosage forms, nitroglycerin is sold in its original amber glass container. Pharmacy staff must not repackage this drug, because it adheres to soft plastic, causing it to lose its effectiveness. The patient should replenish the sublingual tablets every six months, even if unused, and dispose of the remaining tablets.

Nitroglycerin rectal ointment should be dispensed in its original box because the packaging includes dosing markings.

Isosorbide dinitrate (Dilatrate-SR, Isordil) is used for the same purposes as nitroglycerin: the prevention of angina and heart failure.

Isosorbide mononitrate is a nitrate used to treat angina. Isosorbide mononitrate is available as immediate-release and extended-release tablets. Immediate-release isosorbide mononitrate is dosed twice a day, with the doses scheduled seven hours apart. Extended-release tablets are dosed once a day and are scored for splitting.

Side Effects Nitroglycerin can cause severe headaches when a patient first takes it; aspirin or acetaminophen may provide relief. To prevent headaches, the dose of nitroglycerin can be reduced, or if administered as a patch or ointment, it can be placed lower on the body and gradually moved to the chest as the patient acclimates to the medication. Nitroglycerin can also cause orthostatic hypotension when first used, so patients should be advised to move slowly, especially when changing from a sitting or lying position. The drug can also cause flushing. When nitroglycerin must be discontinued, the drug should be tapered and not stopped abruptly.

Both nitroglycerin tablets and the spray may produce a stinging sensation under the tongue.

Contraindications Patients taking nitrates should not take erectile dysfunction drugs, such as avanafil (Stendra), sildenafil (Viagra), vardenafil (Levitra, Staxyn), and tadalafil (Adcirca, Alyq, Cialis). Erectile dysfunction agents also cause vasodilation, and additive effects between these drug classes could lower blood pressure to dangerous levels, with a potentially lethal outcome. Nitrates are contraindicated in patients with a hypersensitivity to organic nitrates. Nitroglycerin is contraindicated in patients with increased intracranial pressure or severe anemia.

Cautions and Considerations Because short-acting dosage forms are designed for immediate absorption, sublingual and buccal (through the cheek) tablets should not be swallowed. Instead, they should be placed in the mouth and allowed to dissolve. Long-acting oral forms are swallowed and should be taken on an empty stomach with a full glass of water.

If a patient does not get relief from chest pain within 5 minutes of taking a dose of short-acting nitroglycerin, emergency medical care (such as 911) should be called, and the patient should repeat the dose. If this second dose is needed, the patient could be experiencing an MI and should be medically evaluated immediately. A total of three doses can be used within a 15-minute time period.

Sublingual nitroglycerin tablets must be kept in their original amber-colored container and protected from light, heat, and moisture. These tablets lose their effectiveness easily in warm and moist conditions. Once the bottle is opened, the tablets are only good for six months, and the date on which it was opened should be written on the container. After six months have passed, the patient should throw away any remaining tablets.

Tolerance to the beneficial effects of nitrates is an additional concern. Tolerance occurs after constant exposure to the drug, resulting in reduced effectiveness of the medication for the patient. Therefore, a drug-free period of at least eight hours a day (usually overnight) is necessary. For example, the transdermal nitrate patch should be removed before bedtime and left off overnight. A new patch should be applied in the morning. The label should instruct the patient in this procedure.

Drug Interactions Nitrates may increase the vasodilatory effects of other vasodilators. The hypotensive effect of other drugs may be heightened with concurrent nitrate use. Phosphodiesterase-5 inhibitors should not be used with nitrates.

Ergot derivatives may decrease the effects of nitrates. Nitrates should not be combined with nitric oxide due to increased risk of methemoglobinemia. Nitrates may enhance the adverse effects of riociguat.

Metabolic Modifiers

Ranolazine (Ranexa) is indicated for the treatment of chronic angina. Ranolazine is a metabolic modifier that helps the heart generate energy more efficiently by allowing the heart to function despite a decrease in oxygen. Ranolazine is used as an adjunct therapy for patients for whom other antianginal drugs do not work. It should be used concurrently with other drugs for the treatment of angina.

Dosage Forms and Administration Ranolazine is produced as an extended-release tablet that cannot be cut or broken in half and must be swallowed whole. It may be taken without regard to meals.

Side Effects Cardiovascular side effects such as hypotension, bradycardia, palpitations, QT prolongation, and edema may occur with ranolazine use. Dizziness, headache, confusion, and syncope have also been reported. Excessive sweating, constipation, tinnitus, and shortness of breath are also side effects.

Contraindications Patients who have liver cirrhosis should not use ranolazine. Other contraindications are related to drug interactions. Concurrent use of drugs that are strong inhibitors of the enzyme cytochrome P450 3A4 CYP3A4 (such as ketoconazole and clarithromycin) or strong inducers of CYP3A4 (such as rifampin, phenobarbital, and St. John's wort) is contraindicated.

Cautions and Considerations Ranolazine may prolong the QT interval. Acute kidney failure has occurred in patients who have kidney dysfunction and use ranolazine. Ranolazine should be used with caution in older adults due to increased risk of adverse events.

Drug Interactions Because ranolazine has many interactions, it is not used as a first-line therapy. It is contraindicated in patients who currently use a strong inhibitor or inducer of CYP3A4. Ranolazine should not be given with simvastatin or digoxin, because it can drastically increase the concentrations of both drugs. Ranolazine may enhance the QT prolongation of other agents that prolong the QT interval.

ACE Inhibitors

ACE inhibitors are commonly used in the treatment of patients with a history of MI or angina. They are addressed in the Hypertension and Drug Treatments section of this chapter.

Anticoagulants

Anticoagulants may be used in the treatment of patients with a history of MI or angina. They are addressed in the clotting disorders section of this chapter.

Beta-Blockers

Beta-blockers are commonly used in the treatment of patients with MI or angina. They are addressed in the Hypertension and Drug Treatments section of this chapter.

Calcium Channel Blockers

Calcium channel blockers may be used in the treatment of patients with a history of MI or angina. They are addressed in the Hypertension and Drug Treatments section of this chapter.

10.5 Heart Failure and Drug Treatments

Heart failure (HF) is a chronic, progressive condition in which the heart is no longer able to pump enough oxygen-rich blood to meet the body's needs. In other words, the heart is unable to keep up with the demands of the body. Symptoms of heart failure include shortness of breath, fatigue, edema, and exercise intolerance.

The goals of therapy for heart failure treatment are to prolong survival, relieve symptoms, improve quality of life, and prevent progression of disease. Most patients are managed with a combination of drugs. Therapy typically includes a medication that inhibits the renin-angiotensin system (such as an ACE inhibitor, ARB, or angiotensin receptor–neprilysin inhibitor) and a beta-blocker. Diuretics are used as needed to help with fluid overload (most commonly a loop diuretic). In certain cases, the combination of hydralazine and a nitrate may be used. Some patients use an aldosterone antagonist or digoxin. Table 10.9 lists common agents used to treat heart failure.

TABLE 10.9 Common Agents for Heart Failure

Generic (Brand)	Pronunciation	Dosage Form	Common Dosage	Dispensing Status
ACE Inhibitors, see Table 10.1				
Aldosterone Antagonists, see Table 15.5				
Angiotensin Receptor Blockers, see Table 10.1				
Angiotensin Receptor–Neprilysin Inhibitor				
sacubitril / valsartan (Entresto)	sak-UE-bi-tril val-SAR-tan	tablet	sacubitril 97 mg / valsartan 103 mg 2 times daily	Rx
Beta-Blockers, see Table 10.1				
Digoxin, see Table 10.5				
Loop Diuretics, see Table 15.5				
Nitrates, see Table 10.9				
Combination Vasodilators				
isosorbide dinitrate/ hydralazine (BiDil)	eye-soe-SOR-bide high-dral-uh-zeen	tablet	20–40 mg isosorbide dinitrate/ 37.5–75 mg hydralazine 3 times a day	Rx

ACE Inhibitors

ACE inhibitors are commonly used in the treatment of patients with heart failure. They are addressed in the Hypertension and Drug Treatments section of this chapter.

Angiotensin Receptor Blockers

Angiotensin receptor blockers may be used in the treatment of patients with heart failure. They are addressed in the Hypertension and Drug Treatments section of this chapter.

Angiotensin Receptor–Neprilysin Inhibitors

Pharm Fact

Sacubitril / valsartan is pronounced sak-UE-bi-tril val-SAR-tan.

Angiotensin receptor–neprilysin inhibitors (ARNIs) are a newer class of drugs used to treat heart failure. Sacubitril is currently the only ARNI available in the United States and is sold as a combination product with the ARB valsartan. Sacubitril is a prodrug that is converted to an active metabolite. The active metabolite ultimately increases diuresis and causes blood vessel dilation. **Sacubitril / valsartan (Entresto)** is the only combination ARNI / ARB available.

Safety Alert

Sacubitril / valsartan is a combination drug that comes in different strengths. Technicians should exercise diligence in selecting the correct strength when working with this medication.

Dosage Forms and Administration Available as a prescription only, sacubitril / valsartan is available in tablet form with several different dose combinations. Technicians should be aware of the dose (sacubitril 24 mg and valsartan 26 mg, sacubitril 49 mg and valsartan 51 mg, and sacubitril 97 mg and valsartan 103 mg).

There are special administration instructions for patients who are using an ACE inhibitor and starting sacubitril / valsartan. Patients must discontinue the ACE inhibitor and wait 36 hours before starting sacubitril / valsartan.

Side Effects Hypotension and orthostatic hypotension are side effects of sacubitril / valsartan. Other side effects include increased potassium levels, increased serum creatinine, dizziness, falling, decreased hematocrit and hemoglobin, angioedema, renal failure, and cough.

Contraindications Sacubitril / valsartan has several contraindications. Hypersensitivity to sacubitril, valsartan, or any component of the formulation contraindicates use. Patients with a history of angioedema should not use sacubitril / valsartan. Sacubitril / valsartan should not be used with (or taken within 36 hours of) an ACE inhibitor. Patients with diabetes should not use sacubitril / valsartan in combination with aliskiren.

Cautions and Considerations Sacubitril / valsartan has a boxed warning for use in pregnancy. Use can cause injury and death to the developing fetus. When pregnancy is detected, sacubitril / valsartan should be discontinued as soon as possible.

Safety Alert

Sacubitril / valsartan has a boxed warning for risk of injury and death to the developing fetus.

Drug Interactions Sacubitril / valsartan may increase the hyperkalemic effects of other medications that increase potassium (such as potassium-sparing diuretics and potassium supplements). Sacubitril / valsartan may also increase the hypotensive effects of other drugs that lower blood pressure.

ACE inhibitors should be avoided in patients using sacubitril / valsartan due to increased risk of angioedema.

Lithium concentrations may be increased in patients using sacubitril / valsartan.

Beta-Blockers

Beta-blockers are commonly used in the treatment of heart failure. They are addressed in the Hypertension and Drug Treatments section of this chapter.

Loop Diuretics

Loop diuretics are commonly used in the treatment of heart failure. This drug class works by inhibiting reabsorption of sodium, chloride, and water in the kidneys, which ultimately results in fast and profound diuresis (urine production). Loop diuretics are addressed in Chapter 15.

Aldosterone Antagonists

Aldosterone antagonists are commonly used in the treatment of heart failure. These agents work by inhibiting the hormone aldosterone, which promotes sodium and water reabsorption in the kidneys. This inhibition ultimately leads to diuresis. Aldosterone antagonists are addressed in Chapter 15.

Digoxin

Digoxin is used for heart failure and as an antiarrhythmic drug. Digoxin is addressed in the Cardiac Arrhythmias and Drug Treatments section of this chapter.

Combination Vasodilators

The combination of hydralazine with a nitrate may be used in patients with heart failure. Both hydralazine and isosorbide dinitrate cause vasodilation. The combination, **isosorbide dinitrate / hydralazine (BiDil)**, has been shown to improve outcomes in patients with heart failure.

Dosage Forms and Administration Isosorbide dinitrate / hydralazine is available as an oral tablet.

Side Effects Side effects include headache, dizziness, chest pain, and weakness.

Contraindications Hypersensitivity to organic nitrates contraindicates use of isosorbide dinitrate / hydralazine. Concomitant use with phosphodiesterase-5 inhibitors and riociguat is also contraindicated.

Cautions and Considerations Severe hypotension may occur with use. Patients with coronary artery disease should use the drug with caution due to the risk of angina and other cardiac abnormalities. The hydralazine component may cause a lupus-like syndrome where patients exhibit symptoms of lupus.

Drug Interactions Isosorbide dinitrate / hydralazine may enhance the blood pressure lowering effects of other antihypertensives. Phosphodiesterase-5 inhibitors should not be used with isosorbide dinitrate / hydralazine. Ergot derivatives may decrease the effects of isosorbide dinitrate / hydralazine. The isosorbide dinitrate component should not be combined with nitric oxide due to increased risk of methemoglobinemia; it may also enhance the adverse effects of riociguat.

10.6 Dyslipidemia, Hypercholesterolemia, Hyperlipidemia, and Drug Treatments

Cholesterol is an odorless, white, waxlike, powdery substance that is present in all foods of animal origin but is not in foods of plant origin. Some cholesterol is essential for good health. It circulates continuously in the blood for use by all body cells. For example, lymphocytes, adrenal cortical cells, muscle cells, and renal cells use cholesterol to make cell membranes and steroid hormones, and the liver uses it to make bile acids. High blood cholesterol is an important risk factor for an MI or a cerebral vascular accident (CVA), otherwise known as a stroke. Consequently, drugs that can lower blood cholesterol levels have come to play an important role in efforts to prevent cardiovascular disease. **Dyslipidemia** is a condition in which levels of atherogenic lipoproteins (protein-lipid complexes that can form abnormal fatty deposits in the arteries) are out of balance, having either increased or decreased. An excessive amount of cholesterol in the blood is known as **hypercholesterolemia**. A related disease is **hyperlipidemia**, a condition in which the levels of one or more lipoprotein levels are elevated.

In the body, the liver is responsible for making new cholesterol when needed and for processing cholesterol from food. The liver puts together packages containing triglycerides (the most common type of fat, in which a molecule of glycerin is bonded to three molecules of fatty acids), cholesterol, and carrier proteins and then releases these molecules into the bloodstream. Because they consist of lipids bound to proteins, these packages are called **lipoproteins**. They are spherical particles with a core of triglycerides and cholesterol, in varying proportions, surrounded by a surface coat of phospholipids (complex lipids containing phosphate). Most blood lipoproteins can be classified as high-density or low-density lipoproteins.

A **high-density lipoprotein (HDL)** absorbs cholesterol and transports the cholesterol back to the liver, after which it is excreted from the body. HDLs are sometimes called *good cholesterol* because elevated levels may reduce the risk for heart disease and stroke.

A **low-density lipoprotein (LDL)** makes up the majority of the body's cholesterol. LDLs are sometimes called *bad cholesterol* because elevated levels may result in plaque buildup in the blood vessels. This buildup can ultimately lead to heart disease or stroke.

A **triglyceride**, a major component of lipoproteins, is a neutral fat synthesized from carbohydrates for storage in adipose (fat) cells. Triglycerides release free fatty acids in the blood. As the lipoproteins circulate, the body draws off triglycerides for energy or storage.

Total cholesterol is a measure of the total amount of cholesterol in the body and is based on HDL, LDL, and triglyceride levels. Total blood cholesterol increases throughout the average person's life. It enhances other risk factors for coronary artery disease. LDLs circulate in the bloodstream to bring needed cholesterol to cells. LDLs not used by cells may be deposited on artery walls, eventually clogging them, as shown in Figure 10.8. The narrowing of arteries due to deposits of cholesterol and fat on their inner surfaces is known as **atherosclerosis**. Atherosclerosis can result in an MI or a stroke. Premature atherosclerosis is a common and significant consequence of dyslipidemia.

Lifestyle modifications are an important part of preventing and treating dyslipidemia. Most patients can achieve an average cholesterol reduction of 10% to 15% through dietary interventions. The major dietary recommendations are to reduce the amount of saturated fats in the diet and increase dietary fiber intake. Physical activity is a lifestyle modification that can also be beneficial.

FIGURE 10.8 Cross Section of Arteries

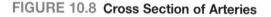

Normal artery

Clogged artery

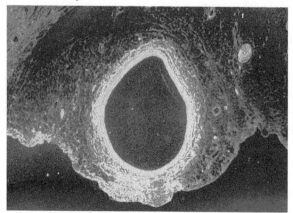
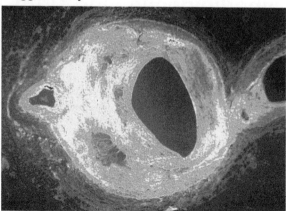

Cholesterol-lowering drugs are always used as an adjunct to lifestyle modifications. Table 10.10 presents the most commonly used lipid-lowering agents. Some medications work better for decreasing LDLs, some for decreasing triglycerides, and others for increasing HDLs.

TABLE 10.10 Commonly Used Antihyperlipidemic Drugs

Generic (Brand)	Pronunciation	Dosage Form	Common Dosage	Dispensing Status
HMG-CoA Reductase Inhibitors (Statins)				
atorvastatin (Lipitor)	a-tor-va-STAT-in	tablet	10–80 mg a day	Rx
fluvastatin (Lescol)	floo-va-STAT-in	capsule, tablet	20–80 mg a day	Rx
lovastatin (Altoprev, Mevacor)	loe-va-STAT-in	tablet	20–80 mg a day	Rx
pitavastatin (Livalo, Zypitamag)	pi-TA-va-sta-tin	tablet	1–4 mg a day	Rx
pravastatin (Pravachol)	prav-a-STAT-in	tablet	40–80 mg a day	Rx
rosuvastatin (Crestor, Ezallor)	roe-soo-va-STAT-in	capsule sprinkle, tablet	5–40 mg a day	Rx
simvastatin (Flolipid, Zocor)	sim-va-STAT-in	oral suspension, tablet	10–40 mg a day	Rx
Fibric Acid Derivatives				
fenofibrate (Antara, Lipofen, TriCor)	fen-oh-FYE-brate	capsule, tablet	130–200 mg a day	Rx
fenofibric acid (Fibricor, Trilipix)	fen-oh-FYE-brik AS-id	capsule	30–160 mg a day	Rx
gemfibrozil (Lopid)	jem-FYE-broe-zil	tablet	600 mg 2 times a day	Rx
Bile Acid Sequestrants				
cholestyramine (Prevalite, Questran, Questran Light)	koe-les-TEER-a-meen	packet, powder	4 g 1–2 times a day	Rx
colesevelam (WelChol)	koe-le-SEV-a-lam	packet, tablet	3.75 g a day	Rx
colestipol (Colestid)	koe-LES-ti-pawl	packet, powder, tablet	2–30 g a day	Rx
ATP Citrate Lyase (ACL) Inhibitor				
bempedoic acid (Nexletol)	BEM-pe-DOE-ik AS-id	tablet	180 mg	Rx
Other Cholesterol-Lowering Agents				
ezetimibe (Zetia)	ee-ZET-e-mib	tablet	10 mg a day	Rx
omega-3 fatty acids (Epanova, Lovaza, Vascepa)	oh-MEG-a-three FAT-tee AS-ids	capsule	1–4 g a day	OTC, Rx

Drugs from different classifications are often prescribed together because they may be synergistic. Combination antihyperlipidemic drugs include the following:

- amlodipine / atorvastatin (Caduet)
- bempedoic acid / ezetimibe (Nexlizet)

- ezetimibe / simvastatin (Vytorin)
- pravastatin / buffered aspirin (Pravigard PAC)

Some drugs negatively affect cholesterol levels, such as by increasing total cholesterol, LDL, or triglycerides or by decreasing HDL. Patients who have hyperlipidemia should avoid such medications. As in other situations, the advantages must be weighed against the disadvantages. Certain drugs may adversely affect lipoproteins:

- amiodarone
- anabolic steroids
- beta-blockers
- corticosteroids
- cyclosporine
- estrogens
- loop diuretics
- progestins
- protease inhibitors
- thiazide diuretics

HMG-CoA Reductase Inhibitors (Statins)

An **HMG-CoA reductase inhibitor**, also known as a *statin*, inhibits the enzyme that catalyzes the rate-limiting step in cholesterol biosynthesis (formation). (HMG-CoA reductase is an abbreviated name for the enzyme.) Statins decrease LDL cholesterol and have beneficial effects on other lipids. Statins are typically first-line therapy for hyperlipidemia. They may also be used to prevent cardiovascular disease in patients with a history of heart disease and in those at risk for heart disease.

Dosage Forms and Administration Statins are available in oral dosage forms. Simvastatin is the only statin also available in an oral suspension.

Studies have shown that fluvastatin, lovastatin, and simvastatin may have a greater cholesterol-lowering effect when taken at night, because most cholesterol is produced when dietary intake is at its lowest (typically overnight).

Safety Alert

High-dose (80 mg) simvastatin may increase patient risk of myopathy and rhabdomyolysis. Therefore, the 80 mg dose of simvastatin should only be used in patients who have been taking simvastatin long term without evidence of toxicity.

Side Effects Side effects of statins include GI upset and headache, which may dissipate with time. Patients who have any unexplained muscle pain or weakness, especially with fever, should report it to their healthcare practitioners immediately. The most serious side effect of all statins is rhabdomyolysis (destruction of muscle accompanied by muscle pain). Liver enzymes should be monitored regularly.

Contraindications Statins are contraindicated in patients with active liver disease or unexplained persistent elevations of liver enzymes. These medications are also contraindicated in patients who are pregnant or breast-feeding.

Pitavastatin and simvastatin should not be taken with cyclosporine.

Lovastatin and simvastatin should not be used with boceprevir, clarithromycin, cobicistat, cyclosporine, erythromycin, gemfibrozil, human immunodeficiency virus (HIV) protease inhibitors, itraconazole, ketoconazole, nefazodone, posaconazole, telaprevir, telithromycin, or voriconazole. Simvastatin should not be used with danazol.

Cautions and Considerations Statins are associated with rhabdomyolysis, a condition characterized by breakdown of muscle tissue that can ultimately lead to acute kidney failure. Myopathy (a muscular disease marked by muscle pain, tender- ness, or weakness) is also related to statin use. Older adults appear to be at increased risk of myopathy.

Liver function abnormalities are associated with statin use. Elevations in liver enzymes may occur and generally appear within the first year of treatment. Caution should be exercised in patients who consume substantial quantities of alcohol, have a history of liver disease, or show signs or symptoms of liver disease. Increases in blood glucose levels may occur in patients using statins. Dose adjustment may be necessary in patients with kidney dysfunction.

Drug Interactions Statins are associated with multiple drug interactions. Bile acid sequestrants may decrease the bioavailability of statins. Fibric acid derivatives may increase the risk of statin side effects. In patients using warfarin, statins may increase the international normalized ratio (INR), a laboratory test that measures the time it takes a patient's blood to clot.

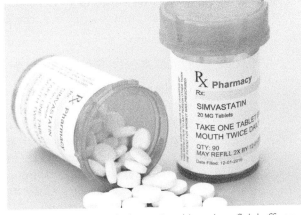

Statins decrease LDL cholesterol and have beneficial effects on other lipids.

Amiodarone, dronedarone, macrolide antibiotics, nefazodone, protease inhibitors, and ranolazine may increase the levels and risk of myopathy of atorvastatin, lovastatin, and simvastatin. Azole antifungals and calcium channel blockers may increase the levels and risk of myopathy of atorvastatin, fluvastatin, lovastatin, and simvastatin. Colchicine may increase the risk of myopathy of atorvastatin, fluvastatin, lovastatin, pravastatin, and simvastatin. Grapefruit juice increases the risk of rhabdomyolysis and myopathy and slows patients' metabolizing of atorvastatin, lovastatin, and simvastatin. Avoidance of grapefruit juice with administration of these drugs is recommended.

Cimetidine may decrease the triglyceride-lowering effect of atorvastatin. Atorvastatin and simvastatin may decrease levels of digoxin.

Put Down Roots

Generic names for fibrates contain the drug stem -*fibr*-.

Fibric Acid Derivatives (Fibrates)

Another class of drugs used to lower high cholesterol, especially high triglycerides, is fibric acid derivatives. A **fibric acid derivative** (or fibrate) lowers LDL cholesterol but more markedly decreases triglycerides. Fibrates may also be used as an alternative to statins when statins cannot be tolerated. The mechanism of action is not fully understood. More information on fibrates can be found in Table 10.10.

Fenofibrate and fenofibric acid are indicated for hypertriglyceridemia, primary hypercholesterolemia, and mixed dyslipidemia. Gemfibrozil is indicated for hypertriglyceridemia and prevention of cardiovascular disease.

Dosage Forms and Administration Fibrates can be taken with or without food. Tablets should be swallowed whole. Capsules should not be opened.

Side Effects Common side effects of fibrates include upset stomach, diarrhea, indigestion, and abdominal cramps. The effects may improve over time and can be diminished by taking the medication with food. Fenofibrate may cause fatigue and muscle aches.

Contraindications Fenofibrate, fenofibric acid, and gemfibrozil are contraindicated in patients with active liver disease, severe kidney dysfunction, and gallbladder disease.

Fenofibrate and fenofibric acid are contraindicated while breast-feeding. Gemfibrozil is contraindicated in patients using repaglinide.

Cautions and Considerations Most patients with gallbladder problems should not use fibrates and fibric acid, and caution should be exercised when fibrates and fibric acid are used in combination with statins because rhabdomyolysis can occur.

Drug Interactions Gemfibrozil may increase the risk of myopathy in patients using statins. It may also increase the adverse effects of ezetimibe.

Bile Acid Sequestrants

Cholesterol is a major precursor to bile acid. A **bile acid sequestrant** forms a nonabsorbable complex with bile acids in the intestines, which is eliminated in the feces. The increased excretion of bile acids results in increased conversion of cholesterol to bile acid. This effectively lowers serum cholesterol levels.

Bile acid sequestrants are indicated for patients with hypercholesterolemia. Colesevelam has additional indications of heterozygous familial hypertriglyceridemia and type 2 diabetes. Cholestyramine has an indication for pruritis associated with partial biliary obstruction.

Dosage Forms and Administration Other medications should be administered at least one hour before or four hours after a bile acid sequestrant.

Cholestyramine is available in oral powder in a large container or oral powder in individual packets. Both should be prepared in a suspension and not taken in dry form. The suspension should not be sipped or held in the mouth for long periods of time due to the risk of tooth discoloration or enamel decay.

Colesevelam is available as a packet that contains granules for oral suspension and as tablets. The granules for oral suspension should not be taken in the dry form. Regardless of the dosage form, colesevelam should be taken with food.

Colestipol tablets should be taken one at a time and swallowed whole with plenty of liquid. Powder forms should not be administered in dry form.

Side Effects Gastrointestinal side effects are common with bile acid sequestrants. Constipation or diarrhea may occur with use. Weakness and flu-like symptoms may also occur.

Contraindications Cholestyramine and colestipol are contraindicated in complete biliary obstruction. Colesevelam should not be used in patients with bowel obstruction, triglyceride levels greater than 500 mg/dL, or history of triglyceride-induced pancreatitis.

Cautions and Considerations Bile acid sequestrants should be used cautiously in patients with a triglyceride level greater than 300 mg/dL because these drugs may further elevate triglyceride levels.

Absorption of fat-soluble vitamins may be decreased in patients using bile acid sequestrants. They should be used with caution in patients with fat-soluble vitamin deficiencies.

Bile acid sequestrants may produce or exacerbate constipation and may cause fecal impaction.

Drug Interactions Bile acid sequestrants may decrease absorption of other drugs taken concurrently. Other drugs should be taken one hour before or six hours after bile acid sequestrants.

ATP Citrate Lyase (ACL) Inhibitors

An **adenosine triphosphate–citrate lyase (ACL) inhibitor** lowers LDL by inhibiting cholesterol synthesis in the liver. ACL works upstream of HMG-CoA reductase in the cholesterol synthesis pathway.

Bempedoic acid (Nexletol) is the only ACL inhibitor currently available in the United States. It is indicated as an adjunct to diet and maximally tolerated statin therapy in adults with heterozygous familial hypercholesterolemia or established cardiovascular disease who require additional LDL lowering.

Dosage Forms and Administration Bempedoic acid is available in oral tablets that are taken once a day with or without food.

Side Effects Side effects of bempedoic acid include upper respiratory tract infection, muscle spasms, hyperuricemia, back pain, abdominal pain or discomfort, bronchitis, pain in extremity, anemia, and elevated liver enzymes.

Contraindications Bempedoic acid has no contraindications.

Cautions and Considerations Bempedoic acid may increase uric acid. Uric acid levels should be monitored, and the medication should be used cautiously in patients with gout.

Tendon rupture has occurred with use of bempedoic acid. Discontinue the drug at the first sign of tendon rupture and avoid use in patients who have a history of tendon disorders or tendon rupture.

Drug Interactions The levels of the statins pravastatin and simvastatin increase with use of bempedoic acid. Avoid doses greater than 40 mg of pravastatin and 20 mg of simvastatin in patients using bempedoic acid.

Other Cholesterol-Lowering Agents

Ezetimibe (Zetia), a cholesterol absorption inhibitor, lowers cholesterol by inhibiting the absorption of cholesterol at the "brush border" of the small intestine (the lining of the small intestine, covered by numerous folds called *microvilli*). This inhibition leads to decreased delivery of cholesterol to the liver. Ezetimibe has the additional benefit of increasing HDL.

Omega-3 fatty acids (Epanova, Lovaza, Vascepa) are used for hypertriglyceridemia. While they are widely available as OTC dietary supplement products, prescription forms are available. Epanova, Lovaza, and Vascepa are omega-3 fatty acid medications indicated for high triglycerides. Vascepa has an additional indication for cardiovascular risk reduction in patients with mild hypertriglyceridemia. The mechanism of action of omega-3 fatty acids is not fully understood. It is thought they decrease liver production of very low-density lipoproteins, which are highly atherogenic.

Dosage Forms and Administration Ezetimibe tablets may be taken without regard to meals. However, administration should occur at least two hours before or at least four hours after bile acid sequestrants.

Omega-3 fatty acids should be administered whole. Lovaza may be taken with or without food. It is recommended patients take Vascepa with food.

Side Effects Side effects of ezetimibe include upper respiratory tract infections, sinusitis, diarrhea, and pain in joints and extremities.

Omega-3 fatty acid use may result in diarrhea, eructation (burping), halitosis (bad breath), or gastrointestinal upset.

Contraindications Hypersensitivity to omega-3 fatty acids contraindicates use. Ezetimibe is contraindicated when used with a statin in patients with active liver disease.

Cautions and Considerations Use ezetimibe with caution in patients with liver or kidney disease.

Gemfibrozil may enhance the adverse effects of ezetimibe.

Omega-3 fatty acids should be used with caution or avoided in patients with fish or shellfish allergies. Bleeding has been reported with use.

Drug Interactions Ezetimibe should not be used with gemfibrozil due to the risk of myopathy. Bile acid sequestrants may decrease the absorption of ezetimibe and dosing should be separated by several hours. Omega-3 fatty acids may increase the effect of anticoagulants.

10.7 Clotting Disorders, Stroke, and Drug Treatments

Thrombin is an enzyme in blood plasma that causes blood clotting. Thrombin reacts with **fibrinogen**, a protein produced in the liver, to create fibrin. **Fibrin**, a protein, arranges into threads that trap circulating platelets, which eventually leads to the formation of a blood clot. Blood clots present a serious and potentially life-threatening problem. **Thrombi** (singular: thrombus) are clots that stay attached to their points of origin, while **emboli** (singular: embolus) are abnormal particles, including clots and air bubbles, that circulate in the blood. Thrombi and emboli develop from abnormalities, such as:

- blood coagulation, resulting in hypercoagulability (excessive coagulation)
- blood flow, leading to stasis (a slowing of the flow of circulating blood)
- platelet adhesiveness, resulting in hypercoagulability
- vessel walls (from damage or surgery)

Venous thrombi usually form in areas of low-velocity blood flow, in areas of surgical or other vein injury, or in large venous sinuses (pockets formed by valves in deep veins). Symptoms of venous thrombi include swelling, discoloration, and pain. A piece of a clot, called an *embolus*, may break off and travel to the lung or cause a sudden blocking of the pulmonary artery; this is known as a **pulmonary embolism (PE)**. Some patients have a **deep vein thrombosis (DVT)**, a condition marked by the formation of a blood clot in one or more deep veins. DVT typically occurs in the legs; a DVT that is proximal (at or superior to [higher than] the knee) is the most serious and may be fatal. DVT has several risk factors:

- age over 40 years
- bed rest for more than four days
- estrogen combined with nicotine
- high-dose estrogen therapy
- major illness
- obesity
- pregnancy
- previous DVT
- surgery
- trauma
- varicose veins

Two classes of drugs—anticoagulants and antiplatelets—are used to reduce the risk of blood clots. An anticoagulant prevents clot formation by inhibiting clotting factors; an antiplatelet reduces the risk of clot formation by inhibiting platelet aggregation (the sticking or clumping together of platelets). Drugs in a third class, thrombolytics, dissolve clots that have already formed.

Cell damage activates a pathway of coagulation, or **clotting cascade** (also referred to as *coagulation cascade*), as shown in Figure 10.9. Each step involves the activation of a factor, which then triggers the next step, until finally a fibrin clot is formed. However, vessel blockage can occur as the result of fat, air, and debris gaining entry into circulation. If any factor along the path is missing, blood may not clot, as occurs in people with hemophilia.

FIGURE 10.9
Clotting Cascade

Each step of the cascade is necessary for the appropriate formation of clots in the body.

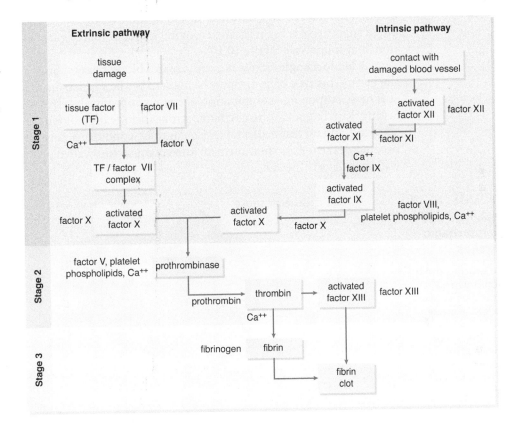

The brain is an oxygen-rich organ and requires a constant supply of oxygenated blood to keep brain tissue alive and functional. A **cerebrovascular accident (CVA)**, commonly known as a **stroke**, is the result of an event that interrupts the oxygen supply to a localized area of the brain. Consequently, a stroke is considered a medical emergency. Stroke can be considered as a finite event, an ongoing event, or a series of prolonged occurrences. A stroke may develop over several hours, days, or months. If the block in blood flow is brief, an individual may experience a **transient ischemic attack (TIA)**, or temporary neurologic changes during a brief period of time. A TIA may be an important warning sign and predictor of imminent stroke.

Symptoms of a stroke come on suddenly and include the following:

- numbness or weakness of the face, arm, or leg (especially on one side of the body)
- confusion and difficulty speaking or understanding speech
- trouble seeing in one or both eyes

- dizziness and loss of balance or coordination
- severe headache with no known cause

There are two major types of strokes: ischemic and hemorrhagic. An **ischemic stroke** occurs when a blood clot obstructs a blood vessel supplying the brain. The stroke can cause cerebral infarction (formation of necrotic tissue in the brain). A hemorrhagic stroke occurs when a blood vessel ruptures, causing cerebral hemorrhage (bleeding in or around the brain).

Ischemic stroke is the most common type of stroke. An ischemic stroke may occur after a newly formed thrombus becomes lodged at its site of origin in a cerebral blood vessel or a blood clot outside the brain disrupts blood flow to the brain. As the lumen (cavity) of the blood vessel narrows and becomes obstructed, blood flow through the vessel slows, diminishes, and in some cases, even ceases. The reduced blood supply to the brain is called cerebral ischemia, and tissue necrosis, called infarction, may follow (see Figure 10.10).

A **hemorrhagic stroke** is a rupture in a blood vessel that supplies an area of the brain. This type of stroke may be marked by the sudden onset of severe headache, stiff neck, stupor, or a combination of these symptoms. Its effects are likely to be long lasting. Risk factors for hemorrhagic stroke include high blood pressure, cigarette smoking, and excessive alcohol intake. In these conditions, tiny vessels in the brain become weakened and may form an **aneurysm**, a thin-walled protrusion in an artery wall that can easily burst.

FIGURE 10.10
Ischemic and Hemorrhagic Strokes

An ischemic stroke occurs when a thrombus becomes lodged in a cerebral blood vessel (left). A hemorrhagic stroke occurs when a vessel ruptures (right).

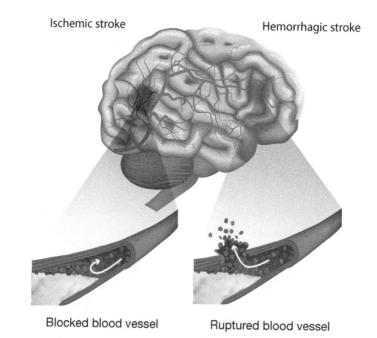

Ischemic stroke

Hemorrhagic stroke

Blocked blood vessel

Ruptured blood vessel

Risk factors for both types of stroke include advanced age, male sex, hypertension, smoking, alcohol abuse, diabetes, and high cholesterol levels. Stroke treatment encompasses preventive and management measures. Antiplatelet therapy, anticoagulant therapy, thrombolytic intervention, cerebrovascular surgery, nonpharmacological therapy, and poststroke management are the most common. Pharmacologic treatment options for TIAs and prevention of initial strokes include antiplatelet and anticoagulant agents.

In the aftermath of a stroke, determination of the cause is critical for establishing optimal poststroke therapy. Antiplatelets, anticoagulants, and thrombolytic agents play important but very different roles in stroke management. For example, treating a hemorrhage with anticoagulant or thrombolytic agents would be detrimental. Antiplatelet agents prevent platelet activation and formation of the platelet plug. Antiplatelet agents are often used to prevent recurrent thrombotic stroke (a type of ischemic stroke) and to prevent initial episodes in high-risk patients.

Thrombotic stroke is an ischemic stroke caused by a blood clot that develops in the brain instead of originating outside the brain. Treatment options for acute thrombotic stroke include anticoagulant agents and thrombolytic agents (see Table 10.11). Anticoagulant agents interfere with the synthesis or activation of the coagulation factors in the blood. Formed clots have the potential to continue to expand and cause greater neurologic damage; anticoagulant agents may prevent existing clots from expanding. Anticoagulant agents are routinely used to treat acute cardioembolic stoke (a stroke resulting from the heart circulating an emboli) and are used for the treatment of DVT and PE as well.

Thrombolytic agents, also known as *thrombolytics* or *fibrinolytics*, differ from anticoagulant agents in one important aspect. Whereas anticoagulant agents can help prevent existing emboli and thrombi from expanding, thrombolytic agents actually dissolve existing thrombi and emboli. Primary indications for thrombolytic therapy include the following:

- acute ischemic stroke
- pulmonary embolism
- acute MI (for the lysis of thrombi in coronary arteries)

Additional information regarding thrombolytics can be found in the Thrombolytics section of this chapter.

Practice Tip

Treatment goals for stroke should include confirming the diagnosis of its cause, evaluating the cause, stabilizing the event, and then establishing a plan to prevent further damage to the brain.

Work Wise

Thrombolytics may be referred to as "clot busters" because they can dissolve blood clots.

TABLE 10.11 Commonly Used Anticoagulants, Antiplatelets, Thrombolytics, and Their Antidotes

Generic (Brand)	Pronunciation	Dosage Form	Common Dosage	Dispensing Status
Anticoagulant Agents				
Direct Thrombin Inhibitors				
bivalirudin (Angiomax)	bye-VAL-i-roo-din	injection	varies; 1.75 mg/kg/hr is common	Rx
dabigatran (Pradaxa)	da-BIG-a-tran	capsule	150 mg	Rx
Heparin and Low-Molecular-Weight Heparins				
dalteparin (Fragmin)	dal-TEP-a-rin	injection	200 units/kg/day divided into 2 doses	Rx
enoxaparin (Lovenox)	ee-nox-a-PAIR-in	injection	1–1.5 mg/kg/day given 1–2 times a day	Rx
heparin or unfractionated heparin (UFH)	HEP-a-rin	injection	IV: doses individualized but often in thousands of units per infusion Subcutaneous: 3,000–5,000 units 2–3 times a day	Rx
Factor Xa Inhibitors				
apixaban (Eliquis)	a-PIX-a-ban	tablet	2.5–10 mg 2 times a day	Rx
edoxaban (Savaysa)	e-DOX-a-ban	tablet	60 mg 1 time a day	Rx

continues

TABLE 10.11 Commonly Used Anticoagulants, Antiplatelets, Thrombolytics, and Their Antidotes—*Continued*

Generic (Brand)	Pronunciation	Dosage Form	Common Dosage	Dispensing Status
fondaparinux (Arixtra)	fon-da-PAIR-i-nux	injection	2.5–10 mg 1 time a day	Rx
rivaroxaban (Xarelto)	ri-va-ROX-a-ban	tablet	2.5–20 mg 1 time a day	Rx
Vitamin K Antagonist				
warfarin	WAR-far-in	tablet	2.5–10 mg a day	Rx
Antidotes				
Antidote for Dabigatran				
idarucizumab (Praxbind)	EYE-da-roo-KIZ-ue-mab	injection	5 g	Rx
Antidote for Heparin				
protamine sulfate	PROE-ta-meen SUL-fate	injection	based on degree of heparin reversal desired	Rx
Antidote for Oral Factor Xa Inhibitors				
andexanet alfa (Andexxa)	an-DEX-a-net AL-fa	injection	varies	Rx
Antidote for Warfarin				
phytonadione, vitamin K (Mephyton)	fye-toe-na-DYE-own	injection	1–10 mg a dose	OTC, Rx
Antiplatelets				
General Antiplatelet Agents				
aspirin (various)	AS-pir-in	capsule, chewable tablet, packet, suppository tablet	325–650 mg every 4–6 hr, not to exceed 4 g a day	OTC, Rx
clopidogrel (Plavix)	kloh-PID-oh-grel	tablet	75 mg a day	Rx
prasugrel (Effient)	PRA-soo-grel	tablet	10 mg a day	Rx
ticagrelor (Brilinta)	tye-KA-grel-or	tablet	90 mg 2 times a day	Rx
Glycoprotein Antagonists				
eptifibatide (Integrilin)	ep-ti-FIB-a-tide	injection	bolus: 180 mcg/kg infusion: 2 mcg/kg/min (up to 15 mg/hr)	Rx
tirofiban (Aggrastat)	tye-roe-FYE-ban	injection	initial dose: 25 mcg/kg infusion: 0.15 mcg/kg/min	Rx
Thrombolytic Agents				
alteplase (Activase)	AL-te-plase	injection	90–100 mg	Rx
tenecteplase (TNKase)	ten-EK-te-plase	injection	30–50 mg	Rx

Direct Thrombin Inhibitors

Direct thrombin inhibitors bind directly to thrombin. They can inhibit circulating thrombin and thrombin that is bound to fibrin. Direct thrombin inhibitors may have a more predictable anticoagulant effect than heparins.

Bivalirudin (Angiomax) is used to treat patients with unstable angina who are undergoing **percutaneous coronary intervention (PCI)**, a nonsurgical procedure in which a catheter is used to place a stent to open blood vessels in the heart. It is a specific and reversible thrombin inhibitor. Bivalirudin is also appropriate for patients with heparin-induced thrombocytopenia who are undergoing PCI. (See the Cautions and Considerations section under Heparin and Low-Molecular-Weight Heparins later in this chapter for information on heparin-induced thrombocytopenia.)

Dabigatran (Pradaxa) is a direct thrombin inhibitor indicated for the treatment and prevention of venous thrombosis and PE and for the prevention of a stroke in nonvalvular atrial fibrillation (atrial fibrillation caused by conditions other than heart valve disorders).

Dosage Forms and Administration Dabigatran is administered orally and can be taken with or without food. Dabigatran is unusual in that it must be stored and dispensed in the original container (either a bottle or blister packs). Once a bottle of dabigatran is open, it must be used within four months.

Safety Alert

Some dosage forms of bivalirudin are prediluted, while others are vials whose contents need to be diluted prior to administration.

Side Effects Common side effects of direct thrombin inhibitors include nausea, headache, back pain, and bleeding due to excessive anticoagulation. Side effects of bivalirudin include hypotension, pain, headache, nausea, bleeding, and back pain. Common side effects of dabigatran include gastrointestinal issues and hemorrhage.

Contraindications Direct thrombin inhibitors are contraindicated in active bleeding. Dabigatran is also contraindicated in patients who have a mechanical prosthetic heart valve.

Cautions and Considerations Direct thrombin inhibitors increase the risk of potentially fatal bleeding. These agents should be discontinued several days prior to surgery, if possible. Patients should report any signs of bleeding to their prescribers and follow instructions regarding laboratory tests.

Safety Alert

Dabigatran carries multiple boxed warnings and must also be dispensed with a Medication Guide.

Dabigatran must be dispensed with an FDA Medication Guide. Dabigatran carries boxed warnings. One warning is for an increased risk of thrombotic events if it is discontinued prematurely. Another is for risk of spinal or epidural hematoma. Older adults should use dabigatran with extreme caution, and other alternatives should be considered due to increased risk of hemorrhage or stroke. Dabigatran should be used cautiously in patients who have kidney impairment; for these individuals, dose adjustment is necessary.

Emergency dabigatran reversal can be achieved with the use of **idarucizumab (Praxbind)**. This agent is reserved for patients who are using dabigatran and require emergency surgery or urgent procedures or have life-threatening or uncontrolled bleeding. Idarucizumab is given intravenously as two 2.5 g doses.

Drug Interactions Direct thrombin inhibitors may enhance the risk of bleeding with other anticoagulants. Concurrent use should be avoided if possible.

Urokinase may enhance the anticoagulant effects of dabigatran. P-glycoprotein inducers (such as carbamazepine, clotrimazole, phenytoin, rifampin, and spironolactone) decrease concentrations of dabigatran; P-glycoprotein inhibitors (such as amiodarone, clarithromycin, dronedarone, itraconazole, ketoconazole, and verapamil) may increase dabigatran concentrations.

More manufacturers are prepackaging drugs so they will not have to be repackaged in the pharmacy. There are several benefits of this practice:

1. It reduces the chance that the drug will be handled inappropriately or exposed to unclean or unsafe environments.
2. It protects light- and moisture-sensitive drugs by allowing them to stay in their original containers.
3. It may reduce confusion for patients taking multiple medications, because the bottle differs from those of other drugs they have received from the pharmacy.
4. It may be safer for the pharmacy technician and pharmacist who dispense the drugs, particularly in the case of teratogenic drugs, which should not be handled by pregnant individuals.

Heparin and Low-Molecular-Weight Heparins

Heparin is a naturally occurring circulatory anticoagulant produced in mast cells (immune system cells). Heparin works by inhibiting clotting factors in the clotting cascade and inactivating thrombin and factor Xa. Heparin does not dissolve a thrombus (clot that stays in place) but will help stabilize the thrombus and prevent emboli (clots that circulate) from breaking off the thrombus and circulating in the blood.

Heparin is indicated for the prevention and treatment of thromboembolic disorders (disorders relating to the blocking of a blood vessel by a particle that has broken off of a thrombus) such as DVT or PE. It is also indicated for the treatment of thrombotic complications associated with atrial fibrillation, for prevention of clotting in arterial and cardiac surgery, and as an anticoagulant for dialysis. Commercially available heparin is derived from porcine (pig) mucosal tissue.

Low-molecular-weight heparins are a class of anticoagulants derived from heparin. A **low-molecular-weight heparin (LMWH)** works similarly to heparin but affects factor Xa more than it affects thrombin. The benefits of LMWHs are that they may present a lower likelihood of bleeding compared with heparin, can be injected subcutaneously (by the patient, if appropriately trained), and have longer half-lives. The longer half-lives of LMWHs allow them to be dosed once or twice a day. LMWHs are usually the anticoagulants of choice for pregnant patients and are used as bridge therapy from IV heparin to oral warfarin. Like commercially available heparin, LMWHs are derived from porcine mucosal tissue.

Dalteparin (Fragmin) is an LMWH used to prevent thromboembolism. **Enoxaparin (Lovenox)**, another LMWH, is used to prevent thrombosis after surgery and to treat DVT with or without pulmonary embolism.

Dosage Forms and Administration Dosage of heparin is measured not in milligrams but in units based on biologic activity; the pharmacy technician must convert units to milliliters to determine the correct volume. Heparin can be given only subcutaneously, usually in the abdomen, or intravenously. This drug must never be administered intramuscularly, because an intramuscular (IM) injection will cause a hematoma (internal pooling of blood).

Safety Alert

Heparin flushes are dilute solutions used to keep IV lines patent. They should not be confused with therapeutic doses of heparin.

LMWH products are available in vials and in prefilled syringes with an attached needle intended for subcutaneous injection. Although doses are fixed by the manufacturer, prescribers sometimes use a dose based on body weight. If a pharmacy technician receives a prescription for a fraction of a dose, or of a mixed dose, it is prudent to check with the prescriber to ensure accuracy.

Dalteparin, like heparin, is dosed in units. Enoxaparin is dosed in milligrams.

Put Down Roots

LMWHs end with the suffix -parin.

Safety Alert

Hospital pharmacy technicians must be very careful to dispense the appropriate syringe and needle for subcutaneous heparin injections. If an IM syringe and needle are dispensed, serious damage can occur. Pharmacy personnel should know which drugs need which syringes.

Side Effects Common side effects of heparin include bruising, bleeding due to excessive anticoagulation, and **thrombocytopenia** (low platelet count). Heparin should be used with caution because hemorrhaging may easily occur.

Side effects of LMWH include bruising, bleeding due to excessive anticoagulation, fever, pain at the injection site, and thrombocytopenia.

Contraindications Heparin should not be used in patients with severe thrombocytopenia or uncontrolled active bleeding. Full-dose heparin should also be avoided when proper coagulation tests cannot be obtained. Hypersensitivity to pork products also contraindicates use.

Concurrent use of LMWHs with other anticoagulants should be avoided.

LMWHs are contraindicated in patients who have a history of heparin-induced thrombocytopenia (see Cautions and Considerations), a hypersensitivity to heparin or pork products, or active major bleeding. Dalteparin is contraindicated in patients who have unstable angina, are experiencing non–Q wave MI, or are undergoing epidural or neuraxial anesthesia who have received prolonged preventive therapy of thromboembolism.

Cautions and Considerations LMWHs have a boxed warning for the risk of epidural or spinal hematoma when undergoing anesthesia or spinal puncture.

Heparin-induced thrombocytopenia (HIT), a potentially fatal immune-mediated reaction caused by heparin or LMWH, is a rare but serious side effect that can be life threatening. It can only be fully detected by laboratory tests but often is preceded by a skin rash. To determine the presence of HIT, patients should report any skin rashes or signs of bleeding to their prescribers right away. Patients who have a history of heparin-induced thrombocytopenia should not use LMWH.

Protamine sulfate is an antidote used to reverse the effects of heparin. It works by combining with heparin to form a complex that does not exert anticoagulant effects. Protamine sulfate is used when a patient is hemorrhaging or has a high risk of hemorrhage. Approximately 1 mg of protamine sulfate neutralizes 100 units of heparin.

LMWHs require dose adjustment in patients who have impaired renal function; they are contraindicated in some cases of severe kidney problems. Patients should inform their prescribers and pharmacists if they know they have kidney disease.

Drug Interactions Heparin and LMWHs may enhance the risk of serious bleeding posed by other anticoagulants. Concurrent use should be avoided, if possible.

Factor Xa Inhibitors

Factor Xa is a clotting factor that is central to coagulation. **Factor Xa inhibitors** are anticoagulants that block the activity of factor Xa and prevent blood clots from developing or getting worse. These drugs can directly or indirectly inhibit factor Xa. See Table 10.11 for more information on factor Xa inhibitors.

The individual drugs within the factor Xa inhibitor class have differing indications. Table 10.12 illustrates the therapeutic uses for each drug.

TABLE 10.12 Indications for Factor Xa Inhibitors

	DVT prophylaxis and PE prophylaxis	DVT treatment and PE treatment	Reduce risk of recurrence of DVT and PE	Reduce risk of stroke and systemic embolism in patients with nonvalvular atrial fibrillation
apixaban	✔	✔	✔	✔
edoxaban		✔		✔
fondaparinux	✔	✔		
rivaroxaban	✔	✔	✔	✔

Dosage Forms and Administration **Apixaban (Eliquis)** and **edoxaban (Savaysa)** may be administered without regard to meals. If patients are unable to swallow whole tablets, tablets may be crushed and suspended in water or juice or mixed with applesauce. **Rivaroxaban (Xarelto)** may be administered with or without food at lower doses (up to 10 mg). Doses of 15 mg or more should be taken with food. Rivaroxaban tablets may be crushed and mixed with applesauce. **Fondaparinux (Arixtra)** is an injectable factor Xa inhibitor that is available as a prefilled syringe. It is for subcutaneous administration and should not be administered intramuscularly. Air bubbles should not be expelled from the syringe before injection.

Side Effects Bleeding is a common side effect of factor Xa inhibitors.

Contraindications Factor Xa inhibitors are contraindicated in active bleeding. Fondaparinux is contraindicated in severe kidney impairment, bacterial endocarditis, and thrombocytopenia associated with a positive test for antiplatelet antibodies in the presence of fondaparinux.

Safety Alert

Factor Xa inhibitors carry multiple boxed warnings.

Cautions and Considerations The oral factor Xa inhibitors—apixaban, edoxaban, and rivaroxaban—must be dispensed with Medication Guides. Factor Xa inhibitors have boxed warnings. One warning is for a risk of spinal or epidural hematomas, which may result in long-term or permanent paralysis. Another warning is for thromboembolic events, which may result from premature discontinuation of these drugs. Edoxaban has an additional boxed warning for reduced efficacy in patients with nonvalvular atrial fibrillation with creatinine clearance of greater than 95 milliliters per minute.

In the case of life-threatening or uncontrolled bleeding, there is a reversal agent for the oral factor Xa inhibitors discussed in this chapter. **Andexanet alfa (Andexxa)** dosing is based on the factor Xa inhibitor used, the dose last taken, and the timing of the most recent dose. Andexanet alfa is an injectable drug and is given as a bolus followed by an infusion.

Factor Xa inhibitors should be used with caution in patients who have kidney impairment; dose reduction is usually required.

Drug Interactions Drugs with anticoagulant properties should be avoided with the use of factor Xa inhibitors, if possible, because of a possible enhanced anticoagulant effect.

The concentrations of apixaban and rivaroxaban may be decreased by St. John's wort and increased by conivaptan and idelalisib. Edoxaban concentrations may be decreased by rifampin.

Vitamin K Antagonists

The clotting cascade involves various factors that ultimately lead to the formation of a fibrin clot. Disruption of specific factors can decrease the body's ability to form clots. Certain factors are considered vitamin K dependent: factors II, VII, IX, and X. Vitamin K antagonists work on these specific factors.

Warfarin, a vitamin K antagonist, affects liver metabolism and prevents production of vitamin K–dependent clotting factors (II, VII, IX, and X). The objective of warfarin therapy is to prevent future clots. As with heparin, warfarin has no effect on existing clots, but it can prevent clot formation, the extension of formed clots, and secondary complications of thrombosis.

Dosage Forms and Administration Warfarin is rapidly and completely absorbed from the GI tract. Minor hemorrhaging (blood loss) may occur, but this is not an indication to stop warfarin therapy. At least three to five days are necessary for warfarin to achieve a therapeutic effect.

Warfarin was previously available as the brand name product Coumadin; now multiple generic formulations are available. For patient safety reasons, all manufacturers of warfarin in the United States use the same color-coding system that corresponds with tablet strength. Table 10.13 illustrates the colors and associated strengths.

Practice Tip

Although many vegetables contain vitamin K, green, leafy vegetables such as kale, spinach, and collard greens have the highest vitamin K content.

TABLE 10.13 Warfarin Tablet Strength and Associated Color

Tablet Strength	Tablet Color
1 mg	Pink
2 mg	Lavender (light purple)
2.5 mg	Green
3 mg	Tan
4 mg	Blue
5 mg	Peach (light orange)
6 mg	Teal (blue green)
7.5 mg	Yellow
10 mg	White

Side Effects The most common side effect of warfarin is bleeding. Other side effects include hair loss, skin lesions, and purple/blue toe syndrome. Signs of bleeding may manifest as blood in the urine or stool; black, tarry stools; bleeding in the mouth or gums; unusual or unexplained bruising; vomiting blood (or material that resembles coffee grounds); and nose bleeds. Patients who experience these side effects should contact their prescribers.

Name Exchange

Warfarin is the generic name for Coumadin.

Contraindications Contraindications to warfarin include hemorrhagic tendencies, recent or potential surgery of the eye or CNS, major regional lumbar block anesthesia or traumatic surgery resulting in large open surfaces, blood dyscrasias, severe uncontrolled hypertension, pericarditis or pericardial effusion, bacterial endocarditis, eclampsia or preeclampsia, threatened abortion, and pregnancy. Warfarin should also not be used in patients with a high potential of medication nonadherence.

Cautions and Considerations Warfarin carries a boxed warning for the risk of major or fatal bleeding and must be dispensed with an FDA Medication Guide.

Warfarin has a **narrow therapeutic index**. This means small differences in dose or blood concentration may lead to serious therapeutic failures or adverse drug events. Patients using warfarin require laboratory monitoring to ensure their blood levels are within its narrow therapeutic index. The **international normalized ratio (INR)**, a blood test that measures how long it takes blood to clot, is used to monitor warfarin therapy. Patients who are prescribed warfarin are encouraged to take their warfarin at the same time each day to maintain steady drug levels in the body. Warfarin is also affected by certain foods. Because it inhibits vitamin K–dependent clotting factors, changes in the amount of vitamin K a patient ingests can affect warfarin activity. All patients, especially those just starting warfarin therapy, should learn about food and drug interactions. Foods high in vitamin K (such as green, leafy vegetables) do not have to be avoided entirely. Patients should simply avoid varying the amount of these foods that they typically eat, whether that be a little or a lot. Wide swings in the amount of vitamin K consumed will affect the activity of oral anticoagulants. Warfarin doses are adjusted according to each patient's typical daily food intake. Alcohol increases warfarin's effects. Patients taking anticoagulant drugs should not drink excessive amounts of alcohol, or bleeding could occur. Moderate alcohol intake (one to two drinks a day) typically does not affect anticoagulation therapy.

Warfarin reversal can be achieved through the use of **phytonadione (Mephyton)**, also known as **vitamin K**. Vitamin K may be ingested orally or administered intramuscularly, intravenously, or subcutaneously. Subcutaneous administration is not preferred. IM or IV administration should be used only when oral dosing is not possible, and doses should be administered slowly. Vitamin K may cause flushing, changes in taste, dizziness, sweating, rapid pulse, and difficulty breathing.

Drug Interactions Warfarin is highly protein bound and metabolized through the liver; therefore, it interacts with many alternative therapies, OTC drugs, and prescription drugs. The drug interactions with warfarin are too numerous to mention here, but some of the most common prescription drugs that interact with warfarin are listed in Table 10.14. Aspirin and NSAIDs affect clotting by changing platelet action, so they generally should not be taken with warfarin or other anticoagulants. (The risk is lower with some of the other anticoagulants, such as heparin and LMWHs.)

TABLE 10.14 Common Drugs That Interact with Warfarin

amiodarone	fluvastatin	rifampin
carbamazepine	gemfibrozil	rosuvastatin
cimetidine	levothyroxine	simvastatin
fenofibrate	lovastatin	sulfamethoxazole
fluconazole	metronidazole	tamoxifen
fluoxetine	phenytoin	voriconazole

Interactions that affect warfarin activity can be serious. A decrease in effectiveness can cause unwanted clots; an increase in effectiveness can cause bleeding. Either way, the results of these interactions can be life threatening. Patients should tell their prescribers and pharmacists about all medications they take so that potential interactions can be identified.

Antiplatelet Agents

An **antiplatelet agent** is a medication that interferes with the chemical reactions that cause platelets to be sticky and aggregate. Table 10.11 includes the most commonly used antiplatelet agents. Antiplatelet agents are used to decrease the risk of stroke, DVT, and clotting associated with cardiovascular blockage. Their specific mechanisms of action vary, but they ultimately decrease platelet adhesion and aggregation. General antiplatelet agents include aspirin, clopidogrel, prasugrel, and ticagrelor.

Dosage Forms and Administration General antiplatelet medications are typically administered orally. The rectal suppository formulation of aspirin is not typically used.

Side Effects Bleeding is the major side effect of antiplatelet drugs. Bleeding may present as blood in the urine or stool, black- or tarry-colored stools, bleeding in the mouth or gums, unusual or unexplained bleeding, vomiting blood or material that looks like coffee grounds, or nosebleeds.

Contraindications See drug-specific sections on contraindications.

Cautions and Considerations As antiplatelets increase the risk of bleeding, they should be discontinued prior to surgeries.

Drug Interactions All antiplatelet drugs can enhance the antiplatelet properties of other drugs that affect platelets. Combination use is not recommended. Concurrent anticoagulant use may increase risk of bleeding.

Aspirin

Aspirin, a commonly used general antiplatelet drug, is covered in depth in Chapter 6.

Clopidogrel

Clopidogrel (Plavix) blocks adenosine diphosphate (ADP, a chemical involved in energy transmission in biologic systems) receptors and thus prevents fibrinogen binding. It also reduces platelet adhesion and aggregation. Clopidogrel is approved to prevent

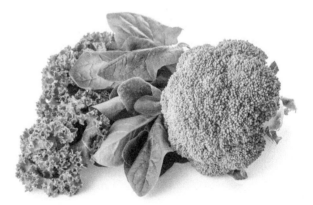

Patients who are taking oral warfarin must consume a consistent amount of green vegetables, such as kale, spinach, broccoli, and brussels sprouts, to prevent a drug-food interaction.

the recurrence of atherosclerotic events such as MI and stroke.

Dosage Forms and Administration Clopidogrel is administered orally and without regard to meals.

Side Effects Refer to the list of antiplatelet drug side effects, noted earlier.

Contraindications Clopidogrel should not be used in patients with active pathologic bleeding such as bleeding caused by a peptic ulcer or intracranial hemorrhage.

Cautions and Considerations Clopidogrel carries a boxed warning specific to patients who are poor CYP2C19 metabolizers. Additionally, clopidogrel must be dispensed with an FDA Medication Guide. In addition to the cautions and considerations noted earlier, clopidogrel must be discontinued at least five days prior to surgery due to the increased risk of bleeding.

Drug Interactions Potentially significant drug interactions exist with clopidogrel. Clopidogrel may increase concentrations of dasabuvir and enzalutamide. Esomeprazole, omeprazole, and pantoprazole may diminish the antiplatelet effects of clopidogrel.

Prasugrel

Prasugrel (Effient) is taken with aspirin to reduce cardiovascular death, MI, and stroke. It is specifically for patients who have undergone PCI. When taken with aspirin, it reduces the risk of an MI. Prasugrel maintains the stent by keeping platelets from sticking together and forming blood clots inside it and the arteries of the heart.

Dosage Forms and Administration Prasugrel must be dispensed and stored in the original container. Prasugrel tablets can be crushed and mixed with water prior to ingestion.

Prasugrel should be stopped at least seven days before surgery.

Side Effects In addition to the antiplatelet drug side effects noted earlier, prasugrel has side effects of hypertension or hypotension, edema, and hyperlipidemia.

Contraindications Contraindications to prasugrel include active bleeding and prior stroke.

Safety Alert

Prasugrel has a boxed warning for the risk of significant or fatal bleeding.

Cautions and Considerations Prasugrel must be dispensed with an FDA Medication Guide. In addition to the cautions and considerations noted earlier, prasugrel has a boxed warning for risk of significant or fatal bleeding. Another warning states that the use of prasugrel is generally not recommended in patients age 75 years or older. Prasugrel should not be used in patients likely to undergo coronary artery bypass surgery.

Drug Interactions Prasugrel may enhance the effect of other drugs that thin the blood. Cangrelor may decrease the antiplatelet effect of prasugrel.

Ticagrelor

Ticagrelor (Brilinta) is used to decrease cardiovascular events in patients who have coronary syndromes or a history of MI. It may also be used to reduce the rate of stent thrombosis in patients who have received a stent for the treatment of an **acute coronary syndrome**, an umbrella term for any sudden obstruction of a coronary artery, reducing blood flow to the heart.

Dosage Forms and Administration Ticagrelor tablets can be crushed and mixed with water prior to ingestion.

Side Effects In addition to the antiplatelet drug side effects noted earlier, ticagrelor may cause shortness of breath. This side effect may decrease with prolonged use.

Contraindications Ticagrelor is contraindicated in active bleeding and in patients with a history of intracranial hemorrhage or severe liver impairment.

Safety Alert

Ticagrelor carries boxed warnings related to increased bleeding risk.

Cautions and Considerations Ticagrelor must be distributed with an FDA Medication Guide. In addition to the cautions and considerations noted earlier, ticagrelor has several boxed warnings. One warning is for increased risk of bleeding (sometimes fatal). Another warning states that maintenance doses of aspirin should not be greater than 100 mg a day due to risk of decreasing ticagrelor efficacy. Ticagrelor should be avoided in patients who require urgent coronary artery bypass grafts.

Ticagreglor must be discontinued at least five days prior to surgery due to the increased risk of bleeding.

Drug Interactions Ticagrelor's activity may be diminished by dexamethasone. Pimozide and simvastatin concentrations may be increased by ticagrelor.

Glycoprotein Antagonists

Another antiplatelet agent is a glycoprotein antagonist. A **glycoprotein antagonist** binds to a receptor on platelets, preventing platelet aggregation as well as the binding of fibrinogen and other adhesive molecules. The action of these antagonists is reversible. Glycoprotein antagonists are indicated for acute coronary syndrome and are administered during invasive procedures to prevent artery closure. Glycoprotein antagonists include **eptifibatide (Integrilin)** and **tirofiban (Aggrastat)**. See Table 10.11.

Dosage Forms and Administration Glycoprotein antagonists should be protected from light. Eptifibatide should be refrigerated until dispensed.

Side Effects The primary side effects of eptifibatide are bleeding and thrombocytopenia. Bleeding and hypersensitivity reactions may occur with tirofiban use.

Contraindications Eptifibatide is contraindicated in patients with active bleeding, a history of a stroke within the last month, a history of a hemorrhagic stroke, severe hypertension, or recent major surgery. It is also contraindicated for hemodialysis and for concurrent administration of another glycoprotein antagonist.

Tirofiban should not be used in patients who have active internal bleeding or severe recent physical trauma, are undergoing a major surgical procedure, or have a history of thrombocytopenia following tirofiban use.

Cautions and Considerations The most common complication of glycoprotein antagonists is bleeding. Eptifibatide should be used with caution in patients who have kidney impairment. Tirofiban may cause thrombocytopenia. Tirofiban doses must be reduced in patients who have kidney impairment.

Glycoprotein antagonists are considered to be high-alert medications by the Institute for Safe Medication Practices. This is due to the heightened risk of causing significant patient harm when used in error.

Drug Interactions Other antiplatelet agents and anticoagulants increase the risk of bleeding with concurrent use of glycoprotein antagonists.

Thrombolytic Agents

A **thrombolytic agent** dissolves clots by binding to the clot protein formed by fibrin. Table 10.11 lists the most commonly used thrombolytic agents. These drugs are recombinant tissue plasminogen activators (tPAs), which are laboratory-made proteins that dissolve blood clots. Thombolytics bind to fibrin in a clot and convert plasminogen (a protein found in the blood that is present in clots) to plasmin, an enzyme. The plasmin degrades the fibrin matrix of the clot, which results in the clot dissolving.

Dosage Forms and Administration Thrombolytics are supplied in the form of a powder to be dissolved in sterile water for injection or in the diluent supplied with the drug for IV use only. While the drug is being reconstituted from the powder, the vial should be gently swirled, never shaken, because shaking can disrupt the thrombolytic agents' molecular structure.

Tenecteplase is incompatible with dextrose, so it should not be used in an IV line containing dextrose 5% in water; the line should be flushed with saline before and after injection.

Safety Alert

Tirofiban (Aggrastat) may be confused with Aggrenox (the brand name for aspirin combined with dipyridamole).

Work Wise

You may hear a thrombolytic referred to as a *tPA*, the acronym for *tissue plasminogen activator*.

Side Effects Side effects include bleeding, arrhythmias, allergy, nausea, vomiting, hypotension, and fever.

Contraindications Thrombolytics have many contraindications. They are all contraindicated in active internal bleeding. Alteplase is contraindicated in patients who have a history of a recent stroke, recent intracranial or intraspinal surgery, recent serious head trauma, or severe uncontrolled hypertension. Tenecteplase should be avoided in patients with a history of stroke or with recent intracranial or intraspinal surgery or trauma, increased risk of intracranial bleeding, or severe uncontrolled hypertension.

Cautions and Considerations Thrombolytics greatly increase the risk of bleeding and hemorrhage. Patients with conditions that increase the risk of bleeding should use them cautiously. These agents should be used with caution in older adults.

Drug Interactions Thrombolytics may increase bleeding when used with other drugs that increase risk of bleeding.

Nitroglycerin may decrease the concentration of alteplase.

10.8 Complementary and Alternative Therapies

Plant sterol esters have been found to significantly lower LDL cholesterol and can be helpful adjuncts to diet and drug therapy for hyperlipidemia. Beta-sitosterol is a plant sterol similar in chemical structure to cholesterol. It is used in several food products, such as margarine and juice, as a neutraceutical for cardiovascular disease. The typical dosage of beta-sitosterol is 800 mg–6 g a day in divided doses with meals. Beta-sitosterol should not be taken with ezetimibe (Zetia), because ezetimibe blocks sitosterol absorption and renders the dose ineffective.

Red yeast rice is a fermented rice product that is used in recipes and in medications to lower cholesterol and improve cardiovascular health. Red yeast rice is available in capsule and tablet form and contains varying amounts of monacolins, agents with HMG-CoA reductase inhibitor activity. Other ingredients in red yeast rice, such as sterols, isoflavones, and monounsaturated fatty acids, also may lower cholesterol. Red yeast rice supplements are usually taken at a dosage of 1,800 mg a day, divided in two doses. Alpha-tocopherol (vitamin E) supplements are used for a variety of conditions, such as cardiovascular disease, cancer, and diabetic neuropathy. The effectiveness of vitamin E for these conditions has not been proven, and there is evidence to suggest that vitamin E may increase the risk of heart failure. However, many individuals take this antioxidant for better health. A total dosage of 400 international units a day has been found to be safe and possibly effective for selected conditions, whereas higher dosages can cause side effects and are associated with poor outcomes.

Garlic contains organosulfur compounds that have antihyperlipidemic, antihypertensive, and antifungal effects. A variety of garlic products and supplements is available, and garlic has been found to be possibly effective in treating atherosclerosis, hypertension, skin fungal infections, and some cancers. The garlic product must contain allicin, the odorous active ingredient produced by crushing garlic cloves. A dosing regimen of 600–1,200 mg a day, divided into three doses, has been used in clinical trials. One clove of fresh garlic a day has also been used. Patients taking warfarin, saquinavir (a drug used to treat HIV), or other protease inhibitors should not take garlic.

Review and Assessment

CHAPTER SUMMARY

Anatomy and Physiology of the Cardiovascular System

- The cardiovascular system (the heart and blood vessels) circulates blood throughout the body, bringing needed oxygen and nutrients to tissues and carrying away carbon dioxide and toxic by-products.

Hypertension and Drug Treatments

- Hypertension (elevated blood pressure) affects about 75 million Americans.

- Family history; smoking; diet and lifestyle choices; kidney disease; decreased pressure or delayed pulse in the lower extremities; obesity; adrenal tumor; and use of drugs such as oral contraceptives, corticosteroids, NSAIDs, decongestants, or appetite suppressants contribute to hypertension.

- Drugs commonly used to treat hypertension include ACE inhibitors, angiotensin receptor blockers (ARBs), calcium channel blockers, diuretics, alpha-blockers, beta-blockers, and direct renin inhibitors.

- ACE inhibitors reduce blood pressure by inhibiting the angiotensin-converting enzyme, preventing the conversion of angiotensin I to angiotensin II, a potent vasoconstrictor.

- Angiotensin receptor blockers (ARBs) reduce blood pressure by blocking angiotensin II at its receptors, preventing constriction of blood vessels. ARBs are less likely to cause coughing than ACE inhibitors are because the angiotensin-converting enzyme, which also breaks down bradykinin, is not inhibited.

- Calcium channel blockers reduce blood pressure by dilating coronary arteries and arterioles, which decreases energy consumption, oxygen requirements, and peripheral vascular resistance to blood flow.

- Beta-blockers compete for the same receptor site as catecholamines and, in turn, inhibit neurotransmitter activity. Beta-blockers may be used for the following cardiovascular conditions: hypertension, angina, atrial fibrillation, heart failure, tachycardia associated with operations, MI, and arrhythmias.

- Beta-blockers may mask symptoms of hypoglycemia; patients with diabetes avoid using these drugs.

Cardiac Arrhythmias and Drug Treatments

- Normal heart rhythm is generated by the sinoatrial (SA) node.

- Various types of arrhythmias show specific patterns on an ECG and are associated with different degrees of danger.

- Pharmaceutical treatment for arrhythmias is directed at preventing these life-threatening conditions by restoring sinus (normal) rhythm.

- The various classes of antiarrhythmic drugs have characteristic electrophysiologic effects on the myocardium and conduction system.

- The classes of drugs used to treat arrhythmias are grouped as class I (membrane-stabilizing agents), class II (beta-blockers), class III (potassium channel blockers), class IV (calcium channel blockers), and others.

- Digoxin (Digitek, Digox, Lanoxin) may be used in managing atrial flutter, atrial fibrillation, and heart failure. The three primary signs of digitalis toxicity are nausea, vomiting, and arrhythmias.

- Digoxin immune Fab (DigiFab) is the antidote for digoxin toxicity.

- Atropine is used to treat bradycardia. It is also used preoperatively to inhibit salivation and secretions.

Angina, Myocardial Infarction, and Corresponding Drug Treatments

- Angina pectoris is chest pain caused by inadequate blood flow to a portion of the heart. The three main types are stable, unstable, and variant.

- Angina is typically treated with beta-blockers, calcium channel blockers, and nitrates. Ranolazine may also be used.

- When heart muscle is deprived of oxygen long enough, the cells die (infarct) causing a myocardial infarction (heart attack).

- Symptoms of an MI include tightness, heaviness, or squeezing sensation in the chest; chest, neck, or jaw pain; chest pain that radiates down the left arm; indigestion or nausea; a sense of impending doom; weakness or fatigue; and sweating.

- Drugs used to treat MI include oxygen, nitroglycerin, and aspirin for acute care. Chronic treatment of MI includes beta-blockers, ACE inhibitors, and medications to treat cholesterol. Calcium channel blockers and nitrates may be used in patients with ischemia.

- Nitrates are drugs commonly used to treat angina; they dilate coronary vessels, allowing more oxygen and nutrients to reach cardiac muscle cells.

- A transdermal nitrate patch should be removed at night to prevent development of tolerance to the drug.

- Patients may experience a severe headache when initiating nitroglycerin therapy.

- Ranolazine is a metabolic modifier used as an adjunct therapy for patients for whom other antianginal drugs do not work.

Heart Failure and Drug Treatments

- Heart failure occurs when the pumping ability of the heart can no longer sustain the oxygen-rich blood flow required to meet the body's needs.

- Therapy to treat the effects of heart failure typically includes an inhibitor of the renin-angiotensin system (such as an ACE inhibitor, ARB, or angiotensin receptor-neprilysin inhibitor) and a beta-blocker. In certain cases, diuretics, aldosterone antagonists, a combination of hydralazine and a nitrate, or digoxin may be used.

- Sacubitril is an angiotensin receptor-neprilysin inhibitor (ARNI) available as a combination product with valsartan. Concurrent ACE inhibitor use is contraindicated with sacubitril / valsartan.

Hyperlipidemia and Drug Treatments

- The liver packages triglycerides, cholesterol, and carrier proteins in spherical particles called *lipoproteins*, which circulate in the blood.

- Drugs are used as an adjunct to proper diet to prevent hyperlipidemia.

- Some combinations of these drugs are synergistic.

- Thiazide diuretics, loop diuretics, and corticosteroids all affect lipoproteins unfavorably.

- Statins are HMG-CoA reductase inhibitors, and their generic names end in -statin.

- Patients taking statins should report any muscle pain or weakness to their healthcare practitioner immediately.

- Fibrates are used to lower triglycerides.

- Bile acid sequestrants are indicated for patients with hypercholesterolemia.

- Ezetimibe is a cholesterol absorption inhibitor and may be used by itself or in combination with other drugs.

- Omega-3 fatty acids are available OTC and by prescription.

Clotting Disorders, Stroke, and Drug Treatments

- Blood clots in the bloodstream (thrombi and emboli) can cause life-threatening pulmonary embolisms and other serious damage.

- Anticoagulants prevent clot formation by affecting clotting factors; antiplatelets reduce the risk of clot formation by inhibiting platelet aggregation.

- A hemorrhagic stroke is caused by a cerebral hemorrhage (bleeding from a ruptured blood vessel). An ischemic stroke is caused by a blood clot in a vessel that supplies the brain, which can cause cerebral infarction (necrotizing of tissue).

- A transient ischemic attack (TIA) can be a predictor of an impending stroke.

- Risk factors for stroke include diabetes, advanced age, male sex, genetic predisposition, smoking, and prior stroke.

- Heparin inactivates thrombin and factor Xa, thereby reducing clot formation; it does not dissolve a clot that has already formed.

- Protamine sulfate is the antidote for heparin.

- Warfarin is a commonly used oral anticoagulant. It has a narrow therapeutic window, and levels should be monitored. Warfarin has many drug interactions. Phytonadione, or vitamin K, is an antidote for warfarin.

- Antiplatelet agents prevent platelet activation and formation of a platelet plug.

- Glycoprotein antagonists are administered during invasive procedures for acute coronary syndrome to prevent artery closure.

- A thrombolytic agent dissolves clots by binding to the clot protein formed by fibrin.

Complementary and Alternative Therapies

- Plant sterol esters may significantly lower LDL cholesterol and can be helpful adjuncts to diet and drug therapy for hyperlipidemia.

- Red yeast rice is a fermented rice product that is used in recipes and in medications to lower cholesterol and improve cardiovascular health.

- Alpha tocopherol (vitamin E) supplements are used for a variety of conditions, such as cardiovascular disease, cancer, and diabetic neuropathy. However, evidence suggests vitamin E may increase the risk of heart failure.

- Garlic contains organosulfur compounds that have antihyperlipidemic, antihypertensive, and antifungal effects.

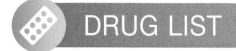

DRUG LIST

Angiotensin-Converting Enzyme (ACE) Inhibitors
benazepril (Lotensin)
captopril
enalapril (Epaned, Vasotec)
enalaprilat
fosinopril
lisinopril (Prinivil, Qbrelis, Zestril)
moexipril
perindopril (Aceon)
quinapril (Accupril)
ramipril (Altace)
trandolapril (Mavik)

Angiotensin Receptor Blockers (ARBs)
azilsartan (Edarbi)
candesartan (Atacand)
eprosartan (Teveten)
irbesartan (Avapro)
losartan (Cozaar)
olmesartan (Benicar)
telmisartan (Micardis)
valsartan (Diovan)

Angiotensin Receptor—Neprilysin Inhibitors
sacubitril / valsartan (Entresto)

Antidote for Dabigatran
idarucizumab (Praxbind)

Antidote for Digoxin Toxicity
digoxin immune Fab (DigiFab)

Antidote for Heparin
protamine sulfate

Antidote for Oral Factor Xa Inhibitors
andexanet alfa (Andexxa)

Antidote for Warfarin
phytonadione, or vitamin K (Mephyton)

Antiplatelets

General Antiplatelet Agents
aspirin (various)
clopidogrel (Plavix)
prasugrel (Effient)
ticagrelor (Brilinta)

Glycoprotein Antagonists
eptifibatide (Integrilin)
tirofiban (Aggrastat)

ATP Citrate Lyase (ACL) Inhibitors
bempedoic acid (Nexletol)

Beta-Blockers (Class II)

Beta-1 Selective (Cardioselective) Beta-Blockers
acebutolol (Sectral)
atenolol (Tenormin)
betaxolol
bisoprolol (Zebeta)
esmolol (Brevibloc)
metoprolol (Kaspargo, Lopressor, Toprol-XL)
nebivolol (Bystolic)

Nonselective Beta-Blockers
labetalol
nadolol (Corgard)
propranolol (Inderal LA, Inderal XL, InnoPran XL)
sotalol (Betapace, Sorine, Sotylize)
timolol

Bile Acid Sequestrants
cholestyramine (Prevalite, Questran, Questran Light)
colesevelam (WelChol)
colestipol (Colestid)

Calcium Channel Blockers (Class IV)

Dihydropyridine Agents
amlodipine (Katerzia, Norvasc)
felodipine (Plendil)
isradipine
nicadipine (Cardene)
nifedipine (Adalat CC, Afeditab, Afeditab CR, Nifediac, Procardia, Procardia XL)
nisoldipine (Sular)

Nondihydropyridine Agents
diltiazem (Cardizem, Cardizem CD, Cardizem LA, Cartia XT, Dilt-XR, Dilacor XR, Matzim LA, Tatzia XT, Tiadylt ER, Tiazac)
verapamil (Calan, Verelan)

Direct Renin Inhibitors
aliskiren (Tekturna)

Direct Thrombin Inhibitors
bivalirudin (Angiomax)
dabigatran (Pradaxa)

Factor Xa Inhibitors
apixaban (Eliquis)
edoxaban (Savaysa)
fondaparinux (Arixtra)
rivaroxaban (Xarelto)

Fibric Acid Derivatives
fenofibrate (Antara, Lipofen, TriCor)
fenofibric acid (Fibricor, Trilipix)
gemfibrozil (Lopid)

Heparin and Low-Molecular-Weight Heparins
dalteparin (Fragmin)
heparin or unfractionated heparin (UFH)
enoxaparin (Lovenox)

HMG-CoA Reductase Inhibitors (Statins)
atorvastatin (Lipitor)
fluvastatin (Lescol)
lovastatin (Altoprev, Mevacor)
pitavastatin (Livalo, Zypitamag)
pravastatin (Pravachol)
rosuvastatin (Crestor, Ezallor)
simvastatin (Flolipid, Zocor)

Membrane-Stabilizing Agents (Class I Antiarrhythmics)
disopyramide (Norpace)
flecainide (Tambocor)
lidocaine
mexiletine
procainamide
propafenone (Rythmol)
quinidine

Metabolic Modifiers
ranolazine (Ranexa)

Other Agents Used to Treat Arrhythmias
atropine
digoxin (Digitek, Digox, Lanoxin)
isoproterenol (Isuprel)

Nitrates

Short-Acting Nitrates
nitroglycerin (GoNitro, Minitran, Nitro-Bid, Nitro-Dur, Nitro-Time, Nitrolingual, NitroMist, Nitrostat, Rectiv)

Long-Acting Nitrates
isosorbide dinitrate (Dilatrate-SR, Isordil)
isosorbide mononitrate

Other Cholesterol-Lowering Agents
ezetimibe (Zetia)
omega-3 fatty acids (Epanova, Lovaza, Vascepa)

Potassium Channel Blockers (Class III Antiarrhythmics)
amiodarone (Nexterone, Pacerone)
dofetilide (Tikosyn)
dronedarone (Multaq)

Thrombolytic Agents
alteplase (Activase)
tenecteplase (TNKase)

Vitamin K Antagonist
warfarin

Vasodilators
hydralazine
isosorbide dinitrate / hydralazine (BiDil)

✓ CHECK YOUR UNDERSTANDING

Take a moment to review what you have learned in this chapter and answer the following questions.

1. Which of the following best describes systolic blood pressure?
   a. the amount of blood in the cardiovascular system
   b. the average amount of pressure when the heart ejects blood and fills
   c. the pressure when the heart ejects blood
   d. the pressure when the heart relaxes and fills

2. Which of the following is *not* a therapeutic indication for ACE inhibitors?
   a. angina
   b. blood clots
   c. heart failure
   d. hypertension

3. Which of the following is a common side effect of ACE inhibitors?
   a. bleeding
   b. dry cough
   c. neutropenia
   d. purple toe syndrome

4. Which of the following ARBs is sensitive to moisture and light and must be dispensed in the original bottle?
   a. azilsartan (Edarbi)
   b. candesartan (Atacand)
   c. olmesartan (Benicar)
   d. telmisartan (Micardis)

5. Which of the following best describes the mechanism by which calcium channel blockers decrease blood pressure?
   a. competing for catecholamine binding sites and blocking beta-receptors in the heart and lungs
   b. directly inhibiting the action of renin
   c. impeding the movement of calcium ions into cardiac muscle cells during depolarization
   d. inhibiting angiotensin-converting enzyme

6. Which of the following best describes the boxed warning for the beta-blockers atenolol, metoprolol, nadolol, propranolol, and timolol?
   a. increased cardiac symptoms with abrupt discontinuation
   b. decreased cardiac symptoms with dosetitration
   c. fetal malformation when used in pregnancy
   d. risk of severe liver disease

7. Which of the following antiarrhythmic drugs may cause leukopenia (low white blood cell count)?
   a. atropine
   b. digoxin
   c. disopyramide
   d. procainamide

8. Which of the following is *not* a boxed warning for amiodarone?
   a. increased risk of heart failure
   b. potential to exacerbate arrhythmias
   c. pulmonary toxicity
   d. risk of severe liver toxicity

9. Which of the following drugs for angina should be dispensed in its original amber glass container?
   a. metoprolol
   b. nitroglycerin
   c. ranolazine
   d. verapamil

10. Which of the following is *not* a drug class that may adversely affect cholesterol levels?
    a. ACE inhibitors
    b. beta-blockers
    c. corticosteroids
    d. thiazide diuretics

11. Which of the following is a caution for the use of statins?
    a. risk of angioedema
    b. risk of dry cough
    c. risk of rhabdomyolysis
    d. risk of worsened asthma

12. Which of the following patient populations should avoid the use of omega-3 fatty acids?
    a. those with fish or shellfish allergies
    b. those with high triglycerides
    c. those with a history of heart attack
    d. those with low HDL

13. Which of the following is the antidote for heparin?
    a. enoxaparin
    b. idarucizumab
    c. protamine sulfate
    d. vitamin K

14. Which of the following is the antidote for warfarin?
    a. enoxaparin
    b. idarucizumab
    c. protamine sulfate
    d. vitamin K

15. Warfarin levels are most affected by which of the following foods?
    a. high sodium chloride-containing foods
    b. vitamin D-containing foods
    c. vitamin K-containing foods
    d. Warfarin levels are not affected by food.

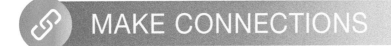

MAKE CONNECTIONS

Take a moment to consider what you have learned in this chapter and respond thoughtfully to the following prompts. Note that some of these activities will require internet access.

1. One of the most common adverse drug events with the use of anticoagulants is bleeding. For this reason, reversal of these drugs is sometimes required. Create a list of each anticoagulant discussed in this chapter and its reversal agent, if it has one.

2. Many cardiovascular system drugs are among the top 200 prescribed drugs. Research a list of the top 200 drugs. Then create a list of drugs in this chapter that are considered top 200 drugs. After you create the list, place the drugs into their respective drug classes.

 The online course includes additional review and assessment resources.

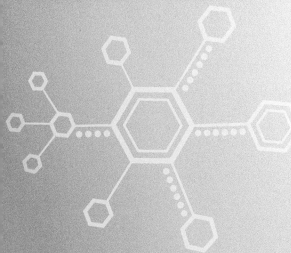

The Respiratory System and Drug Therapy

11

Learning Objectives

1   Describe the anatomy of the respiratory system. (Section 11.1)

2   Differentiate between the main pulmonary diseases. (Section 11.2 through 11.5)

3   Describe the pathophysiology and treatment of asthma. (Section 11.2)

4   Discuss the pathophysiology and treatment of chronic obstructive pulmonary disease. (Section 11.3)

5   Summarize the reemergence of tuberculosis and its associated treatments. (Section 11.5)

6   Describe the mechanism of action and uses of antitussives, expectorants, decongestants, and antihistamines. (Section 11.6)

7   Paraphrase why some drugs are prescribed for their side effects. (Section 11.6)

8   Outline smoking cessation plans and supportive therapy. (Section 11.7)

ASHP/ACPE Accreditation Standards

To view the *ASHP/ACPE Accreditation Standards* addressed in this chapter, refer to Appendix C.

11.1 Anatomy of the Respiratory System

The **respiratory system** contains specific organs that are responsible for obtaining oxygen from the air through inhalation, supplying oxygen to the cells in the body through gas exchange, and removing carbon dioxide from the body via exhalation.

The respiratory system can be divided into the upper respiratory tract and the lower respiratory tract. The upper respiratory tract includes the nose, nasal cavity, mouth, pharynx, and larynx. The lower respiratory tract is made up of the trachea, bronchial tree, alveoli, and lungs. The lower respiratory tract is essential for the exchange of oxygen and carbon dioxide and works with the circulatory system to transport oxygen to the cells of the body while removing carbon dioxide from the body.

The respiratory system is the source of air filtration as air enters the body and assists in the production of sound for speech. Upon inhalation, air flows through the nasal cavity or mouth; the pharynx, larynx, and trachea; and finally through the bronchial tree to the alveoli. The alveoli facilitate the exchange of oxygen and carbon dioxide within the blood. Figure 11.1 shows the upper and lower respiratory tracts, through which air passes and Figure 11.2 shows the exchange of the gases within the alveoli.

The respiratory system contains protective mechanisms to filter air and protect the airways and lungs from harmful substances like dust, bacteria, viruses, and allergens. In the nostrils, hair helps trap large particles like dust. The trachea contains small, hairlike structures called cilia that move in a sweeping motion to help clear out harmful substances. The lining of the respiratory tract contains cells that secrete a protective mucus that helps keep the airway moist and helps to trap and filter waste.

FIGURE 11.1
Upper and Lower Respiratory Tracts

The upper respiratory tract includes structures such as the nose, nasal cavity, mouth, pharynx, and larynx. The lower respiratory tract includes the trachea, lungs, bronchi, and bronchioles.

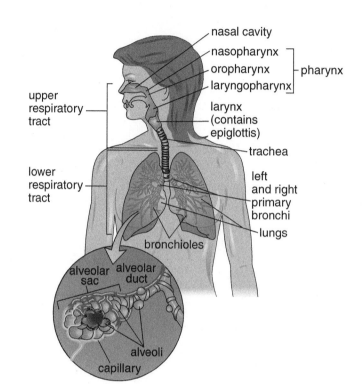

FIGURE 11.2
Exchange of Oxygen and Carbon Dioxide

Oxygen picked up in the lungs is diffused into the red blood cells through the alveoli. Oxygenated red blood cells carry oxygen to all the cells of the body. Carbon dioxide is returned to the lungs through the alveoli to be expelled during exhalation.

Function of the Alveolus in the Lungs

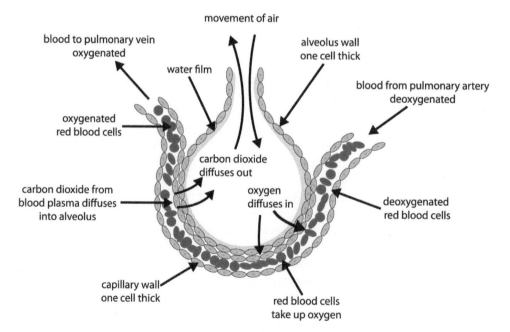

The respiratory diseases covered in this chapter include asthma, chronic obstructive pulmonary disease (COPD), and other related disorders. COPD encompasses two major diseases: emphysema and chronic bronchitis. Other related obstructive diseases include pneumonia, cystic fibrosis, respiratory distress syndrome, tuberculosis, and histoplasmosis. In addition, the lungs are frequently attacked by less severe upper respiratory tract infections, including the common cold. Allergies are also discussed in this chapter because many of the drugs used to treat respiratory conditions are often used to treat allergies. It is important to remember that asthma and allergies are quite different. Smoking, which is closely linked to many respiratory diseases, is also included in this chapter.

11.2 Asthma and Drug Treatments

Asthma is an inflammatory disorder of the airways and causes coughing, wheezing, breathlessness, and chest tightness. It occurs in intermittent attacks that involve a reversible airway obstruction, and it is precipitated by specific triggering events that vary in severity from patient to patient.

In asthma, as a result of the obstructed airways, less oxygen is available to exchange with carbon dioxide, or the surface area available for gas exchange is decreased. Bronchioles, the smallest passageway in the bronchial tree, constrict; mucus production increases; and lung tissue swells (see Figure 11.3), making normal breathing difficult.

Asthma has the following characteristics: reversible small airway obstruction, progressive airway inflammation, and increased airway responsiveness to a variety of endogenous (internal) or exogenous (external or environmental) stimuli. These characteristics translate into recurrent episodes of **wheezing** (a whistling respiratory sound), **dyspnea** (labored or difficult breathing), and cough that have both **acute** (short, severe course) and **chronic** (persisting for a long time) manifestations in most patients.

FIGURE 11.3
Asthmatic Airway

During an asthma attack, the airways "overreact" to produce excess mucus and swelling. The combination of excess mucus and bronchoconstriction decreases airflow.

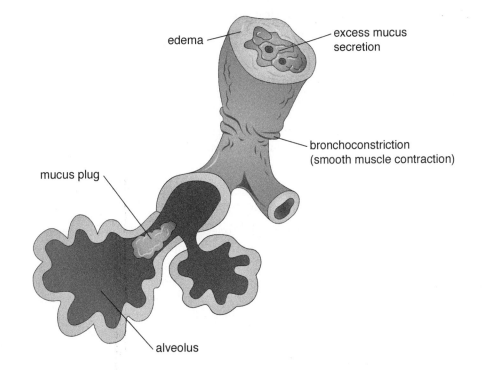

edema

excess mucus secretion

bronchoconstriction (smooth muscle contraction)

mucus plug

alveolus

Asthma differs from normal pulmonary defense mechanisms in its severity of **bronchospasm** (spasmodic contraction of the smooth muscles of the bronchioles, or small airways), apparent failure of normal dilator muscle systems, excessive production of mucus that plugs airways, and presence of sometimes severe long-term inflammatory reactions that may lead to patchy shedding of the linings of small airways.

Asthma is episodic, meaning that times of poor airflow and difficulty with breathing alternate with times of normal function. Acute difficulty with breathing, known as an **asthma attack**, is characterized by hyperreactivity of the airways and bronchospasm, usually in response to allergens or irritants. Common triggers include smoke, dust, exercise, pet dander, cold weather, gastroesophageal reflux disease, colds, and flu. Other potential triggers include medications, exercise, humidity, high temperatures, anxiety, laughing, and certain foods.

Immediately after exposure to a trigger, mast cells in the lung tissue release histamine and other chemical mediators that cause bronchoconstriction and increased mucus production. Edema (swelling) may also result. See Figure 11.3 for an illustration of this process.

Over time, continued release of histamine, bradykinin, prostaglandins, and leukotrienes causes tissues to inflame and airways to constrict and can result in permanent lung tissue damage. Fortunately, in many cases, breathing symptoms and airway constriction can be controlled with proper treatment. Without treatment, lung function can steadily decline.

A commonly used way of assessing the severity of asthma is with an instrument known as a **peak flow meter**, which measures **peak expiratory flow rate (PEFR)**. To establish a patient's PEFR, the patient forcefully blows into the peak flow meter, and PEFR is recorded in liters per minute. Once the patient's personal best PEFR is identified, it can be used to assess future asthmatic episodes with more clarity. A measurement below 50% of a patient's personal best PEFR indicates a medical alert; immediate treatment with a bronchodilator and anti-inflammatory agent is needed, and the patient's healthcare provider should be notified.

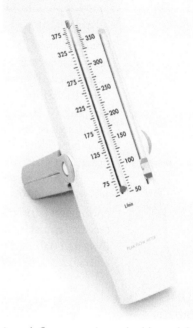

A peak flow meter is a valuable tool for patients to use to measure PEFR and manage symptoms of asthma.

Asthma Management and Drug Therapy

Asthma is categorized into levels of severity (intermittent, mild, moderate, and severe) based on how patients' symptoms affect their ability to sleep at night, continue normal daily activities, and breathe freely. Objective **pulmonary function tests** can be done to assess asthma severity. In addition, if a patient is waking up at night more than twice a month because of asthma symptoms or is using relief medication such as an inhaler more than twice a week, asthma is considered "not controlled." Patients should understand that if their asthma is not controlled, they should seek medical treatment and be sure to adhere to prescribed medication schedules. Drug therapy for asthma includes long-term treatment to prevent exacerbations as well as rescue therapies to help once asthma attack symptoms have begun. Many patients need more than simple rescue therapies. Long-term, steady treatment can improve overall lung function, reduce exacerbations, and decrease the need for short-term relief therapies.

As part of good asthma care, a patient with asthma must learn to manage the disease and its complications and to limit the amount of exposure to irritants that cause airway inflammation. The patient needs to learn what can trigger asthma attacks and how to control those factors. For example, the patient with asthma should avoid contact with smoke as much as possible because smoke is detrimental to patients with asthma. Also, because many people with asthma are allergic to dust mites, patients should follow simple dust mite control steps, including washing sheets and mattress pads at least once a week in hot (130° F or hotter) water. Asthma patients should also obtain a yearly flu vaccination.

Symptoms alone are not always the best measure of respiratory status. For this reason, patients must learn to use a peak flow meter to measure PEFR. The peak flow meter should be used twice a day and the results recorded in a diary as an aid to better management. Often, simply adjusting asthma medications on the basis of the peak flow meter readings helps manage asthma effectively.

Patients with asthma and their caregivers should be aware of the signs and symptoms of **status asthmaticus**, which is a potentially life-threatening condition. An episode of status asthmaticus begins like any other asthma attack, but unlike an ordinary attack, it does not respond to normal management. A patient suffering from such an episode experiences increasing difficulty in breathing and exhibits blue lips and nail beds (cyanosis). The patient may lose consciousness. Status asthmaticus clearly constitutes a medical emergency, and the patient should receive prompt attention. This event may require a visit to the emergency room.

Drug therapy is the mainstay of asthma management. Asthma begins with intermittent attacks and may progress from mild to severe, persistent symptoms. Drug therapy depends on the severity of the disease.

Drug therapy for asthma has two components: quick-relief medications and long-term persistent medications. **Quick relief medication** is used intermittently and provides rapid relief, as needed, when asthma symptoms present or when an asthma attack occurs. **Long-term persistent medications** are used regularly to prevent asthma symptoms or attacks. Pharmacy technicians can help patients treat and prevent asthma attacks by promoting correct use of quick-relief medications and adherence to long-term persistent medications.

An important method of administering asthma medications is by a **metered-dose inhaler (MDI)**—sometimes called a *puffer*—that contains medication and compressed gas. The MDI delivers a specific amount of medication with each activation. The delivery mechanism suspends the medication in particles or droplets that are fine enough to penetrate to the deepest parts of the patient's lungs.

The prescriber usually orders an MDI to be used with a spacer. A **spacer** is attached to the MDI

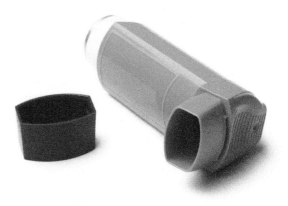

An MDI sprays a controlled amount of drug through the opening when the canister is actuated.

and provides a secondary chamber that holds the drug mist until the patient is ready to breathe. A spacer helps to decrease the amount of spray deposited on the back of the throat and swallowed. It also allows the patient to breathe the mist in at a slower, more effective rate, which, in turn, provides much better penetration of the drug into the lungs. Side effects are reduced because the drug is delivered to the lower portions of the lungs, and fewer particles are left in the mouth and throat to be absorbed. A spacer is extremely useful for children and older adults who may have a hard time coordinating an inhaler. Strong evidence supports the use of spacers.

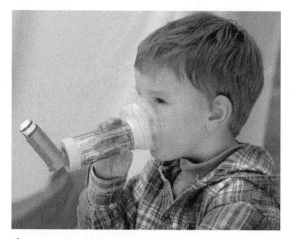

If a spacer is added to an MDI, the medication is more likely to penetrate deep into the lung tissue than if the MDI is used alone. Spacers come with masks (often used by children, as pictured) and without masks.

MDIs need to be shaken well for five seconds before each use and need to be primed before the first use of the device or if the device is dropped or not used for several weeks.

Most patients with asthma have prescriptions for MDIs. Although it may seem easy, the use of an MDI can be difficult and requires the proper technique to administer the medication effectively. The following describes how to use an MDI with a spacer:

1. Inspect the MDI and prime the inhaler, if necessary.
2. Shake the MDI well.
3. Attach the MDI to the spacer.
4. Breathe out completely.
5. Put the mouthpiece of the spacer in your mouth and close your lips around the mouthpiece to form a tight seal.
6. Press down on the canister of the MDI.
7. Take a slow, deep breath and breathe in as much air as you comfortably can.
8. Remove the mouthpiece from your mouth and hold your breath for 10 seconds or as long as comfortably possible.
9. If another puff of the inhaler is needed, wait one minute (except during asthma exacerbations) and repeat. During an asthma exacerbation, you may repeat steps immediately.
10. Rinse the plastic portion of the inhaler and the spacer once a week, and allow the devices to air dry. Patients should always clean the mouthpiece after each use and rinse the mouth if a corticosteroid is used.

If another type of inhaler has been prescribed, the patient should wait five minutes before using it.

The primary difference between an HFA inhaler and a **dry powder inhaler (DPI)** is in its actuation. A patient using an HFA inhaler should breathe in *slowly*, whereas a patient using a DPI should breathe in *quickly*. DPIs do not use gas propellants. Many manufacturers are incorporating asthma drugs into dry-powder devices.

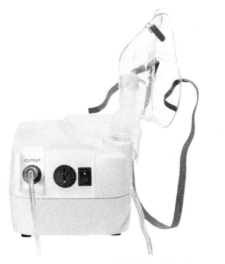

A nebulizer is a common method of administering asthma medication. It is especially effective for children.

Because of the complicated series of steps required to use HFAs and DPIs, they are not recommended for very young children. Asthma medication can be administered to children with a **nebulizer**, a device in which a stream of air flows past a liquid and creates a fine mist, which the patient inhales while breathing normally through a mouthpiece or mask. The drug thus is more likely to be deposited farther into the lungs. This delivery system is quite effective. If not properly cleaned and cared for, however, a home nebulizer can be a source of bronchitis and infections. Therefore, nebulizers should be cleaned regularly. Medications used within MDIs and nebulizers include short-acting beta-2 agonists, corticosteroids, leukotriene inhibitors, mast cell stabilizers, monoclonal antibodies, and xanthine derivatives. Table 11.1 lists the commonly used agents to treat asthma.

TABLE 11.1 Commonly Used Agents to Treat Asthma

Generic (Brand)	Pronunciation	Dosage Form	Common Dosage	Dispensing Status
Short-Acting Beta-2 Agonists				
albuterol* (Accuneb, ProAir HFA, ProAir Respiclick, Proventil HFA, Ventolin HFA)	al-BYOO-ter-awl	aerosol (MDI), nebulizer solution, syrup, tablet	inhalation: 2.5 mg 3–4 times a day via nebulizer MDI: 1–2 puffs 3–4 times a day PO: 2–4 mg 3–4 times a day	Rx
levalbuterol (Xopenex HFA)	lee-val-BYOO-ter-awl	aerosol (MDI), nebulizer solution	inhalation: 0.63–1.25 mg 3 times a day via nebulizer MDI: 2 puffs every 4–6 hr	Rx
metaproterenol*	met-a-proe-TER-e-nawl	syrup, tablet	PO: 10–20 mg 3–4 times a day	Rx
Inhaled Corticosteroids				
beclomethasone (QVAR)	bek-loe-METH-a-sone	aerosol (MDI)	40–160 mcg 2 times a day	Rx
budesonide* (Pulmicort Flexhaler, Pulmicort Respules)	byoo-DES-oh-nide	powder for inhalation, suspension for inhalation	powder: 180–720 mcg 2 times a day suspension: 0.5–1 mg 1 time a day or 0.25–0.5 mg 2 times a day	Rx
ciclesonide (Alvesco)	sye-KLES-oh-nide	aerosol (MDI)	80–320 mcg 2 times a day	Rx
fluticasone* (Flovent, Arnuity Ellipta)	floo-TIK-a-sone	aerosol (MDI), powder for inhalation	MDI 88–880 mcg 2 times a day powder: 100–200 mcg 1 time a day	Rx

continues

TABLE 11.1 Commonly Used Agents to Treat Asthma—*Continued*

Generic (Brand)	Pronunciation	Dosage Form	Common Dosage	Dispensing Status
mometasone (Asmanex HFA, Asmanex Twisthaler)	moe-MET-a-sone	aerosol (MDI), powder for inhalation	110–880 mcg 1–2 times a day	Rx
Combinations				
budesonide / formoterol (Symbicort)	byoo-DES-oh-nide for-MOE-ter-awl	aerosol (MDI)	160/9 mg–320/9 mg 2 times a day	Rx
fluticasone / salmeterol (Advair Diskus, Advair HFA, AirDuo Respiclick)	floo-TIK-a-sone sal-ME-te-role	aerosol (MDI), powder for inhalation	Advair Diskus: 100 mcg/50 mcg–500 mcg/50 mcg 2 times a day Advair HFA: 45 mcg/21 mcg–230 mcg/21 mcg, 2 inhalations 2 times a day AirDuo Respiclick: 55 mcg/14 mcg, 113 mcg/14 mcg or 232 mcg/14 mcg, 2 times a day	Rx
fluticasone / vilanterol (Breo Ellipta)	floo-TIK-a-sone vye-LAN-ter-ol	aerosol (MDI)	100 mcg/25 mcg–200 mcg/25 mcg, 1 puff 1 time a day	Rx
mometasone / formoterol (Dulera)	moe-MET-a-sone for-MOE-ter-awl	aerosol (MDI)	100 mcg/5 mcg–400 mcg/10 mcg 2 times a day	Rx
Leukotriene Inhibitors				
montelukast (Singulair)	mon-te-LOO-kast	chewable tablet, granules, tablet	4–10 mg 1 time a day (4 mg pediatric dose)	Rx
zafirlukast (Accolate)	za-FEER-loo-kast	tablet	10–20 mg 2 times a day (10 mg pediatric dose)	Rx
zileuton (Zyflo)	zye-LOO-ton	tablet	600–1,200 mg 2 times a day	Rx
Monoclonal Antibodies				
benralizumab (Fasenra)	ben-ra-LIZ-ue-mab	injection	SC: 30 mg every 4 weeks for 3 doses, then every 8 weeks	Rx
dupilumab (Dupixent)	doo-PIL-ue-mab	injection	SC (adults): 600 mg for 1 dose; 2 weeks later, 300 mg every other week SC (ages 12–17): weight-dependent dosing; 200–600 mg every 2 weeks depending on weight	Rx
mepolizumab (Nucala)	me-poe-LIZ-ue-mab	injection	SC (adults): 100 mg 1 time every 4 weeks SC (ages 6–11): 40 mg every 4 weeks SC (ages >12 years): 100 mg every 4 weeks	Rx
omalizumab (Xolair)	oh-mah-lye-ZOO-mab	injection	75–375 mg every 2–4 weeks	Rx
reslizumab (Cinqair)	res-LIZ-ue-mab	injection	IV: 3 mg/kg every 4 weeks	Rx
Mast Cell Stabilizer				
cromolyn sodium*	KROE-moe-lin SOE-dee-um	nebulizer solution	20 mg 3–4 times a day	Rx

continues

TABLE 11.1 Commonly Used Agents to Treat Asthma—*Continued*

Generic (Brand)	Pronunciation	Dosage Form	Common Dosage	Dispensing Status
Xanthine Derivative				
theophylline (Elixophyllin, Theo-24, Theochron, Theolair)	thee-OFF-i-lin	capsule, elixir, injection, oral solution, tablet	varies based on patient-specific factors and therapeutic drug levels	Rx

* These products are produced in several dosage forms, such as inhalants, liquids (for use in nebulizers), syrups, and injections. Pharmacists and pharmacy technicians should always carefully read the prescription and select the correct dosage form.

Short-Acting Beta-2 Agonists

Short-acting beta-2 agonists is a drug class that provides quick relief of asthma symptoms. Also known as a *rescue medicine*, a **short-acting beta-2 agonist (SABA)** works by stimulating beta-2 receptors in the lungs and by producing smooth muscle relaxation in the bronchioles. As a result, airway diameter increases, improving the movement of gases into and out of the lungs. SABAs are **bronchodilators**, or agents that relax smooth muscle cells of the bronchioles.

Albuterol (Accuneb, ProAir HFA, ProAir Respiclick, Proventil HFA, Ventolin HFA) is a bronchodilator used in the event of airway obstruction, such as asthma or COPD. It relaxes bronchial smooth muscle by acting on pulmonary beta-2 receptors with little effect on heart rate. Albuterol is administered by inhalation or orally for relief of bronchospasms. The duration of inhaled albuterol is typically three to six hours. **Levalbuterol (Xopenex)** is similar to albuterol. Albuterol contains two chemical forms of albuterol. Levalbuterol only contains the form of albuterol that is thought to induce bronchodilation. **Metaproterenol** is also a bronchodilator for airway obstruction. It has a rapid onset of action (within minutes), a peak effect (in approximately one hour), and a prolonged effect (approximately four hours). Metaproterenol acts primarily on beta-2 receptors, with little or no effect on heart rate.

Dosage Forms and Administration Although oral dosage forms are available, most patients use SABAs by inhaling them into the lungs. Because their effects last for only a few hours, these agents may need to be used multiple times a day. Of the available dosage forms, the handheld MDI and the nebulizer solution are the most frequently prescribed (see Table 11.1).

The pharmacy technician should be alert to the potential for patient overdependence on short-acting beta-2 agonists. If the patient is using more than one canister per month, the pharmacy technician should alert the pharmacist who, in turn, should notify the prescriber. Such overdependence is generally a sign that the patient's asthma is not being adequately controlled and that the prescriber needs to consider alternative treatment regimens. Common SABAs include albuterol, levalbuterol, and metaproterenol.

Side Effects Side effects include tremors and nervousness.

Contraindications Albuterol does not have contraindications. Levalbuterol is contraindicated in patients with a hypersensitivity to albuterol. Metaproterenol does not have contraindications.

Cautions and Considerations Pediatric patients using albuterol MDIs should use spacers if they are under five years of age. For patients younger than four years of age, using a spacer with a face mask may be the best way to deliver the drug. Hypersensitivity reactions have been reported with levalbuterol use. Some formulations of metaproterenol contain benzyl alcohol. Benzyl alcohol is associated with toxicities in neonates.

Drug Interactions SABAs interact with beta-blockers, which are frequently used by people with heart disease. Beta-blockers inhibit the effect of these beta-2 agonist drugs. SABAs and beta-blockers should not be used together; if they must be, prescribers should carefully adjust the doses.

Corticosteroids

Corticosteroids are a class of drugs that act as anti-inflammatory agents to suppress the immune responses. They resemble certain chemicals naturally produced by the adrenal gland and inhibit inflammatory cells by stimulating adenylate cylase. Inhaled corticosteroids may be successful when other drugs are not.

The most common inhaled corticosteroids include budesonide, fluticasone, beclomethasone, and mometasone. Oral steroids include prednisone, hydrocortisone, methylprednisolone (Medrol Dosepak), dexamethasone (Decadron, Dexamethasone Intensol, Dexpak Taperpak), and prednisolone (Flo-pred, Orapred, Pediapred). More information on inhaled corticosteroids can be found in Table 11.1.

Dosage Forms and Administration **Beclomethasone (QVAR)** and **ciclesonide (Alvesco)** are commonly used inhaled corticosteroids and are delivered with an MDI. They should not be confused with DPIs. As with other drugs in this class, patients should be instructed to rinse the mouth after each dose.

Budesonide (Pulmicort Flexhaler, Pulmicort Respules) is a corticosteroid with unique administration techniques. Pulmicort Flexhaler uses a dry-powder, propellant-free inhalant that is breath activated. As a result, some patients find it easier to use. Moreover, the Flexhaler needs to be primed only prior to the initial use rather than before each dose, as is necessary with other corticosteroid inhalers. Inadequate response to budesonide is often the result of improper inhalation technique. Both Pulmicort Flexhaler and Pulmicort Respules are associated with a lower frequency of coughing episodes than other inhaled corticosteroids. Pulmicort Respules was the first formulation of budesonide for use in home nebulizers. This formulation has made it possible to treat children as young as 12 months with budesonide.

Fluticasone (Flovent, Arnuity Ellipta) is the same drug found in the nasal spray Flonase covered later in this chapter in commonly used nasal corticosteroids. For respiratory disorders like asthma, fluticasone is available as an aerosol for inhalation (MDI) and as a DPI. It may be used once or twice daily, depending on the product, and may take up to two weeks to reach maximum benefit.

Mometasone (Asmanex, Asmanex HFA) is a dry powder for inhalation. It should be dosed once daily in the evening or twice daily. The dispenser is called a Twisthaler, and it has a dose counter. When the dose counter gets to 00 or the package has been opened for 45 days, the patient should throw the dispenser away. Pharmacy technicians should write the date opened on the dispenser and make sure the patient knows when to dispose of the drug. Mometasone can be used for prophylactic therapy, but maximum benefit may take two weeks or longer. Mometasone has high potency and little systemic bioavailability.

Side Effects The primary side effects of these drugs, if inhaled, are oral candidiasis (a fungal infection), hoarseness, and dry mouth. This irritation can sometimes lead to episodes of coughing. To reduce the likelihood of these effects, the patient should always be advised to rinse the mouth thoroughly with water after using a corticosteroid inhaler.

Improper technique when using an MDI can result in inadequate response, but this problem can be prevented with proper instruction. It should also be noted that headache is a major side effect of mometasone.

If oral corticosteroids are taken for a long period in a dosage exceeding 10 mg of prednisone a day, they can cause growth of facial hair in female patients, breast development in male patients, "buffalo hump," "moon face," edema, weight gain, and easy bruising. A short-term course of high-dose corticosteroids will not cause these side effects.

Another concern is that corticosteroids may stunt a child's growth. Evidence indicates, however, that inhaled steroids do not affect long-term growth in children. Initially, growth may slow down by a half inch in the first year, but children eventually reach normal adult height. The benefits of controlling asthma may outweigh the risks of achieving normal growth and development.

Patients should always use the lowest effective dose of a corticosteroid. A beta-2 agonist should be added to inhaled corticosteroids if needed to decrease the steroid dose necessary for control. The beta-2 agonist helps open the airway, thus allowing more of the inhaled steroid to reach its site of action in the lungs.

Contraindications Inhaled corticosteroids are contraindicated during acute asthma attacks.

Fluticasone and mometasone powder for inhalation contain lactose and should not be used in those patients with a hypersensitivity to milk proteins or lactose. That same patient population should also avoid the combined products fluticasone / salmeterol, fluticasone / vilanterol, and mometasone / formoterol.

Cautions and Considerations DPIs should not be shaken prior to use. Patients should carefully follow instructions for puncturing the powder packet or capsule and then placing the device in the mouth before forceful inhalation.

Drug Interactions These drugs are cytochrome P450 3A4 (CYP3A4) substrates, and metabolism decreases with concomitant administration with CYP3A4 inhibitors, such as ketoconazole, itraconazole, and ritonavir. Doses must be decreased when patients are using one of these drugs.

Beclomethasone interacts with immunosuppressants, natalizumab, and tacrolimus.

Ciclesonide interacts with aldesleukin, amphotericin, cosyntropin, deferasirox, desmopressin, hyaluronidase, inhaled loxapine, and ritodrine.

Patients who need to take an inhaled corticosteroid with any of these medications should be monitored closely.

Ciclesonide also can enhance effects diuretics have on electrolyte imbalances. This affects both loop diuretics like furosemide and thiazide diuretics like hydrochlorothiazide. Patients should be monitored with laboratory tests when using these medications together.

Leukotriene Inhibitors

Used for long-term control of moderate to severe asthma, leukotriene inhibitors are often prescribed when short-acting beta-2 agonists and inhaled corticosteroids are not adequately controlling breathing symptoms. Leukotrienes increase accumulation of mucus and fluid in the spaces between cells; they also increase vascular permeability, permitting substances to pass through the blood vessels. A **leukotriene inhibitor** blocks either the synthesis of, or the body's inflammatory responses to, leukotrienes. Blocking leukotriene receptors also blocks tissue inflammatory responses. Common leukotriene inhibitors are listed in Table 11.1.

Montelukast

Montelukast (Singulair) is a leukotriene receptor antagonist. This drug is indicated for the prophylaxis and chronic treatment of asthma and is different from other therapies in that it is administered orally. Montelukast has been shown to reduce the incidence of daytime asthma and nocturnal awakenings due to asthma attacks. It can also decrease the need for beta-adrenergic agonists. Unlike the other leukotriene inhibitors, which can be prescribed only for adults or older children, montelukast has been approved for use in children 12 months and older.

Dosage Forms and Administration Montelukast also has the benefit of a once-daily oral dosage, whereas the other leukotriene inhibitors must be dosed two to four times per day. This drug is also approved to treat seasonal allergic rhinitis (inflammation of the nasal membrane). Asthma and allergic rhinitis are treated with the same dose.

Side Effects A headache is the most common side effect associated with the use of montelukast.

Contraindications Montelukast does not have contraindications.

Cautions and Considerations Leukotriene inhibitors are not to be used for reversal of bronchospasm in acute asthma attacks. Leukotriene inhibitors have been associated with liver problems, eosinophilia, vasculitis, and behavioral changes (such as unusual dreams, agitation, anxiety, and hallucinations).

Drug Interactions Gemfibrozil may increase serum concentrations of montelukast.

Zafirlukast and Zileuton

Zafirlukast (Accolate), like montelukast, antagonizes leukotriene receptors, thus reducing edema, mucus, and vascular permeability. It is intended for prophylaxis and long-term treatment in patients five years of age or older. **Zileuton (Zyflo, Zyflo CR)** is a leukotriene inhibitor that reduces the production of leukotrienes rather than blocking leukotriene receptors. It is approved only for patients 12 years of age or older.

Dosage Forms and Administration Both zafirlukast and zileuton are available in tablet form and are taken orally.

Side Effects Side effects are headache, rhinitis, and cough.

Contraindications Zafirlukast and zileuton are contraindicated in patients with liver impairment, and patients using it will need periodic liver tests.

Cautions and Considerations Leukotriene inhibitors are not to be used for reversal of bronchospasm in acute asthma attacks. Leukotriene inhibitors have been associated with liver problems, eosinophilia, vasculitis, and behavioral changes (such as unusual dreams, agitation, anxiety, and hallucinations).

Drug Interactions Zileuton and zafirlukast may enhance the toxic effects of loxapine. Serum concentrations of pimozide, theophylline, and tizanadine may be increased by zileuton use.

Mast Cell Stabilizer

A **mast cell stabilizer** may be used for mild persistent or more severe asthma. A mast cell stabilizer protects mast cell membranes against rupture caused by antigenic substances. As a result, less histamine and fewer leukotrienes and prostaglandins are released in airway tissue. More information can be found in Table 11.1.

The mast cell stabilizer **cromolyn sodium** is a nebulized solution that works topically in the airways. It is a prophylactic drug with no benefit for acute reactions. Cromolyn sodium stabilizes mast cell membranes and directly inhibits other inflammatory cells.

Dosage Forms and Administration The airways must be open before administration, so a bronchodilator is often given first. This drug can be effective, but patient adherence can be problematic. Cromolyn sodium is dosed four times a day, and most patients have difficulty fitting the four doses into their daily routine. Cromolyn sodium is available in other dosage forms for use in other indications, so care must be taken to select the correct one.

Side Effects Cromolyn sodium has an unpleasant taste after inhalation, and side effects include hoarseness, dry mouth, and stuffy nose.

Contraindications Cromolyn sodium is contraindicated during acute asthma attacks.

Cautions and Considerations Use cromolyn sodium with caution in patients with kidney or liver dysfunction.

Drug Interactions Cromolyn sodium has no known drug interactions.

Monoclonal Antibodies

A **monoclonal antibody** is an antibody produced in a laboratory from an isolated specific lymphocyte that produces a pure antibody against a known specific antigen. Monoclonal antibody treatment is an injection-based treatment that is used in addition to inhalers and tablets. These asthma medications are used to help with uncontrolled asthma that has not responded to maximum doses or treatment with other therapies. These types of medications are generally used in patients with allergic asthma or eosinophilic asthma. **Allergic asthma** is asthma exacerbated by airborne allergens. **Eosinophilic asthma** causes individuals to have an increase in eosinophils, a type of white blood cell thought to cause inflammation.

Monoclonal antibodies include **benralizumab (Fasrena)**, **dupilumab (Dupixent)**, and **mepolizumab (Nucala)** and are used for adults and children over 12 years. They are not used for an acute event, as in status asthmaticus or asthma exacerbations. Most of these therapies inhibit interleukin-5 (IL-5), a cytokine that contributes to allergic asthma. **Omalizumab (Xolair)** blocks IgG, an immunoglobulin that is also involved in allergic asthma. These drugs are reserved for cases that have proven difficult to treat with other medications.

Dosage Forms and Administration Benralizumab, mepolizumab, **reslizumab (Cinqair)**, and omalizumab are all injected subcutaneously every two to four weeks. Patients can use these monoclonal antibody therapies at home with an auto-injector. Dupilumab, mepolizumab, omalizumab, and reslizumab may be injected by a healthcare provider in the office once a month.

Side Effects Side effects include injection site reactions, viral infections, sinusitis, headache, and pharyngitis.

Contraindications Benralizumab, dupilumab, and mepolizumab are contraindicated in patients with a known hypersensitivity reaction to these drugs.

Cautions and Considerations Benralizumab, omalizumab, and reslizumab have a boxed warning for hypersensitivity and anaphylactic reactions. These reactions can be immediate or delayed. Live vaccinations should not be given to patients taking dupilumab, as this drug can enhance the adverse effects of live vaccines.

Drug Interactions Omalizumab may increase the toxicities of belimumab and loxapine.

Xanthine Derivative

A **xanthine derivative** is structurally similar to caffeine and causes relaxation of smooth muscle within the airway. This leads to airway dilation and better air movement. Theophylline is the main drug within this class. See Table 11.1 for additional information.

Theophylline (Elixophyllin, Theo-24, Theochron) is a phosphodiesterase inhibitor that reverses early bronchospasm associated with antigens or irritants. Theophylline improves the contractility of the fatigued diaphragm. It can be used as a bronchodilator in reversible airway obstruction due to asthma, chronic bronchitis, or emphysema. Theophylline can also be used for neonatal (the first four weeks after birth) apnea and bradycardia. Blood levels should be maintained at 5 to 20 mcg/mL. Theophylline has many interactions, however, and blood levels can become elevated quickly. Consequently, it is used only for lung disease unresponsive to other drugs.

Dosage Forms and Administration Theophylline is available in a variety of dosage forms, including capsules, an elixir, an oral solution, a solution for injection, and a tablet formulation. For dosage forms administered orally, theophylline should be taken one hour before or two hours after a meal.

Side Effects Common adverse side effects include nausea, vomiting, headache, and insomnia.

Contraindications The premixed injection formulation may contain corn-derived dextrose, and its use is contraindicated in patients with allergies to corn-related products.

Cautions and Considerations Theophylline toxicity is a concern with use. Drug levels should be monitored in all patients using theophylline.

Drug Interactions Drug interactions with theophylline are numerous. Drugs that may interact with theophylline include adenosine; adrenaline-like drugs (e.g., ephedrine, phenylephrine, pseudoephedrine); allopurinol; antiarrhythmic drugs (e.g., mexiletine, propafenone); antiseizure drugs (e.g., carbamazepine, phenobarbital, phenytoin); benzodiazepines (e.g., diazepam, flurazepam); beta-blockers (e.g., propranolol); cimetidine; digoxin; disulfiram; fluvoxamine; interferons; isoproterenol; oral contraceptives; pentoxifylline; rifampin; riociguat; St. John's wort; sulfinpyrazone; tacrine; thiabendazole; ticlopidine; verapamil; and zileuton.

11.3 Chronic Obstructive Pulmonary Disease and Drug Treatments

Chronic obstructive pulmonary disease (COPD) refers to a group of chronic lung diseases that impede airflow and cause breathing difficulty. COPD is a long-term, progressive condition in which airflow is limited by an abnormal inflammatory response.

COPD is irreversible, which means lung function does not significantly improve with administration of bronchodilators. COPD progressively worsens, even with treatment.

On the positive side, COPD is largely preventable. Although some patients are genetically predisposed to developing COPD, most patients with COPD have a history of smoking or exposure to pollution or occupational hazards. Repeated respiratory infections can also contribute to this condition. COPD has several subtypes, including chronic bronchitis and emphysema.

Bronchitis is a condition in which the lining of the bronchial airways becomes inflamed, which obstructs airflow during expiration (see Figure 11.4). This disease is characterized by a cough that produces sputum (phlegm) that may be purulent (containing pus), green, or blood streaked. *Acute bronchitis* is caused by an infection, usually viral; it runs a brief course and is typically terminated by the body's immune responses, often with the aid of antibiotics to prevent or treat secondary bacterial infections. The infection that caused the acute bronchitis generally does not return. *Chronic bronchitis* is a serious disease, defined as excessive production of tracheobronchial mucus sufficient to cause cough with expectoration of at least 30 mL of sputum every 24 hours, for 3 months of the year and for more than 2 consecutive years. Patients usually are overweight, have a barrel chest, and tend to retain carbon dioxide. Most individuals have a morning cough resulting from irritation to the lungs.

Emphysema is characterized by destruction of the tiny alveoli, or air sacs, of the lungs (see Figure 11.1), which results in air accumulation in tissues and organs. Typically, air spaces distal to (farther away from) the terminal bronchioles are enlarged. Inflammation destroys these air sacs, which then lose their ability to expand and contract as well as to pass oxygen into the blood and remove carbon dioxide. In the early stages, shortness of breath occurs only after heavy exercise. As the disease progresses, walking even a short distance can make the patient gasp for air. Patients with emphysema have **tachypnea** (very rapid respiration), which gives them a flushed appearance. Major risk factors are cigarette smoking (which destroys the walls of the lungs), occupational exposure, air pollution, and genetic factors.

FIGURE 11.4
Chronic Bronchitis and Emphysema

Chronic bronchitis and emphysema are the two main types of COPD.

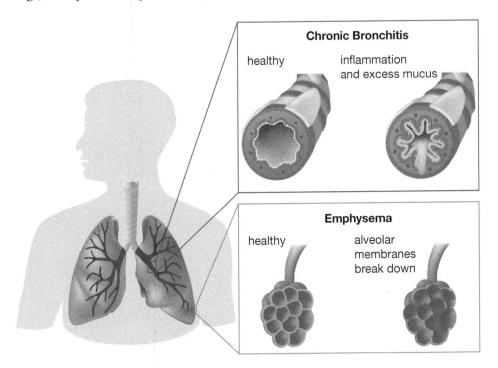

Several factors can contribute to the development of chronic bronchitis. The most prominent factors include cigarette smoke; exposure to occupational dusts, fumes, and environmental pollution; and bacterial infection. Studies of lungs from smoking and nonsmoking subjects clearly demonstrate that those individuals who smoke cigarettes have more bronchial inflammation.

Understanding the treatment for chronic bronchitis and emphysema, requires an understanding of the lungs' natural defense system. When this system is functioning properly, the host defenses of the respiratory tract provide good protection against pathogen invasion, and they remove potentially infectious agents from the lungs. The lungs are normally sterile below the first branch, and when organisms breach this region, infection and inflammation are initiated.

The lung's defenses include a number of different types of cells:

- The ciliary carpet consists of minute hairlike processes, called *cilia*, that move rhythmically to propel fluid or mucus. Any inhaled particles that have become trapped in the fluid are pushed over the inner surface of the airway, then up and out.

- Goblet cells secrete mucus.

- Clara cells, unciliated cells at the branching of the alveolar ducts into the bronchioles, secrete enzymes that break down airborne toxins.

- Epithelial cells produce a protein-rich exudate in the small bronchi and bronchioles.

- Alveolar macrophages help remove dust or microorganisms.

- Type I pneumocytes in the alveolar membranes act as the phagocytes of the lung. They clear waste and organisms from the lung.

- Type II pneumocytes synthesize and secrete surfactant, which lowers the surface tension of pulmonary fluids.

Figure 11.5 demonstrates the locations of various cells in the alveolus and its blood supply.

FIGURE 11.5
Cellular Makeup of an Alveolus

The alveolus contains several types of cells to help defend against pathogen invasion. The alveolus is also where gas exchange takes place.

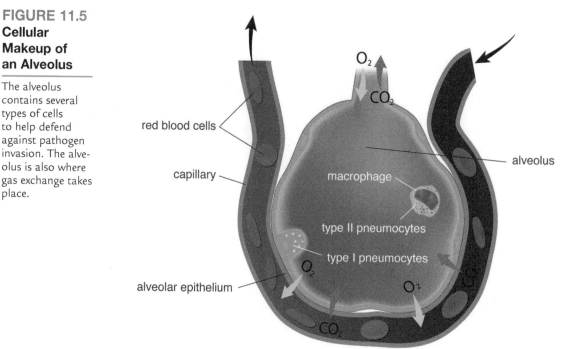

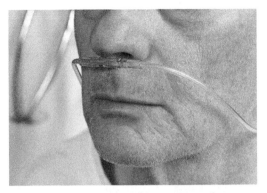
Oxygen can be a key part of the treatment for any patient who has COPD.

Emphysema and chronic bronchitis sometimes occur together, and their pharmacologic treatment is similar. The pharmacologic management of emphysema and bronchitis is still largely empirical, with beta-2 agonists, anticholinergics, and corticosteroids forming the foundation of therapy. Oxygen administration and physical therapy play an important role in treating both lung diseases. In both emphysema and chronic bronchitis, antibiotic therapy is sometimes needed if signs and symptoms of infection are present. Expectorants (discussed in greater detail later in the chapter) are sometimes used to stimulate respiratory secretions and counter dryness, which stimulates irritation and coughing. Drinking large amounts of water helps to break up mucus and enables the patient to cough up secretions; water is the expectorant of choice. Patients with COPD should always be encouraged to get influenza and pneumococcal vaccinations annually because this disease state predisposes them to flu and pneumonia. Table 11.2 identifies the commonly used agents to treat COPD.

TABLE 11.2 Commonly Used Agents to Treat COPD

Generic (Brand)	Pronunciation	Dosage Form	Common Dosage	Dispensing Status
Anticholinergics				
aclidinium (Tudorza Pressair)	a-kli-DIN-ee-um	powder for inhalation	400 mcg 2 times a day	Rx
glycopyrrolate (Lonhala Magnair)	glye-koe-PYE-roe-late	powder for inhalation, nebulizer solution	nebulizer: 25 mcg 2 times a day	Rx
ipratropium (Atrovent)	i-pra-TROE-pee-um	aerosol (MDI), nebulizer solution	MDI: 2 puffs 4 times a day nebulizer: 500 mcg 3–4 times a day	Rx
ipratropium / albuterol (DuoNeb, Combivent Respimat)	i-pra-TROE-pee-um al-BYOO-ter-awl	nebulizer solution, oral inhalation solution	nebulizer: 3 mL treatment 4 times a day oral inhalation solution: 1 inhalation 4 times a day	Rx
revefenacin (Yupelri)	REV-e-FEN-a-sin	nebulizer solution	175 mcg 1 time a day	Rx
tiotropium (Spiriva HandiHaler, Spiriva Respimat)	tye-oh-TROE-pee-um	oral inhalation solution, powder for inhalation	inhale contents of 1 capsule 1 time a day MDI: 2 puffs 1 time a day	Rx
umeclidinium (Incruse Ellipta)	ue-MEK-li-DIN-ee-um	powder for inhalation	1 inhalation 1 time a day	Rx
umeclidinium / vilanterol (Anoro Ellipta)	ue-MEK-li-DIN-ee-um vye-LAN-ter-ol	powder for inhalation	1 inhalation 1 time a day	Rx
Antitrypsin Deficiency Agent				
alpha-1 proteinase inhibitor (Aralast NP, Glassia, Prolastin-C, Zemaira)	AL-fuh-one PRO-tee-nase in-HIB-i-tor	injection	IV: 60 mg/kg 1 time a week	Rx

continues

TABLE 11.2 Commonly Used Agents to Treat COPD—*Continued*

Generic (Brand)	Pronunciation	Dosage Form	Common Dosage	Dispensing Status
Long-Acting Beta-2 Agonists				
arformoterol (Brovana)	ar-for-MOE-ter-awl	nebulizer solution	15 mcg 2 times a day	Rx
formoterol	for-MOE-ter-awl	nebulizer solution	20 mcg 2 times a day	Rx
olodaterol (Striverdi Respimat)	oh-loh-DAT-er-ole	solution for inhalation	2 inhalations 1 time a day	Rx
salmeterol* (Serevent)	sal-ME-te-role	powder for inhalation	1 inhalation 2 times a day	Rx
Mucolytics				
dornase alfa (Pulmozyme)	DOOR-nase AL-fuh	inhalation solution	2.5 mg 1 time a day	Rx
N-acetylcysteine (Mucomyst)	A-seh-til-SIS-teh-een	inhalation solution	20%: 3–5 mL 10%: 6–10 mL as directed by provider	Rx
Phosphodieserase-4 Enzyme Inhibitor				
roflumilast (Daliresp)	roe-FLOO-mi-last	tablet	250–500 mg 1 time a day	Rx
Combination Products for Asthma and/or COPD				
aclidinium / formoterol (Duaklir Pressair)	a-kli-DIN-ee-um for-MOE-ter-awl	aerosol (MDI)	1 inhalation 2 times a day	Rx
budesonide / formoterol (Symbicort)*	byoo-DES-oh-nide for-MOE-ter-awl	aerosol (MDI)	2 inhalations 2 times a day	Rx
fluticasone / salmeterol (Advair Diskus, Advair HFA, AirDuo Respiclick)*	floo-TIK-a-sone sal-ME-ter-awl	aerosol (MDI), powder for inhalation	MDI: 100 mcg/ 50–500 mcg/50 mcg 2 times a day HFA: 2 inhalations 2 times a day	Rx
fluticasone / vilanterol (Breo Ellipta)*	floo-TIK-a-sone vye-LAN-ter-ol	aerosol powder, breath activated	1 inhalation 1 time a day	Rx
fluticasone / umeclidinium / vilanterol (Trelegy Ellipta)*	floo-TIK-a-sone ue-MEK-li-DIN-ee-um vye-LAN-ter-ol	aerosol powder, breath activated	1 inhalation 1 time a day	Rx
glycopyrrolate / formoterol (Bevespi Aerosphere)	GLYE-koe-PIR-oh-late for-MOE-ter-awl	aerosol (MDI)	2 inhalations 2 times a day	Rx
ipratropium / albuterol (Combivent Respimat, DuoNeb)	i-pra-TROE-pee-um al-BYOO-ter-awl	nebulizer solution, oral inhalation solution	nebulizer: 3 mL 4 times a day oral inhalation: 1 inhalation 4 times a day	Rx
mometasone / formoterol (Dulera)	moe-MET-a-sone for-MOE-ter-awl	aerosol (MDI)	2 inhalations 2 times a day	Rx
tiotropium / olodaterol (Stiolto Respimat)	TYE-oh-TROE-pee-um oh-loh-DAT-er-ole	aerosol (MDI)	2 inhalations 1 time a day	Rx
umeclidinium / vilanterol (Anoro Ellipta)	ue-MEK-li-DIN-ee-um vye-LAN-ter-ol	aerosol powder, breath activated	1 inhalation 1 time a day	Rx

* This drug has an FDA indication for COPD and asthma.

Anticholinergics

Used as a first-line treatment for bronchoconstriction related to COPD, **anticholinergic agents** (see Table 11.2) work by inhibiting acetylcholine, a neurotransmitter that stimulates smooth muscle in the lungs to constrict. Anticholinergics are used when long-term bronchodilation is needed. The purpose of these agents is to prevent frequent COPD exacerbations, not to treat acute breathing problems after they begin. These agents improve the quality of life for patients with COPD and can reduce the need for hospitalization.

Side effects of anticholinergics include headache, flushed skin, blurred vision, tachycardia, and palpitations.

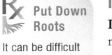

Put Down Roots

It can be difficult to remember which medication is an anticholinergic and which medication is a long-acting beta-2 agonist. The anticholinergic agents that target the respiratory system end in *–ium*. The long-acting beta-2 agonists that are used for respiratory disorders end in *–erol*.

Ipratropium

Ipratropium (Atrovent HFA) blocks the action of acetylcholine in bronchial smooth muscle, causing bronchodilation. It is derived from atropine and is used for prevention, not for acute management. Ipratropium is a short-acting agent and is not absorbed into general circulation when inhaled, so it usually does not cause arrhythmias. It is FDA approved for the treatment of COPD; however, it is sometimes used for emergency treatment of acute asthma exacerbations in combination with other drugs.

Dosage Forms and Administration Ipratropium is available as an aerosol (MDI) and a nebulizer solution.

Side Effects Side effects of anticholinergics include headache, flushed skin, blurred vision, tachycardia, and palpitations.

Contraindications Ipratropium is contraindicated in patients with a hypersensitivity to atropine.

Cautions and Considerations Ipratropium is not indicated for the initial treatment of acute episodes of bronchospasm where rescue therapy is required for a rapid response.

Drug Interactions Ipratropium should not be used with other anticholinergic products. The potential of orally administered potassium chloride to cause ulcers is increased with concurrent use.

Aclidinium

Aclidinium (Tudorza Pressair) is indicated for long-term maintenance treatment of bronchospasm associated with COPD.

Dosage Forms and Administration Aclidinium is available as a DPI with a dose counter. Unlike some other DPIs, aclidinium does not involve loading capsules into an inhaler.

Side Effects Side effects of anticholinergics include headache, flushed skin, blurred vision, tachycardia, and palpitations.

Contraindications Aclidinium does not have any contraindications.

Cautions and Considerations Aclidinium is not for the initial treatment of acute episodes of bronchospasm. The DPI contains lactose and should not be used by patients with severe milk protein allergy.

Drug Interactions Aclidinium should not be used with other anticholinergic drugs. The potential of orally administered potassium chloride to cause ulcers is increased with concurrent use.

Glycopyrrolate

Glycopyrrolate (Lonhala Magnair) is a long-acting anticholinergic used for COPD, including bronchitis and emphysema.

Dosage Forms and Administration Glycopyrrolate comes as a capsule containing a dry powder for oral inhalation. The patient must remove the capsule from a blister pack and insert it into the inhaler device in order to use it.

Side Effects Side effects of anticholinergics include headache, flushed skin, blurred vision, tachycardia, and palpitations.

Contraindications Glycopyrrolate can cause bronchospasm, so it should not be used to treat an acute episode of bronchospasm or rapidly deteriorating COPD. Glycopyrrolate should not be used by patients with lactose insensitivity.

Cautions and Considerations Patients should be cautioned not to swallow the capsule. It should only be used with the inhaler device provided. Glycopyrrolate should be used with caution in patients with glaucoma, urinary retention, benign prostatic hyperplasia (BPH), or heart disease such as arrhythmia.

Drug Interactions Glycopyrrolate should not be used with other anticholinergic products or potassium chloride. Glycopyrrolate can enhance the adverse effects of topiramate, thiazide diuretics, pramlintide, and cannabinoid-containing products. Glycopyrrolate can enhance the anticholinergic and constipating effects of opiate pain medications.

Revefenacin

Revefenacin (Yupelri) is indicated for long-term maintenance treatment of bronchospasm associated with COPD.

Dosage Forms and Administration Revefenacin is used as a nebulizer treatment once a day in combination with short-acting inhaled bronchodilators.

Side Effects The most common side effects for revefenacin include headache, runny nose, back pain, and elevated blood pressure.

Contraindications Revefenacin should not be used to treat an acute episode of bronchospasm or rapidly deteriorating COPD.

Cautions and Considerations Revefenacin should be used with caution in patients with glaucoma, urinary retention, BPH, or heart disease such as arrhythmia.

Drug Interactions Revefenacin should not be used with other anticholinergic products or potassium chloride. It can enhance the adverse effects of topiramate, thiazide diuretics, pramlintide, and cannabinoid-containing products. Revefenacin can enhance the anticholinergic and constipating effects of opiate pain medications.

Umeclidinium

Umeclidinium (Incruse Ellipta) is a long-acting anticholinergic COPD treatment. It is available alone (Incruse Ellipta) or combined with the long-acting beta-2 agonist vilanterol as Anoro Ellipta. Both products are indicated for maintenance treatment of airflow obstruction in patients who have COPD.

Dosage Forms and Administration Umeclidinium is available as a powder for inhalation and dosed once a day.

Side Effects Side effects of anticholinergics include headache, flushed skin, blurred vision, tachycardia, and palpitations.

Contraindications Umeclidinium is contraindicated in patients with a hypersensitivity to milk proteins.

Cautions and Considerations Umeclidinium should not be used for acute episodes of COPD. It should not be started in patients with significantly worsening COPD. Umeclidinium may worsen symptoms in patients with glaucoma and BPH.

Drug Interactions Anticholinergic agents may enhance the anticholinergic effects of umeclidinium. The adverse effects of glucagon may be enhanced with umeclidinium use. The ulcer-causing effects of oral potassium chloride may be enhanced with the use of anticholinergic agents such as umeclidinium.

Tiotropium

Tiotropium (Spiriva Handihaler) is a long-acting anticholinergic and is dosed once daily, although it works for approximately 36 hours. It is indicated only for long-term maintenance therapy for bronchospasms associated with emphysema and chronic bronchitis.

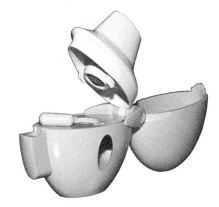

Practice Tip

Tiotropium and some glycopyrrolate formulations are dispensed as a capsule for *inhalation* that is administered using a DPI. Patients can find this confusing and have been reported to erroneously swallow the capsules. Swallowing the capsules will not have the intended therapeutic effect.

Dosage Forms and Administration Tiotropium is provided by the manufacturer in two forms. One is a capsule for inhalation (Spiriva HandiHaler). In this form, one capsule is placed in the HandiHaler, and the button (located on the side of the HandiHaler device) is pressed, which punctures the capsule and allows for the

Tiotropium is available in two dosage formulations. The dry powder inhaler involves inserting a capsule that contains the tiotropium powder into the HandiHaler device. The second formulation is an MDI.

dispersement of powder into the inhaler. After the inhaler is used, the empty capsule should be disposed of in a proper container. The dry powder should not be touched. This drug is sensitive to moisture and heat, and the capsule should not be exposed before the patient is ready to use it. Therefore, the patient needs to know that the package should be peeled back only to the STOP mark. The second form of tiotropium is an MDI (Spiriva Respimat), which is FDA approved for the treatment of asthma.

Side Effects Dry mouth is a common side effect of tiotropium. Side effects of anticholinergics include headache, flushed skin, blurred vision, tachycardia, and palpitations.

Contraindications Tiotropium should not be used by patients who have lactose sensitivity.

Cautions and Considerations Tiotropium capsules are used only with an inhaler device; they should not be swallowed. Patients should take care to follow instructions for puncturing the capsule and inhaling the powder using the inhaler device.

Drug Interactions Tiotropium should not be used with other anticholinergic drugs. The potential of orally administered potassium chloride to cause ulcers is increased with concurrent use.

Antitrypsin Deficiency Agent

Alpha-1 proteinase inhibitor (Aralast NP, Glassia, Prolastin-C, Zemaira), also known as alpha-1 antitrypsin, is a less common therapy indicated for the treatment of emphysema in patients with alpha-1 antitrypsin deficiency. It is an intravenous (IV) drug that works by inhibiting phosphodiesterase-4 (antitrypsin), thereby preventing leukocytes and neutrophils from infiltrating the lungs.

Dosage Forms and Administration Pharmacy technicians should be mindful of infusion rates. Aralast NP and Glassia should be infused at a rate of ≤0.2 mL/kg/minute. Prolastin-C and Zemaira should be infused at approximately 0.08 mL/kg/minute.

Side Effects Side effects include headache, pharyngitis, dizziness, and increased cough.

Contraindications This drug should be used only in patients who have emphysema due to a congenital deficiency of alpha-1 proteinase inhibitor. It is administered once weekly.

Cautions and Considerations Alpha-1 proteinase inhibitor is made from human plasma and therefore carries the risk of transmitting infectious agents. It cannot be mixed with other agents or diluting solutions. Alpha-1 proteinase inhibitor can be infused at home.

Drug Interactions Alpha-1 proteinase inhibitor has no known significant drug interactions.

Long-Acting Beta-2 Agonists

Used for both COPD and asthma, a **long-acting beta-2 agonist (LABA)** works in a way that is similar to the action of short-acting beta-2 agonists (discussed earlier in this chapter). A LABA simply does not have to be administered as frequently. Used more often for COPD, the long-acting agents can also be used for severe asthma. For a list of common long-acting beta-2 agonists, see Table 11.2.

Formoterol (Perforomist) is a long-acting bronchodilator approved for the long-term maintenance treatment of bronchoconstriction in patients with COPD, including bronchitis and emphysema. It is a selective beta-2 agonist, which means that it acts locally in the lungs to relax smooth muscle and inhibit the release of mast cells. It has a faster onset than salmeterol, working within minutes.

Arformoterol (Brovana) is a LABA indicated for long-term COPD therapy. Structurally, it is similar to formoterol; it is the active isomer of formoterol.

Olodaterol (Striverdi Respimat) is another LABA indicated for COPD.

Salmeterol (Serevent) is indicated for maintenance therapy of asthma and COPD. It has a long duration of action, and its onset of action is 30 to 60 minutes.

Dosage Forms and Administration Formoterol is only available as a nebulizer solution. Formoterol must be refrigerated until dispensed. It may be stored at room temperature after dispensing, but it must be discarded after three months if not used. The pharmacy technician must mark on the box the date after which the drug should not be used. This date is either the expiration date or three months after the drug was dispensed, whichever comes first.

Olodaterol is formulated as a soft-mist inhaler that is used once daily.

Salmeterol is taken twice a day. When used for asthma, it should be reserved for individuals who are already receiving anti-inflammatory therapy. Its long duration of action makes it particularly useful for nocturnal symptoms of asthma. Salmeterol is available as a DPI.

Side Effects Common side effects for LABAs include dizziness, heartburn, nausea, and tremors. LABAs can cause cardiac effects, including increased blood pressure and tachycardia. Patients with high blood pressure or heart problems should discuss the side effects of these beta agonists with their physicians before using them.

The most common side effect of formoterol is tremors.

Contraindications LABAs should not be used as monotherapy (use of a single drug to treat a disorder or disease) for patients with asthma. Patients with asthma should always take an inhaled corticosteroid, such as fluticasone, concurrently with the LABA. Even though formoterol has a quick onset, it should not be used to treat acute asthma. Arformoterol is contraindicated in patients with a hypersensitivity to formoterol.

Cautions and Considerations LABAs carry a boxed warning for an increased risk of asthma-related death. Formoterol and arformoterol should not be used in acutely deteriorating patients.

Salmeterol carries an additional boxed warning for the risk of asthma-related hospitalization in pediatric and adolescent patients.

Salmeterol should not be used to treat rescue situations. Improper use of this drug has been implicated in deaths.

Drug Interactions Beta blockers may reduce the effectiveness of LABAs. Tricyclic antidepressants, MAO inhibitors, xanthine derivatives (caffeine, theoromine), and drugs that prolong the QTc interval (e.g., amiodarone, erythromycin, amitriptyline, haloperidol) may increase the effect on the cardiovascular system. The use of steroids and diuretics may increase the risk of hypokalemia and should be used with caution.

Patients should not take salmeterol with other LABAs due to an increased risk of toxicities.

Drugs that should not be used with salmeterol include darunavir, fosamprenavir, indinavir, lopinavir, nelfinavir, and ritonavir.

Mucolytics

Safety Alert

Watch for injectable acetycysteine (Acetadote), which is used to treat acetaminophen toxicity, versus inhalation formulation, which is used as a mucolytic. Both come in vials that look alike, but confusion could result in a serious error.

Name Exchange

Some pharmacy personnel use the name "Mucomyst" to identify a drug as an inhaled mist. Note that Mucomyst is a brand that is no longer on the market.

Another treatment for chronic bronchitis is the use of a **mucolytic** (an agent that destroys or dissolves mucus), such as **N-acetylcysteine**, which breaks apart glycoproteins, thereby reducing viscosity (resistance to flow, or thickness and stickiness) and promoting easier movement and removal of secretions. Another mucolytic, **dornase alfa (Pulmozyme)**, is discussed in the section concerning cystic fibrosis.

Dosage Forms and Administration N-acetylcysteine is available as an inhalation solution and is administered three to four times per day. N-acetylcysteine is also available as an injection for acetaminophen toxicity, but its use for this indication is not discussed in this chapter.

Side Effects Side effects include bronchospasm, bronchitis, nausea, vomiting, and runny nose.

Contraindications N-acetylcysteine has no known contraindications.

Cautions and Considerations Caution should be used in patients with a history of bronchospasm since these patients have an increased risk of hypersensitivity reactions. Acetylcysteine may be confused with acetycholine. Additionally, many may still refer to N-acetylcystine by its trade name Mucomyst, even though it is no longer available. The brand name Mucomyst may be confused with Mucinex.

Drug Interactions N-acetylcysteine has no known significant drug interactions.

Phosphodiesterase-4 Enzyme Inhibitor

Roflumilast (Daliresp), which is a phosphodiesterase-4 enzyme inhibitor made in tablet form, is used to treat severe COPD. It reduces lung inflammation. It should only be used to treat severe COPD, because in less serious cases, the side effects may not outweigh the benefit of the drug. It is an add-on therapy to decrease exacerbations. It also has several interactions with other medications and serious side effects, including mental health problems such as suicidal thoughts.

Dosage Forms and Administration Roflumilast is available in a tablet formulation that is taken daily by mouth.

Side Effects The most frequently reported side effects include diarrhea, nausea, headache, back pain, insomnia, weight loss, dizziness, and decreased appetite. In addition, it is important to know that neuropsychiatric effects such as anxiety, depression, and insomnia have been reported.

Contraindications Roflumilast should not be used in patients with moderate to severe liver impairment.

Cautions and Considerations In addition to the neuropsychiatric effects listed earlier, cases of suicidal behavior or ideation have been reported, and patients should report psychiatric symptoms. Due to the potential for weight loss, patients should monitor their weight regularly.

Drug Interactions Strong inhibitors of CYP3A4, like erythromycin, ketoconazole, fluvaxamine, enaxacin, and cimetidine, can increase roflumilast concentrations and increase adverse reactions. Inducers of CYP3A4, such as rifampicin, phenobarbital, carbamezapine, and phenytoin, should not be used with roflumilast.

Combination Products for Asthma and COPD

To improve patient adherence and ease of administration, several LABAs are available as combination products (see Table 11.2). Pharmacy technicians should keep in mind that combination products have the side effects, contraindications, cautions, and drug interactions of both drugs they comprise.

Aclidinium / formoterol (Duaklir Pressair) is a combination of anticholinergic and LABA indicated for COPD. Patients with milk allergy (lactose intolerance) should not use this product. This inhaler is breath activated, so the patient must close their lips tightly around the mouthpiece and inhale until they hear a click, meaning the full dose has been administered. Patients will know that the inhaler is ready to use when the control window shows green.

Budesonide / formoterol (Symbicort) is a combination MDI containing a corticosteroid and LABA that is indicated for use in both asthma and COPD. It should be used for maintenance treatment and not for the relief of acute bronchospasm. Prior to each

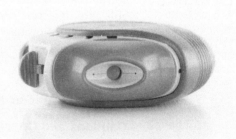

Some DPIs look like a discus and are actuated by breathing in deeply at the opening.

use, the inhaler needs to be shaken. In addition, prior to using the device for the first time, the inhaler needs to be primed by releasing two sprays.

Fluticasone / salmeterol (Advair Diskus, Advair HFA, AirDuo Respiclick) is an anti-inflammatory and beta-2 agonist used for maintenance treatment of asthma and COPD for patients older than 12 years. Fluticasone, a corticosteroid, is a potent vasoconstrictor and anti-inflammatory. Salmeterol is a LABA and relaxes bronchial smooth muscle with little effect on heart rate. Together, the two drugs act synergistically to improve pulmonary function.

Fluticasone / vilanterol (Breo Ellipta) is a corticosteroid and a LABA that is used for both asthma and COPD. The inhaler is breath activated. Each time the cover is removed from the mouthpiece, a dose is prepared, so patients should only take the cover off when they are ready to use the inhaler. This product has several side effects that providers should monitor, including high blood pressure, high blood sugar, headache, sore throat, oral thrush, flu-like symptoms, joint pain, runny nose, pneumonia, upper respiratory tract infection, and fever. Patients should report any of these effects to their provider.

Fluticasone / umeclidinium / vilanterol (Trelegy Ellipta) is another breath-activated inhaler used for COPD. As with fluticasone / vilanterol, a dose of medication is prepared each time the cover is removed. Patients should remove the cover only when they are ready to use the inhaler. This inhaler is intended for long-term treatment and should not be used to treat an acute exacerbation of COPD. As with other corticosteroids, prolonged use may lead to inadequate cortisol production. Discontinuing this medication must be done slowly, not abruptly.

Glycopyrrolate / formoterol (Bevespi Aerosphere) is a combination of an anticholinergic and a LABA used for maintenance treatment of COPD. Prior to use, this inhaler must be primed by releasing four test sprays into the air away from the face and eyes. The inhaler must be reprimed if it hasn't been used for seven days. This inhaler is not intended for rescue treatment of an acute episode of bronchospasm.

Ipratropium / albuterol (Combivent Respimat, DuoNeb) is available as a combination inhaler (Combivent Respimat) and as a solution for nebulizer use (DuoNeb). It is used for COPD patients who require a second inhaler.

Mometasone / formoterol (Dulera) is a combination LABA for maintenance treatment of asthma. Mometasone is the same corticosteroid used in asthma treatment, and it is also used for seasonal allergies, which are discussed later in the chapter. Prior to first use, a mometasone / formoterol inhaler must be primed by releasing four sprays into the air, away from the face and eyes. If it has been more than five days since the last use, the inhaler must be primed again. This product contains a dose counter. Do not remove the drug canister from the actuator, because it may cause inhaler malfunction.

Tiotropium / olodaterol (Stiolto Respimat) is a combination anticholinergic and LABA used for COPD. The inhaler must be primed before first use or if it hasn't been used for more than 21 days. The inhaler should be primed by pointing it toward the ground and spraying it until a cloud appears from the mouthpiece. This product should not be used in patients with heart disease, diabetes, or hyperthyroidism. It should be used with caution in patients with glaucoma, urinary retention, BPH, or history of seizures.

Umeclidinium / vilanterol (Anoro Ellipta) is a dry powder inhaler containing an anticholinergic and LABA used for COPD. The inhaler should not be shaken prior to use. Patients simply remove the cover from the mouthpiece, and a dose is prepared. A click should be heard when the cover is removed—that is the cue to the patient that the dose is ready. If no click is heard, the dose is not ready. Patients should only remove the cover when ready to use it. Like the other combination inhaler products listed here, this inhaler is intended for long-term treatment and should not be used to treat an acute exacerbation of COPD.

11.4 Cystic Fibrosis and Drug Treatments

Cystic fibrosis (CF) is a hereditary disease that involves the gastrointestinal (GI) and respiratory systems. CF can be a fatal disease, with some patients dying in early adulthood. Many health consequences associated with CF are a result of pulmonary manifestations of the disease. GI involvement can be significant. It is due to increased viscosity of secreted mucus, which blocks the bile ducts, and a relative deficiency of pancreatic digestive enzymes. Most patients with CF must take pancreatic enzyme and vitamin supplements so that they can meet their nutritional needs.

Patients with CF experience hypoxia (lack of adequate oxygen), resulting in cyanosis, and in some cases, digital clubbing (enlarged fingertips with loss of normal angle at the nail bed). A patient's respiratory status follows a cyclic pattern, from a state of relative well-being to one of acute pulmonary deterioration. Management of the pulmonary aspect of this disease requires two approaches: respiratory therapy and antibiotic therapy.

Respiratory therapy for CF is referred to as *airway clearance therapy* (ACT). A critical part of ACT is **percussion**, a tapping movement to induce cough and expectoration of sputum from the lungs. In addition to percussion, patients are started on drug treatment at a young age. Drug treatment involves nebulizer therapy with medications that are inhaled to liquefy pulmonary secretions.

Bronchodilators, such as beta-2 agonists and anticholinergics, are used to improve airflow obstruction in CF. Additional agents used to clear airway secretions include inhaled **dornase alfa (Pulmozyme)**, hypertonic saline, and N-acetylcysteine. Oral N-acetylcysteine has an unpleasant taste and odor, and some patients prefer not to use it. In addition to these inhaled medications, patients are also given oral **azithromycin (Zithromax)** and high-dose ibuprofen on a regular basis. These drugs help to prevent infection and have anti-inflammatory effects. More information on azithromycin can be found in Chapter 16.

Antibiotics for Cystic Fibrosis

Antibiotics are used to combat the pathogens that take root in the thickened respiratory mucous secretions present in CF. The infectious organism(s) must be identified so that the appropriate antibiotic can be prescribed. Possible systemic antibiotics given intravenously include amikacin, azithromycin, aztreonam, cefepime, ceftazidime, ciprofloxacin, colistin, doxycycline, gentamicin, imipenem / cilastatin, linezolid, meropenem, piperacillin / tazobactam, tobramycin, and vancomycin. More information on these antibiotics can be found in Chapter 16.

Regular treatment with nebulized antibiotics directed against *Pseudomonas aeruginosa* appears to improve lung function and is recommended for many patients who have CF. Inhaled antibiotics commonly used in the treatment of CF include aztreonam (Cayston) and tobramycin (Bethkis, Kitabis Pak, TOBI, TOBI Podhaler).

Aztreonam (Cayston) is an inhaled antibiotic used to improve respiratory symptoms in patients who have CF. It is for adults and children seven years and older who have certain bacteria in their lungs. Like other antibiotics, even if symptoms improve, it must be used for the full length of the prescription. **Tobramycin (Bethkis, Kitabis Pak, TOBI, TOBI Podhaler)** is an aminoglycoside antibiotic.

Dosage Forms and Administration Aztreonam is available in an inhalation form and injection form, but for use in cystic fibrosis, the inhalation form is used. The aztreonam for inhalation is a powder that must be mixed with a provided diluent prior to nebulization. The reconstituted solution must be used immediately after it is mixed. It may be used only with an Altera nebulizer. Doses must be spaced at least four hours apart.

TABLE 11.3 Commonly Used Agents for Cystic Fibrosis

Generic (Brand)	Pronunciation	Dosage Form	Common Dosage	Dispensing Status
Antibiotics				
azithromycin (Zithromax)	az-ith-roe-MYE-sin	tablet, oral suspension	250–500 mg 1 time a day	Rx
aztreonam (Cayston)	AZ-tree-oh-nam	inhalation solution	75 mg 3 times a day	Rx
tobramycin (Bethkis, Kitabis Pak, TOBI, TOBI Podhaler)	toe-bra-MYE-sin	capsule for inhalation, inhalation solution	capsule for inhalation: 112 mg 2 times a day inhalation solution: 300 mg 2 times a day	Rx
Mucolytic				
dornase alfa (Pulmozyme)	DOOR-nase AL-fa	inhalation solution	2.5 mg 1 time a day	Rx
CFTR Modulators				
ivacaftor (Kalydeco)	eye-va-KAF-tor	tablet oral granules	150 mg 2 times a day	Rx
lumacaftor / ivacaftor (Orkambi)	LOO-ma-KAF-tor eye-va-KAF-tor	tablet oral granules	pediatric dose varies based on age and weight; patients age 12 years and older: 200 mg/125 mg, 2 tablets every 12 hr	Rx
tezacaftor / ivacaftor (Symdeko)	TEZ-a-KAF-tor eye-va-KAF-tor	tablet	pediatric dose varies based on age and weight; patients age 12 years and older: 100 mg/150 mg, 1 tablet in the morning; 1 tablet ivacaftor 150 mg in the evening	Rx
elexacaftor/ivacaftor/ tezacaftor (Trikafta)	el-EX-ah-KAFF-tor eye-va-KAF-tor TEZ-a-KAF-tor	tablet	100 mg/75 mg/50 mg, 2 tablets in the morning; 1 tablet ivacaftor 150 mg in the evening; 12 hr apart	Rx

Tobramycin is available in multiple dosage forms. For use in the management of *Pseudomonas aeruginosa* bacteria in patients with CF, nebulization solutions and a capsule for inhalation are used. Nebulization solutions should be used with the PARI LC PLUS reusable nebulizer. Bethkis requires using the PARI Vios air compressor and Kitabis Pak; TOBI should be used with the DeVilbiss Pulmo-Aide air compressor. The nebulizer solution is inhaled for 15 minutes. The TOBI Podhaler is a DPI with capsules that should be administered by oral inhalation via the Podhaler device, following manufacturer recommendations for use and handling. Capsules should be removed from the blister packaging immediately prior to use and should not be swallowed.

Side Effects Side effects include cough, nasal congestion, wheezing, and nasal passage and throat pain.

Side effects of tobramycin include cough, sore throat, hoarse voice, shortness of breath, throat pain, runny nose, headache, discoloration of sputum, altered sense of taste, bloody nose, and noisy breathing.

Contraindications There are no contraindications to azithromycin and aztreonam therapy. Tobramycin therapy should not be used if a hypersensitivity to tobramycin or other aminoglycosides exists.

Cautions and Considerations Due to the potential for bronchospasm with treatment, a bronchodilator should be given to the patient before treatment with aztreonam.

If multiple different nebulizer treatments are required, the bronchodilator should be administered first, followed by chest physiotherapy, any other nebulized medications, and then tobramycin last.

Drug Interactions No major drug interactions with the inhalation form exist.

Loop diuretics such as furosemide may enhance the nephrotoxic and ototoxic effects of tobramycin. Systemic mannitol should not be used with inhaled tobramycin due to the increased nephrotoxic risk.

Mucolytics for Cystic Fibrosis

Dornase alfa (Pulmozyme) selectively breaks down deoxyribonucleic acid (DNA) in the sputum of CF patients. Patients with cystic fibrosis have very high concentrations of extracellular DNA in their pulmonary sections that has been accumulated in response to infection. By destroying DNA in the mucus, dornase alfa helps reduce secretion viscosity.

Pancreatic Enzymes for Cystic Fibrosis

Because CF affects the GI system and pancreas, most patients must take special vitamins and **pancreatic enzyme supplements** specifically for treatment of CF. These supplements help prevent ductal obstructions and **steatorrhea** (fatty, foul-smelling diarrhea that occurs when dietary fat is not absorbed). They improve growth and life expectancy for children with CF. Several pancreatic enzyme supplements are available. Some common brand names include Creon, Pancreaze, Pertzye, Ultresa, Viokase, and Zenpep. All pancreatic enzyme supplements contain varying amounts of **lipase**, **protease**, and **amylase**. Pancreatic dysfunction also contributes to **malabsorption** (faulty absorption of nutrients), especially of fat-soluble vitamins. Therefore, many patients with CF take supplements containing vitamins A, D, E, and K.

CFTR Modulators

As mentioned previously, cystic fibrosis is a genetic disorder. It is caused by a defect in the cystic fibrosis transmembrane conductance regulator (CFTR) gene responsible for producing the CFTR protein. A defect in the gene can result in no protein, too little protein, or incorrect protein. This faulty gene leads cells to struggle to move salt and water across the cell wall, which can cause a buildup of thick mucus in the lungs and airways.

Significant advancements in the treatment of cystic fibrosis have been made during the past several years. Several gene therapies have been created that target specific gene defects associated with cystic fibrosis rather than treating symptoms like many therapies. **Gene therapy** is the process of altering genes inside the body to treat or prevent disease.

These therapies include **ivacaftor**, **lumacaftor / ivacaftor**, **tezacaftor / ivacaftor**, and **elexacaftor / ivacaftor / tezacaftor**. Table 11.3 identifies these common gene therapies.

Ivacaftor (Kalydeco) is a CFTR potentiator indicated for the treatment of CF in patients age six months and older who have one mutation in the CFTR.

Lumacaftor / ivacaftor (Orkambi) is a CFTR potentiator indicated for the treatment of CF in patients age two years and older who are homozygous for the F508del mutation.

Tezacaftor / ivacaftor (Symdeko) is indicated for the treatment of patients with CF age six years and older who have two copies of the F508del mutation or who have at least one mutation in the CFTR gene that is responsive to tezacaftor / ivacaftor based on in vitro data or clinical evidence.

Elexacaftor / ivacaftor / tezacaftor (Trikafta) is a triple combination therapy approved to treat patients who have at least one F508del mutation in the CFTR gene, the most common cystic fibrosis mutation, estimated to represent 90% of population with cystic fibrosis. It is used in adults and children older than 12 years.

Dosage Forms and Administration CFTR modulators are available in tablet form. Lumacaftor / ivacaftor is available in both tablet and granule form.

Side Effects Side effects of these therapies include headache, nausea, sinus congestion, and dizziness.

Contraindications There are no contraindications for these therapies.

Cautions and Considerations These medications may increase values on liver function tests (LFTs), so monitoring is recommended. Cataracts have been reported in pediatric patients, so monitoring is advised. These therapies should always be taken with food that contains fat, but they should not be taken with food containing grapefruit or Seville oranges.

Drug Interactions Some medications, such as rifampin, rifabutin, carbamazepine, and St. John's wort, can decrease the effectiveness of ivacaftor, lumacaftor / ivacaftor, tezacaftor / ivacaftor, and elexacaftor / ivacaftor / tezacaftor and should not be given. Lumacaftor / ivacaftor can also impact other medications. Immunosuppressant medicines (e.g., sirolimus, tacrolimus, everolimus), certain sedatives (e.g., midazolam, triazolam), antifungals (e.g., itraconazole, voriconazole), and macrolide antibiotics (e.g., erythromycin, clarithromycin) should be avoided. Patients should be counseled that lumacaftor / ivacaftor may decrease the effectiveness of hormonal birth control.

The dosing regimen of tezacaftor / ivacaftor should be adjusted when coadministered with moderate and strong CYP3A4 inhibitors.

Concomitant use of elexacaftor / ivacaftor / tezacaftor with strong CYP3A4 inducers (e.g., rifampin, St. John's wort) is not recommended.

11.5 Other Lung Diseases and Drug Treatments

Many other lung disorders exist in addition to those discussed previously in this chapter. Several measures can be taken to prevent and control lung disease and infection. Not smoking is one way to help prevent lung disease. Avoiding secondhand smoke and air pollution is also important. Influenza and pneumococcal pneumonia often can be prevented with vaccination. Most infections occur when sneezing or coughing exposes people to fluids or droplets that contain bacteria, viruses, or fungi. It has long been thought that respiratory infections are transmitted through inhalation, but recent studies have shown that hand contact is the most frequent culprit. Thus, frequent handwashing and avoiding close contact with infected hosts are the best defense.

TABLE 11.4 Commonly Used Agents for Other Lung Disorders

Generic (Brand)	Pronunciation	Dosage Form	Common Dosage	Dispensing Status
Surfactants				
beractant (Survanta)	ber-AKT-ant	intratracheal suspension	4 mL/kg	Rx
calfactant (Infasurf)	kal-FAK-tant	intratracheal suspension	3 mL/kg	Rx
poractant alfa (Curosurf)	por-AKT-ant AL-fa	intratracheal suspension	2.5 mL/kg	Rx
Antitubercular Agents				
ethambutol	eh-THAM-byoo-tawl	tablet	weight based: 800–1,600 mg 1 time a day	Rx
isoniazid	eye-soe-NYE-a-zid	injection, oral liquid, tablet	300 mg a day	Rx
pyrazinamide	peer-a-ZIN-a-mide	tablet	weight based: 1,000–2,000 mg 1 time a day	Rx
rifampin (Rifadin, Rimactane)	rif-AM-pin	capsule, injection	600 mg a day	Rx
rifapentine (Priftin)	RIF-a-pen-teen	tablet	10–20 mg/kg 1 time a week during continuation phase	Rx
Antifungal Therapy / Histoplasmosis Treatment				
amphotericin B (Abelcet, Ambisome)	am-fuh-TAYR-ih-sin bee	injection	IV: Liposomal AmB: 3 mg/kg/day AmB lipid complex 5 mg/kg/day AmB deoxycholate 0.7–1 mg/kg/day	Rx
itraconazole (Sporanox, Tolsura)	IH-truh-KAH-nuh-zole	capsule, oral solution	Sporanox: 200 mg 3 times a day for 3 days, then 200 mg 2 times a day Tolsura: 130 mg 1 time a day	Rx

Pneumonia

Pneumonia is a common lung infection that affects individuals of all ages. The microorganisms that cause pneumonia gain access to the lower respiratory tract by the following three routes:

- inhalation of aerosolized particles
- entry through the bloodstream
- aspiration of oropharyngeal contents.

Aspiration, which involves inhalation of fluids from the mouth and throat, is a common occurrence in both healthy and ill individuals during sleep. It is the major mechanism by which pulmonary pathogens gain access to the normally sterile lower airways and alveoli.

Pneumonia is treated with antibiotics, depending on the causative organism (see Chapter 16 for information on antibiotics). Patients who get pneumonia from exposure outside of an inpatient facility have **community-acquired pneumonia (CAP)**. Pneumonia that is acquired while an individual is hospitalized or living in a long-term care facility is called **nosocomial pneumonia**. Nosocomial pneumonia is severe and difficult to treat because it is usually caused by pathogens that are more virulent than those that cause CAP. Patients in the hospital setting encounter such pathogens because they are near other sick patients who have these infections.

Respiratory Distress Syndrome

Respiratory distress syndrome (RDS) occurs in neonates (infants) during the first few hours of life. It is characterized by inadequate production of pulmonary **surfactant**: a fluid that, like a soap bubble, lowers the surface tension between the air and alveolar surfaces. This helps keep the lungs and the alveoli open. Lack of surfactant leads to collapse of the alveoli and the inability to obtain enough oxygen. This lack of oxygen can lead to damage to the baby's brain and other organs, so immediate treatment is needed. Prematurity and maternal diabetes are two known causative factors of RDS. If RDS occurs, a replacement surfactant is administered intratracheally.

Table 11.4 lists the replacement surfactant products used to treat RDS.

Beractant (Survanta) is a natural bovine lung extract. Beractant prevents the alveoli from collapsing during expiration by lowering the surface tension between the air and alveolar surfaces. Beractant is used for prophylactic therapy in high-risk infants and for rescue therapy within eight hours of birth.

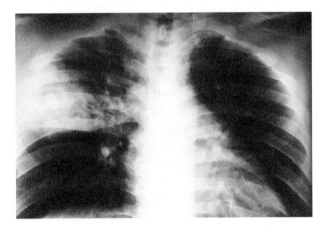

This image is an example of an x-ray of a patient with tuberculosis infection (middle lobe).

Calfactant (Infasurf) is indicated for neonates who are less than 72 hours of age. When taking this drug, infants may require less oxygen than with other RDS drugs. The drug should be stored in the refrigerator. The suspension settles and should be swirled gently but not shaken to redisperse the medication. It is not necessary to warm calfactant before administration. Vials that have been stored unopened at room temperature for less than 24 hours may be safely returned to the refrigerator.

Poractant alfa (Curosurf) may be preferred for very tiny babies because it requires much less fluid than the other RDS drugs and can be administered in one dose. With some of the other drugs, a partial dose must be administered and then another partial dose given two to three hours later.

Dosage Forms and Administration Beractant, calfactant, and poractant alfa are available as suspensions for intratracheal administration.

Side Effects Common side effects include bradycardia, hypotension, endotracheal tube blockage, and oxygen desaturation.

Contraindications These agents have no known contraindications to therapy.

Cautions and Considerations Patients need to be monitored and assessed frequently to modify oxygen and ventilatory support.

Drug Interactions These three agents have no known drug interactions.

Tuberculosis

Tuberculosis (TB) is caused by the bacterium *Mycobacterium tuberculosis*. The disease most commonly affects the lungs, but it may also infect other body tissues and organs. TB is transmitted by respiratory droplets inhaled into the lungs of individuals at risk. Respiratory droplets are produced when infected persons with active TB cough, sneeze, speak, kiss, or spit. Once inhaled, *M. tuberculosis* may spread throughout the body in the bloodstream and in lymphatic fluids. A follicle forms and is surrounded by epithelial cells. The mass may spread or liquefy, forming a cavity filled with fluid and organisms. The fluid may move in the direction of least resistance, spreading organisms and disease within the organ, thereby destroying more tissue (called *fibrosis*). *M. tuberculosis* thrives in areas of high oxygen, so resulting lesions concentrate primarily in the lungs. However, lesions may also occur in bone and kidney tissue.

Tuberculosis is seen primarily in patients with substance abuse disorder, prison populations, immunocompromised individuals, and older adults. It should be included in the differential diagnosis of patients with fever of unknown origin, subacute meningitis, or chronic infection at any site.

Two groups of tuberculosis patients are distinguished by their disease symptoms and antibody production:

- Exposed but showing no disease (latent disease): If time has elapsed since exposure, these patients produce TB antibodies and may have a positive tuberculin skin test (TST). This test result does not mean they have active disease.

- Exposed and having active disease: These patients may or may not produce antibodies, depending on the competence of their immune systems. Significant signs and symptoms of active disease include weight loss, blood in the sputum, night sweats and night fever, chest pain, and malaise.

The agent used for TSTs is **purified protein derivative (PPD)** from killed bacteria. This product is injected intradermally. Individuals who have been exposed to or have the disease show a circular area of hardened tissue (**induration**) at the injection site within 72 hours. A false-negative reaction may occur in individuals recently exposed and in older adults who have delayed-type hypersensitivity. If the reading is positive, the patient should have a chest x-ray taken to check for a lung shadow, which may indicate active disease.

Tuberculosis generally develops slowly and may take as long as 20 years to develop from the time of exposure. The highest incidence of infection occurs one to two years after exposure. Even if the disease is arrested early (4 to 10 weeks after exposure), a patient still has a risk of reactivity for the remainder of that patient's life. The organism can lie dormant for years, until the immune system is depressed, when the organism may reemerge as an active infection. The medical history of the patient should be watched for disease symptoms such as weight loss, fever, night sweats, malaise, and loss of appetite.

The goals of TB therapy are to initiate treatment promptly, convert the sputum culture from positive to negative, achieve cure without relapse, and prevent emergence of drug-resistant strains. The intensive or initial phase of treatment consists of a four-drug regimen, taken for two months. The drugs in this regimen include isoniazid, rifampin, pyrazinamide, and ethambutol. After the intensive treatment phase and a repeat assessment, patients may proceed to the continuation phase of treatment consisting of two drugs, isoniazid and rifampin, taken for four additional months. Table 11.4 describes the most common antitubercular agents. Patients should be given combination therapy with multiple drugs to prevent drug-resistant TB from developing. The most challenging part of TB therapy is that it must be taken for at least six months for full effectiveness.

A strain of *M. tuberculosis* that is highly resistant to many currently used drugs, and therefore very difficult to treat, has emerged. Defined as **multidrug-resistant tuberculosis (MDR TB)**, this strain is a serious health problem. The organisms show resistance to the commonly used therapeutic agents. Risk factors include being exposed to MDR TB, failing to complete TB therapy, being prescribed inappropriate agents, having immune deficiencies, and having a recurrence of TB. Successful therapy for MDR TB may require 18 to 24 months of treatment.

Patient adherence is a major problem in treating TB. The severe side effect profile, the length of time required for treatment, and the number of medications required all contribute to nonadherence. Patients being treated for active TB should avoid alcohol.

Ethambutol

Ethambutol is an antitubercular agent that works by impairing synthesis of the mycobacterial cell wall and is usually well tolerated.

Dosage Forms and Administration Ethambutol is administered as a single daily oral dose.

Side Effects The major side effect is optic neuritis, which is relatively uncommon with standard dosing.

Contraindications Ethambutol should not be used in patients with a known hypersensitivity or known optic neuritis, or in patients unable to report visual changes.

Cautions and Considerations Caution should be used in patients with decreased kidney function and in patients with visual defects like diabetic retinopathy or cataracts.

Drug Interactions Ethambutol decreases the effects of live BCB vaccine. Levels of ethambutol may be increased by various drugs, including aluminum hydroxide.

Isoniazid

Isoniazid is a bactericidal agent that works by inhibiting synthesis of the mycobacterium cell wall.

Dosage Forms and Administration Isoniazid tends to be easily tolerated orally in a single daily dose.

Side Effects Hepatitis is the most serious side effect associated with isoniazid use, and this drug has a boxed warning about this complication. Peripheral neuropathy may also occur. Neuropathy may be minimized with pyridoxine use.

Contraindications Isoniazid should not be used in patients with known hypersensitivity or in patients with severe liver disease.

Cautions and Considerations Isoniazid should be used with caution in patients with liver dysfunction. The risk of hepatitis increases with daily alcohol consumption and coadministration of other drugs metabolized by the liver. Clinical monitoring of liver function should be performed during treatment.

Drug Interactions Isoniazid may increase the levels of numerous agents by affecting intestinal enzyme CYP3A4 metabolism.

Pyrazinamide

Pyrazinamide is a bactericidal agent for TB.

Dosage Forms and Administration Pyrazinamide is available as a tablet and is administered once daily.

Side Effects The most common side effects are nausea and vomiting. Hepatoxicity is also a concern.

Contraindications Pyrazinamide should not be used in patients with known hypersensitivity or active, unstable liver disease.

Cautions and Considerations Use of pyrazinamide may cause hepatic (liver) damage, acute gout, and hypersensitivity. For patients with kidney disease, the dose may need to be reduced and given three times a week.

Drug Interactions Pyrazinamide increases inhibition of GI absorption, and coadministration with pexidartinib should be avoided. Pyrazinamide should not be administered with pretomanid or rifampin as these agents are known to increase the toxicity of pyrazinamide.

Rifampin and Rifapentine

Rifampin (Rifadin, Rimactane) is an antitubercular agent that inhibits bacterial RNA synthesis. Rifampin interferes with oral contraceptives; thus, patients who may become pregnant who are taking this drug must be advised to seek alternative forms of birth control.

Rifapentine (Priftin) has a longer duration of action than rifampin and, therefore, has the advantage of a less frequent administration schedule, leading to improved patient adherence. However, it can still decrease the effectiveness of oral contraceptives like rifampin can. Rifapentine is always used as an adjunctive therapy (a therapy added to the primary therapy).

Dosage Forms and Administration Rifampin is available as an injection or capsule and must be taken on an empty stomach. Rifapentine is available as a tablet.

Side Effects Side effects for these drugs include the discoloration of urine, tears, sweat, and other body fluids, which turn reddish orange. This discoloration can permanently stain soft contact lenses.

Contraindications Rifapentine should not be used in HIV-infected persons taking antiretroviral therapy. Rifampin is contraindicated, or should be used with caution, in patients with HIV infection taking certain antiretroviral agents.

Cautions and Considerations Although rifampin must be taken on an empty stomach, rifapentine must be taken with food. Rifampin and rifapentine interact with a number of drugs. They can decrease concentrations of warfarin, methadone, hormonal contraceptives, and phenytoin. Patients using hormonal contraceptives should use an alternative method of contraception.

Drug Interacations Rifampin and rifapentine have numerous drug interactions due to their effect on intestinal enzyme CYP3A4 metabolism.

Histoplasmosis

Another pulmonary disease, **histoplasmosis**, is caused by a fungus that most commonly occurs in accumulated droppings from bats and various birds, including chickens, pigeons, and starlings. When the fungus-bearing dust is inhaled, spores are transported into the bronchial tubes. The lymphatic tissue reacts to this invasion, and sensitivity develops; as a result, tissue becomes inflamed. This disease is most prevalent in the valleys of the Mississippi and Ohio Rivers.

Histoplasmosis is often referred to as the *summer flu* because it produces flu-like symptoms. Although the disease mimics tuberculosis, most patients recover on their own without treatment. Histoplasmosis is usually self-limiting and is serious only if there are high levels of fungi. If histoplasmosis has disseminated (widely dispersed to other parts of the body), it can be fatal without treatment. More information on antifungals can be found in Chapter 17. Amphotericin B and itraconazole appear to be the only effective drugs for the more serious disseminated form. Surgery may sometimes be indicated.

11.6 Cough, Cold, and Allergy and Corresponding Drug Treatments

The most prevalent form of respiratory tract infection is the **common cold**, which is a mild, self-limited (resolves on its own without treatment) viral infection. Symptoms are readily recognized by the patient and include mild malaise, rhinorrhea (runny nose), sneezing, scratchy throat, fever, and in some cases, itchy eyes. Bacterial sinusitis and otitis media (earaches) are frequent complications necessitating antimicrobial therapy. Antibiotics and sometimes antivirals are used in treating these problems. Viruses are the most common cause of infections in the respiratory system.

Symptoms of some allergies—runny nose and itchy eyes—are the same as those of some colds, so these allergies can be misidentified as a cold. In contrast to the viral cause of the common cold, an allergy results from a state of hypersensitivity induced by exposure to a particular antigen (substance foreign to the body that evokes an immune response). Colds and many allergies are treated with the same medications.

The vast majority of colds are self-limiting, but people seek self-treatment to relieve the symptoms and often to prevent complications. Ordinarily, the common cough and cold are treated with four groups of drugs, either alone or in combination: antitussives, expectorants, decongestants, and antihistamines. Many of these drugs are available as over-the-counter (OTC) products. Offering knowledge of OTC products is a way in which pharmacy technicians can assist individuals who are looking for symptom relief. Technicians can teach patients how to read OTC product labels to find the product that will address their needs. Although recommendations should not be made, technicians can certainly make customers aware of the proper uses and side effects of these drugs.

For the most part, colds can be successfully prevented if a few simple precautions are taken. Colds can be directly transmitted from an infected person to other people when the infected person sneezes or coughs, or they may be passed along indirectly by contact with surfaces such as telephones, doorknobs, or toys. A sneeze or cough should be covered by turning the head and coughing into the elbow, *not the hand*. Many people contract a cold by rubbing their eyes or nose after touching contaminated surfaces or people with colds. Using a telephone right after an infected person has used it

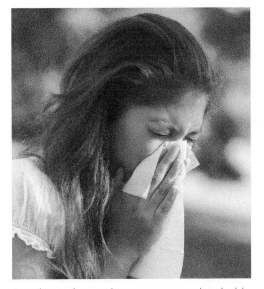

Sneezing and a running nose are associated with the common cold.

is often how a cold is transmitted. In the pharmacy, it is very important to regularly wipe the phones with disinfectant. However, frequent handwashing is the best preventative measure against the common cold—this cannot be stressed enough.

Antitussives

Coughing is a mechanism for clearing the airways of excess secretions and foreign materials, but intense, frequent coughing with lack of sputum production can be bothersome to the patient. In these instances, an antitussive can be therapeutic. An **antitussive** is an agent that suppresses coughing and is indicated when cough frequency needs to be reduced, especially when the cough is dry and nonproductive. The mechanism by which the narcotic and nonnarcotic antitussive agents affect the intensity and frequency of a cough depends on the principal site of action:

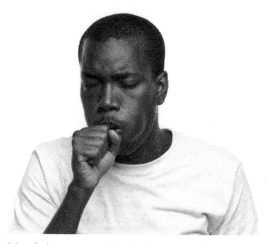

Stimulating receptors in the airways and lungs produces a cough.

(1) central nervous system (CNS) depression of the cough center in the medulla (cough reflex), or (2) suppression of the nerve receptors within the respiratory tract.

The **cough reflex** involves two types of receptors found in the lungs and airways. These receptors, when stimulated, can initiate the events leading to a cough:

- A **stretch receptor** responds to elongation of muscle.
- An **irritant receptor** responds to coarse particles and chemicals.

Theoretically, the cough reflex can be stopped at several points. Antitussive products are designed to act in one or more of the following ways:

- correcting or blocking the irritation of receptors
- blocking transmission to the brain
- increasing the cough center threshold
- blocking the action of the expiratory muscles

Table 11.5 lists the most commonly used antitussive medications.

TABLE 11.5 Commonly Used Agents for Coughs, Colds, and Allergies

Generic (Brand)	Pronunciation	Dosage Form	Common Dosage	Dispensing Status	Controlled Substance Schedule
Antitussive Medications					
benzonatate (Tessalon, Zonatuss)	ben-ZOE-na-tate	capsule	100–200 mg 3 times a day as needed; not to exceed 600 mg a day	Rx	
codeine (various combinations)	KOE-deen	oral liquid	15–30 mg every 6–8 hrs as needed; not to exceed 120 mg a day	behind the counter, Rx	C-II, C-III, or C-V

continues

Generic (Brand)	Pronunciation	Dosage Form	Common Dosage	Dispensing Status	Controlled Substance Schedule
dextromethorphan (Delsym, Robitussin, Triaminic, various brands)	dex-troe-meth-OR-fan	capsule, gel, lozenge, oral liquid, oral strip	regular release: 10–20 mg every 4 hrs or 30 mg every 6–8 hrs Extended release: 60 mg 2 times a day; not to exceed 120 mg a day	OTC, behind the counter	
hydrocodone / chlorpheniramine (TussiCaps, Tussionex)	hye-droe-KOE-done klor-fen-EER-a-meen	capsule, oral solution, oral suspension	varies based on dosage form	Rx	C-II
promethazine / codeine	proe-METH-a-zeen KOE-deen	oral liquid	6.25 mg/10 mg every 4–6 hrs	Rx	C-V
Dextromethorphan Combinations					
dextromethorphan / pseudoephedrine / brompheniramine (Bromfed DM)	dex-troe-meth-OR-fan soo-doe-e-FED-rin brom-fen-EER-a-meen	oral liquid	varies based on dosage form	Rx	
guaifenesin / dextromethorphan (Mucinex DM)	gwye-FEN-e-sin dex-troe-meth-OR-fan	capsule, oral liquid, tablet	varies based on dosage form	OTC	
promethazine / dextromethorphan (Prometh DM, Promethazien DM)	proe-METH-a-zeen dex-troe-meth-OR-fan	oral liquid	varies based on dosage form	Rx*	
Expectorants					
guaifenesin (Mucinex, various brands)	gwye-FEN-e-sin	caplet, capsule granules, oral liquid, syrup, tablet	regular release: 200–400 mg every 4 hr, not to exceed 2.4 g a day extended release: 600–1,200 mg every 12 hr, not to exceed 2.4 g a day	OTC	
Guaifenesin Combinations					
guaifenesin / codeine (Cheratussin AC)	gwye-FEN-e-sin KOE-deen	oral liquid	varies based on dosage form	behind the counter, Rx	C-V
guaifenesin / pseudoephedrine (Mucinex D, Altarussin-PE, Entex T, GoodSense Mucus-D, Maxifed, Poly-Vent IR)	gwye-FEN-e-sin soo-doe-e-FED-rin	tablet	varies based on dosage form	behind the counter	
Decongestants					
oxymetazoline (Afrin, various brands)	ok-see-muh-TAZ-uh-leen	nasal spray	2–3 sprays in each nostril every 12 hr, not to exceed 2 doses a day	behind the counter	
pseudoephedrine (Sudafed, various brands)	soo-doe-e-FED-rin	oral liquid, tablet	IR: 60 mg every 4 to 6 hr XR: 120 mg every 12 hr or 240 mg every 24 hr	behind the counter	

continues

TABLE 11.5 Commonly Used Agents for Coughs, Colds, and Allergies—*Continued*

Generic (Brand)	Pronunciation	Dosage Form	Common Dosage	Dispensing Status	Controlled Substance Schedule
phenylephrine (Neo-Synephrine, Sudafed PE, various brands)	fen-il-EFF-rin	nasal spray, oral liquid, tablet	10 mg every 4 hr, not to exceed 60 mg	OTC	
Pseudoephedrine Combinations					
cetirizine / pseudoephedrine (Zyrtec-D, All Day Allergy-D)	se-TEER-a-zeen soo-doe-e-FED-rin	tablet	1 tablet 2 times a day	behind the counter	
fexofenadine / pseudoephedrine (Allegra-D)	fex-o-FEN-a-deen soo-doe-e-FED-rin	tablet	120 mg 12 hr: 1 tablet 2 times a day; 240 mg 24 hr: 1 tablet 1 time a day	Rx	
guaifenesin / pseudoephedrine (Mucinex D, Alatrussin-PE, Entex T, Maxifed)	gwye-FEN-e-sin soo-doe-e-FED-rin	tablet	varies based on dosage form	behind the counter	
ibuprofen / pseudoephedrine (Advil Cold and Sinus)	eye-byoo-PROE-fen soo-doe-e-FED-rin	liquid-filled capsule, tablet	1–2 tablets every 4–6 hr; not to exceed 6 tablets a day	behind the counter	
ibuprofen / pseudoephedrine-chlorpheniramine (Advil Allergy Sinus, Advil Multi-Symptom Cold)	eye-byoo-PROE-fen soo-doe-e-FED-rin klor-fen-EER-a-meen	tablet	1 tablet every 4–6 hr; not to exceed 6 tablets a day	behind the counter	
loratadine / pseudoephedrine (Alavert Allergy and Sinus D-12, Claritin-D)	lor-AT-a-deen soo-doe-e-FED-rin	tablet	5 mg/120 mg: 1 tablet 2 times a day; 5 mg/ 240 mg: 2 times a day	behind the counter	
naproxen / pseudoephedrine (Aleve-D Sinus and Headache, Sudafed 12 Hour Pressure/Pain)	na-PROX-en soo-doe-e-FED-rin	tablet	1 tablet 2 times a day	behind the counter	
triprolidine / pseudoephedrine (Aprodine, Ed A-Hist PSE, Entre-HIST PSE)	trye-PROE-li-deen soo-doe-e-FED-rin	oral solution, tablet	varies based on dosage form	behind the counter	
Antihistamines					
First Generation					
chlorpheniramine (Chlor-Trimeton, various brands)	klor-fen-EER-a-meen	oral liquid, oral suspension, tablet	IR: 4 mg every 4–6 hours; max daily dose ER: 12 mg every 12 hours; 24 mg max daily dose	OTC	

continues

TABLE 11.5 Commonly Used Agents for Coughs, Colds, and Allergies—*Continued*

Generic (Brand)	Pronunciation	Dosage Form	Common Dosage	Dispensing Status	Controlled Substance Schedule
chlorpheniramine / hydrocodone (Tussionex, TussiCaps)	klor-fen-EER-a-meen hye-droe-KOE-doan	capsule, oral solution, oral suspension	varies based on product	Rx	C-II
clemastine (Dayhist Allergy, Tavist, Tavist Allergy)	KLEM-as-teen	oral liquid, tablet	varies based on product	OTC	
diphenhydramine (Benadryl, various brands)	dye-fen-HYE-dra-meen	capsule, injection, tablet	25 mg every 4 to 6 hr or 50 mg every 6 to 8 hr	Rx OTC	
Second Generation					
azelastine (Astelin, Astepro)	a-ZEL-a-steen	nasal spray	varies based on product	Rx	
cetirizine (Aller-Tec, Alleroff, Zyrtec)	se-TEER-a-zeen	oral liquid, tablet	10 mg 1 time a day	OTC	
desloratadine (Clarinex, Clarinex Reditabs)	des-lor-AT-a-deen	oral liquid, tablet	5–10 mg 1 time a day	Rx	
fexofenadine (Allegra)	fex-o-FEN-a-deen	oral liquid, tablet	1 time a day formulation: 180 mg 1 time a day 2 times a day formulation: 60 mg every 12 hr	OTC	
loratadine (Alavert, Claritin)	lor-AT-a-deen	capsule, oral liquid, tablet	5 mg 2 times a day; 10 mg 1 time a day; max dose 10 mg/day	OTC	
olopatadine (Pataday, Patanase, Patanol)	o-lo-PAT-a-deen	nasal spray, ophthalmic solution	intranasal: 2 sprays into each nostril 2 times a day opthlamic: varies based on product	Rx	
Nasal Corticosteroids					
beclomethasone (Beconase AQ)	bek-loe-METH-a-sone	nasal spray	1–2 sprays in each nostril 2 times a day	Rx	
budesonide (Rhinocort Allergy)	byoo-DES-oh-nide	nasal spray	1–4 sprays in each nostril 1 time a day	Rx	
ciclesonide (Omnaris, Zetonna)	sye-KLES-oh-nide	nasal spray	1–2 sprays in each nostril 1 time a day	Rx	
fluticasone furoate (Flonase Sensimist)	floo-TIK-a-sone fur-OH-ate	nasal spray	2 sprays in each nostril 1 time a day	Rx	
fluticasone propionate (Flonase Allergy Relief)	floo-TIK-a-sone PRO-pee-oh-nate	nasal spray	2 sprays in each nostril 1 time a day	OTC, Rx	
mometasone (Nasonex)	moe-MET-ah-sone	nasal spray	1–2 sprays in each nostril 1 time a day	Rx	
triamcinolone (Nasacort Allergy 24 HR)	trye-am-SIN-oh-lone	nasal spray	1–2 sprays in each nostril 1 time a day	OTC, Rx	

* Dispensing status per federal law. Individual states may have different dispensing statuses.

Codeine

Codeine is the traditional agent used to treat a cough. Codeine is a controlled substance, and its schedule depends on its concentration, its strength, and the other medications used in its combination product. Codeine may be a Schedule II, Schedule III, or Schedule V drug.

Dosage Forms and Administration Codeine-derivative cough suppressants may be available without prescription but are restricted. Many states limit the quantities of these drugs that can be purchased at one time.

Side Effects The most common side effects are nausea, drowsiness, light-headedness, and constipation, especially if the recommended dose is exceeded. Codeine should be taken with food to decrease stomach upset.

Contraindications Contraindications to codeine include respiratory depression, acute or severe asthma, presence of or suspicion of paralytic ileus, and postoperative pain management in children who have undergone tonsillectomy.

Cautions and Considerations Codeine has a boxed warning for respiratory depression and death in children who received codeine after a tonsillectomy or adenoidectomy.

Codeine is also thought to have a drying effect on the respiratory mucosa; this effect would be detrimental to patients with asthma or emphysema.

Drug Interactions Codeine is a CNS depressant, and this effect is additive if taken with other CNS depressants, such as alcohol. Codeine may enhance the constipating effect of eluxadoline.

When used at the recommended dosage, codeine has a low potential for dependency. However, codeine products are frequently misused, so now there are more stringent controls regarding their dispensing. They may be purchased without a prescription in some states, but the purchaser must sign for them, be an adult according to state law, and show identification. The products may be dispensed only by the pharmacist because the pharmacist's initials are required by the patient's signature.

Hydrocodone / Chlorpheniramine

Hydrocodone / chlorpheniramine (TussiCaps, Tussionex, Vituz) is a popular medication. Hydrocodone is a derivative of codeine with many of the same qualities and side effects. It is prescribed for cough and upper respiratory symptoms of allergies and colds. This drug has abuse potential and, therefore, is a Schedule II substance. It has a high potential for psychological and physical dependence. A prescription for this drug should be checked carefully to make sure it is legal.

Dosage Forms and Administration Hydrocodone / chlorpheneriamine is available as a suspension and capsule and is administered twice daily.

Side Effects Side effects include blurred vision, drowsiness, constipation, and mood changes.

Contraindications The extended-release (ER) capsule and suspension should not be used in children younger than six years of age because of the increased risk of fatal respiratory depression.

The oral solution should not be used with or within 14 days of monoamine oxidase inhibitor (MAOI) therapy or in patients who also have narrow-angle glaucoma, urinary retention, severe hypertension, or severe coronary artery disease.

Cautions and Considerations Hydrocodone / chlorpheniramine may cause CNS and respiratory depression. It should be used with caution in older adults. Some formulations contain polysorbate 80 and propylene glycol.

Drug Interactions Hydrocodone / chlorpheniramine interacts with the following drugs: aclidinium, azelastine, conivaptan, eluxadoline, glucagon, MAOIs, paraldehyde, potassium chloride, thalidomide, tiotropium, and umeclidinium. Consequently, concurrent use should be avoided.

Benzonatate

Benzonatate (Tessalon, Zonatuss) is a prescription drug used to treat a nonproductive cough. It locally anesthetizes the stretch receptors in the airways, lungs, and pleura (membrane that lines the thoracic cavity), but it does not affect the respiratory center.

Dosage Forms and Administration Benzonatate is available as an oral capsule. Upon dispensing, benzonatate should have a warning label telling the patient not to chew the capsule, because chewing the drug causes pronounced salivation. Fluid intake is especially encouraged to help liquefy sputum.

Side Effects The main side effects are sedation, headache, and dizziness.

Contraindications This drug is contraindicated in patients who are known to be hypersensitive to benzonatate or related compounds (such as tetracaine).

Cautions and Considerations There are reports of abnormal behavior (mental confusion and hallucinations) with benzonatate use.

Drug Interactions Benzonatate has no known drug interactions.

Dextromethorphan

Dextromethorphan (Delsym) has similar efficacy to codeine; however, it does not have codeine's analgesic properties and does not depress respiration. Further, dextromethorphan acts on the same receptors as codeine, which is why it is a good cough suppressant. Dextromethorphan is a nonopioid derivative of morphine and acts on the cough center to suppress the cough reflex. Dextromethorphan may be the most common nonopioid agent used for cough. If large quantities of dextromethorphan are consumed, it can produce hallucinations; this is known as "robo-tripping," which is popular with teenagers. For this reason, dextromethorphan has become a recreational drug. For states that regulate sales to minors, dextromethorphan purchasers must be 18 years of age or older and be able to show proof of age.

Dosage Forms and Administration Destromethorphan is available as a capsule, gel, lozenge, oral liquid, and oral strip.

Side Effects Common side effects include nausea, vomiting, dizziness, and drowsiness.

Contraindications Dextromethorphan should not be used with an MAOI or within two weeks of discontinuing an MAOI.

Cautions and Considerations Some forms of liquid dextromethorphan contain benzyl alcohol, which can result in neonatal toxicity.

Drug Interactions Dextromethorphan, which is commonly combined with other drugs, interacts with MAOIs. It also interacts with other drugs that affect serotonin levels (such as selective serotonin reuptake inhibitors—SSRIs).

Expectorants

The purpose of an **expectorant** is to enable the patient to rid the lungs and airway of mucus when coughing. Expectorants decrease the thickness and viscosity of mucus, so that a cough will eject mucus and other fluids from the bronchi. Such a cough is called a *productive cough*. Expectorants are used for both dry, unproductive coughs and productive coughs. Table 11.5 lists commonly used expectorants.

Coughing up mucus is easier if the patient is well hydrated. Hydration can be accomplished by drinking six to eight glasses of water a day, which by itself can be as effective as an expectorant. Fluid intake and adequate humidity in the inspired (inhaled) air help liquefy mucus in the respiratory tract and, therefore, are essential in cold therapy.

The most commonly used OTC expectorant is **guaifenesin (Mucinex)**, which is

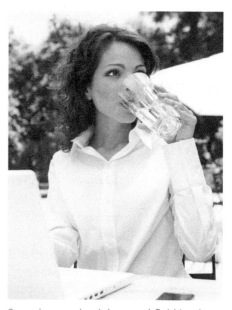

Sometimes maintaining good fluid intake is all that is needed to allow the respiratory tract to clear itself through coughing.

available in many forms. This drug is also frequently combined with other drugs. It is derived from tree bark extract and is a common component of many cough and cold remedies. It loosens phlegm (mucus) and thins bronchial secretions to make coughs more productive and help rid the respiratory tract of mucus. Guaifenesin is especially indicated in patients with a persistent or chronic cough with excessive secretions.

Dosage Forms and Administration Guaifenesin can be taken in caplet, capsule, granule, liquid, syrup, tablet, or sustained-release form.

Side Effects The side effects of guaifenesin include vomiting, nausea, GI upset, and drowsiness.

Contraindications There are no contraindications associated with guaifenesin use.

Cautions and Considerations Some guaifenesin products contain benzyl alcohol (which is implicated in neonatal toxicities) or phenylalanine.

Drug Interactions Guaifenesin has no known significant drug interactions.

Decongestants

Vasodilation of blood vessels in the nasal mucosa allows fluids to leak into these tissues, resulting in swelling and stuffiness. A **decongestant** stimulates the alpha-adrenergic receptors of the vascular smooth muscle, constricting the dilated arteriolar network within the nasal mucosa. This constriction shrinks the engorged mucous membranes, which promotes drainage, improves nasal ventilation, and relieves the feeling of stuffiness. Shrinking the mucous membranes not only makes breathing easier but also permits the sinus cavities to drain. Topical agents are more immediately effective but of shorter duration than systemic agents. Decongestants should not be given to patients who cannot tolerate sympathetic nervous system stimulation. Sympathetic nervous system stimulation increases heart rate and blood pressure and heightens CNS stimulation. Decongestants are often combined with antihistamines in an effort to offset the antihistamine side effect of drowsiness. Most decongestants are OTC drugs.

Following the label directions regarding the frequency and duration of use is very important when using decongestants. Topical nasal application of these drugs over prolonged periods is often followed by a phenomenon called **rhinitis medicamentosa**, more commonly known as *rebound congestion*. It is thought to be caused by severe nasal edema and reduced receptor sensitivity. Patients with this condition use more spray more often, but it is less effective. Patients should be counseled on the use of topical decongestants to prevent rhinitis medicamentosa. Duration of therapy of a nasal decongestant should be limited to three to five days.

Decongestants should be used with caution in older adults and in patients with hypertension, diabetes, or cardiovascular disease. They can be dangerous if overdosed. They directly stimulate the alpha-adrenergic receptors of respiratory mucosa, causing vasoconstriction to relieve congestion. Their mechanism of action also affects blood pressure and the heart.

Table 11.5 describes the most commonly used decongestants. Decongestants can be administered topically or orally. Topical administration takes the form of drops, sprays, and vapors that are applied nasally. Oral administration takes the form of capsules, syrups, and tablets. Administering a decongestant orally distributes the drug through systemic circulation to the vascular bed of the nasal mucosa.

Decongestants are used for temporary symptomatic relief of nasal congestion due to the common cold, upper respiratory allergies, or sinusitis. Decongestants should *not* be taken if the patient is using other sympathomimetic drugs (drugs that stimulate the sympathetic nerves). They should also be avoided if the patient has any of the following conditions:

- diabetes
- heart disease
- uncontrolled hypertension
- hyperthyroidism
- benign prostatic hypertrophy
- Tourette's syndrome

Both oral and topical agents have side effects, which are listed in Table 11.6. Some of these are unpleasant but relatively minor, whereas others can be serious. Side effects differ for oral agents and topical agents.

Work Wise

Spend some time in the cough and cold aisle of a pharmacy near you. Familiarize yourself with the active ingredients of products available for purchase.

TABLE 11.6 Side Effects of Decongestants

Oral Agents	Topical Agents
anxiety	burning sensation
CNS stimulation (can be used to prevent sleep)	contact dermatitis
dizziness	dry mouth
hallucinations	rhinitis medicamentosa
headache	sneezing
increased blood pressure	stinging sensation
increased heart rate	
insomnia	
tremors	

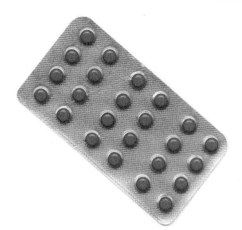

Because pseudoephedrine (pictured above) is a key ingredient in manufacturing methamphetamines, laws have been passed to restrict access to this medication.

Safety Alert

Pharmacy technicians should know the daily purchase limits of products containing pseudoephedrine. At the time of publication, there was a daily limit of 3.6 g per customer, 7.5 g per month per customer for mail order, and 9 g per month per customer at retail stores.

Work Wise

Combinations of ingredients in OTC preparations change frequently without notice to consumers or healthcare professionals. When purchasing any OTC medications, it is important to read the labels.

Pseudoephedrine

Pseudoephedrine (Sudafed, various brands) is a commonly used and effective decongestant. It may be combined with many other drugs. In the past, patients with hypertension were advised to avoid this drug. Current evidence shows that if the hypertension is controlled, by whatever means, then pseudoephedrine is not contraindicated for short-term use. The results of clinical trials cited in the scientific literature indicate that pseudoephedrine works best when combined with an antihistamine.

Pseudoephedrine has strong abuse potential because it is a derivative of ephedrine, which is a controlled substance in some states. In addition, it can be made into methamphetamine. The Combat Methamphetamine Epidemic Act (CEMA) of 2005 was signed into law in 2006 to regulate the quantity or amount of OTC products that can be purchased because of their use in the illegal manufacture of methamphetamine. As a result, the quantity of pseudoephedrine that a consumer may purchase at one time is limited. Products containing pseudoephedrine are kept behind the counter, and the consumer must specifically ask for them and present identification.

Dosage Forms and Administration Pseudoephedrine is available in oral liquid and tablet formulations. It is available as a single agent and in combination with other medications.

Side Effects Common side effects of decongestants are listed in Table 11.6.

Contraindications Pseudoephedrine should not be used with or within two weeks of MAOI therapy.

Cautions and Considerations Chronic use may lead to rebound congestion.

Some formulations contain sodium and should be used with caution in patients following a diet with sodium restrictions. Other formulations contain benzyl alcohol, which is associated with neonatal toxicities.

Drug Interactions Pseudoephedrine should not be used with ergot alkaloids or MAOIs.

Phenylephrine

Phenylephrine (Neo-Synephrine, Sudafed PE, various brands) is used over the counter, primarily to treat symptoms of colds and allergies and itchy, watery eyes. It has replaced pseudoephedrine in many decongestant combinations because it cannot be made into methamphetamine and, therefore, does not require special security measures. Phenylephrine is, however, less effective than pseudoephedrine as a decongestant. Both drugs seem to work better in combination with an antihistamine. Phenylephrine can be administered intravenously to treat hypotension because of the vasoconstriction it causes. It is also used in eye drops and nasal sprays. To prevent rebound congestion, the sprays should not be used more than three days in a row. The eye drops are also used extensively in the treatment of allergies.

Dosage Forms and Administration Phenylephrine is available as a single agent and in combination products.

Side Effects Common side effects of decongestants are listed in Table 11.6.

Contraindications Phenylephrine contraindications include high blood pressure and ventricular tachycardia.

Cautions and Considerations IV phenylephrine has a boxed warning that indicates it should only be used by experienced and adequately trained providers. Phenylephrine should be diluted prior to administration and is known as a *vesicant* (agent that induces blistering). Some phenylephrine products contain sulfites and can, therefore, cause reactions in allergic individuals.

Drug Interactions Phenylephrine should not be used with ergot alkaloids, hyaluronidase, or MAOIs.

Antihistamines

Histamine is a chemical produced by mast cells in the body and is important in the body's immune and inflammatory responses. Mast cells release histamine when the body encounters an antigen. An **antigen** is a molecule that can stimulate or trigger an immune response. Bacteria, viruses, pollen, dander, and even food can activate histamine release. People with allergies have immune systems that overreact to a substance.

The clinical manifestations of histamine release can vary from hives to life-threatening anaphylaxis.

Common allergy or hay fever symptoms include runny nose and watery eyes. These occur because the increase in vascular permeability leads to fluid moving from the capillaries into the tissues. Decreased blood pressure, increased heart rate, and contraction of smooth muscles like bronchi, bronchioles, and the ileum can be found in more severe and life-threatening responses.

Anaphylaxis is a serious or life-threatening allergic response. Anaphylaxis can present with skin and mucosal signs and symptoms such as generalized hives, itching, and swollen lips or tongue; respiratory signs and symptoms like itching throat and ear canal, throat closure, shortness of breath, wheeze, or cough; GI symptoms such as nausea and vomiting; and cardiovascular signs and symptoms such as low blood pressure, rapid heart rate, syncope, and dizziness.

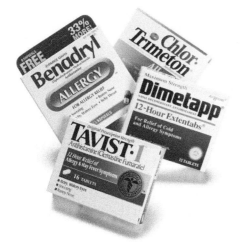

Many antihistamines, such as the ones pictured, are available as OTC products.

Safety Alert

Epinephrine and ephedrine can be easily confused.

Anaphylaxis is also different from a milder allergic reaction in that it involves more than one system in the body (e.g., the cardiac and respiratory systems). These effects are the result of the ability of histamine to affect blood vessels. Histamine increases blood flow, vasodilation, and vascular permeability. In anaphylactic reactions, epinephrine should be administered. Epinephrine is a life-saving medication that is used to treat anaphylaxis.

The histamine response in milder allergic responses can be blocked using **antihistamines**. Two types of antihistamines are available. This chapter discusses antihistamines that block the H_1 receptors in the upper respiratory system. The second type is the H_2 blockers, which affect cells in the GI tract.

Antihistamines (H_1 blockers) act on the H_1 receptors in the body to prevent histamine binding. Antihistamines are used in the following conditions:

- treatment of insomnia
- symptomatic relief of urticarial lesions (hives), edema, and hay fever
- control of cough
- alleviation of vertigo

- alleviation of nausea and vomiting
- relief of serum sickness (hypersensitivity reaction that may occur from several days to three weeks after receiving antisera or following drug therapy)
- control of venom reactions (venom contains histamine and other substances causing histamine release)
- mitigation of the extrapyramidal side effects of antipsychotic medication
- prophylaxis for certain drug reactions
- prophylaxis for certain drug allergies.

Antihistamines are well absorbed in tissues and widely distributed across the blood-brain barrier and placenta. Sedation occurs when they penetrate the blood-brain barrier. People who are pregnant are warned not to take antihistamines because these products can cross the placenta and may adversely affect the fetus. Table 11.5 lists commonly used antihistamines.

First-Generation Antihistamines

First-generation antihistamines for cold and allergy were developed before second-generation varieties. They include chlorpheniramine (used for upper respiratory symptoms), clemastine (used for the common cold and allergies), and diphenhydramine (for allergic reactions and sleep promotion). These drugs, unless combined with a controlled substance, are available OTC and are similar in efficacy.

Chlorpheniramine (Chlor-Trimeton) is available by itself and in combination with other drugs.

Chlorpheniramine / hydrocodone (Tussionex, TussiCaps) is a common and effective treatment for cough. However, it is a drug with a high potential for abuse.

Clemastine (Dayhist Allergy, Tavist, Tavist Allergy) is a first-generation antihistamine used for colds and allergies. Of the first-generation antihistamines, it is the least likely to cause sedation.

Diphenhydramine (Benadryl) is an antihistamine that also has antitussive properties. The main side effect is drowsiness, which is additive if the drug is taken with other CNS depressants.

Dosage Forms and Administration First-generation antihistamines are available as individual products in a variety of dosage forms such as oral liquids, oral suspensions, tablets, capsules, and injections. Many are also available in combination products in different dosage forms for the treatment of allergies and colds.

Side Effects The most common side effects of the currently available antihistamines include anticholinergic responses, hyperactivity (most often in children), and sedation. The anticholinergic responses include dry mouth, drying of the mucosa of the upper respiratory tract, blurred vision, constipation, and urinary retention. Sedation is the most common side effect of antihistamines. Some antihistamines are actually prescribed to induce sleep. In fact, many OTC sleep aids contain the antihistamine diphenhydramine. This effect is synergistic with alcohol use. Dizziness is also a common side effect. The newer drugs on the market have fewer side effects.

Contraindications Contraindications to chlorpheniramine include narrow-angle glaucoma, bladder-neck obstruction, prostate enlargement, acute asthma attacks, stenosing peptic ulcer, and pyloroduodenal obstruction. Clemastine is contraindicated in narrow-angle glaucoma. Diphenhydramine should not be used in patients with acute asthma, in neonates or premature infants, or in people who are breast-feeding.

Cautions and Considerations These medications may cause CNS depression. These drugs should be used with caution in older adults because of the increased risk of confusion, dry mouth, and constipation. Because of these side effects, these drugs are on the Beers Criteria of potentially inappropriate drugs for older adults.

Drug Interactions These drugs may make CNS depressants (such as alcohol and opioids) and anticholinergics more active or effective.

Second-Generation Antihistamines

This drug class includes azelastine, cetirizine, desloratadine, fexofenadine, loratadine, and olopatadine. These agents were developed to provide antihistamine therapy without the unwanted side effects of the first-generation drugs. In general, second-generation antihistamines have fewer CNS side effects and cause less sedation. For these reasons, second-generation antihistamines are popular options for patients compared with their first-generation counterparts. Second-generation antihistamines, however, may cause dry eyes.

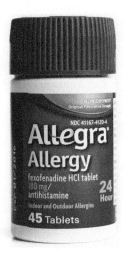

Fexofenadine is sold under the brand name Allegra and is now available as an OTC drug.

Cetirizine, Fexofenadine, Loratadine, and Desloratadine

Cetirizine (Aller-Tec, Alleroff, Zyrtec) is the second-generation antihistamine with the highest potential for drowsiness. It is administered once daily and is available as an OTC product. **Fexofenadine (Allegra)** is a second-generation antihistamine that is generally not as sedating as many of the other antihistamines. Studies have not reported any arrhythmias or other serious reactions in patients who use this drug. **Loratadine (Alavert, Claritin)** has been an OTC drug since 2002, but **desloratadine (Clarinex, Clarinex Reditabs)** does require a prescription. Desloratadine is a long-acting metabolite of loratadine. It has additional anti-inflammatory properties and should not be given with erythromycin or ketoconazole.

Dosage Forms and Administration Second-generation antihistamines are available in tablets, capsules, oral liquids, nasal sprays, and ophthalmic solutions.

Side Effects Side effects include drowsiness, fatigue, and dry mouth.

Contraindications These drugs do not have contraindications.

Safety Alert

Cetirizine may be confused with sertraline (an antidepressant) or stavudine (an antiviral). The brand name Zyrtec may be confused with Zantac (used to treat gastroesophageal reflux disease).

Cautions and Considerations Use cetirizine with caution in patients with renal or hepatic dysfunction. Dose reduction may be required. Use with caution in older adults, as they may be more sensitive to adverse reactions. Fexofenadine should be used with caution in patients with kidney impairment. Dose adjustments may be needed. The oral disintegrating tablet formula of fexofenadine contains phenylalanine. Both loratadine and desloratadine should be used with caution in patients with liver or kidney disease. Pharmacy technicians should be aware that some formulations of loratadine and desloratadine contain benzyl alcohol or phenylalanine.

Drug Interactions These drugs may increase side effects associated with anticholinergic agents and CNS depressants.

Azelastine and Olopatadine

Azelastine (Astelin, Astepro) was the first antihistamine nasal spray. It is indicated in seasonal allergic rhinitis and seems to work as well as the oral antihistamines for

May Cause DROWSINESS

itchy, runny nose and sneezing. It has a bitter taste to many patients. Even though the drug has a low incidence of sedative side effects, the bottle should carry an auxiliary label warning patients of potential drowsiness with the use of this drug. Azelastine is stable for three months after the bottle is opened.

Olopatadine (Pataday, Patanase, Patanol) is a second-generation antihistamine for allergic rhinitis in patients six years and older. This drug is available in nasal and ophthalmic forms, and the nasal form can leave a bitter taste in the mouth. It should be used as rescue therapy for symptoms of allergies. Because it is an antihistamine, it can cause sleepiness.

Dosage Forms and Administration Azelastine is available as a spray. Olopatadine is available in nasal and ophthalmic forms.

Side Effects Side effects include drowsiness, headache, bitter taste (nasal formulations), nose bleeding (nasal formulations), nasal discomfort (nasal formulations), blurred vision (optic formulations), and irritation of the eye (optic formulation).

Contraindications There are no contraindications for the use of azelastine or olopatadine.

Cautions and Considerations Azelastine may cause CNS depression. The ophthalmic product of olopatadine should not be used to treat lens-related irritation. If the patient wears contact lenses, they should remove the lenses prior to administration and wait at least 10 minutes before reinserting them.

Drug Interactions Azelastine may increase the effects of CNS depressants and anticholinergics. Olopatadine has no known drug interactions.

Nasal Corticosteroids

A new group of drugs has emerged to treat allergies: **nasal corticosteroids**. These medications must be used daily for maximum benefit. Administration (spray) should be directed away from the septum to prevent nasal irritation and bleeding. Other side effects of nasal allergy products include cough, sore throat, headache, and runny nose. Typically, these effects are mild and tolerable. Local infections of *Candida albicans* may occur in the nose of patients using nasal corticosteroids on a long-term basis. Nasal corticosteroids are now the most effective monotherapy for allergic rhinitis. These drugs have also shown some value in the treatment of otitis media (earaches) in children. The most commonly prescribed nasal corticosteroids are listed in Table 11.5.

Ciclesonide (Omnaris, Zetonna) is a prodrug that is converted to the active form (desisobutyryl ciclesonide) by an enzyme in the nasal mucosa. This process is known as *target activation*. Theoretically, target activation should reduce side effects; however, systemic exposure is negligible after nasal inhalation. Zetonna, which is not a nasal spray but is inhaled via a nasal inhaler, appears to cause less hoarseness and oral thrush than other nasal steroids because it is dispersed in very small particles.

Fluticasone is used in two different forms. The furoate formulation (**Flonase Sensimist**) is a prescription formulation that provides a fine mist. The propionate formulation (**Flonase Allergy Relief**) is available as an OTC product. The delivery devices differ between the two, so patients may prefer one device over the other.

Mometasone (Nasonex) depresses the release of endogenous (produced in the body) chemical mediators of inflammation (histamine, kinin, and prostaglandins). It reverses the dilation and permeability of vessels in the area and decreases cells' access to the site of injury. Mometasone may be used in children who are over 12 years of age to prevent symptoms of allergic rhinitis.

Beclomethasone (Beconase AQ) and **budesonide (Rhinocort Allergy)** are also available as prescription nasal corticosteroids. **Triamcinolone (Nasacort Allergy 24 HR)** is available as both a prescription and OTC.

Dosage Forms and Administration Nasal corticosteroids are administered intranasally. Patients should use the following instructions to instill these medications:

1. Shake product well before use.
2. Clear nasal passages by either blowing the nose or using a saline irrigation system.
3. Sit in an upright position with the head tilted slightly forward.
4. Close one nostril by pressing it with a finger, and insert the sprayer tip into the other nostril, with the tip pointing away from the nasal septum. Breathe in and depress the applicator to deliver a metered dose.
5. Breathe out from the mouth.
6. Repeat the procedure for the other nostril.

It is not necessary for patients to breathe in quickly or forcefully or to hold their breath. The site of action is in the nose, not deep in the sinuses or lungs. Patients should be aware that postnasal drip may occur and that they may taste the nasally administered medication. Patients should avoid sneezing or blowing their nose just after using the spray.

Side Effects Side effects of nasal allergy products include cough, sore throat, headache, runny nose, nasal irritation, and nasal bleeding.

Contraindications The nasal corticosteroids listed in Table 11.5 do not have contraindications.

Cautions and Considerations To ensure proper dosing, patients should shake these products well before administration. The pharmacy technician should affix an auxiliary label to the drug container to remind patients to shake the container prior to using the medication.

A nasal spray application bottle should be primed when new and whenever it has not been used for a while. **Priming** a nasal spray means that the patient should pump the sprayer a few times away from the face until an even amount of spray exits the applicator.

Drug Interactions Systemic corticosteroids may enhance the hyperglycemic potential of nasal corticosteroids.

11.7 Tobacco Use, Smoking Cessation, and Corresponding Drug Treatment

According to the CDC, smoking causes nearly a half million deaths each year in the United States and increases the risk of death from all causes. Its impact on the respiratory system is especially destructive, resulting in damaged airways and alveoli. In fact, cigarette smoking causes the most cases of lung cancer in the United States and is responsible for nearly 80% of all deaths from COPD. Asthma can also be caused or exacerbated by smoking or by exposure to cigarette smoke. In addition, smoking harms other organs in the body, increasing the risk for heart disease, stroke, cancer, type 2 diabetes mellitus, rheumatoid arthritis, reproductive difficulties, and decreased

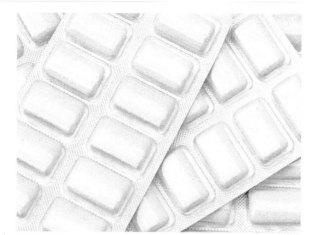
Nicotine replacement therapy is available in multiple forms, including chewing gum.

bone health. On average, cigarette smokers live approximately 15 years less than nonsmokers. Cigarette smoke contains more than 4,000 identified chemical compounds, including at least 43 carcinogens. Lung cancer; leukemia; and cancers of the mouth, pharynx, larynx, esophagus, pancreas, cervix, kidney, and bladder are associated with smoking. Evidence also links smoking with other cancers, such as ovarian, uterine, and prostate. Tobacco is the single largest cause of preventable death.

Environmental (secondhand) tobacco smoke also poses a substantial health threat because it contains all the carcinogens and toxins present in inhaled cigarette smoke. Children living in a household with smokers have a higher risk of respiratory infection, asthma, and middle ear infection than those who live with nonsmokers. Birth defects may be related to the pregnant parent's smoking during pregnancy.

The physical benefits of smoking cessation include a longer life and better health (i.e., decreased risk of lung, laryngeal, esophageal, oral, pancreatic, bladder, and cervical cancers; coronary heart disease; and other diseases aggravated by smoking). A few personal benefits from smoking cessation are listed in Table 11.7.

TABLE 11.7 Personal Benefits from Smoking Cessation

improved performance in athletic endeavors

improved sexual function

better-smelling home, car, clothing, and breath

economic savings

freedom from addiction

healthier babies

improved health

improved self-esteem

improved sense of taste and smell

lack of guilt about exposing others to smoke

opportunity to set a good example for children and young adults

Nicotine, the addictive component of tobacco, is readily absorbed in the lungs from inhaled smoke. Nicotine from smokeless tobacco products, such as chewing tobacco and snuff, is absorbed across the oral or nasal mucosa, respectively. In the body, nicotine is extensively metabolized in the liver and, to a lesser extent, in the kidneys and lungs. One major urinary metabolite, **cotinine**, has a longer half-life (15 to 20 hours) and a tenfold higher concentration than nicotine. Presence of this metabolite indicates that a person is a smoker.

Nicotine and polycyclic aromatic hydrocarbons in cigarette smoke induce the production of hepatic (liver) enzymes responsible for metabolizing caffeine, theophylline, imipramine, and other drugs. Smoking increases plasma cortisol (a major natural glucocorticoid) and catecholamine (sympathomimetic amines, including dopamine, epinephrine, and norepinephrine) concentrations, which affect treatment with adrenergic agonists and adrenergic blocking agents.

Nicotine is an agonist of nicotinic cholinergic receptors with dose-related, pharmacologic effects. These effects include CNS and peripheral nervous system stimulation and depression; respiratory stimulation; skeletal muscle relaxation; dopamine release; peripheral vasoconstriction; and increases in blood pressure, heart rate, cardiac output, and oxygen consumption. Chronic nicotine ingestion leads to physical and psychological dependence. Consequently, smoking cessation results in withdrawal symptoms, usually within 24 hours. These symptoms are listed in Table 11.8.

TABLE 11.8 Symptoms of Nicotine Withdrawal

anxiety	gastrointestinal disturbances
craving for tobacco	headache
decreased blood pressure and heart rate	hostility
depression	increased appetite and weight gain
difficulty concentrating	increased skin temperature
drowsiness	insomnia
frustration, irritability, impatience, restlessness	

Quitting Nicotine

One of the reasons it is so difficult to stop smoking is that nicotine has many properties that reinforce various behaviors. These properties include relaxation, increased alertness, decreased fatigue, improved cognitive performance, and a "reward" effect (pleasure or euphoria). Increased alertness and improved cognitive performance result from stimulation of the cerebral cortex, which can occur at low doses. The "reward" effect, mediated by the limbic system, occurs at high doses.

To combat these properties, smoking cessation treatment involves three main elements: behavior modification, social support from the clinician, and nicotine replacement therapy. Nicotine replacement therapy is recommended as first-line pharmacotherapy for smokers who do not have contraindications to therapy (myocardial infarction in the previous four weeks, serious arrhythmias, severe or worsening angina pectoris). Patients must understand, however, that nicotine replacement therapy is not a substitute for behavior modification and that success is greatest when both are used concomitantly. Individual or group counseling is highly recommended.

The steps in establishing a plan for quitting are as follows:

1. Set a date.
2. Inform family, friends, and coworkers of the decision and request understanding and support.
3. Remove cigarettes from the environment and avoid spending a lot of time in places where smoking is prevalent.
4. Review previous attempts to quit, if applicable, and analyze the factors that caused relapse.
5. Anticipate challenges, particularly during the critical first few weeks.

The key to smoking cessation is total abstinence. Patients should reward themselves for abstaining and avoid situations that serve as smoking triggers. Because drinking alcohol is strongly associated with relapse to tobacco use, smokers should reduce their alcohol consumption or abstain from drinking altogether during the quitting process.

One major reason smokers are reluctant to quit is fear of weight gain. Although weight gain does occur, most smokers gain less than 10 pounds. The weight gain is caused by both increased caloric intake and metabolic adjustments; it can occur even if caloric intake remains constant or is restricted.

Smoking Cessation Agents

The most commonly used agents for smoking cessation are listed in Table 11.9. Patients must be strongly advised to stop smoking when initiating nicotine replacement therapy. Those individuals who continue to smoke may show signs of nicotine excess. The symptoms of nicotine excess are listed in Table 11.10; note that they often overlap with withdrawal symptoms. Dizziness and perspiration are more often associated with excessive nicotine levels; anxiety, depression, and irritability are common symptoms of nicotine withdrawal.

Of the drugs listed in Table 11.7, only Nicoderm CQ, Nicorette, and Nicotrol are approved for OTC purchase. More information on bupropion can be found in Chapter 8.

TABLE 11.9 Commonly Used Agents for Smoking Cessation

Generic (Brand)	Pronunciation	Dosage Form	Common Dosage	Dispensing Status
bupropion (Aplenzin, Forfivo XL, Wellbutrin SR, Wellbutrin XL)	byoo-PROE-pee-on	tablet	150 mg twice a day extended release: 200 mg once a day	Rx
nicotine (Nicoderm CQ, Nicorette, Nicotrol)	NIK-oh-teen	gum, inhaler, lozenge, nasal solution, transdermal patch	varies based on product and patient	OTC, Rx
varenicline (Chantix)	var-EN-i-kleen	tablet	1 mg twice a day	Rx

Nicotine Supplements

Nicotine supplements are used to reduce absorbed nicotine slowly over time, thereby reducing many withdrawal symptoms. They are available in several OTC dosage forms, including gum, inhaler, lozenge, and patch.

Nicotine gum works best for users of smokeless tobacco products. These forms are chewed briefly and then "parked" in the cheek until the craving for nicotine returns. Inhaled forms mimic the use and effects of smoking while eliminating the harmful toxins from inhaling smoke. In the patch form, nicotine is absorbed transdermally and provides the most continuous nicotine delivery. However, this form does not allow the smoker to adjust nicotine exposure throughout the day. Nicotine nasal spray is administered intranasally and results in more rapid absorption compared to oral dosage forms. Its use is limited because of its side effects, such as rhinitis, sneezing, tearing, and nose and throat irritation.

Dosage Forms and Administration Nicotine supplements are available in OTC gum, inhaler, lozenge, and patch. Prescription tablets are also available. The dose of nicotine supplements usually depends on the number of cigarettes smoked daily. Doses should be tapered gradually as nicotine withdrawal symptoms subside.

Side Effects Common side effects for nicotine supplements include mild itching and stinging at the application site (transdermal patch); increased heart rate and blood pressure (gum); and irritation in the mouth, nose, throat, or eyes (nasal spray).

Contraindications Nicotine supplements are contraindicated in patients who smoke after a recent heart attack and in patients who have life-threatening arrhythmias or worsening chest pain. These supplements should be avoided by pregnant patients as well. Nicotine gum should not be used by patients with active temporomandibular joint disease.

Cautions and Considerations Nicotine can increase heart rate and blood pressure. Risk-benefit analysis should be performed for patients who require nicotine replacement and who have concurrent heart disease, hypertension, or arrhythmias. Dental problems may worsen with the gum form of nicotine. Airway irritation may result from the inhaled form of nicotine, and caution must be used in patients with airway disease. Nicotine patches should be used cautiously in patients who are allergic to adhesive tape and in those individuals who have skin problems. Nicotine nasal spray is not recommended for patients with chronic nasal disorders, such as allergy, rhinitis, nasal polyps, or sinusitis.

Drug Interactions Nicotine may enhance cardiac effects related to adenosine use. Cimetidine and varenicline may enhance adverse effects of nicotine.

TABLE 11.10 Symptoms of Nicotine Excess

abdominal pain	headache	perspiration
confusion	hearing loss	visual disturbances
diarrhea	hypersalivation	vomiting
dizziness	nausea	weakness

Bupropion

Bupropion (Aplenzin, Forfivo XL, Wellbutrin SR, Wellbutrin XL) is an antidepressant used to combat the mood changes and emotional instability associated with smoking cessation. It can also reduce cravings for nicotine.

Dosage Forms and Administration Bupropion is available only by prescription.

Side Effects Side effects of bupropion include drowsiness, dizziness, blurred vision, and insomnia. To reduce these effects, patients should avoid drinking alcohol while taking this medication and should take the medication in the morning.

Contraindications Contraindications to bupropion include seizure disorder, history of anorexia or bulimia, abrupt discontinuation of ethanol or sedatives, use of MAOIs, and use of linezolid or IV methylene blue.

Cautions and Considerations When discontinuing bupropion therapy, doses must be tapered to avoid a rebound of depressive symptoms. Patients should not stop taking bupropion abruptly.

As with starting any antidepressant therapy, patients using bupropion should talk with their healthcare provider if they notice symptoms of depression or suicidal ideation. The FDA-approved labeling for bupropion includes a boxed warning that alerts users of bupropion that serious adverse mental health events may occur. Patients should be observed for signs of agitation, hostility, depression, or behavioral changes.

Drug Interactions Bupropion should not be used with MAOIs.

Varenicline

Varenicline (Chantix) blocks nicotine binding to pleasure receptors and reduces the severity of craving and withdrawal symptoms. Smoking while taking Chantix does not provide the same sense of satisfaction. Foods also do not provide as much satisfaction while a patient is taking varenicline, so weight gain is usually not a problem while using this drug for smoking cessation. This advantage is important because weight gain is a common side effect of smoking cessation that causes many patients to resume smoking.

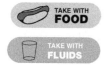

Dosage Forms and Administration Varenicline needs to be started a week before the quit date. It should be taken with food and a full glass of water to help prevent or decrease nausea, which is one of the primary side effects. Varenicline should be taken for 24 weeks, and the patient should attend a smoking cessation program.

Side Effects The most prominent side effect is unusual dreams.

Contraindications Varenicline does not have any contraindications.

Cautions and Considerations The FDA-approved labeling for varenicline includes a boxed warning that alerts users that serious neuropsychiatric events may occur. Patients should be observed for agitation, hostility, depression, and changes in behavior. Patients with suicidal ideation should stop taking varenicline immediately and talk with their healthcare providers.

Drug Interactions Individuals taking varenicline with ethanol, famotidine, inhaled nicotine, intranasal nicotine, nizatidine, ranitidine, tobramycin, or vandetanib should be monitored.

11.8 Complementary and Alternative Therapies

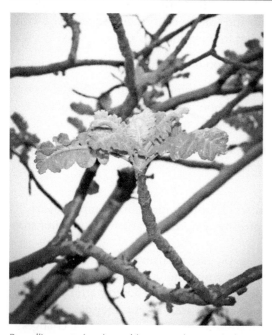

Boswellia serrata is a branching tree whose resin has anti-inflammatory properties.

Boswellia serrata (or Indian frankincense) is a branching tree that is native to India, North Africa, and the Middle East. Its resin possesses anti-inflammatory properties and has been used for centuries to treat chronic inflammatory diseases, such as asthma. Of note, *Boswellia serrata* is for chronic treatment and should be avoided in acute asthma exacerbations. It is usually consumed as the powdered form of the plant resin. In this form, *Boswellia serrata* is usually taken at 300 mg three times a day. The most common GI side effects are diarrhea, stomach pain, and acid reflux. *Boswellia serrata* should be avoided in patients with acid reflux or liver dysfunction.

Choline is a nutrient related to B vitamins. It is naturally consumed through diet (in sources such as egg yolk, liver, peanuts, fish, soybeans, cabbage, and cauliflower) and can be synthesized by the body. Choline may be effective when used orally for management of chronic asthma. Typical choline doses range from 500 to 1,000 mg three times a day. Side effects include decreased blood pressure, nausea, dizziness, and headache.

Yoga is an ascetic discipline in which breath control, simple meditation, and the adoption of bodily postures is practiced for health and relaxation. Yoga may be used to improve symptoms of mild to moderate asthma and COPD. It is generally considered safe in healthy individuals. Patients with intervertebral disk and back ailments, high or low blood pressure, glaucoma, or severe osteoporosis should avoid inverted poses. Certain breathing techniques should be avoided in patients with asthma or COPD.

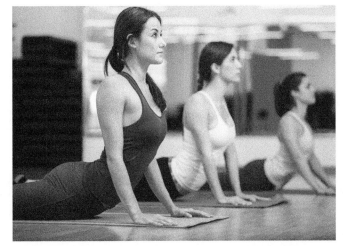

Yoga can benefit patients who have mild to moderate asthma or COPD.

Nasal irrigation describes the flushing of the nasal cavity to remove excess mucus and debris from the nose and sinuses. This practice may effectively relieve allergies and sinusitis. It is generally well tolerated. However, it is important to use clean irrigation dispensers and to use water that is sterile or has been boiled. Patients can purchase kits that include water dispensers and powders for dilution.

Saline nasal spray is a salt-water nasal spray that can also be used to help relieve nasal congestion by helping to loosen secretions. OTC nasal spray formulations are available. The FDA warns of homemade saline nasal sprays made with tap water due to the risk of infections from nonsterile water.

Review and Assessment

CHAPTER SUMMARY

Anatomy of the Respiratory System

- The respiratory system is responsible for obtaining oxygen from the air through inhalation, supplying oxygen to the cells in the body through gas exchange, and removing carbon dioxide from the body via exhalation.

- The respiratory system is divided into the upper respiratory tract (nasal cavity, pharynx, larynx, and trachea) and the lower respiratory tract (lungs and bronchi).

- The respiratory system contains protective mechanisms to filter air and protect the airways and lungs from harmful substances like dust, bacteria, viruses, and allergens.

Asthma and Drug Treatments

- Asthma is a disease in which inflammation causes the airways to tighten; asthma is a reversible condition in that it can improve or be controlled with the use of appropriate medications.

- Asthma is a pulmonary condition with the following characteristics: reversible small airway obstruction, progressive airway inflammation, and increased airway responsiveness to stimuli.

- Drug therapy is the mainstay of asthma management.

- A spacer is recommended for use with an MDI to decrease the amount of spray that is deposited on the back of the throat and then swallowed. It increases drug penetration into the lungs.

- With an HFA inhaler, the patient inhales slowly, whereas with a DPI, the patient breathes in quickly to activate the inhaler.

- Nebulizers are effective delivery systems for children too young to use inhalers.

- Home nebulizers can easily become contaminated if not cleaned properly.

- Short-acting inhaled beta-2 agonists are albuterol, levalbuterol, and metaproterenol.

- Inhaled corticosteroids include beclomethasone, budesonide, ciclesonide, fluticasone, and mometasone. Combination products with inhaled corticosteroids include budesonide / formoterol, fluticasone / salmeterol, fluticasone / vilanterol, and mometasone / formoterol.

- Montelukast (Singulair) is indicated for prophylaxis and chronic treatment of asthma. It is approved for use in adults and children 12 months and older.

- Zafirlukast (Accolate) is a leukotriene receptor antagonist that is used for prophylaxis and long-term treatment in patients five years of age and older. Zafirlukast carries a warning that it can increase theophylline levels.

- Zileuton (Zyflo) is a leukotriene inhibitor that carries warnings about liver toxicity and can increase theophylline levels.

- Cromolyn sodium is a mast cell stabilizer used to treat asthma.

- Benralizumab, dupilumab, mepolizumab, omalizumab, and reslizumab are monoclonal antibodies that can be used to treat severe asthma that is not controlled with other therapies.

- Theophylline interacts with many drugs, so it should be used only when a patient's lung disease is unresponsive to other drugs.

Chronic Obstructive Pulmonary Disease and Drug Treatments

- COPD encompasses emphysema and chronic bronchitis. COPD is irreversible.

- Emphysema is characterized by destruction of the tiny alveoli, or air sacs, of the lungs.

- Chronic bronchitis can be caused by cigarette smoke; exposure to occupational dusts, fumes, and environmental pollution; and bacterial infection.

- Pharmacologic management of bronchitis and emphysema is still largely empirical, and anticholinergics and LABAs are used most frequently.

- Anticholinergics include aclidinium, glycopyrrolate, ipratropium, revenfenacin, tiotropium, and umeclidinium.

- Anticholinergic side effects include headache, flushed skin, blurred vision, tachycardia, and palpitations.

- LABAs include arformoterol, formoterol, indacaterol, olodaterol, and salmeterol. These agents are more frequently used for COPD but may also be used for asthma.

Cystic Fibrosis and Drug Treatments

- Cystic fibrosis (CF) is a hereditary disease that involves the gastrointestinal (GI) and respiratory systems.

- CF can be a fatal disease, with some patients dying in early adulthood.

- Drug therapy for CF involves antibiotic therapy and airway clearance therapy, the latter of which includes the use of inhaled respiratory drugs.

- Gene therapies have been developed to target specific CFTR gene defects in patients with cystic fibrosis.

Other Lung Diseases and Drug Treatments

- Pneumonia is a common lung infection that affects individuals of all ages and is treated with antibiotics.

- Respiratory distress syndrome occurs in neonates and is treated with surfactants.

- The treatment regimen for tuberculosis (TB) depends on whether a patient has active or latent disease.

- Histoplasmosis is often referred to as the *summer flu*. It is usually benign but in rare cases can be life threatening. The only effective drugs for the more serious form are amphotericin B and itraconazole.

Cough, Cold, and Allergy and Corresponding Treatments

- Antitussives, expectorants, decongestants, and antihistamines each have a different mechanism of action and purpose. Most are OTC products.

- Antitussives are indicated to reduce the frequency of a cough, especially when it is dry and nonproductive.

- The cough reflex can be stopped at several points in the reflex pathway.

- Dextromethorphan is the most commonly used OTC antitussive.

- Dextromethorphan may only be sold to individuals who show proof that they are at least 18 years old.

- Expectorants decrease the viscosity of mucus.

- Guaifenesin is the most commonly used OTC expectorant, but drinking several glasses of water may work as well.

- Decongestants stimulate the alpha-adrenergic receptors of the vascular smooth muscle, constricting the dilated arteriolar network and shrinking the engorged mucous membranes. This promotes drainage of the sinus cavities and makes breathing easier. Stimulation of the sympathetic nervous system also increases heart rate and blood pressure and heightens CNS stimulation. Patients sometimes take decongestants to overcome drowsiness. These drugs should not be taken by individuals who cannot tolerate sympathetic stimulation.

- Topical application of decongestants (nasal sprays and drops) can cause rhinitis medicamentosa, or rebound congestion.

- Pseudoephedrine is an effective decongestant, but it may be purchased only in limited quantities. It may only be sold to individuals who show proof that they are least 18 years old.

- Antihistamines are used to alleviate allergic reactions and provide symptomatic relief for the common cold. They prevent histamine from binding to H_1 receptors.

- The most common side effects of antihistamines are sedation and anticholinergic responses (dry mouth, constipation, urinary retention, blurred vision, drying of the mucosa of the upper respiratory tract).

- Many antihistamines are sold over the counter.

- Many OTC sleep medications contain the antihistamine diphenhydramine.

- Second-generation antihistamines may cause fewer side effects.

- The most effective treatment for allergic rhinitis is application of nasal corticosteroids.

Tobacco Use, Smoking Cessation, and Corresponding Drug Treatment

- Benefits of smoking cessation include a longer life and better health. The key to smoking cessation is total abstinence.

- Most nicotine cessation drugs are over the counter.

- Bupropion is an antidepressant used to combat the mood changes and emotional instability associated with smoking cessation. It can also reduce cravings for nicotine.

- Varenicline (Chantix) is a prescription drug that has been successful in helping patients quit smoking.

Complementary and Alternative Therapies

- *Boswellia serrata* possesses anti-inflammatory properties and has been used for centuries to treat chronic inflammatory diseases, such as asthma.

- Yoga may be used to help improve symptoms of mild to moderate asthma.

- Nasal irrigation may be used to help relieve seasonal allergies and sinusitis.

DRUG LIST

Antiasthma Agents

Short-Acting Beta-2 Agonists
albuterol (Accuneb, ProAir HFA, ProAir Respiclick, Proventil HFA, Ventolin HFA)
levalbuterol (Xopenex)
metaproterenol

Inhaled Corticosteroids
beclomethasone (QVAR)
budesonide (Pulmicort Respules, Pulmicort Turbuhaler, Rhinocort Allergy)
budesonide / formoterol (Symbicort)
flunisolide (Aerospan)
fluticasone (Flovent)
fluticasone / salmeterol (Advair Diskus, Advair HFA)
fluticasone / vilanterol (Breo Ellipta)
mometasone (Asmanex, Asmanex HFA)
mometasone / formoterol (Dulera)

Leukotriene Inhibitors
montelukast (Singulair)
zafirlukast (Accolate)
zileuton (Zyflo)

Mast Cell Stabilizer
cromolyn sodium

Monoclonal Antibodies
benralizumab (Fasenra)
dupilumab (Dupixent)
mepolizumab (Nucala)
omalizumab (Xolair)
reslizumab (Cinqair)

Xanthine Derivative
theophylline (Elixophyllin, Theo-24, Theo-chron, Theolair)

Combinations
budesonide / formoterol (Symbicort)
fluticasone / salmeterol (Advair Diskus, Advair HFA)
fluticasone / vilanterol (Breo Ellipta)
ipratropium / albuterol (Combivent Respi-mat, DuoNeb)
mometasone / formoterol (Dulera)

COPD Agents

Anticholinergics
aclidinium / formoterol (Duaklir Pressair)
fluticasone / salmeterol (Advair Diskus, Advair HFA)
fluticasone / vilanterol (Breo Ellipta)
fluticasone / umeclidinium / vilanterol (Trelegy Ellipta)
glycopyrrolate (Lonhala Magnair)
glycopyrrolate / formoterol (Bevespi Aerosphere)
indacaterol / glycopyrrolate (Utibron Neohaler)
ipratropium / albuterol (Combivent Respi-mat, DuoNeb)
revefenacin (Yupelri)
tiotropium / olodaterol (Stiolto Respimat)
umeclidinium / vilanterol (Anoro Ellipta)

Long-Acting Beta-2 Agonists
arformoterol (Brovana)
formoterol (Perforomist)
indacaterol (Arcapta)
olodaterol (Striverdi Respimat)
salmeterol (Serevent)

Phosphodiesterase-4 Enzyme Inhibitors
roflumilast (Daliresp)

Antitrypsin Deficiency Agent
alpha-1 proteinase inhibitor (Aralast NP, Glassia, Prolastin-C, Zemaira)

Cystic Fibrosis Agents

Antibiotics
azithromycin (Zithromax)
aztreonam (Cayston)
tobramycin (Bethkis, Kitabis Pak, TOBI, TOBI Podhaler)

Mucolytics
dornase alfa (Pulmozyme)
N-acetylcysteine (Acetadote)

CFTR Modulators
ivacaftor (Kalydeco)
lumacaftor / ivacaftor (Orkambi)

tezacaftor / ivacaftor (Symdeko)
elexacaftor / ivacaftor / tezacaftor (Trikafta)

Surfactants
beractant (Survanta)
calfactant (Infasurf)
lucinactant (Surfaxin)
poractant alfa (Curosurf)

Tuberculosis Agents
ethambutol (Myambutol)
isoniazid
isoniazid / pyrazinamide / rifampin (Rifater)
pyrazinamide
rifampin (Rifadin)
rifapentine (Priftin)

Antitussives
benzonatate (Tessalon, Zonatuss)
codeine (various combinations)
dextromethorphan (Delsym, various brands)
hydrocodone / chlorpheniramine
    (TussiCaps, Tussionex, Vituz)
promethazine / codeine (Phenergan AC)

Dextromethorphan Combinations
dextromethorphan / pseudoephedrine /
    brompheniramine (Bromfed DM)
guaifenesin / dextromethorphan
    (Mucinex DM)
promethazine / dextromethorphan
    (Prometh DM, Promethazien DM)

Expectorants
guaifenesin (Mucinex, various brands)

Guaifenesin Combinations
guaifenesin / codeine (Cheratussin AC)
guaifenesin / pseudoephedrine (Mucinex D,
    Aldex)

Decongestants
phenylephrine (Neo-Synephrine, Sudafed PE)
pseudoephedrine (Sudafed)

Pseudoephedrine Combinations
cetirizine / pseudoephedrine (Zyrtec-D)
fexofenadine / pseudoephedrine (Allegra-D)
guaifenesin / pseudoephedrine (Mucinex D)
ibuprofen / pseudoephedrine (Advil Cold
    and Sinus)
ibuprofen / pseudoephedrine /
    chlorpheniramine (Advil Allergy Sinus)
loratadine / pseudoephedrine (Alavert

Allergy and Sinus D-12, Claritin-D)
naproxen / pseudoephedrine (Aleve-D Sinus
    and Cold, Sudafed 12 Hour Pressure/
    Pain)
triprolidine / pseudoephedrine (Pseudodine,
    Triacin)

Antihistamines
azelastine (Astelin, Astepro)
cetirizine (Aller-Tec, Alleroff, Zyrtec)
chlorpheniramine (Chlor-Trimeton)
chlorpheniramine / hydrocodone (Tussi-
    Caps, Tussionex, Vituz)
clemastine (Tavist, Tavist Allergy)
desloratadine (Clarinex, Clarinex Reditabs)
diphenhydramine (Benadryl)
fexofenadine (Allegra)
loratadine (Alavert, Claritin)
olopatadine (Pataday, Patanase, Patanol)

Nasal Corticosteroids
azelastine (DermacinRx, Dymista)
beclomethasone (Beconase AQ)
budesonide (Pulmicort Flexhaler, Pulmicort
    Respules, Rhinocort Allergy)
ciclesonide (Omnaris, Zetonna)
fluticasone furoate (Flonase Sensimist)
fluticasone propionate (Flonase Allergy
    Relief)
mometasone (Nasonex)
triamcinolone (Nasacort Allergy 24 HR)

Smoking Cessation Agents
bupropion (Aplenzin, Forfivo, Wellbutrin
    SR, Wellbutrin XL)
nicotine (Nicoderm CQ, Nicorette, Nicotrol)
varenicline (Chantix)

Boxed Warnings
acetylcysteine
benralizumab (Fasenra)
budesonide (Pulmicort Flexhaler, Pulmicort
    Respules, Rhinocort Allergy)
bupropion (Aplenzin, Forfivo XL, Wellbutrin
    SR, Wellbutrin XL)
codeine (various combinations)
fluticasone / salmeterol (Advair Diskus,
    Advair HFA)
isoniazid
isoniazid / pyrazinamide (Rifampin)
long-acting beta-2 agonists
IV phenylephrine

omalizumab (Xolair)
promethazine / codeine (Phenergan AC)
promethazine / dextromethorphan
  (Prometh DM, Promethazien DM)
varenicline (Chantix)
reslizumab (Cinqair)

Medication Guides
  budesonide / formoterol (Symbicort)
  bupropion (Aplenzin, Forfivo XL, Wellbutrin
    SR, Wellbutrin XL)
  fluticasone / salmeterol (Advair Diskus,
    Advair HFA)
  mometasone / formoterol (Dulera)
  omalizumab (Xolair)
  varenicline (Chantix)

✓ CHECK YOUR UNDERSTANDING

Take a moment to review what you have learned in this chapter and answer the following questions.

1. The specific site of gas exchange within the respiratory system is in the
   a. alveoli.
   b. bronchial tree.
   c. larynx.
   d. lungs.

2. Which of the following is the most accurate description of asthma?
   a. viral lung disease that causes coughing, wheezing, breathlessness, and chest tightness
   b. autoimmune disorder that causes coughing, wheezing, breathlessness, and chest tightness
   c. genetic disease that causes coughing, wheezing, breathlessness, and chest tightness
   d. inflammatory disorder of the airways that causes coughing, wheezing, breathlessness, and chest tightness

3. Which asthma medication should be used for the acute relief of bronchospasm?
   a. albuterol
   b. diphenhydramine
   c. fluticasone
   d. montelukast

4. Which of the following is not a risk factor for COPD?
   a. air pollution
   b. high blood pressure
   c. occupational exposure
   d. smoking

5. Which of the following can be used as a first-line treatment for bronchoconstriction related to COPD?
   a. roflumilast
   b. arformoterol
   c. ipratropium
   d. salmeterol

6. Tuberculosis is caused by
   a. *Mycobacterium abscessus.*
   b. *Mycobacterium avium.*
   c. *Mycobacterium tuberculosis.*
   d. *Pseudomonas aeruginosa.*

7. Which of the following are uses of antihistamines?
   a. prophylaxis for certain drug reactions
   b. symptomatic relief of hives and hay fever
   c. treatment of allergies
   d. All answers are correct.

8. Which of the following medications has a limitation on the amount that a consumer may purchase at one time?
   a. benzonatate
   b. clemastine
   c. guaifenesin
   d. pseudoephedrine

9. Which of the following medications would be most appropriate for use to provide symptomatic relief of a runny nose and itchy eyes due to seasonal allergies?
   a. benzonatate
   b. cetirizine
   c. guaifenesin
   d. phenylephrine

10. Which of the following agents may be used for smoking cessation?
    a. bupropion
    b. nicotine
    c. varenicline
    d. All answers are correct.

MAKE CONNECTIONS

Take a moment to consider what you have learned in this chapter and respond thoughtfully to the following prompts. Note that some of these activities will require internet access.

1. Many individuals seek the assistance of pharmacy technicians and pharmacists regarding over-the-counter treatments for allergies and cold symptom relief. Identify situations in which it would be important to involve the pharmacist. Which situations can pharmacy technicians address themselves?

2. How could a pharmacy technician help identify patients with asthma whose disease may not be well controlled? What should a pharmacy technician do in such a situation?

The online course includes additional review and assessment resources.

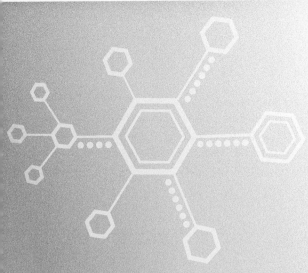

The Gastrointestinal System and Drug Therapy

12

Learning Objectives

1 Describe gastrointestinal (GI) anatomy and physiology. (Section 12.1)

2 Identify drug treatments for GI diseases. (Sections 12.2 to 12.10)

3 Describe gastroesophageal reflux disease and its complications. (Section 12.2)

4 Outline antidiarrheal agents, and explain their mechanisms of action. (Section 12.6)

5 Explain the role of fiber in the digestive process. (Section 12.7)

6 Discuss laxatives and their mechanisms of action. (Section 12.7)

7 Identify the chemoreceptor trigger zone (CTZ), and discuss its role in nausea. (Section 12.9)

8 State the antiemetics that act on the CTZ and their mechanisms of action. (Section 12.9)

9 Describe the measures to prevent and treat hepatitis. (Section 12.10)

ASHP/ACPE Accreditation Standards
To view the *ASHP/ACPE Accreditation Standards* addressed in this chapter, refer to Appendix C.

This chapter will discuss the gastrointestinal (GI) system and its diseases and disorders. Among the GI disorders reviewed are gastroesophageal reflux disease (GERD) and the influence of lifestyle factors on the condition; peptic disease, ulcerative colitis, and Crohn's disease; gallstones and their dissolution; diarrhea, including traveler's diarrhea and infectious diarrhea; and constipation and dietary contributions. Next, the chapter reviews vomiting and explains how the chemoreceptor trigger zone in the brain can initiate it. The chapter concludes with an explanation of the drugs used to treat hepatitis.

12.1 Anatomy and Physiology of the Gastrointestinal System

The **gastrointestinal (GI) system** is the group of organs that processes food and liquids. These actions include **digestion** (breakdown of large food molecules to smaller ones) and **absorption** (uptake of essential nutrients into the bloodstream). The GI system is composed of the **GI tract** (also known as the **alimentary tract**) and a number of supportive organs. The GI tract is a tube that begins in the mouth; extends through the pharynx, esophagus, stomach, small intestine, and large intestine; and ends at the anus (see Figure 12.1). The major function of the GI tract is to convert complex food substances into simple compounds that can be absorbed into the bloodstream and used by the cells of the body. In addition to digestion and absorption, the GI tract also excretes solid waste from the body.

FIGURE 12.1 The Gastrointestinal System

The mouth, esophagus, and stomach are part of the upper GI system, and the intestines, colon, and rectum are part of the lower GI system.

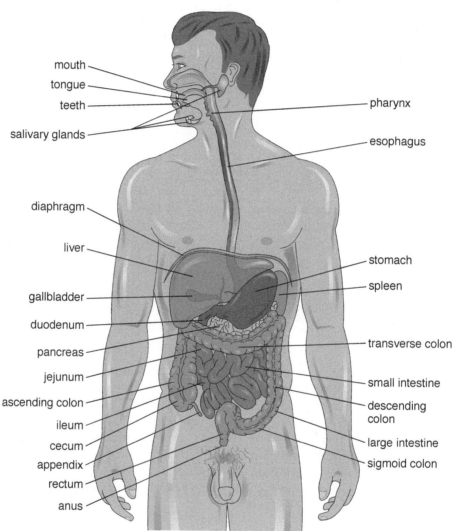

The **stomach** is composed of layers of smooth muscle lined with glands that secrete gastric juice. Gastric juice contains enzymes and hydrochloric acid that help break down food and mucus. From the stomach, contents go to the **small intestine**, where most nutrient absorption takes place. Next, in the **colon**, also called the large intestine, the material that has not been absorbed is exposed to bacteria, which aids in additional digestion. The main role of the large intestine is to absorb water. The **rectum** is the final portion of the large intestine where solid waste is stored until it passes through the anus. It is important to note that the entire GI system is protected by mucous membranes against abrasion and strong digestive enzymes used in the digestion process.

GI transit time, also known as bowel transit time, is the time it takes for material to pass from the mouth to the anus. This time frame is subdivided into gastric emptying time (the time it takes to leave the stomach) and colonic transit time (the time it takes for food to travel through the colon). A shorter GI transit time means that material is moving through the GI tract more quickly and may lead to a decrease in the absorption of nutrients and water. Conversely, if intestinal transit time is slowed, absorption of nutrients and water may increase.

GI transit times vary between individuals and can be affected by the types of foods and amount of water consumed. People who eat more fiber, fruits, vegetables, and whole grains may have shorter transit times compared with those who consume mostly starches and sugars. Medications and certain diseases can also affect the GI transit time. For example, diabetes and certain antidepressants can lead to delayed gastric emptying.

Other components of the GI system include the salivary glands, gallbladder, pancreas, and liver (see Figures 12.1 and 12.2). These organs release secretions that help the body digest food and absorb nutrients. The **salivary glands** produce **Saliva** which provides lubrication for food, makes swallowing easier, and contains enzymes that begin the process of digesting carbohydrates. The **gallbladder** is a pear-shaped organ located below the liver in the upper right abdomen that stores bile. **Bile**, an alkaline fluid, is produced by the liver and aids digestion and absorption of fat and cholesterol from the small intestine. The **pancreas** produces many enzymes that help digest carbohydrates, fats, and proteins. It releases secretions that neutralize the acid from the stomach. In addition to these functions, the pancreas releases important hormones such as insulin and glucagon that help maintain appropriate blood sugar levels in the body.

FIGURE 12.2
Auxiliary Organs of the GI System

Without neutralization by pancreatic secretions, acid from the stomach would damage the small intestine.

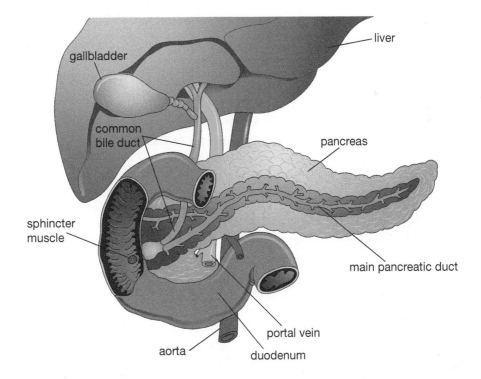

Molecules that are absorbed from the small intestine travel in the blood via the portal vein directly to the liver. The **liver** produces bile and removes harmful substances before they reach general circulation. Before orally administered drugs enter the circulation, they must pass through the liver. The liver metabolizes drugs before they reach their target in the body; this is called the **first-pass effect** (see Figure 12.3).

As described above, gastric acid is important in many processes. It helps digest food and absorption of nutrients. Unfortunately, gastric acidity can contribute to several conditions. Some of these conditions include gastroesophageal reflux disease and peptic ulcer disease.

FIGURE 12.3
Liver Function and First-Pass Effect

The first-pass effect is when the concentration of an orally administered drug is reduced before it reaches systemic circulation because of metabolism by the gut or liver. Alternatives to oral administration are necessary for drugs that will lose their efficacy if they undergo the first-pass effect.

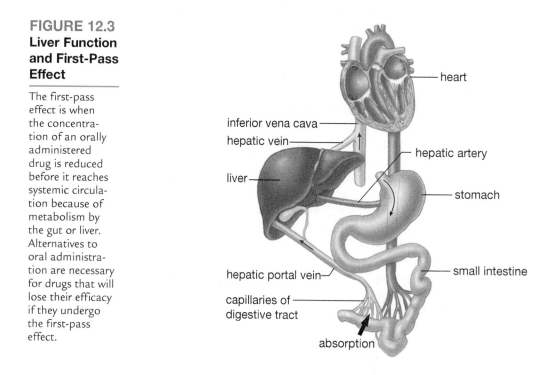

heart

inferior vena cava

hepatic vein

hepatic artery

liver

stomach

hepatic portal vein

small intestine

capillaries of digestive tract

absorption

12.2 Gastroesophageal Reflux Disease and Drug Treatments

Gastroesophageal reflux disease (GERD), also called *heartburn*, is one of the most common GI conditions. Symptoms include a burning feeling or pain behind the sternum (in the upper abdomen and chest) and an acid taste. Patients may also complain of food regurgitation. **Regurgitation** is when swallowed food goes back up through one's throat. GERD patients may have recurrent abdominal pain, which may move about in the **epigastric area**, the region of the upper abdomen immediately below the ribs. They may have nonspecific epigastric discomfort (gnawing or burning) that is worse before meals and may awaken them from sleep.

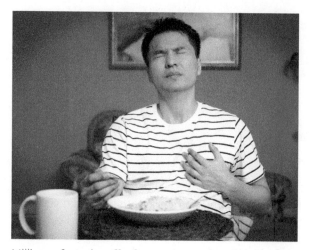

Millions of people suffer from various types of GI ailments, including GERD.

The primary reason for meal-related symptoms of **esophagitis** (inflammation of the esophagus) is the **reflux** (backflow) of acidic stomach contents through an incompetent lower esophageal sphincter. In its normal state, the sphincter is contracted. During swallowing, it relaxes enough to allow the forward passage of food and drink into the stomach; then it contracts again, preventing the reflux of the stomach contents. Heartburn occurs when the sphincter becomes incompetent (unable to keep itself sufficiently contracted). Figure 12.4 shows a normal sphincter retaining the stomach contents and an incompetent sphincter allowing reflux of the stomach contents up into the esophagus.

GERD not only produces bothersome symptoms for patients but also, over time, causes permanent changes in the tissue lining of the esophagus. These changes have been linked to narrowing of the esophagus (esophageal stricture) and esophageal cancers, so repeated bouts of GERD indicate a condition the patient should not ignore. Long-term treatment involves reducing the acidity of the stomach contents to limit damage to the esophagus.

It is important to recognize certain conditions and factors that risk of a compromised lower esophageal sphincter or interfere with the acid production processes within the body and contribute to GERD. Pregnancy, hiatal hernia, obesity, and delayed gastric emptying are conditions that can increase the risk of GERD. In addition, several lifestyle factors and certain foods may aggravate symptoms. Smoking, eating large meals, and eating late at night may contribute. Foods known to trigger reflux symptoms include alcohol, fatty foods, caffeine (e.g., chocolate, coffee, soft drinks and other carbonated beverages, and tea), citric and other acids, gas-producing foods, and certain spices.

Symptomatic relief of mild-to-moderate GERD can be obtained by using a combination of lifestyle modifications and medications. The main premise underlying treatment is that many patients have a lifelong problem. Ideally, persons prone to reflux

**FIGURE 12.4
Function of the Esophageal Sphincter**

(a) The normal esophageal sphincter closes between swallowings.

(b) The incompetent esophageal sphincter does not close completely, allowing the gastric contents (both food and stomach acids) to be ejected upward into the esophagus.

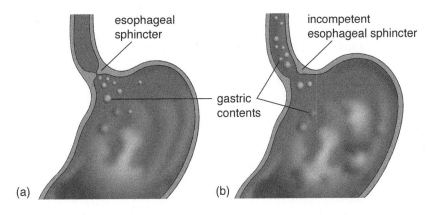

(a) (b)

TABLE 12.1 **Foods and Medications That May Worsen GERD**

Foods	Medications
• alcohol	• alendronate
• caffeine	• anticholinergics
• chocolate	• aspirin
• coffee or soft drinks	• barbiturates
• fatty foods	• dopamine
• garlic	• iron
• onions	• nicotine (from smoking)
• orange juice	• nitrates
• peppermint and spearmint	• nonsteroidal anti-inflammatory drugs (NSAIDS)
• spicy foods	• tetracycline

will adopt preventive behavior, but adherence is difficult to achieve. Patient education remains the cornerstone of therapy. Medications that promote reflux (e.g., theophylline and nifedipine) should be avoided. Patients are typically advised to stop smoking. To reduce discomfort, patients are advised not to lie down for at least three hours after a meal and, if necessary, to sleep with their head propped up.

Although the underlying problems of GERD and GI ulcers relate to damage in the GI tract from stomach acid, most treatments for these conditions do not directly fix this problem. Antacids, proton pump inhibitors (PPIs), and histamine H_2 receptor blockers relieve symptoms of GERD by decreasing acid production in the stomach. However, stomach contents may still be regurgitated into the esophagus or come into contact with an ulcer in the stomach or intestines, but less damage will occur because the gastric juices are not as acidic.

Antacids

Name Exchange

OTC antacids are commonly used products. Technicians may find it helpful to learn the generic and brand names of antacids, as patients often refer to these products by their brand names. Calcium carbonate is commonly known by the brand names Tums or Maalox tablets; calcium carbonate-magnesium hydroxide is sold under the brand names Mylanta Supreme and Rolaids.

Mild-to-moderate GERD (fewer than three episodes per week) can be treated with antacids. **Antacids** are medications used to prevent or correct acidity, especially in the stomach. They contain special ions that react with hydrogen ions in the stomach and neutralize acid. They are effective for only a few hours, so it may be necessary to take these medications after every meal. Antacids are available over the counter (OTC). See Table 12.2 for information on antacids.

Dosage Forms and Administration Antacid therapy has several shortcomings, including low patient adherence and the need for frequent dosing. These medications must be dosed one hour before meals and at bedtime.

Side Effects Common side effects of antacids include constipation, diarrhea, stomach pain, nausea, and vomiting. These effects are generally mild. Calcium- and aluminum-containing antacids tend to cause constipation, whereas magnesium-containing antacids tend to cause diarrhea.

Contraindications There are no contraindications to the use of antacids.

Cautions and Considerations Antacids provide short-term relief for patients with heartburn. Patients requiring repeated or constant use of antacids should see their prescribers and discuss other treatment options. Continuous use of calcium-containing antacids can cause acid hypersecretion, particularly when the medication is discontinued, so long-term use of calcium products should be discouraged.

Antacids must be used with caution in patients with renal failure because aluminum and magnesium can accumulate in the blood. Patients should let their pharmacists or physicians know if they have kidney failure.

Antacid suspensions need to be shaken well before use to ensure adequate mixing of contents and proper dosing.

Drug Interactions Antacids interact with drugs needing an acid environment to be absorbed, which results in decreased absorption and effectiveness (digoxin, phenytoin, isoniazid) and can increase absorption of other drugs leading to toxicity (levodopa). Antacids bind to several other orally administered drugs, decreasing their absorption. For this reason, antibiotics such as isoniazid, quinolones, and tetracyclines should not be taken with antacids. Other interacting medications include iron supplements containing ferrous sulfate and the sulfonylureas (treatment for diabetes). Antacids should be taken more than two hours before or after the other medication.

TABLE 12.2 Commonly Used Agents for GERD

Generic Name (Brand Name)	Pronunciation	Dosage Form	Common Dosages	Dispensing Status
Antacids				
aluminum hydroxide (AlternaGel)	a-LOO-mi-num hye-DROX-ide	oral suspension	PO: 5–30 mL between meals and at bedtime or as directed	OTC
aluminum hydroxide / magnesium carbonate (Gaviscon Extra Strength)	a-LOO-mi-num hye-DROX-ide mag-NEE-zee-um KAR-bon-ate	oral suspension, tablet	varies	OTC
aluminum hydroxide / magnesium hydroxide / simethicone (Mylanta, Maalox [some formulations])	a-LOO-mi-num hye-DROX-ide mag-NEE-zee-um hye-DROX-ide si-METH-i-kone	oral suspension, tablet	varies	OTC
calcium carbonate (Maalox tablets, Tums)	KAL-see-um KAR-bon-ate	capsule, chewable tablet, oral suspension, powder	2–4 tablets with GI distress; max dose 7 g a day	OTC
calcium carbonate / famotidine-magnesium hydroxide (Pepcid Complete)	KAL-see-um KAR-bon-ate fa-MOE-ti-deen mag-NEE-zee-um hye-DROX-ide	tablet	1–2 tablets a day	OTC
calcium carbonate / magnesium hydroxide (Mylanta, Rolaids)	KAL-see-um KAR-bon-ate mag-NEE-zee-um hye-DROX-ide	oral suspension, tablet	tablet and suspension strength varies; max calcium carbonate 7 g a day	OTC
magnesium hydroxide (Phillips' Milk of Magnesia)	mag-NEE-zee-um hye-DROX-ide	oral suspension, tablet	PO: dose varies; up to 4 times a day; max 4,800 mg/day	OTC
Histamine H$_2$ Receptor Antagonists				
cimetidine (Tagamet, Tagamet HB)	sye-MET-i-deen	tablet	400–800 mg 2 times a day	Rx OTC
famotidine (Pepcid, Pepcid AC)	fa-MOE-ti-deen	injection, oral suspension, tablet	20–40 mg 2 times a day	Rx OTC
nizatidine (Axid, Axid AR)	ni-ZAT-i-deen	capsule, oral solution, tablet	150 mg 2 times a day	Rx OTC
Proton Pump Inhibitors				
dexlansoprazole (Dexilant)	deks-lan-SOE-pra-zole	capsule	PO: 30 mg a day	Rx
esomeprazole (Nexium)	es-oh-MEP-ra-zole	capsule, granules, powder for reconstitution	20–40 mg a day	OTC, Rx
lansoprazole (Prevacid)	lan-SOE-pra-zole	capsule, oral suspension, oral disintegrating tablet	15–30 mg a day	OTC, Rx
omeprazole (Prilosec, Prilosec OTC)	oh-MEP-ra-zole	capsule, oral suspension, oral packet, tablet	20–40 mg a day / 20 mg a day	Rx / OTC
omeprazole / sodium bicarbonate (Zegerid)	oh-MEP-ra-zole soe-dee-um by-KAR-bon-ate	capsule, powder for reconstitution	40 mg a day	OTC
pantoprazole (Protonix)	pan-TOE-pra-zole	injection, oral packet, tablet	20 mg a day	Rx

continues

TABLE 12.2 **Commonly Used Agents for GERD**—*Continued*

Generic Name (Brand Name)	Pronunciation	Dosage Form	Common Dosages	Dispensing Status
rabeprazole (Aciphex)	ra-BEP-ra-zole	oral sprinkle capsule, tablet		Rx
Coating Agent				
sucralfate (Carafate)	soo-KRAL-fate	oral suspension, tablet	PO: 1 g 2–4 times a day	Rx
Prostaglandin E Analog				
misoprostol (Cytotec)	mye-soe-PROS-tawl	tablet	PO: 200 mcg 4 times a day	Rx

Histamine H$_2$ Receptor Antagonists

Gastric acid secretion and pepsin (a digestive enzyme) secretion occur in response to histamine, gastrin, foods, stomach distension, caffeine, or cholinergic stimulation. When gastric acid secretion is due to excess histamine release, histamine H2-receptor antagonists can be used. A **histamine H2-receptor antagonist**, also commonly referred to as an H2 blocker, works by blocking the receptors on the stomach's gastric acid–secreting cells and therefore decreases acidity. Similar to antacids, those with heartburn (fewer than three times per week) may use H$_2$ receptor antagonists. All of these antagonists are available in OTC strengths, but some doses are by prescription only. The bedtime dose is the most important dose for H$_2$ receptor antagonists because they can help decrease nighttime acid breakthrough.

Cimetidine (Tagamet, Tagamet HB) is indicated for treating ulcers, gastric hypersecretory states, GERD, postoperative ulcers, and upper GI bleeds and for preventing stress ulcers. It reduces hydrogen ion concentration in gastric secretions by 70%. Four to six weeks of therapy are required for ulcers to heal. Reduced doses are necessary in patients with renal disease. Use may be limited by the quantity of drug interactions. **Nizatidine (Axid, Axid AR)** is used for treating duodenal ulcers and GERD. It may take several days before the nizatidine provides the patient with relief from symptoms. If an antacid is added to the regimen, the doses of the two agents should be taken at least 30 minutes apart. A 100 mg dose of nizatidine is equivalent to approximately 300 mg of cimetidine. Patients should avoid aspirin, alcohol, caffeine, cough and cold preparations, and black pepper and other spices while taking this drug.

Famotidine (Pepcid, Pepcid AC) is used for treating duodenal ulcers, gastric ulcers, stress ulcers, GERD, and hypersecretory conditions. It relieves heartburn, acid indigestion, and sour stomach. The dose should be modified if the patient's kidney function is impaired, and it should be used cautiously in patients taking a calcium channel blocker. **Calcium carbonate-famotidine-magnesium hydroxide (Pepcid Complete)** is indicated for heartburn.

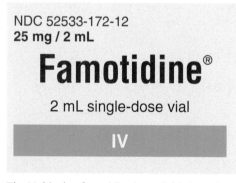

The H$_2$ blocker famotidine is available in oral dosage forms and intravenously (as pictured).

Dosage Forms and Administration All are available in OTC strengths, but some doses are by prescription only. The bedtime dose is the most important dose for H2 receptor antagonists because they can help decrease nighttime acid breakthrough.

Side Effects Side effects of cimetidine include headache, dizziness, drowsiness, diarrhea, agitation, and gynecomastia. Drowsiness is a side effect of nizatidine.

Contraindications A hypersensitivity to other H_2 receptor antagonists contraindicates the use of drugs in this class.

Cautions and Considerations Prolonged treatment (at least two years) may lead to malabsorption of dietary vitamin B12 and its subsequent deficiency.

H2 blockers decrease the absorption of drugs that require an acidic environment to dissolve. Ketoconazole (an antifungal) is an acid-soluble drug that may not be effective if used with H2 blockers. For that reason, an alternative should be sought for patients taking ketoconazole.

Drug Interactions Because it can inhibit the cytochrome P-450 system, cimetidine has many drug interactions. Patients using cimetidine and nizatidine should avoid concurrent use with dasatinib, delavirdine, dofetilide, epirubicin, pazopanib, pimozide, risedronate, or thioridazine.

Famotidine tends to have fewer drug interactions than the other drugs in this class. However, it should still not be prescribed for patients taking dasatinib, delavirdine, pazopanib, or risedronate.

WORKPLACE WISDOM

In April 2020, the FDA ordered that all prescription and OTC ranitidine, an H2 receptor antagonist, be removed from the market due to the investigation of a carcinogenic contaminant. Once a drug recall or withdrawal is announced by the FDA, notification will be provided to the pharmacist from several different sources. Once the notice has been received, the product needs to be removed from the shelves. The recalled medication can be returned to the manufacturer or the reverse distributor. It is important that the medication is removed and the recalls and withdrawals are promptly completed the same day as the notice.

Proton Pump Inhibitors

Acidity in gastric secretions is maintained by an enzyme known as the parietal cell H^+, K^+-ATPase pump (hydrogen ion–potassium ion pump). The term indicates that this enzyme pumps acidic hydrogen ions (H^+)—or protons—into the stomach, pumps nonacidic potassium (K^+) ions out, and uses energy (adenosine triphosphate [ATP]) to do so. A **proton pump inhibitor (PPI)**, a drug that blocks this enzyme, reduces stomach acidity. To work properly, PPIs can-

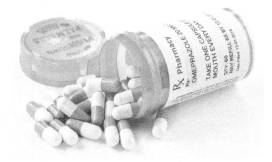

Closeup of concept Omeprazole prescription bottle with capsules.

not be taken on an as needed basis but must be taken daily. PPIs include drugs such as omeprazole and lansoprazole.

Omeprazole (Prilosec, Prilosec OTC) is indicated for the short-term treatment of severe erosive esophagitis, GERD, and hypersecretory conditions. It is also indicated for peptic disease caused by the bacterium *Helicobacter pylori*, in which case it is used in combination with other drugs such as tetracycline, clarithromycin, and an H2 receptor antagonist. **Omeprazole / sodium bicarbonate (Zegerid)** is an OTC medication for the short-term treatment of ulcer and GERD.

Take on an empty stomach

Esomeprazole (Nexium) is the S-enantiomer of omeprazole and is thus very similar to it. Esomeprazole is metabolized more slowly, which leads to higher and more prolonged drug concentrations and longer acid suppression. It relieves heartburn faster than omeprazole and is slightly more effective for healing erosive esophagitis. Esomeprazole is used to treat GERD and in combination with amoxicillin and clarithromycin to treat *Helicobacter pylori (H. pylori)*.

Lansoprazole (Prevacid) has the same mechanism of action and indications as omeprazole. It is used for short-term treatment of ulcers (four weeks) and esophagitis (eight weeks). It is also used in long-term treatment of hypersecretory conditions and Zollinger-Ellison syndrome (hypersecretion from a tumor). H2 blockers and other PPIs can also be used to treat this syndrome

Dexlansoprazole (Dexilant) is the R-enantiomer of lansoprazole. It is indicated for the treatment of GERD for eight weeks and for the treatment of erosive esophagitis for up to six months. The drug has two releases of medicine in one pill. The first is within an hour of taking the drug and the second four to five hours later. To reduce side effects and interactions, dexlansoprazole should be taken with a full glass of water.

Pantoprazole (Protonix) is a prescription-only PPI. Many hospitals have pantoprazole as a preferred proton pump inhibitor because it also has an intravenous (IV) form, which facilitates switching a patient from an IV to an oral dosage form.

Rabeprazole (Aciphex) is a PPI supplied as a delayed-release tablet.

Pharm Fact

Isomers have the same chemical formula, meaning they have the same number and types of atoms, but they have different structures. One type of isomer is an enantiomer, which describes molecules that have the same chemical formula and are mirror images of each other (R- and S-). Lansoprazole and omeprazole are R- and S-enantiomers. Dexlansoprazole is the R-enantiomer of lansoprazole, and esomeprazole is the S-enantiomer of omeprezole.

Dosage Forms and Administration To work properly, PPIs cannot be taken on an as needed basis but must be taken daily before meals. PPIs work best if taken in the morning before eating.

Omeprazole, lansoprazole, and esomeprazole capsules can be opened and mixed with a small amount of applesauce if patients have difficulty swallowing pills. Esomeprazole is also available as a delayed-release oral suspension.

Lansoprazole is available as tablets that are placed on the tongue and allowed to dissolve (oral disintegrating tablets). The dissolved particles must be swallowed without chewing.

Both pantoprazole and rabeprazole are prescription-only medications. Pantoprazole is available as an injection, oral packet, and tablet. Rabeprazole is available in oral sprinkle capsule form and as a tablet.

See Table 12.2 for additional dosage form information.

Side Effects Side effects of PPIs include headache, nausea, vomiting, and diarrhea.

Contraindications A hypersensitivity to one PPI contraindicates the use of all PPIs.

Cautions and Considerations OTC omeprazole should be used for only 14 days. If symptoms have not resolved after two weeks, patients should consult their healthcare practitioners.

Dexlansoprazole should be used with caution in patients who have liver dysfunction.

Some pantoprazole formulations contain polysorbate 80, which can cause hypersensitivity reactions. Safety of pantoprazole in children younger than five years has not been established.

Rabeprazole should be used with caution in patients with severe liver dysfunction.

Drug Interactions PPIs may decrease serum concentrations (the amount of medication in your blood) of clopidogrel. PPIs may decrease the absorption of drugs that need an acidic environment to dissolve. Ketoconazole (an antifungal drug) is an acid-soluble drug that may not work if used simultaneously with PPIs. For that reason, alternatives to PPIs should be sought for patients taking ketoconazole.

Coating Agents

Coating agents adhere to proteins at the ulcer site, forming a protective coat or shield over the ulcer that resists degradation by gastric acid, pepsin, and bile salts. It also inhibits pepsin; exhibits a cytoprotective effect (protecting cells from noxious chemicals); and forms a viscous, adhesive barrier on the surface of the intact intestinal mucosa and stomach.

Sucralfate (Carafate) is a complex of aluminum hydroxide and sulfated sucrose with an affinity for proteins. It is used to treat duodenal ulcers.

Dosage Forms and Administration Sucralfate is dosed every six hours (the duration of the coating action's effectiveness). Patients are often awakened from sleep by the ulcer, so around-the-clock dosing is recommended for the first few days. Once the symptoms of the ulcer are relieved, dosing can be reduced to twice daily for better patient adherence. Sucralfate should be taken on an empty stomach and should not be taken within two hours of other medications.

Side Effects Sucralfate may cause constipation in some patients.

Contraindications Sucralfate does not have contraindications.

Cautions and Considerations Use with caution in patients with renal dysfunction.

Drug Interactions Simultaneous sucralfate administration may decrease the absorption of cimetidine, digoxin, fluoroquinolone antibiotics, ketoconazole, l-thyroxine, phenytoin, quinidine, ranitidine, tetracycline, and theophylline.

Prostaglandin E$_1$ Analogs

As described in more detail in Chapter 6, nonsteroidal anti-inflammatory drugs (NSAIDs) inhibit the production of prostaglandins. This prostaglandin inhibition may lead to gastric ulcers. **Prostaglandin E1 analogs** replace the protective prostaglandins inhibited by NSAIDs.

Misoprostol (Cytotec) is a synthetic prostaglandin E$_1$ analog for NSAID-induced gastric ulcers. In other countries, misoprostol is used for ulcers other than those caused by NSAIDs.

Side Effects The primary side effects of this drug are diarrhea and abdominal pain.

Contraindications Pregnant individuals should not use or handle misoprostol. Misoprostol is also used to induce labor. Patients with prostaglandin allergy are contraindicated from using misoprostol.

Cautions and Considerations Misoprostol is a hazardous agent and should be handled and disposed of appropriately. This drug should not be given to individuals who may become pregnant unless they can comply with effective contraception. Misoprostol may cause abortion, birth defects, or premature birth. Patients should not share their medication with others.

Drug Interactions Antacids may enhance the toxicities of misoprostol. Misoprostol may enhance the therapeutic effects of carbetocin. Misoprostol may enhance the effects of oxytocin.

12.3 Peptic Disease and Drug Treatment

The term **peptic disease** is used to refer to a broad spectrum of disorders of the upper GI tract caused by the action of acid and pepsin. An **ulcer** is a local lesion or lesion of the surface of an organ or tissue. **Peptic ulcers** include gastric ulcers, which form on the lining of the stomach, and duodenal ulcers, which form in the lining of the upper part of the duodenum known as the small intestine (see Figure 12.5). Treatment of ulcers can include H$_2$ antagonists, but most often PPI therapy will be used.

FIGURE 12.5 Peptic Ulcers

Peptic ulcers are erosions of the mucosal lining of the GI tract. PPIs are commonly used to treat these ulcers.

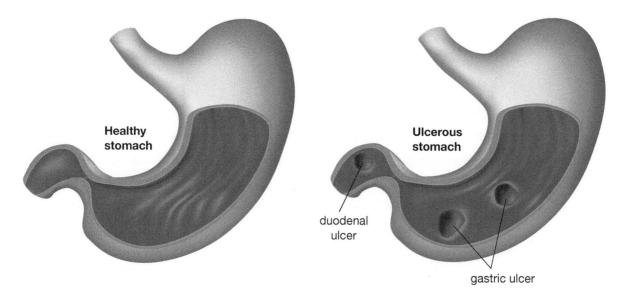

A **gastric ulcer** is a local excavation in the gastric mucosa. These lesions have malignant potential, occur more often in men than women, and become more frequent with aging. They are prevalent in smokers and in certain populations in the Western Hemisphere. Gastric ulcers do not necessarily occur in individuals who are high acid secretors. A family history of gastric ulcers represents a risk factor. As discussed later, a contributing factor for many patients is the presence of the bacterium *H. pylori*.

A **duodenal ulcer** is a peptic lesion situated in the duodenum. Duodenal ulcers occur more frequently in hypersecretors and are more difficult to treat than gastric ulcers because medications are usually absorbed in the stomach before they reach the duodenum.

A **stress ulcer** is another type of ulcer that occurs in the clinical setting in patients who are under severe physiologic stress from serious illness, such as sepsis, burns, major surgery, chronic disease, or chronic infection. Usually, the patient is in the intensive care unit (ICU). Stress ulcers are caused by the breakdown of natural mucosal resistance. The patient usually has no clinical symptoms but can experience acute hemorrhage. Inserting a nasogastric tube yields blood in the aspirate of the stomach contents. Perforations of the stomach wall occur in 8%–18% of patients, with severe pain radiating toward the back. Critically ill patients at high risk for development of a stress ulcer may receive H_2 blockers or proton pump inhibitors (PPIs) prophylactically to prevent an ulcer from developing. If the patient is unable to take enteral medications, intravenous (IV) formulations of these medications may be administered.

NSAIDs such as **ibuprofen** and **aspirin** can cause ulcers (see Table 12.3). These drugs can irritate and erode GI tissue. More importantly, they inhibit production of prostaglandins. Prostaglandins produce inflammation and pain throughout most of the body, but in the stomach, they protect the lining from acid secretion. Prolonged use of NSAIDs removes the protective effects of prostaglandins in the stomach and can result in GI ulceration. When ulceration erodes into a blood vessel, a **GI bleed** can occur. GI bleeds may be asymptomatic for many patients and are particularly dangerous for older adults or those patients who are critically ill. Patients taking long-term NSAIDs, aspirin, and anticoagulation therapy are at high risk for developing ulcers and life-threatening bleeding.

TABLE 12.3 Drugs That May Cause Ulcers

Drug	Adverse Effect
alcohol	irritates the GI tract
aspirin	irritates the GI tract
corticosteroids	reduce the mucosal barrier
iron	causes esophageal ulceration (must be taken with food, milk, or copious amounts of water)
methotrexate	irritates the GI tract, causes ulceration or hemorrhage
NSAIDs (such as ibuprofen, ketorolac, naproxen)	reduce production of prostaglandins
potassium chloride (KCl)	irritates the GI tract

H. Pylori Agents

Research has shown that *H. pylori*, a bacterium, is responsible for the majority of peptic ulcers. It may also play a role in chronic active gastritis and gastric cancer. **Gastritis** is the irritation or inflammation of the stomach lining. If a patient with peptic ulcer disease has a positive (+) test result for *H. pylori*, a multidrug regimen is prescribed (see Table 12.4). These drug combinations treat the ulcer, reduce symptoms, and kill *H. pylori* in the GI tract at the same time. All regimens consist of a PPI or H_2 receptor blocker to heal the ulcer and antibiotics to destroy the bacteria. Combination products are also available.

Bismuth Subcitrate Potassium / Metronidazole / Tetracycline

Bismuth subcitrate potassium / metronidazole / tetracycline (Pylera) is a combination product containing an antacid and two antibiotics and is approved to treat *H. pylori*. It is taken along with a PPI. An advantage of bismuth subcitrate is that it is not a salt of salicylic acid and therefore can be used in people who have an aspirin allergy.

Dosage Forms and Administration Pylera is a prescription-only medication and is available as capsules. Each dose of Pylera includes taking three capsules. Each dose of all three capsules should be taken four times a day, after meals and at bedtime. Patients should drink a full glass of water with each dose. Pylera is combined with a PPI for the morning and evening doses.

TABLE 12.4 Commonly Used *Helicobacter Pylori* Regimens

Proton Pump Inhibitor (PPI)	Plus Antibiotic	Plus Antacid	Brand Names of Combination Products
esomeprazole (Nexium) lansoprazole (Prevacid) omeprazole (Prilosec) pantoprazole (Protonix) rabeprazole (AcipHex)	Clarithromycin* 500 mg 2 times a day Amoxicillin* 1 g 2 times a day or Metronidazole* 500 mg 2 times a day		Prevpac (lansoprazole / amoxicillin / clarithromycin)
PPI listed above	Metronidazole* 250–500 mg 4 times a day	Bismuth subsalicylate (Pepto-Bismol) 525 mg 4 times a day	Pylera (bismuth subcitrate potassium / metronidazole- tetracycline)

*Antibiotics are discussed in detail in Chapter 16.

Side Effects Common side effects include nausea, diarrhea, temporary and harmless darkening of the tongue, and/or black stool.

Safety Alert

Metronidazole and macrodantin (nitrofurantoin, prescribed for urinary tract infections) can be confused with one and the other.

Contraindications A hypersensitivity to bismuth, metronidazole, tetracycline, or any component of the formulation contraindicates the use of this combination product. Patients with severe renal impairment should not use Pylera. Concomitant use with disulfiram or within the previous two weeks, and use with methoxyflurane, alcohol, or products containing propylene glycol, are contraindications. Ingestion of alcohol can cause a severe reaction resulting in nausea, vomiting, and a severe headache. Patients should be advised to not drink alcohol when using this medication.

Cautions and Considerations This product contains a tetracycline and should not be used in pediatric patients. Pylera may cause QT-interval prolongation. Bismuth may be neurotoxic. Patients should be monitored for neurotoxicity.

Drug Interactions Pylera may enhance adverse cardiac effects of other QT-prolonging medications.

Lansoprazole-Amoxicillin-Clarithromycin

Lansoprazole-amoxicillin-clarithromycin (Prevpac) is a combination product containing a PPI and two antibiotics for the treatment of *H. pylori*.

Dosage Forms and Administration This combination product is supplied in individual daily dosage cards to help patients manage the dosing. Each daily card contains two lansoprazole capsules, four amoxacillin capsules, and two clarithromycin film-coated tablets. Treatment is generally 10 to 14 days.

Side Effects Headache, diarrhea, and taste perversion are side effects.

Contraindications Contraindications include severe hypersensitivity to lansoprazole, PPIs, any penicillin or cephalosporin, macrolide antibiotics, or any component of the formulation. Concurrent use with pimozide, cisapride, ergotamine, dihydroergotamine, astemizole, terfenadine, colchicine, lovastatin, or simvastatin contraindicates use. Patients with a history of cholestatic jaundice or hepatic dysfunction with prior clarithromycin use or those individuals with a history of QT-interval prolongation or ventricular arrhythmia should not use Prevpac.

Cautions and Considerations Use with caution in older adults due to an increased risk of cardiac side effects and in patients with renal dysfunction.

Drug Interactions Prevpac may decrease concentrations of clopidogrel. Citalopram, fluticasone-salmeterol, sildenafil, simvastatin, and tamsulosin should not be used concurrently with Prevpac.

12.4 Ulcerative Colitis, Crohn's Disease, and Drug Treatments

Ulcerative colitis and Crohn's disease are inflammatory bowel diseases. Although these diseases differ based on where they are located in the GI tract, both cause chronic diarrhea, vomiting, bloating, fatigue, and abdominal pain. Symptoms flare up unexpectedly, can be mild to severe, and vary widely from person to person. Goals of treatment are to control inflammation and symptoms and then to maintain remission.

Ulcerative colitis involves excessive inflammation of the large intestine or colon. This causes abdominal pain and weight loss as well as diarrhea. The damage tends to be limited to specific portions of the colon or large intestine, and some patients can be cured surgically by removing the affected portion. Months can go by without symptoms (remission) and then symptoms can return (flare up). This disease can be eliminated through a surgical resection, in which physicians remove the diseased part of the colon.

Crohn's disease is an inflammatory bowel disease that causes chronic diarrhea and affects the entire GI tract (from mouth to anus). It also manifests outside the GI tract by penetrating through the intestinal wall and impacting tissues surrounding the gut. It is also different in that it is an autoimmune disease in which the immune system malfunctions and attacks the tissue lining of the entire GI tract. Although surgery is sometimes performed, it cannot cure Crohn's disease. Despite these differences, ulcerative colitis and Crohn's disease share many of the same treatments.

Three main groups of drugs can be used to treat these conditions: corticosteroids, aminosalicylates, and drugs that affect the immune system like disease-modifying antirheumatic drugs (DMARDs) and biologic response modifiers. Recall that DMARDs and biologic response modifiers are discussed in Chapter 6. More information on DMARDs can be found in Chapter 6. Table 12.5 lists the agents commonly used to treat these GI diseases. The location and severity of the disease and whether the goal is to induce remission in a flare or maintain remission determine which therapy is selected.

TABLE 12.5 Commonly Used Agents for Ulcerative Colitis and Crohn's Disease

Generic (Brand)	Pronunciation	Dosage Form	Common Dosage	Dispensing Status
Corticosteroids				
budesonide (Entocort EC)	byoo-DES-oh-nide	capsule, tablet	2 mg 2 times a day	Rx
hydrocortisone (A-Hydrocort, Cortef, Solu-Cortef)	hye-droe-KOR-ti-sone	cream, enema, foam, suppository, tablet	PO: 100–500 mg a day Rectal: apply/instill 2 times a day	Rx
methylprednisolone (A-MethaPred, Depo-Medrol, Medrol, Solu-Medrol)	meth-ill-pred-NISS-oh-lone	tablet	4–48 mg a day	Rx

continues

Generic (Brand)	Pronunciation	Dosage Form	Common Dosage	Dispensing Status
prednisone (Sterapred)	PRED-ni-sone	oral solution, tablet	5–60 mg a day	Rx
Aminosalicylates				
mesalamine (Apriso, Asacol, Canasa, Delzicol, Lialda, Pentasa)	me-SAL-a-meen	capsule, enema, suppository, tablet	PO: dose varies Rectal: 1 time a day	Rx
sulfasalazine (Azulfidine, Sulfazine)	sul-fa-SAL-a-zeen	tablet	2–4 g a day, divided	Rx
Biologic Response Modifiers (see Chapter 6)				
Integrin Receptor Antagonists				
vedolizumab (Entyvio)	VE-doe-liz-yoo-mab	injection	IV initially: 300 mg at weeks 0, 2, and 6; maintenance: 300 mg every 8 weeks	Rx
Interleukin-12 and -23 Antagonist				
ustekinumab (Stelara)	US-tah-kin-yoo-mab	injection	IV initially: 260–520 mg x 1 dose; SC maintenance: 90 mg every 8 weeks	Rx
Immunosuppressant				
azathioprine (Imuran)	ay-za-THYE-oh-preen	tablet	2–3 mg/kg a day	Rx

Corticosteroids

Corticosteroids are used for their anti-inflammatory and immunosuppressive properties. Patients with ulcerative colitis and Crohn's disease typically use corticosteroids orally or intravenously during a disease flare. Several topical formulations are also used. (Refer to Chapter 13 for additional information concerning corticosteroids.)

Dosage Forms and Administration Corticosteroids are available in oral, intravenous, and topical (rectal) formulations.

Side Effects Common side effects of corticosteroids include headache, dizziness, insomnia, and hunger. Taking oral corticosteroids first thing in the morning will lessen the effects of insomnia. Long-term use can affect metabolism in the body and cause facial swelling (typically referred to as "moon facies" or "moon face"), significant weight gain, fluid retention, and fat redistribution to the back and shoulders ("buffalo hump").

Other side effects include high blood pressure, loss of bone mass, electrolyte imbalance, cataracts and glaucoma, and insulin resistance (diabetes). Patients taking corticosteroids for an extended period will need to work with their healthcare practitioners to monitor these effects. If possible, therapy with corticosteroids should be used on a short-term basis and only when needed.

Contraindications Prednisone and methylprednisolone are contraindicated in patients who have systemic fungal infections. Live or live-attenuated vaccines should not be administered when immunosuppressive doses of prednisone are used. Hydrocortisone use is contraindicated in patients with systemic fungal infection, serious infections, and tubercular skin lesions. Contraindications to budesonide include primary treatment of status asthmaticus, acute episodes of asthma, and acute bronchospasm.

Cautions and Considerations Because corticosteroids suppress the immune system, patients taking them are at an increased risk of infection. With prolonged use, corticosteroids have been found to stunt growth in children. Patients who are taking budesonide should be instructed to swallow the capsule whole rather than crush or chew it.

Drug Interactions Corticosteroids may render anticoagulants less effective. Diabetes medications may be less effective when patients are using corticosteroids. Risk of infections with live vaccines increases with concurrent corticosteroid use.

Aminosalicylates

Aminosalicylates are used for both induction and maintenance of remission in patients with Crohn's disease and ulcerative colitis. Although their exact mechanism is unknown, it is thought that aminosalicylates modulate chemical mediators of the inflammatory response. Ulcerative colitis may worsen in patients, particularly children, using aminosalicylates.

Mesalamine

Mesalamine (Apriso, Asacol, Canasa, Delzicol, Lialda, Pentasa) is an aminosalicylate that is available in multiple dosage forms.

Dosage Forms and Administration Mesalamine can be administered orally or rectally. Rectal administration is by enema or suppository. The enema product should be maintained for eight hours or as long as practical; the suppository should be retained for one to three hours.

Side Effects Side effects include upset stomach, headache, arthralgia, and pharyngitis.

Contraindications A hypersensitivity to one aminosalicylate contraindicates the use of all others.

Cautions and Considerations Intolerance or worsening of ulcerative colitis may occur with use. Patients should be monitored for this response. There are reports of hypersensitivity in patients using aminosalicylates. In some cases, this reaction can be rash, and in others, organ involvement occurs (liver, kidney, and heart). Hepatic failure has been reported. Patients with hepatic or renal impairment should be monitored closely when using aminosalicylates. There are reports of myocarditis associated with the use of mesalamine as well.

The enema formulation of mesalamine may contain sulfites. Patients with a sulfite allergy should not use this formulation of mesalamine.

Drug Interactions Mesalamine has no documented drug interactions.

Sulfasalazine

Sulfasalazine (Azulfidine, Sulfazine) is a commonly used aminosalicylate. It is available as an oral product only.

Dosage Forms and Administration Sulfasalazine should be administered in evenly divided doses, preferably after meals. The delayed-release tablets should be swallowed whole, not crushed or chewed.

Side Effects Side effects include upset stomach, headache, arthralgia, and pharyngitis.

Contraindications A hypersensitivity to one aminosalicylate contraindicates the use of all others. Sulfasalazine should be avoided in patients with a sulfa hypersensitivity.

Cautions and Considerations Sulfasalazine may cause a discoloration of urine, perspiration, tears, and semen (orange-yellow).

There are reports of hypersensitivity in patients using aminosalicylates. In some cases, this reaction can be rash, and in others, organ involvement occurs (liver, kidney, and heart). These medications should be used cautiously in patients predisposed to heart conditions. Hepatic failure has been reported. Patients with hepatic or renal impairment should be monitored closely when using aminosalicylates. There are reports of myocarditis associated with the use of sulfasalazine. Use with caution in patients with severe asthma.

Drug Interactions Sulfasalazine may decrease the concentration of cardiac glycosides. The adverse effects of heparin, low-molecular-weight heparin, methotrexate, nitric oxide, and prilocaine may be enhanced by sulfasalazine use.

Biologic Therapies

Safety Alert

Prior to initiating biologic therapies for Crohn's disease and ulcerative colitis, it is recommended that patients be up to date with all immunizations (according to current immunization guidelines).

Patients with moderate to severe Crohn's disease or ulcerative colitis may require biologic therapy. **Biologic therapy** uses parts of the body's natural immune system to treat a condition or disease. In Crohn's disease and ulcerative colitis, biologic therapy helps stop certain proteins from causing inflammation in the GI tract These therapies include biologic response modifiers (see Chapter 6), integrin receptor antagonists, and interleukin-12 and -23 antagonists.

Vedolizumab

Vedolizumab (Entyvio) is an anti-integrin antibody used in both Crohn's disease and ulcerative colitis. Vedolizumab specifically targets integrin proteins in the gastrointestinal tract and is not typically associated with systemic immunosuppression.

Dosage Forms and Administration Vedolizumab is administered by IV infusion.

Side Effects Side effects for vedolizumab include running nose, headache, nausea, fever, fatigue, respiratory tract infection, cough, bronchitis, itching, and pain.

Contraindications There are no known contraindications to vedolizumab.

Cautions and Considerations Infusion-related reactions and hypersensitivity reactions such as dyspnea, bronchospasm, hives, flushing, increased blood pressure and heart rate have been reported with use. Patients are at an increased risk of developing infections, and therapy is not recommended in patients with active, severe infections until resolved. Progressive multifocal leukoencephalopathy (PML), a rare and often fatal infection of the CNS, has occurred.

Drug Interactions Vedolizumab should not be used with anti-TNF agents.

Ustekinumab

Ustekinumab (Stelara) is an interleukin (IL)-12/23 antagonist. Interleukin-12 and interleukin-23 are proteins that contribute to the inflammation process. Ustekinumab blocks the activity of IL-12 and IL-23 and reduces inflammation. Ustekinumab was first approved to treat plaque psoriasis.

Dosage Forms and Administration Ustekinumab is administered as an IV infusion as a single dose for induction therapy and is given as a subcutaneous injection for maintenance treatment. It is available in both a vial and prefilled syringe.

Side Effects Side effects include headache, nausea, vomiting, nasopharyngitis, injection site redness and irritation, bronchitis, itching, urinary tract infections, and sinusitis.

Contraindications Ustekinumab has no contraindications.

Cautions and Considerations Patients are at an increased risk of developing infections. Therapy is not recommended in patients with active, severe infections until resolved. Ustekinumab may increase the risk of malignancy. The needle cover on the prefilled syringe may cause reactions in individuals sensitive to latex.

Drug Interactions Patients taking warfarin or cyclosporine should have these drug concentration levels monitored and doses adjusted as needed.

Immunosuppressants

Medications that suppress the immune system are called **immunosuppressant agents**. These medications may induce response and remission in patients with Crohn's disease or ulcerative colitis. Common side effects of immunosuppressants include sore throat, cough, dizziness, nausea, muscle aches, fever, chills, itching, and headache. These effects are usually mild to moderate. Taking acetaminophen can alleviate some of these effects if they are bothersome.

Azathioprine (Imuran) is an immunosuppressive agent that interferes with nucleic acid synthesis in both normal and precancerous cells. The overall action is suppression of the immune system. This drug is approved to treat severe arthritis and to prevent the rejection of transplanted organs. It is also used as an anti-inflammatory agent in Crohn's disease, ulcerative colitis, and chronic active hepatitis. It is used in patients who have not responded to steroids or aminosalicylates or in those whose disease flares when steroids are withdrawn. It can cause serious but reversible forms of bone marrow depression.

Dosage Forms and Administration Dosing of azathioprine is based on the patient's condition, weight, and response to treatment. It can be taken with food to reduce stomach upset.

Side Effects Side effects unique to azathioprine include arthralgias, rash, alopecia (hair loss), hepatotoxicity, and increased risk of infection.

Contraindications Azathioprine is contraindicated during pregnancy and in patients with rheumatoid arthritis and a history of treatment with alkylating agents.

Cautions and Considerations Azathioprine has a boxed warning for increased risk of malignancy (such as lymphoma). Patients should be warned of this risk prior to starting therapy.

Because immunosuppressants suppress the immune system, patients taking them are at an increased risk of infection. Patients are often instructed to take special precautions to minimize exposure to infection, including wearing face masks, avoiding crowds, and washing their hands frequently.

Drug Interactions Febuxostat may increase concentrations of azathioprine. The side effects of mercaptopurine, natalizumab, and tofacitinib may be enhanced by azathioprine. Toxic effects of azathioprine may be enhanced by pimecrolimus and tacrolimus.

12.5 Gallstones and Drug Treatments

Gallstones are pebble-like structures formed from hardened digestive fluid that can form in the gallbladder and obstruct the **cystic duct** (see Figure 12.6). The cystic duct connects the gallbladder to the common hepatic duct. It then joins the common bile duct. Classic symptoms of gallstones include intense and dull abdominal discomfort. Sweating, nausea, and vomiting are other signs.

FIGURE 12.6
The Gallbladder and Bile Duct

The gallbladder is connected to the common hepatic duct and the common bile duct via the cystic duct.

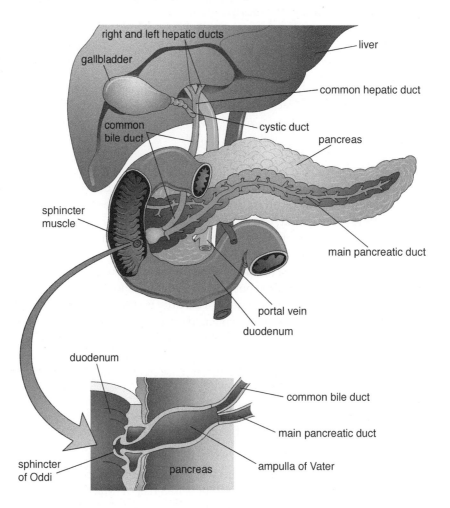

Gallstone Dissolution Agent

Gallstones may be recurrent and are most commonly treated with **cholecystectomy** (surgical removal of the gallbladder). However, there are pharmacologic options. Gallstones can be dissolved with **gallstone dissolution agents**.

Ursodiol

Ursodiol (Actigall) is a naturally occurring bile acid that is administered orally to dissolve cholesterol gallstones in the gallbladder or common bile duct (see Figure 12.6). It decreases the cholesterol content of bile and bile stones by reducing the secretion of cholesterol from the liver and the fractional reabsorption of cholesterol by the intestines. Frequent blood tests are necessary to monitor the drug's effects. Persistent nausea, vomiting, and abdominal pain should be reported. Gallstone dissolution can take several months; for some patients, however, gallstones never dissolve. Even in cases of successful dissolution, recurrence of stones within five years has been observed in 50% of patients.

Dosage Forms and Administration Ursodiol is available as a tablet and is taken two to three times daily. The dose a patient receives is based on weight. It should be taken with food.

Side Effects Common side effects include nausea, diarrhea, constipation, mild stomach pain or discomfort, headache, or dizziness.

Contraindications Ursodiol is contraindicated in patients with complete biliary obstruction. It should not be used in patients with calcified bile stones, as it is ineffective in these cases. Patients who have compelling reasons for cholecystectomy should not receive ursodiol. An allergy to bile acids contraindicates the use of ursodiol.

Cautions and Considerations Gallstone dissolution can take months, and patients should expect a longer period of therapy. Use with caution in patients with liver dysfunction.

Drug Interactions Antacids and bile acid may decrease concentrations of ursodiol. Clofibrate and estrogens may encourage the formation of gallstones and may counteract the benefits of ursodiol.

12.6 Diarrhea and Drug Treatments

 Work Wise

GI disorders are the most common disorders for which patients self-medicate with OTC medications. It is important that pharmacy technicians carefully update the patient profile, including verifying any new OTC medications that a patient is taking.

Diarrhea is defined as excessive, soft, or watery stools. Excessive stool can mean large stool volume or larger number of bowel movements than normal. In diarrhea, increased GI motility leads to frequent bowel movements.

Acute diarrhea is a common condition that can be caused by infections such as traveler's diarrhea and food poisoning as well as certain drugs (see Table 12.6). Infectious causes of diarrhea include bacterial infections such as **salmonella** and *Escherichia coli (E. coli)*, protozoal infections such as giardiasis, or viral infections such as **Norwalk virus** and **rotavirus**. Drugs used to treat infections are discussed in Chapter 16. Chronic diarrhea is less common and can be caused by irritable bowel syndrome, ulcerative colitis, or Crohn's disease.

Diarrhea can be dangerous because it can quickly lead to dehydration. It decreases GI transit time and will impair absorption of drugs, vitamins, nutrients, and toxins. The most commonly used antidiarrheal agents are listed in Table 12.7. Specifically, the antimotility drugs should be used in managing chronic disease states, such as inflammatory bowel disease, postvagotomy diarrhea, and ileostomy. They should not be used to manage short-term, self-limiting diarrhea. These agents can also be hazardous in infectious diarrhea by prolonging fever and delaying clearance of organisms.

TABLE 12.6 Drugs That Can Cause Diarrhea

alcohol	H_2 receptor antagonists
angiotensin-converting enzyme (ACE) inhibitors	magnesium-containing laxatives or antacids
antibiotics	nonsteroidal anti-inflammatory drugs (NSAIDs)
certain chemotherapy agents (fluoropyrimidines, irinotecan)	proton pump inhibitors (PPIs)
digoxin	

TABLE 12.7 Commonly Used Antidiarrheal Agents

Generic (Brand)	Pronunciation	Dosage Form	Common Dosages	Dispensing Status	Controlled Substance Schedule
Adsorbent					
bismuth subsalicylate (Kaopectate, Pepto-Bismol)	BIS-muth sub-sa-LISS-i-late	oral suspension, tablet	2 tablets (262 mg/tab) or 30 mL (17.5 mg/mL) regular strength every 30–60 min as needed; do not exceed 8 doses in 24 hr (16 tablets or 240 mL)	OTC	
Antimotility Drugs					
difenoxin / atropine (Motofen)	dye-fen-OX-in AT-roe-peen	tablet	2 tablets, then 1 tablet after each loose bowel movement or 1 tablet every 3–4 hr as needed; do not exceed 8 tablets in 24 hr	Rx	C-IV
diphenoxylate / atropine (Lomotil)	dye-fen-OX-i-late AT-roe-peen	oral solution, tablet	5 mg (2 tablets or 10 mL) 4 times a day	Rx	C-V
loperamide (Imodium, Imodium A-D)	loe-PAIR-a-mide	capsule, oral solution, tablet	4 mg (2 cap) after first loose bowel movement, then 2 mg (1 cap) after each loose bowel movement; do not exceed 16 mg (8 cap) in 24 hr	OTC	
Drugs for Infectious Diarrhea					
nitazoxanide (Alinia)	nye-tah-ZOX-ah-nide	oral solution, tablet	age 12 and older: 500 mg every 12 hr	Rx	
rifaximin (Xifaxan)	rye-FAX-i-min	tablet	200 mg 3 times a day	Rx	

Adsorbents

Adsorbents are a class of **antidiarrheals**, medications used to slow or stop loose stools (diarrhea). They are thought to work by binding to (and therefore neutralizing) diarrhea-causing toxins. This mechanism of action prevents the adherence of infectious pathogens to the walls of the GI tract.

Bismuth subsalicylate (Kaopectate, Pepto-Bismol) is generally safe to use as an antidiarrheal. This OTC product acts as an adsorbent, instead of reducing GI motility. Bismuth subsalicylate has both antibacterial and antisecretory actions. In addition, it has anti-inflammatory effects, making it beneficial in treating *H. pylori* infection and traveler's diarrhea.

Dosage Forms and Administration Bismuth subsalicylate is available OTC as a chewable tablet and an oral suspension.

Side Effects Bismuth subsalicylate may cause constipation, nausea, vomiting, and darkening of the tongue and/or stools. Taking bismuth subsalicylate with food and plenty of water may relieve nausea symptoms. Although rare, neurotoxic symptoms such as tinnitus (ringing in the ears), confusion, and generalized weakness are also potential side effects. To prevent these more serious side effects, patients should not take excessive doses of bismuth subsalicylate.

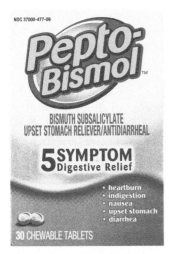

The OTC adsorbent bismuth subsalicylate is sold under the brand name Pepto-Bismol.

Contraindications Bismuth subsalicylate should not be used in patients with a history of severe GI bleeding or coagulation problems. In addition, patients with aspirin hypersensitivity should avoid products containing bismuth subsalicylate because such products may trigger an allergic type of reaction.

Cautions and Considerations Patients should be warned that their tongue and stools might darken while taking this medication. These changes are harmless and temporary. Patients should also be told to stop taking bismuth subsalicylate if they experience confusion, dizziness, or vision changes and to report these problems to their healthcare practitioners.

Bismuth subsalicylate may decrease the effectiveness of tetracycline antibiotics, so patients should not take the two medications concurrently. In addition, bismuth subsalicylate products may enhance the anticoagulant effects of warfarin, thereby increasing a patient's risk of bleeding. To prevent or limit these potential drug interactions, patients should tell their physicians and pharmacists about all prescription and nonprescription products they are taking. Patients with renal failure or gout should consult their healthcare practitioners before using bismuth subsalicylate.

Parents should consult their pharmacists or physicians before giving this product to children. Children and adolescents are at risk of a condition known as Reye's syndrome, a potentially life-threatening disorder caused by salicylate use for viral infections.

Oral suspensions must be shaken well before ingestion to ensure adequate mixing and proper dosing.

Drug Interactions Anticoagulants may increase the risk of bleeding when used with bismuth subsalicylate. Methotrexate concentrations may be increased by bismuth subsalicylate use. Tetracycline levels may decrease with bismuth subsalicylate administration.

Antimotility Drugs

Antimotility drugs for diarrhea work by slowing **peristalsis**, the smooth muscle contractions that propel fecal matter along the colon. Water absorption from the feces is increased as the colon contents spend more time in GI transit. Most of these drugs contain opiates and, therefore, are controlled substances. Recall that long-term use of narcotics for pain leads to constipation; the use of narcotics to control diarrhea is an example of using a drug for its side effects to treat another condition. Drugs in this class include diphenoxylate / atropine, difenoxin / atropine, and loperamide and are not for use in patients younger than two years of age.

Diphenoxylate / Atropine and Difenozin / Atropine

Diphenoxylate / atropine (Lomotil) is a combination of 2.5 mg of diphenoxylate and 0.025 mg of atropine. Diphenoxylate is derived from the narcotic meperidine, which is why the medication is a Schedule V controlled substance. Atropine is added to discourage abuse; it also reduces peristalsis, but in excessive doses, it produces anticholinergic side effects (dry mouth, blurred vision, flushing, and urinary retention).

Dosage Forms and Administration Diphenoxylate / atropine is available as a tablet and oral solution for oral administration. It is taken every 6 hours until control of diarrhea has been achieved, which usually occurs within 48 hours.

Side Effects Additional side effects include constipation, paralytic ileus, respiratory depression, and sedation. Care should be taken in patients who have infectious diarrhea with fever; acute diarrhea; toxic megacolon, which can result in perforation; and advanced liver disease. Both of these drugs slow peristaltic action, which produces bulking of fecal matter.

Contraindications Diphenoxylate / atropine is contraindicated in children younger than two years. This drug is also contraindicated in patients with obstructive jaundice and diarrhea associated with pseudomembranous enterocolitis or enterotoxin-producing bacteria.

Cautions and Considerations Diphenoxylate can cross the blood-brain barrier and cause euphoria, which increases its potential for abuse, and pharmacies must follow state laws regarding controlled substance dispensing. In some states, special restrictions apply to the purchase of these products, and all sales are documented in a logbook.

Opiate derivatives are not appropriate for treating all types of diarrhea. If fever or bloody stool is present, the patient should consult a physician. In addition, if diarrhea continues for 48 hours after use of an opiate derivative, the patient needs further evaluation by a medical professional.

Because opiate derivatives may cause dizziness and drowsiness, patients should be reminded that activities such as driving might not be safe while taking these medications. Patients should be warned to take careful note of the effects of these drugs before attempting such activities.

Drug Interactions Diphenoxylate / atropine may enhance the adverse effects of anticholinergic agents, glucagon, and zolpidem. Central nervous system (CNS) depressant side effects may be increased with concurrent diphenoxylate / atropine use. Diphenoxylate / atropine may enhance the ulcer-causing effects of potassium chloride.

Difenoxin / Atropine

Difenoxin / atropine (Motofen) contains a metabolite of diphenoxylate and is classified as a Schedule IV controlled substance.

Dosage Forms and Administration Difenoxin / atropine is available as a tablet for oral administration. If clinical improvement of diarrhea is not seen in 48 hours, it is not recommended to continue use.

Side Effects The side effect profile and usage are the same as for **diphenoxylate / atropine (Lomotil)**.

Contraindications A hypersensitivity to difenoxin, atropine, or any component of the formulation contraindicates use. Patients with severe liver disease, jaundice, dehydration, or angle-closure glaucoma should not use difenoxin-atropine. This medication is not for use in children younger than two years, patients with diarrhea associated with organisms that penetrate the intestinal mucosa, and patients with pseudomembranous colitis associated with broad-spectrum antibiotics.

Cautions and Considerations Difenoxin / atropine may cause CNS depression. Use with caution in patients with liver or hepatic disease.

Drug Interactions Difenoxin / atropine may enhance the adverse effects of CNS depressants and anticholinergics.

Loperamide

Loperamide (Imodium, Imodium A-D) is a synthetic opioid similar to diphenoxylate. It acts on the intestinal nerves and reduces peristaltic activity, but it does not act on the CNS. Loperamide has been used for prolonged periods (18 months or longer) without loss of efficacy or signs of toxicity.

Dosage Forms and Administration Loperamide is indicated for use in patients two years of age and older. It is available as a tablet, capsule, or oral solution. It is available over the counter for a maximum approved daily dose of 8 mg per day. It is also available as a prescription for a maximum approved dose of 16 mg.

Side Effects Side effects are drowsiness, constipation, and dry mouth. Taking higher than recommended doses of loperamide can result in serious adverse cardiac events, such as torsades de pointes, cardiac arrest, and death.

Contraindications Loperamide should be avoided in children younger than two years and in patients who have abdominal pain without diarrhea.

Cautions and Considerations If diarrhea lasts longer than two days, symptoms worsen, or abdominal swelling or bulging develops, patients should discontinue use and consult a healthcare practitioner.

Drug Interactions Loperamide does not have any major drug interactions.

Drugs for Infectious Diarrhea

Food- and waterborne illnesses can cause significant morbidity and even death. These illnesses result from the ingestion of food or water contaminated with infectious pathogens. Some cases occur domestically, whereas others occur with travel.

Giardia lamblia is a **protozoan** (single-celled animal) that can cause infection (called giardiasis). It is a microscopic parasite that is found worldwide in water. Streams, lakes, wells, and swimming pools can all contain *G. lamblia*. It can also be transmitted through food and person-to-person contact. Symptoms of giardiasis include abdominal cramps, bloating, nausea, and bouts of watery diarrhea.

Traveler's diarrhea (TD) is a condition that poses a significant risk to US citizens who travel to some foreign countries; it is acquired through ingestion of food or water contaminated with bacteria, the most common being the fecal bacterium *E. coli*. TD may affect 30%–70% of travelers after arrival at their destinations. To prevent contamination, travelers should limit their consumption to well-cooked foods, peeled fruits and vegetables, and bottled water. Previously, systemic antibiotics were commonly prescribed, but because of increased antibiotic resistance, this practice is no longer recommended. Most cases of TD resolve on their own within three to five days. Prophylactic antibiotics may be used for travelers who are high risk (such as those who are immunosuppressed) or who are taking critical trips. If prophylaxis is warranted, some physicians recommend taking a quinolone antibiotic (see Chapter 16) and loperamide after the first loose stool.

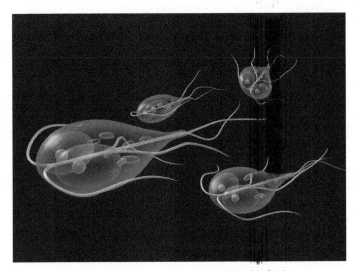

G. lamblia is a protozoan that can cause intestinal infection.

Nitazoxanide

Nitazoxanide (Alinia) is indicated for the treatment of infectious diarrhea caused by the waterborne parasites *G. lamblia* and *Cryptosporidium parvum*. It may be used in patients age one year or older. Nitazoxanide interferes with an enzyme-dependent electron transfer that is essential for anaerobic energy metabolism. Other drugs used against GI parasites are described in a later section of this chapter.

Dosage Forms and Administration Nitazoxanide is available as a tablet and as a powder that is to be mixed with water. Both the powder and oral suspension should be refrigerated. The reconstituted suspension should be discarded after seven days.

Side Effects Nitazoxanide is generally well tolerated, but side effects may include headache, abdominal pain, nausea, or urine discoloration.

Contraindications There are no manufacturer-reported contraindications to the use of nitazoxanide.

Cautions and Considerations Patients with renal or hepatic dysfunction should use nitazoxanide with caution. The safety of this medication has not been established in patients who have human immunodeficiency virus (HIV). Patients who have diabetes should be informed that this drug contains 1.48 g of sucrose per 5 mL.

Drug Interactions There are no known significant interactions with nitazoxanide use.

Rifaximin

Rifaximin (Xifaxan) is indicated for the treatment of TD. Rifaximin works by inhibiting bacterial ribonucleic acid (RNA) synthesis. The significant advantage of this drug is that it is not absorbed into the body, so there is little risk of developing long-term resistance.

Dosage Forms and Administration Rifaximin is available as a tablet for oral use and is indicated for patients 12 years and older. It should not be used in diarrhea complicated by fever or blood in stool.

Side Effects Rifaximin may cause flatulence.

Contraindications Hypersensitivity to rifamycin antibiotics contraindicates use.

Cautions and Considerations Hypersensitivity reactions have occurred with use. Prolonged use may result in bacterial superinfection. Rifaximin should not be used for systemic infections, as it is not efficacious.

Drug Interactions Cyclosporine may increase the concentrations of rifaximin. Rifaximin may diminish the therapeutic effects of sodium picosulfate.

12.7 Constipation and Flatulence and Drug Treatments

Constipation is the opposite of diarrhea. It is characterized by infrequent bowel movements, small stool size, hard stools, or the feeling of incomplete bowel evacuation. Most people pass at least three stools a week, so fewer stools could constitute constipation. However, diagnosis depends on the individual patient. Many episodes of constipation are related to a diet low in fiber or fluid intake. Constipation can also be caused by certain foods or drugs (see Table 12.8). Although many drugs have the potential to cause diarrhea or constipation, the ones most associated with constipation include antacids and pain medications such as opiates. Stress may also exacerbate constipation, whereas light exercise promotes GI motility.

TABLE 12.8 Drugs That May Cause Constipation

- antiemetics
- antihistamines
- calcium- and aluminum-containing laxatives or antacids
- calcium channel blockers
- diuretics
- iron
- nonsteroidal anti-inflammatory drugs (NSAIDs)
- opiates (morphine, hydrocodone, oxycodone, etc.)
- tricyclic antidepressants (TCAs)

Dietary modification and lifestyle changes should accompany pharmacologic treatment of constipation. Adequate dietary intake of fiber (including fruits, vegetables, and whole grains) and regular exercise (even light walking) regulate GI motility. Patients with repeat bouts of constipation should drink plenty of fluids, eat adequate fiber, and exercise regularly.

Drugs that relieve constipation are known as **laxatives**. Typically, laxatives are used only as needed on a short-term basis. Electrolyte abnormalities may occur if laxatives are used too frequently. If patients are regularly using laxatives, they should consult their physicians for a full evaluation.

In addition to oral dosage forms, many laxatives are available as suppositories or enemas. These dosage forms are used for rapid treatment of moderate-to-severe constipation. Rectal suppositories take 15 to 60 minutes to work. They are useful for hospitalized patients who are unable to swallow oral laxatives. Before inserting a rectal suppository, the patient can squat or lie on their side with one leg straight and the other bent. The patient should remove the foil wrapping from the suppository and insert the pointed end first into the rectum (see Figure 12.7). It needs to be inserted far enough into the rectum so that it does not slip out. Afterward, the patient should wash their hands.

FIGURE 12.7 Suppository Insertion

A suppository must be inserted past the rectal sphincter so that it stays in place.

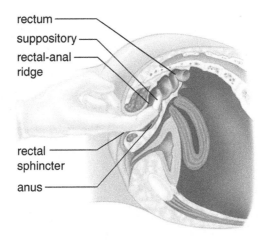

rectum
suppository
rectal-anal ridge
rectal sphincter
anus

An **enema** is a liquid solution that is delivered directly into the rectum. Enemas are used to rapidly empty the bowels prior to surgery or diagnostic procedures, such as a colonoscopy or barium enema. They also can remove excessive fecal matter that is blocking the GI tract. To use an enema, the patient should lie down on their side and bend the knee of the topmost leg with a towel supporting the knee. The enema tip is inserted into the rectum, and the liquid is allowed to drain into the rectum via gravity or by squeezing the bottle. The patient should hold the enema liquid in the rectum for a specific period (2 to 60 minutes, depending on the product) and then defecate normally.

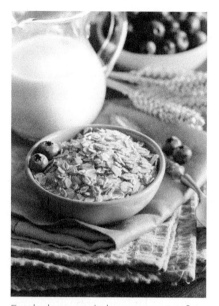

Foods that contain large amounts of fiber include oats and fruit (pictured), as well as beans, vegetables, and flaxseed.

Fiber and Fiber Supplementation

Fiber is defined as the undigested residue of fruits, vegetables, and other foods of plant origin. Fiber can be classified as soluble or insoluble. Soluble fiber is made of carbohydrates that dissolves in water. Examples of foods that contain soluble fiber include beans, peas, fruits, and oats. Insoluble fiber comes from plant cell walls that cannot dissolve in water. Examples of foods that contain insoluble fiber include rye, wheat, and other grains. Total dietary fiber is the sum of both soluble and insoluble fiber. Figure 12.8 illustrates the colon, or large intestine, an organ that depends on dietary fiber to function normally.

Most dietary fiber reaches the colon unaltered; it increases colon content, reduces colon pressure, and increases propulsive motility (forward motion). These effects account for fiber's role in preventing or relieving constipation. Chronic constipation has often been associated with low-fiber diets. It is a common problem among older adults in the United States and other Western countries, but it does not appear to be a problem in less-developed countries.

Extended transit time in the colon permits more water to be absorbed from the GI tract into the body, thus producing smaller, harder stools. Shortening the transit time produces looser, more watery stools because less water is absorbed.

FIGURE 12.8
Large Intestine

The large intestine, also known as the colon, is an organ that depends on dietary fiber for its normal function.

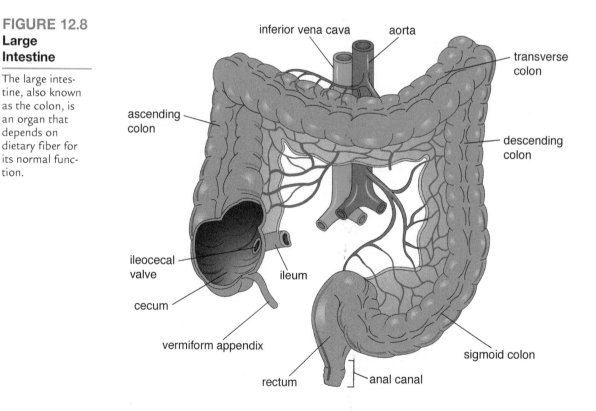

inferior vena cava — aorta — transverse colon — ascending colon — descending colon — ileocecal valve — ileum — cecum — vermiform appendix — sigmoid colon — rectum — anal canal

Insoluble fibers reduce GI transit time. Some soluble fibers, such as psyllium (the common name of a group of plants whose seeds yield fiber), regulate the speed at which waste moves through the colon. Soluble fibers form gels when mixed with water. In the GI tract, they act more like solids than like liquids and thus delay emptying. This action explains why psyllium can be used as an antidiarrheal as well as a laxative. Inactivity or confinement to bed can actually cause constipation when combined with soluble fibers.

The adverse effects of fiber are distension and flatulence, but these symptoms usually subside after the first few weeks of increased fiber consumption. These symptoms may also be associated with esophageal, gastric, or small-bowel or rectal obstruction, especially in patients with intestinal stricture or stenosis. Fiber may also prevent absorption of some drugs and nutrients. Table 12.9 contains information on commonly used agents to treat constipation.

TABLE 12.9 Commonly Used Agents to Treat Constipation

Generic (Brand)	Pronunciation	Dosage Form	Common Dosage	Dispensing Status
Bulk-Forming Laxatives				
methylcellulose (Citrucel, Maltsupex, Unifiber)	meth-il-SELL-yoo-los	powder for solution, tablet	see individual product; taken 3–4 times a day	OTC
polycarbophil (Equalactin, FiberCon, Fiber-Lax, Konsyl Fiber)	pol-i-KAR-boe-fil	chewable tablet, tablet	2 tablets 1–4 times a day	OTC
psyllium (Fiberall, Metamucil)	SIL-ee-um	capsule, oral packet, oral powder for solution	varies based on formulation	OTC
wheat dextrin (Benefiber)	weat DEX-trin	chewable tablet, powder for solution	3 g up to 3 times a day	OTC
Surfactants Laxatives				
docusate (Colace, ex-lax, Surfak)	DOK-yoo-sate	capsule, enema, oral syrup, syrup, tablet	varies based on formulation	OTC
docusate senna (Senokot-S)	DOK-yoo-sate SEN-na	tablet	2 tablets a day	OTC
Osmotic Laxatives				
glycerin (Fleet Glycerin Suppositories)	GLIS-er-in	suppository	1 suppository (2–3 g) for 15 mins 1 time a day	OTC
lactulose (Enulose)	LAK-tu-los	oral solution	10–20 g (15–30 mL) every other day, may increase up to 2 times a day	Rx
magnesium hydroxide (Phillips' Milk of Magnesia)	mag-NEE-zee-um hye-DROX-ide	oral suspension, tablet	tablet: 8 tablets once a day; liquid: 2,400–4,800 mg once per day	OTC
magnesium sulfate (Epsom salts)	mag-NEE-zee-um SUL-fate	granules	5–10 g dissolved in 240 mL of water 1 time a day	OTC
polyethylene glycol 3350 (MiraLax)	pol-ee-ETH-il-een GLYE-kawl 3350	powder for oral solution	8.5–34 g in 240 mL of (8 oz) liquid	OTC

continues

TABLE 12.9 **Commonly Used Agents to Treat Constipation**—*Continued*

Generic (Brand)	Pronunciation	Dosage Form	Common Dosage	Dispensing Status
Stimulant Laxatives				
bisacodyl (Dulcolax, Fleet Bisacodyl Enema)	bis-a-KOE-dil	enema, suppository, tablet	PO: 10–30 mg 1 time a day Rectal: 10 mg suppository or enema 1 time a day	OTC
senna (ex-lax, Fletcher's Laxative, various brands)	SEN-na	chewable tablet, oral solution, syrup, tablet	2–4 tablets (8.6 mg per tablet) or 1–2 tablets (15 mg per tablet) as 1 dose a day or divided 2 times a day	OTC
Antiflatulents				
aluminum hydroxide / magnesium hydroxide / simethicone (Mylanta, Mylanta Maximum Strength)	a-LOO-mi-num hye-DROX-ide mag-NEE-zhum hye-DROX-ide si-METH-i-kone	oral suspension, tablet	tablet: 1–4 tablets up to 4 times a day liquid: 10–20 mL up to 4 times a day	OTC
calcium carbonate / simethicone (Maalox)	kal-SEE-um KAR-bun-ate si-METH-i-kone	tablet	40–125 mg, 4 times a day	OTC
simethicone (Gas-X, Mylicon)	si-METH-i-kone	oral suspension, tablet	40–360 mg 4 times a day	OTC
Bowel Evacuants				
polyethylene glycol 3350 with electrolytes (Colyte, GaviLyte-C, GaviLyte-G, GaviLyte-N, GoLYTELY, MoviPrep, NuLYTELY, TriLyte)	pol-ee-ETH-il-een GLYE-kawl 3350 and ee-LEK-tro-lytes	powder	varies based on formulation	Rx
sodium phosphate (Visicol)	SOE-dee-um FOS-fate	tablet	evening prior to procedure: 3 tablets (last dose will be 2 tablets) every 15 min for a total of 20 tablets day of procedure: Starting 3–5 hr prior to procedure, 3 tablets (last dose is 2 tablets) every 15 min for a total of 20 tablets	Rx
Miscellaneous Agents				
lubiprostone (Amitiza)	loo-bi-PROS-tone	capsule	24 mcg 2 times a day or 8 mcg 2 times a day depending on indication	Rx
methylnaltrexone (Relistor)	meth-il-nal-TREKS-own	injection	12 mcg 1 time a day	Rx

Bulk-Forming Laxatives

Mild constipation can be treated with bulk-forming laxatives. As with dietary fiber, **bulk-forming agents** are poorly absorbed and remain in the GI tract, drawing water and other electrolytes into the GI system. Increased volume in the GI tract triggers peristalsis and facilitates bowel movements. In general, these agents take between one and three days to work. Bulk-forming laxatives work best for preventing constipation rather than as acute treatment. Patients with repeated problems with constipation may consider daily use of a bulk-forming laxative to remain regular. These laxatives may also have beneficial effects in patients who have diabetes or high cholesterol because they absorb fat and reduce glucose. Bulk-forming laxatives are available over the counter.

Methylcellulose (Citrucel, Maltsupex, Unifiber) works by increasing the amount of water in the stool. It can be taken as a powder for solution or as a tablet. The powder for oral solution should be mixed with a cold, noncarbonated beverage.

Polycarbophil (Equalactin, FiberCon, Fiber-Lax, Konsyl Fiber) is a laxative that is available in tablet form and should be taken with plenty of water. Without drinking enough water, polycarbophil may swell and block the esophagus and result in choking. Patients who have difficulty swallowing should not use polycarbophil.

Psyllium (Fiberall, Metamucil) increases non-absorbable bulk to promote soft stools and easy defecation in patients who should avoid straining (e.g., postoperative, postmyocardial infarction, older adults, and pregnant patients). Psyllium is classified as an antidiarrheal as well as a laxative. It absorbs water in the intestine, producing a viscous liquid that promotes peristalsis and reduces transit time. Patients must be active for it to work; as mentioned earlier, psyllium can cause constipation in a bedridden patient. It is also an effective cholesterol-lowering agent.

Wheat dextrin (Benefiber) is a clear fiber supplement. It can be added to beverages or soft foods prior to administration. However, adding it to carbonated beverages is not recommended.

Dosage Forms and Administration Dosage forms and common dosages for bulk-forming laxatives are listed in Table 12.9.

Side Effects Although rare, obstruction of the esophagus or bowels is possible with bulk-forming laxatives. To avoid obstruction, patients should take bulk-forming laxatives with a full glass of liquid (at least eight ounces).

Metamucil is a brand-name product for psyllium.

Contraindications Bulk-forming laxatives are contraindicated in patients with impaired intestinal motility and in patients with intestinal stenosis.

Cautions and Considerations Bulk-forming laxatives should be used with caution in patients with esophageal strictures, ulcers, and intestinal adhesions or who have difficulty swallowing. Products should be taken with at least eight ounces of water to prevent choking or obstruction.

Drug Interactions Because they increase GI motility, bulk-forming laxatives can affect drug absorption. Patients should separate doses of these laxatives from other medications by at least two hours to ensure that other drugs are absorbed properly.

Stool Softeners/Surfactant Laxatives

A **surfactant laxative** is a substance that acts as a detergent, helping fatty and watery components of the intestinal contents to mix, thus making the stool soft and mushy. These laxatives are not as effective for treatment of acute constipation as they are for helping reduce or prevent constipation when it is likely to occur. Surfactant laxatives are typically taken daily.

Docusate (Colace, ex-lax stool softener, Surfak) is a surfactant laxative. Docusate is commonly used and is available over the counter. Docusate is also available as a combination product, **docusate senna (Senokot-S)**.

Dosage Forms and Administration Docusate is available as a capsule, enema, oral liquid, or tablet.

Side Effects Docusate may cause throat irritation (oral formulations), abdominal pain, diarrhea, and intestinal obstruction. Drinking plenty of fluids each day can reduce these effects.

Contraindications Docusate is contraindicated for patients with intestinal obstruction, acute abdominal pain, nausea, or vomiting. This drug should not be used concomitantly with mineral oil.

Cautions and Considerations The oral liquid dosage form has a bitter taste. Taking these products with eight ounces of milk or juice can mask the bad taste. Drinking plenty of fluids while taking surfactants enhances their effects. As with many laxatives, excessive or long-term use may lead to electrolyte imbalance.

Drug Interactions There are no known drug interactions associated with docusate.

Osmotic Laxatives

Osmotic laxatives (for example, **glycerin [Fleet Glycerin Suppositories]**) are organic substances that draw water into the colon and thereby stimulate evacuation of the lower bowel. This mechanism of action allows the retention of nutrients. Glycerin suppositories are a fairly quick, effective method to relieve constipation.

Lactulose

Lactulose (Enulose) is metabolized by bacteria in the colon; this metabolic process reduces fecal pH, reduces absorption of ammonia and toxic nitrogenous substances, and has a cathartic effect (empties the bowel). Lactulose delivers osmotically active molecules to the colon. It is used to prevent and treat hepatic-induced encephalopathy. Normally, the liver removes nitrogen waste by-products that the blood has picked up from the intestines. When the liver is not functioning properly, as in alcohol abuse, these nitrogen by-products build up in the blood, destroying brain cells, which results in encephalopathy. Lactulose is thought to offset this process by reducing ammonia production and increasing absorption from the GI tract.

Dosage Forms and Administration Lactulose is available in a solution form and can be administered orally or rectally. Dosage can vary.

Side Effects The side effects include nausea and vomiting, cramps, diarrhea, and anorexia.

Contraindications Lactulose is not for use in patients requiring a low-galactose diet.

Cautions and Considerations Electrolyte abnormalities can occur with lactulose use. Patients with diabetes should use lactulose with caution, as the product contains lactose and galactose.

Drug Interactions There are no known drug interactions associated with the use of lactulose.

Polyethylene Glycol 3350

Polyethylene glycol 3350 (MiraLax) is an OTC stool softener. This product contains the same active ingredient as GoLYTELY, discussed later in the section on bowel evacuants, but in a much smaller quantity (17 g). It is taken daily to maintain soft stools and to prevent constipation. MiraLax is frequently used in children.

Dosage Forms and Administration Polyethylene glycol 3350 is available as a powder formulation to be mixed with 4 to 8 ounces of liquid and taken by mouth.

Side Effects Side effects include nausea, diarrhea, bloating, and flatulence.

Contraindications There are no contraindications to polyethylene glycol 3350.

Cautions and Considerations Avoid use in patients with bowel obstruction. Use with caution in patients with kidney dysfunction.

Drug Interactions Propylene glycol 3350 may decrease digoxin levels.

Magnesium Hydroxide

Magnesium hydroxide (Phillips' Milk of Magnesia) is a laxative as well as an antacid. Magnesium is supplied as citrate, hydroxide, and sulfate (Epsom salts) forms. Magnesium-containing laxatives promote evacuation of the bowel by causing osmotic retention of fluid, which distends the colon and increases peristaltic activity.

Dosage Forms and Administration Magnesium hydroxide is available as an oral liquid and as a chewable tablet. It should be taken with a full 8 ounce glass of water.

Side Effects Side effects include nausea, diarrhea, bloating, and flatulence.

Contraindications There are no contraindications to magnesium-containing laxatives.

Cautions and Considerations Use with caution in patients with kidney dysfunction, cardiac disease, and preexisting electrolyte abnormalities.

Drug Interactions Magnesium-containing laxatives should not be used in patients taking raltegravir. Magnesium-containing laxatives and products may decrease the concentration of many medications. The following should be administered at least two hours before or six hours after the magnesium dose: digoxin, dolutegravir, gabapentin, erdafitinib, itraconazole, ketoconazole, quinolone antibiotics (e.g., ciprofloxacin, levofloxacin), and tetracycline antibiotics (e.g., doxycycline, minocycline).

Stimulant Laxatives

Acute constipation can be treated with **stimulant laxatives**. These medications work by stimulating parasympathetic neurons that control bowel muscles, thereby enhancing peristalsis and GI motility. To prevent electrolyte imbalances, stimulant laxatives are taken only when needed on a short-term basis. These drugs are commonly used to treat opiate-induced constipation. Serious electrolyte abnormalities are very rare but can occur with chronic use. For this reason, long-term use is not recommended.

Bisacodyl (Dulcolax) and **senna (ex-lax, Fletcher's Laxatives)** are stimulant laxatives. These products are commonly prescribed concurrently for patients who have been taking long-term narcotic pain medications, which can cause constipation. Pharmacy technicians should question any orders for long-term narcotic pain medications that are not accompanied by orders for stimulant laxatives and bring these observations to the attention of a pharmacist.

Dosage Forms and Administration Bisacodyl is available as a tablet for oral use and as a suppository and enema for rectal use. Senna is available as a chewable tablet, oral solution, syrup, and tablet for oral administration.

Side Effects Common side effects of stimulant laxatives include mild abdominal pain, nausea, vomiting, and rectal burning. Patients should take these agents at bedtime to prevent these side effects.

Contraindications Bisacodyl is contraindicated in patients with abdominal pain or obstruction, nausea, or vomiting. Senna should not be taken by patients with intestinal obstruction, acute intestinal inflammation, colitis, ulcerative colitis, appendicitis, and abdominal pain of unknown origin.

Cautions and Considerations Patients should take bisacodyl with a full glass of water on an empty stomach to achieve the best effect. Patients should not ingest dairy products or antacids simultaneously with bisacodyl as they can decrease the drug's effects.

Drug Interactions Antacids may diminish the therapeutic effect of delayed-release bisacodyl tablets by causing the tablets to release the drug before it reaches the large intestine. Gastric irritation and/or cramps may occur.

Miscellaneous Constipation Agents

The agents used for constipation thus far in the chapter are fiber and laxatives. There are, however, other mechanisms of action to treat constipation. One such mechanism involves chloride channels in the gastrointestinal system.

Lubiprostone (Amitiza) is a drug approved for the treatment of chronic idiopathic constipation, opioid-induced constipation, and irritable bowel syndrome with constipation. It is a prostaglandin derivative that activates chloride channels locally in the small intestine, which increases intestinal fluid secretion.

Dosage Forms and Administration Lubirpostone is available in a capsule for oral administration. It should be taken with food and water.

Side Effects Nausea is the primary side effect. Patients may want to take this drug with food to minimize this side effect.

Contraindications Known or suspected bowel obstruction contraindicates use.

Cautions and Considerations **Dyspnea** (shortness of breath) and chest tightness have occurred with lubiprostone use. Patients with moderate-to-severe liver dysfunction should use it with caution.

Drug Interactions Methadone may decrease the therapeutic effect of lubiprostone.

Antiflatulent Agents

Flatulence (stomach or intestinal gas) is a condition that affects many patients. Complaints of excess gas often represent a hyperawareness of or sensitivity to gas.

Intestinal gas is typically caused by the fermentation of undigested food in the colon. Gas can also form when food isn't completely broken down. Other causes of gas include intestinal bacteria changes when taking antibiotics or other medications, poor carbohydrate absorption, swallowed air, and constipation. Food sources of intestinal gas include beans, legumes, cabbage, onions, broccoli, cauliflower, beer, and carbonated drinks.

Simethicone (Gas-X, Mylicon) is an inert silicone polymer for gastric defoaming. By reducing surface tension, the drug causes gas bubbles to break or to coalesce into a foam that can be eliminated more easily by belching or passing flatus. Simethicone relieves flatulence, functional gastric bloating, and postoperative gas pains.

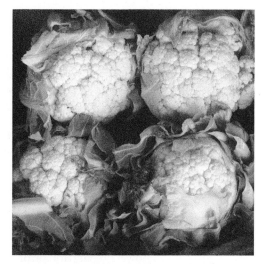

Brassica plants include cauliflower, cabbage, and broccoli, all foods that can cause flatulence.

Dosage Forms and Administration Simethicone is available OTC as chewable tablet or oral liquid. Tablets should be chewed thoroughly prior to swallowing. Dosage recommendations should not be exceeded, especially in children.

Side Effects Simethicone is generally well tolerated.

Contraindications Simethicone does not have contraindications.

Cautions and Considerations Some dosage forms contain benzyl alcohol. These dosage forms should not be used by pediatric patients.

Drug Interactions Simethicone has no known drug interactions.

Bowel Evacuants

In contrast to laxatives, which are used to restore normal bowel function, a **bowel evacuant** is used to cleanse the bowel prior to GI examination (colonoscopy or x-ray with barium enema), or, in rare cases, following ingestion of toxic substances.

Polyethylene Glycol 3350 with Electrolytes

Polyethylene glycol 3350 with electrolytes (Colyte, GaviLyte-C, GaviLyte-G, GaviLyte-N, GoLYTELY, HalfLYTELY, MoviPrep, NuLYTELY, TriLyte) increases the osmolarity of bowel contents, thus drawing large amounts of water into the lumen to flush out the bowel contents.

Dosage Forms and Administration The recommended dose is dissolved in 4 L of fluid. The patient should fast three to four hours prior to administration and for two hours following administration; 240 mL (8 oz) should be consumed every 10 minutes until the solution is gone. The physician or manufacturer usually supplies a printed informational sheet for the patient with explicit instructions. HalfLYTELY is sometimes used instead of GoLYTELY. It consists of 2 L (half the amount of GoLYTELY) of solution that is to be combined with bisacodyl (a stimulant laxative) delayed-release tablets.

Side Effects Side effects include abdominal distention, anal discomfort, nausea, abdominal pain, and vomiting.

Contraindications Ileus, GI obstruction, gastric retention, bowel perforation, toxic colitis, and toxic megacolon all contraindicate the use of polyethylene glycol 3350 with electrolytes.

Cautions and Considerations Serious cardiac arrhythmias have occurred in patients using polyethylene glycol 3350 with electrolytes. Use with caution in patients with renal dysfunction.

Drug Interactions Polyethylene glycol 3350 with electrolytes has no known significant drug interactions.

Sodium Phosphate

Sodium phosphate (Visicol) is indicated for evacuation of the colon and for treating and preventing hypophosphatemia. Like magnesium-containing laxatives, sodium phosphate draws water into the colon. Visicol is a sodium phosphate tablet indicated for bowel preparation prior to colonoscopy.

Dosage Forms and Administration Sodium phosphate tablets are tasteless and can be taken with any clear liquid such as water, lemonade, or ginger ale.

Side Effects This drug has been proven to cause significantly less nausea, vomiting, and bloating than other bowel preparation products.

Contraindications The enema product is contraindicated in patients with kidney impairment, **ascites** (abnormal buildup of fluid in the abdomen), heart failure, known or suspected GI obstruction, or megacolon. Sodium phosphate tablets should not be used in patients with phosphate nephropathy, bowel obstruction or perforation, gastric bypass surgery, toxic colitis, or megacolon.

Cautions and Considerations Sodium phosphate has a boxed warning for the development of acute phosphate nephropathy.

Drug Interactions Drugs with kidney toxicity (such as ACE inhibitors or NSAIDS) increase the nephrotoxic effects of sodium phosphate.

12.8 Other Gastrointestinal Diseases That May Accompany Constipation and Drug Treatments

Low amounts of fiber in the diet not only produce a state of constipation; they can also increase the likelihood that a patient will encounter a number of other GI diseases. Several of these diseases are discussed here.

Diverticular Disease

Diverticular disease occurs when an outpocketing (diverticulum) from the bowel wall forms (diverticulosis) and/or becomes inflamed (diverticulitis; see Figure 12.9). It is believed to result from a deficiency of fiber over time. Vegetarians, whose average daily intake of fiber (40 g) is about twice that of nonvegetarians, have approximately

FIGURE 12.9 Portion of the Colon with Diverticula

In diverticular disease, herniations form along the mucous membranes, and the muscular layers of the colon wall may become inflamed, causing pain.

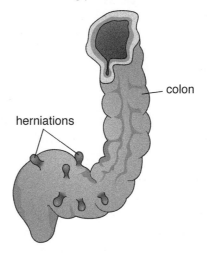

one-third the incidence of diverticular disease. Diverticular disease seems to be related to the predominance of more highly refined carbohydrates and other processed foods in the modern diet. **Colonic segmentation** (in which the colon acts as if it is divided into small parts that move independently of each other rather than contributing to an integrated overall motion) is accompanied by an increase in pressure inside the colon, prolonged GI transit time, and low fecal weight. All of these factors contribute to **herniation** (protrusion through a weakened muscular wall) of the colon lining, with accompanying inflammation and pain. Fiber may reduce the pressure generated in the colon.

Hiatal Hernia

Hiatal hernia is a protrusion through the esophageal hiatus of the diaphragm and is related to chronic constipation. Straining to pass small, firm stools can significantly raise intra-abdominal pressures. Over a period of several years, daily straining to pass stools can force the gastroesophageal junction upward into the thoracic cavity through the **esophageal hiatus** (the opening in the diaphragm through which normally only the esophagus passes).

Irritable Bowel Syndrome

Irritable bowel syndrome (IBS) is the most common of the GI disorders. Many patients with GI complaints are diagnosed with IBS. IBS is a functional disorder in which the lower GI tract does not have the appropriate tone or spasticity to regulate bowel activity. Some evidence also suggests that patients presenting with symptoms of IBS have an abnormal sensitivity to a neurotransmitter within the GI tract. This disorder affects twice as many women as men. Patients with IBS have an increased rate of hospital stays, abdominal surgery, and absenteeism from work. Criteria for diagnosis include the following:

- abdominal distension
- gas
- increased colonic mucus
- irregular bowel habits (diarrhea or constipation more than 25% of the time)
- pain

Hemorrhoids

Hemorrhoids result from pressure exerted on anal veins while straining to pass stool, which causes engorgement of the vascular cushions within the sphincter muscles. Passing a small, hard stool through the anal canal can abrade the overlying mucosa, causing hemorrhoidal bleeding. Prolapse (displacement) of the vascular cushions may occur from rupture of their attachments to the surrounding sphincter. Table 12.10 identifies the most common agents for hemorrhoid treatment.

TABLE 12.10 Commonly Used Hemorrhoidal Agents

Generic (Brand)	Pronunciation	Dosage Form	Dispensing Status
hydrocortisone (Anusol HC, Cortifoam)	hye-droe-KOR-ti-sone	enema, foam, rectal cream, suppository	Rx
nitroglycerin (Rectiv)	nye-troe-GLI-ser-in	rectal ointment	Rx

Hydrocortisone

Hemorrhoids are treated with suppositories, ointments, and, sometimes, surgery. Most medications for hemorrhoids include **hydrocortisone (Anusol HC, Cortifoam)**, a synthetic preparation used to treat inflammation. Modifying the diet by increasing fiber can help prevent hemorrhoids.

Dosage Forms and Administration Hydrocortisone used to treat hemorrhoids is available as an enema, foam, rectal cream, or suppository and by prescription only.

Side Effects Side effects include burning, dryness, or itching of the skin.

Contraindications The rectal enema formulation of hydrocortisone is contraindicated in patients with systemic fungal infections and ileocolostomy during the immediate or early postoperative period. Cortifoam is also contraindicated in patients with obstruction, abscess, perforation, peritonitis, fresh intestinal anastomoses, and extensive fistulas and sinus tracts.

Cautions and Considerations The rectal enema formulation may damage the rectal wall if the applicator is inserted improperly.

Drug Interactions Although hemorrhoidal agents are inserted through the rectal route (considered a systemic route of administration), these drugs are formulated for local activity. However, some systemic absorption may occur through the mucosal lining of the rectum. Hydrocortisone may diminish the therapeutic effects of aldesleukin.

Nitroglycerin

A tear or fissure in the anal canal can also cause pain and bleeding. **Nitroglycerin (Rectiv)**, a vasodilator that causes smooth muscle relaxation, reduces resting pressure on the anal canal and permits healing.

Dosage Forms and Administration A 2%–4% ointment is inserted into the anal canal with the finger. Before instilling nitroglycerin, the patient should place the tube of medication in a container of warm water to soften the tube's contents and allow for an accurate amount of medication to be dispersed. The patient should also don gloves before instillation and wash their hands after the procedure.

Side Effects The primary side effect is headache, and the patient should make sure to take 12-hour breaks from the drug to minimize this effect.

Contraindications Use of phosphodiesterase-5 (PDE-5) inhibitors (such as sildenafil) are contraindicated, as these drugs have been shown to potentiate the hypotensive effects of nitroglycerin. Other contraindications include severe anemia, increased intracranial pressure, and known hypersensitivity to nitrates or nitrites.

Cautions and Considerations Severe hypotension can result from the use of nitroglycerin rectal ointment. Patients with hypotension or those known to be at risk for it should use with caution.

Drug Interactions Antihypertensives and PDE-5 inhibitors may increase the hypotensive effects of nitroglycerin. Aspirin may increase nitroglycerin levels. Heparin's anticoagulant effect may be decreased by the use of nitroglycerin.

12.9 Nausea and Vomiting and Drug Treatments

The vomiting center in the brain is located in the medulla. It receives input from the **chemoreceptor trigger zone (CTZ)** via the vagus nerve or the tenth cranial nerve. The CTZ, which is located below the floor of the fourth ventricle of the brain, receives its input from the cerebral cortex and hypothalamus and also from blood-borne stimuli (such as bacterial toxins and drugs that have access to the brain via the vascular system). The main neurotransmitters that cause nausea and vomiting are acetylcholine, dopamine, histamine, and serotonin.

Vomiting (also referred to as **emesis**) can be initiated in two ways: by stimulating the CTZ, which in turn stimulates the GI tract via the vomiting center; or by stimulating the vagal receptors in the stomach with no CTZ involvement (see Figure 12.10).

**FIGURE 12.10
Chemoreceptor
Trigger Zone
and Vomiting
Center**

The vomiting center in the brain receives input from the chemoreceptor trigger zone (CTZ).

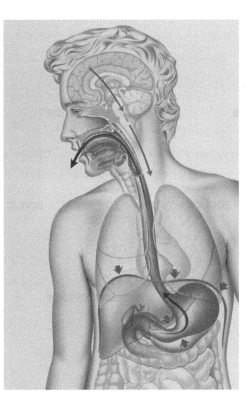

Vomiting can cause dehydration, electrolyte imbalance leading to alkalosis (loss of acid from the body), and possible aspiration pneumonia. It may also cause bradycardia or other arrhythmias resulting from an electrolyte imbalance.

Emesis often results from narcotic intake and is dose related. Morphine and its derivatives stimulate the CTZ. Narcotics also increase the vomiting center's sensitivity to stimuli from the vestibular nuclei of the ear, which is near the vomiting center.

Stimulating the labyrinth system of the inner ear produces impulses that are transmitted via cholinergic and adrenergic tracts to the vestibular nuclei. This is the pathway that commonly underlies car sickness. **Vertigo**, the sensation of the room spinning when one gets up or changes positions, is treated with anticholinergic agents.

An **antiemetic** is a drug that works primarily in the vomiting center to inhibit impulses that travel to the stomach, thus preventing vomiting. Table 12.11 presents the most commonly used antiemetics.

TABLE 12.11 Commonly Used Antiemetic Medications

Generic (Brand)	Pronunciation	Dosage Form	Common Dosages	Dispensing Status
Antihistamines and Anticholinergics				
diphenhydramine (Benadryl)	dye-fen-HYE-dra-meen	capsule, injection, oral solution, tablet	PO: 25–50 mg every 6 hr IM/IV: 10–50 mg	OTC, Rx
dimenhydrinate (Dramamine)	dye-men-HYE-druh-nate	chewable, injection, tablet	50 mg every 4 hr	OTC, Rx
meclizine (Antivert)	MEK-li-zeen	tablet	25–50 mg every 24 hr	Rx
scopolamine (Scopace, Transderm Scop)	scoe-POL-a-meen	injection, transdermal patch	1 patch at least 4 hr prior to exposure, then every 3 days PRN	Rx
Serotonin Receptor Antagonists				
dolasetron (Anzemet)	dol-AS-e-tron	injection, tablet	varies	Rx
granisetron (Kytril)	gra-NI-se-tron	injection, oral solution, tablet, transdermal patch	varies	Rx
ondansetron (Zofran)	on-DAN-se-tron	injection, oral film, oral solution, tablet	varies	Rx
palonosetron (Aloxi)	pa-lone-O-se-tron	injection	varies	Rx
Dopamine Receptor Antagonists: Phenothiazines				
prochlorperazine (Compazine)	proe-klor-PAIR-a-zeen	Injection, suppository, tablet	PO: 5–10 mg every 6–8 hr, IM: 5–10 mg, IV: 2.5–10 mg every 3–4 hr, rectal: 25 mg every 12 hr	Rx
promethazine (Phenergan)	proe-METH-a-zeen	oral solution, suppository, tablet	IM/PO: 12.5–25 mg every 4 hr, rectal: 12.5–25 mg every 12 hr	Rx

continues

TABLE 12.11 **Commonly Used Antiemetic Medications—***Continued*

Generic (Brand)	Pronunciation	Dosage Form	Common Dosages	Dispensing Status
Dopamine Receptor Antagonist: Benzamide				
metoclopramide (Reglan)	met-oh-KLOE-pra-mide	injection, oral solution, tablet	PO: 10 mg IV: 10 mg–20 mg	Rx
Neurokinin-1 Receptor Antagonist				
aprepitant, fosamprepitant (Emend)	ap-REP-i-tant	capsule (aprepitant), injection (fosamprepitant)	varies	Rx

Antihistamines and Anticholinergics

Antihistamines and **anticholinergics** are antiemetics that share a similar chemical structure. They are used to treat mild motion sickness. They work by blocking histamine and acetylcholine, two neurotransmitters in the CTZ and vomiting center (see Table 12.11 for more information).

Dosage Forms and Administration These antiemetics are available in a variety of dosage forms, including injections, topical patches, oral liquids, tablets, and capsules. See Table 12.11 for additional information.

Side Effects Side effects of antihistamine and anticholinergic antiemetics are drowsiness, dry mouth, and urinary retention. Patients who take other medications that also cause drowsiness should be careful because sedation could be excessive. Patients should avoid drinking alcohol and take care when driving until they know how the medication affects them. Patients who have an enlarged prostate should not use anticholinergic antiemetics because they can make urination even more difficult.

In some children, anticholinergic antiemetics have a paradoxical effect, where excitation occurs rather than drowsiness. Parents should be aware of the potential for this side effect.

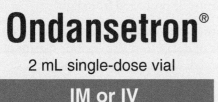

NDC 63323-373-02
4 mg/2 mL (2 mg/2 mL)

Ondansetron®

2 mL single-dose vial

IM or IV

There are times when patients experiencing nausea and vomiting are unable to tolerate oral antiemetics. In these cases, intramuscular or IV administration is used. This label shows the injectable form of the 5-HT3 receptor antagonist ondansetron.

Contraindications Anticholinergic and antihistamine antiemetics should not be given to infants or mothers who are breast-feeding. In addition, patients with glaucoma or those individuals using monoamine oxidase inhibitors (MAOIs) should not take these agents. Contraindications to scopolamine include a hypersensitivity to belladonna alkaloids and narrow-angle glaucoma. The injectable form of scopolamine should not be used repeatedly in patients with chronic lung disease.

Cautions and Considerations Patients who have high blood pressure or heart problems should talk with their prescribers before taking anticholinergic or antihistamine antiemetics.

Drugs with anticholinergic properties will intensify the anticholinergic properties of these drugs.

Serotonin Receptor Antagonists

Work Wise

A few of the 5-HT3 receptor antagonist medications are expensive. For a patient's insurance plan to cover these drugs, the prescriber may need to complete a prior authorization request. As a pharmacy technician, you may be asked to prepare the documentation needed for such a request.

Serotonin (5-HT) receptor antagonists are potent antiemetics used to prevent and treat severe nausea and vomiting associated with chemotherapeutic medications, radiation treatment, or anesthesia. 5-HT receptor antagonists work by blocking serotonin type 3 (5-HT3) receptors in the brain and GI tract. Blocking these receptors stops nausea signals traveling from the brain to the stomach. These powerful antiemetics are prescription-only products (see Table 12.11) that pharmacy technicians in the inpatient and oncology specialty clinics will encounter.

Dolasetron (Anzemet) was designed to be used for the prevention of chemotherapy-induced nausea. 5-HT is released from the GI cells, which stimulates receptors that cause vomiting when chemotherapy is administered. Dolasetron is also used for the prevention of surgery-related nausea. **Granisetron (Kytril)** binds to 5-HT receptors with little or no affinity for dopamine D2, benzodiazepine, or opiate receptors. It blocks the 5-HT receptors both peripherally on vagal nerve terminals and centrally in the CTZ.

Ondansetron (Zofran) blocks 5-HT receptors in either the CTZ or vagal nerve terminals in the small bowel. It is used for chemotherapy-induced emesis. **Palonosetron (Aloxi)** is an injectable 5-HT receptor antagonist that is indicated for chemotherapy-related and postoperative nausea and vomiting. It is injected prior to chemotherapy or surgical procedures.

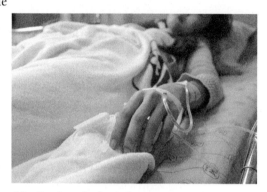

Of saline into the body for treatment.

Dosage Forms and Administration The IV form of dolasetron can be given as an IV push over 30 seconds or diluted in 50 mL of compatible fluid and infused over 15 minutes. Dolasetron can also be diluted in apple or apple-grape juice and taken orally. If given for the prevention of chemotherapy-induced nausea, it should be administered one hour before administration of the chemotherapy agent; if given for postsurgery nausea, it should be given 15 minutes before stopping anesthesia. Dolasetron can also be given to treat postsurgery nausea on an as needed basis. Granisetron is usually given by the IV route. Granisetron must be protected from light.

Side Effects Side effects of serotonin receptor antagonists include headache, constipation, drowsiness, and fatigue. Side effects of dolasetron also include dizziness. Granisetron may cause asthenia (weakness) and diarrhea. Ondansetron can cause either constipation or diarrhea.

Contraindications Dolasetron is contraindicated via the IV route when used for the prevention of chemotherapy-associated nausea and vomiting. Granisetron, ondansetron, and palonosetron do not have contraindications.

Cautions and Considerations Because 5-HT receptor antagonists may cause dizziness and drowsiness, patients should be reminded that activities such as driving may not be safe while taking these medications.

Drug Interactions 5-HT receptor antagonists may enhance the hypotensive effects of apomorphine. 5-HT receptor antagonists may enhance the QT-prolonging effects of other QT-prolonging agents (e.g., TCAs, SSRIs, -*azole* antifungals, and loop diuretics).

Dopamine Receptor Antagonists

Dopamine receptor antagonists include phenothiazines and benzamides. Phenothiazine compounds, related to the typical antipsychotics described in Chapter 8, inhibit the CTZ. **Phenothiazines** are potent antiemetic drugs that work by blocking dopamine and inhibiting the CTZ. They are first-generation antipsychotics when used in higher doses. Pharmacy technicians working in an institutional setting will likely dispense phenothiazines daily because they are frequently ordered in that setting. **Benzamides** cause dopamine antagonism and, at higher doses, 5-HT3 antagonism.

These medications are available in many different dosage forms (see Table 12.11), an important feature because patients with nausea and vomiting may not be able to swallow a pill or oral solution. Patients can receive an intramuscular (IM) or IV injection or a rectal suppository to relieve symptoms.

They act as a sedative, antiemetic, and anticholinergic (causing dry mouth, blurred vision, and urinary retention). Drug-induced movement disorders such as tardive dyskinesia and dystonia (called extrapyramidal symptoms or side effects) are possible with dopamine receptor antagonists, particularly at high doses. **EPS** include uncontrollable movements of the eyes, face, and limbs that may become permanent. Patients, especially older adults, have to be closely monitored for the appearance of EPS. If EPS appear, patients should stop taking the antiemetic. To prevent hypotension, these drugs should not be given by an IV push.

Prochlorperazine

Prochlorperazine (Compazine) is a phenothiazine that can be administered by oral, rectal, IM, or IV routes. It must be used with caution in children and is easily overdosed, precipitating seizures.

Dosage Forms and Administration Prochlorperazine can help with nausea caused by GI disorders. It is available in oral, rectal, IM, and IV formulations.

Side Effects Common side effects include drowsiness, dizziness, blurry vision, headache, dry mouth, nausea, and constipation.

Contraindications Prochlorperazine should not be used in patients with severe CNS depression or coma. In addition, prochlorperazine is contraindicated in pediatric surgery and in children younger than two years or weighing less than 9 kg.

Cautions and Considerations Patients with liver problems cannot eliminate these agents from the bloodstream properly, increasing the risk for EPS effects. Patients should inform their prescribers if they have liver problems so that this risk can be assessed and other therapy chosen if necessary.

Drug Interactions Prochlorperazine can cause QT-interval prolongation and can enhance the effects of other QT-interval prolonging agents (e.g., tricyclic antidepressants [TCAs], SSRIs, and -*azole* antifungals).

Promethazine

Promethazine (Phenergan), a phenothiazine, is a commonly used antiemetic.

Dosage Forms and Administration Promethazine is usually given as an IV push, but if the dose is greater than 100 mg, it should be diluted in the pharmacy to a maximum concentration of 25 mg/mL and infused over 15 to 30 minutes. Suppositories are stored in the refrigerator.

Side Effects Most common side effects include drowsiness, dizziness, and restlessness.

Contraindications Promethazine is contraindicated for patients who are in a coma or experiencing lower respiratory tract symptoms. Promethazine is also contraindicated in children younger than two years and for intra-arterial or subcutaneous administration.

Cautions and Considerations Promethazine has a boxed warning regarding the use of the drug in children younger than two years.

Drug Interactions CNS depressants may enhance the CNS side effects of promethazine. Anticholinergic agents may enhance the anticholinergic side effects of promethazine. Promethazine may enhance the toxic effects of glucagon. The ulcerogenic effects of potassium chloride may be enhanced by promethazine.

Metoclopramide

Metoclopramide (Reglan), a benzamide, is used in **gastric stasis** (lack of stomach motility), GI reflux, and chemotherapy-induced emesis. It inhibits or reduces nausea and vomiting by blocking dopamine receptors in the CTZ. Metoclopramide relieves esophageal reflux by improving the tone of the lower esophageal sphincter and reduces gastric stasis by stimulating motility of the upper GI tract, thus reducing gastric emptying time.

Dosage Forms and Administration Metoclopramide dosing can vary based on indication. When given by injection, doses greater than 10 should be diluted in 50 mL of parenteral solution and infused over 15 to 30 minutes.

Side Effects The side effects are drowsiness, depression, and EPS effects (which are parkinsonian, especially in children). Diphenhydramine is used to reduce the EPS effects. Metoclopramide should not be used longer than 12 weeks.

Contraindications Metoclopramide is contraindicated in patients with GI obstruction, perforation, or hemorrhage; pheochromocytoma; and a history of seizures. It should not be used with other agents that are likely to increase EPS effects.

Cautions and Considerations Metoclopramide has a boxed warning for causing tardive dyskinesia. Metoclopramide should be discontinued in patients with any signs or symptoms of dyskinesia.

Drug Interactions Metoclopramide may increase the adverse effects of antipsychotics, droperidol, and tetrabenazine.

Neurokinin-1 Receptor Antagonists

As the name suggests, neurokinin-1 (NK-1) receptor antagonists work on the NK-1 receptor. The NK-1 receptor is the preferred receptor for substance P, a neuropeptide involved in the induction of nausea and vomiting. The NK-1 receptor antagonists prevent both acute and delayed vomiting.

Aprepitant (Emend) is an oral medication used to treat postoperative and chemotherapy-related nausea. The injectable form of Emend is **fosaprepitant**, which has the same indication.

Dosage Forms and Administration Aprepitant should be administered within three hours prior to surgery or chemotherapy. Fosaprepitant is usually given 30 minutes prior to surgery or chemotherapy.

Side Effects Common side effects of aprepitant and fosaprepitant include fatigue, muscle weakness, and constipation. Hypotension, slow heart rate, diarrhea, GI pain, kidney and liver dysfunction, and blood abnormalities are rare but significant side effects. If a patient experiences severe side effects while taking aprepitant, they should call for medical help immediately.

Contraindications Aprepitant is contraindicated in patients using cisapride or pimozide.

Cautions and Considerations Use with caution in patients with renal impairment.

Drug Interactions Aprepitant may increase the concentration of bosutinib, ibrutinib, ivabradine, lomitapide, naloxegol, olaparib, pimozide, simeprevir, tolvaptan, trabectedin, and ulipristal. Conivaptan, fusidic acid, and idelalisib may increase the serum concentration of aprepitant.

12.10 Hepatitis and Drug Treatments

Hepatitis is a liver disease that has several forms, distinguished by the letters A through G. The three most common (A, B, and C) will be discussed. Each can damage liver cells and cause the liver to become swollen and tender. Some can cause permanent damage. Hepatitis has many causes. Some forms are viral, but others are caused by medications, long-term alcohol use, or exposure to certain industrial chemicals.

Hepatitis A is a viral infection that can be spread from one person to another. It is present worldwide and can be transmitted through blood and body fluids. Incidence has decreased dramatically in the United States since vaccination was targeted in high-risk populations, children in states with high incidence, and infants. Hepatitis A often produces epidemics due to its feces-to-mouth route of transmission. The highest rates occur in children. Treatment is supportive (no drugs, just food and rest). Hepatitis A can be prevented by the hepatitis A vaccine, also known as HAV. If individuals know they have been exposed, they should be protected with immune globulin (IG) within two weeks of exposure. IG can be given by either an IM or IV injection. If it is ordered as an IV injection, it will be written **IVIG**. IG provides passive immunity by increasing the antibody titer and antigen-antibody reaction potential.

Hepatitis B is a virus transmitted parenterally, through bodily fluids, from sexual contact, and perinatally. There are two types of hepatitis B: acute and chronic. *Acute hepatitis B* usually clears up on its own without treatment. The patient develops antibodies that provide lifelong protection. *Chronic hepatitis B*, which is the most dangerous form of hepatitis, continues to be present for six months or more. It can be the cause of serious liver disease, such as cirrhosis or liver cancer. The patient may require a liver transplant. Chronic hepatitis B is treated with antiviral medications, depending on antigens in the blood. The vaccines for hepatitis B, **Engerix-B** and **Recombivax HB**, are given in a three-dose series over six months. Most healthcare workers, including pharmacy technicians, should receive these vaccines. These vaccines are stored in the refrigerator.

Hepatitis C is an infection that cannot be spread from one person to another by casual contact. It is most commonly transmitted through blood transfusions or illicit drug use. The acute form should be treated to prevent the disease from becoming chronic. It can progress to liver fibrosis and end-stage liver disease. The virus genotype is determined in patients who have hepatitis C. There are several genotypes, with type 1 being the most common. Treatments for type 1 and treatments that can be used for all genotypes are included in the following sections.

Hepatitis B and Hepatitis C Agents

Prevention of hepatitis is achieved through vaccination. Anyone who works in a hospital must be vaccinated against hepatitis B. The Centers for Disease Control and

Prevention now recommends that travelers who are going to endemic areas or who are otherwise high-risk patients should be vaccinated against hepatitis B in two to three doses over the six months prior to travel. They should also receive a hepatitis A vaccine two to four weeks before travel. It is sometimes recommended that babies and school-children have the hepatitis B vaccine with their other immunizations. Anyone who is immunocompromised should also be vaccinated against hepatitis. Table 12.12 lists the drugs used to treat hepatitis B or C.

TABLE 12.12 Most Commonly Used Agents to Treat Hepatitis B or C

Generic (Brand)	Pronunciation	Dosage Form	Common Dosage	Dispensing Status
entecavir (Baraclude)	en-TEK-a-vir	oral liquid, tablet	0.5 to 1 mg a day	Rx
peginterferon alfa-2a (Pegasys)	peg-in-ter-FEER-on AL-fa 2A	injection	SC: 180 mcg each week	Rx
ledipasvir / sofosbuvir (Harvoni)	le-DIP-as-vir soe-FOSS-bue-vir	tablet	1 tablet a day	Rx
sofosbuvir (Sovaldi)	soe-FOS-bue-vir	tablet	1 tablet a day	Rx
ribavirin (Copegus, Moderiba, Rebetol, Ribasphere, Ribasphere RibaPak, Virazole)	rye-ba-VYE-rin	capsule, oral solution, tablet	500–600 mg 2 times a day	Rx
Nucleoside Reverse Transcriptase Inhibitors (NRTIs)				
lamivudine (Epivir, Epivir-HBV)	la-MIV-yoo-deen	oral solution, tablet	100 mg a day	Rx
tenofovir alafenamide (Vemlidy)	te-NOE-fo-veer te-NO-fo-veer al a FEN a mide	tablet	25 mg a day	Rx
tenofovir disoproxil fumarate (Viread)	te-NOE-fo-veer dye-soe-PROX-il FUE-ma-rate	oral powder, tablet	300 mg a day	Rx
Chronic Hepatitis C Treatments				
elbasvir / grazoprevir (Zepatier)	ELB-as-vir and graz-OH-pre-vir	tablet	1 tablet a day	Rx
glecaprevir / pibrentasvir (Mavyret)	glec-A-pre-vir and pi-BRENT-as-vir	tablet	3 tablets a day	Rx
ombitasvir-paritaprevir / ritonavir / dasabuvir (Viekira Pak)	om-BIT-as-vir par-i-TA-pre-vir rit-OH-na-vir da-SA-bue-vir	tablet	PO: ombitasvir / paritaprevir / ritonavir 2 tablets every morning with dasabuvir 1 tablet 2 times a day	Rx
simeprevir (Olysio)	sim-E-pre-vir	capsule		Rx
sofosbuvir / velpatasvir (Epclusa)	soe-FOS-bue-vir and vel-PAT-as-vir	tablet	1 tablet a day	Rx

Entecavir

Entecavir (Baraclude) is indicated for the treatment of chronic hepatitis B. It blocks an enzyme responsible for replication of the virus in the body. The major advantage of entecavir is that it can be used in HIV-positive patients.

Dosage Forms and Administration Entecavir is taken once a day on an empty stomach—that is, two hours before or after eating.

Side Effects The most common side effects include headache, fatigue, dizziness, and nausea.

Contraindications There are no contraindications for the use of entecavir.

Cautions and Considerations There are three boxed warnings associated with entecavir. The first is for lactic acidosis, severe liver enlargement, and fatty liver. Use entecavir with caution in patients with risk factors for liver disease. The second boxed warning is for severe exacerbation of hepatitis B upon drug discontinuation. Patients should be monitored for several months after stopping treatment. The third boxed warning is for HIV resistance to some antiretrovirals in patients using entecavir with unrecognized or untreated HIV.

Drug Interactions Entecavir's adverse effects may be enhanced by ganciclovir, ribavarin, and valganciclovir.

Lamivudine

Lamivudine (Epivir, Epivir-HBV) is a nucleoside reverse transcriptase inhibitor (NRTI) that is used for the treatment of hepatitis B. Lamivudine is also used to treat HIV (see Chapter 17). However, because there are more potent viral suppressors, the use of lamivudine is decreasing. Lamivudine must be taken exactly as prescribed. It has the fewest side effects of any of the NRTIs.

Dosage Forms and Administration For the treatment of hepatitis B, lamivudine is administered once daily with or without food.

Side Effects The most common reported adverse effects include headache, nausea, malaise and fatigue, nasal signs and symptoms, diarrhea, and cough.

Contraindications There are no contraindications to the use of lamivudine.

Cautions and Considerations Lamivudine is indicated to treat HIV and chronic hepatitis B. When used for the treatment of hepatitis B, lamivudine has several boxed warnings. The first warning is about product selection. The hepatitis B product (Epivir-HBV) should not be used to treat HIV. The second warning is about medication discontinuation. After therapy stops, patients should be monitored closely for hepatitis exacerbations. The third boxed warning addresses HIV resistance. Healthcare practitioners need to be aware that HIV resistance may emerge when patients who have hepatitis B and an undiagnosed HIV infection use lamivudine. Lamivudine may precipitate pancreatitis.

Drug Interactions Emtricitabine and lamivudine should not be used together. Ganciclovir, ribavarin, and valganciclovir may enhance the toxic effects of lamivudine.

Peginterferon Alfa-2a

Pegylated interferon is a class of drugs that includes Pegylated interferon-alpha-2a, Pegylated interferon-alpha-2b, and Pegylated interferon-beta-1a. **Peginterferon alfa-2a (Pegasys)** is interferon linked to a high-molecular-weight branched polyethylene glycol (PEG) molecule. This linkage increases the half-life, allowing once-weekly dosing. It is indicated for patients who have hepatitis C and chronic hepatitis B. The advantage of peginterferon alfa-2a over regular interferon is its long half-life.

Dosage Forms and Administration The prefilled syringes should be stored in the refrigerator. They can safely be left out for 24 hours, but no longer. The drug should be injected subcutaneously into the abdomen or thigh, using a different site each time to prevent tissue damage or irritation.

Side Effects The most common side effects include fatigue, headache, myalgia, and fever.

Contraindications Contraindications to the use of peginterferon alfa-2a include a hypersensitivity to other interferons, autoimmune hepatitis, and decompensated cirrhosis. It should not be used in neonates and infants because the formulation includes benzyl alcohol. When combined with ribavirin, peginterferon alfa-2a is contraindicated in individuals who are pregnant or have a partner who is pregnant.

Cautions and Considerations Peginterferon alfa-2a has a boxed warning for causing or aggravating fatal or life-threatening neuropsychiatric, autoimmune, ischemic, and infectious disorders. Therapy should be discontinued immediately in patients with signs or symptoms of these disorders.

Drug Interactions Peginterferon alfa-2a may enhance the adverse effects of clozapine, telbivudine, and zidovudine.

Ribavirin

Ribavirin (Copegus, Moderiba, Rebetol, Ribasphere, Ribasphere RibaPak, Virazole) can be used for the treatment of respiratory syncytial virus (RSV) infections as well as hepatitis C. Ribavirin inhibits the replication of RNA and DNA in the virus.

Dosage Forms and Administration Ribavirin is administered by inhalation for RSV and orally for hepatitis C. For hepatitis C, it should always be taken concurrently with interferon therapy.

Side Effects Ribavirin is known to cause bothersome side effects, including anxiety, emotional lability, irritability, fatigue, fever, headache, injection-site inflammation/reaction, myalgia, nausea, and rigor.

Contraindications Ribavirin is contraindicated in patients who have hemoglobinopathies (such as sickle-cell anemia), individuals who are or who may become pregnant, individuals whose partners are pregnant, patients using didanosine, and patients who have renal impairment.

Cautions and Considerations Ribavirin has several boxed warnings. The first warning states that ribavirin monotherapy is not effective for the treatment of chronic hepatitis C. It should be used in combination with other therapies. Another warning is for the risk of hemolytic anemia, which may result in worsening cardiac disease. A third boxed warning focuses on the severe teratogenic and embryocidal effects associated with the use of ribavarin. Ribavirin should not be used in individuals who are pregnant or whose partners are pregnant. Extreme measures to prevent pregnancy should be taken during therapy (by the patient and the patient's partners) and for six months after therapy.

Drug Interactions Ribavirin may enhance the adverse effects of didanosine. Ribavirin may decrease the effect of live vaccines.

Ledipasvir / Sofosbuvir

Ledipasvir, a nonstructural protein 5A (NS5A) inhibitor, is available as a combination product **ledipasvir / sofosbuvir (Harvoni)**. **Sofosbuvir (Sovaldi)**, a nonstructural protein 5A (NS5B) inhibitor, is also available by itself.

Dosage Forms and Administration The regimen and duration of treatment depends on the HCV genotype and the patient population. The sofosbuvir-only product needs to be taken in combination with other drugs.

Side Effects Common adverse reactions to both drugs are fatigue and headache.

Contraindications There are no contraindications to either drug or the combination product.

Cautions and Considerations Significant drug interactions may exist, and screening should occur prior to starting either drug. These drugs should be prescribed by an experienced healthcare practitioner. The ledipasvir / sofosbuvir combination product may contain lactose. Use with caution in patients with lactose intolerance.

Drug Interactions Sofosbuvir blood levels can be decreased by carbamazepine, oxcarbazepine, phenobarbital, phenytoin, and Saint-John's-wort.

Tenofovir

Tenofovir (Viread, Vemlidy) is a nucleotide reverse transcriptase inhibitor (NRTI) that is used to treat hepatitis B and HIV (see Chapter 17). Tenofovir's limiting toxicity is renal dysfunction.

Dosage Forms and Administration Tenofovir can be dosed once daily without regard to food.

Side Effects Other side effects include dizziness, depression, skin rash, and dyslipidemia.

Contraindications Tenofovir does not have contraindications.

Cautions and Considerations Tenofovir carries two boxed warnings. One is for the risk of lactic acidosis and severe hepatomegaly. The other is for the risk of severe and acute exacerbation of hepatitis B upon discontinuation. Kidney toxicity is a concern with tenofovir use. Patients should not take other drugs that could also damage the kidneys while using tenofovir. Use should be discontinued in patients who experience subsequent decline in renal function.

Drug Interactions Adefovir may decrease the effectiveness of tenofovir. Tenofovir may increase levels of adefovir. Concomitant use is not recommended.

Elbasvir / Grazoprevir

Elbasvir / grazoprevier (Zepatier) is a combination product used in the treatment of chronic hepatitis C genotype 1 or 4 infection. Zepatier is indicated for use with ribavirin in certain patients.

Dosage Forms and Administration Prior to therapy initiation, all patients should be tested for hepatitis B infection. Elbasvir / grazoprevir is taken once daily with or without food. The duration of treatment depends on the patient population and ranges from 12 to 16 weeks.

Side Effects The most common side effects include fatigue, headache, and nausea.

Contraindications Contraindications include hypersensitivity to any component of the combination product and severe hepatic impairment. Other contraindications are related to drug interactions. Concurrent use of drugs that inhibit organic anion transporting polypeptides 1B1/3, and concurrent use of strong inducers of cytochrome

P-450 3A4 and efavirenz are contraindicated. Phenytoin, carbamazepine, rifampin, atazanavir, darunavir, lopinavir, saquinavir, tipranavir, and Saint-John's-wort are specific drug interactions.

Cautions and Considerations Zepatier contains a boxed warning of an increased risk of reactivation of hepatitis B infection. Liver toxicity is a concern with use. Increases in the liver enzyme ALT can be seen; therefore, testing is recommended at certain intervals during therapy.

Drug Interactions There are many drug interactions with this combination product. See the Contraindications section for specific drugs that should never be used.

Glecaprevir / Pibrentasvir

Glecaprevir / pibrentasvir (Mavyret) is a combination product used in the treatment of chronic hepatitis C. It can treat genotypes through 6.

Dosage Forms and Administration Glecaprevir / pibrentasvir is dosed one daily and should be taken with food.

Side Effects The most commonly reported side effects include headache and fatigue.

Contraindications Contraindications include hypersensitivity to any component of the combination product and severe hepatic impairment. It should not be taken with atazanvir or rifampin.

Cautions and Considerations Mavyret contains a boxed warning of an increased risk of reactivation of hepatitis B infection. Liver toxicity is a concern with use.

Drug Interactions Mavyret should not be taken with carbamazepine, efavirenz, and Saint-John's-wort.

Ombitasvir / Paritaprevir / Ritonavir / Dasabuvir

 TAKE WITH FOOD

Ombitasvir / paritaprevir / ritonavir / dasabuvir (Viekira Pak) is a combination product used for the treatment of chronic hepatitis C infection.

Dosage Forms and Administration Each fixed-dose tablet contains ombitasvir 12.5 mg, paritaprevir 75 mg, and ritonavir 50 mg; these are copackaged with dasabuvir 250 mg tablets. Viekira Pak should be administered with a meal. Adverse reactions include headache, fatigue, and nausea. Vierkira XR is also available and is an extended-release formulation of the Viekira Pak that is taken once daily.

Side Effects The most common side effects include fatigue, nausea, itching, insomnia, and weakness.

Contraindications Contraindications include hypersensitivity to any component of the combination product and severe hepatic impairment. Other contraindications are related to drug interactions. Concurrent use of drugs that are highly dependent on cytochrome P-450 3A4 for clearance, concurrent use of strong inducers of cytochrome P-450 3A4 and 2C8, or strong inhibitors of 2C8 are contraindicated. Alfuzosin, carbamazepine, ergot derivatives (dihydroergotamine, ergonovine, ergotamine, and methylergonovine), efavirenz, ethinyl estradiol-containing products, gemfibrozil, lovastatin, midazolam (oral), phenobarbital, phenytoin, pimozide, rifampin, sildenafil (when used for the treatment of pulmonary arterial hypertension), simvastatin, Saint-John's-wort, and triazolam are specific drug contraindications.

Cautions and Considerations Elevation of hepatic enzymes has occurred with use. Individuals using ethinyl estradiol products (often oral contraceptives) are at an increased risk. Ritonavir, a component of the product, is also used to treat HIV. HIV resistance to ritonavir may occur in patients using Viekira Pak with undiagnosed or untreated HIV. Use with caution in patients with moderate liver impairment.

Drug Interactions There are many drug interactions with this combination product. See the Contraindications section for specific drugs that should never be used with Viekira Pak.

Simeprevir

Simeprevir (Olysio) is a protease inhibitor for the treatment of chronic hepatitis C. It is not meant to be used as monotherapy; simeprevir should be used in combination with other agents.

Dosage Forms and Administration Simeprevir should be taken with food.

Side Effects Common adverse effects include rash and photosensitivity.

Contraindications No contraindications have been reported by the manufacturer.

Cautions and Considerations Simeprevir doses should not be missed. Skipped doses may lead to viral resistance. Simeprevir should not be used in patients with moderate-to-severe hepatic dysfunction.

Drug Interactions Simeprevir may increase concentrations of bosutinib, cisapride, pazopanib, other protease inhibitors, topotecan, and vincristine. Conivaptan, cyclosporine, erythromycin, fusidic acid, idelalisib, ledipasvir, and milk thistle may increase the concentrations of simeprevir. Saint-John's-wort may decrease the serum concentrations of simeprevir.

Sofosbuvir / Velpatasvir

Sofosbuvir / velpatasvir (Epclusa) is a combination product indicated for the treatment of chronic hepatitis C. It treats all genotypes.

Dosage Forms and Administration Epclusa is given as one tablet by mouth once daily with or without food. In certain patients, Epclusa may be used with ribavirin.

Side Effects The most commonly reported adverse side effects include headache and fatigue.

Contraindications Epclusa should not be coadministered with amiodarone; medications that induce p-glycoprotein; or inducers of CYP2B6, CYP2C8, or CYP3A4. Example drug interactions include Rifampin, Saint-John's-wort, carbamazepine, phenytoin, and efavirenz.

Cautions and Considerations Epclusa contains a boxed warning of an increased risk of reactivation of hepatitis B infection.

Drug Interactions Rifampin, Saint-John's-wort, carbamezepine, and other inducers of P-glycoprotine and/or moderate to strong inducers of CYP2B6, CYP2C8, and CYP3A4 may decrease the effect of sofosuvir / velpatasvir. Coadministration of amioarone, topotecan, carbamazepine, phenytoin, phenobarbital, rifabutin, rifampin, refapentine, efavirenze, and tipranavir / ritonavir is not recommended. Acid reducing agents like antacids, H2-receptor antagonists, and PPIs can decrease velpatasvir concentrations; if necessary, these drugs should be separated from sofosbuvir / velpatasvir administration.

12.11 Complementary and Alternative Therapies

Shiatsu acupressure or massage has been used to treat nausea. Shiatsu acupressure involves finger pressure at certain points along the body.

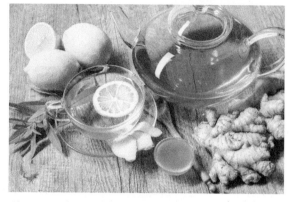

Ginger may be used for nausea.

Ginger (*Zingiber officinale*) can be used to reduce nausea associated with surgery, vertigo, and motion sickness. It also has demonstrated benefits in pregnant individuals with morning sickness, but it has not undergone rigorous safety testing in this patient population. The mechanism of action of ginger is still poorly defined, but it may exert its effects by blocking 5-HT in the same way that other antiemetics do. The standard dose for preventing nausea and vomiting is 500 to 1,000 mg. Ginger may cause heartburn, gas, bloating, mouth and throat irritation, and diarrhea. Because ginger has anti-platelet effects, its use should be avoided in patients taking aspirin, warfarin, or other anticoagulants.

Probiotics are products that contain live cultures of yeast or bacteria. They are used as nonpharmacologic adjunctive treatment for diarrhea, constipation, *H. pylori* infection, and antibiotic-induced diarrhea. They may even be used to treat diarrhea associated with rotavirus, Crohn's disease, ulcerative colitis, and IBS. Probiotic organisms are not pathogenic and are commonly available in capsules, powders, beverages, and yogurts, some of which need to be refrigerated to keep the microorganisms alive. These products are used to colonize the GI tract with beneficial organisms for digestion and regular GI motility. The probiotic organisms compete with harmful bacteria, hopefully replacing or displacing them. They may enhance the immune response to pathogenic organisms and break down toxins. Patients with poor immune system function should not use probiotic products. Doses vary based on the product and indication.

Lactobacilli are Gram-positive bacteria that are normal flora of the human GI tract. Common lactobacilli products contain *Lactobacillus acidophilus*, *Lactobacillus helveticus*, *Lactobacillus bulgaricus*, and *Lactobacillus rhamnosus*. Lactobacilli products are taken each day, divided into three or four doses. They are usually well tolerated with few side effects, the most common of which are gas and bloating.

Saccharomyces boulardii (*S. boulardii*) is a yeast organism that lives in the human GI tract. Florastor is the brand name of a product that is used to prevent antibiotic-associated diarrhea. Typically, 250–500 mg of Florastor is taken two to four times a day. *S. boulardii* can cause gas, bloating, and constipation.

Bifidobacteria agents are not as well studied as lactobacilli and *S. boulardii* products. However, they might be effective for diarrhea associated with a variety of causes. Doses vary with products and indications. As with other probiotics, bifidobacteria are well tolerated in general but have the potential to cause gas and bloating.

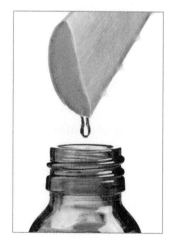

Aloe ingested orally is used to treat constipation.

Aloe ingested orally may be used to treat patients with constipation. It appears to work as a stimulant laxative. Dosing may range from 40 to 170 mg of dried juice. Caution is advised when taking aloe supplements, as adverse effects, including diarrhea and drug interactions, are possible. Aloe supplements should not be used by individuals who are pregnant or breast-feeding, unless directed by a healthcare practitioner.

Review and Assessment

CHAPTER SUMMARY

Gastrointestinal System

- The GI tract is a tube that begins in the mouth; extends through the pharynx, esophagus, stomach, small intestine, and large intestine; and ends at the anus.

- The digestive and absorptive processes take place in the GI tract.

- Mucous membranes protect the entire digestive system against abrasion and strong digestive chemicals.

Gastrointestinal Diseases

- Gastroesophageal reflux disease (GERD) is commonly known as *heartburn*. Alcohol, nicotine, and caffeine exacerbate GERD.

- Antacids can be used to treat GERD; they neutralize the acidic stomach contents so that, if reflux does occur, the contents will be less irritating to the esophageal lining.

- H_2 blockers can be used to treat GERD. The bedtime dose of the H_2 blockers is the most important one. PPIs may also be used for GERD.

- The three types of ulcers are *gastric ulcer*, *duodenal ulcer*, and *stress ulcer*.

- There are drug regimens for the treatment of the bacterium *H. pylori*, which contributes to the development of ulcers.

- Gastritis is an irritation and superficial erosion of the stomach lining. Ulcerative colitis is an inflammation of the large bowel.

- Azathioprine (Imuran) is used to treat GI diseases as well as other autoimmune diseases.

- Mesalamine (Apriso, Asacol, Canasa, Delzicol, Lialda, Pentasa) and sulfasalazine (Azulfidine, Sulfazine) are used to treat ulcerative colitis.

  Sulfasalazine (Azulfidine, Sulfazine) decreases inflammatory response in the colon. It can change the color of urine and stain soft contact lenses.

- Ursodiol (Actigall) is used to dissolve gallstones, but it can take several months.

Diarrhea

- Diphenoxylate-atropine (Lomotil) is a combination drug and a controlled substance used to treat diarrhea.

- Loperamide (Imodium) may be as effective as diphenoxylate-atropine and is available over the counter.

Constipation and Flatulence

- Dietary fiber increases colon content and propulsive motility.

- Chronic constipation is often associated with low-fiber diets.

- Aluminum hydroxide-magnesium hydroxide-simethicone is a gastric defoaming antiflatulent agent. It reduces surface tension, causing bubbles to be broken or to coalesce into a foam that can be eliminated more easily by belching or passing flatus.

- Constipation can be relieved with bulk-forming laxatives, surfactant laxatives, osmotic laxatives, and stimulant laxatives.

- Patients taking opioids should take a stimulant laxative.

- Constipation and lack of dietary fiber increase the likelihood of other diseases, including diverticular disease, hiatal hernia, and hemorrhoids.

Nausea and Vomiting

- The chemoreceptor trigger zone (CTZ), when stimulated, may trigger vomiting.

- Some antiemetics bind to serotonin (5-HT) receptors to prevent nausea.

Hepatitis

- Hepatitis A, hepatitis B, and hepatitis C are the most common hepatitis viruses.

- Hepatitis C can be transmitted only through blood and body fluids.

- Vaccines have been developed to prevent infection by hepatitis A and hepatitis B but not hepatitis C.

DRUG LIST

GERD

Antacids
aluminum hydroxide (AlternaGel)
aluminum hydroxide / magnesium carbonate (Gaviscon Extra Strength)
aluminum hydroxide / magnesium hydroxide-simethicone (Mylanta)
calcium carbonate (Maalox, Tums)
calcium carbonate / famotidine-magnesium hydroxide (Pepcid Complete)
magnesium hydroxide (Phillips' Milk of Magnesia)

Histamine H$_2$ Receptor Antagonists
cimetidine (Tagamet, Tagamet HB)
famotidine (Pepcid, Pepcid AC)
nizatidine (Axid, Axid AR)
ranitidine (Zantac, Zantac 75)

Proton Pump Inhibitors
dexlansoprazole (Dexilant)
esomeprazole (Nexium)
lansoprazole (Prevacid)
omeprazole (Prilosec, Prilosec OTC)
omeprazole / sodium bicarbonate (Zegerid)
pantoprazole (Protonix)
rabeprazole (Aciphex)

Coating Agent
sucralfate (Carafate)

Prostaglandin E Analog
misoprostol (Cytotec)

H. pylori

Antibiotics
amoxicillin (Amoxil, Trimox)
clarithromycin (Biaxin)
metronidazole (Flagyl, Flagyl IV)

Combinations
bismuth subcitrate / metronidazole-tetracycline (Pylera)
lansoprazole / amoxicillin / clarithromycin (Prevpac)

Gastrointestinal Diseases

Aminosalicylates
mesalamine (Apriso, Asacol, Canasa, Delzicol, Lialda, Pentasa)
sulfasalazine (Azulfidine, Sulfazine)

Corticosteroids
budesonide (Entocort EC)
hydrocortisone (A-Hydrocort, Cortef, Solu-Cortef)
methylprednisolone (A-MethaPred, Depo-Medrol, Medrol, Solu-Medrol)
prednisone (Sterapred)

Immunosuppressant
azathioprine (Imuran)

Gallstone Dissolution Agent
ursodiol (Actigall)

Antidiarrheals

Adsorbent
bismuth subsalicylate (Kaopectate, Pepto-Bismol)

Antimotility Drugs
difenoxin / atropine (Motofen)
diphenoxylate / atropine (Lomotil)
loperamide (Imodium, Imodium A-D)

Drugs for Infectious Diarrhea
nitazoxanide (Alinia)
rifaximin (Xifaxan)

Antiflatulent Agents
aluminum hydroxide-magnesium hydroxide / simethicone (Mylanta, Mylanta Maximum Strength)
calcium carbonate / simethicone (Maalox)
simethicone (Gas Aid, Mylicon Drops)

Bowel Evacuants
polyethylene glycol 3350 with electrolytes (Colyte, GaviLyte-C, GaviLyte-G, GaviLyte-N, GoLYTELY, HalfLYTELY, MoviPrep, NuLYTELY, TriLyte)
sodium phosphate (Visicol)

Bulk-Forming Laxatives
methylcellulose (Citrucel, Maltsupex, Unifiber)
polycarbophil (Equalactin, FiberCon, Fiber-Lax, Konsyl Fiber)
psyllium (Fiberall, Metamucil, Perdiem Fiber Therapy)
wheat dextrin (Benefiber)

Osmotic Laxatives
glycerin (Fleet Glycerin Suppositories)
lactulose (Enulose)
magnesium hydroxide (Phillips' Milk of Magnesia)
magnesium sulfate (Epsom Salts)
polyethylene glycol 3350 (MiraLax)

Stimulant Laxatives
bisacodyl (Dulcolax)
senna (ExLax, Fletcher's Castoria, various brands)

Surfactant Laxatives
docusate (Colace, Ex-Lax Stool Softener, Surfak)
docusate-senna (Senokot-S)

Miscellaneous
lubiprostone (Amitiza)
methylnaltrexone (Relistor)

Hemorrhoidal Agent
hydrocortisone (Anusol HC, Cortifoam)
nitroglycerin (Rectiv)

Antiemetic Medications

Antihistamines and Anticholinergics
diphenhydramine (Benadryl)
meclizine (Antivert, Dramamine)
scopolamine (Scopace, Transderm Scop)

Serotonin Receptor Antagonists
dolasetron (Anzemet)
granisetron (Kytril)
ondansetron (Zofran)
palonosetron (Aloxi)

Phenothiazines
prochlorperazine (Compazine)
promethazine (Phenergan)

Other Antiemetic Medications
aprepitant, fosaprepitant (Emend)
metoclopramide (Reglan)

Hepatitis Drugs
entecavir (Baraclude)
hepatitis B vaccine (Engerix B, Recombivax HB)
immune globulin (Gamunex)
lamivudine (Epivir, Epivir-HBV)
ledipasvir / sofosbuvir (Harvoni)
ombitasvir / paritaprevir / ritonavir / dasabuvir (Viekira Pak)
peginterferon alfa-2a (Pegasys)
ribavirin (Copegus, Moderiba, Rebetol, Ribasphere, Ribasphere RibaPak, Virazole)
simeprevir (Olysio)
sofosbuvir (Sovaldi)
tenofovir (Viread)

Boxed Warnings
bismuth subcitrate-metronidazole / tetracycline (Pylera)
entecavir (Baraclude)
immune globulin (Gamunex)

lamivudine (Epivir, Epivir-HBV)
peginterferon alfa-2a (Pegasys)
metoclopromide (Reglan)
metronidazole (Flagyl)
misoprostol (Cytotec)
promethazine (Phenergan)
ribavirin (Copegus)
sodium phosphate (Visicol)
tenofovir (Viread)

metoclopramide (Reglan)
peginterferon alfa-2a (Pegasys)
ribavirin (Copegus, Moderiba, Rebetol,
    Ribasphere, Ribasphere RibaPak, Virazole)

✓ CHECK YOUR UNDERSTANDING

Take a moment to reflect on what you have learned in this chapter and answer the following questions.

1. A most common cause of gastritis is
   a. food.
   b. alcohol.
   c. medicine.
   d. stress.

2. Which of the following drugs commonly causes gastric ulcers?
   a. antacids
   b. aspirin
   c. omeprazole
   d. famotidine

3. Which drug is a laxative that stimulates peristalsis and GI motility?
   a. Carafate
   b. Cytotec
   c. Dulcolax
   d. Prevacid

4. Which drug is a coating agent?
   a. Axid
   b. Carafate
   c. Cytotec
   d. Prevacid

5. Which antidiarrheal is a controlled substance?
   a. Alinia
   b. Imodium
   c. Lomotil
   d. loperamide

6. Which drug is used to treat GERD?
   a. Actigall
   b. Dulcolax
   c. Imuran
   d. Protonix

7. Which drug is used to treat Crohn's disease?
   a. Actigall
   b. aspirin
   c. cyclizine
   d. sulfasalazine

8. Which drug is used to treat gallstones?
   a. Actigall
   b. Azulfidine
   c. Imuran
   d. Rowasa

9. Which drug should not be touched by a pregnant technician?
   a. Actigall
   b. Cytotec
   c. Imuran
   d. Rowasa

10. Hepatitis C is transmitted through
    a. *Anopheles* mosquitos.
    b. blood.
    c. fecal-oral route.
    d. sweat.

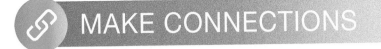

MAKE CONNECTIONS

Take a moment to consider what you have learned in this chapter and respond thoughtfully to the following prompts. Note that some of these activities will require internet access.

1. How are you preparing to study the gastrointestinal diseases for the certification exam? Be sure to be able to describe how and what medications are used to treat the various conditions in this chapter. Consider familiarizing yourself with the over-the-counter medications in an outpatient or retail pharmacy.

2. What experiences have you had working as part of a team? How might you apply those experiences to working as a pharm tech?

 The online course includes additional review and assessment resources.

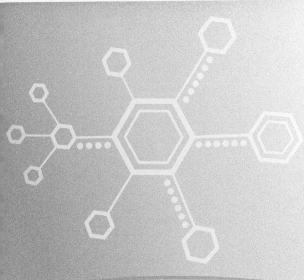

The Endocrine System and Drug Therapy 13

Learning Objectives

1 Describe the physiologic processes of the endocrine system. (Section 13.1)

2 Summarize the concept of hormones and how they regulate the body. (Section 13.1)

3 Explain the treatments for disorders of the thyroid. (Section 13.2)

4 List commonly used corticosteroids. (Section 13.3)

5 Summarize diabetes and the proper treatment and care of patients with diabetes. (Section 13.4)

6 Identify the classes of drugs used to treat diabetes. (Section 13.4)

7 Describe how the medications used to treat diabetes work. (Section 13.4)

ASHP/ACPE Accreditation Standards

To view the *ASHP/ACPE Accreditation Standards* addressed in this chapter, refer to Appendix C.

The endocrine system regulates a number of functions to keep the body in balance as well as to control complicated processes such as those involved in reproduction. The same hormones the endocrine system uses to trigger activity may also be used to treat patients. The pharmacologic agents used in these treatments include thyroid preparations, calcium, corticosteroids, and medications for diabetes.

13.1 Anatomy and Physiology of the Endocrine System

The **endocrine system** consists of ductless glands and other structures that secrete hormones directly into the bloodstream. A **hormone** is a secretion released by an endocrine gland into the circulatory system that has a specific regulatory effect on organs and other tissues. Endocrine glands include the pineal, pituitary, thyroid, parathyroid, thymus, adrenal, and reproductive glands as well as the pancreatic duct and the hypothalamus (see Figure 13.1). The cell, tissue, or organ affected by a hormone is called its **target**. Through the work of hormones, the endocrine system maintains homeostasis within the body by regulating the physiologic functions involved in normal daily living and in times of stress.

FIGURE 13.1
Endocrine System

Endocrine glands release hormones directly into the bloodstream, where they travel throughout the body to trigger responses in specific target tissues.

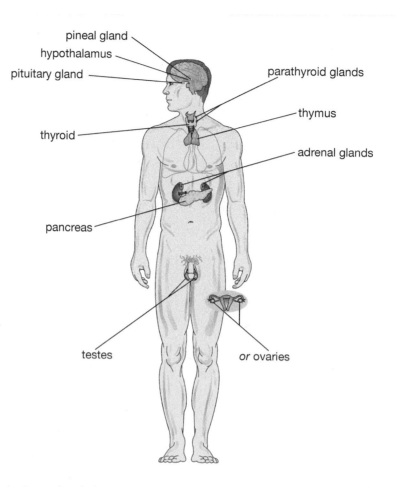

pineal gland
hypothalamus
pituitary gland
parathyroid glands
thymus
thyroid
adrenal glands
pancreas
testes
or ovaries

The pituitary gland plays a leading role in the endocrine system because its hormones regulate several other endocrine glands as well as a number of body activities, as shown in Figure 13.2. The endocrine system produces two types of hormones: steroid hormones and nonsteroid hormones. A **steroid hormone** is a messenger that passes directly into the cells of the target organ. Cortisol is one example of a steroid hormone. It is produced by the adrenal gland and released in response to stress and a low concentration of glucose in the blood.

A **nonsteroid hormone** does not have the ability to penetrate cells. Instead, it binds to receptors on a cell membrane to activate secondary messengers within the cell. Adrenaline, also known as *epinephrine*, is one example of a nonsteroid hormone. When adrenaline is released in response to an immediate stressor (e.g., the anticipation of danger), it produces the **fight-or-flight response**, the body's physical preparation to either escape or do battle when faced with danger.

The endocrine system secretes hormones at a rate that keeps their level in the blood almost constant. The body can do this because it receives continuous feedback from its systems, known as a **feedback mechanism**. **Negative feedback** occurs when the level of hormone in the blood or the level of a chemical it affects moves above or below a desired range. When this occurs, hormone production is lowered or raised in the opposite direction to bring the blood level of the hormone or the chemical it affects back into the appropriate range.

Positive feedback is rare. In positive feedback, the presence of the hormone or chemical it affects promotes the production of more of that hormone or chemical until some other input stops it. Positive feedback does not result in keeping the hormone or chemical within a particular range.

FIGURE 13.2
Pituitary Hormones

The pituitary gland plays a key role in regulation of the thyroid, adrenal glands, and hormones within the kidney.

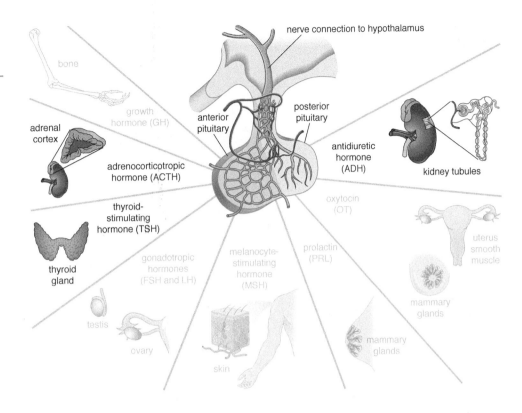

The disorders discussed in this chapter relate to the thyroid, adrenal glands, and pancreas. Disorders that relate to reproductive and growth hormones are discussed in Chapter 14. The thyroid is located in the throat and responds to thyroid-stimulating hormone (TSH). The adrenal glands are located on the top of the kidneys and are responsible for producing catecholamines (such as epinephrine) and steroid hormones (such as cortisol). Finally, the pancreas and its specialized cells are responsible for producing insulin and glucagon, key hormones that assist the body in the management of glucose.

Thyroid Gland

Pharm Fact

Calcitonin, a hormone that regulates calcium and phosporus in the body, is also made by the thyroid.

The **thyroid gland**, shown in Figure 13.3, produces hormones that stimulate various body tissues to increase their metabolic activity. Two of these hormones, **triiodothyronine (T_3)** and **thyroxine (T_4)**, are stored as thyroglobulin, which the thyroid cells must break down before T_3 and T_4 can be released into the bloodstream. T_3 and T_4 are usually bound to protein molecules. Thyroid hormones are only active when they are not bound to protein in the blood. T_3 is more physiologically active than T_4. The feedback mechanism that controls the thyroid is called the *hypothalamic-pituitary axis*. Chemical transmitters from the hypothalmus gland located just above the pituitary, called *hypothalmus releasing factors*, regulate the pituitary gland in a stress response. This stress response system for the body signals the pituitary gland to produce thyroid-stimulating hormone (TSH), which in turn stimulates the thyroid to produce T_3 and T_4 (see Figure 13.4). These hormones build up in circulating blood and slow the pituitary gland's production and release of TSH. For a patient with signs of hormonal imbalance, measuring the amount of serum TSH can help determine whether the thyroid is functioning normally; in some instances, other tests for T_3 and T_4 may be needed. It is also important to note that some peripheral conversion of T_4 to T_3 occurs in the tissues.

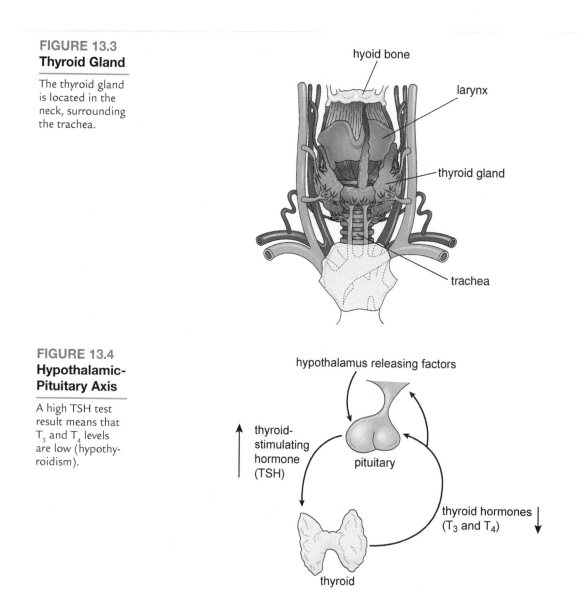

FIGURE 13.3
Thyroid Gland

The thyroid gland is located in the neck, surrounding the trachea.

hyoid bone

larynx

thyroid gland

trachea

FIGURE 13.4
Hypothalamic-Pituitary Axis

A high TSH test result means that T_3 and T_4 levels are low (hypothyroidism).

hypothalamus releasing factors

thyroid-stimulating hormone (TSH)

pituitary

thyroid hormones (T_3 and T_4)

thyroid

Adrenal Glands and Corticosteroids

The adrenal glands are located on the top of the kidneys. The adrenal medulla, or inner portion of an adrenal gland, functions like the sympathetic nervous system and produces catecholamines such as epinephrine (adrenaline) and norepinephrine. The adrenal cortex, or outer portion, produces several types of steroid hormones. Each such hormone, known as a **corticosteroid**, has its own combination of **glucocorticoid** (involved in cholesterol, fat, and protein metabolism) and **mineralocorticoid** (involved in regulating electrolyte and water balance) activity. The principal adrenal steroid hormone is cortisol. It is responsible for **gluconeogenesis** (conversion of fatty acids and proteins to glucose), anti-inflammatory reactions, stimulation of fat deposition, and sodium and water retention (steroids are necessary for mineral retention). The adrenal cortex also produces various sex hormones.

As with the thyroid hormones, the production of cortisol and other steroids begins in the hypothalamic-pituitary axis. The hypothalamus produces corticotropin-releasing factor (CRF), which stimulates the pituitary gland to produce adrenocorticotropic hormone (ACTH), which in turn enters the bloodstream and travels to the adrenal cortex, where it stimulates the release of cortisol into the blood. Through a feedback mechanism, the rising cortisol levels slow the action of the hypothalamus in producing and releasing CRF. Steroid production follows a **circadian** rhythm (regular recurrence in cycles of 24 hours). As Figure 13.5 shows, steroid production peaks in the morning, and the low point occurs close to midnight.

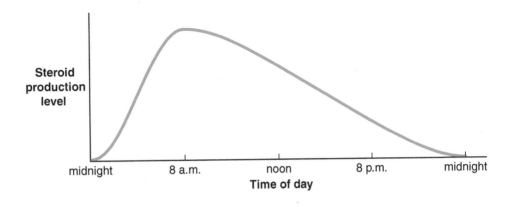

FIGURE 13.5
Steroid Production

Steroid production follows a circadian rhythm, with a peak in the morning and a low point around midnight.

Pancreas

The pancreas contains groups of specialized cells, called *islets of Langerhans*, that produce insulin. **Insulin** helps cells burn glucose for energy and bind with cell membrane receptors to allow glucose uptake, enhances the transport of amino acids and their incorporation into proteins, increases ion transport into tissues, and inhibits fat breakdown. Thus, in addition to having other metabolic roles, insulin is critical in maintaining blood glucose levels.

13.2 Thyroid Disorders and Drug Treatments

The thyroid gland produces the hormones triiodothyronine (T_3) and thyroxine (T_4), which stimulate various body tissues to increase their metabolic activity. The two most common thyroid disorders are hypothyroidism and hyperthyroidism. *Hypothyroidism* refers to conditions in which the production of thyroid hormones is below normal. *Hyperthyroidism*, in contrast, refers to the body's production an excess of thyroid hormones. Both conditions can be treated. See Table 13.1 for a list of common agents for treating thyroid disorders.

TABLE 13.1 Commonly Used Agents for Thyroid Disorders

Generic (Brand)	Pronunciation	Dosage Form	Dispensing Status
Thyroid Replacement Agents			
levothyroxine (Euthyrox, Levo-T, Levothyroid, Levoxyl, Synthroid, Tirosint, Unithroid)	lee-voe-thye-ROX-een	capsule, injection, oral solution, tablet	Rx
liothyronine (Cytomel, Triostat)	lye-oh-THYE-roe-neen	injection, tablet	Rx
thyroid desiccated (Armour Thyroid, Nature-Throid)	THYE-roid DES-i-kay-ted	tablet	Rx
Antithyroid Agents			
methimazole (Tapazole)	meth-IM-a-zole	tablet	Rx
propylthiouracil (PTU)	proe-pil-thye-oh-YOOR-a-sil	tablet	Rx

Hypothyroidism and Thyroid Replacement Therapy

Safety Alert

Levothyroxine and levofloxacin (an antibiotic) can be misread for each other. Tall man lettering, such as in *levoFLOXacin*, can be useful to help differentiate them.

Hypothyroidism refers to conditions in which the production of thyroid hormones is lower than normal. The causes of hypothyroidism include surgical removal of the thyroid and defects in thyroid function due to autoimmune destruction of the gland or radioactive iodine therapy. Pituitary dysfunction or an abnormality in the hypothalamus can also cause thyroid failure. Symptoms of hypothyroidism include tiredness, lethargy, hair loss, weight gain, changes in sleep, depressed mood, and increased appetite. Congenital (at birth) hypothyroidism may arise in infants and is often caused by an iodine deficiency in the pregnant parent's diet during pregnancy. It can cause severe impairment of mental growth and is marked by a thick tongue, lethargy, lack of response to commands, and short stature. It can be corrected if treated in the first 6 to 12 months of life.

Thyroid replacement therapy is indicated for hypothyroid states and thyroid cancer. In the absence of natural hormones, thyroid hormone replacement is required. Although thyroid hormones increase metabolism, replacement therapy should not be used to treat obesity. Drugs commonly used to treat hypothyroidism are listed in Table 13.1. Hypothyroidism causes increased sensitivity to numerous drugs. Thyroid replacement agents and their effects on a patient's metabolism may require adjustments in the dosages of other medications. Due to the nature of this type of dosing, common dosages are not listed in Table 13.1.

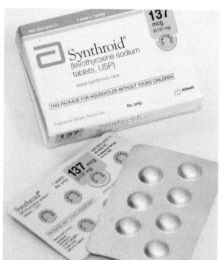

Levothyroxine is available as a generic drug or as the brand product Synthroid.

Levothyroxine (Euthyrox, Levo-T, Levothroid, Levoxyl, Synthroid, Tirosint, Unithroid) is synthetic T_4. It is recommended for chronic hypothyroidism therapy. Levothyroxine may alter the protein binding of other drugs, so the technician should check the patient profile for drugs currently being taken.

Generic and brand name levothyroxine products are therapeutically equivalent, and they are now AB rated according to the FDA (that is, shown by studies to be bioequivalent, as a generic should be to the corresponding brand-name drug). One clinical study showed that switching products does not cause problems, but it is usually undesirable to switch brands once a patient has become stable. Some prescribers are concerned that the small FDA-allowable compositional differences between brand and generic levothyroxine products could affect blood levels. All patients taking thyroid hormones should undergo TSH tests periodically as well as approximately six weeks after changes in dosage or brands. Once a patient is stable on a brand, the prescriber will typically write **dispense as written (DAW)** on the prescription, which means it is for that brand name only. Most pharmacy computer programs automatically switch all drugs to a generic; when the switch happens with this drug, which may be frequent, technicians may need to switch the drug back to the brand if indicated by the prescriber.

Liothyronine (Cytomel, Triostat) is synthetic T_3. It may be used for hypothyroidism and management of goiter.

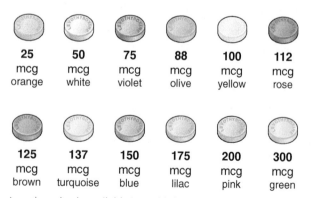

| 25 mcg orange | 50 mcg white | 75 mcg violet | 88 mcg olive | 100 mcg yellow | 112 mcg rose |

| 125 mcg brown | 137 mcg turquoise | 150 mcg blue | 175 mcg lilac | 200 mcg pink | 300 mcg green |

Levothyroxine is available in multiple strengths, each with a different color.

Dosage Forms and Administration Levothyroxine is available as a capsule, injection, and tablet. Liothyronine is available as an injection and tablet. **Thyroid desiccated (Armour Thyroid, Nature-Throid)** is available in tablet form only.

Side Effects Common side effects of thyroid hormone products are primarily those associated with dosing of thyroid hormones that is too high. These effects include heart palpitations or arrythmias, increased blood pressure, racing pulse, flushing, anxiety, irritability, fatigue, headache, heat intolerance, insomnia, hair loss, sweating, weight loss, diarrhea, stomach cramps, fever, and difficulty breathing. Reduced fertility and elevated liver enzymes are less obvious signs of excess thyroid hormones. Rarer side effects include angina, heart attack, and seizure. To avoid these effects, lab tests are used to monitor the levels of thyroid hormones in the blood so that the dose can be adjusted downward if needed.

Contraindications Levothyroxine use and liothyronine use are contraindicated in the presence of an acute heart attack, untreated hyperthyroidism, or uncorrected adrenal insufficiency. Thyroid desiccated, which contains beef and pork products, should not be used in patients with a hypersensitivity to beef or pork.

The injection form of liothyronine should not be used in patients who are undergoing artificial rewarming due to hypothermia.

Cautions and Considerations Thyroid hormones have a boxed warning saying they should not be used for the treatment of obesity or for weight loss.

Serious and potentially life-threatening toxic effects can occur with higher doses, especially in patients with normal levels of thyroid hormones. Patients should be reminded to get regular blood tests to check thyroid hormone levels. Various thyroid hormone brands may contain slightly different amounts, enough for changes in therapy to be experienced by individual patients. Once one brand of a thyroid hormone is chosen, the patient should continue receiving that brand at each refill. Levothyroxine can have cardiovascular side effects, so patients should immediately report any chest pain, increased pulse, palpitations, heat intolerance, or excessive sweating. In overdose, it can cause "too rapid" a correction and, therefore, a risk of cardiotoxicity and hyperthyroidism.

Drug Interactions Aluminum-containing products may decrease concentrations of levothyroxine when taken within four hours of taking levothyroxine.

Bile acid sequestrants, calcium-containing products, magnesium-containing products, and multivitamins may decrease the concentrations or all thyroid replacement therapies. Thyroid products should not be taken at the same time as bile acid sequestrants.

Carbamazepine, ciprofloxacin, estrogen products, fosphenytoin, iron salts, phenytoin, rifampin, and selective serotonin reuptake inhibitors (SSRIs) may decrease the efficacy of thyroid hormones. Tricyclic antidepressants may enhance the cardiotoxic effects of thyroid agents.

Orlistat, raloxifene, and sevelamer may decrease concentrations of levothyroxine. Thyroid products may increase the patient's metabolism of theophylline. Warfarin's anticoagulant effect may be enhanced by thyroid products.

Hyperthyroidism

Hyperthyroidism, also called *thyrotoxicosis*, describes an excessive level of thyroid hormones. This condition is less common than hypothyroidism. Common causes of hyperthyroidism include **Graves' disease**, thyroid nodules or tumors, and pituitary nodules or tumors.

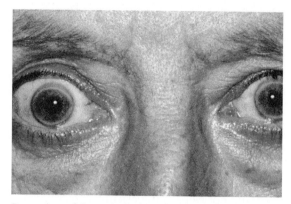

Protrusion of the eyeballs, known as *exophthalmos*, is a symptom of hyperthyroidism.

Symptoms of hyperthyroidism are varied, the most prominent being weight loss and hair loss. Adults with hyperthyroidism may have heart problems due to prolonged hyperactivity caused by the excessive hormone levels. Another prominent symptom is **exophthalmos**, a condition in which fat collects behind the eyeball, causing the eyeball to protrude and making it difficult to close the eye. This condition can cause corneal ulceration.

Hyperthyroidism in children is managed with surgery and hormone replacement therapy. In adults, surgery is indicated for malignant lesions, esophageal obstruction, failure of thyroid therapy, or large multinodular goiters.

Thyroid storm is a dangerous condition that presents clinical features similar to those of hyperthyroidism, but more exaggerated. Thyroid storm is a life-threatening medical emergency. It commonly lasts approximately three days, although symptoms may persist for an additional eight days. Treatment includes IV fluids, antipyretics, cooling blankets, and sedation. Antithyroid drugs are given in large doses when thyroid storm is suspected. Table 13.1 presents the most commonly used antithyroid agents for hyperthyroidism.

Treatment for hyperthyroidism usually involves surgery, which removes or reduces the malfunctioning gland, or **radioiodine ablation**, which destroys the thyroid gland via radioactive iodine. Afterward, **oral thyroid supplementation** is given to artificially provide adequate hormone levels. Propylthiouracil and methimazole are sometimes used for short-term suppression of thyroid hormones until surgery or radioactive iodine ablation can be performed.

Methimazole (Tapazole) is used for the treatment of hyperthyroidism in patients for whom surgery or radioactive iodine therapy is not appropriate. It may also be used to treat hyperthyroid symptoms in patients awaiting thyroidectomy or radioactive iodine therapy.

Propylthiouracil (PTU) blocks the synthesis of T_3 and T_4 and the conversion of T_4 to T_3. This drug is used for palliative treatment of hyperthyroidism, as adjunctive therapy to improve hyperthyroidism in preparation for surgical treatment, and for management of thyroid storm.

Name Exchange

Propylthiouracil is commonly abbreviated by prescribers as PTU. Technicians may see the drug listed this way in prescriptions.

Dosage Forms and Administration Both agents are available as tablets. Administration of propylthiouracil is preferred over methimazole in thyroid storm. The recommended doses should not be exceeded.

Side Effects Both propylthiouracil and methimazole cause altered taste and mild **alopecia** (hair loss). Bone marrow depression with fever, sore throat, and malaise can occur and can be serious. An autoimmune reaction and a warfarin-like anticoagulant reaction can also occur. Patients should notify the prescriber or pharmacist in the event of fever, sore throat, unusual bleeding or bruising, headache, or general malaise.

Contraindications Methimazole and propylthiouracil do not have contraindications.

Cautions and Considerations Propylthiouracil carries a boxed warning for liver toxicity, which may be fatal in some cases. If propylthiouracil is being used for chronic therapy, the following parameters should be monitored: CBC with differential, prothrombin time (PT), liver function tests, thyroid function tests (T_4, T_3, and TSH), and periodic blood cell counts.

Methimazole use is also associated with liver toxicity. In addition, it is associated with increased bleeding, bone marrow suppression, and dermatitis. Patients taking this drug should be monitored for hypothyroidism, T_3 and T_4 levels, complete blood count (CBC) with differential, and liver function (baseline and as needed).

Drug Interactions Methimazole and propylthiouracil may decrease the anticoagulant effects of warfarin.

The adverse effects of clozapine may be exacerbated by methimazole and propylthiouracil.

13.3 Adrenal Glands and Drug Treatments

The adrenal cortex (the outside portion of an adrenal gland) produces corticosteroids. The isolation of the corticosteroid cortisol **(hydrocortisone)** marked a milestone in medicine. Clinical trials in rheumatoid arthritis produced dramatic results, and researchers soon found that cortisone, another corticosteroid, improves symptoms in an amazing number of disease states. Further research led to the development of other corticosteroids—**prednisone (Prednisone Intensol, Rayos), methylprednisolone (Depo-Medrol, Medrol, Solu-Medrol)**, and **dexamethasone (DoubleDex, MAX Care-Pak, TopiDex, Decadron, DexPak, TaperDex, Dexabliss)**—that have greater anti-inflammatory potency and less effect on renal sodium resorption. These drugs are used as anti-inflammatory or immunosuppressive agents in treating a variety of diseases, including those of hematologic, allergic, inflammatory, neoplastic, or autoimmune origin. Adrenal gland disorders include Cushing's syndrome (an excess of cortisol production) and Addison's disease (a deficiency of corticosteroids). Table 13.2 identifies corticosteroids commonly used to treat adrenal gland disorders.

TABLE 13.2 Commonly Used Corticosteroids

Generic (Brand)	Pronunciation	Dosage Form	Dispensing Status
betamethasone (Celestone)	bay-ta-METH-a-sone	injection	Rx
budesonide (Entocort EC, Uceris)	byoo-DES-oh-nide	capsule, tablet	Rx
cortisone	KOR-ti-sone	tablet	Rx
dexamethasone (DoubleDex, MAX Care-Pak, TopiDex, Decadron, DexPak, TaperDex, Dexabliss)	dex-a-METH-a-sone	elixir, injection, oral solution, tablet	Rx
hydrocortisone (Cortef, Solu-Cortef)	hye-droe-KOR-ti-sone	injection, tablet	Rx
methylprednisolone (Depo-Medrol, Medrol, Solu-Medrol)	meth-ill-pred-NISS-oh-lone	injection, tablet	Rx
prednisolone (Medrol DosePak, Pediapred, Veripred, Orapred ODT)	pred-NISS-oh-lone	oral disintegrating tablet, oral solution, oral suspension, tablet	Rx
prednisone (Prednisone Intensol, Rayos)	PRED-ni-sone	oral solution, tablet	Rx

Cushing's Syndrome

Cushing's syndrome is caused by an overproduction of cortisol or excessive administration of corticosteroids over an extended period. It may also be caused by tumors in the adrenal glands. Patients have a protruding abdomen; a round, puffy face; and fat deposits above the shoulder blades. The fat distribution may not change even with cessation of corticosteroid therapy.

Surgery is used most often to remove tumors causing Cushing's syndrome. Sometimes cytotoxic or chemotherapy drugs are used to treat the tumor and suppress corticosteroid production. (See Chapter 20 for more information on chemotherapeutic agents.)

Addison's Disease

Addison's disease is a life-threatening deficiency of glucocorticoids and mineralocorticoids that is treated with daily administration of a corticosteroid. The symptoms of Addison's disease include the following:

- debilitating weakness
- hyperkalemia (abnormally high concentration of potassium in the blood)
- hyperpigmentation of skin, produced by increased melanin production, typically on the nipples, at creases in the skin, on the lips, and inside the mouth
- low levels of serum sodium and glucose
- reduced blood pressure
- weight loss

Corticosteroid Therapy

Acute adrenal deficiency can be life threatening and is treated with IV fluids and systemic corticosteroids. Systemic corticosteroids replace corticosteroids in a deficiency. They are also used for a variety of other conditions, particularly for their immunosuppressant and anti-inflammatory properties. Systemic corticosteroids may be used for asthma, autoimmune disorders, and hypersensitivity and allergic reactions.

Dosage Forms and Administration Corticosteroids are available in many dosage forms: tablets, syrups, injections, inhalants, eye drops, creams, ointments, lotions, suppositories, and others. They are commonly packed in dose packs. For example, the Medrol Dosepak contains twenty-one 4 mg tablets. On the first day, the patient takes a loading dose; the dose decreases each day thereafter, as described on the package.

Side Effects Common side effects of corticosteroids include headache, dizziness, insomnia, and hunger. Taking corticosteroids in the morning may lessen these effects, especially insomnia. Long-term or excessive use can affect normal metabolism in the body and cause symptoms of steroid overproduction. Severe effects include high blood pressure, loss of bone mass (osteoporosis), electrolyte imbalance, cataracts or glaucoma, and insulin resistance (diabetes). Patients taking corticosteroids for long periods need special monitoring to prevent or treat these effects.

Contraindications Dexamethasone use is contraindicated in systemic fungal infections and cerebral malaria. Contraindications to hydrocortisone include serious infections (except septic shock or tuberculous meningitis) and skin lesions of viral, fungal, or tubercular origin. Injectable hydrocortisone should not be administered intramuscularly in patients with idiopathic thrombocytopenic purpura or via the intrathecal route.

Cautions and Considerations Patients should not stop taking corticosteroids abruptly. Untoward and life-threatening effects can occur if a patient who has been taking chronic corticosteroids discontinues them suddenly. Because these medications can suppress the immune system if taken in large doses, patients taking them may be at an increased risk for infection. Growth and development must be monitored closely in children taking corticosteroids for long periods because these drugs have the potential to stunt growth. Corticosteroids may cause gastrointestinal events, including gastritis, ulcer formation, and gastrointestinal bleeding.

Drug Interactions Corticosteroids may render anticoagulants less effective. Diabetes medications may be less effective when patients are using corticosteroids. Risk of infections with live vaccines increases with concurrent corticosteroid use.

Aprepitant, azole antifungals, and protease inhibitors may increase corticosteroid levels. Carbamazepine, phenytoin, and rifampin may decrease corticosteroid levels.

Adverse reactions of other immunosuppressants may increase the adverse effects of corticosteroids. The fluid-retaining side effects of androgens are enhanced by corticosteroids. Quinolones used with corticosteroids increase the risk of tendon rupture.

13.4 Diabetes and Drug Treatments

The pancreas contains groups of specialized cells, called *islets of Langerhans*, that produce insulin. **Diabetes** is a disease characterized by high blood glucose due to insufficient levels of insulin. If left untreated, diabetes can cause a range of serious conditions and, eventually, death.

In persons with diabetes, either the secretion of insulin from the pancreas or the use of insulin within the body is inadequate, which leads to excessive blood glucose levels. The normal blood glucose level is around 100 mg/dL. At elevated levels, the kidneys are not able to reabsorb the excess, and glucose spills into the urine. Levels consistently above 140 to 160 mg/dL are associated with long-term effects of diabetes. An elevated blood sugar level is known as **hyperglycemia**.

Diabetes can damage all major organ systems and can be devastating if left untreated. Over time, diabetes can destroy eyesight, kidneys, and peripheral circulation. Uncontrolled diabetes can result in blindness, a need for dialysis, and amputation of limbs. Although approximately 20% of persons older than 60 years have diabetes, some estimates suggest that only half of those with diabetes in the United States are diagnosed.

Symptoms of diabetes include the following:

- frequent infections
- glycosuria (presence of glucose in the urine)
- hunger and thirst
- increased urination (polyuria) and nocturia (excessive urination at night)
- numbness and tingling
- slow wound healing (hyperglycemia inhibits activity of neutrophils, a type of white blood cell)
- visual changes (blurry vision)
- nausea and vomiting
- weight loss, irritability, and ketoacidosis
- fatigue

Although acute **hypoglycemia**, in which a patient's blood glucose level falls below 70 mg/dL, is the more dangerous condition, chronic hyperglycemia, in which blood glucose remains above 180 mg/dL, can result in long-term complications that can destroy quality of life. If diabetes goes unchecked, the patient is at risk of developing the following complications:

- Retinopathy, the leading cause of blindness in the United States. In **diabetic retinopathy**, the blood vessels of the retina, at the back of the eye, become damaged, resulting in insufficient blood supply. The vessels' rupture causes loss of sight.

- **Diabetic neuropathy**, which results in a lack of blood flow to nerves, leaving them unable to function. Symptoms include pain that ranges from dull and aching to sharp and stabbing.

- Vascular problems that lead to atherosclerosis of peripheral coronary and cerebrovascular vessels. The decreased blood flow causes neuropathy and slows healing, especially in the feet and legs. Wounds that fail to heal may result in a need for amputation.

- Dermatologic issues that are often expressed as boils, acne, or fungal infections.

- Nephropathy, or kidney damage, which occurs in 10%-21% of patients with diabetes and is the primary cause of end-stage renal disease.

Types of Diabetes and Treatment

The four types of diabetes are type 1, type 2, gestational, and secondary diabetes. **Type 1 diabetes** occurs most commonly in children and young adults, but it may occur at any age. The average age of patients when first diagnosed with type 1 diabetes is 11 years old. Patients with type 1 diabetes are insulin dependent and have no ability to produce their own insulin. Type 1 diabetes is only treatable with insulin. This group comprises 5%-10% of patients with diabetes.

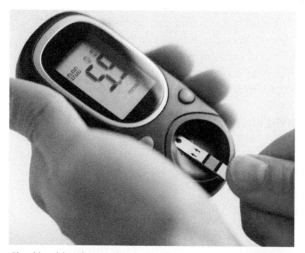

Checking blood sugar levels is a daily component of maintaining health while living with diabetes. Although this task has been part of diabetes care since the mid-1960s, today's meters require less blood and are less painful.

Type 2 diabetes comprises 80%-90% of diabetes cases. Most patients diagnosed with type 2 diabetes are over 40 years of age. Patients with type 2 diabetes have insulin resistance, which means that the cells within tissues are less sensitive to the effects of insulin. A relative insulin insufficiency (impaired insulin secretion) can also occur. Ultimately, glucose is not absorbed into cells in the body in response to insulin. Glucose remains elevated in the blood stream, resulting in long-term complications. Diabetes is associated with metabolic syndrome, which includes lack of physical activity, obesity, high cholesterol, and high blood pressure.

Gestational diabetes occurs during pregnancy due to insulin resistance caused by elevated hormones. Onset occurs during the second and third trimesters. Gestational diabetes poses multiple health risks for both the mother and developing child. Gestational diabetes can be treated with exercise, healthy eating, and insulin. Usually, it disappears after the birth of the baby, but 30%-40% of patients who have gestational diabetes develop type 2 diabetes in 5 to 10 years.

Secondary diabetes is caused by drugs. Among these drugs are oral contraceptives, beta-blockers, diuretics, calcium channel blockers, glucocorticoids, and phenytoin. Secondary diabetes may cease when the drug causing it is discontinued.

The goal of diabetes treatment is to approximate nondiabetic physiology as closely as possible. Treatment consists of healthy eating, exercise, and medications. Blood glucose monitoring is very important to prevent both acute and long-term complications and to guide treatment for reaching target fasting blood glucose goals. To prevent long-term complications, diabetes should be controlled to maintain fasting blood glucose levels between 80 and 130 mg/dL. Patients with type 1 diabetes must receive insulin. Patients with type 2 diabetes may be able to control the disease through healthy eating and exercise alone, but commonly they have to add a drug therapy. Cases of diabetes that are difficult to control may be referred to as *brittle*.

General treatment guidelines for a patient with any type of diabetes include the following:

- attention to healthy eating
- blood pressure control
- adherence to medication regimen
- control of hyperlipidemia
- daily foot inspections
- increased physical activity
- learning to recognize hypoglycemia
- monitoring progress at home through blood glucose testing
- monitoring progress at the doctor's office with **glycosylated hemoglobin (A1c)**, a test that measures the level of hemoglobin A1c in the blood as a means of determining the average blood sugar concentrations for the preceding two to three months—shown as A1c, HbA1c
- engaging in patient education
- prompt treatment of all infections
- setting individual goals

Agents used to treat diabetes include insulin, glucagon-like peptide 1 (GLP-1) receptor agonists, dipeptidyl peptidase-4 (DPP-4) inhibitors, metformin, sodium-glucose linked transporter-2 inhibitors, insulin secretagogues (sulfonylureas and meglitinides), and thiazolidinediones (TZDs). Table 13.3 presents a list of agents commonly used to treat diabetes. It should be noted that insulin does not have a standard common dosage; instead, dosage is determined by the requirements of the individual patient.

TABLE 13.3 Commonly Used Agents to Treat Diabetes

Generic (Brand)	Pronunciation	Dosage Forms	Common Dosage	Dispensing Status
Rapid-Acting Insulin				
inhaled insulin (Afrezza)	in-HAILD IN-soo-lin	powder for inhalation	individualized to patient	Rx

continues

TABLE 13.3 Commonly Used Agents to Treat Diabetes—*Continued*

Generic (Brand)	Pronunciation	Dosage Forms	Common Dosage	Dispensing Status
Rapid-Acting Insulin				
insulin aspart (Fiasp, NovoLog, NovoLog Mix 70/30)	IN-soo-lin AS-part	injection	individualized to patient	Rx
insulin glulisine (Apidra)	IN-soo-lin GLOO-lis-een	injection	individualized to patient	Rx
insulin lispro (Admelog, Humalog, Lyumjev)	IN-soo-lin LYE-sproe	injection	individualized to patient	Rx
Short-Acting Insulin				
regular insulin (Humulin R, Myxredlin, Novolin R, Novolin R Flexpen, Novolin R Relion)	RE-gyoo-lar IN-soo-lin	injection	individualized to patient	OTC
Intermediate-Acting Insulin				
neutral protamine Hagedorn (NPH) insulin (Humulin N, Humulin 70/30, Humulin 70/30 Kwikpen, Novolin N, Novolin 70/30, Novolin 70/30 Flexpen, Novolin 70/30 Relion)	NUU-trahl pro-teh-meen HAG-eh-dorn IN-soo-lin	injection	individualized to patient	OTC
regular insulin U-500 (Humulin R U-500, Humulin R U-500 Kwikpen)	RE-gyoo-lar IN-soo-lin	injection	individualized to patient	Rx
Long-Acting Insulin				
insulin degludec (Tresiba, Tresiba FlexTouch)	IN-soo-lin DEG-lu-dek	injection	individualized to patient	Rx
insulin detemir (Levemir)	IN-soo-lin DET-e-meer	injection	individualized to patient	Rx
insulin glargine (Basaglar KwikPen, Lantus, Lantus SoloStar, Semglee, Toujeo Max SoloStar, Toujeo SoloStar)	IN-soo-lin GLAR-jeen	injection	individualized to patient	Rx
Premixed Insulin				
insulin NPH / regular 70/30 (Humulin 70/30, Humulin 70/30 Kwikpen, Novolin 70/30, Novolin 70/30 Flexpen, Novolin 70/30 Relion)	IN-soo-lin NPH / RE-gyoo-lar	injection	individualized to patient	Rx
insulin lispro protamine / lispro 75/25 (Humalog 75/25)	IN-soo-lin LYE-sproe PRO-tah-meen / LYE-sproe	injection	individualized to patient	Rx

continues

TABLE 13.3 **Commonly Used Agents to Treat Diabetes**—*Continued*

Generic (Brand)	Pronunciation	Dosage Forms	Common Dosage	Dispensing Status
insulin aspart protamine / aspart 70/30 (Novolog 70/30)	IN-soo-lin AS-part PRO-tah-meen / AS-part	injection	individualized to patient	Rx
Premixed Insulin				
insulin lispro protamine / lispro 50/50 (Humalog 50/50)	IN-soo-lin LYE-sproe PRO-tah-meen / LYE-sproe	injection	individualized to patient	Rx
Glucagon-Like Peptide 1 (GLP-1) Receptor Agonists				
albiglutide (Tanzeum)	al-bi-GLOO-tide	injection	30 mg a week	Rx
dulaglutide (Trulicity)	doo-la-GLOO-tide	injection	0.75–1.5 mg a week	Rx
exenatide (Byetta)	ex-EN-a-tide	injection	5–10 mcg a week	Rx
exenatide ER (Bydureon)	ex-EN-a-tide ee-rr	injection	2 mg a week	Rx
liraglutide (Victoza)	lir-a-GLOO-tide	injection	0.6–1.8 mg a day	Rx
lixisenatide (Adlyxin)	lix-i-SEN-a-tide	injection	10–20 mcg a day	Rx
pramlintide (SymlinPen)	PRAM-lin-tide	injection	15–120 mcg before meals	Rx
semaglutide (Ozempic, Rybelsus)	sem-a-GLOO-tide	injection, tablet	0.25–1 mg a week	Rx
Dipeptidyl Peptidase-4 (DPP-4)				
alogliptin (Nesina)	al-oh-GLIP-tin	tablet	25 mg a day	Rx
linagliptin (Tradjenta)	lin-a-GLIP-tin	tablet	5 mg a day	Rx
saxagliptin (Onglyza)	sax-a-GLIP-tin	tablet	2.5–5 mg a day	Rx
sitagliptin (Januvia)	si-ta-GLIP-tin	tablet	100 mg a day	Rx
Metformin and Combination Products				
metformin (Fortamet, Glumetza, Riomet, Riomet ER)	met-FOR-min	oral solution, tablet	500–2,000 mg a day	Rx
alogliptin / metformin (Kazano)	al-oh-GLIP-tin met-FOR-min	tablet	12.5 mg/500 mg or 1 g 2 times a day	Rx
canagliflozin / metformin (Invokamet, Invokamet XR)	kan-a-gli-FLOE-zin met-FOR-min	tablet	100 mg/1 g a day	Rx
dapagliflozin / metformin (Xigduo XR)	dap-a-gli-FLOE-zin met-FOR-min	tablet	5 mg/500 mg a day	Rx
empagliflozin / metformin (Synjardy, Synjardy XR)	emp-a-gli-FLOE-zin met-FOR-min	tablet	15 mg/2 g a day	Rx
ertugliflozin / metformin (Segluromet)	er-too-gli-FLOE-zin met-FOR-min	tablet	15 mg/2 g a day	Rx
glipizide / metformin	GLIP-i-zide met-FOR-min	tablet	10 mg/2 g a day	Rx
glyburide / metformin	GLYE-byoo-ride met-FOR-min	tablet	20 mg/2 g a day	Rx
linagliptin / metformin (Jentadueto, Jentadueto XR)	lin-a-GLIP-tin met-FOR-min	tablet	5 mg/2 g a day	Rx

continues

TABLE 13.3 **Commonly Used Agents to Treat Diabetes**—*Continued*

Generic (Brand)	Pronunciation	Dosage Forms	Common Dosage	Dispensing Status
pioglitazone / metformin (Actoplus Met)	pye-oh-GLIT-a-zone met-FOR-min	tablet	15 mg/850 mg a day	Rx
Metformin and Combination Products				
saxagliptin / metformin (Kombiglyze XR)	sax-a-GLIP-tin met-FOR-min	tablet	2.5 mg/1 g a day	Rx
sitagliptin / metformin (Janumet)	sit-a-GLIP-tin met-FOR-min	tablet	100 mg/2 g a day	Rx
dapagliflozin / metformin / saxagliptin (Qternmet XR)	dap-a-gli-FLOE-zin met-FOR-min sax-a-GLIP-tin	tablet	10 mg / 5 mg / 2 g a day	Rx
empagliflozin / metformin / linagliptin (Trijardy XR)	emp-a-gli-FLOE-zin met-FOR-min lin-a-GLIP-tin	tablet	25 mg / 5 mg / 2 g a day	Rx
Sodium-Glucose Linked Transporter-2 (SGLT-2) Inhibitors				
canagliflozin (Invokana)	kan-a-gli-FLOE-zin	tablet	100–300 mg a day	Rx
dapagliflozin (Farxiga)	dap-a-gli-FLOE-zin	tablet	5–10 mg a day	Rx
empagliflozin (Jardiance)	em-pag-gli-FLOE-zin	tablet	10–25 mg a day	Rx
ertugliflozin (Steglatro)	er-too-gli-FLOE-zin	tablet	5–15 mg a day	Rx
Sulfonylureas				
glimepiride (Amaryl)	GLYE-me-pye-ride	tablet	2–4 mg a day	Rx
glipizide (Glucotrol, Glucotrol XL)	GLIP-i-zide	tablet	5–10 mg a day	Rx
glyburide (DiaBeta, Glynase)	GLYE-byoo-ride	tablet	5–10 mg a day	Rx
Meglitinide				
nateglinide (Starlix)	na-TEG-li-nide	tablet	60–120 mg before meals	Rx
Thiazolidinediones (TZDs)				
pioglitazone (Actos)	pye-oh-GLIT-a-zone	tablet	15–30 mg a day	Rx
rosiglitazone (Avandia)	roe-zi-GLIT-a-zone	tablet	4–8 mg a day	Rx
Miscellaneous Products				
becaplermin (Regranex)	be-KAP-ler-min	gel	varies	Rx
glucagon	GLOO-kah-gone	injection (IM, IV, SC)	1 mg	Rx

Insulin

The human body normally produces insulin at certain rates in order to maintain steady glucose concentrations in the blood. These rates are called a *basal rate* and a *bolus rate* (see Figure 13.6). **Basal insulin** is slowly released throughout the day and night to allow energy for basic cellular function. In contrast, **bolus insulin** is released at mealtimes to react with glucose entering the body from food intake. When insulin is given by injection, the goal is to mimic this natural physiologic insulin production. For patients with type 1 diabetes, multiple injections each day of combination basal and bolus insulins are necessary to achieve physiologic insulin dosing. Patients with type 2 diabetes may be given insulin using a similar physiologic dosing schedule or as one injection of long-acting insulin at bedtime in addition to oral medications.

FIGURE 13.6 Normal Glucose Production

The timing of bolus insulin released with meals is called *prandial*, which means "with meals."

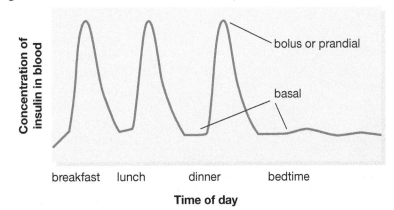

Based on the duration of their pharmacological action, insulin products are classified as rapid acting, short acting, intermediate acting, or long acting (see Figure 13.7). The differences are related to the molecular structure of insulin. **Rapid-acting insulin** begins to work in approximately 10 minutes and, for practical purposes, lasts as long as 2 hours. It is administered just before meals to reduce **prandial** (mealtime) elevations in blood glucose. **Short-acting insulin** begins to work in around 30 minutes and lasts up to 4 hours in most cases. It is also taken prior to meals. **Intermediate-acting insulin** begins to be effective in 30 to 60 minutes and lasts 6 to 8 hours in most cases. It is used either one or two times a day. **Long-acting insulin** works for approximately 24 hours and is injected one time a day.

FIGURE 13.7 Insulin Classifications and Their Effects

Insulin products are classified as rapid acting, short acting, intermediate acting, or long acting. This figure identifies the average time and concentration of each product.

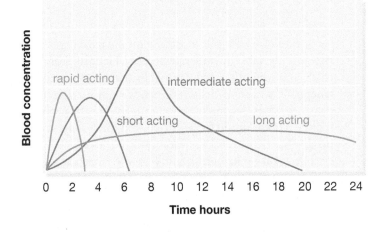

Dosage Forms and Administration Insulin is available in a **vial** (container that holds medicine) for use with a syringe and in a **self-injector pen** (a syringe that only needs to pierce the skin to pump medicine into the body). Insulin pumps are also available. An **insulin pump** delivers insulin through a tiny tube inserted just under the skin. These pumps can be programmed to deliver just the right amount of insulin each hour of the day for an individual patient. The tube must be reinserted every three days. Pumps eliminate the need for multiple injections a day but must be well understood

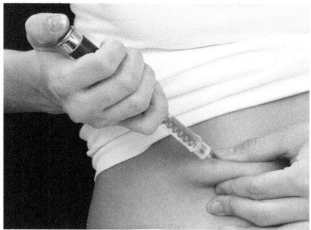

A patient can use self-injector pens to administer their own insulin.

and properly maintained to work effectively. Inhaled insulin is also available and does not require injection.

Insulin should not be injected into an area of the body that will receive a rigorous workout. The injection site should be rotated frequently because decreased subcutaneous fat can lead to lipoatrophy (loss of fat) at the injection site. Figure 13.8 illustrates the method of rotating insulin administration sites. Insulin enters the blood best from the abdomen, then the arms and legs, and last the buttocks.

Other side effects are rare but can include lipodystrophy (fat accumulation or depletion at the injection site). This effect can be largely avoided by rotating injection sites.

FIGURE 13.8
Rotation of Administration Sites for Insulin

The numbers in the figure indicate the order in which each region should be used for the injection of insulin. The boxes within the regions indicate a single injection site. After injecting all the first boxes in each region, the patient injects the second box in each region, working sequentially through the entire series.

Table 13.4 lists the most commonly used types of insulin. Most insulin formulations are available by prescription only. Neutral protamine Hagedorn (NPH) insulin and the U-100 strength of regular insulin are usually available without a prescription. In an emergency situation, insulin does not require a prescription, but the person dispensing the drug needs documentation to make sure the correct insulin is dispensed. Some states require a prescription for a syringe, and many states require proof of need. Some insulin products are clear, and some are cloudy. If manually mixing two kinds of insulin into one syringe, the clear insulin should be pulled into the syringe first.

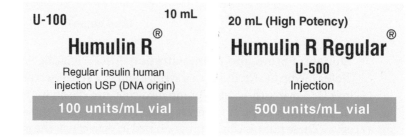

Regular insulin is available in three concentrations: 100 units/mL, 300 units/mL, and 500 units/mL. Pharmacy technicians should exercise particular caution to ensure they are dispensing the correct concentration. Errors can be fatal.

TABLE 13.4 Profiles of Common Insulin Products

Generic (Brand)	Onset of Action	Maximum Peak and Duration	Appearance
Rapid-Acting Insulin			
insulin human inhalation (Afrezza)	1–5 min	12–15 min; 3–4 hr	colored cartridge
insulin aspart (Fiasp, NovoLog, NovoLog Mix 70/30)	2–5 min (Fiasp) 10–15 min (NovoLog)	1–2 hr; 4 hr	clear
insulin glulisine (Apidra)	5 min	1 hr; 2 hr	clear
insulin lispro (Admelog, Humalog, Lyumjev)	10–15 min	1–2 hr; 4 hr	clear
Short-Acting Insulin			
regular insulin U-100 (Humulin R, Myxredlin, Novolin R, Novolin R Flexpen, Novolin R Relion)	30 min	4 hr; 8 hr	clear
Intermediate-Acting Insulin			
neutral protamine Hagedorn (NPH) insulin (Humulin N, Humulin 70/30, Humulin 70/30 Kwikpen, Novolin N, Novolin 70/30, Novolin 70/30 Flexpen, Novolin 70/30 Relion)	1 hr	6–8 hr; 24 hr	cloudy
regular insulin U-500 (Humulin R U-500, Humulin R U-500 Kwikpen)	30 min	8 hr; 24 hr	clear
Long-Acting Insulin			
insulin degludec (Tresiba, Tresiba FlexTouch)	1 hr	9 hr; 25 hr	clear
insulin detemir (Levemir)	1 hr	9 hr; 36 hr	clear
insulin glargine (Basaglar KwikPen; Lantus; Lantus SoloStar; Semglee; Toujeo Max SoloStar; Toujeo SoloStar)	1 hr	none; 24–36 hr	clear
Premixed Insulin			
insulin NPH / regular 70/30 (Humulin 70/30, Humulin 70/30 Kwikpen, Novolin 70/30, Novolin 70/30 Flexpen, Novolin 70/30 Relion)	30–60 min	2–10 hr; 18–24 hr	cloudy
insulin lispro protamine / lispro 75/25 (Humalog 75/25)	10–30 min	1–6 hr; 14–24 hr	cloudy
insulin aspart protamine / aspart 70/30 (Novolog 70/30)	10–30 min	1–6 hr; 14–24 hr	cloudy
insulin lispro protamine / lispro 50/50 (Humalog 50/50)	10–30 min	1–6 hr; 14–24 hr	cloudy
insulin degludec / liraglutide (Xultophy)	1 hr	9 hr; 25 hr	clear

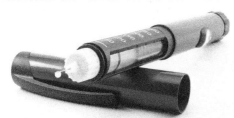

Insulin pens were developed to improve adherence to medication regimens by making injection quicker and easier.

Degludec, detemir, glargine, and regular insulin U-300 or regular insulin U-500 should not be mixed with any other type of insulin. All insulins must be stored in the pharmacy refrigerator.

Manufacturers have developed insulin pens for the easy administration of insulin. Each pen consists of a disposable needle and a syringe of insulin. Insulin pens are available in various shapes and forms, and most are very simple to use.

Regular insulin U-100 (Humulin R, Myxredlin, Novolin R, Novolin R Flexpen, Novolin R Relion) may be administered subcutaneously, intramuscularly, or intravenously. This is the only type of insulin that may be administered intravenously. **Regular insulin U-500 (Humulin R U-500, Humulin R U-500 Kwikpen)** should only be administered subcutaneously.

Uniquely, **insulin human inhalation (Afrezza)** is administered by inhalation. It is available in cartridges of various colors.

Insulin aspart (Fiasp, NovoLog, NovoLog Mix 70/30) is a rapid-acting insulin analog. It is made by substituting aspartic acid for one of the amino acids in insulin. NovoLog is similar to Humalog, but Humalog contains the amino acid lysine. Fiasp (faster insulin aspart) is a faster-acting insulin aspart with onset of appearance in the bloodstream beginning approximately 2 to 5 minutes after administration. This is due to the addition of niacinamide (vitamin B_3) in the formulation. Both forms of insulin aspart may be used with an insulin pump. Each dose should be injected before meals for Novolog and at the start of meals or within 20 minutes after starting a meal for Fiasp.

Insulin glulisine (Apidra) is another rapid-acting insulin. It is available in vials and in pens and can be injected immediately before or after meals.

Safety Alert

Lispro and Lantus are often confused.

Insulin lispro (Admelog, Humalog, Lyumjev) is a rapid-acting insulin, so patients can inject it immediately before or after meals. This allows the dose to be adjusted depending on the amounts and types of foods eaten. In addition, blood glucose can be tested, and then the drug can be dosed accordingly. Insulin lispro may be used with a pump to maintain proper blood glucose levels. It is available in two concentrations: 100 units/mL and 200 units/mL. The 100 units/mL formulation is available in vials and insulin pens; the 200 units/mL formulation is available in insulin pens only.

Neutral protamine Hagedorn (NPH) insulin (Humulin N, Humulin 70/30, Humulin 70/30 Kwikpen, Novolin N, Novolin 70/30, Novolin 70/30 Flexpen, Novolin 70/30 Relion) is an intermediate-acting insulin. NPH insulin can be used alone or in combination with other insulins, such as regular insulin. NPH insulin appears cloudy.

Name Exchange

Technicians may hear other healthcare practitioners refer to insulin glargine more frequently by the brand name Lantus.

Insulin glargine (Basaglar KwikPen, Lantus, Lantus SoloStar, Semglee, Toujeo Max SoloStar, Toujeo SoloStar) is a synthetic type of long-acting insulin. It differs from human insulin by three amino acids. Insulin glargine is associated with less nocturnal hypoglycemia and weight gain than conventional insulin. Because it precipitates when injected in subcutaneous tissue, insulin glargine may cause pain at the injection site. The precipitation causes the insulin to be absorbed slowly and to maintain a relatively constant blood level over 24 hours. There is no noticeable peak in action, and insulin glargine more closely approximates physiologic insulin release than other insulins do. It cannot be mixed with any other insulin. Insulin glargine is available in two concentrations: 100 units/mL and 300 units/mL. The 100 units/mL product is available under the brand name Lantus (in both vials and pens), and the 300 units/mL product is available as Toujeo SoloStar (only as a pen).

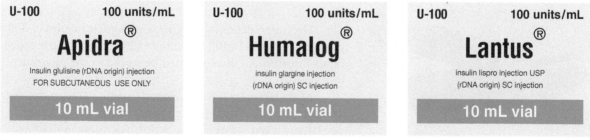

Insulin is available in various types.

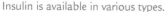

Insulin detemir (Levemir) is also classified as a long-acting insulin. Insulin detemir is used as a basal insulin. It may require administration two times a day. Insulin detemir is available in vials and insulin pens.

Insulin degludec (Tresiba, Tresiba FlexTouch), the newest long-acting insulin available, comes in two concentrations: 100 units/mL and 200 units/mL. Technicians must be alert to select the proper concentration. Selecting the wrong concentration could result in serious adverse effects, including death.

Dosage Forms and Administration All insulin products must be stored in the refrigerator until dispensed or used by the patient.

Side Effects The most common "side effect" of insulin is hypoglycemia. However, although it is often listed as a side effect, hypoglycemia is, in fact, the intended effect of insulin. However, someone using insulin is at an increased risk of developing serious hypoglycemia when doses are too high or meals are skipped. If blood glucose concentrations drop lower than 40 mg/dL, loss of consciousness and brain damage can occur. Diabetic coma is life threatening if not treated immediately. Symptoms of serious hypoglycemia include shakiness, headache, blurred vision, dizziness, confusion, irritability, hunger, and tiredness.

Other side effects are rare but can include lipodystrophy (fat accumulation or depletion at injection site). This effect can be largely avoided by rotating injection sites.

Contraindications Insulin human inhalation is contraindicated in patients with chronic lung disease, such as asthma or chronic obstructive pulmonary disease (COPD). Injectable forms of insulin have no contraindications.

Cautions and Considerations Most hospitalizations and emergency room visits for patients with type 1 diabetes result from hypoglycemic events, so the risk of hypoglycemia cannot be overemphasized. Patients must be instructed to recognize and treat low blood glucose when it occurs. Family members of an individual who uses insulin should be taught how to administer glucagon. This medication is given when the patient is unconscious because of hypoglycemia and cannot self-treat by ingesting a food or beverage containing sugar.

The different types of insulin are packaged in boxes that are similar in appearance and contain similar volumes of the drug, which can cause confusion.

Inhaled insulin has a boxed warning for acute bronchospasm in patients with chronic lung disease. Most insulin products have a concentration of 100 units of insulin per mL, which means one 10 mL bottle of insulin has 1,000 units. Insulin is dispensed in milliliters but administered in units, and pharmacy technicians must determine how long the insulin will last for each patient.

More concentrated insulin products (200 units/mL, 300 units/mL, and 500 units/mL) are available. Pharmacy technicians should take great care to ensure these are not given to patients in place of the 100 units/mL dose, as this mistake could be fatal. Xultophy (combination of degludec and liraglutide) requires a Medication Guide to be given to patients when dispensing.

All insulin products must be stored in the refrigerator until dispensed or used by the patient. Once insulin warms to room temperature, the protein begins to degrade. Therefore, patients should keep insulin vials or pens in the refrigerator until they use them. Once opened, most insulin vials expire in 28 to 30 days. Most insulin pens are also good for one month after opening, but a few expire in 14 days. It is not considered counseling to make the patient aware of these dates, because drug storage does not require the judgment of the pharmacist. If exposed to extreme heat or cold, insulin can become degraded. Patients should protect insulin from heat (for instance, they should avoid keeping it in a car during the summer) and from freezing temperatures.

Patients who are traveling by plane should keep insulin with them in a carry-on bag because air cargo areas on planes may not be climate controlled. Finally, patients should discard any insulin package that contains clumps or appears frosty.

Drug Interactions Insulin may enhance the hypoglycemic effects of other agents used for diabetes. Beta-blockers and salicylates may enhance the hypoglycemic effects of insulin. Thiazide diuretics may decrease the efficacy of insulin.

Glucagon-Like Peptide 1 (GLP-1) Receptor Agonists

A **glucagon-like peptide 1 (GLP-1) receptor agonist**, also known as an *incretin mimetic*, mimics the endogenous incretin hormones and **glucose-dependent insu-linotropic polypeptide**, which are produced in response to the arrival of glucose from the intestines. GLP-1 agonists have multiple physiologic effects. First, incretin and incretin mimetics facilitate the proper timing and function of phase I and phase II insulin response. **First-phase insulin secretion** refers to the immediate burst of insulin that occurs with, or even slightly before, the first bite of food. **Second-phase insulin secretion** refers to the continued but somewhat slower release of insulin in the hours after eating. In type 2 diabetes, both phase I and phase II insulin responses are blunted. Second, incretins and incretin mimetics inhibit glucagon production in the pancreas that otherwise promotes an undesirable increase in blood glucose. Third, incretins have some effect on appetite by producing **satiety**, a sensation of fullness and satisfaction. Many patients experience significant and sustained weight loss on GLP-1 agonists. (Other medications to treat diabetes—such as insulin, sulfonylureas, and thiazolidinediones—are associated with weight gain.) Incretin mimetic drug therapies are used most often in combination with other medications to treat type 2 diabetes. They also reduce the risk of cardiovascular disease.

Abiglutide (Tanzeum), dulaglutide (Trulicity), exenatide (Byetta), exenatide ER (Bydureon), liraglutide (Victoza), lixisenatide (Adlyxin), and **semaglutide (Ozempic, Rybelsus)** are injectable products that mimic the action of GLP-1. Because GLP-1 is released only when glucose is introduced into the blood-stream, hypoglycemia between meals does not occur. Like GLP-1, then, these drugs do not carry a risk of causing low blood glucose levels.

Pramlintide (SymlinPen) mimics **amylin**, a hormone coproduced with insulin that reduces glucagon production, slows gastric emptying, and produces satiety. This incretin mimetic can be used by patients with type 1 diabetes to supplement insulin. The addition of pramlintide to an insulin regimen can dramatically reduce the amount of insulin a patient has to take. Pramlintide is injected 30 minutes prior to each meal or snack that contains at least 30 g of carbohydrate.

Injectable incretin mimetic products must be stored in the refrigerator until dispensed. Once these products reach room temperature, they begin to degrade. Injectable incretin products are good at room temperature for only 30 days. Therefore, patients should keep these products in the refrigerator until they begin using them and then leave the product at room temperature until they are done using them. Patients should protect these products from temperature extremes.

Dosage Forms and Administration GLP-1 agonists are available as injections.

Side Effects Common side effects of GLP-1 drugs include nausea, vomiting, diarrhea, dizziness, fatigue, and headache. Nausea is common at the beginning of therapy but diminishes over time. Side effects can be minimized by beginning treatment at a low dose and increasing the dose slowly. Timing injections immediately before eating can reduce nausea, vomiting, and upset stomach. Over a period of several weeks, the patient

R꒰
Put Down Roots

Note the common drug stems for this class of drugs: *–glutide* or *–natide.*

can move the time of injection further ahead of eating until reaching 30 to 60 minutes prior to a meal.

Contraindications Contraindications for exenatide ER and liraglutide include a patient or family history of medullary thyroid carcinoma and multiple endocrine neoplasia type 2. Pramlintide use is contraindicated in patients with gastroparesis or hypoglycemia unawareness.

Cautions and Considerations A Medication Guide should be given to patients when GLP-1 drugs are dispensed. Exenatide use has been associated with pancreatitis (inflammation of the pancreas). Patients should stop taking exenatide immediately and seek medical attention if they experience persistent or serious abdominal pain, especially if it is accompanied by vomiting. Liraglutide and semaglutide each have a boxed warning for thyroid tumor risk, which is very rare but serious.

If pramlintide is given with insulin, the patient can be at serious risk for low blood glucose levels, and signs and symptoms can appear within three hours of taking the medications. Blood glucose levels should be checked before and after the injection. In addition, patients should be instructed on how to treat low blood glucose when it occurs. Pramlintide has a boxed warning for patients with type 1 diabetes as it can cause severe hypoglycemia.

Drug Interactions Androgens and corticosteroids may increase the hypoglycemic effects of all diabetes medications. All diabetes medications may enhance the hypoglycemic effects of other diabetes medications.

Exenatide may decrease the effectiveness of oral contraceptives.

Dipeptidyl Peptidase-4 (DPP-4) Inhibitors

Put Down Roots

The generic name of GLP-1 drugs all end in *–gliptin*.

Alogliptin (Nesina), linagliptin (Tradjenta), saxagliptin (Onglyza), and **sitagliptin (Januvia)** are oral DPP-4 inhibitors. A **dipeptidyl peptidase-4 (DPP-4) inhibitor** slows the inactivation of incretin hormones, thereby allowing them to persist longer and produce beneficial effects. Satiety does not seem to be as pronounced with DPP-4 inhibitors, so weight loss is not usually an added benefit.

Dosage Forms and Administration DPP-4 inhibitors are available as oral tablets and are taken one time a day without regard to food.

Side Effects Common side effects of DPP-4 inhibitors include headache, nasopharyngitis (runny nose and sore throat), and upper respiratory tract infection. The reason for these unusual side effects is not fully understood.

Contraindications DPP-4 inhibitors should not be used in patients with pancreatitis.

Cautions and Considerations Doses of DPP-4 inhibitors are cleared by the kidneys, so they must be adjusted for patients with kidney disease. Patients with kidney problems should alert their prescribers so that proper dosing is ordered.

Drug Interactions DPP-4 inhibitors may enhance the adverse effects of other diabetes medications and angiotensin-converting enzyme (ACE) inhibitors.

Metformin (Biguanide)

Initial drug therapy for type 2 diabetes is usually **metformin (Fortamet, Glumetza, Riomet, Riomet ER)**. This drug is the only biguanide available, which is used alone or in combination with other agents. Metformin works by inhibiting excess hepatic glucose production, a process that normally occurs at a slow rate overnight.

Metformin also increases insulin sensitivity in muscle and other body tissues. Dosage Forms and Administration Metformin is typically taken two to three times a day with food or meals. When treatment begins, a low dose is prescribed to prevent upset stomach, abdominal cramps, and diarrhea. Slowly, the dose is increased. Metformin can take as long as three weeks to reach full effect. It usually does not cause hypoglycemia unless it is taken in combination with other agents for diabetes. In addition, metformin can promote mild weight loss (five to six pounds) and improve cholesterol profiles. The best time to test blood glucose when taking metformin is in the morning, just after waking. See Table 13.3 for metformin products. Metformin is paired with other antidiabetic agents into several combination products, which are listed in Table 13.3 but are not discussed in this text.

Side Effects Common side effects of metformin include upset stomach, abdominal cramps, nausea, diarrhea, flatulence, and a metallic taste in the mouth. These effects can be diminished or avoided by taking the medication with food and increasing the dose slowly. Over time, these side effects decrease.

Serious but rare side effects include **lactic acidosis**, a potentially fatal condition that requires medical care and hospitalization. This side effect can usually be avoided if patients stop taking metformin when they are severely ill or hospitalized. The risk for lactic acidosis increases under the following circumstances:

- severe dehydration or altered fluid balance
- excessive alcohol consumption
- liver or kidney impairment (or the taking of other drugs that contribute to impairment)
- sepsis (a serious, acute infection in the bloodstream that requires IV antibiotics)
- unstable or acute heart failure.

Contraindications Metformin is contraindicated for patients who have kidney dysfunction, liver problems, or heart failure because these conditions raise the risk for lactic acidosis. Metformin should also be avoided in the presence of shock, sepsis, or metabolic acidosis. This medication should also not be used in patients 80 years of age or older unless they have normal kidney function. The dose generally should not be increased to the maximum dose in adults over 80.

Cautions and Considerations Metformin contains a boxed warning for increased risk of lactic acidosis. Patients who are taking metformin should temporarily discontinue the medication when undergoing procedures in which contrast dye or iodine substances are used. Such patients are usually instructed to stop taking metformin the day before the procedure and to resume the medication 48 hours after the procedure. Drug interactions between these substances and metformin can precipitate kidney failure and lactic acidosis. The combination products that contain metformin and ertugliflozin (Segluromet) and lilnagliptin (Jentadueto, Jentadueto XR) require that patients receive Mediation Guides when dispensed.

Drug Interactions The lactic acidosis side effect of metformin may be exacerbated by other drugs that can cause lactic acidosis (such as alcohol, carbonic anhydrase inhibitors, or topiramate).

**Put Down
Roots**

The generic drug names of SGLT-2 inhibitors all end in –*gliflozin*.

Sodium-Glucose Linked Transporter-2 (SGLT-2) Inhibitors

Sodium-glucose linked transporter-2 (SGLT-2) inhibitors, such as **canagliflozin (Invokana)**, **dapagliflozin (Farxiga)**, **empagliflozin (Jardiance)**, and **ertugliflozin (Steglatro)** are a class of new medications used for type 2 diabetes (see Table 13.3). A **sodium-glucose linked transporter-2 (SGLT-2) inhibitor** works by blocking the reabsorption of glucose that the kidneys filter out of the bloodstream, thus increasing the excretion of glucose in the urine. SGLT-2 inhibitors are also prescribed to reduce the risk of cardiovascular disease in patients with diabetes.

Patients taking SGLT-2 inhibitors can experience urinary tract infections and genital fungal infections such as yeast infections. Patients who have a history of these types of infections prior to taking these medications should talk with their healthcare prescribers before taking SGLT-2 inhibitors. Some patients have experienced low blood pressure or high potassium blood levels from taking these drugs.

Contraindications The use of canagliflozin, dapagliflozin, empagliflozin, and ertugliflozin is contraindicated for patients with severe kidney impairment or end-stage renal disease as well as for patients who are on dialysis.

Cautions and Considerations SGLT-2 inhibitors are not for use in patients with type 1 diabetes. They may cause hypotension. This effect may be pronounced in adults age 65 and older and in patients who have kidney dysfunction or are using antihypertensive drugs. Kidney toxicity is a concern with use of SGLT-2 inhibitors. Hyperkalemia may occur with use. Patients using SGLT-2 inhibitors are at increased risk of certain fungal infections. These drugs should be used with caution in patients with kidney or liver impairment.

Drug Interactions SGLT-2 inhibitors are associated with many drug interactions, only some of which are covered in this text.

Diabetes medications, androgens, and beta-blockers increase the risk of hypoglycemia of other blood glucose lowering products. Loop diuretics may diminish the therapeutic effects of diabetes agents.

SGLT-2 inhibitors can heighten the potassium-increasing effects of other drugs that increase potassium (such as ACE inhibitors, aliskiren, angiotensin receptor blockers, eplerenone, heparin, and potassium-sparing diuretics).

Carbamazepine, efavirenz, fosphenytoin, phenobarbital, phenytoin, primidone, and rifampin may decrease the serum concentration of canagliflozin.

Canagliflozin may increase the hypotensive effects of loop diuretics. Pimozide levels may be increased by canagliflozin.

**Put Down
Roots**

To recognize a meglitinide, look at the ending. They end in –*glinide*.

Insulin Secretagogues

An agent that stimulates insulin production from the pancreas to directly lower blood glucose levels is known as an **insulin secretagogue**. A **sulfonylurea** is an insulin secretagogue, as is a **meglitinide**. Sulfonylureas include **glimepiride (Amaryl)**, **glipizide (Glucotrol, Glucotrol XL)**, and **glyburide (DiaBeta, Glynase)**. **Nateglinide (Starlix)** is a meglitinide.

Dosage Forms and Administration Sulfonylureas and meglitinides differ in their onset and duration of action. Sulfonylureas can take 30 minutes or more to start working and can last for 8 hours or longer. Meglitinides act within 10 minutes and last around 2 hours. Sulfonylureas are used alone or in combination with other agents to treat type 2 diabetes. They are taken before breakfast each day and sometimes again before dinner. Meglitinides are used in combination with other agents to treat type 2 diabetes. They are taken just before eating and provide an extra boost of insulin for a specific meal. Table 13.3 provides information on common sulfonylureas and meglitinides.

Safety Alert

Quinolone antibiotics and diabetes medications can interact and cause serious hypoglycemia. Pharmacy technicians should always watch for these two drugs when dispensing.

Side Effects Low blood glucose reactions (hypoglycemia) are the most common side effect of these medications. Symptoms of hypoglycemia include shakiness, headache, blurred vision, dizziness, confusion, irritability, hunger, and tiredness. Hypoglycemia tends to occur when a patient takes the medication but then skips a meal or does more physical activity than usual. Patients can avoid this effect by refraining from skipping meals and from omitting a dose when they anticipate eating significantly less than usual. Other side effects include nausea, diarrhea, and constipation.

Contraindications All sulfonylureas and meglitinides are contraindicated in the presence of diabetic ketoacidosis. Glipizide, glyburide, and nateglinide should not be used to treat type 1 diabetes. In addition, glyburide use is contraindicated with bosentan use.

Safety Alert

Technicians must be careful not to confuse Glucotrol and Glucotrol XL.

Cautions and Considerations Because sulfonylureas and meglitinides increase the risk of hypoglycemia, patients should be informed of the symptoms of low blood glucose and know how to treat it. Patients should monitor their blood glucose level at home regularly and whenever they feel their level may be low. The best times to check blood glucose when taking sulfonylureas are first thing in the morning before eating (fasting) and then occasionally before other meals during the day. The best time to check blood glucose when taking meglitinides is one to two hours after meals. Patients with liver or kidney disease may not be able to take sulfonylureas, depending on the agent chosen. Patients with either of these conditions should talk with their prescribers before taking one of these agents.

Safety Alert

Technicians must be careful not to confuse glyburide and glipizide.

Drug Interactions Diabetes medications, androgens, and beta-blockers increase the risk of hypoglycemia of other blood glucose lowering products. Loop diuretics may diminish the therapeutic effects of diabetes agents.

Sulfonylureas may enhance the adverse effects of alcohol (flushing is commonly seen). Cimetidine and fluconazole may increase the serum concentrations of sulfonylureas.

Calcium channel blockers, estrogens, isoniazid, nicotinic acid, and phenothiazines may decrease the blood glucose lowering effects of meglitinides. Chloramphenicol, cyclosporine, probenecid, sulfonamides, and warfarin may increase the hypoglycemic effects of meglitinides.

Put Down Roots

The generic drug names of TZDs all end in –glitazone.

Thiazolidinediones (TZDs)

A **thiazolidinediones (TZD)**, also known as a **glitazone**, is used in combination with metformin or a sulfonylurea to treat type 2 diabetes (see Table 13.3). The TZDs—**pioglitazone (Actos)** and **rosiglitazone (Avandia)**—work by directly increasing insulin sensitivity in cells of the body. TZDs connect with intracellular receptors to stimulate production of more insulin receptors. This process can take weeks or months to occur; thus, onset of effect is not immediate. The best time to check blood glucose levels when using TZDs is first thing in the morning before eating (fasting), and occasionally after meals during the day.

Common side effects of TZDs include fluid accumulation (edema) and weight gain. If patients notice rapid weight gain or swelling, especially with shortness of breath, they should talk with their prescribers right away.

Rare but serious effects include liver toxicity and macular edema (swelling of the eye, resulting in distorted vision). If patients experience unexplained nausea, vomiting, abdominal pain, fatigue, or dark urine, they should report these symptoms to their healthcare prescribers. Regular blood tests are conducted to monitor liver function.

Patients with diabetes should see an eye doctor annually for an eye examination in which their pupils are dilated and their retinas are examined.

Contraindications Because TZDs can cause fluid retention and edema, pioglitazone and rosiglitazone therapies should not be initiated in patients with New York Heart Association (NYHA) class III or class IV heart failure.

Cautions and Considerations TZDs can worsen heart failure, and they have a boxed warning regarding this issue. Patients with heart failure should not take TZDs. Patients with edema or heart problems may not be good candidates for TZD therapy. In some patients with fertility problems, TZDs increase ovulation and pregnancy rates. Patients who are sexually active but do not want to become pregnant should use a contraceptive to prevent pregnancy. When dispensing pioglitazone, patients should receive a Medication Guide.

Drug Interactions Diabetes medications, androgens, and beta-blockers increase the risk of hypoglycemia of other blood glucose lowering products. Loop diuretics may diminish the therapeutic effects of diabetes agents.

Rosiglitazone should not be used with insulin because of the increased risk of fluid retention, heart failure, and hypoglycemia.

Miscellaneous Products

Patients and their caregivers may also have use of other agents, such as glucagon for insulin toxicity and becaplermin for diabetic ulcers. **Glucagon** is a natural hormone released by the pancreas which stimulates the liver to produce glucose for release into the blood stream. Glucagon is used when too much insulin has been administered and the blood glucose is so low that the patient loses consciousness. It is available as an administration kit for injection. Family members and caregivers should be trained on how to use and inject glucagon, as the patient will be unable to self-inject when needed.

Patients with diabetes must take very good care of their feet, which are particularly vulnerable to infections. Diabetic ulcers (open wounds that are typically slow to heal) are the leading cause of foot and leg amputation and a leading reason for hospital admissions among patients with diabetes. Patients should be instructed to avoid the use of OTC foot products unless otherwise directed by a physician. They should be instructed to moisturize their feet daily to prevent the skin from cracking. They should also keep nails trimmed to prevent ingrown toenails. It is common for patients with diabetes to have neuropathies of the legs. This sensation can be very painful, or the patient may feel total numbness in the extremities. With numbness, patients can injure their feet and not even be aware of it, which in turn can lead to serious infections.

Becaplermin (Regranex), a gel listed in Table 13.3, is a recombinant human platelet–derived growth factor that speeds the healing of lower-extremity diabetic ulcers. Some studies have shown that this drug, which acts locally and has very little systemic effect, can increase the incidence of complete healing of diabetic foot ulcers. If a wound treated with becaplermin does not decrease in size by 30% within 10 weeks or heal within 20 weeks, use of this drug should be reassessed.

Complementary and Alternative Therapies

Some people with hormonal disorders use complementary or alternative medicine in addressing them.

Chromium is an essential trace element that some people have used for diabetes prevention and treatment. Claims of its effectiveness are somewhat controversial, in that patients should not expect dramatic reductions in blood glucose levels from taking it. Patients with diabetes have been found to be deficient in chromium, but little definitive evidence is available to verify that correcting chromium deficiency is beneficial for improving blood glucose levels. Typical doses range from 200 to 1,000 mg a day. Side effects are rare but may include headache, insomnia, diarrhea, and hemorrhage. Patients with kidney or liver disease should not take chromium.

Cinnamon is often taken for type 2 diabetes. One initial study showed potential benefits, but all subsequent trials have shown that cinnamon has little effect on blood glucose levels. Although manufacturers of cinnamon products claim benefits, patients should know that taking cinnamon may not produce any noticeable effect on their blood glucose or hemoglobin A1c results. Patients with liver disease probably should not take cinnamon, because it has the potential to exacerbate hepatic conditions.

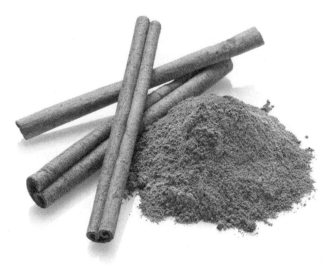

Although studies on its benefits have shown cinnamon has little effect on blood glucose levels, it may be used by patients with diabetes.

Review and Assessment

CHAPTER SUMMARY

Anatomy and Physiology of the Endocrine System

- The endocrine system maintains the body's homeostasis by regulating physiologic functions involved in normal daily living and stress.

- The tissue affected by a hormone is called the *target*.

- The endocrine system is composed of glands, including the adrenal glands, thyroid, and pancreas.

- Regulation of hormone synthesis is achieved via an intricate negative feedback mechanism.

Thyroid Disorders and Drug Treatments

- The thyroid gland produces hormones that stimulate various body tissues to increase their metabolic activity.

- Thyroid replacement therapy should not be used to treat obesity.

- Hypothyroidism is treated with levothyroxine (Euthyrox, Levo-T, Levothyroid, Levoxyl, Synthroid, Tirosint, Unithroid), liothyronine (Cytomel, Triostat), or thyroid desiccated (Armour Thyroid, Nature-Throid).

- Hyperthyroidism is treated with propylthiouracil and methimazole (Tapazole).

Adrenal Glands and Drug Treatments

- Corticosteroids are used as immunosuppressants and anti-inflammatories and in treating diseases of hematologic, allergic, neoplastic, or autoimmune origin.

- Cushing's syndrome is caused by cortisol overproduction, excessive administration of corticosteroids over an extended period, or adrenal gland tumors.

- Addison's disease is a deficiency of glucocorticoids and mineralocorticoids.

- Corticosteroids have many adverse effects, some of which can be severe. Patients taking them for long periods of time need to be monitored.

Diabetes and Drug Treatments

- The four types of diabetes are type 1, type 2, gestational, and secondary.

- Type 1 diabetes patients must take insulin. Type 2 diabetes patients may be able to control the disease through diet and exercise, but often they have to add drug therapy (including insulin). Gestational diabetes usually goes away after the baby's birth, but the patient who gave birth is at high risk of developing type 2 diabetes. Secondary (drug-induced) diabetes may cease when the drug is discontinued.

- Acute hypoglycemia is dangerous, but chronic hyperglycemia, involving blood glucose above 180 mg/dL, has devastating complications. Retinopathy, neuropathy, nephropathy, and vascular and dermatologic complications can affect the quality and length of life.

- Most insulins require a prescription, although in an emergency situation, insulin may not require a prescription. Some states require a prescription for syringes.

- Insulin lispro (Admelog, Humalog, Lyumjev) is a rapid-onset insulin, so patients can inject it immediately before or after meals.

- Insulin glargine (Basaglar KwikPen, Lantus, Lantus SoloStar, Semglee, Toujeo Max SoloStar, Toujeo SoloStar) is a long-acting insulin that provides a constant concentration over 24 hours. It more closely approximates physiologic insulin release than other insulins do.

Complementary and Alternative Therapies

- Chromium is an essential trace element that some people have used for diabetes prevention and treatment. Little evidence for its effectiveness in reducing blood glucose levels is available.

- Cinnamon is sometimes taken for type 2 diabetes. One initial study showed potential benefits, but all subsequent trials have shown that cinnamon has little effect on blood glucose levels.

DRUG LIST

Thyroid Preparations

Drugs to Treat Hypothyroidism
levothyroxine, (Euthyrox, Levo-T, Levothyroid, Levoxyl, Synthroid, Tirosint, Unithroid)
liothyronine (Cytomel, Triostat)
thyroid desiccated (Armour Thyroid, Nature-Throid)

Drugs to Treat Hyperthyroidism
methimazole (Tapazole)
propylthiouracil

Corticosteroids
betamethasone (Celestone)
budesonide (Entocort EC)
cortisone
dexamethasone (DoubleDex, MAX Care-Pak, TopiDex, Decadron, DexPak, TaperDex, Dexabliss)
hydrocortisone (Cortef, Solu-Cortef)
methylprednisolone (Depo-Medrol, Medrol, Solu-Medrol)

prednisolone (Medrol DosePak, Pediapred, Veripred, Orapred ODT)
prednisone (Prednisone Intesol, Rayos)

Agent for Diabetic Ulcers
becaplermin (Regranex)

Agents for Diabetes

Rapid-Acting Insulin
insulin human inhalation (Afrezza)
insulin aspart (Fiasp, NovoLog, NovoLog Mix 70/30)
insulin glulisine (Apidra)
insulin lispro (Admelog, Humalog, Lyumjev)

Short-Acting Insulin
regular insulin U-100 (Humulin R, Myxredlin, Novolin R, Novolin R Flexpen, Novolin R Relion)

Intermediate-Acting Insulin
neutral protamine Hagedorn (NPH) insulin (Humulin N, Humulin 70/30, Humulin 70/30 Kwikpen, Novolin N, Novolin

70/30, Novolin 70/30 Flexpen, Novolin
70/30 Relion)
regular insulin U-500 (Humulin R U-500,
Humulin R U-500 Kwikpen)

Long-Acting Insulin
insulin degludec (Tresiba, Tresiba
FlexTouch)
insulin detemir (Levemir)
insulin glargine (Basaglar KwikPen, Lantus,
Lantus SoloStar, Semglee, Toujeo Max
SoloStar, Toujeo SoloStar)

Premixed Insulin
insulin NPH / regular 70/30
(Humulin 70/30, Humulin 70/30 Kwikpen,
Novolin 70/30, Novolin 70/30 Flexpen,
Novolin 70/30 Relion)
insulin lispro protamine / lispro 75/25
(Humalog 75/25)
insulin aspart protamine / aspart 70/30
(Novolog 70/30)
insulin lispro protamine / lispro 50/50
(Humalog 50/50)

*Glucagon-Like Peptide 1 (GLP-1) Receptor
Agonists*
albiglutide (Tanzeum)
dulaglutide (Trulicity)
exenatide (Byetta)
exenatide ER (Bydureon)
liraglutide (Victoza)
lixisenatide (Adlyxin)
pramlintide (SymlinPen)
semaglutide (Ozempic, Rybelsus)

Dipeptidyl Peptidase-4 (DPP-4) Inhibitors
alogliptin (Nesena)
linagliptin (Tradjenta)
saxagliptin (Onglyza)
sitagliptin (Januvia)

Metformin
metformin (Fortamet, Glumetza, Riomet,
Riomet ER)

Metformin Combinations
alogliptin / metformin (Kazano)
canagliflozin / metformin (Invokamet,
Invokamet XR)
dapagliflozin / metformin (Xigduo XR)

empagliflozin / metformin (Synjardy,
Synjardy XR)
ertugliflozin / metformin (Segluromet)
glipizide / metformin
glyburide / metformin
linagliptin / metformin (Jentadueto,
Jentadueto XR)
pioglitazone / metformin (Actoplus Met)
saxagliptin / metformin (Kombiglyze XR)
sitagliptin / metformin (Janumet)
dapagliflozin / metformin / saxagliptin
(Qternmet XR)
empagliflozin / metformin / linagliptin
(Trijardy XR)

*Sodium-Glucose Linked Transporter-2
(SGLT-2) Inhibitors*
canagliflozin (Invokana)
dapagliflozin (Farxiga)
empagliflozin (Jardiance)
ertugliflozin (Steglatro)

Sulfonylureas
glimepiride (Amaryl)
glipizide (Glucotrol, Glucotrol XL)
glyburide (DiaBeta, Glynase)

Meglitinide
nateglinide (Starlix)

Thiazolidinediones (TZDs)
pioglitazone (Actos)
rosiglitazone (Avandia)

Boxed Warnings
alogliptin / metformin (Kazano)
canagliflozin / metformin (Invokamet,
Invokamet XR)
dapagliflozin / metformin (Xigduo XR)
dapagliflozin / metformin / saxagliptin
(Qternmet XR)
empagliflozin / metformin (Synjardy,
Synjardy XR)
empagliflozin / metformin / linagliptin
(Trijardy XR)
ertugliflozin / metformin (Segluromet)
glipizide / metformin
glyburide / metformin
insulin human inhalation (Afrezza)
levothyroxine (Euthyrox, Levo-T,
Levothyroid, Levoxyl, Synthroid, Tirosint,
Unithroid)

linagliptin / metformin (Jentadueto, Jentadueto XR)
liothyronine (Cytomel, Triostat)
liraglutide (Victoza)
metformin (Glucophage)
metformin / sitagliptin (Janumet)
pioglitazone (Actos)
pioglitazone / metformin (Actoplus Met)
pramlintide (SymlinPen)
propylthiouracil
repaglinide / metformin (Prandimet)
rosiglitazone (Avandia)
saxagliptin / metformin (Kombiglyze XR)
semaglutide (Ozempic, Rybelsus)
sitagliptin / metformin (Janumet)
thyroid desiccated (Armour Thyroid, Nature-Throid)

Medication Guides
alogliptin (Nesina)
alogliptin / metformin (Kazano)
canagliflozin (Invokana)
canagliflozin / metformin (Invokamet, Invokamet XR)
dapagliflozin (Farxiga)
dapagliflozin / metformin (Xigduo XR)
dapagliflozin / metformin / saxagliptin (Qternmet XR)
degludec / liraglutide (Xultophy)

dulaglutide (Trulicity)
empagliflozin (Jardiance)
empagliflozin / metformin (Synjardy, Synjardy XR)
empagliflozin / metformin / linagliptin (Trijardy XR)
ertugliflozin (Steglatro)
ertugliflozin / metformin (Segluromet)
exenatide (Bydureon, Byetta)
linagliptin (Tradjenta)
linagliptin / metformin (Jentadueto, Jentadueto XR)
insulin human inhalation (Afrezza)
liraglutide (Victoza)
lixisenatide (Adlyxin)
metformin / ertugliflozin (Segluromet)
metformin / lilnagliptin (Jentadueto, Jentadueto XR)
metformin / sitagliptin (Janumet)
pioglitazone (Actos)
pioglitazone / metformin (Actoplus Met)
pramlintide (SymlinPen)
rosiglitazone (Avandia)
saxagliptin (Onglyza)
saxagliptin / metformin (Kombiglyze XR)
semaglutide (Ozempic, Rybelsus)
sitagliptin (Januvia)
sitagliptin / metformin (Janumet)

✓ CHECK YOUR UNDERSTANDING

Take a moment to review what you have learned in this chapter and answer the following questions.

1. Thyroid hormone tablets have standardized colors corresponding to strength. Which of the following colors represents a 100 mcg tablet?
   a. green
   b. pink
   c. yellow
   d. white

2. Which of the following classes of drugs can enhance the effects of thyroid medication?
   a. serotonin reuptake inhibitors
   b. anticoagulants
   c. antiseizure agents
   d. tricyclic antidepressants

3. Which of the following conditions is one in which the production of corticosteroids is excessive?
   a. Addison's disease
   b. Cushing's syndrome
   c. type 1 diabetes
   d. type 2 diabetes

4. Which of the following corticosteroids is available in an injectable form?
   a. cortisone
   b. methylprednisolone
   c. prednisolone
   d. prednisone

5. Which of the following medications would a patient with type 1 diabetes be most likely to use?
   a. linagliptin
   b. metformin
   c. glimepiride
   d. glulisine

6. Which of the following insulins works the fastest once injected?
   a. Levemir
   b. Humulin R
   c. Humalog
   d. Fiasp

7. Which of the following medications used to treat diabetes is given as an injection?
   a. dulaglutide
   b. saxagliptin
   c. nateglinide
   d. empagliflozin

8. Which of the following medications for diabetes must be stopped 48 hours in advance of a procedure involving contrast dye so as to avoid the development of lactic acidosis?
   a. alogliptin
   b. metformin
   c. glipizide
   d. dapagliflozin

9. Which of the following classes of drug therapy for diabetes works by blocking the reabsorption of glucose that the kidneys filter out of the bloodstream?
   a. sulfonylureas
   b. dipeptidyl peptidase-4 inhibitors
   c. incretin mimetics
   d. sodium-glucose linked transporter-2 inhibitors

10. Which of the following drugs is contraindicated in a patient with heart failure?
    a. alogliptin
    b. exenatide
    c. insulin glulisine
    d. pioglitazone

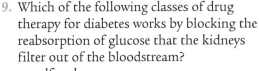

MAKE CONNECTIONS

Take a moment to consider what you have learned in this chapter and respond thoughtfully to the following prompts. Note that some of these activities will require internet access.

1. A patient taking prednisone comes to the pharmacy complaining of insomnia. The patient states that she takes this medication at bedtime. Describe the circadian rhythm for release of natural steroid production. What time of day might be a better time for the patient to take prednisone so that it doesn't interfere with her sleep?

2. Describe the major differences between type 1 and type 2 diabetes and how the treatments differ.

 The online course includes additional review and assessment resources.

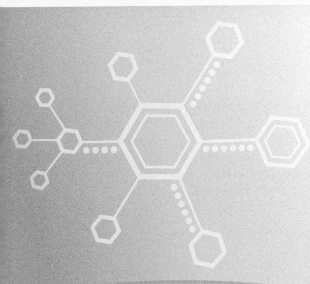

The Reproductive System and Drug Therapy

14

Learning Objectives

1 Summarize the concept of hormones and how they regulate the body. (Section 14.1)

2 Discuss sex hormones and their physiologic functions. (Section 14.1)

3 Outline the concept and applications of hormone replacement therapy. (Section 14.2)

4 Describe sexual dysfunction and the options for management. (Section 14.3)

5 Distinguish the various formulations of oral contraceptives. (Section 14.4)

6 Outline the drugs used urgently during labor and delivery. (Section 14.5)

7 Describe the treatments used to treat growth disorders. (Section 14.6)

ASHP/ACPE Accreditation Standards
To view the *ASHP/ACPE Accreditation Standards* addressed in this chapter, refer to Appendix C.

The endocrine system regulates a number of functions to keep the body in balance as well as to control complicated processes such as those involved in reproduction. This chapter covers the part of the endocrine system responsible for reproduction and sex hormones. The pharmacologic agents used in treatments related to the reproductive system include oral contraceptives, hormone replacement therapy, gender-affirming care options, drugs used during labor and delivery, and growth hormones.

14.1 The Reproductive System and Related Hormones

The reproductive system and related hormones are considered part of the endocrine system. Within the endocrine system, the pituitary gland plays a leading role because its hormones regulate several other glands, especially the testes and ovaries, which are responsible for reproduction. Sex hormones are controlled by pituitary hormones, particularly follicle-stimulating hormone (FSH) and luteinizing hormone (LH) (see Figure 14.1). The pituitary hormones travel in the bloodstream to the ovaries and testes. There, they stimulate specific cells to produce additional hormones and release them into the blood.

Regulation of hormone synthesis by a particular gland is achieved via an intricate negative feedback mechanism involving that gland and the hypothalamic-pituitary axis. Negative feedback is the mechanism in which feedback from the body's systems keeps blood levels of a hormone or a chemical within a certain range. Through this negative feedback mechanism, the pituitary gland senses increased sex hormone levels and then slows the secretion of the releasing factors by the hypothalamus.

FIGURE 14.1
Pituitary Hormones

The pituitary gland plays a key role in growth, onset of puberty, and reproductive cycles.

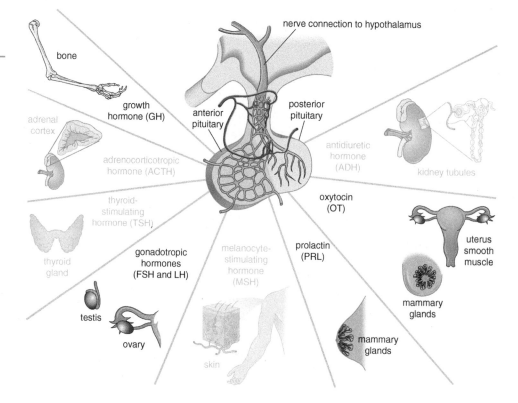

People of all genders produce sex hormones; however, these hormones are produced in different amounts and have different effects depending in part on which sex organs a person possesses. Sex hormones, including certain androgens, estrogens, and progestins, stimulate the development of secondary sex characteristics and promote the growth and maintenance of the reproductive system.

Androgen

An **androgen** is a hormone that promotes the development and maintenance of typically masculine physical characteristics. Androgens are produced by the sex organs, testes and ovaries, as well as by the adrenal glands and peripheral fat tissue. In females, androgrens are largely converted into other types of hormones, but in males, they are responsible for the development of the reproductive system and secondary sex characteristics. An important androgen is **testosterone**, which is produced by the Leydig cells in the testes. Pituitary hormones travel in the bloodstream to the testes, where they stimulate the Leydig cells to produce testosterone and release it into the blood. Through a feedback mechanism, the increased testosterone levels then slow the secretion of the releasing factors by the hypothalamus.

Testosterone is responsible for initiating sperm production and for behavioral characteristics (for example, aggressiveness). It is required during adulthood for the maintenance of libido, sexual potency, fertility (sperm production), muscle mass and strength, fat distribution, bone mass, and erythropoiesis (red blood cell production).

Estrogen

Estrogen is a group of hormones that are formed primarily in the ovaries from androgenic precursors and produce typically feminine secondary sex characteristics. When the hypothalamic-pituitary axis releases FSH to the ovaries, it stimulates estrogen production for approximately the first 14 days in each reproduction cycle of about 28 days. As estrogen builds up in the bloodstream, a feedback mechanism reduces the activity of the hypothalamus in producing and releasing the gonadotropin-releasing hormone (GnRH).

Estrogen compounds are the growth hormones of reproductive tissue in females. In addition, they share some actions of androgens on the skeleton and other tissues. Estrogen causes endometrial growth, increased cervical mucus, cornification (thickening and maturing) of vaginal mucosa, growth of breast tissue (ducts and fat deposits), increased closure of the growth plates in bones, sodium retention, carbohydrate metabolism, and calcium utilization.

Estrogen is used for contraceptive formulations (discussed at length later in this chapter), relief of menopausal symptoms, gonadal failure, and prostatic cancer.

Progesterone

Progesterone is responsible for controlling the preparation of the uterus for a fertilized ovum. It is produced during days 14 through 28, approximately, of the reproduction cycle. Progesterone is important for maintaining pregnancy once fertilization and implantation of the ovum have occurred.

Progestins are a group of synthetic forms of progesterone. Both progesterone and estrogen prevent ovulation. Progesterone achieves this by inhibiting the secretion of LH, whereas estrogen suppresses the secretion of FSH, thereby blocking follicular development and ovulation.

Progestin is used primarily in oral contraceptive pills and to prevent uterine cancer in postmenopausal women who take hormone replacement therapy. Types of progestin include levonorgestrel, medroxyprogesterone, norethindrone, and norgestimate. Generally, progestin is offered in combination with estrogen. Another important use is the treatment of menstrual dysfunction, such as irregular cycles, protracted uterine bleeding, dysmenorrhea, amenorrhea, and endometriosis. It is believed that poorly cycling estrogens may promote enlargement of the **endometrium** (the inner membrane of the uterus). Treatment with a progestin lowers the incidence of endometrial enlargement. Progestin alone does not promote menstrual bleeding, but in patients who either have endogenous estrogen or are treated first with estrogen, cyclic treatment with progestin helps to restore normal cycling.

Put Down Roots

To understand the function of progesterone, break down the word into its roots: *pro-*, meaning "forward" or "forth"; *gest-*, meaning "gestation"; and *-sterone*, meaning "steroid hormone."

14.2 Hormone Replacement Therapy

Hormone replacement therapy (HRT) relieves symptoms of a deficiency in sex hormones. Such deficiency is usually caused as part of the natural aging process but can be associated with other conditions as well. As ovarian and testes function declines with age, symptoms related to sexual function can occur, as well as other symptoms related to the functions that sex hormones regulate and maintain. **Hormone therapy** can also be used to augment sexual characteristics or to support gender identity and transition.

TABLE 14.1 Common Agents Used for Hormone Replacement Therapy

Generic (Brand)	Pronunciation	Dosage Form	Common Dosages	Dispensing Status
Testosterone Only				
testosterone (Androderm, AndroGel, Aveed, Axiron, Depo-Testosterone, Fortesta, Testopel)	tes-TOS-te-rone	buccal mucoadhesive, injection, nasal gel, pellet for implant, transdermal gel, transdermal patch, transdermal solution	buccal: 30 mg 2 times a day intranasal: 11 mg 3 times a day injection: 50–400 mg 1 time every 1–4 weeks implant: 150–450 mg every 3–6 months transdermal patch: 2–6 mg per day transdermal gel: 70–100 mg per day transdermal solution: varies	Rx, C-III
Estrogen Only				
conjugated estrogen (Premarin)	CON-ju-gate-ed ES-troe-jen	injection, tablet	0.3 or 0.625 mg a day	Rx
estradiol (Alora, Climara, Dotti, Elestrin, Estrace, Estring, EstroGel, Evamist, Femring, Menostar, Minivelle, Vagifem, Vivelle-Dot)	es-tra-DYE-awl	cream, emulsion, gel, injection, intramuscular oil, patch, tablet, transdermal solution, vaginal ring	variable depending on dosage form and indication	Rx
Progestin Only				
progesterone (Crinone, Endometrin, First-Progesterone, Prometrium)	pro-JES-te-rone	capsule, cream, gel, injection, vaginal suppository	PO: 200–400 mg a day vaginal: 45–90 mg a day	Rx
Estrogen / Progestin				
conjugated estrogen / medroxyprogesterone (Premphase, Prempro)	CON-ju-gate-ed ES-troe-jen me-DROX-ee-pro-JES-te-rone	tablet	0.625 mg a day	Rx
estradiol / drospirenone (Angeliq)	es-tra-DYE-awl droe-SPY-re-nown	tablet	1 mg estradiol/0.5 mg drospirenone a day	Rx
estradiol / levonorgestrel (Climara Pro)	es-tra-DYE-awl lee-voe-nor-JES-trel	transdermal patch	0.25–0.5 mg/day applied 2 times a week	Rx
estradiol / norethindrone (Activella, CombiPatch)	es-tra-DYE-awl nor-eth-IN-drone	tablet, transdermal patch	0.5 mg estradiol/0.14 mg norethindrone per day applied 2 times a week	Rx
estradiol / norgestimate (Prefest)	es-tra-DYE-awl nor-JES-ti-mate	tablet	1 mg estradiol/0.9 mg norgestimate a day	Rx
ethinyl estradiol / norethindrone (Activella, Amabelz, Angeliq, Bijuva, Femhrt, Fyavolv, Jinteli, Lopreeza, Mimvey, Prefest, Premphase, Prempro)	ETH-in-il es-tra-DYE-awl nor-eth-IN-drone	tablet	2.5–5 mg estradiol/0.5–1 mg norethindrone a day	Rx

TABLE 14.2 Gender-Affirming Therapy

Generic (Brand)	Pronunciation	Dosage Form	Common Dosages	Dispensing Status
Masculinizing Hormone Therapy				
testosterone (Androderm, AndroGel, Aveed, Axiron, Depo-Testosterone, Fortesta, Testopel)	tes-TOS-te-rone	gel, cream, patch	varies depending on dosage form and indication	Rx
testosterone cypionate (Depo-Testosterone)	tes-TOS-te-rone SI-pe-oh-nate	injection	50–400 mg every 2–4 weeks	Rx
testosterone enanthate (Xyosted)	tes-TOS-te-rone i-NAN-thate	implant, intranasal gel, injection, oral capsule, transdermal cream, transdermal gel	varies depending on dosage form and indication	Rx
Feminizing Hormone Therapy				
estradiol (Alora, Climara, Dotti, Elestrin, Estrogel, Evamist, Menostar, Minivelle, Vivelle-Dot)	es-tra-DYE-awl	gel, cream, patch	0.25 mg a week	Rx
estradiol (Estrace)	es-tra-DYE-awl	tablet	0.5–2 mg a day	Rx
estradiol cypionate (Depo-Estradiol)	es-tra-DYE-awl SI-pe-oh-nate	injection	1–5 mg every 3–4 weeks	Rx
estradiol valerate (Delestrogen, Natazia)	es-tra-DYE-awl VA-le-rate	injection, oral tablet	varies depending on dosage form and indication	Rx
progesterone (Crinone, Endometrin, EC-RX Progesterone, Prometrium)	pro-JES-te-rone	oral capsule, transdermal cream, vaginal gel, vaginal insert	200–400 mg a day	Rx
Antiandrogen				
spironolactone (Aldactone, Carospir)	speer-on-oh-LAK-tone	oral suspension, tablet	25–300 mg a day	Rx

Male Hypogonadism

Hypogonadism is a condition in which the body's sex glands produce few or no hormones. In male hypogonadism, the testes do not secrete sufficient androgens, and the usual development of muscle, facial hair, genitals, and voice is altered. Symptoms include breast enlargement, muscle loss, and decreased libido. If hypogonadism is secondary to brain tumors, additional symptoms may include headache, visual disturbances, and breast discharge. Hypogonadism in males is usually treated with testosterone.

Testosterone (Androderm, AndroGel, Aveed, Axiron, Depo-Testosterone, Fortesta, Testopel) is typically delivered through transdermal systems or patches.

Dosage Forms and Administration Testosterone is available in multiple dosage forms and is used in a variety of ways depending on whether it is being used as hormonal replacement, gender-affirming care, or to treat erectile dysfunction.

When administered orally, testosterone undergoes extensive first-pass metabolism (when the liver metabolizes and deactivates a drug before it reaches the bloodstream) in the gastrointestinal tract and liver. To overcome this problem, intramuscular injections are given biweekly. Transdermal dosage forms overcome some of the drawbacks associated with oral and intramuscular administration. Applying transdermal testosterone in the evening provides a serum testosterone concentration that mimics the natural circadian (on a 24-hour cycle) secretion of the hormone.

Androderm and AndroGel are applied to a fleshy area of the back, abdomen, or upper arm. The usual starting dosage for Androderm is two patches applied every evening (approximately every 24 hours). Patients should be cautioned not to use the same site more than once every seven days. The system may be worn while taking a shower or bath. When using the patch, virilization of a sex partner is unlikely, because the occlusive outer film prevents the partner from coming in contact with the drug. The application site should be allowed to dry before dressing. Patients should wash their hands with soap and water after handling this drug. AndroGel should be applied once daily, preferably in the morning, to clean, dry, intact skin. These drugs increase libido and sexual potency within weeks or months and also improve the patient's sense of well-being.

Side Effects Common side effects of testosterone include increased hair growth on the body, baldness, skin rash, acne, nausea, enlarged breasts, changes in mood, changes in sex drive, increased blood pressure, and headache. Testosterone can cause prolonged erections. Erections lasting longer than four hours indicate a need to seek immediate medical care. Patients experiencing any of the following should contact their healthcare provider: chest pain, shortness of breath, unusual changes in mood or behavior, swelling of ankles or feet, rapid weight gain, seizure, painful urination, numbness or tingling (especially on one side of the body), dark urine, or yellowing of the skin.

Adverse effects may occur with testosterone, particularly if the patient's dose is too high. Testosterone can cause **hirsutism** (abnormal hairiness) and acne. Hepatoxicity and abnormally high levels of red blood cells are rare but serious adverse effects. Other adverse effects from androgen therapy include oily skin, ankle edema, priapism (frequent or prolonged, painful penile erections), and **gynecomastia** (breast enlargement, with or without tenderness). Use of a low initial dosage in **nonvirilized** males (in other words, those lacking typically masculine secondary sex characteristics) mimics the natural increase in serum testosterone concentration during puberty. It produces **virilization** gradually, which minimizes the adverse effects of androgens, especially priapism. Gynecomastia is the result of the conversion of testosterone to estradiol (E2) through peripheral pathways. Males with hepatic cirrhosis are predisposed to gynecomastia.

Contraindications Patients with a history of breast or prostate cancer should not take testosterone. Testosterone is contraindicated in patients with polycythemia, heart failure, blood clotting disorder or history of blood clots, liver disease, or kidney disease. It is also contraindicated in patients who are pregnant or breast-feeding.

Cautions and Considerations Testosterone must be used with caution in patients with diabetes, high cholesterol, or high blood pressure.

Topical testosterone carries a boxed warning for virilization in children exposed to these products. Testosterone gel and topical solution products must be dispensed with a Medication Guide.

Drug Interactions Testoterone should not be taken with sodium fusidate because it can affect liver function.

Female Hypogonadism and Menopause

The rate of estrogen production declines with age, triggering the onset of menopause. **Menopause** is defined as the cessation of menses for one year. **Perimenopause**, a period of time prior to menopause, is characterized by a gradual loss of ovarian function and irregular bleeding before termination of menses. Perimenopause and menopause are accompanied by a change in the site, amount, and pattern of estrogen production.

Symptoms of estrogen reduction include irregular bleeding and irregular menstrual cycles. **Vasomotor** symptoms, which affect the constriction and dilation of blood vessels, may also appear. Commonly known as *hot flashes*, occurrences of vasomotor instability start in the face and move down over the body; the severity is related to the rate of estrogen decline. Other symptoms of estrogen reduction can include atrophic vulvovaginitis, characterized by excessive vaginal dryness; **dyspareunia** (painful intercourse); and infections (due to a dryness-related reduction in the number of lactobacilli that produce protective acids). Estrogen depletion also leads to a reduction in the amount of glycogen to be metabolized, an increase in pH of the vaginal area, and loss of lubrication, causing urethral and bladder atrophy. Additional effects of perimenopause and menopause can include insomnia, irritability, depression, and other mood changes.

As ovarian function declines with age, androstenedione, produced in the adrenal cortex, becomes the primary source of estrogen, and estrone becomes the dominant circulating estrogen. Because the naturally occurring concentration of androstenedione and the efficiency of its conversion may vary considerably among patients experiencing perimenopause or menopause, HRT is often provided during perimenopause to ease the transition into menopause. A small amount of additional estrogen continues to be produced through the metabolism of adrenal steroids to estradiol in peripheral fat tissue. Depending on body fat, some people experiencing perimenopause or menopause may not need estrogen replacement. Estrogen is also effective in preventing bone loss, lowering cholesterol levels, and improving the color and turgor (firmness) of skin.

Table 14.1 presents some of the most commonly used supplements for hormone therapy for the symptoms of perimenopause and menopause. It is important for technicians to know that even if these medications have the exact same ingredients, they cannot be interchanged. The doses differ slightly in each.

Patients taking any form of estrogen, whether it is in contraceptives or hormone therapy, should be aware that smoking is associated with greater morbidity, especially in patients over 35 years of age. Estrogen therapy and smoking increase the risk of blood clots, which increases the risk of deep vein thrombosis (discussed in Chapter 10).

It is recommended that HRT be used only to manage the vasomotor symptoms of perimenopause and menopause, and its use should be limited to the shortest duration possible. Hormone therapy is also associated with some risk of breast cancer. For this reason, some practitioners do not prescribe estrogen to patients who have had breast cancer or who have a family history of breast cancer.

Whether or not to use HRT is a decision for the patient and their physician. The advantages and disadvantages are different for each patient depending on that patient's family history and physical condition. If a patient who has been on HRT for a long time chooses not to continue, hormones should be tapered off.

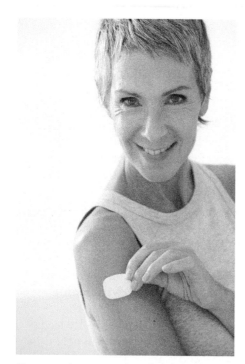

Hormone therapy can be administered via different dosage forms. Patches, as pictured, are one such dosage form.

Estrogen-Only Hormone Therapy Products

A **conjugated estrogen (Premarin)** is an estrogen of equine origin. In fact, the brand name comes from the source, which is pregnant mares' urine.

Estradiol (Alora, Climara, Dotti, Elestrin, Estrace, Estring, EstroGel, Evamist, Femring, Menostar, Minivelle, Vagifem, Vivelle-Dot) is bioidentical to human hormones. It is produced in many shapes and forms, none of which is interchangeable.

Dosage Forms and Administration Topical estrogen may be safer than pills because it avoids first-pass metabolism through the liver. Vivelle-Dot, a small patch, is placed on the abdomen for three and a half days. Elestrin is a gel that is contained in a pump and should be applied over the entire upper arm and shoulder area.

Estring and Femring contain the medication in a ring that is inserted in the vagina. The ring releases an initial burst of estradiol, followed by a tapered, low dose for a 90-day period. Insertion of the ring is similar to using a diaphragm. If removed, the ring should be rinsed in lukewarm water before reinsertion. This drug relieves symptoms of weak pelvic muscles without releasing significant systemic concentrations of estradiol. Therefore, it is not used for vasomotor symptoms or for the prevention of osteoporosis. A patient with an intact uterus also needs a progestin product to prevent endometrial hyperplasia.

Evamist is a topical estrogen spray in a metered-dose pump. The initial dose is one spray a day. Subsequently, the dose is titrated to relieve symptoms but should not exceed two or three sprays a day. Evamist is applied to the inside of the forearm at the same time each day. The spray should be allowed to dry for a few minutes. Sunscreen should be applied before the spray; if applied after, it decreases the effectiveness of the spray.

Estrogen-only hormone therapy products come in a variety of dosage forms and vary in their administration.

Side Effects Common side effects of estrogen hormone therapy include dizziness, abdominal pain or bloating, diarrhea, nausea, headache, breast tenderness, vaginal discharge, fluid retention, hair loss, and depression. These effects may subside with continued therapy. Sometimes, hormone replacement therapy can cause patches of darkened skin on the face, called **melasma**. Patients should inform their prescribers about these effects so that necessary dose changes can be made. Some patients find that specialty or extemporaneously compounded forms of estrogen, with or without progesterone, produce fewer side effects.

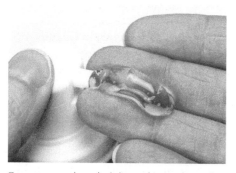

Estrogen can be administered transdermally. The product pictured is a gel that is applied topically.

Contraindications Contraindications to estrogens include a known or suspected history of breast cancer; estrogen-dependent malignancy; undiagnosed abnormal genital bleeding; active deep vein thrombosis, pulmonary embolism (PE), or a history of these conditions; active arterial thromboembolic disease or a history of this condition; liver impairment or disease; and pregnancy.

Cautions and Considerations Estrogen-only hormone replacement has several boxed warnings. It may increase the risk of endometrial cancer in patients with an intact uterus. Estrogen-only therapy is also associated with cardiovascular disorders and dementia.

Drug Interactions Estrogen derivatives may diminish the therapeutic effect of anastrozole, anticoagulants, and somatotropin. Estrogen may decrease the serum concentration of simeprevir.

Progestin Hormone Therapy Products

Progesterone (Crinone, Endometrin, First-Progesterone, Prometrium) is used for amenorrhea (absence of menstruation) and for the prevention of endometrial hyperplasia in patients with an intact uterus using estrogen therapy.

Dosage Forms and Administration Progesterone products come in a wide variety of dosage forms to suit patient needs.

Side Effects Headache, dizziness, and depression are commonly reported side effects.

Contraindications Contraindications to progesterone include undiagnosed abnormal vaginal bleeding; history of deep vein thrombosis or PE; history of arterial thromboembolic disease; history of or suspected malignancy of a breast or the genitals; liver dysfunction or disease; history of ectopic pregnancy; and pregnancy.

Cautions and Considerations Progesterone has several boxed warnings. It has a warning about increased risk of breast cancer and a second warning regarding the risk of dementia. A third warning indicates that HRT should be used for the shortest duration at the lowest effective dose possible.

Drug Interactions Progesterone may diminish the therapeutic effects of anticoagulants and diabetes agents. Colchicine, doxorubicin, pazopanib, rivaroxaban, silodosin, topotecan, and vincristine concentrations may be increased by progesterone. Ulipristal may diminish the effects of progesterone.

Estrogen / Progestin Hormone Therapy Products

Combination therapy with an estrogen product and a progestin is used if a patient has an intact uterus. In the normal cycle, high levels of estrogen before ovulation cause cells in the uterine lining to multiply. Estrogen can cause the same effect when given for HRT, leading to endometrial hyperplasia, which may progress to uterine cancer. A progestin counteracts these effects. Therefore, patients with an intact uterus should receive both an estrogen and a progestin. If progestin therapy can be avoided, however, the risk of side effects from HRT medication decreases tremendously.

Conjugated estrogen / medroxyprogesterone (Premphase, Prempro) contains the same estrogens as Premarin with the addition of a progestin. Each Prempro tablet contains both estrogen and progestin. The contents of Premphase depend on the day of therapy. Tablets for the first 14 days contain estrogen only (tablets are maroon), and the subsequent 14 tablets contain both estrogen and progestin (tablets are blue).

Ethinyl estradiol / norethindrone (Activella, Amabelz, Angeliq, Bijuva, Femhrt, Fyavolv, Jinteli, Lopreeza, Mimvey, Prefest, Premphase, Prempro) contains a combination of hormones commonly used in oral contraceptives but at a lower dosage.

Estradiol / drospirenone (Angeliq) is available as an oral tablet. Drospirenone is a progestin with antiandrogen activity. For this reason, estradiol / drospirenone may result in decreased acne.

Estradiol / levonorgestrel (Climara Pro) is provided by the manufacturer as a patch. It may decrease the intensity and number of hot flashes, night sweats, and vaginal dryness associated with menopause. The patch is stored at room temperature and is applied once a week.

Estradiol / norgestimate (Prefest) is available as a tablet containing 1 mg of estradiol and 0.9 mg of norgestimate.

Estradiol / norethindrone (CombiPatch) is a matrix transdermal in which the drugs are incorporated within an adhesive matrix layer and released continuously. **Estradiol / norethindrone (Activella)** is the tablet form of this drug combination. Activella is indicated for symptoms of menopause and vulvar atrophy and for the prevention of osteoporosis. It also decreases total cholesterol but at the expense of decreased high-density lipoprotein (HDL) levels. Activella is used to control moderate to severe vasomotor symptoms of menopause.

Dosage Forms and Administration Combination estrogen and progestin products are available as oral tablets and as dermal paches. While oral tablets are taken daily, the patches are removed and reapplied weekly.

The patch should be applied twice a week to a smooth, fold-free area of dry skin on the abdomen and should be worn continuously. It should be stored in the refrigerator before dispensing.

Side Effects Common side effects of combination estrogen and progestin include headache, upset stomach, bloating, swelling, acne, and breast tenderness as well as changes in menstrual flow and bleeding, weight, and sex drive. Rare but serious side effects include depression, severe abdominal pain, yellowing of skin or eyes, rash, extreme fatigue, fever, or dark-colored urine. If any of these effects occur, the patient should seek medical care.

Contraindications Contraindications to estrogen / progestin products include unusual genital bleeding; history of breast cancer; known or suspected estrogen-dependent tumor; active thrombosis; liver impairment or disease; known or suspected pregnancy; and kidney insufficiency.

Safety Alert

Estrogens plus progestin therapy carries a boxed warning. This combination should not be used to prevent cardiovascular disease or dementia.

Cautions and Considerations Estrogen plus progestin therapy is associated with cardiovascular disease and dementia. Breast cancer risk may be increased in patients using these products. Estrogen plus progestin therapies carry boxed warnings for these reasons.

Drug Interactions Estrogen derivatives may diminish the therapeutic effect of anastrozole, anticoagulants, and somatotropin. Estrogen may decrease the serum concentration of simeprevir.

Progesterone-containing agents may diminish the therapeutic effects of anticoagulants and diabetes agents. Colchicine, doxorubicin, pazopanib, rivaroxaban, silodosin, topotecan, and vincristine concentrations may be increased by progesterone-containing products. Ulipristal may diminish the effects of progesterone-containing products.

Gender-Affirming Hormone Therapy

Transgender and gender diverse people experience a gender identity that differs from the sex they were assigned at birth, which is typically limited to male or female. Gender identity is an inwardly experienced concept involving how individuals perceive themselves and what they call themselves related to gender. Gender may be outwardly marked by expressions through clothing, hairstyle, behavior, or even vocal inflections. Some transgender and gender diverse individuals may seek to align their internal

Work Wise

Transgender and gender diverse individuals sometimes avoid or delay medical care due to fear of rejection or mistreatment by healthcare providers. Maintaining a professional and nonjudgmental work environment helps all patients feel comfortable seeking care.

experience of gender more closely with their outward appearance through a process called **gender transition**. Gender transition can include social transition, which may include changes in clothing, name, or pronouns, as well as physical transitions, which may include gender-affirming hormone therapy or other medical or surgical interventions. Many individuals also seek community support, mental health support, or both as they navigate major life changes as part of their transition or cope with experiences of discrimination. Counseling is often required by individuals' care providers or insurance plans to access gender-affirming care. The goal of gender-affirming hormone therapy is to acquire secondary sex characteristics that are aligned with an individual's gender identity. These agents are included in Table 14.2.

Masculinizing hormone therapy involves terminating menstruation and inducing the development of typically masculine secondary sex characteristics in individuals who were assigned female at birth. Testosterone is traditionally used, most commonly through subcutaneous or intramuscular injections; transdermal patches, creams, or gels; or subcutaneous pellets. In masculinizing therapy, the use of testosterone is typically sufficient to suppress the body's estrogen production. Using testosterone typically produces facial and body hair growth, increased muscle mass, redistribution of body fat, loss of menses, enlargement of the clitoris, and a deepened voice. An important note is that testosterone therapy alone does not prevent pregnancy, even with the cessation of menses. Side effects may include oily skin, acne, vaginal atrophy, weight gain, sleep apnea, or polycythemia (the production of too many red blood cells). The transdermal treatments can cause skin irritation, and patients must be careful to avoid unintended transference to women, nonbinary adults who would not want contact with this drug, children, or pets through direct contact to the area of application.

Feminizing hormone therapy involves suppressing the effects of androgens and inducing the development of typically feminine secondary sex characteristics in individuals who were assigned male at birth. This is typically achieved by a combination of estrogen and an antiandrogen, and some regimens may also include progesterone. Estradiol is the estrogen that is typically used in oral and sublingual tablets; subcutaneous and intramuscular injections; and transdermal patches, creams, and gels. Use of estradiol typically results in changes in body fat distribution, softening of the skin and decreased oiliness, breast growth, and thinning and slowed growth of facial and body hair. Unlike masculinizing therapy, feminizing therapy does not have any effect on the pitch of an individual's voice; patients seeking changes to voice pitch may use speech therapy or vocal coaching. Side effects may include decreased muscle mass, declines in libido and erections, shrinking of the testes and decreased sperm production, or weight gain. There may be an increased risk of venous thromboembolism (blood clots) with estradiol in patients with co-occurring risk factors; in these situations, transdermal estradiol is the preferred formulation.

Spironolactone (Aldactone, Carospir) is a commonly used antiandrogen. It can produce decreased hair growth, muscle mass, and sperm production, as well as breast growth, redistribution of body fat, and voice changes. Side effects can include skin rash or itching, decreased sexual desire, diarrhea, nausea, vomiting. There may be an increased risk of electrolyte imbalance, liver disease, and changes in blood cells.

14.3 Sexual Dysfunction and Drug Treatments

Sexual dysfunction is a change in an individual's sexual function that prevents the enjoyment of sexual activity. The sexual response cycle usually includes excitement, plateau, orgasm, and resolution. Dysfunction can occur at any phase of the response cycle.

TABLE 14.3 Common Agents Used to Treat Sexual Dysfunction

Generic (Brand)	Pronunciation	Dosage Form	Common Dosages	Dispensing Status
Phosphodiesterase-5 Inhibitors				
avanafil (Stendra)	av-AN-a-fil	tablet	100–200 mg a day	Rx
sildenafil (Revatio, Viagra)	sil-DEN-a-fil	tablet	25–100 mg a day	Rx
tadalafil (Adcirca, Alyq, Cialis)	tah-DAL-a-fil	tablet	5–10 mg a day	Rx
vardenafil (Levitra, Staxyn)	var-DEN-a-fil	tablet	10 mg a day	Rx
Other Agents				
alprostadil (Caverject, Edex, Muse)	al-PROS-ta-dil	injection, urethral pelle	varies depending on patient and dosage form	Rx
flibanserin (Addyi)	flib-AN-ser-in	tablet	100 mg 1 time a day at bedtime	Rx

Erectile Dysfunction

Erectile dysfunction (ED) (a chronic inability to achieve a penile erection or to maintain one until ejaculation) has many causes, including testosterone deficiency, alcoholism, cigarette smoking, psychological factors, and medications. ED may also be referred to as *impotence*. Testosterone can be used for ED in combination with other medications listed in Table 14.3. The agents listed below, particularly alcohol, are known to cause ED.

- alcohol
- amphetamines
- antidepressants (some)
- antihypertensives
- corticosteroids
- estrogens
- H$_2$ blockers
- haloperidol
- lithium
- opioids

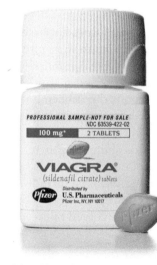

Sildenafil is sold under the brand name Viagra.

Phosphodiesterase-5 Inhibitors

The drugs most frequently used to treat ED are the phosphodiesterase-5 (PDE-5) inhibitors. In fact, they are usually listed among the top 50 drugs dispensed in pharmacies today. Although PDE-5 inhibitors are the best-known options, other treatment options are available for patients to consider. However, the routes of administration for these products are not as convenient as the oral route of PDE-5 inhibitors.

A **phosphodiesterase-5 (PDE-5) inhibitor** works by enhancing the relaxant effect of nitric oxide released in response to sexual stimulation. This allows an erection to occur naturally by relaxing the smooth muscle of penile vasculature, increasing the flow of blood into the penis. PDE-5 inhibitors have, for the most part, replaced other drugs used for ED. They have many interactions with other drugs, most notably a potentially lethal interaction with nitrates (nitroglycerin, isosorbide dinitrate, and isosorbide mononitrate) used to treat ischemic heart disease, as described in Chapter 10. Taking PDE-5 inhibitors with nitrates can dangerously lower blood pressure, and this effect can last for several hours.

Sildenafil (Revatio, Viagra) should be taken at least one hour before sexual activity. Sildenafil can cause temporary vision disturbances, headache, and indigestion.

Vardenafil (Levitra, Staxyn) has the same side effect profile as sildenafil, but it is often prescribed when sildenafil proves ineffective.

Tadalafil (Adcirca, Alyq, Cialis) is sometimes called the "weekender" because it is effective for 36 hours. Peak plasma levels of the drug are obtained in two hours. It has a faster onset and longer duration than the other PDE-5 inhibitors.

Avanafil (Stendra) appears to have enhanced PDE-5 selectivity compared to the other PDE-5 inhibitors and a more rapid onset of action, and its absorption is not significantly affected by food.

Dosage Forms and Administration PDE-5 inhibitors are taken orally. Sildenafil and avanafil are taken anywhere from 15 minutes to an hour prior to sexual activity. Vardenafil is a rapidly dissolving tablet, which allows it to be used immediately prior to sexual activity. Tadalafil continues to work for 36 hours, so it can be taken up to a day or two before sexual activity.

Put Down Roots

An easy way to identify a PDE-5 inhibitor is to look at the ending of the drug name. The names of PDE-5 inhibitors end with -*afil*.

Safety Alert

Use of PDE-5 inhibitors with nitrates or alpha blockers should be avoided, as the combination can cause a life-threatening drop in blood pressure.

Side Effects Common side effects of PDE-5 inhibitors include headache, flushing, nausea, blurred vision, stuffy or runny nose, back pain, and muscle pain. These effects may subside with use. Patients should speak with their provider if these effects are bothersome.

Contraindications PDE-5 inhibitors are contraindicated in patients who take nitrates or alpha-blockers. Combining PDE-5 inhibitors with these other drugs can cause a dramatic drop in blood pressure, which can be life-threatening.

Phosphodiesterase inhibitors are contraindicated in patients with low blood pressure, uncontrolled high blood pressure, heart disease, history of stroke, and some cardiac arrhythmias.

Cautions and Considerations Patients taking other medications for blood pressure should discuss them with their prescribers before taking PDE-5 inhibitors. Drinking alcohol while taking a PDE-5 inhibitor can worsen its effects on blood pressure. Patients should be discouraged from smoking or drinking alcohol for a few hours before sexual activity when taking one of these drugs. Patients taking a PDE-5 inhibitor may experience increased heart rate, dizziness, and headache.

Drug Interactions All PDE-5 inhibitors interact with several other medications. Most notably, they have a potentially lethal interaction with nitrates (nitroglycerin, isosorbide dinitrate, and isosorbide mononitrate) used to treat ischemic heart disease. Patients should ensure that their pharmacists and prescribers know all the medications and OTC dietary supplements they take to avoid any dangerous interactions. Pharmacy technicians can help by obtaining thorough medication histories for patients who bring in prescriptions for PDE-5 inhibitors. Sildenafil has major drug interactions with erythromycin and some antifungal medications.

Alprostadil

Alternative treatment options for ED are available. One of these options is alprostadil **(Caverject, Edex, Muse)**. Considered a second-line choice of therapy for ED, alprostadil is a prostaglandin that works as a vasodilator, relaxing smooth muscle in the vasculature of the penis. Alprostadil is injected into the base of the penis or inserted as a pellet into the urethra.

Dosage Forms and Administration Caverject and Edex are penile injections, and MUSE (medicated urethral system for erection) is a urethral suppository. Caverject is administered as an injection into the corpora cavernosa on the sides of the penis (hence the name). The manufacturer provides Caverject as a kit that contains six syringes and single-dose vials of freeze-dried powder for reconstitution and administration. The vials should be refrigerated until dispensed, but they may be kept at room temperature for up to three months. In the Caverject Impulse dual-chamber syringe system, the powder and water are stored in separate chambers in the prefilled syringe. The plunger must be rotated before injection. MUSE comes with a small plastic applicator that inserts a micropellet of alprostadil into the urethra. MUSE works quickly, usually within 10 minutes. It should be refrigerated unless it will be used within 14 days.

Side Effects Side effects of alprostadil include penile pain and urethral burning. High doses can cause hypotension and dizziness.

Contraindications Alprostadil is contraindicated with Sickle cell disease, clotting disorders, multiple myeloma and leukemia.

Cautions and Considerations MUSE can cause vaginal burning and itching in a sexual partner.

Drug Interactions Eluxadoline may increase levels of alprostadil by decreasing metabolism.

Sexual Dysfunction

Sexual dysfunction is marked by persistent, recurrent problems with sexual arousal and response. Many people experience sexual dysfunction at some point in their lives. Sexual dysfunction can take different forms, including decreased desire, reduced arousal, anorgasmia (inability to achieve orgasm), and pain.

Treatment should be directed at the causes of sexual dysfunction, which are often multifactorial. Nonpharmacological options such as counseling, lifestyle changes, and the use of vaginal lubricants and moisturizers may provide relief. Use of testosterone and antidepressants (see Chapter 8) may also improve sexual function.

There is only one FDA-approved drug used to treat sexual dysfunction in pre-menopausal patients, **flibanserin (Addyi)**. Flibanserin works by modulating the neurotransmitters serotonin, dopamine, and norepinephrine and has been shown to increase sexual desire. As with other drugs that affect neurotransmitters, it may take six to eight weeks before improvement is noticed.

Dosage Forms and Administration Flibanserin is available as a 100 mg tablet that is taken one time a day before sleep to mitigate certain side effects.

Side Effects The most serious side effects of flibanserin are hypotension and fainting. Other common effects associated with flibanserin include fatigue, dizziness, headache, nausea, and sedation.

Contraindications Contraindications to flibanserin include concomitant alcohol use, liver impairment, and concomitant use of drugs that strongly inhibit its metabolism.

Safety Alert

Flibanserin carries a boxed warning about use with alcohol. This combination can increase risk of severe low blood pressure and fainting.

Cautions and Considerations Flibanserin has boxed warnings for increased risk of severe hypotension and loss of consciousness in patients with liver impairment and those using alcohol concurrently. Due to these adverse effects, flibanserin is part of an FDA-required Risk Evaluation and Mitigation Strategy (REMS) program for prescribers and pharmacies. REMS programs use risk minimization strategies beyond professional labeling to ensure that the benefits of certain drugs outweigh the risks. Flibanserin must also be dispensed with a Medication Guide.

CNS depression may result from flibanserin. Patients should be cautioned about performing tasks that require them to be mentally alert.

Little is known about adverse effects on patients who take flibanserin while pregnant or breast-feeding, and it is not recommended to treat these populations.

Drug Interactions Flibanserin has multiple drug interactions. It should not be used with alcohol, azelastine, bosutinib, conivaptan, fusidic acid, idelalisib, orphenadrine, paraldehyde, pazopanib, silodosin, thalidomide, topotecan, or vincristine.

14.4 Contraception and Drug Treatments

Pharmacology plays an important role in family planning today. Medications can factor into patients' decisions to become or avoid becoming pregnant, help them successfully carry a child to term, and ease the pain of childbirth.

Contraception is any practice that serves to prevent pregnancy during sexual activity. These practices can be either nonpharmacologic or pharmacologic. Contraceptive methods that are nonpharmacologic include abstinence and natural birth control. Contraceptive methods that are pharmacologic include oral contraceptives; various barrier products, such as external and internal condoms; transdermal and vaginal contraceptives; and various injections, implants, and intrauterine devices. Because of the pharmacology foundation of this textbook, the pharmacologic methods of contraception are discussed in depth in this section.

Choosing a method of contraception is a personal decision, and individuals must consider several factors, including rates of effectiveness, ease of use, and adherence requirements. Patients should understand that rates of effectiveness for preventing pregnancy reported in product labeling refer to "perfect use." These rates are only achieved when the patient follows instructions exactly. If a product is difficult to use or undesirable for a particular patient, adherence and the effectiveness of the product will not be ideal. Perfect use is not representative of actual use in many cases, and all products have some failures, even if such failures are rare.

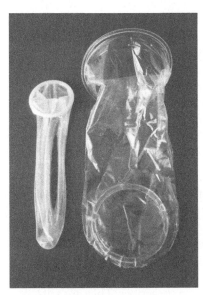

The external (formerly "male") condom (left) and internal (formerly "female") condom (right) are barrier methods of contraception. Both devices are OTC products that prevent sperm from entering a vagina.

Barrier Contraception

Barrier birth control products are used when intercourse is anticipated. These products form a physical barrier that prevents sperm from entering the uterus through the cervix. To be effective, the products are put in place prior to intercourse, left there for a specific amount of time, and then removed. Barrier products do not alter normal ovulation, cervical mucus, or endometrial lining formation. Patients should understand that rates of effectiveness for contraception methods are only achieved when the patient follows instructions exactly.

External Condoms

The **external condom** is placed over the erect penis before it enters the vagina. External condoms were formerly referred to as *male condoms*. Condoms collect ejaculate (semen and sperm) and prevent sperm from coming into contact with the vagina or cervix. Ejaculate material is removed along with the condom. Condoms are the only birth control method that also prevents or lowers the risk of transmission of sexually transmitted infections (STIs), also referred to as *sexually transmitted diseases (STDs)*. Latex and polyurethane condoms provide the best protection because they are impermeable. Other than latex allergy and skin irritation, no apparent side effects are typically associated with condom use.

Latex allergy is a contraindication to latex condom use. If an individual or their partner has a latex allergy, they should use polyurethane condoms.

Difficulty in getting the proper fit, keeping the condom on during the entire sexual activity, and maintaining an erection while wearing a condom have been reported as problems that decrease the ease of use and effectiveness of condoms. Concurrent use of external and internal condoms is not recommended because friction between the condoms can cause them to break.

Water-based lubricants such as K-Y Jelly and Astroglide can be used with latex condoms. However, oil-based lubricants can cause condoms to break and are not recommended for use with condoms. Some other vaginal products and medications can contain oil-based ingredients such as butoconazole or mineral oil. Therefore, patients using these therapies should abstain from intercourse or ensure their partners use polyurethane condoms until the therapy is completed.

Internal Condoms

The **internal condom** is inserted into the vagina before sexual activity to form a physical barrier between the penis and the vagina. Internal condoms were formerly referred to as *female condoms*. The internal condom is made of nitrile material instead of latex, and it is inserted up to eight hours before sexual activity. When used properly, the condom holding the ejaculate is removed after intercourse. Condoms are the only contraception method that also prevents or lowers the risk of STI transmission. Few if any side effects are typically associated with the use of internal condoms.

The internal condom is not contraindicated in any specific patient population. This type of condom can be used as an alternative barrier method when one of the partners has a latex allergy.

To maintain the effectiveness of an internal condom, partners must ensure that the penis does not slip between the vagina and the outer surface of the condom and that the outer ring does not get pushed inside the vagina. Although the internal condom can be removed at any time after intercourse, it is most effective when removed before standing to avoid spilling semen. To remove the condom, the outer ring is twisted to seal it, and then the condom is pulled out.

Patients should be aware that concurrent use of external and internal condoms is not recommended, as friction between the condoms can cause them to break. Finally, patients should understand that the internal condom is more expensive than the external condom and has a slightly lower rate of effectiveness at preventing pregnancy.

Diaphragms and Cervical Caps

The **diaphragm** and the **cervical cap** are made of rubber, latex, or silicone and are bordered by a rounded ring that fits over the cervix inside the vagina. They form a barrier that covers the cervical opening and prevents sperm from entering the uterus and traveling to the fallopian tubes. A diaphragm is larger than a cervical cap and covers a larger area over the cervix. These products work best when used with a **spermicide** that kills sperm cells on contact. Diaphragms and cervical caps are prescription items that must be fitted or sized to the internal anatomy by a prescriber. They are self-inserted prior to sexual intercourse and left in place for at least six hours after sexual intercourse. Some individuals experience more frequent urinary tract infections when using diaphragms or cervical caps. This effect is thought to be related to changes in the normal vaginal flora from exposure to the spermicide that is used along with these devices. Use of a diaphragm without a spermicide, however, diminishes its effectiveness at preventing pregnancy. Therefore, to reduce the incidence of urinary tract infections, it is recommended that individuals urinate before inserting these devices and again right after intercourse.

Diaphragms and cervical caps used with spermicide may cause irritation, burning, or itching of mucous membranes. If irritation, burning, or rash from the spermicide continues, an alternative form of contraceptive should be considered.

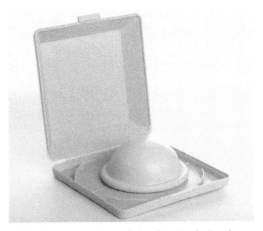
A diaphragm, as pictured, is a barrier device that fits over the cervix.

The diaphragm should not be used by individuals who have an allergy to latex or spermicide, frequent urinary tract infections, or a history of toxic shock syndrome. Some anatomic differences (such as uterine prolapse) can make it difficult to get a proper fit for a diaphragm and preclude some patients from being able to use one. To be most effective, diaphragms and cervical caps should be used with nonoxynol cream or gel. Patients with hypersensitivity to nonoxynol-9 should avoid products with spermicide.

Diaphragms and cervical caps do not protect against transmission of STIs. These contraceptives are meant to be reused, but they must be thoroughly cleaned with mild soap and water and properly stored after each use. In addition, patients should be refitted for a diaphragm or cervical cap after pregnancy, miscarriage, abortion, pelvic surgery, or significant weight loss or gain because the shapes of the uterus and vagina change.

Hormonal Contraceptives

Pharmacologic contraception involves manipulating hormones to prevent ovulation and to change the texture of cervical mucus. These drugs contain ethinyl estradiol (a synthetic estrogen), one of several synthetic progestins, or both. An **oral contraceptive (OC)** that contains synthetic estrogens works by suppressing production of LH, the hormone that triggers ovulation. OCs that contain progestins suppress LH production and thicken cervical mucus, making movement difficult for sperm.

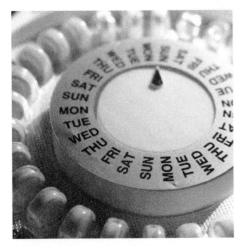
A variety of birth control pills is available.

OCs are taken at the same time each day to maintain a steady and elevated hormone level. Depending on the product chosen, patients begin therapy on the first day of their menstrual flow, the first Sunday after their menstrual flow begins, or whenever desired. Regardless of the product, backup contraception, such as a barrier method, must be used to prevent pregnancy for at least the first seven days of therapy, if not for the entire first cycle.

Hormonal contraceptives also include emergency contraception; oral, transdermal, vaginal, injectable, and implantable contraceptives; and intrauterine devices. Table 14.4 identifies the commonly used hormonal contraceptives.

TABLE 14.4 Commonly Used Hormonal Contraceptives

Generic (Brand)	Pronunciation	Dosage Form	Dosage Frequency	Dispensing Status
Combination Oral Contraceptives				
ethinyl estradiol / desogestrel (Apri, Azurette, Bekyree, Caziant, Cyred, Cyred EQ, Emoquette, Enskyce, Isibloom, Juleber, Kalliga, Kariva, Mircette, Pimtrea, Reclipsen, Similiya, Velivet, Viorele, Volnea)	ETH-in-il es-tra-DYE-awl des-oh-JES-trel	tablet	1 time a day	Rx
ethinyl estradiol / drospirenone (Beyaz, Gianvi, Jasmiel, Lo-Zumandimine, Loryna, Nikki, Ocella, Safyral, Syeda, Tydemy, Yasmin 28, Yaz, Zarah, Zumandimine)	ETH-in-il es-tra-DYE-awl droh-SPYE-re-none	tablet	1 time a day	Rx
ethinyl estradiol / ethynodiol diacetate (Kelnor, Zovia)	ETH-in-il es-tra-DYE-awl e-thye-noe-DYE-awl dye-AS-e-tate	tablet	1 time a day	Rx
ethinyl estradiol / levonorgestrel (Afirmelle, Altavera, Amethia, Amethyst, Ashlyna, Aubra, Aviane, Ayuna, Camrese, Chateal, Daysee, Delyla, Enpresse, FaLessa, Falmina, Fayosim, Introvale, Jaimiesse, Jolessa, Kurvelo, Larissia, Lessina, Levonest, Levora, Lillow, LoJaimiesse, LoSeasonique, Lutera, Marlissa, Orsythia, Portia, Quartette, Rivelsa, Seasonique, Setlakin, Simpesse, Sronyx, Trivora, Vienva)	ETH-in-il es-tra-DYE-awl LEE-voe-nor-jes-trel	tablet	1 time a day	Rx
ethinyl estradiol / norethindrone (Alyacen, Aranelle, Balziva, Briellyn, Cyclafem, Dasetta, Leena, Necon, Nortrel, Philith, Pirmella, Vyfemla, Wera)	ETH-in-il es-tra-DYE-awl nor-ETH-in-drone	tablet	1 time a day	Rx
ethinyl estradiol / norgestimate (Estarylla, Femynor, Mili, Mono-Linyah, Previfem, Sprintec, Tri Femynor, Tri-Estarylla, Tri-Linyah, Tri-Lo-Estarylla, Tri-Lo-Marzia, Tri-Lo-Mili, Tri-Lo-Sprintec, Tri-Mili, TriNessa, Tri-Previfem, Tri-Sprintec, Tri-VyLibra, VyLibra)	ETH-in-il es-tra-DYE-awl nor-JES-ti-mate	tablet	1 time a day	Rx
ethinyl estradiol / norgestrel (Cryselle-28, Elinest, Low-Orgestrel)	ETH-in-il es-tra-DYE-awl nor-JES-trel	tablet	1 time a day	Rx
Progestin-Only Oral Contraceptive				
norethindrone (Camila, Deblitane, Errin, Generess FE, Heather, Incassia, Jencycla, Kaitlib Fe, Layolis FE, Lyza, Nora-Be, Norlyda, Norlyroc, Ortho-Micronor, Sharobel, Tulana, Wymza Fe)	nor-ETH-in-drone	tablet	1 time a day	Rx

continues

TABLE 14.4 **Commonly Used Hormonal Contraceptives**—*Continued*

Generic (Brand)	Pronunciation	Dosage Form	Dosage Frequency	Dispensing Status
Emergency Contraceptives				
levonorgestrel (Plan B, Plan B One-Step, Aftera, EContra One-Step, My Choice, My Way, New Day, Opcicon One-Step, Preventeza, React, Take Action)	LEE-voe-nor-jes-trel	tablet	1 dose within 72 hr of unprotected intercourse with optional second dose 12 hr later	OTC, Rx
ulipristal (Ella)	yoo-li-PRISS-tal	tablet	1 dose within 72 hr of unprotected intercourse	Rx
Transdermal Contraceptives				
ethinyl estradiol / norelgestromin (Xulane)	ETH-in-il es-tra-DYE-awl nor-el-JES-troe-min	patch	applied 1 time a week for 3 weeks, and then left off for 1 week	Rx
levonorgestrel / ethinyl estradiol (Twirla)	LEE-voe-nor-jes-trel ETH-in-il es-tra-DYE-ole	patch	applied 1 time a week for 3 weeks, and then left off for 1 week	Rx
Vaginal Contraceptive				
ethinyl estradiol / etonogestrel (EluRyng, NuvaRing)	ETH-in-il es-tra-DYE-awl ee-toe-noe-JES-trel	vaginal ring	inserted and left in for 3 weeks, removed for 1 week	Rx
Injectable Contraceptive				
medroxyprogesterone (Depo-Provera, Depo-SubQ Provera 104, Provera)	me-DROKS-ee-proe-JES-te-rone	injection	IM: 150 mg every 3 months Sub-Q: 104 mg every 3 months	Rx
Implantable Contraceptive				
etonogestrel (Nexplanon)	ee-toe-noe-JES-trel	implant	inserted in upper arm by healthcare provider once every 3 yr	Rx
Intrauterine Devices				
intrauterine copper contraceptive (Paragard)	in-TRAH-yoo-teer-in COP-ur con-TRAH-sep-tiv	intrauterine implant	inserted by healthcare provider, 8–10 yr	Rx
levonorgestrel (Kyleena, Liletta, Mirena, Skyla)	LEE-voe-nor-jes-trel	intrauterine implant	inserted by healthcare provider, 5–6 yr	Rx

Oral Contraceptives

OCs contain either a combination of estrogen and progestin or progestin only (see Table 14.4). Combination OCs come in monophasic, biphasic, and triphasic dosing regimens. Monophasic regimens contain the same dose each day throughout the menstrual cycle, whereas biphasic and triphasic regimens increase the dosage once or twice during a cycle. The color of the tablet usually changes as the dose changes.

Many contraception products are available and used as extended oral regimens. Such products involve taking a steady dose for 84 days before allowing a hormone-free week, during which menstruation occurs. In effect, patients experience bleeding only once every three or four months. Although concern about endometrial thickening exists, such a regimen works well for patients who have menstrual cycle–related migraines, severe premenstrual symptoms, endometriosis, or polycystic ovarian syndrome. Prescribers occasionally order a similar extended regimen of monophasic oral contraceptives.

OCs are among the most frequently prescribed pharmaceutical agents in the United States. For these products to be optimally effective with the lowest frequency of side effects, patients should be well informed as to their proper use.

Ethinyl estradiol / desogestrel (Apri, Azurette, Bekyree, Caziant, Cyred, Cyred EQ, Emoquette, Enskyce, Isibloom, Juleber, Kalliga, Kariva, Mircette, Pimtrea, Reclipsen, Similiya, Velivet, Viorele, Volnea) contains a type of progestin classified as third generation. Third-generation progestins are thought to have less androgen activity.

Ethinyl estradiol / drospirenone (Beyaz, Gianvi, Jasmiel, Lo-Zumandimine, Loryna, Nikki, Ocella, Safyral, Syeda, Tydemy, Yasmin 28, Yaz, Zarah, Zumandimine) contains a progestin that is known as a spironolactone analog. Drospirenone has mineralocorticoid activity as well as progestin activity, so it works as a potassium-sparing diuretic, thereby potentially reducing the risk of sodium and fluid retention and weight gain.

Ethinyl estradiol / ethynodiol diacetate (Kelnor, Zovia) contains a first-generation progestin. Ethynodiol diacetate may exhibit estrogen-like activity.

Ethinyl estradiol / levonorgestrel (Afirmelle, Altavera, Amethia, Amethyst, Ashlyna, Aubra, Aviane, Ayuna, Camrese, Chateal, Daysee, Delyla, Enpresse, FaLessa, Falmina, Fayosim, Introvale, Jaimiesse, Jolessa, Kurvelo, Larissia, Lessina, Levonest, Levora, Lillow, LoJaimiesse, LoSeasonique, Lutera, Marlissa, Orsythia, Portia, Quartette, Rivelsa, Seasonique, Setlakin, Simpesse, Sronyx, Trivora, Vienva) contains a second-generation progestin. Levonorgestrel has androgen-like properties. This may result in adverse effects such as lowering high-density lipoprotein concentrations.

Ethinyl estradiol / norethindrone (Alyacen, Aranelle, Balziva, Briellyn, Cyclafem, Dasetta, Leena, Necon, Nortrel, Philith, Pirmella, Vyfemla, Wera) contains a first-generation progestin and is a commonly prescribed OC.

Norethindrone (Camila, Deblitane, Errin, Generess FE, Heather, Incassia, Jencycla, Kaitlib Fe, Layolis FE, Lyza, Nora-Be, Norlyda, Norlyroc, Ortho-Micronor, Sharobel, Tulana, Wymza Fe) is a progestin-only contraceptive. This means it does not contain an estrogen component. Progestins act to prevent pregnancy by inhibiting the secretion of LH, which causes egg release; causing thickening of the cervical mucus to impede the entry of sperm; and altering the uterine lining to prevent implantation of a fertilized egg. Therefore, progestins can be used as contraceptives by themselves without additional estrogens.

Ethinyl estradiol / norgestimate (Estarylla, Femynor, Mili, Mono-Linyah, Previfem, Sprintec, Tri Femynor, Tri-Estarylla, Tri-Linyah, Tri-Lo-Estarylla, Tri-Lo-Marzia, Tri-Lo-Mili, Tri-Lo-Sprintec, Tri-Mili, Tri-Previfem, Tri-Sprintec, Tri-VyLibra, VyLibra) contains a third-generation progestin with fewer androgenic effects.

Dosage Forms and Administration These hormonal contraceptives are taken orally on a daily basis. The dose should be taken at the same time each day to be most effective. Patients should pay particular attention to the instructions for missed doses. In many cases, missed doses can result in loss of effectiveness for contraception, and other barrier methods must be used to prevent pregnancy for the remainder of the menstrual cycle.

Side Effects Common side effects of oral contraceptives include weight gain, nausea, vomiting, bloating, increased appetite, fatigue, breast tenderness or enlargement, headaches, and edema (fluid retention). These effects tend to subside with continued use but can be a reason to stop or change therapy if bothersome. Patients should discuss these effects with their prescribers. Breakthrough bleeding (blood flow in the middle of a menstrual cycle) can occur, especially at the start of therapy. If it continues, the patient should talk with their prescriber. An increase in blood pressure can occur in the first few months of OC therapy. Serious side effects can include blood clots, heart attacks, and strokes. Smoking increases the risk of these effects. Patients should speak with their provider about their health and family history to assess their own potential risks for these effects. Patients with clotting disorders or a family history of clotting disorders may not be able to take oral contraceptives.

Contraindications Patients with clotting disorders should not take OCs, because these agents can increase the formation of blood clots. Blood clots may be fatal, depending on their location and severity. Patients who have disorders that affect potassium levels, such as kidney disease, liver dysfunction, or adrenal insufficiency, should not take ethinyl estradiol / drosperinone. Patients with heart or cerebrovascular disease should not take OCs. Drospirenone has actions similar to the diuretic spironolactone and can adversely affect potassium levels.

Cautions and Considerations Patients with a history of breast, endometrial, ovarian, or cervical cancer should discuss the risks and benefits of OCs with their healthcare practitioners. Some controversy exists about whether OCs increase the risk of cancer in these organs, so patients should make informed decisions about their own care.

The advantage of products containing only progestin is that the lower hormone dose reduces side effects, such as headaches and elevated blood pressure. These products are commonly used in patients for whom OCs are typically not appropriate (such as patients who have high blood pressure, heart disease, or a blood clotting disorder or are older than 35 years of age, especially those who smoke). Smoking in conjunction with hormone therapy increases the risk of heart attack, blood clots, and stroke.

Patients with high blood pressure should be encouraged to use other methods of contraception, if possible. The most serious adverse effect of OCs is the development of cardiovascular complications, such as heart attack, stroke, or other forms of thromboembolic disease.

Many OC products are on the market. All OC products have special packaging and dispensing regulations. These regulations state that all patients, upon receipt of their prescriptions, must receive a patient information leaflet that has been approved by the FDA.

The disadvantage of products containing only progestin is that missed doses affect failure rate more quickly than contraceptives containing estrogen. If a dose of a progestin-only pill is missed by more than three hours, the patient should take it as soon as they remember and should use a backup birth control method, such as condoms, for at least 48 hours.

Technicians should remind patients that oral contraceptives do not prevent transmission of STIs. To avoid transmission, patients must use a barrier method.

Drug Interactions Other medications, herbal preparations, and supplements can interact with oral and other hormonal contraceptives and reduce their effectiveness. Table 14.5 describes various drug interactions. Patients may need to use additional or alternative methods of contraception to prevent pregnancy while taking interacting medications. Alternative methods of birth control should be continued until the entire menstrual cycle is complete, even if this goes beyond when therapy with the interacting drug is finished.

TABLE 14.5 Hormonal Contraceptive Interactions

Class	Drug(s)	Type of Interaction
antibiotics	erythromycin, griseofulvin, penicillins, rifampin, tetracyclines	may decrease OC effectiveness; interfere with enterohepatic cycling and recycling of estrogen, which can cause a fluctuation in hormone levels
anticonvulsants	carbamazepine, felbamate, phenobarbital, phenytoin, primidone	decrease OC action through increased metabolism of hormones
antifungals	fluconazole, itraconazole, ketoconazole	may decrease OC action (see *antibiotics*)
benzodiazepines	alprazolam, chlordiazepoxide, diazepam, flurazepam, triazolam	metabolism of benzodiazepines that undergo oxidation may be decreased, increasing central nervous system (CNS) effects
bronchodilators	theophylline	theophylline metabolism may be decreased, increasing side effects of bronchodilators
corticosteroids	hydrocortisone, methylprednisolone, prednisolone, prednisone	effects of corticosteroids may be increased owing to inhibition of metabolism by OC
tricyclic antidepressants (TCAs)	amitriptyline, imipramine	TCA metabolism may be decreased, increasing its side effects

 Work Wise

Emergency contraceptives may be colloquially referred to as the *morning-after pill*. Legal age requirements for taking emergency contraception vary from state to state.

Emergency Contraceptives

In the event of unprotected sex, administration of an **emergency contraceptive** may prevent pregnancy if medications are taken quickly, up to 120 hours after unprotected sex. These medications cannot interfere with a pregnancy after implantation; that is why timing is so important. Emergency contraception is not intended to be used as a primary method of contraception.

Various options exist for emergency contraception. Products containing levonorgestrel, **ulipristal (ella)**, and estradiol plus levonorgestrel are used. Levonorgestrel products include Plan B, Plan B One-Step, Aftera, EContra One-Step, My Choice, My Way, New Day, Opcicon One-Step, Preventeza, React, and Take Action. One-pill products including Plan B One-Step and Take Action, are OTC products with no age restrictions for purchase. Ulipristal (ella) is available by

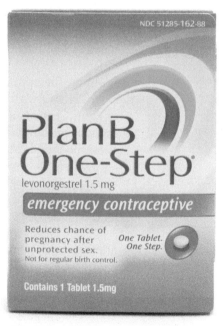

Plan B One-Step is an example of emergency contraception.

prescription only. Two-pill products such as Plan B are available by prescription. Estradiol plus levonorgestrel is not sold in a form specific to emergency contraception. This method uses commercially available oral contraceptives at increased doses.

Dosage Forms and Administration Emergency contraception is taken orally within one to five days after having unprotected sex. Most forms of emergency contraception are most effective if taken within one day of unprotected sex and lose effectiveness the longer the individual waits to take it.

Side Effects Nausea and vomiting are the most common side effects of emergency contraceptives. Antiemetic medication (meclizine or metoclopramide) can be given prior to the emergency contraceptive to reduce these side effects. If a patient vomits within three hours of taking emergency contraception, the medication should be taken again along with an antiemetic medication to reach its full effectiveness. Headache, dizziness, and abdominal pain are also possible.

Contraindications Levonorgestrel and ulipristal are contraindicated in pregnant individuals. Ulipristal should not be taken when breast-feeding. If ulipristal must be administered, then breast milk will need to be pumped and discarded for up to three days after taking the medication. Even conditions that would typically make long-term oral contraception use dangerous (clotting disorders and cardiovascular or liver disease) are not contraindicated in the short-term use of emergency contraception.

Cautions and Considerations Some medications that affect liver function can alter the effectiveness of emergency contraception. These medications may include antiseizure and antiretroviral (human immunodeficiency virus [HIV]) agents.

Drug Interactions Oral contraceptive drug interactions can be found in Table 14.5, and they refer to emergency contraceptives as well.

Ulipristal levels may be decreased by barbiturates, bosentan, efavirenz, felbamate, griseofulvin, oxcarbazepine, St. John's wort, and topiramate.

Transdermal Contraceptives

A **transdermal contraceptive** uses a stick-on patch to deliver a combination of estrogen and progesterone in a steady supply through the skin (see Table 14.4). As is true for oral contraceptives, the hormones that are delivered alter the menstrual cycle and prevent follicle maturation and ovulation. They also thicken cervical mucus, making it difficult for sperm to pass through the cervix. These agents include **ethinyl estradiol / norelgestromin (Xulane)** and **levonorgestrel / ethinyl estradiol (Twirla)**.

Dosage Forms and Administration One patch is applied each week for three weeks and then left off for one week while menstruation occurs. The patch should be replaced the same day of the week. It is placed on a clean, dry, intact area of skin on the buttock, abdomen, upper outer arm, or upper torso (not the breasts). The area of patch application should be rotated.

Side Effects Common side effects of transdermal contraceptives are similar to those of oral contraceptives and include breast tenderness, headache, irritation at the application site, nausea, menstrual cramps, and abdominal pain. These effects tend to subside with continued use. If these effects remain bothersome, an alternative contraceptive agent should be tried.

Contraindications As with all estrogen and progesterone hormone products, the benefits and risks of therapy must be weighed. Hormone therapy can increase the risk of cardiovascular events, stroke, and blood clots. Risk of blood clots is especially high for patients 35 years and older who smoke. These hormones can exacerbate depression and migraine headaches. Patients with these conditions should discuss use of hormone contraception with their healthcare practitioners.

Safety Alert

Transdermal contraceptives carry boxed warnings.

Cautions and Considerations Transdermal contraceptives carry a boxed warning for increased risk of cardiovascular disease in patients who smoke, especially those over 35 years old. Ethinyl estradiol and levonorgestrel combination patch products also have a boxed warning about the contraindication in obesity.

If the patch detaches (fully or partially) from the skin, it should be reapplied if possible. If detachment lasts for less than a day, no backup birth control is needed. If detachment lasts longer than a day, then nonhormonal methods of birth control such as a barrier method should be used for seven days. If the patch cannot be reapplied, a new patch should be used, and backup contraception should be used for seven days. A new cycle then begins, and the day to change the patch must be altered.

Drug Interactions See Table 14.5 for drug interactions.

Vaginal Contraceptives

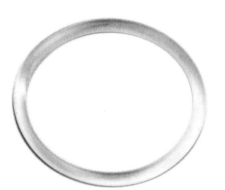

The **vaginal ring, ethinyl estradiol / etonogestrel (EluRyng, NuvaRing)**, is a combination contraceptive that contains synthetic estrogen and progesterone.

Dosage Forms and Administration The ring is inserted into the vagina, where the hormones are absorbed through the vaginal mucosa. This device is left in place for three weeks and then removed for a week while menstruation occurs.

The soft, flexible vaginal ring is compressed and inserted into the vagina to prevent ovulation.

Side Effects Common side effects of the vaginal ring include headache, nausea, vaginal secretion, vaginitis, bloating, cramps, and weight gain. Use of the vaginal ring may be associated with fewer side effects than experienced with oral contraceptives, presumably because the ring delivers a lower hormonal dose to a localized area. Side effects may subside with continued use. If the effects continue to be bothersome, patients should discontinue therapy and talk with their prescribers.

Contraindications The vaginal ring should not be used in patients with breast cancer or other estrogen- or progestin-dependent tumors, liver tumors or disease, pregnancy, or undiagnosed uterine bleeding. Patients at high risk of arterial or venous thrombosis (such as those with cerebrovascular disease, coronary artery disease, diabetes mellitus with vascular disease, deep vein thrombosis, pulmonary embolism, migraines, uncontrolled hypertension, or inherited coagulopathies and those over the age of 35 who smoke) should not use the vaginal ring.

Safety Alert

The vaginal ring carries a boxed warning for increased risk of cardiovascular disease.

Cautions and Considerations When stored in a pharmacy, vaginal rings such as the NuvaRing must be kept in the refrigerator to maintain their potency until patients pick up their prescribed products. Patients should be directed to keep their vaginal rings in the refrigerator until they plan to use them.

The vaginal ring carries a boxed warning for increased risk of cardiovascular disease in patients who smoke, especially those over 35 years old.

Drug Interactions See Table 14.5 for drug interactions.

150 mg per mL

Depo-Provera ®
Contraceptive Injection
IM

1 mL prefilled syringe (single dose)

Injectable Contraceptives

Medroxyprogesterone (Depo-Provera, Depo-SubQ Provera 104, Provera) works by inhibiting ovulation, thickening cervical mucus, and changing the endometrium to inhibit implantation.

Dosage Forms and Administration Medroxyprogesterone is an intramuscular injection given in the deltoid or gluteus maximus every three months. It is administered by a healthcare practitioner. The subcutaneous injection form is also administered by a health care provider in the back of the arm.

Side Effects Common side effects of medroxyprogesterone injection include menstrual irregularity, abdominal pain, weight changes, dizziness, headache, weakness, fatigue, and nervousness. Also possible are decreased libido, inability to achieve orgasm, pelvic pain, backache, breast pain, leg cramps, hair loss, depression, bloating, nausea, rash, insomnia, edema, hot flashes, acne, sore joints, and vaginitis. Patients should understand the risks of these potential side effects along with the benefits when choosing this long-term contraception option. Because the drug is long acting, these effects are unavoidable once they occur and will probably continue for three months.

Contraindications Patients with clotting disorders should not take medroxyprogesterone because it can increase the formation of blood clots. In addition, patients with heart or cerebral vascular disease should not take systemic contraceptive medications. A clot in a coronary or cerebral artery could be fatal.

Safety Alert

Medroxyprogesterone carries a boxed warning for bone mineral density loss.

Cautions and Considerations Medroxyprogesterone has a boxed warning related to bone mineral density loss, so it is not recommended for long-term use.

Medroxyprogesterone should not be used if conception has already occurred. For this reason, the patient may be required to take a pregnancy test before administration. It can take weeks for a normal menstrual cycle to resume after using medroxyprogesterone.

Drug Interactions Medroxyprogesterone may diminish the effectiveness of anticoagulants, diabetes medications, and aripiprazole.

Medroxyprogesterone's effectiveness may be decreased by acitretin, aprepitant, atazanavir, barbiturates, bile acid sequestrants, carbamazepine, darunavir, efavirenz, fosphenytoin, griseofulvin, lamotrigine, mifepristone, mycophenolate, phenytoin, and ulipristal.

Medroxyprogesterone may increase the blood clotting effects of tranexamic acid.

Implantable Contraceptives

Etonogestrel (Nexplanon) is an implant placed just under the skin on the inner upper arm and replaced every three years to prevent pregnancy. This product must be inserted by a healthcare practitioner. It works by inhibiting ovulation, thickening the cervical mucus, and changing the endometrium to inhibit implantation.

Dosage Forms and Administration Implantable contraceptives must be inserted by a qualified healthcare provider. This involves a provider visit during which an incision is made and the implantable device is inserted. Some bruising can be expected in the days after insertion.

Side Effects Common side effects of etonogestrel include changes in menstrual bleeding, weight gain, and mood swings. Other potential side effects include upper respiratory tract infection, vaginitis, breast pain, acne, and abdominal pain. These effects, if particularly bothersome, can be sufficient reason to have the implant removed.

Contraindications Etonogestrel should not be used if conception has already occurred. For this reason, the patient may be required to take a pregnancy test before insertion of the implant. Patients with clotting disorders should not take etonogestrel because it can increase the formation of blood clots. In addition, patients with heart or cerebrovascular disease should not take systemic contraceptive medications. A clot in a coronary or cerebral artery could be fatal.

Cautions and Considerations Because this product is a long-term option for contraception, patients should understand the risks and potential complications of using this drug. It can take three to four weeks for ovulation to resume after removing this implant.

Drug Interactions Etonogestrel may diminish the effectiveness of anticoagulants and diabetes medications.

The effectiveness of etonogestrel may be decreased by acitretin, aprepitant, atazanavir, barbiturates, bile acid sequestrants, carbamazepine, darunavir, efavirenz, fosphenytoin, griseofulvin, lamotrigine, mifepristone, mycophenolate, phenytoin, and uliprista.

Intrauterine Devices

An **intrauterine device (IUD)** is placed into the uterus by a healthcare practitioner and may stay in place for up to 10 years, depending on the product. There are several types of IUDs on the market. Some IUDs contain **levonorgestrel (Kyleena, Liletta, Mirena, Skyla)**, a hormone that alters the endometrium to prevent implantation; other IUDs contain **copper (Paragard)**.

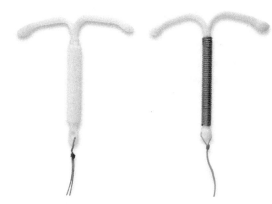

Although the exact mechanism of action is not fully understood, IUDs primarily prevent pregnancy by impeding fertilization. The presence of the IUD device in the uterus causes an inflammatory response that is toxic to sperm and ova and impairs implantation.

Dosage Forms and Administration IUDs are a device (see photo) that is surgically placed into the uterus by a healthcare provider.

Side Effects Side effects of IUDs can include spontaneous abortion (miscarriage), septicemia, pelvic infection, perforation of the uterus, vaginitis, abnormal menstrual bleeding, anemia, pain, cramping, backaches, and tubal damage. These effects can be serious and should be fully discussed and understood before patients choose this contraception method.

IUDs can contain hormones (pictured left) or copper (pictured right).

Contraindications Patients with an abnormal or distorted uterine shape, active pelvic inflammatory disease, endometriosis, Wilson's disease, or unexplained uterine bleeding should not use IUDs. Patients with breast cancer should not use an IUD that contains an active hormone (levonorgestrel). Patients with an allergy for copper should not use copper-containing IUDs.

Cautions and Considerations IUDs should not be used if conception has already occurred. For this reason, the patient may be required to take a pregnancy test before administration. An IUD is a long-term but reversible option for contraception.

Drug Interactions Copper IUDs do not contain drugs and are not associated with interactions.

Hormonal IUDs may decrease the effectiveness of other drugs, including anticoagulants and medications that lower blood glucose.

Heavy Menstrual Bleeding

If a patient's period involves a blood loss greater than 80 mL, it may be considered heavy menstrual bleeding. Many prescribers treat this with nonsteroidal anti-inflammatory drugs (NSAIDs) or an oral contraceptive to decrease cramps and bleeding. Heavy menstrual bleeding is usually caused by too little progesterone. Drugs to treat heavy menstrual bleeding are described in Table 14.6.

TABLE 14.6 Drugs to Treat Heavy Menstrual Bleeding

Generic (Brand)	Pronunciation	Dosage Form	Dosage Frequency	Dispensing Status
estradiol valerate / dienogest (Natazia)	es-tra-DYE-ole VAL-er-ate dye-EN-oh-jest	tablet	1 time a day	Rx
tranexamic acid (Lysteda)	tran-eks-AM-ik AS-id	injection, tablet	PO: 2–3 times a day SC: first 5 days of cycle	Rx

Estradiol valerate / dienogest (Natazia) reduces blood loss by about 50% and is the first OC approved to treat this problem. It has antiandrogenic effects. The drug requires a four-phase regimen. Estradiol is decreased as dienogest is increased during the cycle to prevent breakthrough bleeding. This regimen has four estrogen-only tablets each cycle instead of the hormone-free period of other oral contraceptives.

Tranexamic acid (Lysteda) is a synthetic antifibrinolytic drug. It prevents the binding of fibrin (a protein involved in the clotting of blood) and plasmin (an enzyme that dissolves the fibrin of blood clots) in a reversible manner. This drug should be taken for five days during menstruation. Any vision changes should be reported immediately because such symptoms could signal clotting within the retina.

Dosage Forms and Administration Estradiol valerate / dienogest is taken orally one time a day. Tranexamic acid is taken orally two or three times a day or injected for the first five days of menstrual bleeding. Oral dosage forms should not be crushed or chewed. Tranexamic acid should not be taken for longer than five days.

Side Effects Side effects of estradiol / dienogest are similar to those described earlier in this chapter for oral contraceptives. Taking it after the evening meal or at bedtime can reduce nausea.

Side effects of tranexamic acid include nausea, vomiting, diarrhea, and muscle pain. Serious side effects include changes in eyesight, fainting, coughing up blood, pain in the groin or calf, and swelling or weakness in the arms or legs. These effects suggest a blood clot could be forming. Patients experiencing these effects should seek care immediately.

Contraindications Estradiol / dienogest is contraindicated in breast cancer or other estrogen- or progestin-dependent tumors, liver disease, pregnancy, undiagnosed abnormal uterine bleeding, and patients at high risk of arterial or venous thrombotic disease.

Tranexamic acid injection is contraindicated in patients with acquired defective color vision, active blood clotting, and subarachnoid hemorrhage. Oral tranexamic acid should not be used in patients with active thromboembolic disease or risk of thrombosis, or with concurrent use of combination OCs.

Cautions and Considerations Patients with a history of breast, endometrial, ovarian, or cervical cancer should discuss the risks and benefits of estradiol / dienogest with their healthcare practitioners. Some controversy exists about whether

Safety Alert

These agents carry a boxed warning for increased risk of cardiovascular disease in patients who smoke.

estradiol / dienogest increases patients' risk for these types of cancer, so patients should make informed decisions about their own care.

Tranexamic acid is associated with visual defects. If visual changes are noted, patients should discontinue use. Clotting has been reported with tranexamic acid use.

Estradiol valerate / dienogest and tranexamic acid carry a boxed warning for increased risk of cardiovascular disease in patients who smoke, especially those over the age of 35.

Drug Interactions Estradiol / dienogest interactions are the same as those for OCs and can be found in Table 14.5.

OCs and tretinoin may increase the thrombotic effects of tranexamic acid.

14.5 Pregnancy, Childbirth, and Drug Treatments

Childbirth poses dangers to both the pregnant parent and child, and death or serious injury is not uncommon. Even during relatively uncomplicated deliveries, childbirth may be extremely painful for the person giving birth. With the advent of modern medicine and pharmaceutical products, pregnant patients and their healthcare providers have numerous tools at their disposal. For uncomplicated deliveries, pregnant patients may choose not to use drugs, though they are available to control pain. For emergency situations, however, drugs are necessary. If labor ceases, use of a drug that induces labor could prevent the need for a caesarean section (C-section). If a C-section is performed, other drugs are involved. If uncontrolled bleeding occurs, drugs are usually indicated. Table 14.7 lists the drugs most commonly used during childbirth.

TABLE 14.7 Common Agents Used during Childbirth

Generic (Brand)	Pronunciation	Dosage Form	Common Dosage	Dispensing Status
Induction Agents				
dinoprostone (Cervidil, Prepidil, Prostin E2)	dye-noe-PROST-oan	vaginal gel, vaginal insert, suppository	individualized to patient	Rx
misoprostol (Cytotec)	mye-soe-PROS-tawl	tablet	individualized to patient	Rx
oxytocin (Pitocin)	ox-i-TOE-sin	injection	individualized to patient	Rx
Tocolytic Agents				
indomethacin (Indocin, Tivorbex)	in-doe-METH-a-sin	capsule, oral suspension, suppository	individualized to patient	Rx
magnesium sulfate	mag-knee-ZEE-um SUL-fate	injection	individualized to patient	Rx
nifedipine (Procardia)	nye-FED-i-peen	capsule, tablet	individualized to patient	Rx

Work Wise

Pharmacy technicians may not counsel patients on how to use a pregnancy test. If there are any questions, technicians should refer patients to the pharmacist.

Pregnancy Tests and Pregnancy

Detecting a pregnancy early allows a pregnant individual to make informed lifestyle decisions and seek appropriate healthcare resources for an optimal outcome. Critical organ systems develop during the first month of embryogenesis; these systems are affected by components of the pregnant individual's diet (such as vitamins and caffeine) and environment (such as smoking) and by their medications. Early confirmation of pregnancy allows for earlier prenatal care, earlier detection of an ectopic pregnancy (a potentially life-threatening condition), and more time for counseling and consideration of alternatives.

Pregnancy tests detect **human chorionic gonadotropic (hCG)**, a hormone produced by the cell mass that forms after the fertilized egg develops and starts to form an embryo and placenta. Because hCG levels can be measured as early as six to eight days after conception, a person can test for pregnancy after the first day of a missed menstrual period (depending on the test used). All currently marketed tests detect hCG with monoclonal antibodies (MCAs) specific for the hormone. A chromogen-reactive enzyme linked to one of the antibodies changes color in the presence of hCG, indicating pregnancy. MCA tests provide results in one to five minutes. These tests differ in the time and number of steps required to complete them, the clarity of instructions, and the ease with which their results can be determined. Consumers generally achieve better than 95% accuracy with home pregnancy tests. Brand names of pregnancy tests include First Response, e.p.t., and Clearblue.

To use a pregnancy test properly, a patient should take the following steps:

1. Check the expiration date.
2. Read the instructions twice.
3. Wait the recommended number of days after the first day of their last menstrual period.
4. Collect the sample from the first morning urine.
5. If the urine is collected in a container, the container should be clean. A plastic or waxed paper cup should not be used.
6. If the test cannot be done immediately, the urine should be refrigerated. The patient should be sure to set the container of urine in a room-temperature location 20 to 30 minutes before the test is performed.
7. If the test is positive, the patient should make an appointment to see a doctor.
8. If the test is negative, the patient should wait three to five days. If menstruation does not begin, they should perform the test again. If the second test is negative and menstruation has not started, the patient should see a doctor.

False-negative test results can occur due to chilled urine, chilled test reagents, diluted urine, or high-dose pancreatic enzyme replacement. False-positive results can occur due to collecting the urine in a waxed paper cup, an undetected miscarriage or recent abortion, or elevated levels of hCG (e.g., due to a tumor).

Sexually active individuals who may have the ability to become pregnant should make sure they get the daily requirements of folic acid, iron, and calcium. It is common for a person to become pregnant but to remain unaware of the pregnancy for some time, and these three substances are very important in the formation of a fetus. Folic acid prevents neural tube defects; iron prevents anemia, preterm delivery, and low birth weight in infants; and calcium is important for bone development.

Drugs Used to Slow Labor

A drug used to slow labor is called a **tocolytic agent**. Very few tocolytic agents are available. These agents are considered specialty use.

Indomethacin (Indocin, Tivorbex) is a prostaglandin inhibitor and NSAID used as a tocolytic agent. Prostaglandin normally stimulates uterine contractions and causes cervical ripening (softening to permit delivery). Prostaglandin inhibitors inhibit the synthesis of prostaglandins.

Magnesium sulfate is used to prevent seizures in preeclampsia or eclampsia (caused by hypertension) during pregnancy. It has a tocolytic effect (slows uterine contraction) and is also used frequently for this purpose.

Nifedipine (Procardia) is a calcium channel blocker (see Chapter 12) used as a tocolytic agent. It relaxes smooth muscle.

Dosage Forms and Administration Tocolytic agents are administered and monitored closely by a healthcare provider, usually in an inpatient setting. Nifedipine is available as a soft capsule that contains 10 or 20 mg of nifedipine. The capsule is punctured and placed under the tongue so that the drug is absorbed more quickly.

Side Effects Side effects of tocolytic agents include dizziness, headache, and nausea. Nifedipine and magnesium sulfate may cause flushing. Nifedipine can also cause heartburn and peripheral edema.

Contraindications Indomethacin is contraindicated in pregnant patients with bleeding disorders, hepatic or renal impairment, or gastrointestinal ulcers. Magnesium sulfate should not be used in patients with myasthenia gravis or neuromuscular disorders.

Safety Alert

Indomethacin has a boxed warning about increased risk of gastrointestinal bleeding, heart attack, and stroke.

Cautions and Considerations Indomethacin, like other NSAIDs, contains multiple boxed warnings related to cardiovascular and gastrointestinal risks. Indomethacin is contraindicated in patients with a history of hypersensitivity, urticaria, and asthma. Magnesium sulfate has severe consequences when used in error. It is a high-alert drug, so special care must be taken when dispensing this intravenous drug. Nifedipine is contraindicated in patients with hypersensitivity to calcium channel blockers.

Drug Interactions NSAIDs, nifedipine, and magnesium interact with several other medications, some of which are contraindicated in pregnancy. Orders for these medications to slow labor should be checked carefully by the pharmacist to assure safe and effective use.

Drugs Used to Induce Labor

Safety Alert

An order for oxytocin might be confused for oxygen.

Labor induction is the process of stimulating uterine contractions to speed the onset of labor. Inducing labor may be indicated in pregnancies that last longer than 39 weeks, prelabor rupture of membranes, fetal demise, diabetes in the pregnant person, and delivery of twins. Both pharmacologic and nonpharmacologic strategies may be used.

Dinoprostone (Cervidil, Prepidil, Prostin E2) promotes cervical ripening in patients when there is medical or obstetrical indication for the induction of labor. Prepidil is a gel that is packaged in a syringe. Prostin E is a suppository in a foil wrapper. Cervidil is a vaginal insert with a string attached so that it can be removed at the appropriate time.

Misoprostol (Cytotec) is also used for cervical ripening. It is a prostaglandin E analog and is also used for labor induction. The tablets are usually cut into halves or quarters and inserted into the vagina. Pregnant women should not touch misoprostol because it can induce premature labor.

Oxytocin (Pitocin) is a synthetic duplicate of a natural hormone secreted by the posterior lobe of the pituitary gland. The hormone stimulates the contraction of uterine smooth muscle at term, when uterine muscle is most sensitive to the hormone. Such a drug is called an **oxytocic agent**. Side effects for the pregnant patient may include vomiting, irregular heart rate, tachycardia, and postpartum bleeding. The child may experience bradycardia, arrhythmias, and jaundice. This drug should be used as a last resort.

Dosage Forms and Administration These medications may be self-administered or applied by a healthcare provider, depending on where the patient is in the progression of labor and delivery.

Side Effects Side effects of these products vary and will be monitored by the patient's healthcare provider.

Contraindications Dinoprostone is contraindicated in cases where vaginal delivery is contraindicated.

Misoprostol should not be given to patients with hypersensitivity to prostaglandins.

Oxytocin is contraindicated in pregnant patients with unfavorable fetal positions, fetal distress, hypertonic or hyperactive uterus, or contraindications to vaginal delivery. It is also contraindicated in emergencies in which surgical intervention is preferred and adequate uterine activity fails to achieve progress.

Safety Alert

Each of these agents carry boxed warnings and should be used with extreme caution.

Cautions and Considerations Dinoprostone has boxed warnings to be used only by an experienced physician and to adhere strictly to dosage recommendations.

Misoprostol also carries boxed warnings. It can result in abortion, premature birth, or birth defects. It should not be used to reduce the risk of NSAID-induced ulcers in patients of childbearing potential.

Oxytocin has a boxed warning that it should not be used for elective induction of labor.

Drug Interactions Dinoprostone may enhance the adverse effects of carbetocin and oxytocin.

Antacids may enhance the adverse effects of misoprostol.

Misoprostol may enhance the adverse effects of oxytocin agents. Oxytocin may cause QT prolongation and should be used cautiously with other agents that may prolong the QT interval.

14.6 Growth Disorders and Drug Treatments

Growth rates vary by sex and age throughout childhood. Growth delay may be caused by various factors, including family growth patterns, genetic disorders, malnutrition, systemic or chronic illness, psychosocial stress, or a combination of these. In addition, growth delay may be due to an endocrine deficiency. Thyroxine, cortisol, insulin, and growth hormone all affect skeletal and somatic growth.

Nonendocrine-related disorders that can cause growth delay include intrauterine growth retardation, chromosomal defects, abnormal growth of cartilage or bone, poor nutrition, and a variety of systemic diseases. Some patients show a variation from normal growth (constitutional growth delay); these patients include those who are small for their age and those who have delay in skeletal growth, in the onset of puberty, and in adolescent development. Another type of growth delay is a family trait (in other words, it is inherited). These patients are shorter than their peers but are comparable in height with other family members and grow at a parallel rate. Puberty occurs at the expected time and progresses as usual. However, adult height is short.

Growth Hormone

From childhood to adulthood, **growth hormone (GH)** plays a fundamental role in metabolism. Measurements of height and weight over time serve as an index of physical and emotional health. Growth failure is a well-recognized disorder of childhood. In many children, a deficiency of endogenous growth hormone causes retardation of growth, which may be treated with exogenous hormone replacement.

Growth hormone is a mixture of peptides (short protein molecules) from the anterior pituitary gland released in response to **growth hormone–releasing factor (GHRF)**. The major component is the peptide somatotropin. The pituitary releases GH in response to stimulation by GHRF, a neuropeptide secreted by the hypothalamus. GH release occurs irregularly throughout the day and during sleep stages III and IV (the deepest stages of non-REM sleep). GH stimulates the growth of skeletal muscle and connective tissue. It increases the rate of protein synthesis and fatty acid mobilization from adipose tissue and decreases the rate of glucose utilization. It is inhibited by glucocorticoids, obesity, depression, progesterone, hypokalemia, and altered thyroid function.

Growth Hormone Deficiency

Growth hormone deficiency, a disorder that occurs when the pituitary gland does not produce enough growth hormone, affects 1 in 5,000 children. Among the known causes are intracranial infection (from tuberculosis and meningitis), skull fracture, radiation, and cancer. This disorder can be treated by the administration of somatropin or other growth promotion agents.

Name Exchange

Pharmacy personnel should be careful not to confuse somatotropin (growth hormone) and somatropin (the drug).

Somatropin

Originally, **somatotropin** (as GH is called when produced naturally by the human body) was recovered from the pituitaries of human cadavers, a process that required 20 to 30 cadavers to obtain sufficient hormone to treat one patient. Today, the drug **somatropin (Genotropin, Humatrope, Omnitrope, Saizen, Serostim, Zomacton, Zorbtive)** is supplied through recombinant DNA technology. Genetic material from human cells is inserted into microorganisms, which then reproduce with the added genes and produce the hormone. The hormone is recovered, purified, and packaged. Table 14.8 presents the synthetic human growth hormone most commonly used as a growth-promotion agent.

TABLE 14.8 Commonly Used Synthetic Human Growth Hormone

Generic (Brand)	Pronunciation	Dosage Form	Dispensing Status
somatropin (Genotropin, Humatrope, Omnitrope, Saizen, Serostim, Zomacton, Zorbtive)	soe-ma-TROE-pin	injection	Rx

GH replacement therapy is most successful when begun at a young age. That is, the younger the patient at the time of GH treatment, the greater the height that may be achieved through replacement. Bone age and the extent of epiphyseal fusion at the time of treatment also influence the eventual response to GH. GH treatment is minimally effective if employed after ages 15 to 16 in males or 14 to 15 in females. Approximately 80%–90% of patients who receive GH experience "catch up" growth. Maximum increases in growth occur within the first 6 to 12 months of therapy, with a decline in response after that. GH therapy should be continued throughout childhood and adolescence to prevent slowing of growth velocity. When epiphyseal closure has occurred, little further response takes place. Treatment duration usually ranges from 2 to 10 years. GH has not been effective for patients under the following conditions: short stature among other family members; growth retardation associated with psychosocial dwarfism; steroid-induced short stature; Down syndrome; bone and cartilage disorders; or renal, GI, or cardiac disease.

Dosage Forms and Administration Growth hormone is administered by a healthcare professional.

Side Effects Common side effects of growth hormone include joint and muscle pain, swelling, and breast tissue growth. Growth hormone is also associated with type 2 diabetes, carpal tunnel syndrome, and some forms of cancer. Patients should speak with their healthcare provider to discuss the risks and benefits.

Contraindications Somatropin is contraindicated in pediatric patients with closed epiphyses, progression or recurrence of any underlying intracranial lesion or actively growing intracranial tumor, acute critical illness, acute respiratory failure, evidence of active malignancy, or active diabetes-related retinopathy. Patients with Prader-Willi syndrome who are obese, have a history of airway obstruction, or have a respiratory impairment also should not receive somatropin.

Cautions and Considerations Somatropin should be used with caution in patients with diabetes or with risk factors for impaired glucose tolerance. Insulin sensitivity may be decreased.

Intracranial hypertension has been reported with somatropin use. Fluid retention may also occur with use.

Scoliosis may progress in patients using somatropin who experience rapid growth.

Some somatropin formulations may contain benzyl alcohol. Large amounts of benzyl alcohol may be associated with neonatal gasping syndrome.

Hypothyroidism has been observed in less than 5% of treated patients. Thyroid supplementation is unnecessary, however, unless the patient has thyroid deficiency during treatment. The hypothyroidism appears to result from a change in the conversion of thyroxine or thyroid-controlling hormone rather than a true deficiency.

Drug Interactions Somatropin may decrease the hypoglycemic effect of diabetes medications. Cortisone and prednisone effectiveness may be diminished by somatropin use. Estrogen derivatives may decrease the effectiveness of somatropin.

14.7 Complementary and Alternative Therapies

Hormonal disorders are often treated with complementary and alternative medicine.

Soy, also known as *isoflavone* or **phytoestrogen**, is a plant source of protein used to treat several conditions. In the United States, it is used most frequently for hot flashes associated with menopause. Soy is a source of fiber and protein found most commonly in milk and dairy substitutes. It can be obtained from dietary sources alone or from a combination of food and oral supplements. It has estrogenic effects that can be beneficial for menopausal symptoms, diabetes, high cholesterol, osteoporosis, kidney disease, and, possibly, breast cancer prevention. Soy is usually well tolerated but can cause upset stomach, diarrhea, constipation, bloating, nausea, and even insomnia in some cases. It can also worsen migraine headaches, especially for patients whose headaches are related to hormonal fluctuations of the menstrual cycle.

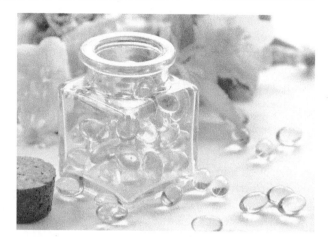

Evening primrose oil is available as a liquid and capsules, as pictured.

Black cohosh is a plant product with estrogenic effects used for menopausal symptoms such as hot flashes. It is sometimes used in combination with St. John's wort for psychological symptoms that may be associated with menopause, such as depression and mood swings. Studies have not produced standard dosing, so success varies. Side effects of black cohosh include upset stomach, rash, headache, dizziness, weight gain, cramping, breast tenderness, and vaginal spotting (bleeding). Some concern exists about black cohosh and liver disease because some patients have experienced symptoms similar to those of hepatitis after taking black cohosh. Patients with liver disease and those who are pregnant or breast-feeding should avoid black cohosh.

Evening primrose oil is sometimes used to reduce symptoms of menopause or premenstrual syndrome. However, studies have found mixed results and do not currently support its effectiveness for these conditions. Evidence for the use of evening primrose oil for osteoporosis is also mixed. It is considered safe to take, and few side effects have been reported.

Wild yam, also called *Mexican yam*, contains a phytoestrogen similar to soy, and it has mild estrogenic effects. It is applied topically or ingested orally as a tincture. Some patients use it for menopausal symptoms such as hot flashes. Published research does not recommend a formulation or dose that is consistently effective. Ingestion of large amounts can cause vomiting. More research is needed to determine the clinical usefulness of wild yam.

Review and Assessment

CHAPTER SUMMARY

The Reproductive System and Related Hormones

- Progestins are used primarily in oral contraceptive pills and to prevent uterine cancer in postmenopausal patients taking hormone replacement therapy (HRT).

Hormone Replacement Therapy

- Testosterone undergoes extensive first-pass metabolism in the gastrointestinal tract and liver after oral administration. To overcome this problem, various testosterone derivatives and innovative dosage forms have been developed.

- The side effects of progestin are acne, depression, fatigue, and weight gain.

- The side effects of estrogen include dizziness, abdominal pain or bloating, diarrhea, nausea, headache, breast tenderness, vaginal discharge, fluid retention, hair loss, and depression.

- The decision to take HRT for menopausal symptoms is personal and requires consultation between the patient and their physician. The advantages must be weighed against the disadvantages, taking into consideration family history and physical condition.

- Gender transition can include social transition (such as changes in clothing, name, or pronouns); as well as physical transitions, which may include gender-affirming hormone therapy or other medical or surgical interventions.

Sexual Dysfunction

- Erectile dysfunction (ED) has many causes, including testosterone deficiency, alcoholism, cigarette smoking, medications, and psychological factors.

- The following drugs may cause ED: alcohol, amphetamines, antidepressants, antihypertensives, corticosteroids, estrogens, H_2 blockers, haloperidol, lithium, and opiates.

- ED is treated primarily with the phosphodiesterase-5 inhibitors sildenafil (Viagra), tadalafil (Cialis), and vardenafil (Levitra).

- Sexual dysfunction can take different forms, including decreased desire, reduced arousal, anorgasmia (inability to achieve orgasm), and pain.

- Fibanserin is a drug used for sexual dysfunction.

Contraceptives and Drug Treatments

- The advantages of oral contraceptives include ease of use, high efficacy rate, and relative safety.

- Most oral contraceptives are a combination of estrogen and progestin. They suppress ovulation by interfering with the production of hormones that regulate the menstrual cycle. They also alter the cervical mucus to prevent penetration of sperm, and they change the composition of the endometrium to inhibit implantation. The progestin-only pills rely on the effects of progestin on the cervical mucus and endometrium. They also inhibit the secretion of LH, which causes egg release.

- Patients should not smoke while taking oral contraceptives.

- Many forms of contraceptives are on the market. They are available in pill form, patches, vaginal rings, injections, implants, and intrauterine devices.

- Emergency contraceptives are available over the counter and by prescription.

- Oral contraceptives can interact with the following classes of drugs: antibiotics, anticonvulsants, antifungals, benzodiazepines, bronchodilators, corticosteroids, lipid-lowering agents, and tricyclic antidepressants (TCAs).

Pregnancy, Childbirth, and Drug Treatments

- Pregnancy tests detect the presence of the hormone human chorionic gonadotropin (hCG).

- Agents are available to slow labor and induce labor.

Growth Disorders

- Measurement of height and weight over time serves as an index of physical and emotional health. A deficiency of growth hormone causes growth failure.

- Human growth hormone is manufactured with recombinant DNA technology.

- Once epiphyseal closure has occurred, little further response to GH treatment can be expected.

Complementary and Alternative Therapies

- Plant products such as soy, black cohosh, and wild yams have varying estrogenic effects that may be beneficial for menopausal symptoms.

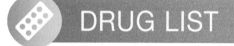 # DRUG LIST

Drugs to Treat Erectile Dysfunction
alprostadil (Caverject, Edex, Muse)
avanafil (Stendra)
fibanserin (Addyi)
sildenafil (Viagra)
tadalafil (Cialis)
testosterone (Androderm, AndroGel, Aveed, Axiron, Depo-Testosterone, Fortesta, Testopel)
vardenafil (Levitra)

Hormone Replacement Therapy Products

Testosterone-Only Hormone Therapy Product
testosterone (Androderm, AndroGel, Aveed, Axiron, Depo-Testosterone, Fortesta, Testopel)

Estrogen-Only Hormone Therapy Products
conjugated estrogen (Premarin)
estradiol (Alora, Climara, Dotti, Elestrin, Estrace, Estring, EstroGel, Evamist, Femring, Menostar, Minivelle, Vagifem, Vivelle-Dot)

Projestin-Only Hormone Therapy Product
progesterone (Crinone, Endometrin, First-Progesterone, Prometrium)

Estrogen / Progestin Hormone Therapy Products
conjugated estrogen / medroxyprogesterone (Premphase, Prempro)
estradiol / drospirenone (Angeliq)
estradiol / levonorgestrel (Climara Pro)
estradiol / norethindrone (Activella, CombiPatch)

estradiol / norgestimate (Prefest)

ethinyl / estradiol / norethindrone (Activella,
Amabelz, Angeliq, Bijuva, Femhrt,
Fyavolv, Jinteli, Lopreeza, Mimvey, Prefest,
Premphase, Prempro)

Masculinizing Hormone Therapy

testosterone cypionate (Depo-Testosterone)

testosterone enanthate (Xyosted)

testosterone (AndroGel, Fortesta, Testim,
Vogelxo, Androderm)

testosterone (Testopel)

Feminizing Hormone Therapy

estradiol (Alora, Climara, Dotti, Elestrin,
Estrace, Estring, EstroGel, Evamist,
Femring, Menostar, Minivelle, Vagifem,
Vivelle-Dot)

estradiol (Estrace)

estradiol cypionate (Depo-Estradiol)

estradiol valerate (Delestrogen)

progesterone (Prometrium)

Antiandrogen

spironolactone (Aldactone)

Contraceptives

Combination Oral Contraceptives

ethinyl estradiol / desogestrel (Apri,
Azurette, Caziant, Cyclessa, Desogen,
Emoquette, Enskyce, Kariva, Mirecette,
Orth-Cept, Reclipsen, Solia, Velivet,
Viorele)

ethinyl estradiol / drospirenone (Beyaz,
Gianvi, Loryna, Nikki, Ocella, Syeda,
Vestura, Yasmin 28, Yaz, Zarah)

ethinyl estradiol / ethynodiol diacetate
(Kelnor, Zovia)

ethinyl estradiol / levonorgestrel (Altavera,
Amethia, Amethyst, Aviane, Camrese,
Enpresse, Falmina, Introvale, Jolessa,
Lessina, Levora, Lutera, Lybrel, Marlissa,
Myzilra, Orsythia, Portia, Quasense,
Quartette, Seasonique, Trivora)

ethinyl estradiol / norethindrone (Alyacen,
Aranelle, Balziva, Briellyn, Cyclafem,
Dasetta, Leena, Necon, Nortrel, Philith,
Pirmella, Vyfemla, Wera)

ethinyl estradiol / norgestimate
(MonoNessa, Ortho-Cyclen, Ortho-
TriCyclen, Ortho-TriCyclen Lo, Previfem,
Sprintec, TriNessa, Tri-Previfem,
Tri-Sprintec)

ethinyl estradiol / norgestrel (Cryselle 28,
Elinest, Low-Ogestrel, Norgestrel, Ogestrel,
Ovral)

Progestin-Only Oral Contraceptive

norethindrone (Camila, Errin, Heather,
Jolivette, Lyza, Micronor, Nora-BE,
Nor-QD)

Emergency Contraceptives

levonorgestrel (Plan B, Plan B One-Step,
Next Choice, Next Choice One Dose, Take
Action)

ulipristal (ella)

Other Hormonal Contraceptives

ethinyl estradiol / etonogestrel (NuvaRing)

ethinyl estradiol / norelgestromin (Ortho
Evra)

levonorgestrel / ethinyl estradiol (Twirla)

medroxyprogesterone (Depo-Provera,
Provera)

Implantable Contraceptive

etonogestrel (Implanon)

Intrauterine Devices

copper (Paragard)

levonorgestrel (Liletta, Mirena, Skyla)

Drugs Used for Heavy Menstrual Bleeding

estradiol / dienogest (Natazia)

tranexamic acid (Lysteda)

Drugs for Pregnancy and Childbirth

dinoprostone (Cervidil, Prepidil,
Prostin E)

indomethacin (Indocin, Tivorbex)

magnesium sulfate

misoprostol (Cytotec)

nifedipine (Procardia)

oxytocin (Pitocin)

Synthetic Human Growth Hormones

somatropin (Genotropin, Humatrope,
Omnitrope, Saizen, Serostim, Zomacton,
Zorbtive)

Boxed Warnings

alprostadil (Caverject)

conjugated estrogen (Cenestin, Enjuvia,
Premarin)

conjugated estrogen / medroxyprogesterone
(Premphase, Prempro)

dinoprostone (Cervidil, Prepidil, Prostin E)

estradiol (Alora, Climara, Divigel, Elestrin,

Estrogel, Estring, Evamist, Femring, Menostar, Minivelle, Vivelle, Vivelle-Dot)
estradiol / drospirenone (Angeliq)
estradiol / levonorgestrol (Climara Pro)
estradiol / norethindrone (Activella, CombiPatch)
estradiol / norgestimate (Prefest)
estropipate (Ogen, Ortho-Est)
ethinyl estradiol (Estinyl)
ethinyl estradiol / desogestrel (Apri, Azurette, Caziant, Cyclessa, Desogen, Emoquette, Enskyce, Kariva, Mirecette, Orth-Cept, Reclipsen, Solia, Velivet, Viorele)
ethinyl estradiol / drospirenone (Gianvi, Loryna, Nikki, Ocella, Safyral, Syeda, Vestura, Yasmin 28, Yaz, Zarah)
ethinyl estradiol / ethynodiol diacetate (Kelnor, Zovia)
ethinyl estradiol / etonogestrel (NuvaRing)
ethinyl estradiol / levonorgestrel (Traditional: Altavera, Amethyst, Aviane, Enpresse, Falmina, Lessina, Levora, Lutera, Lybrel, Marlissa, Myzilra, Orsythia, Portia, Trivora; Extended combinations: Amethia, Camrese, Introvale, Jolessa, Quasense, Quartette, Seasonique)
ethinyl estradiol / norethindrone (Alyacen, Aranelle, Balziva, Briellyn, Cyclafem, Dasetta, Leena, Necon, Nortrel, Philith, Pirmella, Vyfemla, Wera)
ethinyl estradiol / norgestimate (MonoNessa, Ortho-Cyclen, Ortho-TriCyclen, Ortho-TriCyclen Lo, Previfem, Sprintec, TriNessa, Tri-Previfem, Tri-Sprintec)
ethinyl estradiol / norgestrel (Cryselle 28, Elinest, Low-Ogestrel, Norgestrel, Ogestrel, Ovral)
flibanserin (Addyi)
levonorgestrel (Next Choice, Norplant, Norplant II, One Step, Plan B)
medroxyprogesterone (Depo-Provera, Provera)
misoprostol (Cytotec)
oxytocin (Pitocin)
progesterone (Crinone, Endometrin, First-Progesterone Prometrium)
testosterone (Androderm, AndroGel, Aveed, Axiron, Depo-Testosterone, Fortesta, Testopel)

Medication Guides
flibanserin (Addyi)
testosterone (Androderm, AndroGel, Aveed, Axiron, Depo-Testosterone, Fortesta, Testopel)

✓ CHECK YOUR UNDERSTANDING

Take a moment to review what you have learned in this chapter and answer the following questions.

1. Which of the following hormones promotes development and maintenance of typically masculine physical characteristics?
   a. estrogen
   b. phosphodiesterase
   c. progesterone
   d. testosterone

2. Which of the following drugs is contraindicated in patients who take nitrates?
   a. tadalafil
   b. estradiol / drospirenone
   c. norethindrone
   d. oxytocin

3. Which of the following drugs is used to induce labor?
   a. somatropin
   b. misoprostol
   c. alprostadil
   d. estradiol

4. Which of the following drugs is found in both NuvaRing and Nexplanon?
   a. levonorgestrel
   b. etonogestrel
   c. medroxyprogesterone
   d. norethindrone

5. A patient with a history of a blood clotting disorder should not take which of the following drugs?
   a. flibanserin
   b. phosphodiesterase-5 inhibitor
   c. ethinyl estradiol / levonorgestrel
   d. somatropin

6. Which of the following drug classes does not interact with oral contraceptives?
   a. anticonvulsants
   b. antibiotics
   c. tricyclic antidepressants
   d. antihypertensives

7. Which of the following is a barrier method of birth control that covers the cervical opening and prevents sperm from entering the uterus?
   a. external condom
   b. internal condom
   c. diaphragm
   d. vaginal ring

8. Which of the following drugs can be used to suppress effects of androgens during gender-affirming therapy?
   a. estradiol valerate
   b. progesterone
   c. spironolactone
   d. levonorgestrel

9. Which of the following drug combinations is *not* found in *oral* contraceptives?
   a. ethinyl estradiol / drosperinone
   b. ethinyl estradiol / norgestrel
   c. ethinyl estradiol / desogestrel
   d. ethinyl estradiol / etonogestrel

10. Which of the following is available in a transdermal patch dosage form?
    a. conjugated estrogen
    b. estradiol / levonorgestrel
    c. progesterone
    d. vardenafil

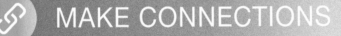

MAKE CONNECTIONS

Take a moment to consider what you have learned in this chapter and respond thoughtfully to the following prompts. Note that some of these activities will require internet access.

1. A patient requests a refill of their oral contraceptive while dropping off a new prescription for amoxicillin. The pharmacist wants you to let her know when the patient arrives so she can counsel on proper use of these medications together. Why?

2. Why should patients limit the length of use of estrogen hormone replacement therapy in treating symptoms of menopause? Is the same precaution applicable for a patient who has had a hysterectomy? Explain why or why not.

The online course includes additional review and assessment resources.

The Renal System and Drug Therapy

Learning Objectives

1 Describe the anatomy and physiology of the renal system. (Section 15.1)

2 Describe renal system dysfunction and assessment of renal function. (Section 15.2)

3 List antibiotics used to treat urinary tract infections. (Section 15.3)

4 Describe the indication, dosage and administration, side effects, contraindications, and cautions and considerations of phenazopyridine. (Section 15.3)

5 List agents used to treat urinary incontinence and describe their dosage and administration, side effects, contraindications, and cautions and considerations. (Section 15.4)

6 Compare and contrast alpha-blockers and 5-alpha-reductase inhibitors for the treatment of benign prostatic hyperplasia. (Section 15.5)

7 Describe chronic kidney disease. (Section 15.6)

8 Describe drug classes commonly used for adjunct therapy in the treatment of chronic kidney disease and list their dosage and administration, side effects, contraindications, and cautions and considerations. (Section 15.6)

9 State common causes of anemia. (Section 15.7)

10 Identify commonly used erythropoietin-stimulating agents and their boxed warnings. (Section 15.7)

11 List oral and parenteral iron supplements and list their dosage and administration, side effects, contraindications, and cautions and considerations. (Section 15.7)

12 Summarize drug classes commonly used to treat patients who have advanced chronic kidney disease and are undergoing dialysis. (Section 15.8, 15.9)

13 State commonly used immunosuppressants prescribed for patients who have end-stage chronic kidney disease and have undergone kidney transplantation. (Section 15.9)

14 List complementary and alternative therapies used for the treatment of renal disorders. (Section 15.10)

ASHP/ACPE Accreditation Standards

To view the *ASHP/ACPE Accreditation Standards* addressed in this chapter, refer to Appendix C.

The kidneys, ureters, bladder, and urethra are components of the **renal system**, also known as the *urinary system*. Because the renal system is responsible for filtering and eliminating waste products from the body, any disorders of the renal system can upset the body's delicate balance and result in many serious health problems. In addition to filtering waste products, the renal system filters most drugs and their metabolites, which makes this body system of utmost importance when studying pharmacology.

Therefore, patients who have impaired renal function are also at risk for drug accumulation and toxicity and must undergo regular laboratory blood tests to ensure that their drug levels remain within a therapeutic range.

This chapter addresses disorders related to the renal system, including urinary tract infections, incontinence, benign prostatic hyperplasia, kidney disease (acute, chronic, and end-stage), anemia, and kidney transplant. Drug therapy for the renal system is varied. Some drugs, such as urinary analgesics, antimuscarinics, erythropoietin-stimulating agents, phosphate binders, and calcimimetics, are more specific to the renal system. Other drugs—such as alpha-blockers; 5-alpha-reductase inhibitors; diuretics; iron, folic acid, and vitamin D supplements; and immunosuppressants—are used for indications in various body systems.

15.1 Anatomy and Physiology of the Renal System

The renal system (see Figure 15.1), also called the *urinary system*, is responsible for filtering and clearing metabolic by-products and waste products from the blood while maintaining the body's proper fluid, pH, and electrolyte balance. If these waste products are not eliminated from the body, they build up and become toxic.

FIGURE 15.1
The Renal System

The renal system includes the kidneys, important organs that maintain the balance of water, electrolytes, and acids and bases in extracellular fluid.

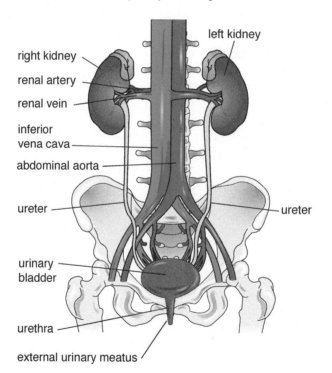

right kidney
renal artery
renal vein
inferior vena cava
abdominal aorta
ureter
urinary bladder
urethra
external urinary meatus
left kidney
ureter

The kidneys are the primary organs for this waste **filtration** process, commonly referred to as **elimination**. Blood flows through the kidneys, which filter these waste products and produce **urine**, a modified filtrate of plasma. Urine formation is essential for normal body function because it enables the blood to reabsorb necessary nutrients, water, and electrolytes. Large molecules, such as plasma proteins, cannot cross the glomerular basement membranes (the barrier that separates the vasculature from the urinary space) to be filtered from the blood, whereas small molecules—such as water, ions, and glucose—do pass through the membranes to be reabsorbed later into the blood.

In the process of urine formation, the kidneys regulate the following metabolic functions:

- volume of blood plasma, which contributes significantly to the regulation of blood pressure
- concentration of waste products in the blood
- concentration of electrolytes in plasma, such as sodium (Na^+), potassium (K^+), bicarbonate (HCO_3^-), calcium (Ca^{2+}), and phosphate (PO_4^{3-})
- acid-base balance (pH) of plasma
- regulation of necessary hormones such as renin, erythropoietin, and vitamin D

After the kidneys perform their filtering function, the ureters transport the urine to the urinary bladder. There, the urine is held until voided, when the urine exits the body through the urethra.

Kidneys

A **kidney** is one of two bean-shaped organs which are located in the upper abdominal region. Although the kidneys are in the abdominal region, they are not inside the peritoneal cavity, where the stomach, pancreas, and intestines are located. On the tops of the kidneys sit the adrenal glands, which are part of the endocrine system, not the renal system. Hormones released by the adrenal glands regulate physiologic functions of several body systems. (To learn more about the adrenal glands, see Chapter 13.)

The blood is filtered by the kidneys. The **renal artery**, which branches off of the abdominal aorta, brings blood into the kidneys. The filtered blood returns to the bloodstream via the **renal vein**. The **renal cortex** is the outer layer of a kidney and is responsible for filtration. The **renal medulla**, in the body of each kidney, also performs filtration. Both the renal cortex and the renal medulla are made up of microscopic nephrons. A **nephron** is the functional filtering unit of the kidney (see Figure 15.2).

FIGURE 15.2
Anatomy of the Kidney

The kidney contains about 2 million microscopic nephrons, which produce urine and maintain constancy in the body's internal environment.

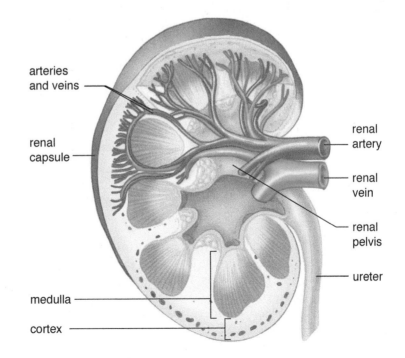

A normal human kidney contains approximately 2 million microscopic nephrons (see Figure 15.3). The nephrons work to produce urine and thereby maintain constancy in the body's internal environment. The renal tubules of the nephrons produce urine through three processes: filtration, reabsorption, and secretion. The role that individual nephrons play in these processes is outlined below.

FIGURE 15.3
Anatomy of a Nephron

Each part of the microscopic-sized nephron performs one or more of the following functions: filtration; reabsorption; and secretion of select electrolytes, fluids, and other substances.

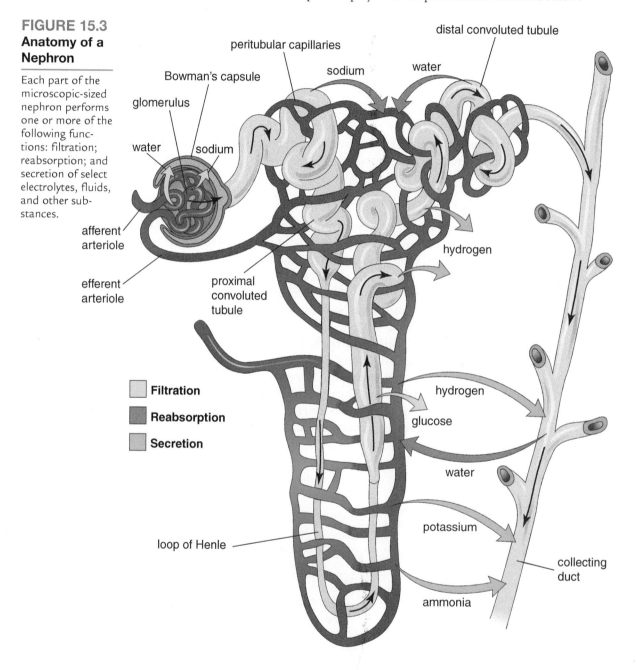

Blood containing fluid and waste products enters the nephron through the afferent arteriole into the Bowman's capsule. Here, the capillaries are tightly folded, forming the **glomerulus**. The tight folding in the glomerulus and the small amount of space inside the capsule create the high pressure that forces fluid and other substances out of the blood. **Glomerular filtration** is the initial step in urine production and the maintenance of fluid balance. Large molecules, such as proteins, are not filtered out in the glomerulus, but most fluids and other smaller substances are. Blood leaves the Bowman's capsule via the efferent arteriole. **Filtrate**, the fluids and by-products filtered from the blood in the glomerulus, continues through the nephron.

The filtrate passes through the distal and proximal convoluted tubules and the **loop of Henle**, a long, U-shaped structure from which water and salts are reabsorbed into the blood (see Figure 15.3). As filtrate passes through these structures, molecules are selectively exchanged between the tubules, loop of Henle, and surrounding capillaries through several mechanisms. Some substances are reabsorbed into the blood through simple diffusion. Others are exchanged between the blood and filtrate through **secretion**, an active transport process. Still others move across the membranes due to force of pressure, which is another way to describe filtration. Those substances that are filtered out of the blood or secreted into the filtrate (but do not reenter the blood) are then eliminated from the body as urine.

Proper urine production and maintenance of fluid balance rely on the tubular reabsorption and secretion processes. **Reabsorption** is the process by which substances are pulled back into the blood after waste products have been removed during the formation of urine. In fact, reabsorption of water and sodium into the blood is essential for maintaining good hydration. When the kidneys are not functioning correctly, the proper balance of reabsorption and secretion is not maintained; as a result, toxins build up in the blood and begin to poison the body.

Ureters and Urinary Bladder

A **ureter** is one of two paired muscular ducts that extend from the renal pelvis (see Figure 15.2) to the urinary bladder. The main function of the ureters is to move urine from the kidneys to the urinary bladder. This movement is facilitated by smooth muscle contraction in the walls of the ureters.

The **urinary bladder** is located in the pelvic region. This organ collects and holds urine until the fluid exits the body during urination. The bladder is made of stretchy epithelial and smooth muscle cells (see Figure 15.4), which allow it to expand and hold up to 1 L of fluid. However, the functional capacity of the bladder (the volume held before voluntary voiding) is much smaller: approximately 300–400 mL in adults.

FIGURE 15.4
Anatomy of the Bladder

Although the bladder can hold up to 1 L of urine, stretch receptors typically trigger the urge to urinate when only 30%–40% of that volume has accumulated.

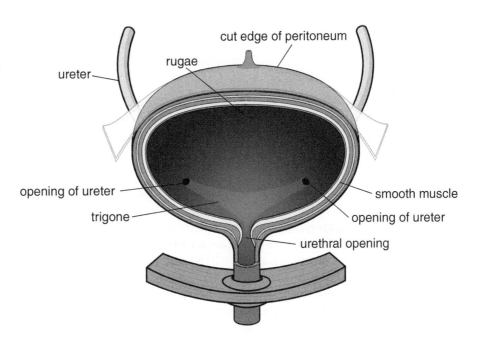

Once urine flows down the ureters and into the urinary bladder, the **internal urethral sphincter**, an involuntary muscle, relaxes as the bladder fills to allow urine into the urethra. The **external urethral sphincter**, a voluntary muscle, holds the urine in the bladder before it exits the body. A **detrusor muscle** is smooth muscle in the bladder that contracts to help push urine out. When the bladder is full and distended, stretch receptors sense the pressure and cause the detrusor muscles in the bladder to contract and the internal and external urethral sphincter to relax. Urine is pushed out, and the bladder empties. This urination process is called **micturition**.

15.2 Renal Function and Pharmacokinetics

Recall that pharmacokinetics is the study of how drugs are absorbed, distributed, and eliminated from the bloodstream. One of these phases, elimination, is highly dependent on renal function. Consequently, assessment of a patient's renal function is critical to prescribing appropriate medication dosing.

Renal System Dysfunction

When the kidneys are not functioning properly, the right balance of reabsorption and secretion is not maintained. Toxins build up in the blood and start to poison the body. This dysfunction can cause a number of side effects and problems for patients. Patients who are experiencing kidney failure have edema; vomiting; weakness; and **anuria**, or an inability to produce urine. Those patients who are experiencing **acute kidney disease** have a rapid reduction in kidney function, which may be caused by renal ischemia, trauma, pregnancy, extracellular volume depletion, hemorrhage, surgery, or shock. As a result of this reduction in kidney function, patients accumulate toxic nitrogen and other waste products. **Uremia** is the clinical syndrome resulting from renal dysfunction. In this syndrome, excessive products of protein metabolism (e.g., urea) are retained in the blood, and the toxic condition produced is marked by nausea, vomiting, vertigo, seizures, and coma.

Dysfunction within the ureters or urinary bladder also causes problems for the patient. When the ureters or urinary bladder fail to work properly, a patient may experience urinary retention or incontinence. **Urinary retention** occurs when the kidneys produce urine, but the micturition process does not function properly, and consequently, urine accumulates in the bladder. This problem is a malfunction of the bladder. The inability to control the external urethral sphincter, thus allowing urine to leak out of the bladder, is called **urinary incontinence**.

Assessment of Renal Function

Assessment of renal function is an important part of patient care. **Glomerular filtration rate (GFR)**, the volume of blood that passes through glomeruli each minute, is considered the optimal way to assess renal function. However, the process of measuring GFR is costly and time consuming. For this reason other markers are more commonly used to assess kidney function.

Laboratory blood tests are used to diagnose and monitor renal function. The most common tests are **blood urea nitrogen (BUN)** and **serum creatinine (SCr)**. When renal function is impaired, the elimination of urea, nitrogen, and creatinine (a by-product of muscle metabolism) is also impaired, and the concentrations of these substances increase in the blood. The results of these tests vary according to age, weight, and gender, as well as other factors such as exercise. However, the results of BUN and SCr blood tests are good markers for a patient's renal function.

Work Wise

Learning health-care jargon is an important communication skill. Abbreviations used to describe renal function are pronounced in different ways. For example, the abbreviations *BUN* and *GFR* are generally pronounced by saying the letters individually. The abbreviation *CrCl* is generally spoken by saying "creatinine clearance."

Typically, the normal range for BUN is 7–20 mg/dL. The normal range for SCr is 0.5–1.5 mg/dL. SCr can be used to calculate **creatinine clearance (CrCl)**. CrCl is the volume of blood plasma cleared of creatinine per minute. Compared to measuring GFR, CrCl is a faster and more cost-effective way to assess kidney function. A low CrCl (<60 mL/min) is a sign of impaired renal function. CrCl estimates the level of renal function while taking into account such factors as age, ideal body weight, and sex. A common formula used by prescribers and pharmacists to calculate CrCl is the **Cockcroft and Gault equation**:

$$\text{Male patients: CrCl in mL/min} = \frac{(140 - \text{age}) \times \text{weight in kg}}{(\text{SCr in mg/dL} \times 72)}$$

$$\text{Female patients: CrCl in mL/min} = \frac{(140 - \text{age}) \times \text{weight in kg} \times 0.85}{(\text{SCr in mg/dL} \times 72)}$$

Although other formulas for estimating renal function exist, the Cockcroft and Gault equation is used most often when adjusting drug dosing for renal impairment. For example, the dose is decreased or the interval between doses is increased for many drugs when CrCl drops below 30 mL/min or 60 mL/min.

Nephrotoxicity and Renal Dosing

Because of the importance of the kidneys to the pharmacokinetic process, prescribers need to be especially mindful of lowering medication doses for a patient who has impaired renal function. Dose adjustment often depends on the degree of renal dysfunction present. Some drugs need dose adjustment only in the case of severe renal failure, whereas others cannot be used even in mild kidney impairment.

Drug accumulation in a patient's blood can lead to serious side effects and toxicities. Certain drugs can also cause **nephrotoxicity**, or direct damage to kidney tissue. Nephrotoxicity is usually reversible; however, if it is not addressed quickly, this condition can cause renal failure. For that reason, a patient who is taking a drug that is considered nephrotoxic or potentially nephrotoxic under certain conditions (such as dehydration) must be closely monitored. Examples of nephrotoxic drugs include nonsteroidal anti-inflammatory drugs (NSAIDs), amphotericin B, contrast media (dye for imaging procedures), aminoglycosides, and the antineoplastic drugs cisplatin and carboplatin.

15.3 Urinary Tract Infection and Drug Treatments

A **urinary tract infection (UTI)** occurs when bacteria, most often *Escherichia coli* (*E. coli*), enter the opening of the urethra and multiply. A UTI is classified according to its anatomic location in the urinary tract: **cystitis** is a lower urinary tract infection, and **pyelonephritis** is an upper urinary tract infection.

A UTI usually begins in the lower urinary tract (urethra and bladder) and, if not treated, progresses to the upper urinary tract (ureters and kidneys). Even when the urinary tract is healthy, bacteria may enter. In a UTI, many more microorganisms than normal are found. The presence of bacteria in the urine combined with localized symptoms are considered diagnostic indicators of a UTI. Urination may be difficult or painful, and blood may appear in the urine. Fever is also a common symptom for a patient who has a UTI.

Community-acquired UTIs account for more than 5 million physician visits yearly. The highest incidence of UTIs occurs in sexually active females. Incidence is related to the ability of *E. coli* intestinal bacteria to colonize the vagina. The close proximity of the vaginal opening to the urethra allows bacteria to ascend the short urethra and gain access to the bladder. UTIs become a problem for males age 50 and older because of prostatic obstruction (obstruction of the prostate), catheter use, or surgery.

A UTI is typically treated with an antibiotic. This therapy is often accompanied by the use of a urinary analgesic (see Table 15.1). Antibiotics are covered in greater detail in Chapter 16.

TABLE 15.1 Commonly Used Agents for the Treatment of a UTI

Generic (Brand)	Pronunciation	Dosage Form	Common Dosage	Dispensing Status
Antibiotics, see Chapter 16				
Urinary Analgesic				
phenazopyridine (Azo Urinary Pain Relief, Pyridium)	fen-az-oh-PEER-i-deen	tablet	200 mg 3 times a day	OTC

Antibiotics

Treatment for a UTI may involve a single dose of an antibiotic or a 3- to 14-day regimen, depending on the extent of infection and the agent selected. In some instances, a UTI can recur or persist despite antibiotic treatment. If several infections occur in sequence, an antibiotic may be prescribed for 6 to 12 months to prevent recurrence. Female patients with recurrent UTIs may be instructed to urinate and take one dose of an antibiotic immediately after sexual intercourse.

Although antibiotics are covered in further detail in Chapter 16, antibiotics commonly used in the treatment of a UTI include the following:

- **amoxicillin**
- **amoxicillin / clavulanate (Augmentin)**
- **ciprofloxacin (Cipro)**
- **fosfomycin (Monurol)**
- **levofloxacin**
- **nitrofurantoin (Furadantin, Macrobid, Macrodantin)**
- **sulfamethoxazole / trimethoprim (Bactrim, Bactrim DS, Sulfatrim)**.

Specific information regarding the dosage and administration, side effects, contraindications, and cautions and considerations of these medications can be found in Chapter 16.

Urinary Analgesics

Patients' UTI symptoms typically respond to antibiotic therapy within several days. However, patients may continue to experience pain, burning, urgency, frequency, and other discomforts arising from the lower urinary tract during this period. For that reason, prescribers may also order an over-the-counter (OTC) **urinary analgesic** to relieve these discomforts. **Phenazopyridine (Azo Urinary Pain Relief, Pyridium)** is a commonly used urinary analgesic for the treatment of UTIs. This medication is also indicated for symptomatic relief from trauma, surgery, endoscopic procedures, and the passage of catheters related to the lower urinary tract.

Dosage Forms and Administration Phenazopyridine may be taken without regard to meals. Duration of therapy is typically two days, as needed.

Side Effects Headache and stomach cramps are the most common side effects associated with phenazopyridine. In addition, the use of phenazopyridine can turn the urine orange, which may be alarming to patients. Patients should be informed of this harmless side effect prior to taking this medication and should be warned that this colored urine may stain clothing.

Contraindications Phenazopyridine is contraindicated in patients who have kidney disease or liver disease.

Cautions and Considerations Acute renal failure has been reported with phenazopyridine use and is typically accompanied by hemolytic anemia. Patients should be aware that phenazopyridine is an analgesic and does not have antimicrobial properties. Consequently, this medication is used concurrently with an antibiotic.

Drug Interactions The adverse effects of local anesthetics and sodium nitrite may be enhanced by phenazopyridine use.

Phenazopyridine's adverse effects may be enhanced by concurrent use of dapsone and nitric oxide.

15.4 Urinary Incontinence and Drug Treatments

Recall that urinary incontinence is the involuntary loss of urine. The prevalence of incontinence correlates with age, with one-third of adults (ages 18 through 64) and one-half of older adults (ages 65 and above) affected by this disorder. The two common types of urinary incontinence are urge incontinence (also called *overactive bladder*) and overflow incontinence. Patients with **urge incontinence** experience a sudden need to urinate that is difficult to delay. **Overflow incontinence** is marked by the involuntary release of urine when the bladder becomes overly full, even if individuals feel no urge to urinate.

The primary symptoms of urinary incontinence are urgency, frequency, and pain. These symptoms can also affect patients' lifestyles by limiting travel or creating anxiety over the ability to find or access a bathroom when necessary. To treat urinary incontinence, prescribers order medications such as an antimuscarinic or a beta-3 adrenergic agonist (see Table 15.2). They also recommend behavioral techniques, such as pelvic muscle exercises and bladder training, that patients can do to address this condition.

TABLE 15.2 Commonly Used Agents for the Treatment of Urinary Incontinence

Generic (Brand)	Pronunciation	Dosage Form	Common Dosage	Dispensing Status
Anticholinergics (Antimuscarinics)				
darifenacin (Enablex)	dar-i-FEN-a-sin	tablet	7.5 mg a day	Rx
fesoterodine (Toviaz)	fes-oh-TER-oh-deen	tablet	4–8 mg a day	Rx

continues

Generic (Brand)	Pronunciation	Dosage Form	Common Dosage	Dispensing Status
oxybutynin (Ditropan, Gelnique, Oxytrol)	ox-i-BYOO-ti-nin	oral syrup, tablet, transdermal gel, transdermal patch	PO: 5 mg–30 mg 1–3 times a day transdermal gel: 1 sachet or 1 pump a day transdermal patch: 3.9 mg patch applied every 3–4 days	Rx
solifenacin (Vesicare)	sol-i-FEN-a-sin	tablet	5 mg a day	Rx
tolterodine (Detrol)	tole-TAIR-oh-deen	capsule, tablet	2–4 mg a day	Rx
trospium (Sanctura)	TROSE-pee-um	capsule, tablet	immediate release: 20 mg 2 times a day XR: 60 mg a day	Rx
Beta-3 Adrenergic Agonist				
mirabegron (Myrbetriq)	mir-a-BEG-ron	tablet	25–50 mg a day	Rx

Anticholinergics (Antimuscarinics)

In some types of urinary incontinence, patients experience abnormal bladder contractions. The abnormal bladder contractions are associated with the action of the chemical messenger acetylcholine. An **anticholinergic** inhibits acetylcholine. Specifically, an **antimuscarinic** works by inhibiting acetylcholine in the nerves that control involuntary bladder contraction and emptying. These agents relax smooth detrusor muscles. Commonly prescribed antimuscarinics and their dosage forms are listed in Table 15.2.

Dosage Forms and Administration **Darifenacin (Enablex)**, **fesoterodine (Toviaz)**, **solifenacin (Vesicare)**, and **oxybutynin (Ditropan, Gelnique, Oxytrol)** tablets should not be chewed, crushed, or divided but should be swallowed whole. **Tolterodine (Detrol)** extended-release capsules should not be chewed, crushed, or opened but should be swallowed whole. **Trospium (Sanctura)** should not be taken on an empty stomach but should be administered in the morning with water at least one hour prior to a meal.

Oxybutynin is unique among the antimuscarinics in that it is available in a variety of dosage forms. In addition to being available as tablets, oxybutynin is available as an oral syrup, transdermal gel, and transdermal patch. Oral liquids should be measured with a dosing syringe, spoon, or cup. Oxybutynin transdermal gel (Gelnique) is available in a bottle with a pump or in premeasured sachets (packets). Gelnique should be applied to clean, dry, intact skin on the abdomen, thighs, or upper arms, or shoulders. This gel should *not* be applied to recently shaved skin. The application site should be rotated, and the hands should be washed after administration. The treated area should be covered with clothing after the gel has dried to prevent transfer of medication to others. In addition, patients should be instructed to not bathe, shower, or swim for one hour after gel application.

The oxybutynin patch (Oxytrol) comprises three layers: a backing film that protects the middle adhesive and drug layer, the adhesive and drug layer, and a release liner that is pulled off prior to application. Oxytrol is applied twice a week to dry, intact skin on the abdomen, hip, or buttock. The site should be rotated with each application, and a patch should not be reapplied to the same site within seven days. The transdermal patch should be stored away from humidity and moisture at room temperature.

Side Effects Common side effects associated with antimuscarinics include dry mouth, constipation, blurred vision, and urine retention. The effects may improve over time but may not completely disappear. Drinking plenty of water or sucking on hard candy may help alleviate dry mouth. Staying hydrated or using a stool softener may help with constipation. The oxybutynin patch minimizes the side effects of dry mouth and constipation, possibly because the transdermal patch is constantly releasing the drug.

Other side effects of antimuscarinics include hallucinations, drowsiness, and GI upset. If patients experience abdominal pain, eye pain, or difficulty with urination, they should consult their prescribers.

Contraindications Antimuscarinics are contraindicated in patients who have gastric retention or narrow-angle glaucoma.

Cautions and Considerations Antimuscarinics may take several weeks to begin working. These medications should be used with caution in older adults. This patient population may be particularly susceptible to adverse effects such as hallucinations, dry mouth, blurred vision, and constipation.

Darifenacin has a specific consideration. This medication must be protected from light.

Drug Interactions The urinary incontinence agents have anticholinergic side effects that may potentiate side effects of other drugs with anticholinergic properties, such as ipratropium and scopolamine.

Beta-3 Adrenergic Agonists

Beta-3 adrenergic agonists are approved to treat certain types of urinary incontinence. A **beta-3 adrenergic agonist** works by relaxing the detrusor muscles during urine storage. This muscle relaxation increases the capacity of the bladder. **Mirabegron (Myrbetriq)** is the only beta-3 adrenergic agonist available for use in the United States.

Dosage Forms and Administration Mirabegron is available only in oral tablets. These tablets can be administered without regard to meals. Doses of mirabegron should be decreased in patients who have liver or kidney impairment.

Side Effects Common side effects associated with this beta-3 adrenergic agonist include hypertension, tachycardia, headache, dizziness, constipation, dry mouth, diarrhea, UTI, back pain, nasopharyngitis, and flu-like symptoms.

Contraindications There are no contraindications for the administration of mirabegron.

Cautions and Considerations Mirabegron is not recommended for use in patients who have uncontrolled hypertension due to reported dose-related increases in blood pressure. It should be used cautiously in patients who have controlled hypertension, as exacerbations of hypertension have been reported. The risk of urinary retention may be increased, so mirabegron should be used cautiously in patients who have bladder obstruction. Mirabegron use is not recommended in patients who have severe liver impairment or end-stage renal disease.

Drug Interactions Mirabegron inhibits CYP2D6 and, therefore, increases the levels of drugs that are metabolized by CYP2D6. For example, levels of metoprolol, despiramine, doxirubicin, and tamoxifen may be increased with mirabegron use. If a mirabegron user is to start digoxin, the lowest possible digoxin dose should be used.

15.5 Benign Prostatic Hyperplasia and Drug Treatments

Benign prostatic hyperplasia (BPH) is one of the most common prostatic diseases among older male patients. This abnormal enlargement of the prostate gland appears to occur with aging as well as with a combination of certain pathophysiologic influences (see Figure 15.5). An enlarged prostate becomes a problem when it obstructs urine outflow from the bladder.

Increasing evidence shows that nonsurgical interventions, especially drug therapy, may be effective as primary treatment for selected patients who have BPH. Alpha-blockers and 5-alpha-reductase inhibitors represent promising and innovative approaches to pharmacologic management of BPH (see Table 15.3).

FIGURE 15.5
Male Urinary System

Male patients who have BPH may find they have frequent bladder infections due to urinary retention.

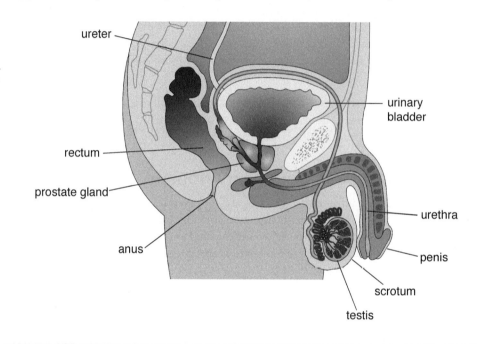

TABLE 15.3 Commonly Used Agents for the Treatment of BPH

Generic (Brand)	Pronunciation	Dosage Form	Common Dosage	Dispensing Status
Alpha-Blockers				
alfuzosin (Uroxatral)	al-FYOO-zoe-sin	tablet	10 mg a day	Rx
doxazosin (Cardura, Cardura XL)	dox-AY-zoe-sin	tablet	4–8 mg a day	Rx
tamsulosin (Flomax)	tam-SOO-loe-sin	capsule	0.4–0.8 mg a day	Rx
terazosin	ter-AY-zoe-sin	capsule	10–20 mg a day	Rx
5-Alpha-Reductase Inhibitors				
dutasteride (Avodart)	du-TAS-tur-ide	capsule	0.5 mg a day	Rx
dutasteride / tamsulosin (Jalyn)	du-TAS-tur-ide tam-SOO-loe-sin	capsule	0.5 mg/0.4 mg a day	Rx
finasteride (Propecia, Proscar)	fin-AS-tur-ide	tablet	5 mg a day	Rx

Put Down Roots

Many generic drug names of alpha-blockers end in -*osin*.

Alpha-Blockers

The oral formulations of certain alpha-blockers are used to treat patients who have BPH, especially those who also have hypertension. These two conditions are a common combination in older male patients. In addition to treating BPH, alpha-blockers are sometimes prescribed to assist in the passage of kidney stones lodged in the ureters.

Recall that **alpha-blockers** work by inhibiting the alpha-1 receptors in the prostate gland and bladder, as well as in blood vessels in the rest of the body. As a result, alpha-blockers relax urethral sphincters and prostatic smooth muscle, which enhances urinary outflow from the bladder. Commonly used alpha-blockers for the treatment of BPH include **alfuzosin (Uroxatral)**, **doxazosin**, **tamsulosin (Flomax)**, and **terazosin**.

Two alpha-blockers have additional indications. Prazosin has an indication for the treatment of hypertension, and the immediate-release formulation of terazosin also has an indication for the treatment of hypertension.

Dosage Forms and Administration Alfuzosin is a long-acting tablet and is dosed once a day. It should be taken immediately following a meal at the same time each day. Patients should be instructed to swallow the tablet whole and not to split, chew, or crush the tablet. The coating of the tablet must remain intact for alfuzosin to be released at the appropriate rate.

The immediate-release formulation of doxazosin has an indication for the treatment of hypertension, as designated by the FDA. In addition, the dosing instructions for doxazosin depend on whether the formulation is an extended-release tablet or an immediate-release tablet. Extended-release tablets should be swallowed whole with the morning meal and should not be split, crushed, or chewed. Immediate-release tablets can be administered in the morning or evening.

Tamsulosin capsules should be administered 30 minutes after a meal and at the same time each day. These capsules should be swallowed whole.

Terazosin capsules should be taken at the same time each day.

Side Effects Common side effects of alpha-blockers include dizziness, drowsiness, fatigue, headache, fainting, and **orthostatic hypotension**, which is a drop in blood pressure that causes dizziness when transitioning from sitting or lying down to standing up. Rising slowly from a seated or lying position can alleviate this effect.

Ejaculation disorders are also commonly associated with the use of alpha-blockers. These disorders include diminished ejaculation, in which a lower volume of semen is ejaculated through the penis, and retrograde ejaculation, in which semen is not ejaculated through the penis but enters the bladder. Other sexual side effects of alpha-blockers are rare but serious. One such effect is **priapism**, a prolonged and painful erection. If this condition occurs, patients should seek medical attention immediately to prevent permanent damage and impotence.

Contraindications Alfuzosin is contraindicated in patients who have moderate to severe liver insufficiency and in individuals who are taking itraconazole, ketoconazole, or ritonavir. These medications may increase the blood levels of alfuzosin.

The other alpha-blockers discussed here do not have contraindications.

Cautions and Considerations Alpha-blockers can have a **first-dose effect**, whereby blood pressure drops dramatically and may cause dizziness or fainting. Patients are often observed closely during the first dose to monitor for this effect. Repeated blood-pressure measurements may be required for four to six hours after taking the first dose. Consequently, patients should be careful about driving or operating machinery until they know how the medication affects them.

These agents must be used with caution in patients who have gastrointestinal (GI) disorders, liver disease, or kidney impairment. Alpha-blockers can exacerbate GI motility (movement) disorders. Patients should inform their prescribers if they have any of these conditions before taking alpha-blockers.

Drug Interactions Alpha-blockers may enhance the hypotensive effects of other drugs that lower blood pressure. For example, the hypotensive effects of beta-blockers may be increased when used with alpha-blockers. Only one alpha-blocker should be used at a time due to the increase in side effects when two or more are used. Cimetidine may exaggerate the hypotensive effects of tamsulosin.

5-Alpha-Reductase Inhibitors

Pharm Fact

In addition to treating BPH, finasteride (Propecia, Proscar) may be used to treat male-pattern hair loss.

Like alpha-blockers, 5-alpha-reductase inhibitors are prescribed for the treatment of BPH. A **5-alpha-reductase inhibitor** works by inhibiting the conversion of testosterone into its active form, dihydrotestosterone (DHT), in the prostate gland, hair follicles, and other androgen-sensitive tissues. Impeding this process reduces the size of the prostate because prostate tissue growth is dependent on testosterone, an androgen. Although blocking testosterone altogether would reduce prostate size, the side effects of reduced androgen production in the body are undesirable for most patients. With this class of drugs, only DHT production is blocked, thereby reducing prostate size while allowing adequate levels of testosterone to remain in the bloodstream.

Two 5-alpha-reductase inhibitors have slight differences in their mechanism of action. **Dutasteride (Avodart)** blocks 5-alpha-reductase enzymes type 1 and type 2. In contrast, **finasteride (Propecia, Proscar)** inhibits only type 2. A combination drug, **dutasteride / tamsulosin (Jalyn)**, is used to treat an enlarged prostate in male patients who have BPH.

Safety Alert

Proscar (a brand name of finasteride, which is used for BPH) and Prozac (the brand name of the antidepressant fluoxetine) can easily be confused. The FDA and the Institute for Safe Medication Practices (ISMP) recommend tall man lettering for Prozac (PROzac) to help distinguish the drug from other sound-alike and look-alike medications.

Dosage Forms and Administration Dutasteride may be administered with or without food. This medication is available in capsules, which should be swallowed whole. Chewing or opening these capsules may result in the capsule contents irritating the mouth or throat. If contact is made with a leaking capsule, the contact area should be washed immediately with soap and water.

Finasteride is available in tablets and may be administered with or without food. It may take a minimum of six months of therapy to determine whether finasteride adequately treats BPH. Finasteride tablets have a protective coating. If the tablets are crushed or broken, there is a risk of drug absorption through the skin. People who are pregnant or of childbearing potential should avoid touching crushed or broken tablets due to the risk of fetal toxicity.

Side Effects Common side effects associated with 5-alpha-reductase inhibitors include decreased libido, erectile dysfunction, and ejaculation disorders. Hypotension may also occur. Another side effect of using these medications is **gynecomastia**, or breast enlargement in male adults or children. If this effect is bothersome, patients should speak with their prescribers to determine if drug therapy should be discontinued.

Contraindications Use of dutasteride, dutasteride / tamsulosin, and finasteride is contraindicated in pediatric patients, patients of childbearing potential, and pregnant patients. In addition, dutasteride / tamsulosin should not be used in combination with other 5-alpha-reductase inhibitors or tamsulosin.

Cautions and Considerations Because 5-alpha-reductase inhibitors block an active form of testosterone production, these medications could be harmful to a developing fetus. In addition, these medications have the potential to be absorbed through

Safety Alert

Dutasteride and finasteride should not be handled by people who are pregnant or may become pregnant due to their potential for absorption and subsequent risk to a developing fetus.

the skin, posing another risk to a fetus. For that reason, people who are pregnant or of childbearing potential should wear gloves if handling broken tablets or opened capsules to prevent measurable absorption. They should also avoid contact with semen from a partner who has been exposed to 5-alpha-reductase inhibitors. This exposure may occur through use of the drug or skin absorption of the drug. The combination drug dutasteride / tamsulosin should not be handled by people who are pregnant or may become pregnant, as this medication causes birth defects.

Another caution for the use of 5-alpha-reductase inhibitors involves a possible link between the use of these medications and an increase in the incidence of fast-growing prostate cancers that are more likely than others to metastasize. Ongoing research continues to pursue this relationship to provide more definitive guidance for healthcare practitioners.

Patients who have taken dutasteride / tamsulosin should not donate blood for at least six months after discontinuing the drug. Patient adherence to this time frame prevents the administration of dutasteride to a transfusion recipient who is pregnant or of childbearing potential.

Drug Interactions Dutasteride levels may be increased by cimetidine, clarithromycin, erythromycin, isoniazid, itraconazole, ketoconazole, and nefazodone. Dutasteride levels may be decreased by carbamazepine, rifamycin derivatives, and St. John's wort. Finasteride does not have known significant drug interactions.

15.6 Chronic Kidney Disease and Drug Treatments

Kidney disease, or renal disease, can be acute or chronic. **Acute kidney failure**, also known as *acute kidney injury* and *acute renal failure*, is a decrease in kidney function that occurs over hours, days, or weeks. If supportive care is provided and the cause of failure resolved, kidney function may return to normal. If the decrease in function is sufficiently severe, acute kidney disease can be life threatening and may result in some degree of permanent damage.

Chronic kidney disease (CKD), on the other hand, involves progressive damage to kidney tissue, resulting in the death of this tissue over time. Common causes of CKD include diabetes and untreated hypertension. CKD is more common than acute kidney disease and cannot be reversed. As it worsens, it can be categorized into stages that guide the approach and degree of urgency for treatment (see Table 15.4). Drug therapies such

TABLE 15.4 Stages of Chronic Kidney Disease

Stage	GFR (mL/min/1.73 m²)	Description
1	≥ 90	normal kidney function; urine findings, structural abnormalities, or a genetic trait indicative of kidney disease
2	60–89	mildly reduced kidney function; urine findings, structural abnormalities, or a genetic trait indicative of kidney disease
3a	45–59	moderately reduced kidney function
3b	30–44	moderately reduced kidney function
4	15–29	severely reduced kidney function
5	< 15	end-stage renal disease (sometimes called *renal failure* and *end-stage kidney disease*)

as diuretics and other renal protective medications can help slow the progression of the disease in early stages, but in later stages, these agents are of no use. Eventually, in end-stage renal disease, dialysis and kidney transplantation are the only means of treatment.

Acute kidney disease typically improves or reverses as its cause is resolved. Therefore, drug treatment for acute kidney disease is limited and short term. CKD is more frequently treated with medication. Therapy is aimed at reestablishing an appropriate intravascular fluid volume and pressure and treating underlying problems.

Preventing and treating complications of CKD are important in disease-state management. Common complications of CKD include volume overload and hypertension. Volume overload is a frequent concern in patients who have a GFR of less than 15 mL/min/1.73 m² and is often managed with a combination of dietary sodium restriction and diuretic therapy. Hypertension management is essential to preventing kidney disease progression. In order to decrease blood pressure, angiotensin-converting enzyme (ACE) inhibitors and angiotensin receptor blockers (ARBs) are given initially. (To learn more about ACE inhibitors and ARBs, refer to Chapter 10.)

After the administration of antihypertensive agents, diuretic therapy begins. A **diuretic** is a substance that increases the volume of urine output. The primary purpose of using diuretics is to rid the body of excess fluid and electrolytes. Diuretics are most often used as **adjunct therapy** (therapy used together with the primary treatment) to improve urine output in patients who have kidney disease, to reduce blood volume in patients who have hypertension, or to treat edema. In addition, the effectiveness of certain drugs may be enhanced with diuretic therapy.

Table 15.5 presents the diuretics most commonly used for CKD. Some diuretics, such as thiazide diuretics and potassium-sparing diuretics, tend to be used more often for treating hypertension. Other diuretics, such as loop diuretics, are used more frequently for treating kidney failure or reducing edema. Carbonic anhydrase inhibitors are typically used in patients who have edema as well as acid-base balance issues. Combinations of these diuretic classes may be used in certain cases of kidney failure to maximize urine output.

WORKPLACE WISDOM

While most diuretics act directly in the nephrons, their actions extend beyond the renal system. In fact, one of the most common indications for the use of diuretics is hypertension (elevated blood pressure), a disorder related to the cardiovascular system. Thiazide diuretics, in particular, are used to treat hypertension. Patients who have heart failure, another cardiovascular disorder, are often prescribed loop diuretics for chronic use. Edema, mountain sickness (altitude sickness), and ascites (abnormal accumulation of serous fluid in the abdomen) are other indications for diuretics. More information regarding the cardiovascular indications for diuretic use is provided in Chapter 10.

TABLE 15.5 Commonly Used Agents for the Adjunct Treatment of CKD

Generic (Brand)	Pronunciation	Dosage Form	Common Dosage	Dispensing Status
Carbonic Anhydrase Inhibitor				
acetazolamide (Diamox Sequels)	a-seet-a-ZOLE-a-mide	capsule, injection, tablet	250–375 mg a day or every other day	Rx
Loop Diuretics				
bumetanide (Bumex)	byoo-MET-a-nide	injection, tablet	individualized to patient	Rx
ethacrynic acid (Edecrin, Sodium Edecrin)	eth-a-KRIN-ik AS-id	injection, tablet	individualized to patient	Rx
furosemide (Lasix)	fur-OH-se-mide	injection, oral solution, tablet	individualized to patient	Rx
torsemide (Demadex)	TORE-se-mide	tablet	individualized to patient	Rx
Potassium-Sparing Diuretics				
amiloride	a-MIL-oh-ride	tablet	5–20 mg a day	Rx
eplerenone (Inspra)	ep-LAIR-a-none	tablet	25–50 mg a day	Rx
spironolactone (Aldactone, CaroSpir)	speer-on-oh-LAK-tone	oral suspension, tablet	25–200 mg a day	Rx
triamterene (Dyrenium)	trye-AM-ter-een	capsule	200–300 mg a day	Rx
Thiazide and Thiazide-Related Diuretics				
atenolol / chlorthalidone (Tenoretic)	a-TEN-oh-lawl chlor-THAL-i-doan	tablet	50–100 mg/25 mg	Rx
bisoprolol / hydrochlorothiazide (Ziac)	bis-OH-proe-lawl hye-droe-klor-oh-THYE-a-zide	tablet	20 mg/12.5 mg a day	Rx
chlorothiazide (Diuril, Sodium Diuril)	klor-oh-THYE-a-zide	injection, oral suspension, tablet	250–100 mg a day	Rx
chlorthalidone	klor-THAL-i-doan	tablet	12.5–25 mg a day	Rx
hydrochlorothiazide, HCTZ	hye-droe-klor-oh-THYE-a-zide	capsule, tablet	12.5–50 mg a day	Rx
indapamide	in-DAP-a-mide	tablet	1.25–2.5 mg a day	Rx
lisinopril / hydrochlorothiazide (Prinzide, Zestoretic)	lyse-IN-oh-pril hye-droe-klor-oh-THYE-a-zide	tablet	10–80 mg/12.5–50 mg a day	Rx
losartan / hydrochlorothiazide (Hyzaar)	loe-SAR-tan hye-droe-klor-oh-THYE-a-zide	tablet	50–100 mg/12.5–25 mg a day	Rx
metolazone (Zaroxolyn)	me-TOLE-a-zone	tablet	2.5–20 mg a day	Rx
triamterene / hydrochlorothiazide (Dyazide, Maxzide)	trye-AM-ter-een hye-droe-klor-oh-THYE-a-zide	capsule, tablet	37.5–75 mg/25–50 mg a day	Rx

Carbonic Anhydrase Inhibitors

Carbonic anhydrase inhibitors may be used as adjunct therapy in the treatment of CKD. A carbonic anhydrase inhibitor works in the nephrons by increasing excretion of bicarbonate ions, which carry sodium, potassium, and water into the urine. In addition, carbonic anhydrase inhibitors increase urine volume and change urine pH from acidic to alkaline.

Acetazolamide (Diamox Sequels) is a commonly used carbonic anhydrase inhibitor (see Table 15.5). Acetazolamide treats edema. This medication is also indicated for the treatment of acute mountain sickness, glaucoma, periodic paralysis, and seizures.

Dosage Forms and Administration Acetazolamide capsules are extended release, whereas the tablets are immediate-release. Oral acetazolamide may be taken with food to decrease GI upset. Acetazolamide is also available as an injection.

Side Effects Common side effects associated with acetazolamide include **tinnitus** (ringing in the ears), tingling, nausea, vomiting, diarrhea, drowsiness, and changes in taste. Oral acetazolamide may cause an alteration in taste or leave a bitter flavor in the mouth.

Contraindications Acetazolamide should not be used in patients who have a hypersensitivity to sulfonamides. Patients who have a sulfa allergy may have cross-reactivity when using carbonic anhydrase inhibitors. If patients experience a rash while taking one of these agents, they should notify their prescribers immediately. Other contraindications include liver disease or insufficiency, decreased sodium or potassium levels, adrenocortical insufficiency, cirrhosis, hyperchloremic acidosis, and severe kidney disease or dysfunction (such as renal failure and anuria, a condition in which patients are not producing urine). Long-term use of acetazolamide to treat narrow-angle glaucoma is also contraindicated. In addition, acetazolamide should not be used concurrently with aspirin due to enhanced toxicity of the carbonic anhydrase inhibitor.

Cautions and Considerations Increases and decreases in blood glucose may occur with the use of acetazolamide. Consequently, prescribers exercise caution when prescribing this medication for patients who have diabetes and monitor these patients closely. Electrolyte imbalances (such as low sodium or low potassium) may also occur with acetazolamide use.

Drug Interactions Carbonic anhydrase inhibitors, in general, have additional cautions. The use of more than one carbonic anhydrase inhibitor is not recommended, and the adverse effects of these medications may be enhanced by the concurrent use of salicylates.

Loop Diuretics

A **loop diuretic** works by inhibiting reabsorption of sodium, chloride, and water in the ascending loop of Henle. This unique site of action produces fast and profound diuresis (urine production). Sodium, chloride, magnesium, calcium, and potassium are all excreted quickly and efficiently with the use of a loop diuretic. For that reason, loop diuretics are used to pull fluid out of the body rapidly. Typically, these agents are used to treat swelling and fluid accumulation due to heart or kidney failure.

Common loop diuretics used as adjunct therapy during the treatment of CKD are listed in Table 15.5. These loop diuretics include **bumetanide (Bumex)**, **ethacrynic acid (Edecrin, Sodium Edecrin)**, **furosemide (Lasix)**, and **torsemide (Demadex)**. Furosemide is particularly frequently prescribed (see Figure 15.6). The specific indications for the various loop diuretics can be found in Table 15.6.

FIGURE 15.6
Medication Label for Furosemide

Furosemide is a commonly used loop diuretic. It is available as an oral medication (as pictured) and as an injectable.

NDC 0000-0000-000

Store at 20° to 25° C (68° to 77° F) Protect from moisture. PROTECT FROM LIGHT.

Furosemide
Tablets

40 mg

30 Tablets

Rx Only

TABLE 15.6 FDA Indications for Commonly Used Loop Diuretics

FDA Indication	Bumetanide (Bumex)	Ethacrynic Acid (Edecrin, Sodium Edecrin)	Furosemide (Lasix)	Torsemide (Demadex)
acute pulmonary edema		X	X	
edema associated with heart failure, hepatic disease, or kidney disease	X	X	X	X
hypertension	X		X	X
short-term management of ascites		X		

Pharm Fact

The brand name for furosemide is Lasix. This brand name was designed to indicate its approximate duration of action: *La* (an abbreviated form of "lasts") + *six* (representing six hours) = *Lasix*.

Dosage Forms and Administration Bumetanide injection may be used intravenously or intramuscularly.

Ethacrynic acid injection should only be used intravenously and infused slowly. If a second dose is needed, the injection site should be rotated. Intramuscular or subcutaneous injections of ethacrynic acid are not recommended due to local pain and irritation.

The oral form of furosemide should be given in two doses a day at a six- to eight-hour interval. The rationale for this dosing interval is to prevent **nocturia**, or excessive nighttime urination.

Torsemide is available as a tablet that may be taken with or without food.

Side Effects The side effects of loop diuretics include hypotension, dizziness, headache, skin rash, hair loss (alopecia), GI upset, diarrhea, and constipation. Patients should be reminded to rise slowly from seated or lying positions to help with decreases in blood pressure and dizziness. In addition, oxotoxicity (production of adverse effects on organs or nerves involved in hearing or balance) has been reported with oral and IV torsemide use.

Contraindications The use of loop diuretics is contraindicated in patients who have anuria. Bumetanide and torsemide should not be used in patients who are experiencing hepatic coma. Bemetanide should also not be used by patients who have severe electrolyte depletion. Ethacrynic acid should not be used in patients who have a history of severe watery diarrhea with use and should not be used in infants.

Cautions and Considerations Because loop diuretics deplete potassium levels in the body, patients often take potassium supplements with these diuretics to maintain proper electrolyte balance. Cases of ototoxicity have been reported with loop diuretic use and are associated with rapid injection, severe kidney dysfunction, and concomitant use of other ototoxic drugs (such as aminoglycosides).

Name Exchange

A *boxed warning*, displayed on a prescription drug's package insert, is the official term to refer to a serious or life-threatening risk associated with the use of that drug. However, you may also hear pharmacy personnel use the term *black box warning*.

Certain loop diuretics have special cautions and considerations. Bumetanide and furosemide have boxed warnings for a risk of profound electrolyte depletion with excessive dosing. Careful medical supervision is required in patients using these drugs.

Drug Interactions Loop diuretics enhance the ability of other antihypertensives to decrease blood pressure. Concurrent use of NSAIDs may decrease the efficacy of loop diuretics.

Potassium-Sparing Diuretics

Potassium-sparing diuretics (listed in Table 15.5) are used primarily to treat hypertension and edema and, consequently, may serve as adjunct therapy in the treatment of CKD. A **potassium-sparing diuretic** works by blocking the exchange of potassium for sodium that takes place in the collecting duct and the connecting tubules (tubules that connect the distal convoluted tubule to the collecting duct). This inhibition is done either directly (in the case of amiloride and triamterene) or indirectly by interfering with aldosterone activity (eplerenone, spironolactone). Water follows sodium and is thus excreted along with sodium ions without depleting the body's potassium, which may happen with thiazide and loop diuretics.

Amiloride and Triamterene

Amiloride and **triamterene (Dyrenium)** are two commonly used potassium-sparing diuretics. They are pharmacologically similar and work by directly blocking sodium channels. They do not have aldosterone action. Triamterene / hydrochlorothiazide is a widely used combination diuretic. This drug is discussed in more detail in the Thiazide and Thiazide-Related Diuretics section.

Side Effects Potassium retention is a side effect associated with all potassium-sparing diuretics. Other side effects include GI upset, headache, confusion, and drowsiness. Triamterene, however, has a unique side effect: blue-green discoloration of urine. Patients should be informed of this side effect and be warned that discolored urine may stain clothing.

Contraindications Potassium-sparing diuretics should not be used in the presence of elevated serum potassium, kidney insufficiency or impairment, or anuria.

Amiloride should not be used in patients who are taking other drugs that increase potassium, such as potassium supplements. This medication also should not be used in patients who have diabetic nephropathy.

Triamterene has specific contraindications. This medication should not be used in patients who have severe liver disease and should not be administered concurrently with other potassium-sparing agents.

Cautions and Considerations Potassium-sparing agents can cause hyperkalemia (high potassium levels) because they promote potassium retention. Patients who have been prescribed potassium-sparing diuretics must undergo periodic laboratory tests to monitor for this effect and should avoid salt substitutes and foods containing high amounts of potassium (such as bananas). In addition, patients who are taking drugs that increase potassium levels, such as ACE inhibitors, are particularly at risk for hyperkalemia. Consequently, this class of diuretics should be administered with caution in this patient population.

Drug Interactions Potassium-sparing diuretics should be administered with caution in patients using drugs that increase potassium (such as ACE inhibitors and ARBs).

Eplerenone and Spironolactone

Eplerenone (Inspra) is indicated for patients who have hypertension and for those who have symptomatic heart failure following acute myocardial infarction (MI). **Spironolactone (Aldactone, CaroSpir)** is used primarily to treat hypertension, heart failure, **hyperaldosteronism** (a condition in which the body produces too much aldosterone), and ascites (see Figure 15.7). Spironolactone is sometimes used to treat hormonal acne related to pregnancy, the menstrual cycle, or falling estrogen levels.

Eplerenone and spironolactone are also categorized as aldosterone antagonists. Whereas amiloride and triamterene directly block the aldosterone-sensitive sodium channels, an **aldosterone antagonist** works by inhibiting aldosterone. **Aldosterone** promotes sodium and water reabsorption in the distal convoluted tubule and collecting duct of the nephron. Eplerenone is more specific than spironolactone in its affinity for aldosterone.

FIGURE 15.7
Medication Label for Spironolactone

Spironolactone is a potassium-sparing diuretic that is available as a tablet and oral suspension.

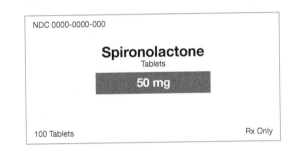

NDC 0000-0000-000

Spironolactone
Tablets

50 mg

100 Tablets   Rx Only

Dosage Forms and Administration Eplerenone tablets may be taken with or without food. Spironolactone is available as a tablet and an oral suspension, both of which may also be taken with or without food.

Side Effects Potassium retention, GI upset, headache, confusion, and drowsiness are side effects related to potassium-sparing diuretics. A specific side effect associated with aldosterone antagonists is gynecomastia. If bothersome, this effect may limit therapy because there is no treatment for it other than to stop taking the drug.

Contraindications Potassium-sparing diuretics should not be used in the presence of elevated serum potassium, kidney insufficiency or impairment, or anuria.

Eplerenone and spironolactone have a shared contraindication: neither drug should be used in patients who have Addison's disease. These medications also each have specific contraindications associated with their use. Eplerenone contraindications include concomitant use of drugs that strongly inhibit cytochrome P450 3A4 (CYP3A4), such as ketoconazole, itraconazole, clarithromycin, and ritonavir. In patients who have hypertension, the following are contraindications for eplerenone: impaired kidney function, type 2 diabetes with microalbuminuria, and concomitant use of potassium supplements or other potassium-sparing diuretics. Spironolactone is contraindicated with concomitant eplerenone use.

Cautions and Considerations Patients who are prescribed potassium-sparing agents must undergo periodic laboratory tests to monitor for hyperkalemia and should avoid salt substitutes and foods containing high amounts of potassium (such as bananas).

Drug Interactions These diuretics must be administered with caution in patients who are taking ACE inhibitors or other drugs that increase potassium levels.

Thiazide and Thiazide-Related Diuretics

Thiazide and thiazide-related diuretics are indicated for the treatment of edema and hypertension. They may also be used as adjunct therapy in patients who have CKD. Some of these medications include **chlorothiazide (Diuril, Sodium Diuril); chlorthalidone; hydrochlorothiazide, HCTZ; indapamide; metolazone (Zaroxolyn)**, and combination **triamterene / hydrochlorothiazide (Dyazide, Maxzide)**, a combination potassium-sparing diuretic and thiazide diuretic used for the treatment of hypertension and edema in patients with low potassium or for whom low potassium levels could be dangerous. Other combinations are available. **Atenolol / chlorthalidone (Tenoretic)** is a cardioselective beta-blocker combined with a diuretic that is used to treat hypertension. **Bisoprolol / hydrochlorothiazide (Ziac)** is a beta-blocker combined with a diuretic. **Lisinopril / hydrochlorothiazide (Prinzide, Zestoretic)** is a combination ACE inhibitor and thiazide diuretic used for the treatment of hypertension, heart failure, and acute MI. **Losartan / hydrochlorothiazide (Hyzaar)** is an ARB combined with a thiazide diuretic used for the treatment of hypertension and stroke risk reduction. These commonly prescribed thiazide and thiazide-related diuretics are listed in Table 15.5.

These diuretics have similar potencies but may differ in onset, peak, and duration of action.

Thiazide and thiazide-related diuretics work by blocking a molecular pump that pulls sodium and chloride back into the blood from the distal convoluted tubule. Therefore, the use of thiazides and thiazide-related diuretics promotes sodium and water excretion in the urine, lowers the sodium level in the blood, and reduces vasoconstriction. The increased sodium concentrations in the urine lead to an increased exchange of potassium for sodium, so potassium is also lost.

Dosage Forms and Administration Chlorthalidone should be taken with food or milk early in the day. With multiple doses, the last dose should be taken no later than 6:00 p.m. to prevent nocturia.

Chlorothiazide is available in oral and injectable forms. The injection should only be given via the IV route.

Hydrochlorothiazide is only available in an oral form and may be taken once or twice a day.

Indapamide should be administered in the morning to prevent nocturia and may be taken with food or milk if GI upset occurs.

Metolazone should be taken with food early in the day to prevent nocturia; the last dose should be taken no later than 6:00 p.m.

Side Effects Side effects associated with thiazide diuretics include hypokalemia. For that reason, patients should be told to ingest potassium (bananas, orange juice, citrus fruits) daily. Other side effects of these diuretics include hypomagnesemia (deficiency of magnesium in the blood), hyperuricemia (excess of uric acid in the blood), hyperglycemia (excess of sugar in the blood), and hypercalcemia (excess of calcium in the blood). Metolazone may increase patients' sensitivity to sunlight.

Contraindications Thiazide diuretics are related to sulfonamide drugs and, therefore, are contraindicated in patients who have a hypersensitivity to sulfonamides. These medications are also contraindicated in patients who have anuria.

Metolazone has an additional contraindication. This oral diuretic should not be administered to patients who are experiencing hepatic coma or precoma.

Cautions and Considerations Thiazide diuretics deplete the body's potassium levels, which is essential for effective cardiac function. Consequently, patients often take potassium supplements with these diuretics to maintain proper electrolyte balance.

Safety Alert

Hyzaar, the brand name for losartan / hydrochlorothiazide, is easily confused with Cozaar, the brand name for losartan only. For that reason, pharmacy technicians should ensure that prescriptions for Hyzaar include both losartan (the ARB component) *and* hydrochlorothiazide.

Name Exchange

Hydrochlorothiazide is a commonly used thiazide diuretic. Healthcare practitioners often refer to hydrochlorothiazide by its abbreviation: *HCTZ*.

Drug Interactions Thiazide diuretics can interact with alcohol, which may contribute to decreased blood pressure. For that reason, patients should use caution when drinking alcohol while taking these medications. Thiazides also interact with drugs used to treat diabetes, resulting in increased blood glucose levels. However, this interaction is not a concern if a low-dose drug regimen is followed. Because thiazide diuretics may interact with corticosteroids and lithium, these medications are not typically used concurrently. Further, thiazide and thiazide-related diuretics may increase the QT-prolonging effects of dofetilide. Prolonged QT intervals can ultimately lead to cardiac death.

FIELD NOTES

It is estimated that nearly half of older adults use at least five prescription drugs. These medications may be prescribed by different providers and filled at different pharmacies. This practice, known as *polypharmacy*, has been linked to preventable health problems and unnecessary deaths, according to an article from Kaiser Health News. The path to drug overuse can be progressive. For example, an older adult may be taking an antihypertensive to treat high blood pressure. The use of this medication may, in turn, result in that individual developing swollen ankles. The individual is then prescribed a diuretic to treat the swollen ankles, which, in turn, causes a potassium deficiency. To treat this deficiency, the older adult is then prescribed a potassium supplement, which results in the individual experiencing nausea. The nausea is then treated with another medication, which causes the individual to feel confused, which is, in turn, treated with more medication. Eliminating duplicate medications, assessing for drug interactions, and reviewing medicine regimens for appropriate dosing may reduce the incidence of polypharmacy.

15.7 Anemia and Drug Treatments

Anemia is a condition characterized by a lower-than-normal number of healthy red blood cells (RBCs) or low levels of hemoglobin, a protein in RBCs. Hemoglobin (Hgb) and hematocrit (HCT) are markers for the laboratory blood tests used to diagnose anemia. When Hgb and HCT values fall below normal ranges, anemia is suspected. Further diagnostic measures and iron studies may be used to determine the cause of anemia.

The most common cause of anemia is inadequate production of RBCs. This condition may result from reduced **erythropoietin**, a hormone secreted by the kidneys that stimulates the production of RBCs. CKD reduces the kidney's ability to make erythropoietin, thus impeding **erythropoiesis**, the production of RBCs. To counter this reduction in erythropoietin, erythropoietin-stimulating agents are prescribed to treat this underlying cause of anemia (see Table 15.7).

A lower RBC count may also be caused by iron or vitamin B deficiencies. If nutrient deficiency is found to be the cause of anemia, supplemental iron or vitamin B therapies, shown in Table 15.7, are prescribed. However, sometimes multiple factors contribute to anemia, making therapy more complicated. For example, a patient may have anemia secondary to a deficiency in multiple nutrients. In this case, therapy is targeted at restoring these specific nutrients to optimal levels.

TABLE 15.7 Commonly Used Agents for the Treatment of Anemia

Generic (Brand)	Pronunciation	Dosage Form	Common Dosage	Dispensing Status
Erythropoietin-Stimulating Agents				
darbepoetin alfa (Aranesp)	dar-be-POE-e-tin AL-fa	injection	varies	Rx
epoetin alfa (Epogen, Procrit, Retacrit)	eh-POE-e-tin AL-fa	injection	varies	Rx
Oral Iron Supplements				
ferrous fumarate (Femiron, Ferrocite, Hemocyte)	FER-us FYOO-ma-rate	tablet	100–200 mg elemental iron a day in divided doses	OTC, Rx
ferrous gluconate (Ferate, Fergon)	FER-us GLOO-koe-nate	tablet	100–200 mg elemental iron a day in divided doses	OTC
ferrous sulfate (Ferosol, FeroSul, Slow Iron)	FER-us SUL-fate	capsule, elixir, oral drops, syrup, tablet	100–200 mg elemental iron a day in divided doses	OTC, Rx
Parenteral Iron Supplements				
ferumoxytol (Feraheme)	fer-ue-MOX-i-tol	injection	510 mg × 2 doses, separated by 3 to 8 days	Rx
iron dextran (Infed)	EYE-ern DEX-tran	injection	100 mg a dose	Rx
iron sucrose (Venofer)	EYE-ern SOO-krose	injection	100 mg a dose	Rx
sodium ferric gluconate (Ferrlecit)	SOE-dee-um FERR-ic GLOO-ko-nate	injection	125 mg a dose	Rx
B Vitamins				
folic acid, vitamin B_9 (various brands)	FOE-lik AS-id, VYE-ta-min B-nine	injection, tablet	0.4–5 mg a day	OTC, Rx
cyanocobalamin, vitamin B_{12} (various brands)	sye-an-oh-koe-BAL-a-min, VYE-ta-min B-twelve	injection, nasal solution, oral lozenge, sublingual liquid, sublingual tablet, tablet	100–2,000 mcg a day	OTC, Rx

Pharm Fact

Epoetin alpha (Epogen, Procrit, Retacrit) works by stimulating the production of RBCs and is the manufactured form of erythropoetin, which naturally occurs in the human body.

Erythropoietin-Stimulating Agents

Patients who have CKD often are deficient in erythropoietin. An **erythropoietin-stimulating agent (ESA)** is used to induce RBC production by activating the release of reticulocytes (a **reticulocyte** is an immature RBC).

ESAs are indicated to treat anemia caused by CKD or by the administration of chemotherapy to patients who have cancer. Two commonly prescribed ESAs are **darbepoetin alfa (Aranesp)** and **epoetin alfa (Epogen, Procrit, Retacrit)**, also known as erythropoietin. Epoetin alfa has two additional indications: anemia due to the use of zidovudine in patients who are infected with human immunodeficiency virus (HIV) and reduction of allogeneic RBC transfusion in patients who are undergoing elective, noncardiac, nonvascular surgery.

Dosage Forms and Administration The preferred route of administration for epoetin alfa and darbepoetin alfa is the subcutaneous route. However, the IV route of administration should be used for patients who have CKD and are undergoing hemodialysis.

Side Effects The side effects of using ESAs include hypertension, peripheral edema, shortness of breath, cough, seizures, increased risk of blood clots, and allergic reactions.

Contraindications Both darbepoetin alfa and epoetin alfa are contraindicated in patients who have uncontrolled hypertension or pure red cell aplasia (a rare condition in which patients lack the precursors to RBCs). Epoetin multidose vials contain benzyl alcohol, which is contraindicated in neonates and infants as well as in pregnant or breast-feeding patients.

Cautions and Considerations ESAs have several boxed warnings regarding their use. One warning is for the risk of serious cardiovascular events, thromboembolic events, stroke, and death. Another warning is specific to patients who have CKD. In these patients, the use of ESAs is associated with a greater risk of death, serious cardiovascular problems, and stroke when used to elevate Hgb levels to more than 11 g/dL. A third warning relates to shortened overall survival and increased risk of tumor progression in patients who have breast, non–small cell lung, head and neck, lymphoid, or cervical cancer. ESAs must be dispensed with Medication Guides.

Drug Interactions ESAs may stimulate the blood clotting effects of lenalidomide (a drug used in the treatment of multiple myeloma and myelodysplastic syndromes) and thalidomide (a drug used in the treatment of multiple myeloma and of complications associated with leprosy). Therapy should be monitored in patients using ESAs with either drug.

Oral and Parenteral Iron Supplements

Iron is used alone to treat iron-deficiency anemia or in combination with ESAs to treat anemia associated with CKD. The process of replacing iron is called **iron supplementation**. This process can take up to six months to replenish iron stores and produce normal RBCs with adequate hemoglobin content. Table 15.7 lists commonly used iron supplements.

Iron supplements may be administered orally or parenterally. An **oral iron supplement** is an iron supplement that is taken by mouth. Oral supplements include **ferrous fumarate (Femiron, Ferrocite, Hemocyte), ferrous gluconate (Ferate, Fergon)**, and **ferrous sulfate (Ferosol, FeroSul, Slow Iron)**. The dosage of these iron supplements is based on the amount of elemental iron required.

Parenteral iron supplements include **ferumoxytol (Feraheme), iron dextran (Infed), iron sucrose (Venofer)**, and **sodium ferric gluconate (Ferrlecit)**. These iron supplements are available by prescription only and are administered intravenously, which allows a more rapid restoration of iron levels than oral iron supplements do.

The indications for parenteral iron products vary slightly. Table 15.8 lists the FDA-approved indications for each drug.

Dosage Forms and Administration Oral ferrous fumarate, ferrous gluconate, and ferrous sulfate should be administered with water or juice. The vitamin C in juice increases iron absorption. If GI upset occurs with the administration of these oral iron supplements, the supplements can be taken on an empty stomach or with food. If food must be coadministered, patients should avoid consuming cereals, dietary fiber,

TABLE 15.8 FDA Indications of Commonly Used Parenteral Iron Supplements

Parenteral Iron Supplement	FDA Indication
ferumoxytol (Feraheme)	iron deficiency in adults who have CKD or adults who do not tolerate or respond to oral iron supplements
iron dextran (INFeD)	iron deficiency (when oral iron supplementation is not adequate or not possible)
iron sucrose (Venofer)	iron deficiency in CKD
sodium ferric gluconate (Ferrlecit)	iron deficiency in hemodialysis patients receiving supplemental epoetin therapy

tea, coffee, eggs, and milk due to decreased iron absorption. The tablet and capsule forms of iron supplements should be swallowed whole and should not be crushed, chewed, split, divided, or opened.

In addition, oral iron products should not be taken with antacids or other acid-reducing medications because absorption of iron will be decreased. These oral iron supplements should also not be taken with tetracycline or fluoroquinolones because iron binds to these antibiotics and reduces their effectiveness at fighting infection.

Ferumoxytol, iron dextran, iron sucrose, and sodium ferric gluconate are administered intravenously. Iron dextran may also be administered intramuscularly. During parenteral iron administration, patients should be reclined or semi-reclined. These injections can be administered diluted or undiluted, with the exception of ferumoxytol; this medication must be diluted with normal saline or dextrose 5% in water (D$_s$W) prior to administration.

Side Effects GI side effects may occur with the use of oral iron supplements. These side effects include nausea, vomiting, constipation, and diarrhea. Stools may also appear darker in color.

Parenteral iron therapy is associated with side effects such as hypotension, rash, dizziness, itching, edema, and fever. Ferumoxytol and iron dextran, in particular, may cause hypersensitivity reactions, including anaphylaxis.

Contraindications Use of oral iron supplements is contraindicated in hemochromatosis and hemolytic anemias.

Iron dextran is contraindicated in any anemia not associated with iron deficiency.

Cautions and Considerations Oral iron supplements can pose a poison risk to children. Iron overdose in children can be fatal, and doses do not have to be extremely large to cause significant problems. Patients should be instructed to keep oral iron supplements in childproof packaging and out of the reach of children.

Parenteral iron preparations should be avoided in patients who have active systemic infections. Documentation of allergenic cross-reactivity for parenteral iron is limited. However, there is a possibility of cross-reactivity between parenteral iron products.

Two of the parenteral iron supplements have boxed warnings. Ferumoxytol has a warning for hypersensitivity reactions and anaphylaxis. Symptoms such as hypotension, syncope, and cardiorespiratory arrest may occur with use. Emergency resuscitation equipment and personnel trained in the management of anaphylaxis should be present during administration of ferumoxytol and for 30 minutes after administration. Patients' pulse and blood pressure readings should be monitored during this time.

Safety Alert

The ISMP considers iron dextran a high-alert medication. High-alert medications are those medications that pose a heightened risk of causing significant harm when used in error.

Like ferumoxytol, iron dextran has a boxed warning for risk of hypersensitivity reactions and anaphylaxis. This risk may be increased by concurrent use of ACE inhibitors. Anaphylactic-type reactions, including fatalities, have followed the administration of iron dextran. Consequently, emergency resuscitation equipment and personnel trained in the management of anaphylaxis should be present during administration. A test dose of iron dextran should be administered prior to the first therapeutic dose. If no signs or symptoms of hypersensitivity follow the test dose, the full therapeutic dose may be given.

Healthcare practitioners should be aware that ferumoxytol use may alter the appearance of magnetic resonance imaging (MRIs) for up to three months. In addition, healthcare practitioners should know that iron dextran is considered a high-alert medication by the Institute for Safe Medication Practices (ISMP).

Some formulations of sodium ferric gluconate contain benzyl alcohol. Benzyl alcohol may be fatally toxic to neonates.

Drug Interactions Oral iron has many drug interactions. Iron absorption is decreased by calcium supplements and medications that decrease the acidity of the GI tract (such as proton pump inhibitors). Iron may decrease the absorption of medications such as fluoroquinolones and doxycycline.

Drugs that decrease blood pressure may enhance the hypotensive effects of parenteral iron. Dimercaprol may enhance the nephrotoxic effects of injectable iron preparations.

Patients using ACE inhibitors may experience heightened adverse effects with iron dextran preparations.

In addition, the effects of certain medications may be exacerbated by the use of parenteral iron supplements. For example, the concurrent use of dimercaprol and parenteral iron supplements may enhance nephrotoxicity, and the concurrent use of antihypertensives and parenteral iron supplements may result in dramatic hypotensive effects.

B Vitamins

Folate-deficiency anemia is anemia caused by a lack of folic acid in the blood. **Folic acid**, also known as *vitamin B₉*, helps the body make RBCs. Folate-deficiency anemia is more likely to occur in patients who do not consume enough foods rich in folic acid (such as green, leafy vegetables). Other causes of this type of anemia include overconsumption of alcohol; GI system diseases (such as celiac disease); certain medications, such as methotrexate; and pregnancy. Folic acid, both oral and injectable, is indicated for the treatment of folate-deficiency anemia. **Vitamin B₁₂**, also known as cobalamin, is naturally occurring in many animal products such as meat, fish, poultry, eggs, and milk.

Vitamin B₁₂ deficiency can cause anemia. This type of anemia is more likely to occur in patients with inadequate dietary intake of vitamin B₁₂ (such as strict vegetarians or vegans) and those with decreased stomach absorption of vitamin B₁₂ (such as those with pernicious anemia or a history of stomach or bariatric surgery). Vitamin B₁₂, commonly in the form of cyanocobalamin, is used to treat vitamin B₁₂ deficiency anemias.

Dosage Forms and Administration Oral formulations of folic acid may be administered without regard to meals. Injectable formulations may be given undiluted or diluted in normal saline or D₅W. Oral cyanocobalamin may be taken with or without food. Oral lozenges should be allowed to dissolve in the mouth, and sublingual tablets should be allowed to dissolve under the tongue before swallowing. Depending on the formulation, injectable cyanocobalamin may be given diluted or undiluted.

Side Effects Abdominal cramps, diarrhea, rash, sleep disorders, irritability, confusion, and nausea are side effects of folic acid. Hypersensitivity reactions have occurred with the use of injectable folic acid. Oral cyanocobalamin is associated with nausea, headache, and diarrhea. Nasal dosage forms are associated with headache, infection, and runny nose. Reported side effects of injectable cyanocobalamin include weakness, headache, and hypersensitivity reactions.

Contraindications Oral and injectable folic acid do not have contraindications. Sensitivity to vitamin B_{12} contraindicates cyanocobalamin use.

Cautions and Considerations Folic acid should not be used alone in patients who have anemias that are also due to vitamin B_{12} deficiency. These patients should have supplemental vitamin B_{12} therapy. In addition, folic acid use may decrease the serum concentrations of phenytoin, fosphenytoin, or phenobarbital.

Some injectable formulations of folic acid contain benzyl alcohol, which may be fatally toxic to neonates. Other formulations contain aluminum. Toxic aluminum concentrations may be seen with high doses, prolonged use, or renal dysfunction. Patients with Leber disease (a hereditary optic nerve disorder) may experience worsening optic atrophy with vitamin B_{12} use. Those with severe anemia that is treated intensely with vitamin B_{12} may experience hypokalemia and sudden death.

Drug Interactions Folic acid may enhance the adverse effects of fluorouracil. Folic acid may decrease the therapeutic effects of raltitrexed and concurrent use should be avoided.

Folic acid may decrease the levels of phenobarbital, phenytoin, primidone, and sulfadoxine. Sulfasalazine may decrease levels of folic acid. Chloramphenicol and colchicine may decrease the effects of cyanocobalamin.

15.8 Advanced Chronic Kidney Disease and Dialysis Therapies

Treatment for advanced stages of CKD often includes dialysis or kidney transplant. **Dialysis** is an artificial method of filtering blood and correcting the electrolyte imbalances caused by kidney failure. It has two common types: hemodialysis and peritoneal dialysis. **Hemodialysis** is accomplished by diverting blood flow through a machine that mechanically filters the blood and then returns it to the body (see Figure 15.8). **Peritoneal dialysis** is accomplished by putting **dialysate** (a fluid that draws toxins from the body into itself) into the abdominal cavity and leaving it there for a certain period—typically, a few hours (see Figure 15.9). During this time, toxins and electrolytes diffuse into the dialysate fluid from the many capillaries in the abdominal cavity.

Dialysis can be a lifesaving intervention. However, it is not without adverse effects. Patients who have CKD and are undergoing dialysis therapy may experience imbalances in electrolytes and hormones, such as phosphorus, calcium, and parathyroid hormone. Consequently, these patients must have their electrolyte and hormone levels monitored. Depending on the results of laboratory tests, patients may require drug therapy to balance these levels. Drugs commonly used in patients who are undergoing dialysis can be found in Table 15.9.

FIGURE 15.8
Hemodialysis

In hemodialysis, a patient is connected to a machine in a dialysis center and must remain at the center for several hours.

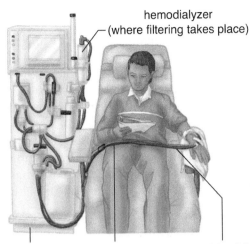

hemodialyzer
(where filtering takes place)

hemodialysis machine | unfiltered blood flows to hemodialyzer | filtered blood flows back to body

FIGURE 15.9
Peritoneal Dialysis

In peritoneal dialysis, a patient has the freedom to receive treatment at home, at work, or while traveling.

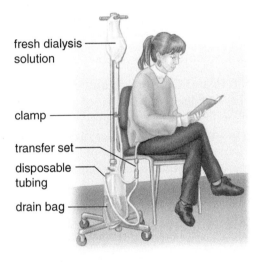

fresh dialysis solution

clamp

transfer set

disposable tubing

drain bag

TABLE 15.9 Commonly Used Agents for Dialysis Therapies

Generic (Brand)	Pronunciation	Dosage Form	Common Dosage	Dispensing Status
Phosphate Binder				
sevelamer (Renagel, Renvela)	se-VEL-a-mer	oral packet, tablet	varies based on serum phosphorus levels	Rx
Vitamin D Supplement				
calcitriol (Rocaltrol)	kal-si-TRYE-ole	capsule, injection, ointment, oral solution	IV: 0.5–3 mcg 3 times a week oral: 0.25–1 mcg a day	Rx
Calcimimetic				
cinacalcet (Sensipar)	sin-a-KAL-set	tablet	30–180 mg a day	Rx

Phosphate Binders

Phosphorus is not removed efficiently in patients who have CKD and are undergoing dialysis. For this reason, a combination of dietary phosphorus restrictions and medications to prevent phosphate absorption, called *phosphate binders*, may be used. A **phosphate binder** binds to dietary phosphorus in the GI tract and forms phosphate compounds that cannot be absorbed. Ultimately, the phosphate compounds are excreted in the feces.

A variety of phosphate-binding agents is available. **Sevelamer (Renagel, Renvela)** is commonly used. This medication binds phosphate in the intestinal lumen (cavity), limiting its absorption. The drug has the ability to decrease serum phosphate concentrations without altering calcium, aluminum, or bicarbonate concentrations.

Dosage Forms and Administration Sevelamer is available as a powder and as tablets. Patients with a swallowing disorder may need to use the powder packet for oral suspension due to the risk of esophageal tablet retention. Tablets should be swallowed whole and not chewed, crushed, or divided. Crushed or divided tablets will rapidly expand in water or saliva and may present a choking hazard.

Side Effects Sevelamer may cause vomiting, nausea, diarrhea, and GI upset. Sevelamer hydrochloride (Renagel) has the specific side effect of metabolic acidosis.

Contraindications Bowel obstruction contraindicates sevelamer use.

Cautions and Considerations Sevelamer should be used with caution in patients who have GI disorders. The use of this drug may also cause bowel obstruction or bowel perforation.

In addition, sevelamer use may decrease the absorption of various vitamins, such as vitamin B_9 (folic acid), vitamin D, vitamin E, and vitamin K. Serum calcium, bicarbonate, and chloride concentrations should be monitored during sevelamer therapy.

Other considerations are specific to the salt forms of sevelamer. Renagel, a hydrochloride salt, may induce metabolic acidosis. Renvela has the advantage of being a carbonate salt, which serves as a buffer and may be better tolerated. These two products should not be interchanged without prescriber approval.

Drug Interactions Sevelamer can interfere with the absorption of other drugs. For example, it may decrease the concentration of calcitriol, cyclosporine, levothyroxine, mycophenolate, quinolone antibiotics, or tacrolimus. Therefore, patients should take other medications at least one hour before or three hours after the administration of this drug.

Vitamin D Supplements

In normally functioning kidneys, **vitamin D** is converted to its biologically active form. Vitamin D has many responsibilities in the body, including regulating calcium, phosphorus, and parathyroid hormone levels.

When kidney function declines, the ability to activate vitamin D decreases. Without active vitamin D, calcium and phosphorus levels in the body become abnormal. To compensate for these abnormal levels, the parathyroid glands secrete parathyroid hormone. Parathyroid hormone ultimately leads to increased calcium in the blood (pulling from bone stores). Excess calcium in the bloodstream is problematic because it can deposit in soft tissues and lead to calcification. If the arteries leading to the heart, for example, become calcified, blood flow may be reduced, and a heart attack may occur. Calcification of the lungs may lead to difficulty breathing, and calcification of joints may lead to pain. Excess parathyroid hormone can also be harmful by causing secondary hyperparathyroidism, which can lead to problems with bones.

One way to prevent the electrolyte and hormone imbalances caused by inadequate active vitamin D is to supplement with the active form of vitamin D. **Calcitriol (Rocaltrol)** is one such drug that is indicated to treat secondary hyperparathyroidism in patients who have CKD. Calcitriol is also indicated for patients who have hypoparathyroidism or pseudohypoparathyroidism.

Dosage Forms and Administration Oral dosage forms of calcitriol include capsules and an oral solution, and these formulations may be administered without regard to food. IV calcitriol may be administered as a bolus dose through a catheter at the end of hemodialysis.

Side Effects Hypercalcemia, headache, skin rash, increased urination, urinary tract infection, and nausea are common side effects of calcitriol use.

Contraindications Contraindications for calcitriol include hypersensitivity to other vitamin D products, hypercalcemia, and vitamin D toxicity.

Cautions and Considerations Calcitriol use may lead to excessive vitamin D. Products that contain vitamin D (such as multivitamins, vitamin D supplements, and vitamin D analogs) may increase the risk of vitamin D toxicity. Excessive vitamin D may also lead to suppression of parathyroid hormone, increased calcium in the urine, increased serum phosphate levels, bone disease, or hypercalcemia. Due to the risk of hypercalcemia, calcium levels should be monitored closely in patients using calcitriol.

Other causes of hypercalcemia may include the use of thiazide diuretics and abrupt dietary changes, such as an increased intake of dairy products. Patients should maintain adequate dietary (supplemental) calcium for a clinical response to vitamin D. For patients who have a tendency to develop hypercalcemia, low doses of calcium or no supplementation may be necessary.

Oral calcitriol formulations may contain potential allergens such as coconut oil, palm seed oil, or tartrazine. The IV calcitriol formulations may contain aluminum. Toxic aluminum concentrations may be seen with high doses, prolonged use, or kidney dysfunction. This risk is higher in premature neonates.

Drug Interactions Calcitriol is metabolized by CYP3A4. Drugs that induce metabolism (such as carbamazepine and phenytoin) or inhibit metabolism (such as clarithromycin and ketoconazole) may alter calcitriol levels. Calcitriol may increase the levels of aluminum hydroxide, magnesium salts, and sucralfate. For that reason, concurrent therapy is not advised. Bile acid sequestrants, such as cholestyramine, may decrease the levels of calcitriol.

Calcimimetics

A class of drug known as *calcimimetics* lowers parathyroid hormone and calcium levels by increasing the parathyroid gland's sensitivity to calcium in the blood. **Cinacalcet (Sensipar)** is a commonly used **calcimimetic** indicated for the treatment of primary and secondary hyperparathyroidism. It also has an indication for the treatment of parathyroid carcinomas.

Dosage Forms and Administration Cinacalcet should be administered with food or shortly after a meal. Tablets should be administered whole and should not be chewed, crushed, or divided.

Side Effects Nausea and vomiting are the most frequent adverse effects associated with cinacalcet use. **Hypocalcemia**, or lower-than-normal levels of calcium in the blood, may also occur with the use of this calcimimetic.

Contraindications Cinacalcet is contraindicated in patients who have hypocalcemia.

Cautions and Considerations Cinacalcet should only be used by patients who have CKD and are undergoing dialysis. Patients' calcium levels should be monitored during cinacalcet therapy to avoid hypocalcemia, a potentially dangerous condition that can increase the likelihood of seizures.

Drug Interactions Cinacalcet is partially metabolized by CYP3A4, creating a potential for related drug interactions. Inhibitors of 3A4, such as ketoconazole, may increase levels of cinacalcet. Inducers of 3A4, such as phenytoin, may decrease cinacalcet levels. Cinacalcet may increase the concentrations of aripiprazole, atomoxetine, brexpiprazole, doxorubicin, eliglustat, iloperidone, metoprolol, pimozide, tamoxifen, thioridazine, tricyclic antidepressants, and vortioxetine. It may decrease the effects of codeine and tamoxifen.

15.9 End-Stage Chronic Kidney Disease and Kidney Transplantation

Kidney transplantation is the treatment of choice for end-stage (stage 5) CKD. This process involves surgically implanting a kidney from a living or deceased donor into a recipient. Kidney transplantation is one of the most common transplant operations in the United States.

Potential kidney transplant recipients undergo an evaluation to determine if they are eligible candidates for the procedure. If so, they are placed on a **national waiting list**. Waiting list priority depends on key factors such as the type of kidney problem, disease severity, and likelihood of transplant success. Kidney transplantation takes approximately three hours. After the procedure, patients can expect to stay in the hospital for several days. Procedure recovery time varies, but the average period is six months.

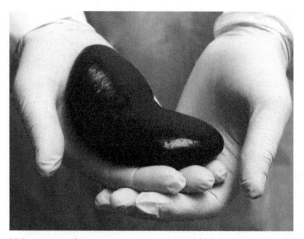

kidney transplant surgery concept. real kidney is in hands of transplant surgeon. cadaver, donor kidney. International Kidney Day Holiday

Almost all patients who undergo kidney transplantation require maintenance immunosuppression with renal transplant drugs to help prevent organ rejection. A **renal transplant drug** is a medication that assists the body in accepting a transplanted kidney. Organ rejection occurs when an organ recipient's immune system recognizes the donor organ as foreign. The recipient's immune system then attempts to attack the donated organ.

At the time of transplant, powerful induction drugs (immunosuppressive therapy aimed to reduce the risk of transplant rejection) are given. For treatment after the immediate transplant period, maintenance renal transplant immunosuppressants are used (see Table 15.10). Glucocorticoids, discussed in Chapter 13, may also be used.

TABLE 15.10 Commonly Used Immunosuppressants for Renal Transplant

Generic (Brand)	Pronunciation	Dosage Form	Common Dosage	Dispensing Status
cyclosporine (Gengraf, Neoral, Sandimmune)	SYE-kloe-spor-een	capsule, injection, oral solution	varies	Rx
mycophenolate mofetil (CellCept)	my-koe-FEN-oh-late MOE-fe-til	capsule, injection, oral suspension, tablet	varies	Rx
mycophenolic acid (Myfortic)	my-koe-fen-AW-lik AS-id	delayed-release capsule	varies	Rx
tacrolimus (Astagraf XL, Envarsus XR, Prograf)	ta-KROE-li-mus	capsule, granules, injection, ointment, oral packet, tablet	varies	Rx

Immunosuppressants

Safety Alert

Mycophenolate mofetil and mycophenolic acid are similar drugs. However, they are not the same, nor are they interchangeable. Double-check prescriptions for either of these drugs to make sure that patients receive the correct formulation.

An **immunosuppressant** is a drug that strategically suppresses the body's immune system. This action is advantageous for organ transplantation because it can help prevent organ rejection. A variety of immunosuppressants are used for kidney transplant patients.

Cyclosporine (Gengraf, Neoral, Sandimmune) is an immunosuppressant indicated for the prevention of transplant rejection. Cyclosporine works by inhibiting interleukin-2 and other cytokines (immunoregulatory proteins) secreted by lymphocytes (a type of white blood cell). Cyclosporine has a small therapeutic window, and blood levels of this drug should be monitored closely.

Mycophenolate is an immunosuppressant indicated for preventing the body from rejecting a kidney transplant. It is available in two forms: **mycophenolate mofetil (CellCept)** and **mycophenolic acid (Myfortic)**. Both forms of mycophenolate block the proliferation of lymphocytes.

Tacrolimus (Astagraf XL, Envarsus XR, Prograf) is an immunosuppressant similar to cyclosporine and is indicated for the prevention of transplanted organ rejection. It suppresses cellular immunity by inhibiting lymphocytes.

Dosage Forms and Administration The oral solution formulation of cyclosporine should not be consumed out of a plastic or a Styrofoam cup. Cyclosporine binds to plastic and Styrofoam, so using these types of containers may result in receiving a smaller dose than intended. Cyclosporine also should not be taken with grapefruit juice, which can increase levels of this immunosuppressant.

Mycophenolate mofetil is available for both oral and IV administration. When preparing mycophenolate mofetil for IV use, technicians should make sure to use only D_5W as a diluent. Mycophenolic acid is available for oral administration only.

Side Effects Common side effects of immunosuppressants include sore throat, cough, dizziness, nausea, muscle aches, fever, chills, itching, and headache. Most of the time, these effects are mild to moderate. Taking acetaminophen can alleviate some of these effects if they are bothersome. Close follow-up care with a healthcare practitioner is necessary for many years after kidney transplantation.

Contraindications Cyclosporine is contraindicated in patients who have a hypersensitivity to polyoxyethylated castor oil. CellCept, a brand name for mycophenolate mofetil, should not be used in patients who have a hypersensitivity to polysorbate 80. Tacrolimus does not have contraindications.

Cautions and Considerations Cyclosporine has several boxed warnings. One warning states that its different formulations are not bioequivalent and should not be used interchangeably. Other warnings include increased risks of hypertension; infections; and malignancies such as lymphomas, kidney impairment, and skin cancer. An additional boxed warning states that patients who are taking cyclosporine should be supervised only by experienced healthcare practitioners.

Mycophenolate has several boxed warnings as well. One warning states that mycophenolate mofetil and mycophenolic acid are not interchangeable. A second warning is for increased risk of congenital malformations and first-trimester pregnancy loss when used by pregnant patients. Other warnings address the risk of infections and of malignancies (such as lymphoma and skin cancer). An additional boxed warning states that only experienced healthcare practitioners should be supervising patients who are taking mycophenolate. Mycophenolate mofetil and mycophenolic acid must be dispensed with Medication Guides.

Tacrolimus has boxed warnings for increased risk of infection and possible development of malignancies such as lymphoma. Another warning states that only experienced healthcare practitioners should be supervising patients taking tacrolimus. Extended-release tacrolimus (Astragraf XL, Envarsus XR) has a boxed warning for increased mortality in female liver transplant recipients. Use of extended-release tacrolimus is not indicated for liver transplantation. In addition, Astagraf XL formulation must be dispensed with an FDA Medication Guide.

Patients taking immunosuppressants are at an increased risk of infection. For that reason, patients are instructed to take special precautions to minimize exposure to infection, such as by wearing face masks and avoiding crowded public areas. Frequent handwashing to prevent disease is always recommended. Patients should also be instructed on precautions concerning appropriate handling and disposal of immunosuppressants because these drugs are considered hazardous agents.

Drug Interactions Immunosuppressants have many drug interactions. The following paragraphs discuss these interactions but address only drugs that should *not* be used concurrently with each immunosuppressant. Immunosuppressants may also enhance the adverse effects of live vaccines and should not be used concurrently with them.

Cyclosporine may increase the concentrations of aliskiren, atorvastatin, bosutinib, cholic acid, dronedarone, lovastatin, pimozide, pitavastatin, silodosin, simeprevir, simvastatin, topotecan, and vincristine. Cyclosporine levels may be increased by conivaptan, crizotinib, idelalisib, and mifepristone. Cyclosporine levels may be decreased by enzalutamide. Eplerenone and potassium-sparing diuretics may enhance the hyperkalemic effect of cyclosporine. Foscarnet and tacrolimus may enhance the nephrotoxic effects of cyclosporine. Cyclosporine may enhance the adverse effects of natalizumab, pimecrolimus, and tofacitinib.

Mycophenolate concentrations may be decreased by bile acid sequestrants, cholestyramine, natalizumab, rifamycin derivatives, and tacrolimus. Pimecrolimus may enhance mycophenolate's adverse reactions.

Tacrolimus may increase the levels of bosutinib, pazopanib, silodosin, topotecan, and vincristine. This immunosuppressant may also enhance the adverse effects of clozapine, cyclosporine, and tofacitinib. Conversely, certain drugs affect tacrolimus levels in the body as well as the adverse effects associated with this immunosuppressant. Tacrolimus levels may be increased by conivaptan, crizotinib, and idelalisib. Tacrolimus levels may be decreased by enzalutamide. The adverse effects of tacrolimus may be enhanced by eplerenone, foscarnet, mifepristone, natalizumab, pimecrolimus, potassium-sparing diuretics, sirolimus, and temsirolimus.

Orally administered tacrolimus cannot be taken with antacids. Alcohol can increase the rate of release of the extended-release formulation of tacrolimus.

Practice Tip

Pharmacy technicians should consult a pharmacist or other drug information specialist for specific drug interaction queries related to the use of immunosuppressants.

Immunosuppressants; drugs used for cancer therapy; and some antiviral drugs, hormone agents, and bioengineered drugs may be considered hazardous drugs (HDs). Healthcare workers, including pharmacy technicians and pharmacists, who prepare or handle HDs may be exposed to these drugs in the workplace. Exposure to HDs, particularly repeated exposures, can lead to adverse effects. Some of these effects are mild, such as skin rashes; other effects are more serious, such as infertility, leukemia, and cancer. The risks typically depend on the HD's toxicity and the healthcare worker's degree of exposure to it.

Pharmacy technicians can protect themselves from unnecessary exposure by donning personal protective equipment, commonly referred to as *PPE*, and by closely following protocols for the handling of HDs. For more information, pharmacy technicians can visit the National Institute for Occupational Safety and Health (NIOSH) website at https://www.cdc.gov/niosh/index.htm. The NIOSH website provides information regarding PPE and the safe handling of HDs.

15.10 Complementary and Alternative Therapies

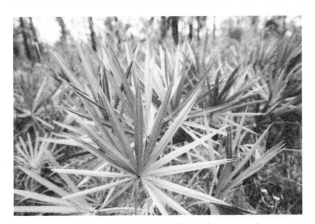

Saw palmetto supplements come from the saw palmetto plant and may be used to treat BPH.

Saw palmetto is used to treat BPH symptoms, such as frequent or painful urination as well as urinary hesitancy and urgency. Clinical studies have shown that this herbal treatment may have efficacy similar to that of finasteride in reducing these symptoms. Saw palmetto is thought to inhibit 5-alpha-reductase, which prevents conversion of testosterone to DHT. It has some anti-inflammatory effects but does not reduce prostate-specific antigen levels (blood tests that screen for prostate cancer). Saw palmetto's side effects are mild and include dizziness, headache, nausea, vomiting, constipation, and diarrhea. Drug interactions with anticoagulants and some hormone therapies are possible. Patients should inform their prescribers and pharmacists if they take saw palmetto. Typical doses are 160 mg twice a day or 320 mg once a day. Saw palmetto teas do not generally provide a high-enough dose to be effective.

Cranberry juice is used for the prevention of recurrent UTIs. Some clinical trials suggest that daily ingestion of 16 ounces of unsweetened cranberry juice is effective in preventing UTIs in pregnant, hospitalized, and older female patients. Although initially thought to acidify urine, cranberry juice is now believed to work by adhering to bacterial cells and preventing them from attaching to the inner walls of the bladder. Cranberry juice does not release bacteria that have already adhered to the bladder wall, so it does not treat an active UTI. Although side effects are few, cranberry juice, when consumed in large quantities, can cause GI upset and diarrhea. Cranberry juice can interact with warfarin, so patients drinking this beverage on a regular basis or in large amounts should inform their healthcare practitioners.

Review and Assessment

CHAPTER SUMMARY

Anatomy and Physiology of the Renal System

- The renal system is responsible for clearing waste products from the blood while maintaining proper fluid, pH, and electrolyte balance.

- The main function of the kidneys is to maintain the balance of water, electrolytes, and acids and bases in the body.

- The kidneys form urine, which is essential for normal body function.

- Ureters transport urine from the kidneys to the urinary bladder.

Renal Function and Pharmacokinetics

- When the kidneys are not functioning correctly, the proper balance of reabsorption and secretion is not maintained, and toxins build up in the blood.

- Patients who are experiencing acute kidney disease have a rapid reduction in kidney function and accumulate toxic nitrogen and other waste products.

- Uremia is the clinical syndrome resulting from renal dysfunction.

- Dysfunction within the ureters or urinary bladder may cause urinary retention or incontinence.

- Kidney function can be assessed via laboratory measurements (BUN and SCr) and calculated estimates (such as CrCl).

- Due to the kidneys' importance to the pharmacokinetic process, prescribers need to be especially mindful of lowering medication doses for a patient who has impaired renal function.

- Certain drugs are toxic to the kidneys; this nephrotoxicity is usually reversible if addressed quickly. Patients using drugs that are toxic to the kidneys should be closely monitored.

Urinary Tract Infection

- A UTI occurs when bacteria, most often *Escherichia coli* (*E. coli*), enter the opening of the urethra and multiply.

- UTIs are typically treated with an antibiotic, often accompanied by a urinary analgesic.

- Phenazopyridine, an OTC urinary analgesic, is used to treat the signs and symptoms associated with UTIs, including pain, burning, urgency, frequency, and other discomforts.

Urinary Incontinence

- Urinary incontinence often affects older adults.

- Commonly used agents for treating urinary incontinence include antimuscarinics and beta-3 adrenergic agonists.

- Antimuscarinics work by inhibiting acetylcholine in the nerves that control involuntary bladder contraction and emptying.

- Common side effects associated with anti-muscarinics include dry mouth, constipation, blurred vision, and urine retention.

- Beta-3 adrenergic agonists, such as mirabegron, work by relaxing the detrusor muscles during urine storage.

- Common side effects associated with mirabegron include hypertension, tachycardia, headache, dizziness, constipation, dry mouth, diarrhea, UTI, back pain, nasopharyngitis, and flu-like symptoms.

Benign Prostatic Hyperplasia

- BPH commonly affects older males.

- Alpha-blockers, which are used to treat BPH, relax urethral sphincters and prostatic smooth muscle, enhancing urinary outflow from the bladder.

- The use of alpha-blockers is associated with dizziness, fatigue, orthostatic hypotension, and priapism.

- 5-alpha-reductase inhibitors treat BPH by inhibiting the conversion of testosterone to DHT, thus reducing the size of the prostate.

- Common side effects associated with 5-alpha-reductase inhibitors include decreased libido, erectile dysfunction, ejaculation disorders, and gynecomastia.

- 5-alpha-reductase inhibitors should not be handled during pregnancy.

Chronic Kidney Disease

- CKD involves progressive damage to kidney tissue, resulting in the death of this tissue over time.

- CKD is classified by stage (stage 1–stage 5); the higher the stage, the more severe the kidney dysfunction.

- A common complication of CKD is volume overload, which is treated with diuretics.

- Another common complication of CKD is hypertension, which is treated with antihypertensive agents such as ACE inhibitors and ARBs.

- The primary purpose of diuretics is to rid the body of excess fluid and electrolytes.

- Diuretics include carbonic anhydrase inhibitors, loop diuretics, potassium-sparing diuretics, thiazide and thiazide-related diuretics, and multiple combination products.

- Common side effects associated with acetazolamide, a carbonic anhydrase inhibitor, include tinnitus (ringing in the ears), tingling, nausea, vomiting, diarrhea, drowsiness, and changes in taste.

- Side effects of using loop diuretics include hypotension, dizziness, headache, skin rash, hair loss (alopecia), GI upset, diarrhea, and constipation.

- Potassium-sparing diuretic use is associated with potassium retention, GI upset, headache, confusion, drowsiness, and gynecomastia.

- Side effects associated with thiazide and thiazide-related diuretics include hypokalemia, hypomagnesemia, hyperuricemia, hyperglycemia, and hypercalcemia.

Anemia

- Anemia is a condition characterized by a lower-than-normal number of healthy RBCs or low levels of hemoglobin.

- CKD reduces the kidney's ability to make erythropoietin, impeding erythropoiesis, the production of RBCs.

- Erythropoietin-stimulating agents (ESAs) are used to induce RBC production by activating the release of reticulocytes.

- The side effects of ESAs include hypertension, peripheral edema, shortness of breath, cough, seizures, increased risk of blood clots, and allergic reactions.

- ESAs have several boxed warnings. One is for the risk of serious cardiovascular events, thromboembolic events, stroke, and death. Another, specifically for patients with CKD, is for greater risk of death, serious cardiovascular problems, and stroke when used to elevate Hgb levels above 11 g/dL. A third relates to shortened overall survival and increased risk of tumor progression in patients with breast, non–small cell lung, head and neck, lymphoid, or cervical cancers.

- Iron supplements are available in oral and injectable formulations and are used to treat iron-deficiency anemia.

- Oral iron supplementation may have side effects such as nausea, vomiting, constipation, and diarrhea; parenteral iron supplementation is associated with side effects such as hypotension, rash, dizziness, itching, edema, and fever.

- Folate-deficiency anemia is caused by a lack of folic acid in the blood; consequently, folic acid is used to treat this type of anemia.

- Abdominal cramps, diarrhea, rash, sleep disorders, irritability, confusion, and nausea are side effects of folic acid.

- Vitamin B_{12} deficiency may result in anemia; vitamin B_{12}, typically in the form of cyanocobalamin, is used for this type of anemia.

Dialysis Therapies

- Treatment for advanced stages of CKD often includes dialysis, which is an artificial method of filtering blood and correcting the electrolyte imbalances caused by kidney failure.

- Dialysis has two common types: hemodialysis and peritoneal dialysis.

- Hemodialysis is accomplished by diverting blood flow through a machine that mechanically filters the blood and then returns it to the body.

- Peritoneal dialysis is accomplished by putting dialysate (a fluid that draws toxins from the body into itself) into the abdominal cavity and leaving it there for a certain period.

- Because electrolyte and hormone levels may fluctuate during dialysis therapy, they must be monitored closely. Patients may require drug therapy to balance these levels.

- Phosphate binders, vitamin D supplements, and calcimimetics are commonly used in patients undergoing dialysis.

- Phosphate binders bind to dietary phosphorus to remove it efficiently in patients who have CKD.

- Side effects of phosphate binders include vomiting, nausea, diarrhea, and GI upset.

- Vitamin D supplements help to prevent the electrolyte and hormone imbalances caused by inadequate active vitamin D in patients who have CKD.

- Side effects associated with vitamin D supplements include hypercalcemia, headache, skin rash, increased urination, UTI, and nausea.

- Calcimimetics lower parathyroid hormone and calcium levels by increasing the parathyroid gland's sensitivity to calcium in the blood.

- Nausea, vomiting, and hypocalcemia are the most frequent adverse effects associated with the use of calcimimetics.

Kidney Transplantation

- Kidney transplantation is the treatment of choice for end-stage (stage 5) CKD.

- Close follow-up care with a healthcare practitioner is necessary for many years after kidney transplantation.

- Almost all patients who undergo kidney transplantation require immunosuppressants to help prevent organ rejection.

- Patients taking immunosuppressants are at an increased risk of hypertension, infection, and malignancies such as lymphomas.

- Common side effects of immunosuppressants include sore throat, cough, dizziness, nausea, muscle aches, fever, chills, itching, and headache.

- Immunosuppressants have several boxed warnings and drug interactions.

Complementary and Alternative Therapies

- Saw palmetto is sometimes used for the treatment of BPH.

- Some clinical trials suggest that daily ingestion of cranberry juice may help prevent UTIs.

DRUG LIST

Urinary Tract Infections

Antibiotics

amoxicillin
amoxicillin / clavulanate (Augmentin)
ciprofloxacin (Cipro)
fosfomycin (Monurol)
levofloxacin
nitrofurantoin (Furadantin, Macrobid, Macrodantin)
sulfamethoxazole / trimethoprim (Bactrim, Bactrim DS, Sulfatrim)

Urinary Analgesic

phenazopyridine (Azo-Urinary Pain Relief, Pyridium)

Urinary Incontinence

Anticholinergics (Antimuscarinics)

darifenacin (Enablex)
fesoterodine (Toviaz)
oxybutynin (Ditropan, Gelnique, Oxytrol)
solifenacin (Vesicare)
tolterodine (Detrol)
trospium (Sanctura)

Beta-3 Adrenergic Agonist

mirabegron (Myrbetriq)

BPH Agents

Alpha-Blockers

alfuzosin (Uroxatral)
doxazosin (Cardura, Cardura XL)
tamsulosin (Flomax)
terazosin

5-Alpha-Reductase Inhibitors

dutasteride (Avodart)
dutasteride / tamsulosin (Jalyn)
finasteride (Propecia, Proscar)

Chronic Kidney Disease

Carbonic Anhydrase Inhibitor

acetazolamide (Diamox Sequels)

Loop Diuretics

bumetanide (Bumex)
ethacrynic acid (Edecrin, Sodium Edecrin)
furosemide (Lasix)
torsemide (Demadex)

Potassium-Sparing Diuretics

amiloride
eplerenone (Inspra)
spironolactone (Aldactone, CaroSpir)
triamterene (Dyrenium)

Thiazide and Thiazide-Related Diuretics

atenolol / chlorthalidone (Tenoretic)
bisoprolol / hydrochlorothiazide (Ziac)
chlorothiazide (Diuril, Sodium Diuril)
chlorthalidone
hydrochlorothiazide, HCTZ
indapamide
lisinopril / hydrochlorothiazide (Prinzide, Zestoretic)
losartan / hydrochlorothiazide (Hyzaar)
metolazone (Zaroxolyn)
triamterene / hydrochlorothiazide (Dyazide, Maxzide)

Anemia

Erythropoietin-Stimulating Agents
    darbepoetin alfa (Aranesp)
    epoetin alfa (Epogen, Procrit, Retacrit)

Oral Iron Supplements
    ferrous fumarate (Femiron, Ferrocite, Hemocyte)
    ferrous gluconate (Ferate, Fergon)
    ferrous sulfate (Ferosol, FeroSul, Slow Iron)

Parenteral Iron Supplements
    ferumoxytol (Feraheme)
    iron dextran (Infed)
    iron sucrose (Venofer)
    sodium ferric gluconate (Ferrlecit)

B Vitamins
    folic acid, vitamin B_9 (various brands)
    cyanocobalamin, vitamin B_{12} (various brands)

Dialysis

Phosphate Binder
    sevelamer (Renagel, Renvela)

Vitamin D Supplement
    calcitriol (Rocaltrol)

Calcimimetic
    cinacalcet (Sensipar)

Renal Transplant

Immunosuppressants
    cyclosporine (Gengraf, Neoral, Sandimmune)
    mycophenolate mofetil (CellCept)
    mycophenolic acid (Myfortic)
    tacrolimus (Astagraf XL, Envarsus XR, Prograf)

Medication Guide
    ciprofloxacin (Cipro)
    darbepoetin alfa (Aranesp)
    epoetin alfa (Epogen, Procrit, Retacrit)
    levofloxacin
    mycophenolate mofetil (CellCept)
    mycophenolic acid (Myfortic)
    tacrolimus (Astragraf XL formulation)

✔ CHECK YOUR UNDERSTANDING

Take a moment to review what you have learned in this chapter and answer the following questions.

1. Which renal system organ is the primary filter for clearing waste products from the blood while maintaining proper fluid, pH, and electrolyte balance?
   a. bladder
   b. kidneys
   c. liver
   d. ureters

2. Which drug class is considered nephrotoxic?
   a. cephalosporins
   b. loop diuretics
   c. nonsteroidal anti-inflammatory drugs
   d. thiazide diuretics

3. What common side effect is associated with the use of phenazopyridine?
   a. constipation
   b. cough
   c. edema
   d. orange-colored urine

4. Which anticholinergic (antimuscarinic) must be protected from light?
   a. darifenacin (Enablex)
   b. fesoterodine (Toviaz)
   c. oxybutynin (Ditropan, Gelnique, Oxytrol)
   d. solifenacin (Vesicare)

5. What drug class includes mirabegron (Myrbetriq)?
   a. alpha-blockers
   b. antimuscarinics
   c. beta-3 adrenergic agonists
   d. immunosuppressants

6. What side effect is associated with the use of alpha-blockers?
   a. edema
   b. neutropenia
   c. orthostatic hypotension
   d. urine discoloration

7. Carbonic anhydrase inhibitors have cross-reactivity in patients with allergies to which drug class?
   a. ACE inhibitors
   b. loop diuretics
   c. penicillins
   d. sulfa drugs

8. Which boxed warning is associated with bumetanide and furosemide?
   a. adrenocortical insufficiency
   b. decreased sodium or potassium levels
   c. profound electrolyte depletion
   d. severe kidney disease or dysfunction

9. Which drug class includes chlorthalidone (Hygroton)?
   a. aldosterone inhibitors
   b. carbonic anhydrase inhibitors
   c. potassium-sparing diuretics
   d. thiazide and thiazide-related diuretics

10. Which boxed warning does *not* apply to ESAs?
    a. risk of serious cardiovascular events, thromboembolic events, stroke, and death
    b. greater risk of death, serious cardiovascular problems, and stroke when elevating Hgb levels to more than 11 g/dL in patients who have chronic kidney disease
    c. shortened overall survival and increased risk of tumor progression in patients who have breast, non–small cell lung, head and neck, lymphoid, or cervical cancer
    d. profound electrolyte depletion

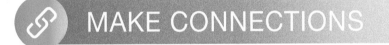

MAKE CONNECTIONS

Take a moment to consider what you have learned in this chapter and respond thoughtfully to the following prompts. Note that some of these activities will require internet access.

1. Diuretics are commonly used drugs and, consequently, appear on top 200 drug lists. For that reason, pharmacy technicians in both community pharmacies and institutional settings are likely to encounter diuretics. To familiarize yourself with the various diuretics, create a table listing each diuretic class discussed in this chapter and its side effects.

2. Oral iron supplements are commonly used to treat iron-deficiency anemia. Most oral supplements are OTC drugs, which makes these medications cost effective and easily accessible. However, oral iron supplements can pose a poison risk to children and can be fatal. Use internet resources to research oral iron overdoses in children. Include the dose ingested and ways to keep oral iron supplements safe from children.

 The online course includes additional review and assessment resources.

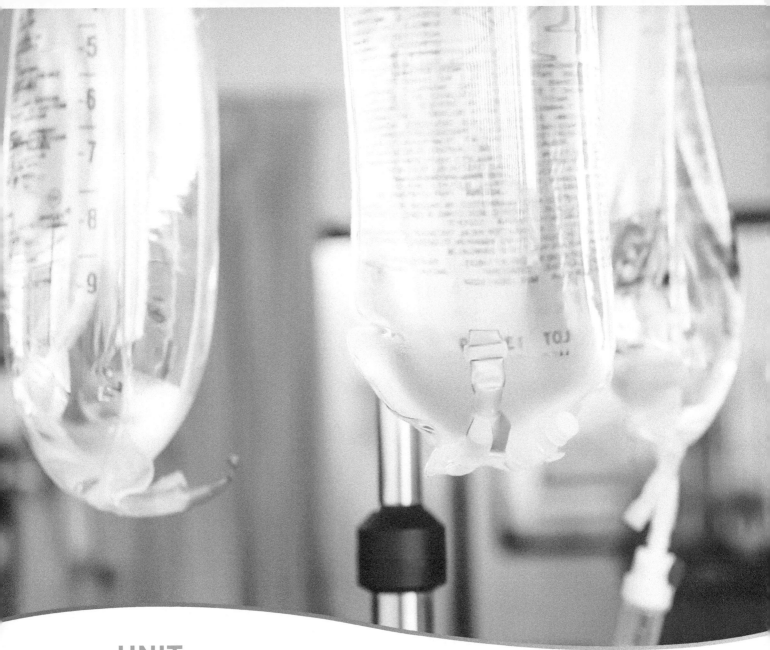

UNIT

3 Pharmacology and Multisystems

Chapter 16 The Immune System, Bacterial Infections, Fungal Infections, and Drug Therapy

Chapter 17 The Immune System, Viral Infections, and Drug Therapy

Chapter 18 Pain, Anesthesia, and Drug Therapy

Chapter 19 Nutrition, Fluids, Electrolytes, and Drug Therapy

Chapter 20 Cancer and Drug Therapy

The Immune System, Bacterial Infections, Fungal Infections, and Drug Therapy

16

Learning Objectives

1 Identify the major organs and cells involved in the immune response. (Section 16.1)

2 Describe the differences between the innate and adaptive immune systems. (Section 16.1)

3 Define *antigen* and *antibody*. (Section 16.1)

4 Identify the major types of antibiotics by drug class. (Sections 16.2, 16.7)

5 Determine which auxiliary labels to use when dispensing major types of antibiotics and antifungals. (Sections 16.3, 16.6, 16.7)

6 Discuss storage requirements for liquid antibiotics. (Section 16.4)

7 List common ophthalmic antibiotics. (Section 16.5)

8 Describe treatments for common sexually transmitted infections. (Section 16.6)

9 Define therapeutic effects, side effects, contraindications, and administration routes of major antibiotics and antifungals. (Sections 16.3, 16.6, 16.7)

10 Use appropriate antibiotic and antifungal general drug terminology in written and oral communication. (Sections 16.3, 16.7)

11 Describe the differences between bacteria and fungi. (Section 16.7)

ASHP/ACPE Accreditation Standards
To view the *ASHP/ACPE Accreditation Standards* addressed in this chapter, refer to Appendix C.

The immune system is a complex network of barriers, organs, and molecules that have evolved over millions of years to work together to defend the body against invading pathogens. Before the 20th century, infection was the most common cause of death in the United States. The development of antibiotics, antifungals, and vaccines has helped treat and prevent infections caused by pathogens.

This chapter describes the immune system and explains the use of antimicrobial agents in treating bacterial and fungal infections that commonly afflict this system. It covers various bacteria and fungi and the typical infections they cause. The number of antimicrobial drugs is large and varied; however, knowing these drugs will be useful because pharmacy technicians often work with them. Antibiotics are frequently dispensed for community-acquired infections, which account for more outpatient visits to physicians than any other medical condition. Antibiotics are also used for infections acquired in hospital or institutional settings (nosocomial infections).

16.1 Anatomy and Physiology of the Immune System

The **immune system** is a complex system made up of specialized organs, ducts, cells, and proteins that work together to help fight infection. The immune system is responsible for protecting and defending the body from foreign particles and pathogens and from internal mechanisms that can cause the body to turn against itself.

Organs that are part of the immune system include the bone marrow, thymus, lymphatic system, and spleen, as shown in Figure 16.1. The bone marrow and thymus are the sites where the cells used by the immune system are produced. **Bone marrow**, which is the spongy material inside bones, is what produces the white blood cells needed to fight infection (B cells and T cells), red blood cells needed to carry oxygen, and platelets needed to help blood clot. The thymus also monitors blood content and produces T cells, or T lymphocytes. The **lymphatic system** is a network of tubes throughout the body. It is made up of lymph nodes, which can trap microbes; lymph vessels, which carry the fluid of the lymphatic system to help cleanse the body's tissues; and white blood cells.

The **spleen** is an organ that filters blood and removes microbes and damaged red blood cells. It can also make some antibodies and lymphocytes.

FIGURE 16.1
The Immune System

Organs within the immune system include the bone marrow, thymus, lymphatic system, and spleen.

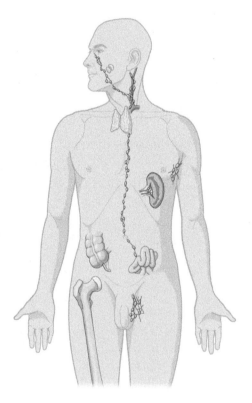

Without an immune system, pathogens could enter the body and cause infection. A **pathogen** is a microorganism, such as a bacterium or virus, that can cause infection or disease. The introduction of a pathogen triggers the body's immune system.

The immune system is typically divided into two categories: the innate immune system and the adaptive immune system. Both are important in protecting against infection.

The Innate Immune System

The **innate immune system** can be thought of as the immune system a person is born with. It orchestrates the body's automatic response to pathogens. This innate immune response provides **nonspecific immunity**, or *innate immunity*. The innate immune system's first line of defense includes the skin, the lungs' mucous lining, and stomach acid, which together serve as a barrier that helps protect an individual from pathogens. If pathogens get past a barrier, the innate immune system deploys its second line of defense, sending inflammatory cells to the site of infection and activating the complement system. The **complement system** is a collection of proteins called *complements* that trigger one another in a chain reaction that complements, or enhances, immunity. The complement system's proteins attract inflammatory cells, mark some bacteria for destruction by phagocytes, kill other pathogenic microbes, and promote the clearance (removal from the body) of immune complexes, which are combined antigen-antibody molecules. The innate immune system reacts similarly to all pathogens.

To work properly the innate immune response requires a variety of white blood cells, including neutrophils, mast cells, basophils, dendritic cells, eosinophils, macrophages, and natural killer cells. Neutrophils, the most abundant type of white blood cell, are usually the first type of cell to respond to an infection. They are responsible for **phagocytosis**, the process by which phagocytes engulf and often destroy pathogens and other particulate matter. Mast cells release chemicals that induce inflammation; two of these chemicals, histamine and heparin, also help with wound healing. Basophils also release histamine. Dendritic cells are antigen-presenting cells, or cells that detect antigens on pathogens and then transport those pathogens to lymphocytes, another type of white blood cell. Lymphocytes are discussed below with the adaptive immune system. Eosinophils secrete toxic proteins and other substances that kill bacteria and parasites. Macrophages move between blood vessels and tissues to invade pathogens; they contain receptors that detect microbes and destroy them through phagocytosis. Natural killer cells do not attack pathogens directly; however, they are able to destroy cells that are infected with pathogens.

The Adaptive Immune System

The **adaptive immune system** can be thought of as the *acquired* immune system because it learns and remembers specific pathogens it has encountered. The adaptive immune system provides long-lasting protection and defense against recurring infections. B cells and T cells, the two main types of lymphocytes, are the primary cells used in the adaptive immune system.

B cells produce antibodies. An **antibody** is a *Y*-shaped protein that recognizes and then binds to a specific type of antigen after the immune system has been exposed to that antigen. An **antigen** is a molecule or molecular structure, often found on the surface of pathogens (such as pathogenic bacteria and viruses), that causes the immune system to produce antibodies against it. Antigens can be thought of as identification tags that tell the body they are a foreign substance and a potential threat to that body. Antibodies are created after the first exposure of an antigen to the immune system. Once exposure has occurred and antibodies for a specific antigen exist, the body can use those antibodies to respond to future attacks by the antigen.

T cells work with other cells to attack a pathogen and can be divided into two types: T-helper cells and killer T cells. T-helper cells are also known as *CD4+* cells because they express CD4 protein on their surface. T-helper cells do not target and kill an invading pathogen, but they are vital to the immune response because they help orchestrate that response and coordinate the attack. Killer T cells find and destroy

Pharm Fact

Antibodies do not destroy a pathogen, but they alert other processes so the pathogen can be destroyed.

infected cells and tumors. When abnormalities occur within the immune system, autoimmune disorders, allergic diseases, and immunodeficiencies can result.

16.2 Bacterial Infections

Bacteria are single-celled organisms that live in almost all environments. For example, many bacteria can be found on the skin, in the mouth, and in the gastrointestinal tract at all times. The vast majority of these organisms only cause disease when they grow uncontrollably or enter the bloodstream. Other bacteria are **pathogenic**, or able to cause an infection or disease when they enter the body through the eyes, nose, or mouth or through bites or wounds on the skin.

When bacteria penetrate body tissues, they sometimes establish an infection. A **bacterial infection** is a condition in which bacteria grow in body tissues and cause tissue damage to the host either by their presence or by toxins they produce. These toxins cause many of the symptoms experienced when an infection is present. The immune system fights back to destroy the bacteria, usually resulting in fever and inflammation. The immune system can often overcome simple infections, but more serious infections may require the assistance of antibiotics to kill the invading bacteria.

The general signs that an infection may be bacterial are a fever of 101° F or higher and elevated white blood cell count ($>12,000/mm^3$). The onset of fever alone, however, is not diagnostic of a bacterial infection. Fevers may also be caused by self-limiting viral illnesses and some types of malignancy and autoimmune disorders. In many situations, symptoms or physical findings are necessary to explain a fever.

Although humans have known of the existence of infectious diseases for thousands of years, it was not until the 19th century that a major cause—bacteria—was identified through the work of Louis Pasteur and other scientists. By the early 20th century, researchers had isolated and identified the organisms that cause cholera, syphilis, bubonic plague, gonorrhea, leprosy, and other illnesses. Once these bacteria were identified, physicians and scientists could begin researching how to kill or treat them.

In 1907, German physician Paul Ehrlich patented the drug arsphenamine as a treatment for syphilis. Although this drug marked a breakthrough in the treatment of a major infectious disease, it was not until 1936 that the first true antibiotic, sulfanilamide (a sulfonamide), was discovered. While the discovery and use of sulfanilamide was valuable and important, this antibiotic did not treat all infections. When penicillin became widely available in the 1940s, physicians finally had a powerful weapon to use against several common infections, including strep throat, pneumonia, and syphilis. Today, a wide variety of antibiotics are used to combat bacterial infections. Each antibiotic is effective against specific types of bacteria.

Work Wise

Bacteria names are often abbreviated in the workplace. For example, technicians may hear *Streptococcus pneumoniae* called "Strep. pneumo." *Clostridium difficile* can be called "C. diff," and *Escherichia coli* is often referred to as "E. coli."

Types of Bacteria

Determining the appropriate antibiotic to use against specific bacteria requires laboratory testing. A sample of material obtained from the infected area is stained, observed under a microscope, and classified according to characteristics that help determine which drug to prescribe. These characteristics include whether the bacteria need oxygen to live, what shape they have (see Figure 16.2), what arrangement they are in, and the thickness of their cell walls.

One characteristic used to classify bacteria is whether they need oxygen in order to survive. Bacteria are either **aerobic**, which means they need oxygen, or **anaerobic**, meaning they can survive in an environment void of oxygen. Bacteria are also classified by their shape, which can be spherical, rod shaped, or spiral shaped (see Figure 16.2). The arrangement of cells is considered as well. If bacterial cells grow in chains or lines, their name begins with *strep*. If they grow in clusters, their name begins with *staph*. If they grow in pairs, their name begins with *diplo*. For instance, *Staphylococcus aureus*, a common bacteria found on the skin, is round and grows in clusters like grapes. See Table 16.1 for more information.

FIGURE 16.2 Characteristic Bacterial Shapes

Spherical bacteria (a) are called *cocci*. Rod-shaped bacteria (b) are called *bacilli*. Spiral-shaped bacteria (c) are called *spiral*. *Streptococcus pyogenes*, the bacteria that cause strep throat, are round and grow in chains.

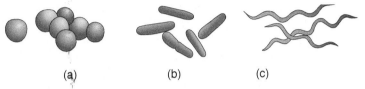

(a)   (b)   (c)

TABLE 16.1 Common Bacterial and Associated Infections

Bacteria	Shape	Associated Infection(s)
Aerobic		
Gram-Positive		
Bacillus anthracis	bacilli	anthrax
Corynebacterium diphtheriae	bacilli	diphtheria
Enterococcus faecalis *Enterococcus faecium*	cocci	intestinal infection urinary tract infection (UTI)
Gardnerella vaginalis *	bacilli	vaginal infections
Lactobacillus species (spp.)	bacilli	vaginal infections
Listeria monocytogenes	bacilli	meningitis
Staphylococcus aureus, other *Staphylococcus* spp.	cocci	skin infection endocarditis
Streptococcus pneumoniae *Streptococcus pyogenes (Group A)*	cocci	pneumonia, respiratory tract infection (RTI) strep throat
Gram-Negative		
Bordetella pertussis	coccobacilli	pertussis
Enterobacter spp. *Escherichia coli*	bacilli	intestinal infection
Haemophilus influenzae	bacilli	RTI
Helicobacter pylori	bacilli	stomach ulcers
Klebsiella spp.	bacilli	intestinal infection
Neisseria meningitidis *Neisseria gonorrhea*	cocci	meningitis gonorrhea
Proteus spp.	bacilli	intestinal infection
Pseudomonas aeruginosa	bacilli	various difficult-to-treat infections

continues

TABLE 16.1 Common Bacterial and Associated Infections—*Continued*

Bacteria	Shape	Associated Infection(s)
Salmonella typhi	bacilli	typhoid fever
Shigella spp.	bacilli	intestinal infection
Vibrio cholerae	comma-shaped bacilli	cholera
Yersinia pestis	bacilli	plague
Anaerobic		
Gram-Positive		
Clostridium tetani	bacilli	tetanus
Clostridium perfringens	bacilli	gangrene
Clostridium botulinum	bacilli	botulism
Clostridium difficile	bacilli	intestinal infection
Peptostreptococcus, Streptococcus	cocci	dental infection
Gram-Negative		
Bacteroides fragilis	bacilli	abdominal infection, sepsis
Miscellaneous		
Treponema pallidum	spirochete	syphilis
Mycoplasma pneumonia *Legionella* spp.	atypical	RTI, pneumonia
Gram-Negative		
Borrelia burgdorferi	spirochete	Lyme disease

*Note that some of these entries are gram-variable, meaning they can appear as gram-positive or gram-negative.

Finally, bacteria are said to be either Gram-positive or Gram-negative. This classification comes from a staining technique named after its developer, Hans Christian Joachim Gram. In this technique, a purple stain called *crystal violet* is applied to the bacteria, and then they are viewed under a microscope. **Gram-positive bacteria** have a thick cell wall that absorbs this stain and appears purple. **Gram-negative bacteria** have a thin cell wall that does not absorb this stain and appears pink. Knowing whether the cell walls are thick or thin is necessary to identify the best antibiotic treatment.

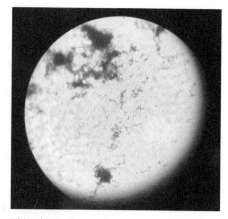

This photo shows Gram-positive bacteria through a microscope.

Antibiotic Selection

An **antibiotic** is a chemical substance with the ability to kill or inhibit the growth of bacteria. In developing antibiotics, the challenge is to find a way to kill the invading organism without harming the patient receiving treatment. This mission is easier to accomplish against bacteria than against other kinds of pathogens because many biological processes are unique to bacteria and not shared by humans. Antibiotics work by gaining access to the inside of the bacterial cell and interfering with these unique biological processes in one of six ways:

- preventing folic acid synthesis (sulfonamides)
- impairing cell-wall formation (penicillins and cephalosporins)
- blocking protein formation (macrolides, tetracyclines, and aminoglycosides)
- interfering with deoxyribonucleic acid (DNA) formation (quinolones)
- disrupting cell membranes (daptomycin)
- disrupting DNA structure (metronidazole)

Physicians and other healthcare providers prescribe antibiotics based on the type of pathogen suspected of causing the infection, the antibiotic's spectrum of activity, and the location of the pathogen. An antibiotic's **spectrum of activity** is the range of bacteria against which it is effective. For example, penicillin can treat Gram-positive, aerobic bacteria, so it can be used against *Streptococcus pyogenes*, a Gram-positive, aerobic bacteria that causes strep throat. To identify a bacteria and facilitate the choice of drug treatment, a sample or swab of the bacteria is taken from the patient and grown in culture in a laboratory. Then, various antibiotics are tested on the culture to determine which drug has the best effect on the pathogen. This laboratory test is called a **culture and sensitivity (C&S) test**. The amount of a drug needed to inhibit growth of a bacteria is called its **minimum inhibitory concentration (MIC)**; MIC results are often reported along with the C&S results.

When a patient has a serious or life-threatening infection, antibiotic treatment must begin immediately; healthcare providers cannot wait for laboratory tests to confirm what type of bacteria is causing the infection. In this situation, the patient is given a **broad-spectrum antibiotic**, which is effective against multiple organisms. This approach of using a medication to treat a patient before the specific microorganism causing their infection is identified is called **empirical treatment**.

A **nosocomial infection**, or healthcare-associated infection (HAI), is one that is acquired while the patient is in a hospital or nursing home. Nosocomial infections are often drug resistant and difficult to treat. In these cases, the common first choice of therapy cannot be used, because the bacteria are already known to be resistant. Because these infections can be serious and even life threatening, aggressive antibiotics may be warranted. In these situations, broad-spectrum drugs are started empirically, and therapy is modified based on C&S results.

The choice of route of administration for antibiotic therapy depends on the site and severity of the infection as well as the bacteria suspected of causing it. In most cases, antibiotics are best given at even intervals throughout the day. For children, antibiotics are often dosed for an entire day, based on the child's weight, but are administered in divided doses. Doses provided in this text are presented as general guides for recognizing when a prescribed dose is out of the ordinary. Always refer to the package insert or other reliable sources to verify proper dosing and double-check dose calculations for children.

An antibiotic may be either a **bactericidal agent**, which kills the invading bacteria, or a **bacteriostatic agent**, which inhibits the growth or multiplication of bacteria. It is preferable to start antibiotic treatment after the bacteria have been identified by culturing. The outcome of antibiotic treatment can be evaluated in two ways: (1) by the clinical response, meaning the extent to which signs and symptoms have disappeared, or (2) by the microbiologic response, meaning the extent to which the organism has been eradicated. Bacterial infections are contagious until antibiotics have been administered for 24 to 48 hours. Viral infections are not treated with antibiotics.

Antibiotic Side Effects and Dispensing Issues

The parenteral forms of antibiotics should be mixed exactly as directed by the manufacturers. If mixed inappropriately, the drugs can be ineffective or may cause tissue or vein irritation, renal failure, or even death. When dispensing oral forms of these drugs, it is important to swab the counting tray with alcohol before placing a new drug on the tray to prevent cross contamination, especially with penicillin and sulfa drugs. For example, if a tray used to dispense sulfa is not wiped down before another drug is placed on the tray, sulfa particles could stick to the new drug and cause an adverse reaction in a patient who is allergic to sulfa.

Most antibiotics are taken on an empty stomach because food slows absorption of the drug. However, some antibiotics can cause extreme gastrointestinal (GI) upset, and the manufacturer may recommend that these drugs be taken with food. It is important for technicians to follow the prompts on the computer or the patient handouts to use the appropriate auxiliary label for "take with food" or "take on an empty stomach."

It is also important to know that antibiotic agents can interfere with the action of birth control medication and reduce the effectiveness of hormonal contraceptives. Patients should be made aware of this and be warned to use backup contraception for the duration of their menstrual cycle.

To maintain consistent drug serum levels, ideally antibiotics should be administered around the clock. An IV administration route can facilitate around-the-clock dosing for very ill patients. Otherwise, spacing the dosage evenly throughout the day suffices to maintain a relatively constant drug serum level.

Antimicrobial Resistance

TAKE ALL OF THIS MEDICATION

When choosing appropriate drug therapy, prescribers must also take into account **antibiotic resistance**. Bacteria have the ability to develop defense mechanisms that resist or inactivate antibiotics used on them. For instance, many bacteria that cause common respiratory tract infections (RTIs) are now resistant to the most frequently used drugs, like amoxicillin. Three of the most critical highly resistant organisms are *Pseudomonas aeruginosa*, *Acinetobacter baumannii*, and *Enterobacteriaceae* species. Antibiotic resistance is a growing problem as we use more and more of these common drugs. If a patient develops an infection that is resistant to the most powerful

antibiotics, no therapy exists to treat it, a grim situation that can cause death. To help prevent antibiotic resistance, prescribers must be mindful of using appropriate antibiotics only when necessary.

A pharmacy technician's role in preventing the overuse of antibiotics is to ensure that all antibiotic prescriptions display an auxiliary label on the bottle that advises the patient to take all the medication. Because prescriptions for antibiotics have begun to stipulate dose loading on the front end, the patient should be instructed

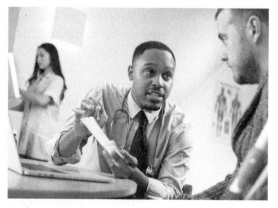
A physician informs his patients of the risk of developing antibiotic resistance.

Pharm Fact

Pharmacy personnel play a key role in preventing antibiotic resistance by reminding patients to take all the prescribed medication.

that, after the initial dose of such a prescription, successive doses will be smaller. In any event, it is important that the patient complete the prescribed course of medication and not save or share any of the medication.

16.3 Antibiotic Drugs and Their Mechanisms of Action

Before the 1930s, systemic bacterial infections could not be effectively treated with drugs. Infections were often treated topically with an **antiseptic** (a substance that kills or inhibits the growth of microorganisms). An antiseptic should not be confused with a **disinfectant**, which is an agent used to kill microorganisms on nonliving objects. Topical products, however, are not safe to be used systemically. With the discovery of sulfonamides in the 1930s, a new era began. Since that time, several additional classes of antibiotics have been discovered. All drugs in each class of antibiotics have some similarities in their molecular structure. See Table 16.2 for a list of common antibiotic drugs.

TABLE 16.2 Common Antibiotic Drugs

Generic (Brand)	Pronunciation	Dosage Form	Common Dosage	Dispensing Status
Sulfonamides and Nitrofurantoin				
nitrofurantoin (Macrobid, Macrodantin)	nye-troe-fyoor-AN-toyn	capsule, oral liquid	adult: 50–100 mg 1–4 times a day pediatric: 5–6 mg/kg/day in divided doses	Rx
sulfamethoxazole / trimethoprim (Bactrim, Bactrim DS, Septra, Septra DS)	sul-fa-meth-OX-a-zole trye-METH-oh-prim	injection (IV), oral suspension, tablet	varies depending on age and infection treated	Rx
Penicillins				
Aminopenicillins				
amoxicillin (Amoxil, Moxatag)	a-mox-i-SIL-in	capsule, chewable tablet, oral suspension, tablet	adult: 250–875 mg 2–3 times a day pediatric: 20–90 mg/kg/day in divided doses	Rx
ampicillin	am-pi-SIL-in	capsule, injection, oral suspension	pediatric: 50–100 mg/kg/day divided every 6 hr, oral dose IM/IV: dose varies by age of patient; typical doses range in hundreds of milligrams a day in divided doses PO: 250–500 mg 4 times a day	Rx
Natural Penicillins				
penicillin G (Pfizerpen)	pen-i-SIL-in G	injection	dose varies by age of patient; typical doses range from thousands to millions of units a day in divided doses	Rx
penicillin V potassium	pen-i-SIL-in V poh-TAS-ee-um	solution, tablet	adult: 125–250 mg every 6–8 hr pediatric: 25–50 mg/kg/day in divided doses	Rx
Antistaphylococcal Penicillins				
dicloxacillin	dye-klox-a-SIL-in	capsule	adult: 125–250 mg every 6 hr pediatric: 12.5 mg/kg/day in divided doses	Rx
nafcillin	naf-SIL-in	injection	1,000–2,000 mg every 4 hr	Rx

continues

TABLE 16.2 Common Antibiotic Drugs—*Continued*

Generic (Brand)	Pronunciation	Dosage Form	Common Dosage	Dispensing Status
Antistaphylococcal Penicillins				
oxacillin	ox-a-SIL-in	injection, solution	adult: 500–2,000 mg every 4–6 hr pediatric: 50–100 mg/kg a day in divided doses IV: dose varies by age of patient; typical doses range in hundreds of milligrams a day in divided doses	Rx
Combination Penicillins				
amoxicillin / clavulanate (Augmentin, Augmentin XR)	a-mox-i-SIL-in klav-yoo-LAN-ate	chewable tablet, oral suspension, tablet	adult: 250–500 mg every 8–12 hr pediatric: 20–45 mg/kg/day in divided doses	Rx
ampicillin / sulbactam (Unasyn)	am-pi-SIL-in sul-BAK-tam	injection	adult: 1.5–3 g every 6 hr pediatric: 100–200 mg/kg/day in divided doses	Rx
piperacillin / tazobactam (Zosyn)	pi-PER-a-sil-in ta-zoe-BAK-tam	injection	adult: 3.375 g every 6 hr pediatric: varies by age and weight of patient; usually given multiple times a day	Rx
ticarcillin / clavulanate	tye-kar-SIL-in klav-yoo-LAN-ate	injection	varies by age of patient; typical doses range in hundreds of milligrams a day in divided doses	Rx
Cephalosporins				
First Generation				
cefazolin (Ancef, Kefzol)	sef-AZ-oe-lin	injection	250 mg to 1 g taken every 6, 8, or 12 hr (dosing depends on type of infection being treated); also given before or during surgical procedures	Rx
cephalexin (Keflex)	sef-a-LEX-in	capsule, oral suspension, tablet	adult: 250–750 mg every 6 hr pediatric: 25–50 mg/kg/day in divided doses	Rx
Second Generation				
cefaclor	SEF-a-klor	capsule, oral suspension, tablet	adult: 250 mg every 8 hr or 375–500 mg every 12 hr pediatric: 20–40 mg/kg/day divided every 8–12 hr	Rx
cefotetan	SEF-oh-tee-tan	injection	500 mg–3 g every 12 hr	Rx
cefoxitin (Mefoxin)	SEF-ox-ih-tin	injection	1–2 g every 6–8 hr; also given before or during surgical procedures	Rx
cefuroxime (Ceftin, Zinacef)	se-fyoor-OX-eem	injection, oral suspension, tablet	IM/IV: 750 mg to 1.5 g every 8 hr; also given before or during surgical procedures PO: adult: 250–1,000 mg 2 times a day pediatric: 20–30 mg/kg/day in divided doses 2 times day	Rx

continues

TABLE 16.2 Common Antibiotic Drugs—*Continued*

Generic (Brand)	Pronunciation	Dosage Form	Common Dosage	Dispensing Status
Third Generation				
cefdinir	SEF-di-neer	capsule, oral suspension	adult: 300–600 mg every 12–24 hr pediatric: 7 mg/kg every 12 hr or 14 mg/kg every 24 hr	Rx
cefiderocol (Fetroja)	SEF-i-DER-oh-kol	injection	IV: 2 g every 8 hr	Rx
cefditoren (Spectracef)	sef-de-TOR-en	tablet	200–400 mg 2 times a day	Rx
cefixime (Suprax)	SEF-icks-eem	capsule, chewable tablet, oral suspension, tablet	adult: 400 mg/day pediatric: 8 mg/kg/day	Rx
cefotaxime (Claforan)	sef-oh-TAX-eem	injection	pediatric: 50–224 mg/kg/day divided every 4–6 hr IM: 0.5–1 g single dose IM/IV: 1–2 g every 4–12 hr depending on severity of infection	Rx
cefpodoxime	sef-poe-DOX-eem	oral suspension, tablet	adult: 100–200 mg 2 times a day pediatric: 10 mg/kg/day divided every 12 hr	Rx
ceftazidime (Fortaz, Tazicef)	SEF-tay-zi-deem	injection	adult: 1–2 g every 8–12 hr pediatric: 30–50 mg/kg every 8–12 hr	Rx
ceftibuten (Cedax)	sef-TYE-byoo-ten	capsule, oral suspension	adult: 400 mg 1 time a day pediatric: 9 mg/kg/day	Rx
ceftriaxone (Rocephin)	sef-trye-AX-one	injection	adult: 1–2 g 1 or 2 times a day pediatric: 50–75 mg/kg single dose or divided (max dose: 2 g/day)	Rx
Fourth Generation				
cefepime (Maxipime)	SEF-e-peem	injection	adult: 1–2 g every 8–12 hr pediatric: 50 mg/kg every 8–12 hr	Rx
Fifth Generation				
ceftaroline (Teflaro)	SEF-tare-oh-leen	injection	600 mg every 12 hr	Rx
Carbapenems				
doripenem (Doribax)	dore-i-PEN-em	injection	500 mg every 8 hr	Rx
ertapenem (Invanz)	er-ta-PEN-em	injection	1,000 mg 1 time a day	Rx
imipenem / cilastatin (Primaxin)	i-mi-PEN-em sye-la-STAT-in	injection	250–1,000 mg every 6–8 hr	Rx
meropenem (Merrem)	mer-o-PEN-em	injection	500–1,000 mg every 8 hr	Rx
meropenem / vaborbactam (Vabormere)	mer-o-PEN-em VAY bo meer	injection	4 g every 8 hr	Rx
Monobactam				
aztreonam (Azactam, Cayston)	AZ-tree-oh-nam	injection, oral inhalation product	500–2,000 mg every 6–12 hr	Rx

continues

TABLE 16.2 Common Antibiotic Drugs—*Continued*

Generic (Brand)	Pronunciation	Dosage Form	Common Dosage	Dispensing Status
Lincosamide				
clindamycin (Cleocin)	klin-da-MYE-sin	capsule, cream, foam, gel, injection, lotion, oral solution, suppository, tablet, topical solution	IM/IV: 600–2,700 mg/day in divided doses PO (adult): 150–300 mg every 6 hr PO (pediatric): 8–20 mg/kg/day in 3–4 divided doses topical: varies depending on product; usually given 1–2 times a day	Rx
Macrolides				
azithromycin (Zithromax, Z-Pak, Zmax, Zithromax Tri-Pak)	aye-ZITH-roe-mye-sin	injection, ophthalmic solution, oral suspension, tablet	IV: 500 mg/day for 2–10 days, depending on type of infection PO (adult): 250–500 mg/day for 3–5 days PO (pediatric): varies by age, weight, and type of infection	Rx
clarithromycin (Biaxin, Biaxin Filmtab, Biaxin XL Filmtab, Biaxin XL Pac)	kla-RITH-roe-mye-sin	oral suspension, tablet	adult: 250–500 mg every 12 hr pediatric: 15 mg/kg/day divided every 12 hr	Rx
erythromycin (EES, EryC, EryPed, Ery-Tab, Erythrocin, Pediazole)	eh-rith-roe-MYE-sin	capsule, gel, injection, ophthalmic ointment, oral suspension, pledget, solution, tablet	varies depending on age of patient and type of infection; usually given 3–4 times a day	Rx
Aminoglycosides				
amikacin	am-i-KAY-sin	injection	varies	Rx
gentamicin (Garamycin, Gentak, Gentasol, Gentopic)	jen-ta-MYE-sin	injection, ophthalmic ointment, ophthalmic solution	varies	Rx
tobramycin (TOBI, Tobrex)	toe-bra-MYE-sin	injection, ophthalmic ointment, ophthalmic solution, nebulizer solution	varies	Rx
Tetracyclines				
doxycycline (Adoxa, Oracea, Vibramycin)	dox-i-SYE-kleen	capsule, injection, oral liquid, tablet	100–200 mg 2 times a day	Rx
minocycline (Minocin, Solodyn)	mi-noe-SYE-kleen	capsule, injection	100 mg every 12 hr	Rx
tetracycline	te-tra-SYE-kleen	capsule, oral liquid, tablet	250–500 mg 2–4 times a day	Rx

continues

TABLE 16.2 Common Antibiotic Drugs—*Continued*

Generic (Brand)	Pronunciation	Dosage Form	Common Dosage	Dispensing Status
tigecycline (Tygacil)	tye-gi-SYE-kleen	injection	100 mg once, then 50 mg every 12 hr	Rx
Fluoroquinolones (Quinolones)				
ciprofloxacin (Cetraxal, Ciloxan, Cipro, Otiprio)	sip-roe-FLOX-a-sin	injection, oral liquid, ophthalmic drops and ointment, otic solution, otic suspension, tablet	IV: 200–400 mg every 12 hr PO (adult): 250–750 mg every 12 hr PO (pediatric): 6–20 mg/kg every 8–12 hr	Rx
levofloxacin	lee-voe-FLOX-a-sin	injection, oral liquid, tablet	250–750 mg a day	Rx
moxifloxacin (Avelox, Moxeza, Vigamox)	mox-i-FLOX-a-sin	injection, ophthalmic solution, tablet	IV/PO: 400 mg a day opthalmic: 1 drop 2–3 times a day	Rx
Miscellaneous Antibiotics				
daptomycin (Cubicin)	DAP-toe-mye-sin	injection	6–10 mg/kg 1 time a day	Rx
linezolid (Zyvox)	li-NE-zoh-lid	injection, oral liquid, tablet	600 mg every 12 hr	Rx
metronidazole (Flagyl, MetroCream, MetroGel, MetroLotion, Noritate Cream, Nuvessa, Vandazole)	me-troe-NYE-da-zole	capsule, injection, tablet, topical cream, topical gel, topical lotion, vaginal gel	250–750 mg every 8–24 hr	Rx
vancomycin (Vancocin)	van-koe-MYE-sin	capsule, injection	500–1,000 mg every 6–12 hr	Rx

Safety Alert

Doses identified in this text are presented as general guides. Always refer to the package insert or other reliable sources to verify proper dosing.

TAKE WITH **FOOD**

TAKE WITH **FLUIDS**

Do not drink alcoholic beverages when taking this medication

Sulfonamides and Nitrofurantoin

Sulfonamides, or sulfa drugs, are among the oldest antibiotics on the market and are effective against a broad spectrum of microorganisms. A **sulfonamide** is bacteriostatic and works by blocking bacteria from making folic acid, which is necessary for their survival. Although humans can absorb folic acid from food, bacteria cannot and thus must make folic acid.

Sulfonamides are commonly used for the following:

- UTIs
- otitis media (middle ear infections), especially in children
- lower respiratory tract infections
- prophylaxis in *Pneumocystis carinii* pneumonia in immunocompromised patients

Sulfa drugs are used most often to treat urinary tract infections (UTIs). The most common sulfa drug is a combination containing sulfamethoxazole and trimethoprim. **Sulfamethoxazole / trimethoprim (Bactrim, Bactrim DS, Septra, Septra DS)** is especially good for UTIs caused by *Escherichia coli*. Sulfa drugs are also used to treat community-acquired methicillin-resistant *Staphylococcus aureus* (MRSA) skin infections and as a prophylaxis against *Pneumocystis carinii* pneumonia, a common deadly lung infection in patients who have end-stage acquired immunodeficiency syndrome (AIDS).

Like sulfa drugs, **nitrofurantoin (Macrobid, Macrodantin)** is used to treat UTIs (see Figure 16.3). Its mechanism of action is not well understood, but its spectrum of activity is similar to that of sulfonamides. It works best if taken with food and plenty of fluids. Table 16.2 lists dosing information for a common sulfonamide and for nitrofurantoin. Nitrofurantoin may be an appropriate alternative in patients with a UTI who are unable to use sulfa drugs.

FIGURE 16.3
Macrobid Label

Nitrofurantoin is sold under several names, including Macrobid.

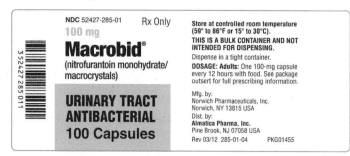

Dosage Forms and Administration It is important that a patient taking sulfa drugs maintain an adequate fluid intake of six to eight glasses a day. The technician should always place an auxiliary label on sulfonamides and related drugs reminding the patient to drink lots of water or other fluids.

Due to the incidence of sulfa drug allergies, technicians should be careful to wipe down counting trays containing sulfa in an effort to prevent cross contamination of the next drug used on the tray.

Side Effects Sulfa drugs in use today cause fewer allergic reactions than older sulfa drugs did. The most common side effect is a rash. Other side effects include nausea, drug fever (often confused with a recurrent fever from the infection), vomiting, jaundice, blood complications (acute hemolytic anemia, agranulocytosis, and aplastic anemia), and kidney damage. **Stevens-Johnson syndrome**—a reaction that can be fatal, marked by large red blotches on the skin—can occur. If a rash occurs, the patient should stop taking the drug immediately. Sulfa drugs should have an auxiliary label warning patients to avoid the sun, which can cause severe skin rashes. Sulfonamides can crystallize in the urine and deposit in the kidneys, resulting in a painful, dangerous condition.

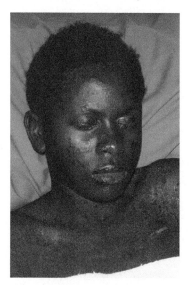

Stevens-Johnson syndrome, a potentially fatal reaction, can occur with the use of sulfa drugs.

☼ Avoid
SUN EXPOSURE

Nitrofurantoin use may also cause nausea or vomiting. A unique side effect is urine discoloration (nitrofurantoin makes the urine appear brown). Patients should be alerted to this harmless but sometimes alarming effect. Nitrofurantoin may cause false urine glucose tests.

Contraindications Sulfamethoxazole / trimethoprim is contraindicated in patients with a history of drug-induced immune thrombocytopenia, with megaloblastic anemia (a below-normal concentration of erythrocytes or hemoglobin in the blood) due to folate deficiency, or with marked liver or kidney dysfunction, and in infants younger than two months of age.

Contraindications to nitrofurantoin include anuria (producing no urine), oliguria (having little urine), significant impairment of kidney function, and history of jaundice or hepatic dysfunction associated with prior nitrofurantoin use. It is also contraindicated in pregnant patients at term; during labor and delivery, or when the onset of labor is imminent; and in neonates younger than one month of age.

TAKE WITH FOOD

Cautions and Considerations Taking sulfa drugs with food can help alleviate the common side effects of nausea and vomiting. Sulfa allergy is common, so pharmacy technicians should always inquire about drug allergies when dispensing a sulfa drug.

Administering nitrofurantoin with food may improve absorption and decrease side effects.

Drug Interactions Sulfamethoxazole / trimethoprim may cause a condition called **long QT syndrome** (or **QT prolongation**) when combined with other drugs that lengthen the QT interval. Long QT syndrome is a heart rhythm disorder that can cause a life-threatening cardiac **arrhythmia** (varying or irregular heartbeat). Drugs that prolong the QT interval and increase risk of this disorder include antiarrhythmic agents (such as amiodarone, disopyramide, dofetilide, procainamide, quinidine, and sotalol), chlorpromazine, cisapride, dolasetron, droperidol, mefloquine, moxifloxacin, tacrolimus, and ziprasidone. Sulfamethoxazole / trimethoprim may decrease the effectiveness of live vaccines when coadministered.

Nitrofurantoin use may decrease the effectiveness of the antibiotic norfloxacin. Concurrent alcohol use should be avoided because of the risk of CNS depression.

Do not drink alcoholic beverages when taking this medication

Penicillins

Safety Alert

Penicillin is not the same drug as penicillamine, which is an immunosuppresant drug.

The **penicillin** drug class was one of the first groups of antibiotics used in the treatment of bacterial infections. These antibiotics are obtained from the mold *Penicillium chrysogenum*. Penicillins, which come in many types (amino-, natural, antistaphylococcal, extended-spectrum, and combination penicillins), primarily treat infections caused by Gram-positive bacteria (see Table 16.1). They kill bacteria by inhibiting the formation of bacterial cell walls. A bacterium's weakened cell wall allows an excessive amount of water to enter the bacterium through osmosis. The cell increases in size and lyses (bursts), as the cell membrane cannot contain the cell contents. Human cells do not have rigid cell walls; therefore, they are not affected by penicillins. Some bacteria, however, are resistant to penicillins because the pathogens produce an enzyme called **beta-lactamase**, which destroys the beta-lactam ring present in the molecular structure of all penicillins. This action renders the drug inactive. For this reason, some penicillin products are available as a combination of penicillin with a **beta-lactamase inhibitor** (an agent that inhibits beta-lactamase). Table 16.2 lists commonly used penicillins.

Penicillin is most active against growing and reproducing bacteria—generally Gram-positive aerobes and anaerobes. Penicillin and penicillin derivatives are among the drugs of choice for the following conditions:

- abscesses
- beta-hemolytic streptococcus
- meningitis
- otitis media
- pneumonia
- respiratory tract infections
- streptococcal pharyngitis
- tooth and gum infections
- sexually transmitted infections (STIs; including syphilis and gonorrhea)
- endocarditis (heart valve infection) due to streptococci

Penicillin and other antibiotics have also been shown to reduce the risk of disease and death in patients with subacute bacterial endocarditis, an inflammation of the lining of the heart and its valves. These patients are at risk any time a body cavity is invaded.

Preventative dosing, or prophylaxis, with penicillins may be recommended when a patient with certain conditions undergoes any kind of surgical procedure, including higher risk dental procedures. **Amoxicillin (Amoxil, Moxatag)** is often used for patients who can take oral medication. In the case of penicillin allergy, cephalexin, clindamycin, azithromycin, or clarithromycin may be used.

Dosage Forms and Administration Oral penicillins work best when taken on an empty stomach, but if stomach upset occurs, they can be taken with food. Technicians should advise patients to avoid taking these medications with acidic beverages, such as fruit juice, or carbonated drinks, such as cola products, because the acid in these beverages can deactivate the drug. Patients should be instructed to shake oral suspensions well before every dose. Most of these suspensions must also be refrigerated. Suspensions prepared with water are good for only 14 days from the mixing date. Any medication left over after treatment should be disposed of properly.

Side Effects Common side effects of penicillins include stomach upset and diarrhea. Taking them with food can help with these side effects; however, this may decrease absorption. Other rare but more severe side effects include mental disturbances, seizures, kidney damage, and bleeding abnormalities. These particular side effects tend to occur more often at higher doses and when the doses are administered by IV infusion.

Contraindications Most penicillin contraindications are associated with hypersensitivity. If a person has a true hypersensitivity to one type of penicillin, use of the others is contraindicated. **Amoxicillin / clavulanate (Augmentin)** is contraindicated in patients with liver dysfunction or severe renal impairment.

Cautions and Considerations **Penicillin G benzathine** carries a boxed warning that it is not for IV use. Cardiopulmonary arrest and death have occurred, and the product should only be administered by deep IM injection.

Many patients who are allergic to penicillin are also allergic to cephalosporins, another class of antibiotics that inhibits cell-wall formation. Therefore, pharmacy technicians should always inquire about all drug allergies when taking a patient's medication history or when preparing to administer penicillins or cephalosporins.

Although IV preparations are often used in conjunction with other antibiotics (such as aminoglycosides, for difficult infections), they should not be mixed in the same IV bag.

Some bacteria have become resistant to **methicillin**, an older penicillin used for difficult staphylococcal infections. The antistaphylococcal penicillins (also called *penicillinase-resistant penicillins*) have largely replaced it in practice. **Methicillin-resistant *Staphylococcus aureus* (MRSA)** infections are resistant to all antistaphylococcal penicillins, and consequently, few drugs can treat them. Special precautions are used to protect against the spread of this bacteria to other patients. For instance, access to an affected patient's hospital room is restricted, and anyone who enters must don protective gear such as a gown, mask, and gloves.

Drug Interactions Antibiotics such as penicillins may reduce the efficacy of oral contraceptives. While rare, contraceptive failure may occur, and patients should use backup contraception during therapy and until their next cycle of contraception is started. Penicillins may increase the risk of bleeding when used with anticoagulants such as heparin or warfarin. Live vaccine effectiveness may decrease with penicillin use; coadministration should be avoided.

Cephalosporins

Antibiotics in the **cephalosporin** family have a mechanism of action similar to that of penicillins, but they differ in their antibacterial spectrum, resistance to beta-lactamase, and pharmacokinetics. Cephalosporins are one of the most used antibiotics because they cover a wide range of organisms and have lower toxicity than other antibiotics with the same coverage. Research now suggests that of persons reporting a penicillin allergy, only 10–15% have evidence of a skin test–confirmed allergy. In those with a positive penicillin skin test, only 2% have evidence of a skin test–confirmed allergy to cephalosporin. Most computerized drug profile systems place penicillin and cephalosporin in the same category; therefore, if someone has an allergy to either, the computer system will indicate that the patient is allergic to both. Cephalosporins are divided into five groups, each of which is called a **generation**. In general, first-generation cephalosporins work best on Gram-positive bacteria. Activity against Gram-negative bacteria increases through the subsequent generations.

The first-generation cephalosporins are similar to the penicillinase-resistant penicillins. They are used for mild to moderate **community-acquired** (not acquired in a hospital or nursing home) infections in ambulatory patients. They can all be taken by mouth except **cefazolin (Ancef, Kefzol)**, which is only administered via IV or IM injection. IV and IM injections require longer needles than subcutaneous (under the skin) injections.

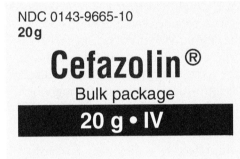

NDC 0143-9665-10
20 g

Cefazolin®
Bulk package
20 g • IV

Cefazolin is a first-generation cephalosporin that is injectable and can be administered intravenously or intramuscularly.

Second-generation cephalosporins have increased activity, especially against *Haemophilus influenzae*, an important pathogen in the pediatric group. Second-generation cephalosporins are used for otitis media in children and for respiratory and urinary tract infections. Most can be dosed orally; **cefuroxime (Ceftin, Zinacef)** also has IV and IM forms.

The third-generation cephalosporin drugs are active against a wide spectrum of Gram-negative organisms and are used in severe infections.

They are manufactured in a variety of dosage forms. Because of their long half-life, they are also used in ambulatory patients, especially children, with dosing done before and after school. **Ceftibuten (Cedax), cefdinir, cefditoren (Spectracef), cefixime (Suprax)**, and **cefpodoxime** are orally active third-generation cephalosporins. **Cefotaxime (Claforan), ceftazidime (Fortaz, Tazicef)**, and **ceftriaxone (Rocephin)** are available only in injectable forms. Injection of ceftriaxone may be painful, so this agent is often mixed with lidocaine to diminish the discomfort. It is used frequently in emergency department settings, and it is also used to treat STIs.

Cefepime (Maxipime) is an injectable fourth-generation cephalosporin and is considered to have broad-spectrum coverage. It is used for treating pneumonia, urinary tract infections, and **sepsis** (a systemic inflammatory response to an infection, usually a blood-borne bacterial infection) caused by Gram-negative organisms. Cefepime is considered as effective as the third-generation cephalosporin ceftazidime, but it is more cost-effective because cefepime is given two times a day, whereas ceftazidime is dosed two or three times a day. Because of their activity against *Pseudomonas aeruginosa*, both are used for hospital-acquired infections.

Ceftaroline (Teflaro) is a fifth-generation cephalosporin. It has activity similar to that of ceftriaxone, with the benefit of being effective against MRSA.

Do not drink alcoholic beverages when taking this medication

Cephalosporins are among the drugs of choice for the following conditions:

- dental work, oral infections: oral dosage form, first and second generation
- heart and pacemaker procedures (surgical prophylaxis): cefazolin
- intra-abdominal infections: cefoxitin, cefotetan
- meningitis: parental dosage form, third generation
- neurosurgical operations (surgical prophylaxis): cefazolin
- obstetric and gynecologic (OB-GYN) procedures and surgery (surgical prophylaxis): cefazolin
- orthopedic surgery (surgical prophylaxis): cefazolin
- upper respiratory tract and sinus infections: oral dosage form, second generation
- UTIs: parental dosage form, third generation

Dosage Forms and Administration Several of the cephalosporin drugs have noteworthy dispensing issues. Patients with diabetes who are prescribed cefdinir in oral suspension form must be informed of its high sugar content (2.86 g per teaspoon). Cefpodoxime is available in an oral suspension. With the exception of cefdinir and cefixime, which may be stored at room temperature, oral suspensions of cephalosporins must be refrigerated following reconstitution. A dropper, spoon, or oral syringe with milliliter and teaspoon markings should be dispensed with these drugs.

Most cephalosporin oral liquid dosage forms are suspensions and should be shaken well before every dose. This is because the active drug granules have a tendency to settle to the bottom of the bottle. Shaking also provides even dosing throughout the regimen. These drugs are reconstituted in the pharmacy. When a suspension is prepared with sterile water, it usually expires 14 days after mixing.

Side Effects Cephalosporins share the same side effects as penicillins; a few have also been known to initiate unique toxic reactions. They generally are associated with a lower frequency of toxicity than many other antibiotics.

Common side effects of cephalosporins include nausea, vomiting, diarrhea, headache, and dizziness. Most of the time, these effects are tolerable. Other rare but more severe side effects include mental disturbances, seizures, heart palpitations, and bleeding abnormalities. These rarer side effects tend to occur more frequently at higher doses and when the drugs are administered intravenously. Some of the more serious side effects can be worsened by alcohol intake, so patients should avoid alcohol while taking a cephalosporin.

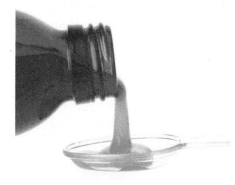

Most oral liquid forms of cephalosporins are available as suspensions and should be shaken well before use.

Contraindications Cephalosporins are contraindicated in patients with a hypersensitivity to other cephalosporins. Ceftriaxone should not be used in neonates with elevated bilirubin levels or who are receiving IV calcium-containing products. Cefditoren is contraindicated in patients with milk-protein hypersensitivity or carnitine deficiency. Cefepime is contraindicated in patients with penicillin or beta-lactam hypersensitivity.

Cautions and Considerations Allergic reactions to cephalosporins are common. Many patients who are allergic to penicillin may also be allergic to cephalosporins. Therefore, technicians should always inquire about all drug allergies when taking a patient's medication history or when preparing to administer cephalosporins or penicillins.

Some cephalosporins should be taken with food, and others should be taken on an empty stomach. For example, cefditoren should be taken with food but not with antacids. Refer to the package insert to verify proper instructions with regard to food.

Some of the products in this class can be taken twice a day instead of three times a day. This feature may be advantageous for parents with children in daycare or school, where it may be difficult to administer medications in the middle of the day.

Drug Interactions Technicians should warn patients against drinking alcohol with a cephalosporin or within 72 hours of cephalosporin use because it can cause acute alcohol intolerance. Cephalosporins may increase the activity of the anticoagulant warfarin. Loop diuretics (such as furosemide) should be used with caution in patients taking cephalosporins because of an increased risk of nephrotoxicity (toxicity that causes damage to the kidneys). Ceftriaxone should not be used in neonates receiving any calcium-containing products. Ceftriaxone use may also increase cyclosporine levels.

Carbapenems and Monobactams

The carbapenem and monobactam drug classes are grouped together here because they differ only slightly in their molecular structure from penicillins and cephalosporins. These drug classes kill bacteria by inhibiting the formation of the cell wall. A **carbapenem** is used for mixed infections that have both Gram-positive and Gram-negative bacteria; a **monobactam** is used primarily for Gram-negative bacterial infections. Both drug classes are used in special situations for serious healthcare-associated infections (HAIs) or nosocomial infections. Carbapenems include doripenem, ertapenem, imipenem, and meropenem. Aztreonam is a monobactam.

Carbapenems and monobactams are among the drugs of choice for the following conditions:

- intra-abdominal infections
- complicated skin and skin structure infections
- complicated UTIs

Imipenem / cilastatin (Primaxin) is a carbapenem drug with excellent in vitro and in vivo activity against Gram-positive and Gram-negative bacteria. Its side effects are similar to those of other beta-lactams except that seizures seem to occur more frequently. The carbapenem **meropenem (Merrem)** has similar coverage, but meropenem is less likely to cause seizures. It is approved for bacterial meningitis and intra-abdominal infections.

Meropenem / vaborbactam (Vabomere) is a carbapenem drug designed to have improved activity against klebsiella pneumoniae carbapenamase (KPC)-producing bacteria. KPC-producing bacteria are highly drug resistant Gram-negative bacilli that are difficult to treat and associated with high morbidity and mortality. Meropenem / vaborbactam is approved for use in the treatment of complicated urinary tract infections, including pylonephritis.

Doripenem (Doribax) inhibits cell-wall synthesis and kills bacteria. It is indicated for intra-abdominal infections and UTIs.

Ertapenem (Invanz) is an injectable carbapenem administered one time a day. It is approved for severe community-acquired infections.

A monobactam, **aztreonam (Azactam, Cayston)**, is also being used to treat serious infections, including sepsis, intra-abdominal infections, peritonitis, skin and soft tissue infections, and infections of the urinary tract. Aztreonam is active only against aerobic, Gram-negative bacteria. The advantage of this drug is its low likelihood of cross-allergenicity with other beta-lactams. Patients should notify their physician immediately if skin rash, redness, or itching develops.

Dosage Forms and Administration A common dose of doripenem is made by reconstituting 500 mg with 10 mL of NS or sterile water for injection and gently shaking to create a suspension. Next, the suspension is inspected visually for any foreign matter. Then, the suspension is withdrawn using a syringe and needle and added to an infusion bag containing 100 mL of NS or D_5W. The expiration of doripenem in an NS infusion bag is 12 hours at room temperature and 72 hours under refrigeration. Doripenem in a D_5W infusion bag expires after 4 hours at room temperature or 24 hours refrigerated.

The carbapenems are available for IV administration. Aztreonam, the only available monobactam, is commonly administered intravenously for serious infections. An inhalation formulation of aztreonam is available for use in patients with cystic fibrosis.

Side Effects Side effects of carbapenems include skin rash, headache, anemia, and pain. Aztreonam inhalation can cause sore throat, cough, nasal congestion, wheezing, fever, and chest discomfort. The IV form of aztreonam may cause neutropenia, increased liver enzymes, and skin rash.

Contraindications Hypersensitivity to one carbapenem contraindicates use of other agents in the class. IM use of ertapenem is contraindicated in patients with a hypersensitivity to amide-type anesthetics. Aztreonam does not have contraindications.

Cautions and Considerations Seizures have been reported during treatment with carbapenems. These reactions occurred most commonly in patients with CNS disorders such as a history of seizures and in patients with renal impairment. Carbapenems require dosage adjustment in patients with kidney dysfunction. Aztreonam has rare cross-allergenicity with penicillins, cephalosporins, and carbapenems and should be used with caution in patients with a history of beta-lactam hypersensitivity. Aztreonam requires dosage adjustment in patients with renal impairment.

Drug Interactions The CNS side effects of carbapenems may be potentiated (activated or exacerbated) by concurrent cyclosporine use. Using ganciclovir with carbapenems may result in seizures. Carbapenems may decrease levels of the antiseizure medication valproic acid.

Lincosamides and Macrolides

Erythromycin is the oldest macrolide antibiotic, having been discovered in the 1950s. Erythromycin is still used today, but since its discovery, other macrolides have been synthesized.

Lincosamides are among the drugs of choice for:

- acne
- dental work
- anaerobic pneumonia
- bone infections
- bowel infections
- vaginal infections
- intra-abdominal infections

Macrolides are among the most commonly prescribed drugs for the following illnesses and other specific bacteria:

- sexually transmitted infections
- group A beta-hemolytic *Streptococcus*
- influenza
- Legionnaires' disease
- *Mycoplasma pneumoniae*
- *Streptococcus pneumoniae*

Members of the **lincosamide** and **macrolide** drug classes work by blocking bacteria's ability to produce needed proteins for survival. At low doses, these drugs are bacteriostatic, but at high doses, they can be bactericidal.

Clindamycin (Cleocin), the most commonly prescribed lincosamide, is used to treat infections caused by organisms including anaerobes such as *Staphylococcus aureus, Streptococcus pneumoniae,* and *Streptococcus pyogenes.* Clindamycin is used for bone and joint infections, gynecologic infections, intra-abdominal infections, sepsis, and skin and soft tissue infections.

Macrolides have a broad spectrum of activity: they work against many Gram-positive and some Gram-negative bacteria. Macrolides are used mainly to treat respiratory tract infections and pneumonia. They are also used with other drugs to treat infection caused by *Helicobacter pylori*, the bacteria found in association with stomach ulcers.

Clarithromycin (Biaxin) and **azithromycin (Zithromax)** are second-generation macrolides. Azithromycin is a commonly prescribed antibiotic and has an unusually short and convenient duration of therapy of 3 to 5 days relative to other antibiotics, which are usually taken for 7 to 14 days. See Table 16.2 for additional dosing information. An azithromycin Z-Pak is dispensed differently than most antibiotics. On the first day, the patient takes a **loading dose** (a large initial dose that rapidly brings blood concentration to a therapeutic level) of 500 mg. Maintenance doses of 250 mg one time a day are then taken on days 2 through 5, although this regimen can vary depending on the type of infection. There is also a three-pack of 500 mg tablets that should be taken one time a day over a three-day period. Zmax is an extended-release powder for oral suspension that delivers a full treatment in one dose. It comes in 1 g and 2 g packages and is approved to treat community-acquired pneumonia.

Dosage Forms and Administration Clindamycin is available in oral, injectable, topical, and suppository forms. When used for acne, clindamycin is often dispensed topically.

Erythromycin is available for topical use in gel/jelly, pad, and solution formulations. It is also available for ophthalmic use as an ointment. Oral formulations include tablets (regular, enteric coated, and delayed release) and capsules. Azithromycin is available as an IV formulation, ophthalmic solution, and as a tablet and oral suspension.

Side Effects Common side effects of lincosamides and macrolides include stomach upset, nausea, vomiting, heartburn, abdominal pain, and diarrhea. The most serious side effect of clindamycin is pseudomembranous colitis, a *Clostridioides difficile* overgrowth that inflames the large intestine and makes its innermost layer slough off, often causing watery or bloody diarrhea. If patients develop diarrhea, the drug must be discontinued. To reduce these effects, patients should take lincosamides and macrolides with food. If abdominal pain or diarrhea is severe, patients should seek medical attention immediately, because such pain could indicate a serious problem.

Liver toxicity has also occurred with the use of erythromycin. Patients with prior liver problems should not take this medication. If **jaundice** (yellowing of skin and eyes) occurs with erythromycin use, medical attention should be sought immediately.

NDC 52584-870-21
9,000 mg / 60 mL

Cleocin Phosphate®

Clindamycin injection, USP
Bulk package

150 mg / mL • IM or IV

Clindamycin (Cleocin) has injectable (as pictured), oral, and topical dosage forms.

Contraindications Clindamycin is contraindicated in patients with a hypersensitivity to other lincosamides.

Hypersensitivity to one macrolide contraindicates use of all other macrolides. Azithromycin and clarithromycin are contraindicated in patients with liver dysfunction associated with prior use. Other contraindications to clarithromycin include a history of QT prolongation, a history of ventricular cardiac arrhythmia, and concomitant use with colchicine in patients with liver or kidney impairment. Clarithromycin and erythromycin are contraindicated in patients who are taking cisapride, pimozide, ergotamine, dihydroergotamine, simvastatin, lovastatin, or astemizole.

Cautions and Considerations Clindamycin has a boxed warning because it can cause severe and possibly fatal colitis.

Safety Alert

Clindamycin may cause severe and potentially fatal colitis. Clindamycin carries a boxed warning for this reason.

Drug Interactions Macrolides, especially erythromycin and clarithromycin, have many drug interactions. It is important for the pharmacy technician to help the pharmacist maintain an accurate drug list for patients using them. Some of the effects caused by these interactions can be severe. For example, macrolides should not be given with QT-prolonging agents such as antiarrhythmics and tricyclic antidepressants due to the increased risk of QT interval prolongation. Diltiazem should not be used with macrolides. Methadone and macrolides may lead to life-threatening arrhythmias. Clarithromycin interacts with several HIV medications, including some protease inhibitors (covered in Chapter 17). Concurrent use increases clarithromycin levels and decreases the protease inhibitor level. Efavirenz and etravirine should not be used with clarithromycin. Clarithromycin should not be used with colchicine due to increased plasma concentrations of colchicine and the risk of toxicity. Clarithromycin should not be used with alpha-adrenergic blockers. Azithromycin should not be administered with aluminum- or magnesium-containing antacids due to decreased absorption, making azithromycin less effective.

Clindamycin should not be used concurrently with erythromycin due to decreased erythromycin effectiveness. Concurrent use of clindamycin with neuromuscular blockers like cisatracurium may enhance the neuromuscular blocking effects.

Aminoglycosides

Members of the **aminoglycoside** drug class kill bacteria by blocking their ability to make proteins essential for survival. Aminoglycosides are often used in conjunction with other antibiotics, such as penicillins, cephalosporins, and vancomycin. Aminoglycosides work synergistically with these other drug classes. **Synergistic drug therapy** is drug therapy using two or more drugs together because they employ different mechanisms of action that work better together than either drug works alone. In this case, penicillins, cephalosporins, and vancomycin inhibit cell wall synthesis and help increase the ability of the aminoglycoside to get through the bacteria cell wall and inhibit bacteria protein synthesis. The aminoglycosides gentamicin and tobramycin are also used topically to treat bacterial eye infections.

Many healthcare institutions have instituted extended-interval aminoglycoside dosing (EIAD) for the IV formulations of these drugs. With EIAD, an aminoglycoside is administered one time a day instead of multiple times a day. The side effects of aminoglycosides can be serious, and less frequent exposure to the drug seems to help reduce its toxic effects. Special nomograms (dosing algorithms) are used for dosing in these situations. Common aminoglycosides and their routes of administration are listed in Table 16.2.

Aminoglycosides are commonly used for:

- life-threatening infections caused by Gram-negative aerobes
- sepsis
- infections in patients with a compromised immune system
- peritonitis

Dosage Forms and Administration Aminoglycosides are often dosed based on weight or therapeutic drug levels. Because of this, pharmacy technicians preparing these drugs should be aware that doses will vary.

Side Effects Side effects of aminoglycosides can include nephrotoxicity and ototoxicity. With proper monitoring of blood levels and laboratory tests, these effects can be avoided or minimized. However, these side effects limit the use of aminoglycosides to the treatment of difficult infections.

Contraindications Cross-sensitivity may exist among aminoglycosides; therefore, hypersensitivity to one aminoglycoside contraindicates the use of others.

Cautions and Considerations Aminoglycosides carry boxed warnings. One warning is for toxicities associated with use (nephrotoxicity and ototoxicity). Another warns that patients using aminoglycosides should be carefully monitored by healthcare personnel. Aminoglycosides should be avoided in pregnancy due to increased risk of fetal harm. Aminoglycosides have been known to cause **neuromuscular blockade** (the blocking of neuromuscular transmission) in some cases. If a patient complains of muscle weakness, difficulty breathing, numbness, tingling, twitching, or seizures, the drug should be discontinued. Patients with muscular disorders, such as myasthenia gravis or Parkinson's disease, should not be given aminoglycosides. Caution must be used if aminoglycosides are given after surgery, because they may interact with neuromuscular blockers, a class of drugs used in many surgical procedures.

Although aminoglycosides are often used in conjunction with other antibiotics such as cephalosporins or penicillins, they should not be mixed in the same IV infusion bag. Ophthalmic preparations should be kept as sterile as possible. Patients should be instructed not to touch the tip of the applicator to the eye or other surfaces during medication administration.

Drug Interactions The risk of kidney toxicity increases when aminoglycosides are used concurrently with nonsteroidal anti-inflammatory drugs (NSAIDs). Coadministration with loop diuretics may increase the risk of ototoxicity.

Pharm Fact

Hospital pharmacists often play a key role in dosing aminoglycoside antibiotics for patients.

Safety Alert

Aminoglycosides have boxed warnings for the risk of nephrotoxicity and ototoxicity. Another boxed warning states aminoglycosides should be carefully monitored by healthcare personnel.

NDC 6332-3017-302
20 mg / 2 ml

Gentamicin
Pediatric

IM or IV • 2 ml single-dose vial

Gentamicin is an aminoglycoside that is used in pediatric and adult patients.

Put Down Roots

It is easy to recognize aminoglycosides by looking at their names. The aminoglycosides end in the suffix -*cin*.

Tetracyclines

Another class of drugs for bacterial infections is tetracyclines. A **tetracycline** is a broad-spectrum bacteriostatic drug that inhibits protein synthesis within bacterial cells. Consequently, tetracyclines require a functioning immune system to cure an infection. Tetracycline antibiotics include **doxycline (Adoxa, Oracea, Vibramycin), minocycline (Adoxa, Oracea, Vibramycin), tetracycline**, and **tigecycline (Tygacil)**.

Tetracyclines are among the drugs of choice for:

- acne
- anthrax
- chronic bronchitis
- Lyme disease
- *Mycoplasma pneumoniae* infections (walking pneumonia)
- *Rickettsia* infections (Rocky Mountain spotted fever)
- some sexually transmitted infections, such as chlamydia

Do not take with ANTACIDS

℞ **Put Down Roots**

If the name of the generic form of a drug ends in *-cycline*, it is highly likely it is a tetracycline antibiotic.

Dosage Forms and Administration Most drugs that reach their expiration date lose effectiveness. Tetracyclines are unique in that after expiration, they can degrade to toxic substances and may cause kidney failure. Therefore, pharmacy technicans should always diligently check expiration dates on tetracyclines. Patients should be alerted to complete drug courses, and if any drug remains, they should dispose of them and not save them for future use.

Side Effects Common side effects of tetracyclines include stomach upset, nausea, and vomiting. Tetracyclines should be taken with plenty of water to avoid gastric irritation. They are best taken without food on an empty stomach. Doxycycline and minocycline, however, may be taken with food if gastric irritation occurs, but they should not be taken with dairy products or antacids. Tetracyclines also cause photosensitivity. Patients should be informed that their skin will burn faster when exposed to the sun and that a skin rash may develop. When taking a tetracycline, patients should apply sunscreen and other protection (sun-protective clothing) when spending time outside.

Contraindications Hypersensitivity to one tetracycline contraindicates the use of other tetracyclines.

Cautions and Considerations Tetracyclines chelate (bind) with metals and ions, including calcium, aluminum, magnesium, and zinc. When this occurs, these medications cannot be absorbed into the bloodstream. Patients should avoid food, drink, and other products that contain these substances (such as cheese, milk, antacids, and laxatives).

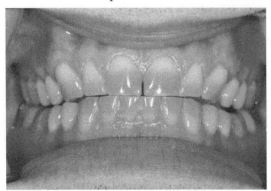

This photo shows permanent tooth discoloration due to tetracycline use.

With this drug class, patients should be warned to avoid the sun because the tetracyclines can cause photosensitization.

Tetracyclines also accumulate in teeth and bones and can cause permanent discoloration and enamel hypoplasia (a condition in which it remains in an immature state). Consequently, children younger than eight and pregnant or breast-feeding individuals cannot use tetracyclines due to the potential for permanent tooth damage in the individual, fetus, or child.

Tetracyclines break down over time and become toxic. Therefore, expired tetracyclines should be discarded properly and never be saved for future use.

Drug Interactions Tetracyclines should not be administered with aluminum-, calcium-, magnesium-, or zinc-containing products (such as antacids) due to decreased absorption. Tetracyclines should not be used with systemic acitretin due to increased risk of pseudomotor cerebri (high pressure in the fluid around the brain). Digoxin levels may increase when digoxin is used concurrently with a tetracycline.

Fluoroquinolones (Quinolones)

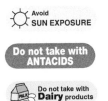

Avoid SUN EXPOSURE

Do not take with ANTACIDS

Do not take with Dairy products

Members of the **fluoroquinolone** (also called **quinolone**) drug class kill bacteria by inhibiting the enzyme that helps DNA to coil. If DNA cannot coil, it is rendered useless, and the cell dies because it cannot function. Quinolones have strong, rapid bactericidal activity against Gram-negative bacteria and some Gram-positive bacteria. Table 16.2 lists the most commonly used quinolones.

Quinolones are among the drugs of choice for the following conditions:

- bone and joint infections
- eye infections
- serious RTIs
- serious UTIs

Quinolones also have a special use as treatment for anthrax, a potential bio-terrorism agent.

Because of overprescribing, resistance to quinolones has developed. Therefore, their use is discouraged in ordinary and frequently seen infections. Quinolones should be reserved for more serious and difficult-to-treat Gram-negative bacterial infections.

Safety Alert

Cipro can be mistakenly read as Ceftin (cefuroxime).

Put Down Roots

Quinolones are easy to recognize because they share a common ending: -floxacin.

Safety Alert

Ciprofloxacin and cephalexin can look very much alike, depending on the handwriting.

Safety Alert

Quinolones carry boxed warnings for the risk of tendon inflammation and rupture. There is a boxed warning that applies to myasthenia gravis patients (increased muscle weakness). Quinolones must also be dispensed with a Medication Guide.

Dosage Forms and Administration Quinolones are available in IV, ophthalmic, oral, otic, and topical forms. If a patient using ciprofloxacin is switched from oral to IV, dose adjustments must be made. For example, a 250 mg oral dose of ciprofloxacin corresponds to a 200 mg IV dose. The doses of levofloxacin and moxifloxacin are usually the same whether given orally or intravenously.

Side Effects Common side effects of quinolones include nausea, vomiting, dizziness, diarrhea, and a bitter or unpleasant taste in the mouth. If the patient cannot tolerate these effects, different antibiotics will need to be chosen. Taking quinolones with food does not necessarily reduce these effects. These drugs also cause photosensitivity, so patients should wear sunscreen when outside. Less common but serious side effects include liver toxicity and alterations in glucose metabolism. Prolongation of the QT interval has occurred with quinolone use. QT prolongation is a syndrome associated with an increased risk of life-threatening cardiac arrhythmia. Consequently, drugs that prolong the QT interval (such as quinolones) may not be the best choice for patients with heart problems.

Contraindications Quinolones should not be used during pregnancy. Ciprofloxacin is contraindicated with concurrent administration of tizanidine.

Cautions and Considerations Quinolones carry boxed warnings for a risk of tendon inflammation and rupture and, in patients with myasthenia gravis, for increased muscle weakness. Changes in mental function and seizures have been reported with quinolones, especially ciprofloxacin. If a patient is exhibiting confusion, agitation, dizziness, hallucinations, insomnia, nightmares, or paranoia, use of the drug should be stopped, and the patient should seek medical attention immediately. Quinolones are associated with joint malformation and usually should not be used in children. Quinolones are also associated with photosensitivity, so patients should avoid excessive sun exposure. Quinolone drugs must be dispensed with a Medication Guide. The FDA mandates that Medication Guides be issued with certain drugs to make certain that information is communicated to prevent adverse effects, to ensure that patients are making informed decisions about serious side effects, or to communicate essential adherence instructions.

Drug Interactions Pharmacy technicians should be aware that many drugs interact with quinolones. Quinolones may inhibit clearance of caffeine and theophylline, leading to increased blood levels of those substances. Quinolones may prolong QT intervals and may enhance the QT interval–prolonging effects of other drugs. Quinolones should not be taken with antacids, dairy products, or calcium-fortified juices, because their absorption will be reduced.

Miscellaneous Antibiotics

Antibiotics that do not belong to the drug classes already listed include metronidazole, linezolid, daptomycin, and vancomycin.

Metronidazole

The drug **metronidazole (Flagyl, MetroCream, MetroGel, MetroLotion, Noritate Cream, Nuvessa, Vandazole)** is an antibiotic in the **nitroimidazole** class that is effective against fungi and protozoa as well as bacteria. Such capability is unusual, because the cells of fungi and protozoa are much more similar to those of humans than to those of bacteria.

Metronidazole is among the drugs of choice for the following conditions:

- amoebic dysentery
- bacterial vaginosis
- *Clostridium difficile* infections
- *Giardia* infections
- *Helicobacter pylori* ulcers
- intestinal infections
- rosacea
- sexually transmitted infections, including *Trichomonas* infections

Work Wise

The antibiotic metronidazole is pronounced "me-troe-NYE-da-zole."

Dosage Forms and Administration The dosage forms of metronidazole are capsules, IV, tablets, topical, and vaginal. The topical and vaginal forms are easily confused. The vaginal form has an applicator. Technicians should check to be sure which form the prescriber wants if there is any doubt.

Side Effects The most common side effects of metronidazole are headache, anorexia, vomiting, diarrhea, and abdominal cramps. Taking metronidazole with food can help alleviate these effects. A metallic taste in the mouth and urine discoloration may also occur.

Contraindications Metronidazole is contraindicated in patients with a hypersensitivity to nitroimidazole derivatives. This medication is also contraindicated in the first trimester of pregnancy, with use of disulfiram within the past two weeks, and with use of alcohol (or alcohol-containing products) during therapy or within three days of therapy discontinuation.

Cautions and Considerations Metronidazole carries a boxed warning for possible carcinogenicity. Because of this, unnecessary use should be avoided.

One of the most important things to remember about metronidazole is that it interacts with alcohol to cause a severe reaction. Patients can become quite ill with nausea, vomiting, flushing, sweating, and headache if they ingest any alcohol while taking metronidazole or within three days after stopping the medication. Some cough medicines and other over-the-counter (OTC) products have alcohol in them. Patients should be warned not to consume these products (in addition to alcoholic beverages) when taking metronidazole.

Drug Interactions Metronidazole should be avoided, when possible, when patients are using QT interval–prolonging agents. Mebendazole and ritonavir may enhance the toxic effects of metronidazole. Metronidazole may increase the serum concentrations of warfarin, and increased monitoring should occur when the two are used together.

Linezolid

Like other members of its class, **linezolid (Zyvox)**, the first **oxazolidinone** approved by the FDA, inhibits bacterial protein synthesis.

Linezolid may be used to treat the following:

- MRSA infections
- vancomycin-resistant *Enterococcus* (VRE) infections
- other Gram-positive infections

Dosage Forms and Administration Linezolid must be protected from light. Its dosage forms are IV, oral liquid, and tablet. The IV form comes in an IV bag. It should be administered alone and not through a line that is administering other drugs. Linezolid is not suitable for simultaneous administration because it has many physical incompatibilities and may precipitate in the line.

Side Effects Side effects associated with linezolid include headache, diarrhea, decreased hemoglobin, leukopenia, and thrombocytopenia.

Contraindications Linezolid should not be used with monoamine oxidase inhibitors (MAOIs) or within 14 days of taking them.

Cautions and Considerations Myelosuppression (such as anemia) has been reported in patients using linezolid. Caution should be exercised in patients who have preexisting myelosuppression or are using other drugs that cause myelosuppression. Optic neuropathy has been reported in patients treated for longer than 28 days. Serotonin syndrome may occur when linezolid is used with other serotonergic drugs.

Drug Interactions Linezolid may increase the toxic effects of alcohol, which should not be used concurrently. MAOIs should be avoided because of increased adverse effects. Linezolid may decrease patients' metabolism of the triptan medications used for migraines. The effectiveness of live vaccines decreases with linezolid use, and vaccine use should be postponed until three days after linezolid cessation.

Daptomycin

Daptomycin (Cubicin) is classified as a **cyclic lipopeptide**. This drug class works by binding to bacterial membranes and causing cell membrane depolarization, ultimately leading to an inhibition of DNA and RNA synthesis. Bacterial death follows.

Daptomycin may be used for the following conditions:

- complicated skin and skin structure infections
- *Staphylococcus aureus* blood infections

Dosage Forms and Administration Daptomycin comes as a powder in a vial for reconstitution. Daptomycin should not be reconstituted with dextrose-containing solutions (such as D_5W). Instead, NS or lactated Ringer's solution should be used.

Side Effects The most common side effects reported with daptomycin use include anemia, diarrhea, vomiting, and constipation. Chest pain, peripheral edema, skin rash, and respiratory side effects may also occur.

Contraindications Daptomycin does not have contraindications.

Cautions and Considerations Daptomycin use may result in eosinophilic pneumonia, and use must be discontinued immediately if it develops. Anaphylaxis has been reported with use. Daptomycin may be associated with myopathy and peripheral neuropathy. Use cautiously in patients with kidney dysfunction.

Drug Interactions HMG-CoA reductase inhibitors (commonly called statins) may enhance the adverse effects of daptomycin.

Vancomycin

A single drug in a class by itself is **vancomycin (Vancocin)**. Its mechanism is not fully understood, but it probably works by inhibiting cell-wall formation. Vancomycin has antimicrobial activity against Gram-positive bacteria and is used primarily to treat MRSA infections; in fact, it is the drug of choice. Unfortunately, some enterococci are resistant to vancomycin; these are called vancomycin-resistant *Enterococcus* (VRE).

FIGURE 16.4
Medication Label for Vancomycin

The name *vancomycin* was derived from the word *vanquish*, meaning "to defeat." When this drug was discovered in the 1950s, it was used to combat penicillin-resistant *Staphylococcus aureus*. Today, vancomycin is used to treat MRSA and is most frequently administered via the IV route.

NDC 45932-0028-1 IMPORTANT: READ INSERT FOR PRECAUTIONS AND DIRECTIONS BEFORE USE.
Vancomycin Hydrochloride for Injection, USP
Sterile, Lyophilized. **Preservative Free.**
*Each vial contains: Vancomycin hydrochloride equivalent to 500 mg vancomycin.
Usual Adult Dosage: 2 g daily in divided doses.
500 mg*/vial
For Intravenous Use
Dilute contents of the vial with 10 mL Sterile Water for Injection. **Prior to reconstitution,** store at 20° to 25°C (68° to 77°F) [see USP Controlled Room Temperature].
MUST BE FURTHER DILUTED BEFORE USE. SEE INSERT.
After reconstitution, this vial may be stored in a refrigerator for 96 hours without significant loss of potency. Made in Denmark.
Rx only
Manufactured by: Xellia Pharmaceuticals ApS
0 12345-679-12 0 xxxxxx-A Lot xxxxxx EXP MM-YYYY

Vancomycin is most frequently administered intravenously because the oral form is poorly absorbed into the bloodstream (see Figure 16.4). The oral dosage form is used only for infections that are localized within the intestines. Intravenous doses range between 500 mg and 2 grams a day in divided doses.

Vancomycin is among the drugs of choice for:

- MRSA infections
- endocarditis
- *Clostridium difficile* infections

Dosage Forms and Administration Vancomycin is typically administered intravenously. One gram of vancomycin for IV use is diluted in at least 250 mL of fluid.

Even though the drug-to-diluent ratio is 1 gram to 200 mL, it is always best to mix this drug in a larger amount of fluid than the minimum required. This tactic helps prevent the drug from being infused too quickly and the patient from experiencing red man syndrome (a syndrome associated with vancomycin infusion that results in flushing and redness in the neck and face, rash, and hypotension).

Side Effects Vancomycin may display **nephrotoxicity** (toxicity that causes damage to the kidneys) and **otoxicity** (which causes tinnitus, hearing loss, and balance problems). With proper monitoring of blood levels and laboratory tests, kidney and hearing damage can be avoided or minimized. However, these side effects limit vancomycin's use to the treatment of difficult infections.

Contraindications Vancomycin does not have contraindications.

Cautions and Considerations Vancomycin must be administered slowly (usually over 60 minutes or more) to avoid red man syndrome.

Drug Interactions Vancomycin may decrease the effectiveness of live vaccines. Oral vancomycin should not be coadministered with bile acid sequestrants because of diminished vancomycin effect.

16.4 Storage of Liquid Antibiotics

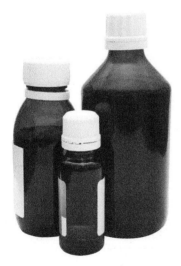

Liquid medications require extra attention because some must be refrigerated and others must not.

Many antibiotics are available as oral suspensions, a powder drug that must be reconstituted with water prior to dispensing. After reconstitution, some need refrigeration and some may be stored at room temperature. This is important information the technician should pass on to the patient or caregiver. It is *not* counseling, and no professional judgment is required. Drug storage does not require the technician to make a decision—the drug is either refrigerated or stored at room temperature—and it is a valuable and necessary piece of information for the patient to have. Because many medications do not require refrigeration but many others do, patients are often confused. Manufacturers have made an effort to minimize the number of drugs that need refrigeration. Table 16.3 helps simplify this issue for pharmacy technicians.

The flavors of these liquid drugs may be changed to suit a patient's taste. It is usually a pharmacy technician who makes this suggestion and changes a flavor. This feature of liquid drugs has made a difference in adherence in the pediatric population.

TABLE 16.3 Storage and Flavors of Reconstituted Liquid Antibiotics

Generic (Brand)	Refrigerate?	Standard Flavor Additive
amoxicillin (Amoxil)	yes	mixed berry
amoxicillin / clavulanate (Augmentin, Augmentin XR)	yes	orange
ampicillin	yes	bubble gum

continues

Generic (Brand)	Refrigerate?	Standard Flavor Additive
azithromycin (Zithromax, Zithromax Tri-Pak, Zithromax Z-Pak)	no	cherry
cefaclor	yes	strawberry
cefdinir	no	strawberry
cefixime (Suprax)	no	strawberry
cephalexin (Keflex)	yes	berry
ciprofloxacin (Cipro)	no	strawberry
clarithromycin (Biaxin)	no	fruit
clindamycin (Cleocin)	no	fruit
doxycycline (Vibramycin)	no	raspberry
erythromycin (EES, EryPed)	depends on formulation	orange
linezolid (Zyvox)	no	orange
penicillin	yes	fruit
sulfamethoxazole / trimethoprim (Bactrim, Septra, Sulfatrim)	no	grape or cherry
tetracycline	no	fruit

16.5 Ophthalmic Antibiotics

Some of the antibiotics discussed in this chapter have an ophthalmic (eye) dosage form. In contrast, very few antibiotics have an otic (ear) form, because the ophthalmic forms are also often used for ear conditions. However, otic (ear) medications are never used in the eye, since it would be extremely painful for the patient. This is because otic medicines are not manufactured with the same **pH** (acidity/alkalinity) as those for the eye. Table 16.4 lists antibiotic ophthalmic medications.

Because ophthalmic medications must have the same pH as the eye and because of the extreme sterility demanded in the manufacturing process for ophthalmics, eye drops are very expensive, especially the newer ones. Insurance companies often reject them in favor of less expensive eye drops. In such cases, technicians should let the prescriber know which eye drops are available and which the insurer is most likely to cover.

TABLE 16.4 **Commonly Used Ophthalmic Antibiotics**

Generic (Brand)	Pronunciation	Dosage Form	Common Dosage	Dispensing Status
azithromycin (AzaSite)	az-ith-roe-MYE-sin	drops	dosage varies	Rx
bacitracin	bas-i-TRAY-cin	ointment	½-inch strip in the affected eye(s) 1–3 times a day	Rx
ciprofloxacin (Ciloxan)	sip-roe-FLOKS-a-sin	drops, ointment	dosage varies	Rx

continues

TABLE 16.4 **Commonly Used Ophthalmic Antibiotics—***Continued*

Generic (Brand)	Pronunciation	Dosage Form	Common Dosage	Dispensing Status
erythromycin (Ilotycin)	e-rith-roe-MYE-sin	ointment	½-inch strip in the affected eye(s) up to 6 times a day as directed by provider	Rx
gatifloxacin (Zymaxid)	gat-i-FLOKS-a sin	drops	dosage varies	Rx
gentamicin (Gentak, Genoptic)	jen-ta-MYE-sin	drops, ointment	drops: 1–2 drops in the affected eye(s) every 4 hr; dosage may be increased to as much as 2 drops every hr ointment: ½-inch strip in the affected eye(s) 2–3 times a day	Rx
moxifloxacin (Vigamox, Moxeza)	moks-i-FLOKS-a-sin	drops	1 drop in the affected eye(s) 3 times a day for 7 days	Rx
ofloxacin (Ocuflox)	oh-FLOKS-a-sin	drops	days 1–2: 1–2 drops in the affected eye(s) every 2–4 hr days 3–7: 1–2 drops 4 times a day	Rx
sulfacetamide (Bleph-10)	sul-fa-SEE-ta-mide	drops, ointment	drops: 1–2 drops in the affected eye(s) every 2–3 hr initially ointment: ½-inch strip in the affected eye(s) 4 times a day and at bedtime	Rx
tobramycin (Tobrex)	toe-bra-MYE-sin	drops, ointment	drops: 1–2 drops in the affected eye(s) every 4 hr ointment: ½-inch strip in the affected eye(s) every 8–12 hr	Rx

16.6 Sexually Transmitted Infections and Drug Treatments

Most genital-system infections are transmitted by sexual activity; therefore, they are called *sexually transmitted infections (STIs)*. They were formerly known as *STDs* and *venereal diseases*. Ways to avoid STIs are to abstain from sexual contact or to be in a long-term, mutually monogamous relationship with a partner who has been tested and is known to be uninfected. Barrier contraceptives are known to help limit exposure to STIs, but use errors and product failures may occur. One of the most severe STIs, acquired immunodeficiency syndrome (AIDS), is caused by human immunodeficiency virus (HIV). HIV/AIDS and other viral STIs are discussed in Chapter 17. STIs of bacterial origin are discussed in the following sections.

Chlamydia

If untreated, an infection by *Chlamydia trachomatis* can progress to cause serious reproductive and other health problems with both short-term and long-term consequences. Chlamydia is known as the "silent" disease, because many people with chlamydia have no symptoms. It can occur in the rectum from anal intercourse and in the throat from oral sex. Chlamydial infections often occur with gonorrhea. Partners are frequently reinfected if their sex partners are not treated. Chlamydia can be easily treated and cured with antibiotics.

Gonorrhea

Gonorrhea is caused by *Neisseria gonorrhoeae*. The organism attaches to mucosal cells in the oropharyngeal area, eyes, joints, rectum, and genitalia. The infection causes inflammation and leukocytes (white blood cells) to move into the area, which results in the production of pus. Some patients experience painful urination and pus discharge from the penis. Complications can include urethral scarring with partial blockage of the urethra. Blockage of the vas deferens, the sperm-carrying duct, results in sterility. The disease is more insidious in individuals with a uterus, a cervix, fallopian tubes, or ovaries. In these patients, gonorrhea may cause abdominal pain due to pelvic inflammatory disease (PID), which involves extensive infection of these organs. Scarring in the fallopian tubes may block movement of ova; if a blockage is total, an ectopic pregnancy or sterility may result.

In any patient, untreated gonorrhea can cause a systemic infection involving the heart, meninges (membranes that surround the brain and spinal cord), eyes, pharynx, or joints. If a newborn's eyes are infected, blindness can result. In most states, erythromycin or silver nitrate solution is applied to the eyes of newborns as a prophylactic. If the person who gave birth to the newborn is known to be infected, the infant is given penicillin intramuscularly.

Gonorrhea infection can be acquired at any point of sexual contact, including the pharynx and anus. Recovery does not confer immunity, and reinfection is possible. Penicillin was once frequently used for gonorrhea, but due to resistance, a combination of a cephalosporin (such as ceftriaxone) and a macrolide (such as azithromycin) is now common. The *Chlamydia trachomatis* microorganism is commonly found with *Neisseria gonorrhoeae*, so patients who may have gonorrhea typically are also tested for chlamydia.

Syphilis

Syphilis is caused by *Treponema pallidum*, a spirochete bacteria that moves with a corkscrew-like action. A long incubation time (time from exposure to clinical onset) allows the sexual partners of an infected patient to be traced and treated before symptoms are apparent. Incubation averages three weeks, with symptoms typically appearing between two weeks and several months following infection. A syphilis infection develops in three stages: the primary stage, the secondary stage, and the late or tertiary stage. It can also be congenital.

Primary-Stage Infection

A primary-stage syphilis infection typically produces a **chancre**, a small, usually painless ulcer with a hard base, at the site of infection. Usually, the lesion heals in a few weeks. Individuals with a cervix may be unaware of the infection if the chancre is on the cervix. In patients with a penis, the chancre may be in the urethra. Fluids from the sore are highly infectious. If the infected patient does not receive treatment during this stage, the infection will progress to the secondary stage.

Secondary-Stage Infection

A secondary-stage syphilis infection may produce skin rashes, patchy hair loss, malaise, or mild fever. Symptoms subside after a few weeks, and the disease becomes latent. During the latent phase, syphilis is still in the body despite one having no signs or symptoms.

Late or Tertiary-Stage Infection

A tertiary-stage syphilis infection usually occurs after an interval of at least 10 years. Lesions appear as rubbery masses of tissue in many organs and sometimes on the skin. The infection may cause extensive damage, including deafness, blindness, CNS lesions, or perforation of the roof of the mouth, resulting from a hyperimmune reaction to the remaining spirochetes. Because symptoms in the first two stages are not disabling, patients often enter the latent period without receiving medical attention.

Congenital Syphilis

Congenital syphilis occurs in newborns as a result of infection crossing the placenta into the fetus. Neurologic damage to the fetus results if pregnancy occurs during the tertiary stage. Pregnancy during the primary or secondary stage is likely to result in a stillbirth.

Other Sexually Transmitted Infections

Two other sexually transmitted infections, nongonococcal urethritis and vaginitis, play a major role in public health. Nongonococcal urethritis may be caused by catheters or chemical agents; some cases are acquired sexually. Symptoms, which can be mild in some individuals, may include genital discharge, burning while urinating, and itching. In patients with a uterus, cervix, fallopian tubes, or ovaries, symptoms are more likely to be serious; the infection may also cause abdominal pain or abnormal bleeding and can progress to PID.

Vaginitis, an inflammation of the vagina caused by infection, allergic reaction, or hormone deficiency, is characterized by vaginal discharge and odor. It can be caused by any of several organisms or by other factors. Vaginitis due to *Gardnerella vaginalis* results from interaction between that organism and an anaerobic bacteria in the vagina, neither of which alone can produce the disease. It is characterized by a frothy discharge with fishy odor and a vaginal pH between five and six. Vaginitis may also be caused by *Trichomonas vaginalis*, a parasite normally found in individuals of any sex. *T. vaginalis* causes an infection if vaginal acidity is disturbed. Common signs and symptoms include profuse yellowish or light-cream-colored discharge with a disagreeable odor that causes irritation, burning, and itching.

Agents for Treating Sexually Transmitted Infections

Safety Alert

Bicillin L-A and Bicillin C-R (which is penicillin G benzathine combined with penicillin G procaine) are frequently dispensed in place of each other. However, the procaine in Bicillin C-R makes it shorter acting. The longer-acting Bicillin L-A is needed for syphilis.

Table 16.5 presents the most commonly used agents for sexually transmitted infections. Many of these medications were introduced in Section 16.2.

Azithromycin (Zithromax, Zithromax Tri-Pak, Zithromax Z-Pak) is provided by the manufacturer in several forms. The powdered form is approved for administration as a one-time dose to treat some sexually transmitted bacterial infections, such as certain stages of syphilis and gonococcal infections.

Ceftriaxone (Rocephin) is used frequently, especially against penicillinase-producing bacteria.

Doxycycline (Doryx, Doxy, Vibramycin) is used to treat lymphogranuloma venereum, which is caused by *Chlamydia trachomatis*.

Metronidazole (Flagyl, Flagyl ER, MetroGel Vaginal, Nuvessa, MetroGel, MetroCream) is used to treat *Gardnerella vaginalis* (formerly called *Haemophilus vaginalis*) infections. It is important that the patient complete the full course of treatment.

Tetracycline (Sumycin) can be used to control *Chlamydia trachomatis*, which frequently occurs with gonorrhea. Tetracycline and **erythromycin (ERY-C, Ery-Tab, Erythrocin)** are both effective against chlamydia.

Penicillin G benzathine (Bicillin L-A) is used to treat syphilis. It is especially effective during the primary stage. Penicillin is administered in low concentration, but it is appropriate treatment because the spirochete bacteria that causes syphilis grows slowly. This agent is effective for approximately two weeks.

TABLE 16.5 Commonly Used Antibacterial Agents for STIs

Generic (Brand)	Pronunciation	Dosage Form	Common Doses	Dispensing Status
azithromycin (Zithromax, Zithromax Tri-Pak, Zithromax Z-Pak)	az-ith-roe-MYE-sin	injection (IV), oral liquid, tablet	PO: 1–2 g 1 time a day depending on infection	Rx
ceftriaxone (Rocephin)	sef-trye-AKS-one	injection	IM: 250 mg for one dose	Rx
doxycycline (Doryx, Doxy, Vibramycin)	dox-i-SYE-kleen	capsule, injection (IV), oral liquid, tablet	100 mg 2 times a day for 7 days	Rx
erythromycin (ERY-C, Ery-Tab, Erythrocin)	er-ith-roe-MYE-sin	capsule, injection, oral liquid, tablet, topical ointment, topical pads, topical solution	500 mg 4 times a day for 7 days OR erythromycin ethylsuccinate 800 mg 4 times a day for 7 days	Rx
metronidazole (Flagyl, Flagyl ER, MetroGel Vaginal, Nuvessa, MetroGel, MetroCream)	me-troe-NYE-da-zole	capsule, injection (IV) tablet, topical cream, topical gel, topical lotion	PO: 500 mg 2 times a day for 7 days topical: 0.75% 1 time a day vaginally for 5 days	Rx
penicillin G benzathine (Bicillin L-A)	pen-i-SIL-in G BENZ-a-theen	injection (IM)	<1 year syphilis duration: 2.4 million units as a single dose late latent, tertiary syphilis: 2.4 million units 1 time a week for 3 doses	Rx
tetracycline (Achromycin V)	te-tra-SYE-kleen	capsule	250–500 mg 4 times a day	Rx

16.7 Fungi, Fungal Diseases, and Drug Treatments

A **fungus** is a single-celled organism similar to an animal cell and to a green plant cell. All three are **eukaryotic** (have a defined nucleus), in contrast to bacteria, which are **prokaryotic** (lack a defined nucleus). Fungi (plural of fungus, pronounced FUN-jye) include mushrooms, yeasts, and molds. They are distinguished from green plants by the absence of chlorophyll, the substance that gives plants their green color, and by the fact that they reproduce via spores. Fungus cells are distinguished from animal cells and bacterial cells by the presence of a unique rigid cell wall. All eukaryotic cells have similar molecular machinery for performing life functions such as making proteins, replicating DNA, and storing and releasing energy. This machinery is different from the corresponding machinery in prokaryotic cells. Therefore, the antibiotics discussed earlier in this chapter that work against bacteria do not work against fungi, and a drug that can kill a fungus is likely to be toxic to a human as well. Still, there are some differences between human and fungal cells that can be used as the basis for antifungal drugs. For example, human cell membranes contain cholesterol, a type of lipid found in animal cells that is a key constituent of cell membranes and a precursor to hormone production; the cell membranes of fungi instead contain **ergosterol**, another lipid unique to fungi.

Usually, fungal infections are topical and mild. **Dermatophyte** fungi, or fungi of the skin, cause some of the most frequent and ordinary infections, such as athlete's foot and ringworm. *Candida*, another common fungus, causes vaginal yeast infections and oral thrush. However, when a fungus gains entry to the bloodstream or cannot be destroyed because of immunodeficiency, it can cause serious systemic infection. Table 16.6 lists common fungi and related infections.

TABLE 16.6 Examples of Fungal Organisms and the Resulting Infections

Organism	Fungal Infection	Description of Infection
Aspergillus	aspergillosis	inflammation in the skin, lungs, or bones
Blastomyces	blastomycosis	infection begins from inhalation through the lungs; produces tumors in the skin and other body tissues
Candida (yeast)	candidiasis	usually a superficial infection of the mucous membranes, but sometimes systemic
Coccidioides	coccidioidomycosis	known as valley fever and endemic to the western United States, Mexico, and South America; an acute but benign self-limiting respiratory tract infection in its primary form, but a virulent, severe disease of the viscera, CNS, and lungs in its secondary form; sometimes misdiagnosed as lung cancer
Cryptococcus	cryptococcosis	invasion of CNS most commonly seen in immunocompromised patients
Histoplasma	histoplasmosis	usually asymptomatic infection resulting from inhalation of spores, but can cause acute pneumonia

Systemic fungal diseases are most likely to develop in patients whose immune systems are depressed by disease, drug therapy (for example, the use of corticosteroids or antineoplastics), or poor nutrition. Patients at risk for fungal infections include those who have recently received transplants and are receiving immunosuppressive medications, those with IV catheters, and those with certain cancers or human immunodeficiency virus (HIV). Fungi can also cause systemic infections of the body organs and tissues, such as the lungs, brain and central nervous system (CNS), and blood.

Some antifungal agents prevent the synthesis of ergosterol, a building block for fungal cell membranes. Because human cell membranes use cholesterol instead of ergosterol, they are affected minimally by antifungals. Other antifungal agents act by inhibiting fungal cytochrome P450, which is different from human cytochrome P450, so these

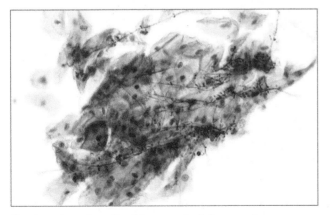

Fungi, such as these *Candida*, are unicellular organisms responsible for several systemic diseases.

medications have little effect on human cells but destroy the cells of the fungi. Some antifungals are available in topical dosage forms and are now available OTC. These topical agents are covered in Chapter 5.

Used with certain antimicrobial agents, **pulse dosing** is a type of dosing regimen that produces escalating antimicrobial levels early in the dosing interval, followed by a prolonged dose-free period. This type of dosing is sometimes used for fungal nail infections. With this type of regimen, patients take a higher dose for one week, followed by three weeks off of the drug. The cycle is then repeated. Because the drug persists in the nail for several months, this regimen works as well as continuous daily dosing. In addition, patients take much less drug, the treatment is safer, and it costs less.

Antifungal drugs are dispensed as topical, IV, and systemic agents. Even though the topical agents seem relatively mild compared to other antifungal agents, serious side effects have been reported. Close attention to the dosing regimen is needed to avoid overdosing. Table 16.7 lists the most commonly used antifungals.

TABLE 16.7 Commonly Used Antifungals

Generic (Brand)	Pronunciation	Dosage Form	Common Dosage	Dispensing Status	Indications
Azoles					
butoconazole (Gynazole-1)	bew-toe-KON-a-zole	vaginal cream	1 time a day for 1–3 days	OTC, Rx	vaginal
clotrimazole (Lotrimin AF, Trivagizole 3)	kloe-TRIM-a-zole	cream, lozenge, topical solution, vaginal cream and suppository	PO: dissolve in mouth 5 times a day topical: 2 times a day for 2–4 weeks vaginal: 1 time a day for 3–7 days	OTC, Rx	skin, nails, oral thrush, and vaginal
clotrimazole / betamethasone (Lotrisone)	kloe-TRIM-a-zole bay-ta-METH-a-sone	cream, lotion	2 times a day for 4 weeks	Rx	skin and nails
fluconazole (Diflucan)	floo-KON-a-zole	injection, oral suspension, oral tablet	IV: varies depending on infection PO: 150 mg in 1 dose for vaginal infections, 200–800 mg/day for systemic infections	Rx	various
itraconazole (Onmel, Sporanox)	i-tra-KON-a-zole	capsule, oral solution, tablet	200–400 mg/day	Rx	various
ketoconazole (Extina, Nizoral, Zolegel)	kee-toe-KON-a-zole	cream, foam, gel, shampoo, tablet	200–400 mg a day for 2–4 weeks topical: 1 time a day	Rx	skin and nails, systemic
miconazole (Desenex, Lotrimin, Micatin, Monistat, Oravig)	mye-KON-a-zole	lotion, ointment, powder, solution, spray, suppository, tablet, topical cream, vaginal cream	topical: 2 times a day for 2 weeks vaginal: 1,200 mg at bedtime for 1 day, 200 mg/day for 3 days, 100 mg/day for 7 days Oral (buccal): 50 mg to upper gum 1 time a day	OTC	skin, nails, and vaginal

continues

TABLE 16.7 Commonly Used Antifungals—*Continued*

Generic (Brand)	Pronunciation	Dosage Form	Common Dosage	Dispensing Status	Indications
posaconazole (Noxafil)	poe-sa-KON-azole	injection, oral suspension, tablet	100–400 mg 2–3 times a day	Rx	various
tioconazole (Vagistat-1)	tee-oh-KON-a-zole	vaginal ointment	1 application at bedtime for 1 day	OTC	vaginal
voriconazole (Vfend)	vor-i-KON-a-zohl	injection, oral suspension, tablet	IV: 4–6 mg/kg every 12 hr PO: 200 mg every 12 hr	Rx	various
Echinocandins					
caspofungin (Cancidas)	kas-poe-FUN-jin	injection	70 mg initial dose, then 50 mg/day	Rx	systemic
micafungin (Mycamine)	mye-ka-FUN-gin	injection	preventative: 50 mg/day active treatment: 150 mg/day	Rx	systemic
Polyenes					
amphotericin B (Abelcet, AmBisome)	am-foe-TER-i-sin BEE	injection	individualized to patient and disease	Rx	systemic
amphotericin B lipid complex (Abelcet)	am-foe-TER-i-sin BEE LIP-ed com-PLEX	injection	individualized to patient and disease	Rx	systemic
amphotericin B liposomal (AmBisome)	am-foe-TER-i-sin BEE LYE-poh-sohm-al	injection	individualized to patient and disease	Rx	systemic
nystatin	nye-STAT-in	oral suspension, tablet	500,000–1 million units 3 times a day	Rx	oral thrush
nystatin (Nyamyc, Nystop)	nye-STAT-in	cream, ointment, powder	2 times a day until lesions heal	Rx	skin and nails
Miscellaneous Agents					
butenafine (Lotrimin Ultra, Mentax)	bew-TEN-a-feen	cream	1 time a day for 2 weeks	OTC, Rx	skin and nails
ciclopirox (Loprox, Penlac)	sye-KLO-pie-rox	cream, gel, lotion, nail lacquer, shampoo, topical suspension	depends on dosage form and site of infection but can take up to 12 weeks for cure	Rx	skin and nails
flucytosine (Ancobon)	floo-SYE-toe-seen	capsule	50–150 mg/kg/day in divided intervals every 6 hr	Rx	systemic
griseofulvin (Grifulvin V, Gris-PEG)	gri-see-oh-FUL-vin	capsule, oral suspension, tablet	varies depending on age and weight of patient (4 weeks for athlete's foot, 4–6 months for nail infections)	Rx	skin and nails
terbinafine (Lamisil AT)	TER-bin-a-feen	cream, spray	1 time a day for 1–2 weeks	OTC	skin and nails

Azoles

Antifungals ending in the suffix *-azole* are in the **azole** family and are generally well tolerated. Members of the azole family interfere with fungal cytochrome P450 and inhibit the formation of the fungal cell wall.

Butaconazole (Gynazole-1) is used for the treatment of vulvovaginal candidiasis.

Clotrimazole is especially effective against oral candidiasis.

Fluconazole (Diflucan) is metabolized through the cytochrome P450 system. The oral form is used for vaginal and oral candidiasis, whereas the IV form should be reserved for patients unable to tolerate oral therapy.

Itraconazole (Sporanox) is especially useful for fungal infections of the nails.

Ketoconazole (Extina, Nizoral, Zolegel) has the same side effect profile as most of the other antifungal agents.

Miconozole (Desenex, Lotrimin, Micatin, Monistat, Oravig) is available for the treatment of mild *oropharyngeal candidiasis*, *vulvovaginal candidiasis*, and various skin and mucous membrane fungal infections.

Posaconazole (Noxafil) has different uses depending on its dosage form. The tablet and intravenous forms are used for invasive *Candida* and *Aspergillus* infections. The suspension form of posaconazole, which is cherry flavored, may be used for oropharyngeal infections and for systemic infections.

Voriconazole (Vfend) is an alternative to amphotericin B for life-threatening fungal infections.

Dosage Forms and Administration Butaconazole is supplied as a vaginal cream to be administered intravaginally using the applicator supplied with the medication.

Clotrimazole is supplied as a troche (a small lozenge), topically for skin and nail infections **(Lotrimin AF)**, and vaginally **(Trivagizole 3)**.

Itraconazole is available in capsules and oral solution. Patients should take itraconazole capsules with a fatty meal or acidic drink to improve absorption, but capsules should not be taken within two hours of taking antacids or histamine-2 (H2) receptor blockers. Capsules should not be substituted for the oral solution, because the solution is more readily absorbed.

Oral ketoconazole comes in a tablet dosage form. This drug is also available topically.

Miconazole is available in oral and topical formulations. The oral formulation is a buccal tablet applied to the upper gums.

Oral dosage forms of posaconazole should be administered with food.

Voriconazole can be started intravenously and switched to an oral dose. IV voriconazole must be infused over one to two hours and should not be infused simultaneously with any other products. Voriconazole must be reconstituted and used immediately.

Side Effects When azoles are ingested orally, nausea, vomiting, abdominal pain, and diarrhea are the most frequently reported side effects. Topically applied azoles are associated with application-site reactions such as burning, discomfort, edema, and pain.

The most common side effects of fluconazole are headache, rash, and GI upset.

Itraconazole and ketoconazole are particularly likely to cause stomach symptoms. Because itraconazole can be toxic to the liver, patients should report any unusual nausea, vomiting, jaundice, or changes in the stool to their healthcare provider immediately.

Ketoconazole side effects are dose dependent and include nausea, anorexia, and vomiting.

Voriconazole is associated with transient vision changes (such as seeing flashes of light or having sensitivity to light), visual hallucinations, alopecia, nail changes or loss, and skin rash. Voriconazole has serious side effects such as liver toxicity and blurred vision. Patients taking this drug should not drive at night.

Contraindications Azoles are contraindicated with concurrent use of quinidine; benzodiazepines such as alprazolam, chlordiazepoxide, clonazepam, diazepam, and triazolam; dofetilide; pimozide; and statins such as lovastatin, simvastatin, and atorvastatin. Miconazole is contraindicated in patients with milk-protein allergy.

Cautions and Considerations Ketoconazole carries boxed warnings regarding hepatotoxicity that could result in liver transplantation, adrenal insufficiency (decreased production of corticosteroids), and the potential for QT prolongation when administered with dofetilde, quinidine, pimozide, cisapride, methadone, dysopyramide, drondarone, and ranolazine.

Itracanzole also has boxed warnings. One warning is due to severe drug interactions. Itraconazole should not be used with methadone, disopyramide, dofetilide, dronedarone, quinidine, ergot alkaloids, ergotamine, methylergometrine, irinotecan, lurasidone, oral midazolam, pimozide, triazolam, felodipine, nisoldipine, ranolazine, eplerenone, cisapride, lovastatin, simvastatin, ticagrelor, colchicine, fesoterodine, telithromycin, or solifenacin.

Itraconazole's other boxed warning emphasizes that itraconazole should not be used to treat fungal nail infections in patients who have ventricular dysfunction such as heart failure.

Fluconazole may cause QT prolongation, and caution should be exercised when using it with other medications that can cause arrhythmia.

Drug Interactions Azole antifungals are associated with multiple drug-drug interactions. See the Contraindications section for a listing of drug interactions. Azole antifungals decrease the activity of the probiotic *Saccharomyces boulardii*.

Echinocandins

The generic names of drugs belonging to the **echinocandin** class of antifungals end in the suffix *-fungin*. Echinocandins include caspofungin and micafungin. Echinocandins work by inhibiting the synthesis of β-(1,3)-D-glucan, which is an integral component of the fungal cell wall.

Caspofungin (Cancidas) was the first echinocandin commercially available. It is only available in IV form for the treatment of invasive *Aspergillus* and *Candida* in patients who are unresponsive to other therapies, such as amphotericin B or itraconazole. Caspofungin seems to cause fewer hypersensitivity reactions than the other drugs in this class.

Micafungin (Mycamine) is used to treat patients with an *Aspergillus* or *Candida* infection.

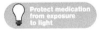

Dosage Forms and Administration Micafungin should be reconstituted and mixed with either NS or D_5W. After the diluent is injected into the vial, it should be gently swirled but not shaken. Once reconstituted, the micafungin preparation is good for 24 hours at room temperature and must be protected from light.

Side Effects The echinocandins are injectable and may result in infusion and hypersensitivity reactions, including rash, redness, hypotension, and—in some cases—angioedema. Pain at the injection site is another potential side effect.

Contraindications Micafungin and caspofungin do not have contraindications.

Cautions and Considerations The echinocandins are associated with anaphylaxis and histamine-related reactions. Use should be discontinued immediately if anaphylaxis occurs.

Drug Interactions Echinocandins decrease the activity of the probiotic *Saccharomyces boulardii*. Cyclosporine may increase toxic effects of caspofungin. Rifampin may decrease the concentrations of caspofungin. Micafungin may increase drug levels of pimozide, and concurrent use is not recommended.

Polyenes

The **polyene** antifungal class includes **amphotericin B lipid complex (Abelcet)**, **amphotericin B liposomal (AmBisome)**, and **nystatin**. Amphotericin B binds to ergosterol, a sterol in the cell membranes of fungi. This alters cell-wall permeability (the ability of a material to allow molecules or ions to pass through it), allowing electrolytes and other substances to leak out. While amphotericin B has a higher attraction to ergosterol in the cell walls of fungi, it can also bind to cholesterol in a human cell and cause toxicity. Amphotericin B is particularly toxic to the liver and kidneys. Thus, its use is reserved for the most serious and life-threatening fungal infections. Nystatin is an antifungal that can be used topically and systemically.

Abelcet and AmBisome are lipid complex injectable forms of amphotericin B that are associated with less kidney toxicity. These drugs are administered by IV infusion. They are indicated for treating aspergillosis and any type of progressive fungal infection in patients intolerant to amphotericin B. A wide range of side effects similar to those of amphotericin B has been reported.

Nystatin is most often used in liquid form to swish and swallow. It is given commonly to patients with **oral candidiasis**, also known as *thrush*, an infection in the mouth caused by yeast-like fungi of the genus *Candida*.

Dosage Forms and Administration Amphotericin B should be infused slowly to help prevent fever, chills, nausea, vomiting, and headache. This drug is also available in an IV liposome dosage form, in which the drug molecules are surrounded by a layer of oil or fat (see Figure 16.5). This protective layer decreases the drug's ability to come into direct contact with body tissues and thus reduces its toxic effects. Amphotericin B should not be mixed or "piggybacked" with other drugs. To avoid precipitation, it should not be mixed with normal saline. **Normal saline (NS)** is a sterile IV or irrigation solution containing a concentration of 0.9% sodium chloride in water. Amphotericin B is usually mixed in D_5W and stored in the refrigerator; it must be infused within six hours of being mixed. Antiemetic substances (agents that prevent or eliminate nausea and vomiting; covered in Chapter 12), can reduce the severity of nausea and vomiting.

FIGURE 16.5
Liposome Dosage Form

Amphotericin B's liposomal dosage form was developed to reduce toxicity and infusion-related reactions. The liposome is made of phosopholipids and cholesterol with amphotericin inserted into it. The liposome keeps its structure until it reaches the fungal cell. At that point, the drug is released into the cell membrane.

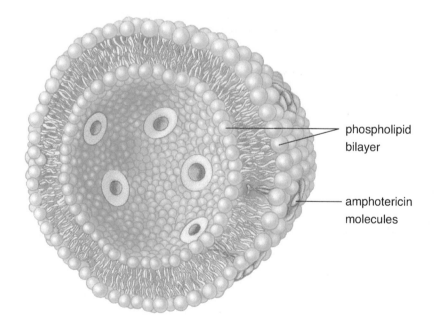

phospholipid bilayer

amphotericin molecules

If the patient does not have a central venous catheter, the IV site should be changed frequently, as phlebitis (inflammation of a vein) is common with administration of this drug.

Side Effects Amphotericin B is associated with bothersome side effects in addition to nephrotoxicity and hepatotoxicity. Its side effects include fever, chills, shaking, and headache. Prophylaxis with acetaminophen, an antihistamine such as diphenhydramine, or both is often necessary to alleviate or prevent infusion-related side effects. Potassium, calcium, and magnesium stores are often depleted. Anemia (a below-normal concentration of erythrocytes or hemoglobin in the blood) is also common.

Oral nystatin is associated with diarrhea, nausea, stomach pain, and vomiting. Topical nystatin is associated with hypersensitivity reactions. Because nystatin is available in oral and topical formulations, it is important to ensure the correct product is selected.

Contraindications Amphotericin B and nystatin do not have contraindications.

Cautions and Considerations Reports of anaphylaxis are associated with amphotericin B use, and infusions should be supervised. If patients exhibit signs of anaphylaxis, administration should be discontinued immediately.

Drug Interactions Amphotericin B should not be used with foscarnet. Nystatin diminishes the effects of the probiotic *Saccharomyces boulardii*.

Miscellaneous Antifungals

Other antifungals include the topical products **butenafine (Lotrimin Ultra, Mentax)**, **ciclopirox (Loprox, Penlac)**, and **terbinafine (Lamisil AT)**. **Flucytosine (Ancobon)** and **griseofulvin (Grifulvin V, Gris-PEG)** are systemic.

Dosage Forms and Administration Contraceptive failure is possible with griseofulvin use, and alternative nonhormonal contraception should be used. Griseofulvin liquid should be protected from light.

Side Effects Butenafine is associated with burning, contact dermatitis, erythema, irritation, pruritus, and stinging. Ciclopirox, which is applied topically, is associated with acne, alopecia, contact dermatitis, dry skin, skin burning, eye pain, and headache. Terbinafine may cause headache, skin rash, diarrhea, dyspepsia, and nasopharyngitis.

Flucytosine is associated with rash; leukopenia; thrombocytopenia; GI symptoms such as nausea, diarrhea, and vomiting; and hepatic side effects. Side effects of griseofulvin include dizziness, fatigue, skin rash, photosensitivity, and diarrhea. Griseofulvin may enhance toxic effects of alcohol. Concurrent use is not recommended.

Contraindications Griseofulvin is contraindicated in patients who are pregnant or have liver failure or porphyria. Butenafine, ciclopirox, flucytosine, and terbinafine do not have contraindications.

Cautions and Considerations Flucytosine carries a boxed warning to use extreme caution in patients with renal dysfunction. The agent should be used only in combination with other antifungals to prevent development of resistance. Patients with bone marrow depression or hematologic disease, or who are undergoing therapy that causes bone marrow suppression, should use flucytosine with caution.

Griseofulvin should be discontinued if granulocytopenia occurs. Penicillin and griseofulvin have a potential for cross-sensitivity. Severe skin reactions have been reported with griseofulvin use; it is recommended that patients discontinue therapy and seek emergency medical care if severe skin reactions occur.

Depression has been reported with terbinafine use. Patients should contact their healthcare practitioners immediately if they experience any signs and symptoms of depression.

Drug Interactions Systemic antifungals may diminish the therapeutic effect of the probiotic *Saccharomyces boulardii*, and concurrent use should be avoided. Butenafine and ciclopirox do not have known drug interactions.

Terbinafine may increase serum concentrations of pimozide and thioridazine, and concurrent use should be avoided. It may decrease levels of tamoxifen.

Flucytosine, when combined with drugs that cause bone marrow suppression (like azathioprine and gancilovir interferon), increase the risk of bone marrow suppression.

16.8 Complementary and Alternative Therapies

Pharm Facts

Echinacea and zinc are also common alternative therapies for viral infections, such as colds.

Some complementary and alternative therapies that may be used for infections include echinacea and zinc. Patients who are using a complementary or alternative therapy should tell their healthcare providers, pharmacists, and pharmacy technicians. **Echinacea (Echinacea purpurea)** is an herb some patients use to treat the common cold, RTIs, and even vaginal yeast infections. Some claim that echinacea reduces the severity and length of symptoms. Echinacea does not cure infections, but it may be used to augment drug therapy. Some studies indicate that echinacea increases phagocytosis, the process by which the immune system cells "eat up" foreign cells such as bacteria. It also enhances lymphocyte activity. Echinacea products contain various concentrations of this herbal remedy. A standard dose has not been established. However, for echinacea to have a chance of being effective, patients must use it multiple times a day and initiate its use at the very first signs of infection. Dosing is typically heaviest during the first 5 days of infection and continues for up to 10 days.

Zinc is a necessary nutrient. One important role zinc plays is to help with immune function. Some have tried to use supplemental zinc to shorten the length of colds and enhance wound healing. Additional research needs to be done, but some evidence suggests there may be a benefit in individuals with low levels of zinc. There is no established dose for zinc. Most people obtain an adequate amount of zinc in their diet. Side effects may include increased heart rate, agitation, vomiting, and nausea. The use of intranasal zinc has led to the loss of smell, in some cases long term or permanently.

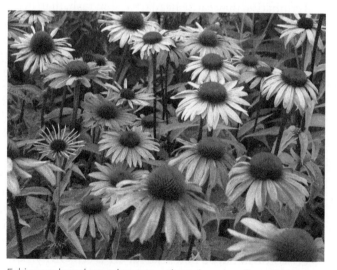

Echinacea-based complementary therapies come from *Echinacea purpurea*, the purple coneflower plant. Some people use echinacea for the common cold.

Review and Assessment

CHAPTER SUMMARY

Anatomy and Physiology of the Immune System

- The immune system is a complex system made up of different organs, ducts, cells, and proteins that work together to help fight infection.

- The bone marrow, thymus, lymphatic system, and spleen are major organs of the immune system.

- The innate and adaptive immune systems both play a key role in fighting infection.

- Specific white blood cell types that are critical to the innate immune response include neutrophils, mast cells, basophils, dendritic cells, eosinophils, macrophages, and natural killer cells.

- B cells and T cells are the primary cells used in the adaptive immune system and are the two main types of lymphocytes.

- Antibodies recognize antigens and then mark them for attack by other proteins and cells.

- Antigens are substances such as bacteria or viruses that cause antibodies to be formed. Antigens can be thought of as identification tags that tell the body that they or the cells they are on are a foreign substance and a potential threat to the body.

Bacterial Infections

- Bacteria are single-celled organisms that occur in almost all environments. When they penetrate body tissues, they can establish areas of infection.

- An infection is the growth of bacteria or other pathogens in body tissues, causing tissue damage and eliciting an immune response.

- General signs of infection that suggest a bacterial origin are fever (101° F or greater) and a high white blood cell count ($>12,000/mm^3$). The onset of fever alone is not diagnostic of bacterial infection.

- Bacteria can be classified by oxygenation needs (aerobic or anaerobic), shape, arrangement of cells, and Gram-stain result (positive or negative). Classification directs antibiotic selection.

- An antibiotic works in one of six ways: (1) preventing folic acid synthesis, (2) impairing cell-wall formation, (3) blocking protein formation, (4) interfering with DNA formation, (5) disrupting cell membranes, or (6) disrupting DNA structure.

- The outcome of antibiotic treatment can be evaluated in two ways: (1) by the clinical response, meaning the extent to which signs and symptoms have disappeared, or (2) by the microbiologic response, meaning the extent to which the organism has been eradicated.

- A bactericidal agent kills bacteria.

- A bacteriostatic agent inhibits the growth or multiplication of bacteria.

- Bacterial infections are contagious until antibiotics have been taken for 24 to 48 hours.

- Antibiotics may interfere with the effectiveness of contraceptives.

Antibiotic Drugs and Their Mechanisms of Action

Sulfonamides and Nitrofurantoin

- Nitrofurantoin may be an acceptable alternative to sulfa drugs for UTIs.

- Sulfonamides are used in the treatment of UTIs, otitis media, lower respiratory tract infections, and prophylaxis of *Pneumocystis carinii* pneumonia in immunocompromised patients.

- Patients taking sulfonamides should be told to drink six to eight glasses of water a day to keep the urine dilute and avoid crystallization of the drug in the urine. They should be told to avoid exposure to sunlight and to stop taking the drug immediately and notify their healthcare practitioner if a rash appears (the most common side effect of the sulfas).

Penicillins

- Penicillins come in many types and are primarily used for the treatment of Gram-positive infections.

- Penicillins are bactericidal in that they kill bacteria by preventing them from forming the rigid wall needed for survival. Human cells do not have rigid cell walls and are, therefore, unaffected by penicillin.

- Some bacteria are resistant to penicillins because they produce an enzyme called *beta-lactamase*. Beta-lactamase renders penicillins inactive.

- Penicillins should not be taken with fruit juices or colas because the acids in them could deactivate the drug. A common side effect of penicillins is diarrhea.

Cephalosporins

- Cephalosporins have a mechanism of action similar to that of penicillins but a different antibacterial spectrum.

- Patients allergic to penicillins may also be allergic to cephalosporins, and vice versa. Most computerized drug profile systems place penicillins and cephalosporins in the same category; if a patient has an allergy to either, the computer will probably indicate they are allergic to both.

- The first-generation cephalosporins are similar to the antistaphylococcal penicillins, with limited Gram-negative coverage. The second-generation cephalosporins have broader coverage, especially against *H. influenzae*. The third generation is active against a wide spectrum of Gram-negative organisms. The fourth-generation cephalosporin is considered "broad spectrum," with both Gram-negative and somewhat less Gram-positive coverage. The fifth-generation cephalosporin, ceftaroline, has coverage against MRSA.

Carbapenems and Monobactams

- Carbapenems and monobactams are drugs that are structurally similar to penicillins and cephalosporins. They kill bacteria by inhibiting cell-wall formation.

- Carbapenems are used for mixed Gram-positive and Gram-negative infections. Monobactams, in contrast, are used only for Gram-negative bacteria.

Lincosamides and Macrolides

- Lincosamides and macrolides can be bacteriostatic (at low doses) and bactericidal (at high doses). They work by blocking bacteria's ability to produce proteins needed for survival.

- Clindamycin, a lincosamide, carries a boxed warning because it can cause severe and possibly fatal colitis. Its use should be reserved for treatment of serious infections for which use of other antimicrobials is inappropriate.

- Azithromycin is a commonly used macrolide available in various formulations.

- Macrolides, in particular clarithromycin and erythromycin, have many drug interactions. It is important for the pharmacy technician to help the pharmacist maintain accurate drug lists for patients using them.

Aminoglycosides

- Aminoglycosides are used to treat very serious infections. They work by blocking a bacteria's ability to make proteins essential for survival.

- Nephrotoxicity and ototoxicity are concerns with aminoglycoside use. Drug blood levels and other laboratory measurements are used to minimize these potentially harmful effects.

Tetracyclines

- Tetracyclines are bacteriostatic and inhibit protein synthesis within bacterial cells.

- Tetracyclines are best taken on an empty stomach. Doxycyine and minocycline may be taken with food but not dairy products or antacids.

- Children, pregnant individuals, and individuals who breast-feed should not take tetracyclines.

- Technicians should always check the expiration date on tetracyclines. It can be dangerous to dispense one of these drugs if it is out of date.

Fluoroquinolones

- Fluoroquinolones, also called *quinolones*, are antibiotics with strong, rapid bactericidal activity against Gram-negative bacteria and some Gram-positive bacteria. They work by interfering with DNA coiling.

- They are often used for bone and joint infections, eye infections, and serious RTIs and UTIs.

- Quinolones should not be used during pregnancy.

Miscellaneous Antibiotics

Metronidazole

- Metronidazole is unusual in that it is effective against bacteria, fungi, and protozoa.

- Metronidazole use is associated with a metallic taste and urine discoloration.

- Metronidazole interacts significantly with alcohol to cause a severe reaction. Patients can become quite ill with nausea, vomiting, flushing, sweating, and headache if they ingest any alcohol while taking metronidazole or within three days of stopping the medication.

Linezolid

- Linezolid works by inhibiting bacterial protein synthesis and is used for MRSA, VRE, and other Gram-positive infections.

- Linezolid may increase the toxic effects of alcohol and should not be used concurrently.

Daptomycin

- Daptomycin works by inhibiting bacterial DNA and RNA synthesis. It is used for complicated skin and skin structure infections and for *Staphylococcus aureus* blood infections.

- Daptomycin comes as a powder for reconstitution and should not be mixed with dextrose-containing solutions.

Vancomycin

- Vancomycin is an antibiotic with activity against Gram-positive bacteria and is used primarily to treat MRSA infections.

- Vancomycin can be ototoxic and nephrotoxic.

- Vancomycin is usually administered intravenously and must be diluted before use.

Storage of Liquid Antibiotics

- After reconstitution, some antibiotics need to be stored in the refrigerator, whereas others may be kept at room temperature.

- Pharmacy technicians may give patients information about whether a drug must be refrigerated—it is not counseling.

Ophthalmic Antibiotics

- Ophthalmic dosage forms may be used in the ear, but otic dosage forms should never be put in the eye.

- Ophthalmic antibiotics are very expensive because of stringent manufacturing requirements. Technicians often need to know which antibiotics are less expensive in order to advise the prescriber.

Sexually Transmitted Infections

- Most genital-system infections are transmitted by sexual activity.

- Chlamydia, gonorrhea, syphilis, nongonococcal urethritis, and vaginitis can all be treated with antibiotics.

Fungi, Fungal Diseases, and Drug Treatments

- A fungus is a single-celled organism that has similarities to both animal and green plant cells.

- Drugs that fight bacterial infections are generally not effective for fungal infections.

- A fungal infection can range from topical and mild to systemic and severe.

Polyenes

- Polyene antifungals include amphotericin B and nystatin.

- Amphotericin B is injectable and can be toxic to the liver and kidneys. It is reserved for serious fungal infections.

- Nystatin can be used topically and systemically.

Azoles

- Azoles inhibit the formation of the fungal cell wall.

- When azoles are used orally, common side effects include nausea, vomiting, abdominal pain, and diarrhea.

- Drug interactions are a concern when patients are using azoles with other medications.

Echinocandins

- Caspofungin and micafungin are echinocandins that are used to treat patients with an *Aspergillus* or *Candida* infection.

- Echinocandins are associated with hypersensitivity reactions.

Complementary and Alternative Therapies

- Patients may use echinacea and zinc to prevent and treat infections.

DRUG LIST

Ophthalmics
azithromycin (AzaSite)
bacitracin
ciprofloxacin (Ciloxan)
erythromycin (Ilotycin)
gatifloxacin (Zymaxid)
gentamicin (Genoptic, Gentak, Gentasol, Gentopic)
moxifloxacin (Vigamox, Moxeza)
ofloxacin (Ocuflox)
sodium sulfacetamide (Bleph-10)
tobramycin (Tobrex)

Sulfonamides and Nitrofurantoin
nitrofurantoin (Macrobid, Macrodantin)
sulfamethoxazole / trimethoprim (Bactrim, Bactrim DS, Septra, Septra DS)

Penicillins
amoxicillin (Amoxil, Moxatag)
amoxicillin / clavulanate (Augmentin, Augmentin XR)
ampicillin
ampicillin / sulbactam (Unasyn)
dicloxacillin
methicillin
nafcillin
oxacillin
penicillin G (Pfizerpen)
penicillin V potassium
piperacillin / tazobactam (Zosyn)
ticarcillin / clavulanate

Cephalosporins
cefaclor
cefazolin (Ancef, Kefzol)
cefdinir
cefditoren (Spectracef)
cefepime (Maxipime)
cefiderocol (Fetroja)
cefixime (Suprax)
cefotetan
cefotaxime (Claforan)
cefoxitin (Mefoxin)
cefpodoxime
ceftaroline (Teflaro)
ceftazidime (Fortaz, Tazicef)
ceftibuten (Cedax)

ceftobiprole
ceftriaxone (Rocephin)
cefuroxime (Ceftin, Zinacef)
cephalexin (Keflex)

Carbapenems
doripenem (Doribax)
ertapenem (Invanz)
imipenem / cilastatin (Primaxin)
meropenem (Merrem)
meropenem / vaborbactam (Vabormere)

Monobactam
aztreonam (Azactam, Cayston)

Lincosamide
clindamycin (Cleocin)

Macrolides
azithromycin (Zithromax, Z-Pak, Zmax, Zithromax Tri-Pak)
clarithromycin (Biaxin)
erythromycin (EES, EryC, EryPed, Ery-Tab, Erythrocin, Pediazole)

Aminoglycosides
amikacin
gentamicin (Garamycin, Gentak, Gentasol, Gentopic)
tobramycin (TOBI, Tobrex)

Tetracyclines
doxycycline (Adoxa, Doryx, Doxy, Oracea, Vibramycin)
minocycline (Minocin, Solodyn)
tetracycline
tigecycline (Tygacil)

Fluoroquinolones (Quinolones)
ciprofloxacin (Cetraxal, Ciloxan, Cipro, Otiprio)
levofloxacin
moxifloxacin (Avelox, Moxeza, Vigamox)

Miscellaneous Antibiotics
daptomycin (Cubicin)
linezolid (Zyvox)
metronidazole (Flagyl, MetroCream, MetroGel, MetroLotion, Noritate Cream, Nuvessa, Vandazole)
vancomycin (Vancocin)

Agents for Treating STIs

azithromycin (Zithromax)

ceftriaxone (Rocephin)

doxycycline (Doryx, Doxy, Vibramycin)

erythromycin (ERY-C, Ery-Tab, Erythrocin)

metronidazole (Flagyl, MetroCream, MetroGel, MetroLotion, Noritate Cream, Nuvessa, Vandazole)

penicillin G benzathine (Bicillin L-A)

tetracycline

Azoles

butoconazole (Gynazole-1)

clotrimazole (Lotrimin AF, Trivagizole 3)

clotrimazole / betamethasone (Lotrisone)

fluconazole (Diflucan)

itraconazole (Sporanox)

ketoconazole (Nizoral)

miconazole (Desenex, Lotrimin, Micatin, Monistat)

posaconazole (Noxafil)

tioconazole (Vagistat-1)

voriconazole (Vfend)

Echinocandins

caspofungin (Cancidas)

micafungin (Mycamine)

Polyenes

amphotericin B (Abelcet, AmBisome)

amphotericin B liposomal (AmBisome)

amphotericin B lipid complex (Abelcet, Amphotec)

nystatin (Nyamyc, Nystop)

Miscellaneous Antifungals

butenafine (Lotrimin Ultra, Mentax)

ciclopirox (Loprox, Penlac)

griseofulvin (Grifulvin V, Gris-PEG)

terbinafine (Lamisil AT)

Boxed Warnings

amikacin

clindamycin (Cleocin)

ciprofloxacin (Cipro)

flucytosine (Ancobon)

gentamicin (Garamycin, Gentak, Gentasol, Gentopic)

ketoconazole (Nizoral)

itraconazole (Sporanox)

levofloxacin (Levaquin)

metronidazole (Flagyl, MetroCream, MetroGel, MetroLotion, Noritate Cream, Nuvessa, Vandazole)

moxifloxacin (Avelox)

penicillin G benzathine

tobramycin (TOBI, Tobrex)

Medication Guides

ciprofloxacin (Cetraxal, Ciloxan, Cipro, Otiprio)

levofloxacin

moxifloxacin (Avelox, Moxeza, Vigamox)

ofloxacin (Ocuflox)

✓ CHECK YOUR UNDERSTANDING

Take a moment to review what you have learned in this chapter and answer the following questions.

1. It is especially important that a person taking sulfonamides
   a. avoid the sun and drink lots of water.
   b. avoid drinking alcohol.
   c. get sufficient rest and avoid the sun.
   d. take the medication with food.

2. The most common side effect of sulfa drugs is
   a. drowsiness.
   b. rash.
   c. dry mouth.
   d. diarrhea.

3. Penicillin should be taken with
   a. cola.
   b. water.
   c. fruit juice.
   d. milk.

4. Which drug is effective against anthrax?
   a. gentamicin
   b. azithromycin
   c. penicillin
   d. doxycycline

5. Which of the following should the patient avoid taking with dairy?
   a. tetracycline
   b. penicillin
   c. azithromycin
   d. cephalexin

6. Which drugs may be associated with tendon injuries?
   a. metronidazole
   b. levofloxacin
   c. amoxicillin / clavulanate
   d. cephalexin

7. Which drug has a large amount of sugar in the oral liquid dosage form?
   a. cefpodoxime
   b. cefdinir
   c. cefaclor
   d. amoxicillin / clavulanate

8. Clindamycin has a boxed warning for
   a. colitis.
   b. heart disease.
   c. pancreatic cancer.
   d. liver impairment.

9. Which drug is a lipid complex that is less toxic than the older IV form of the drug?
   a. Cefepime
   b. meropenem
   c. Abelcet
   d. gentamicin

10. Which two antifungals come in an IV dosage form?
    a. fluconazole and amphotericin B
    b. fluconazole and griseofulvin
    c. griseofulvin and amphotericin B
    d. clotrimazole and ketoconazole

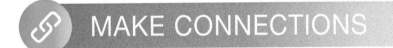 MAKE CONNECTIONS

Take a moment to consider what you have learned in this chapter and respond thoughtfully to the following prompts. Note that some of these activities will require internet access.

1. A parent picks up amoxicillin for their child. It is dosed three times a day. The parent asks whether they need to send the drug to school for the middle-of-the-day dose. Can a technician answer this question? Why or why not?

2. A patient presents a prescription for metronidazole. It is for the patient and their partner. The pharmacist is on the phone, and the patient wants to leave. Can the technician counsel the patient on the use of alcohol and the importance of abstaining from sex for a certain period? Why or why not? How might a technician best handle this situation?

 The online course includes additional review and assessment resources.

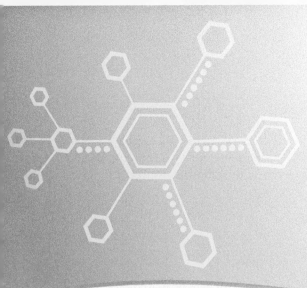

The Immune System, Viral Infections, and Drug Therapy

17

Learning Objectives

1. Explain the differences between bacteria, fungi, and viruses and why the drugs used to treat them must have different mechanisms of action. (Section 17.1)

2. Differentiate antiviral and antiretroviral drugs by their indications, therapeutic effects, side effects, dosages, and administration. (Sections 17.2 and 17.3)

3. Use antiviral and antiretroviral terminology correctly in written and oral communication. (Sections 17.2 and 17.3)

4. Identify drugs used for HIV and understand their synergism. (Section 17.3)

5. Describe the importance of immunization. (Section 17.4)

6. Identify common vaccines and their side effects. (Section 17.4)

ASHP/ACPE Accreditation Standards

To view the *ASHP/ACPE Accreditation Standards* addressed in this chapter, refer to Appendix C.

Viruses are often confused with bacteria and fungi, but they are vastly different entities. Viruses are treated with drugs that have markedly different mechanisms of action from those that treat bacteria or fungi. If left untreated, viral infections may be harmful or even deadly.

Preventive strategies are preferred for viruses and other infectious diseases that are difficult to treat. The administration of vaccines provides prophylaxis for diseases that have a high risk of mortality or cause significant illness. Vaccination, often called *immunization*, is a way to boost the immune system in advance of exposure to disease-causing pathogens that impact public health.

17.1 Viruses and Viral Infections

A **virus** is an infectious agent that is much smaller than a bacterium and differs from a bacterium in many ways. For instance, a virus is not a whole-cell organism. It consists of segments of genetic material (DNA or RNA) surrounded by a capsid, or protein shell. A virus can be thought of as a piece of information with the sole purpose of replicating itself. It cannot, however, replicate on its own; it must attach itself to a host cell in order to replicate. After attaching to a host cell, the virus injects information or instructions into that cell to tell it to make copies of the virus. The host cell's normal function is halted, and the cell releases newly formed viruses. These viruses then invade other cells.

This process continues as the infection spreads. Viruses can infect a spectrum of cells including animal, plant, and bacterial cells. In humans, viruses are among the most common infectious agents and are spread by one of the following routes:

- direct contact
- ingestion of contaminated food or water
- inhalation of airborne particles
- exposure to contaminated body fluids or equipment

An individual virus particle, a **virion**, consists of a core of genetic material—either deoxyribonucleic acid (DNA) or ribonucleic acid (RNA)—and a protein shell, known as a **capsid**, that surrounds and protects the nucleic acid. Depending on the virus, the capsid may be covered with a membrane called an **envelope**, which carries surface proteins that attach to the host cell's receptors. A virus without an envelope covering the capsid is called a **naked virus**.

Stages of Viral Infection

Within the body, viral infection takes place at the cellular level in the following stages:

1. **Attachment:** An individual virus, or virion, attaches to cell receptors.
2. **Penetration:** With the majority of viruses, the virion penetrates the cell as the cell membrane indents and closes around it in a process called *endocytosis*. The virion escapes into the cytoplasm of the cell.
3. **Uncoating:** The virion sheds its capsid and presents its DNA or RNA to the cell nucleus.
4. **Replication and Assembly:** The virion's DNA or RNA converts the host cell's nuclear activity to viral activity, causing the cell to rapidly produce new viral particles. (The energy of the host cell is used to infect the cell and make more viruses.)
5. **Release:** The duplicated viruses are released from the host cell.

When a virus's DNA or RNA takes over host-cell nuclear activity, it synthesizes viral nucleic acid and protein, which leads to the production of more virus particles. The infected host cell may become so damaged that it disintegrates, releasing bursts of mature virions. If the host cell is not destroyed, it releases virions slowly. If the original virion was is not a naked virus, each newly created virion acquires its envelope from the nuclear or cell membrane of the host during the release process. See Figure 17.1 for an illustration of this process. All virus-infected cells have some cellular characteristics that differ from those of uninfected cells. These differences provide opportunities for medications to target and block viral division with medications without affecting normal cells.

Significant Viral Infections

Influenza, hepatitis B, and human immunodeficiency virus (HIV) infections are common and significant illnesses caused by viral infections. **Influenza** (commonly referred to as *the flu*) is caused by the influenza virus. Its symptoms are more severe than those of the common cold and include a rapid onset of malaise (vague discomfort and tiredness), myalgia (muscle pain), headache, chills, and fever. Patients with

FIGURE 17.1 Stages of Viral Infection

The following figure describes the life cycle of a virus and how it causes an infection.

LIFE CYCLE OF VIRUSES

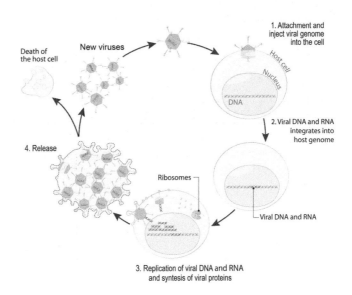

shortness of breath, wheezing, purulent (consisting of pus) or bloody sputum, fever persisting for more than seven days, or severe muscle pain should be advised to seek medical attention. Patients at high risk for complications secondary to influenza include adults aged 65 and older; patients with cardiovascular disease, renal disease, diabetes, or respiratory conditions such as asthma; and **immunocompromised** patients, or those individuals who have a deficient immune system response. Immunocompromised patients include patients with HIV or who have recently received organ or tissue transplants. Annual vaccinations for these patient populations are recommended.

Hepatitis, an inflammation of the liver, is a viral infection that has various types (referred to as *A* through *G*). Hepatitis can range from a very benign disease to a serious illness leading to death. Although hepatitis is discussed in Chapter 12, some of the drugs presented in this chapter are also used to treat hepatitis B.

Advancements in HIV treatments have changed the trajectory for people living with HIV or AIDS. In the past, an HIV diagnosis usually indicated an early death, but today, with the proper medications and adherence to therapies, HIV is viewed as a chronic disease. Adherence to a medication regimen is a critical factor in treatment success. This can be challenging for patients because most regimens include at least three medications, and they can have a complicated dosing schedule. While manufacturers have combined some of these drugs into a single pill, counseling and monitoring for patient adherence are important services a pharmacy team can deliver. Medications to treat HIV have many drug interactions, so it is important that the pharmacy team monitor and check for interactions.

Classification of Viral Infections

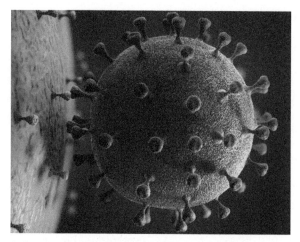

A virus surrounds a cell. A virus does not have all the components of a cell and requires the metabolic and genetic resources of a living cell to replicate itself.

Viral infections are classified in several ways. One classification is based on the duration, or length of time, the viral particles have been in a patient's body and the severity of the symptoms or illness they have caused. Another classification measures the extent of the infection within the body or the parts of the body that are affected. Viral infections can also be classified by the virions' size and shape, genetic makeup (DNA or RNA), host, or induced pathogenic characteristics.

Viral Duration and Severity

Within the classification of viral duration and severity, there are three categories: acute, chronic, and slow. An **acute viral infection** quickly resolves and leaves no latent infection. Examples include the common cold, influenza, and various other respiratory tract viruses. A **chronic viral infection** has a protracted (lengthy) course with long periods of remission interspersed with reappearance; a herpesvirus infection is an example. A **slow viral infection** maintains a progressive course over months or years, causing cumulative damage to body tissues, ultimately ending in the host patient's death. HIV is an example of a slow viral infection.

Extent of Viral Infection

When healthcare providers evaluate the extent of a viral infection, they must determine whether the infection is local or generalized. A **local viral infection** affects tissues of a single system, such as the respiratory tract, the skin, or an eye. A **generalized viral infection** has spread or is spreading to other tissues by way of the bloodstream or the tissues of the central nervous system (CNS).

Latent Viruses

Even after the symptoms of the acute stage of an infection have ceased, it is possible for a virus to lie dormant and undetectable in a cell; this is known as **latency**. Later, under certain conditions and possibly years after the initial breakout or transmission of infection, the virus may reproduce and again behave as an infectious agent, causing cell damage. Herpesviruses and HIV can both behave in this manner. Some viruses of this kind can transform normal cells into cancer cells.

Virus and Host-Cell Interaction

A virus can have several damaging effects on a host cell. It can alter the structure of the host cell; incorporate itself into the genetic material of the host cell, thus becoming part of its nucleic acid pool; divide when the host cell divides; or kill the host cell.

Most viruses possess several antigens on their surfaces that stimulate host cells to produce immunoglobulins. An **immunoglobulin** is a type of antibody that is produced mainly by white blood cells (WBCs) called *B lymphocytes*. An immunoglobulin that matches a viral protein may prevent the virus from attaching to a cell receptor and may destroy the virus. T lymphocytes may also become sensitive to viral antigens, at which time they release chemicals to kill the virus or stimulate other cells, such as macrophages, to destroy the virus or virus-infected cells.

A significant response of some virus-infected cells is the production of interferons, a type of protein. An **interferon** exhibits antiviral activities that are host specific but not virus specific. Interferons induce the production of hundreds of other proteins. Some of these proteins disrupt various stages of viral replication, including the synthesis of viral RNA. Other proteins help prevent viral spread to neighboring uninfected cells. Although interferons are produced in response to viral infection, they are encoded in the host cell's DNA. Therefore, interferons are host specific that is, interferon molecules made by human cells work only in human cells.

17.2 Antiviral Agents (Nonretroviral)

Bacterial infections are easier to treat with medication than are viral infections. Because antibiotics often disrupt a cellular process unique to the invading bacterial strain, they can be administered without harming the patient. In contrast, viruses use the host's own cellular processes to function and replicate themselves. As a result, medications that block the life cycle of a virus are often toxic to the patient, much more so than antibiotics and in much the same way as chemotherapy agents for cancer. An **antiviral drug** is one that has been formulated to seek out a virus and prevent its replication in body fluids or in host cells without interfering with normal cell function. Table 17.1 presents an overview of the most commonly used antiviral agents. HIV and antiretroviral drugs are discussed later in this chapter.

Therapeutic Uses of Antiviral Agents

Antiviral agents are used to treat the following viral infections:

- herpesvirus infections
    - ~ herpes simplex virus type 1 (HSV-1)
    - ~ herpes simplex virus type 2 (HSV-2)
    - ~ varicella zoster (chicken pox and shingles)
    - ~ cytomegalovirus (human herpesvirus type 5)
- influenza
- respiratory syncytial virus (RSV)

TABLE 17.1 Commonly Used Antiviral Agents

Generic (Brand)	Pronunciation	Dosage Form	Common Dosage	Dispensing Status
Antiherpes Agents				
acyclovir (Avaclyr, Sitavig, Zovirax)	ay-SYE-kloe-veer	buccal tablet, capsule, injection, ointment, ophthalmic ointment, oral suspension, tablet, topical cream	oral herpes (cold sores): Buccal: 50 mg single dose Chicken pox (pediatric): PO (pediatric): ≥2 years and ≤40 kg: 20 mg/kg 4 times a day PO (pediatric): >40 kg: 800 mg 4 times a day Topical: varies by age, product, and indication	Rx

continues

TABLE 17.1 Commonly Used Antiviral Agents—*Continued*

Generic (Brand)	Pronunciation	Dosage Form	Common Dosage	Dispensing Status
acyclovir (Avaclyr, Sitavig, Zovirax)	ay-SYE-kloe-veer	buccal tablet, capsule, injection, ointment, ophthalmic ointment, oral suspension, tablet, topical cream	Genital herpes (acute): IV: 5 mg/kg 3 times a day for 5–7 days, followed with oral therapy for a minimum of 10 days total treatment PO: 200 mg 5 times a day or 400 mg 3 times a day for 7–10 days Genital herpes (chronic suppression): PO: 400 mg 2 times a day for 1 year Herpes zoster (shingles) and chicken pox (adult): IV: 10 mg/kg 3 times a day for 7–10 days PO: 800 mg 5 times a day for 7–10 days	Rx
famciclovir (Famvir)	fam-SYE-kloe-veer	tablet	Genital herpes (acute): 1,000 mg 2 times a day for 1 day Genital herpes (chronic suppression): 250 mg 2 times a day for 1 year Herpes labialis (cold sores): 1,500 mg single dose Herpes zoster (shingles): 500 mg every 8 hr for 7 days	Rx
valacyclovir (Valtrex)	val-ay-SYE-kloe-veer	tablet	Genital herpes (acute): 1 g 2 times a day for 10 days Genital herpes (chronic suppression): 1 g a day Herpes labialis (cold sores): 2 g every 12 hr for 1 day Herpes zoster (shingles): 1 g 3 times a day for 7 days	Rx
valganciclovir (Valcyte)	val-gan-SYE-kloh-veer	oral solution, tablet	Cytomegalovirus treatment: 900 mg 2 times a day for 21 days, then 900 mg a day for maintenance Cytomegalovirus prophylaxis posttransplant: 900 mg a day	Rx
Anti-Influenza Agents				
baloxavir marboxil (Xofluza)	ba-LOX-a-veer mar-BOX-el	tablet	40–80 kg: 40 mg single dose >80 kg: 80 mg single dose	Rx
oseltamivir (Tamiflu)	oh-sel-TAM-i-veer	capsule, oral suspension	PO (adult): 75 mg 2 times a day for 5 days PO (pediatric): varies by age and weight of patient	Rx
peramivir (Rapivab)	per-RAM-i-veer	injection	12 mg/kg: up to 600 mg single dose	Rx
zanamivir (Relenza)	zan-AM-e-veer	powder for inhalation	10 mg (2 inhalations) 2 times a day	Rx
Other Antiviral Agents				
ribavirin (Virazole)	rye-ba-VYE-rin	capsule, oral solution, powder for inhalation, tablet	RSV: continuous aerosolization: 6 g administered over 12 to 18 hr per day for 3 to 7 days Intermittent aerosolization: 2 g over 2 hr 3 times a day for 3 to 7 days	Rx
palivizumab (Synagis)	pah-li-VIZ-yoo-mab	injection	100 mg/mL	Rx

Antiherpes Agents

Although there are more than 100 various strains of herpesvirus, only a small proportion is regularly found in humans. The most common herpesvirus infections in humans are caused by HSV-1, HSV-2, and varicella-zoster virus. HSV-1 is associated with oral herpes (and sometimes genital herpes). **Oral herpes**, also known as *cold sores* or *fever blisters*, are painful, fluid-filled lesions most commonly located around the mouth, chin, and upper lip. HSV-2 is associated with genital herpes. **Genital herpes** may appear as lesions that cause a burning sensation below the waist, most commonly around the genitals or rectum. Varicella-zoster virus causes chicken pox (varicella) and shingles (herpes zoster). Antiviral agents for herpesvirus are commonly used to prevent and treat outbreaks.

Acyclovir

Acyclovir (Avaclyr, Sitavig, Zovirax) acts by interfering with viral DNA synthesis. It is used to treat genital herpes in certain patients, herpes zoster (shingles), and varicella (chicken pox). The intravenous (IV) form is considered the drug of choice for herpes encephalitis. The dosage regimen changes depending on the type of infection being treated and the patient's status. Both short- and long-term side effects have been reported. Acyclovir can be used for suppression of herpes in patients who have had multiple outbreaks.

Dosage Forms and Administration Acyclovir is available in buccal form, capsule, injection, ointment, opthalmic ointment, oral suspension, tablet form, and topical cream. The injection is for IV administration only and should be administered over at least 1 hour. Dosages vary based on indication.

Safety Alert

Acyclovir may be confused with famciclovir, ganciclovir, Retrovir, valacyclovir, or valganciclovir. Dosing and indications may help distinguish between these medications.

Side Effects The most common side effects include nausea, vomiting, diarrhea, and malaise. Acyclovir may also cause CNS side effects such as confusion, hallucinations, and seizures; higher acyclovir doses and administration to patients with renal failure increase the risk of these CNS side effects.

Contraindications Acyclovir is contraindicated in patients with a hypersensitivity to valacyclovir.

Cautions and Considerations Acyclovir should be used with caution in older adults due to its CNS side effects. Renal failure has been reported with acyclovir use. Dehydration, preexisting renal disease, and nephrotoxic drugs increase risk. Patients should be adequately hydrated when taking acyclovir.

Drug Interactions Acyclovir use may diminish the therapeutic effect of varicella and herpes zoster vaccines. Foscarnet may enhance the nephrotoxic effect of acyclovir.

Famciclovir

Famciclovir (Famvir) is used to manage acute herpes zoster (shingles), to treat recurrent herpes simplex in immunocompromised patients, and to treat genital herpes. The primary side effects are nausea and headache. The advantage of this drug is that it can be dosed less frequently than acyclovir. It is a **prodrug**, which is a compound that must be metabolized in the body to form an active pharmacologic agent. The active compound after the biotransformation of famciclovir is penciclovir.

Dosage Forms and Administration Famciclovir is available in tablet form.

Side Effects Famciclovir use is associated with headache, nausea, diarrhea, and fatigue.

Contraindications Famciclovir is a prodrug (a compound that is chemically converted to another active compound after administration) of penciclovir; therefore, penciclovir allergy contraindicates famciclovir use.

Cautions and Considerations Famciclovir contains milk products and should be used prudently by patients with milk-product sensitivities.

Drug Interactions Famciclovir may diminish the therapeutic effect of varicella and herpes zoster vaccines.

Valacyclovir

Valacyclovir (Valtrex) is used to treat herpes zoster in immunocompetent adults and to treat genital herpes. It shortens the duration of postherpetic neuralgia (burning pain that continues after a shingles rash has resolved). It is better absorbed than acyclovir, and once absorbed, it is converted to acyclovir in the liver and digestive tract. The end result is higher levels of acyclovir in the blood. Prescriptions for valacyclovir generally are for shorter periods and require fewer pills per day than those for acyclovir.

Dosage Forms and Administration Valacyclovir is available as a tablet and should be taken with plenty of water and within 48 hours of the onset of the zoster rash.

Side Effects Valacyclovir has CNS side effects, such as confusion, hallucinations, and seizures. Other side effects include nausea, vomiting, diarrhea, and constipation.

Contraindications Valacyclovir is a prodrug for acyclovir and should not be used in patients with a hypersensitivity to acyclovir.

Cautions and Considerations Valacyclovir should be used with caution in older adults due to its CNS side effects. Caution should be used in patients with renal impairment, the elderly, and/or those receiving nephrotoxic agents since acute renal failure may occur.

Work Wise

Gancilcvoir and valganciclovir are considered hazardous drugs so it is important to follow handling precautions as outlined in the pharmacy's workplace policies and procedures.

Drug Interactions Foscarnet may enhance the nephrotoxic effects of valacyclovir, and the combination should be avoided. Valacyclovir use may diminish the therapeutic effect of varicella and herpes zoster vaccines.

Valganciclovir

Valganciclovir (Valcyte) is an oral prodrug for **ganciclovir (Vitrasert)**. When working with valganciclovir, it is important to follow precautions appropriate for chemotherapy drugs (see Chapter 20).

Dosage Forms and Administration Valganciclovir is available as a tablet and oral solution. It should be taken with food. Broken or crushed tablets must not be handled. As with hazardous drugs, damaged tablets should be disposed of in special containers. Valganciclovir has a boxed warning regarding its mutagenic properties. Therefore, pregnant patients and pharmacy staff should not handle this drug.

Safety Alert

Valganciclovir has boxed warnings regarding hematolologic toxicity, impairment of fertility, fetal toxicity, and mutagenic properties.

Side Effects Side effects associated with valganciclovir include hypertension, headache, insomnia, diarrhea, vomiting, tremors, fever, and increased serum creatinine.

Contraindications Valganciclovir is a prodrug for ganciclovir and should not be used in patients with a hypersensitivity to ganciclovir.

Cautions and Considerations Valganciclovir has two boxed warnings. The first concerns reports of severe leukopenia, neutropenia, anemia, thrombocytopenia, pancytopenia, bone marrow suppression, and aplastic anemia. Patients with certain low levels of neutrophils, platelets, or hemoglobin should not use valganciclovir. Immunosuppressed patients also should not use valganciclovir.

The other boxed warning concerns valgancyclovir's effects on reproduction. Valganciclovir may temporarily or permanently impair fertility in patients of any gender. It is also associated with birth defects and cancer. Individuals who may become pregnant should use effective contraception during and for 30 days after valganciclovir treatment. Patients who have the ability to produce sperm should use barrier contraception during treatment and for 90 days after therapy. Pregnant pharmacy technicians should avoid directly handling valganciclovir.

Drug Interactions Valganciclovir may enhance the toxic effects of the antibiotic imipenem, including the risk of seizure. It may also enhance the toxic effects of reverse transcriptase inhibitors (with the exception of stavudine).

Anti-Influenza Agents

Influenza, or flu, is a contagious viral infection of the respiratory system. There are different types of influenza, with type A and type B being the most common. Type A and type B cause seasonal flu, which affects up to 20% of Americans annually. Common symptoms include fever, fatigue, aches, and chills. For most people, influenza infections self-resolve. However, in others, influenza infections can be deadly. Young children, older adults, residents of nursing homes, pregnant individuals, and individuals with chronic illness are all at an increased risk for developing complications of influenza. Anti-influenza agents are used to prevent or treat influenza in high-risk patients.

Antiviral treatments for influenza generally work best if started within 48 hours of symptom onset. These medications can reduce fever and flu symptoms. Because influenza viruses change over time, it is important for prescribers to review information on drug susceptibility patterns for the circulating virus strains prior to prescribing an anti-influenza medication.

Baloxavir Marboxil

Baloxavir marboxil (Xofluza) works differently than oseltamivir, zanamivir, and peramivir. Baloxavir marboxil prevents flu virus replication by inhibiting polymerase acidic endonuclease, which is needed for viral gene transcription. Baloxavir is indicated for the treatment of influenza type A or B in people 12 years of age or older.

Dosage Forms and Administration Baloxavir marboxil is taken as a single-dose tablet by mouth, and it must be started within 48 hours of symptom onset.

Side Effects Baloxavir marboxil may cause diarrhea, bronchitis, nasopharyngitis, headache, and nausea.

Contraindications Baloxavir marboxil does not have contraindications.

Cautions and Considerations Influenza viruses change over time, so it is important for prescribers to review information on drug susceptibility patterns for the circulating virus strains prior to prescribing. Hypersensitivity reactions like anaphylaxis, angioedema, erythema, and urticaria (hives) have been reported.

Drug Interactions Live influenza vaccine effectiveness decreases with concomitant baloxavir marboxil use.

Oseltamivir

Safety Alert

Tamiflu, the brand name of oseltamivir, may be confused with FluMist, the nasal influenza vaccine.

Oseltamivir (Tamiflu) is an inhibitor of the enzyme neuramindase, which helps stop the enzyme from releasing viral particles into the plasma of infected cells. Oseltamivir is indicated for the treatment or prevention of influenza type A and type B. Therapy must be initiated within 48 hours of symptom onset. Food generally improves tolerance, so it is best to take oseltamivir orally at breakfast and dinner. Oseltamivir has been shown to decrease the duration of the flu by up to three days.

Dosage Forms and Administration Oseltamivir is used for the treatment and prophylaxis of influenza. Oseltamivir is ideally administered within 48 hours of symptom onset. If the pharmacy is out of stock of this medication, the technician should help the patient find another pharmacy that has stock.

Side Effects Oseltamivir may cause vomiting, nausea, abdominal pain, and diarrhea. Less common side effects include nosebleeds and eye infections.

Contraindications Oseltamivir does not have contraindications.

Cautions and Considerations Oseltamivir should be used cautiously in patients with cardiovascular disease, hepatic impairment, or renal impairment.

Some oseltamivir formulations contain benzyl alcohol, which has been associated with toxic reactions (potentially fatal) in neonates. Use of these formulations should be avoided in the neonatal population.

The oral suspension contains sorbitol, which may cause diarrhea.

Drug Interactions Live influenza vaccine effectiveness decreases with concomitant oseltamivir use.

Peramivir

Peramivir (Rapivab), which has an IV dosage form, is an inhibitor of the enzyme neuraminidase, which helps stop the enzyme from releasing viral particles into the plasma of infected cells. It is indicated for the treatment of acute uncomplicated influenza type A and type B (not requiring hospitalization) in patients 18 years of age or older who have been symptomatic for no more than two days. Most often, peramivir is used in patients unable to tolerate oral anti-influenza agents.

Dosage Forms and Administration Peramivir is available as an IV infusion.

Side Effects Peramivir may cause diarrhea.

Contraindications Peramivir does not have contraindications.

Cautions and Considerations Peramivir may increase the risk of serious skin reactions, including erythema multiforme and Stevens-Johnson syndrome. Patients with influenza should be monitored for these and for signs of abnormal behavior, since they may be at increased risk of hallucinations and delirium early in their illness.

Drug Interactions Live influenza vaccine effectiveness decreases with concomitant peramivir use.

Zanamivir

Zanamivir (Relenza) is indicated for the treatment and prophylaxis of influenza type A and type B. Therapy with zanamivir must be initiated within 48 hours of symptom onset. If the pharmacy is out of stock of this medication, the technician should help the patient find another pharmacy that has stock.

Dosage Forms and Administration Zanamivir is inhaled using a breath-activated plastic device called a *disk inhaler*. The recommended dosage is 10 mg (two inhalations) every 12 hours. If the patient is also using a bronchodilator, they should be instructed to use the bronchodilator immediately prior to the administration of zanamivir. Zanamivir is sometimes prescribed as a prophylactic, especially in nursing homes and other group settings.

Side Effects Headache, throat or tonsil discomfort, and cough are side effects of zanamivir use.

Contraindications Zanamivir is contraindicated in patients with a hypersensitivity to milk protein.

Cautions and Considerations Zanamivir contains milk products and should be used prudently by patients with milk-product sensitivities.

Drug Interactions Live influenza vaccine effectiveness decreases with concomitant zanamivir use.

Other Antiviral Agents

RSV, or respiratory syncytial virus, causes acute respiratory illness. RSV is the most common cause of lower respiratory tract infections in infants. Pediatric patients with RSV often present with difficulty breathing, bronchitis, or pneumonia. Adults with RSV have similar symptoms. While other therapies, such as bronchodilators and corticosteroids, are traditionally used first, the antiviral agents palivizumab and ribavirin may also be effective.

Palivizumab

Palivizumab (Synagis) is a monoclonal antibody used to prevent serious lung infections in children and babies caused by RSV. It is used in high risk babies and children born prematurely or who have other medical problems like congenital heart issues.

Dosage Forms and Administration Palivizumab is administered by IM injection. The first injection is given prior to the beginning of RSV season. Monthly doses are then administered during the RSV season.

Side Effects The most common side effects of palivizumab are fever and rash.

Contraindications Palivizumab does not have contraindications.

Cautions and Considerations Palivizumab has caused anaphylactic and hypersensitivity reactions. Like other IM injections, caution should be used in administering the medication to patients with thrombocytopenia other coagulation disorders. Palivizumab may interfere with some immunological-based RSV diagnostic tests.

Drug Interactions Palivizumab has no known drug interactions.

Ribavirin

Ribavirin (Virazole) is useful in treating viral infections and may be useful in treating patients with RSV.

Dosage Forms and Administration Ribavirin comes in multiple dosage forms. For RSV, it typically has an inhaled dosage form, but it can be used orally for other indications. Ribavirin is absorbed systemically from the respiratory tract following inhalation. Absorption of the inhaled form depends on respiratory factors and the drug delivery system.

Side Effects Ribavirin has the serious side effect of hemolytic anemia, which may worsen underlying cardiac disease and lead to fatal and nonfatal heart attacks. Patients with heart disease should avoid using ribavirin. The most common side effects are fatigue, headache, and insomnia. Nausea and anorexia can also occur.

Contraindications Ribavirin is contraindicated in individuals who are pregnant, individuals whose partners are pregnant, patients with hemoglobinopathies, patients with autoimmune hepatitis, and patients who are also taking didanosine.

Safety Alert

Ribavirin carries boxed warnings for teratogenic and embryocidal effects, worsening of cardiac disease due to increased risk of hemolytic anemia, use as monotherapy for hepatitis C treatment, and sudden respiratory deterioration in pediatric patients.

Cautions and Considerations Ribavirin has several boxed warnings. When used orally, ribavirin may cause hemolytic anemia, which may worsen underlying cardiac disease. When taken for hepatitis C, ribavirin should not be used as monotherapy. In pediatric patients, ribavirin use may result in sudden respiratory deterioration.

Another boxed warning exists for pregnant individuals because of ribavirin's significant teratogenic and embryocidal effects. Its use should be avoided in individuals who are pregnant. Individuals who may become pregnant and whose partners are undergoing ribavirin therapy should use two contraceptive methods. Pregnant pharmacy technicians should avoid directly handling ribavirin.

Lastly, the inhaled product also carries a boxed warning. Caution with the inhalation product should be exercised in patients on mechanical ventilation due to a risk that ribavirin could precipitate in the respiratory equipment.

Drug Interactions Ribavirin may increase serum concentrations of azathioprine. Ribavirin may enhance the toxic effects of didanosine, so the combination should be avoided. Live influenza vaccine effectiveness decreases with concomitant ribavirin use.

17.3 HIV/AIDS and Antiretroviral Agents

Safety Alert

One of the biggest challenges in treating HIV is patient difficulty adhering to the drug regimen due to problematic side effects and complex dosing.

A **retrovirus** is a virus that inserts genetic information from its RNA into host cells' DNA. Retroviruses use an enzyme called **reverse transcriptase** to convert their RNA into DNA. They then incorporate that DNA into host cells' DNA, which allows these viruses to replicate.

Human immunodeficiency virus (HIV) is a retrovirus transmitted in body fluids that causes acquired immunodeficiency syndrome (AIDS) by attacking T lymphocytes. There are two main types of the HIV virus, HIV-1 and HIV-2. HIV-1 is the most common type and is found all over the world. HIV-1 and HIV-2 are both retroviruses and have similar effects on the body, but they are genetically different. This means that not all treatments will be effective for both types. HIV attaches to receptors on the surface of a **CD4 cell** (CD4 cells are important infection-fighting cells in the body's immune response). HIV then fuses with the CD4 cell membrane, which allows HIV to enter the host cell. Once inside the CD4 host cell, HIV releases and uses reverse transcriptase to convert its genetic material from RNA to DNA. HIV also releases **integrase**, an enzyme that integrates that DNA into the DNA of the host CD4 cell. In other words, HIV genetic material combines with the host cell's genetic material and is able to replicate along with the host cell. Newly formed immature HIV pushes out of the host CD4 cell and releases protease, an enzyme that promotes the assembly of viral parts into intact HIV and allows HIV virions to be infectious. Patients with advanced and severe forms of HIV develop **acquired immunodeficiency syndrome (AIDS)**. In patients with AIDS, even simple infections that normally would not cause any significant problems can become deadly because of the destruction of the CD4 cells from the HIV infection.

Work Wise

Many ineffective herbal products and remedies are promoted as "miracle cures" and sold to patients with HIV and AIDS. These products do not cure these diseases. Technicians should encourage patients to talk with their healthcare practitioners about herbal products they want to take.

An **antiretroviral** is a drug that limits the progression of HIV or other retrovirus infections. The cadre of antiretroviral drugs used against HIV and AIDS saves lives, but these agents have numerous severe side effects and drug interactions, making them difficult medications to tolerate. Various antiretrovirals can be combined into therapy called a **cocktail** to take advantage of the effects of synergistic drug therapy. By attacking the viral replication process in multiple stages, a cocktail can destroy more of the virus.

Although antiretrovirals can reduce the number of viruses in the body to almost undetectable levels, patients must continue to take the drugs throughout their life to prevent progression of the illness and death. They must follow medication instructions carefully to receive optimal effect.

The classes of drugs used to treat HIV include nucleoside reverse transcriptase inhibitors (NRTIs), nonnucleoside reverse transcriptase inhibitors (NNRTIs), protease inhibitors (PIs), integrase strand transfer inhibitors (INSTIs), fusion inhibitors, CCR5 antagonists, post-attachment inhibitors (PAIs), and pharmacokinetic enhancers. Figure 17.2 identifies where within the HIV life cycle these agents take effect.

A patient with HIV generally takes a combination of three or more antiviral drugs from two different classes, such as two NRTIs plus an INSTI, two NRTIs plus an NNRTI, or two NRRTs plus a PI with a pharmacokinetic enhancer. Some of these cocktails are available packaged into a single tablet; among these are Atripla, Biktarvy, Dovato, Stribild, Triumeq, and Truvada. Patients new to treatment may start with one of these combination pills. The selection of the initial regimen is individualized and based on efficacy, potential for pregnancy, pill burden (number of tablets and other dosage forms a patient takes each day), drug-drug interaction potential, cost, comorbid conditions, and resistance testing. Over time, the virus develops resistance to various antiviral agents, so patients change drug treatments periodically. Medication adherence is important in helping prevent treatment resistance.

FIGURE 17.2 Drugs Treatments Impacting the HIV Life Cycle

Drugs for the treatment of HIV work at various phases of the HIV life cycle.

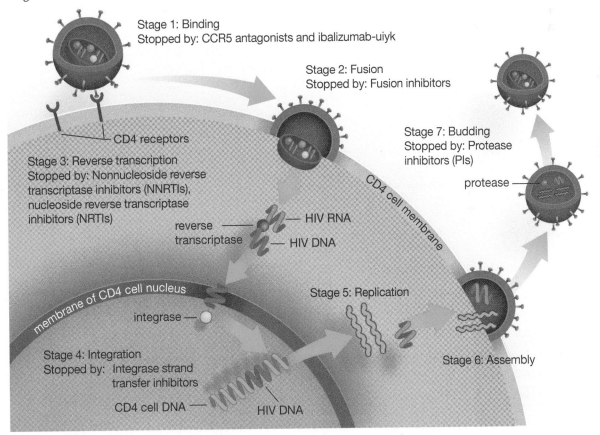

Nucleoside Reverse Transcriptase Inhibitors

A **nucleoside reverse transcriptase inhibitor (NRTI)** works by inhibiting reverse transcriptase. This action prevents the formation of a DNA copy of viral RNA, thus preventing the virus from multiplying or hiding itself within a host cell. Figure 17.2 (see above), illustrated where NRTIs work in the HIV life cycle. Table 17.2 provides

TABLE 17.2 Commonly Used Antiretroviral Agents

Generic (Brand)	Pronunciation	Dosage Form	Common Dosage	Dispensing Status
Nucleoside Reverse Transcriptase Inhibitors (NRTIs)				
abacavir (Ziagen)	a-BAK-a-veer	oral solution, tablet	600 mg a day	Rx
abacavir / lamivudine (Epzicom)	a-BAK-a-veer la-MIV-ue-deen	tablet	600 mg/300 mg a day	Rx
abacavir / lamivudine / zidovudine (Trizivir)	a-BAK-a-vir la-MIV-ue-deen zye-DOE-vyoo-deen	tablet	300 mg/150 mg/300 mg a day	Rx
efavirenz / emtricitabine / tenofovir (Atripla)	e-fa-VEER-ens em-trye-SYE-ta-bean ten-OE-foe-veer	tablet	600 mg/200 mg/300 mg a day	Rx
emtricitabine (Emtriva)	em-trye-SYE-ta-bean	capsule, oral solution	PO (capsule): 200 mg a day PO (solution): 240 mg a day	Rx
emtricitabine / tenofovir disoproxil fumarate (Truvada)	em-trye-SYE-ta-bean ten-OE-foe-veer dye-soe-PROX-il FUE-ma-rate	tablet	200 mg/300 mg a day	Rx
emtricitabine / tenofovir alafenamide (Descovy)	te-NO-fo-veer al-a-FEN-a-mide	tablet	200 mg/25 mg a day	Rx
emtricitabine / tenofovir alafenamide (Descovy)	te-NO-fo-veer al-a-FEN-a-mide	tablet	200 mg/25 mg a day	Rx
lamivudine (Epivir)	la-MIV-yoo-deen	oral solution, tablet	100 mg a day	Rx
lamivudine / zidovudine (Combivir)	la-MIV-yoo-deen zye-DOE-vue-deen	tablet	150 mg/300 mg 2 times a day	Rx
stavudine (Zerit)	STAV-yoo-deen	capsule, powder for oral solution	30–40 mg every 12 hr	Rx
tenofovir disoproxil fumarate (Viread)	te-NO-fo-veer dye-soe-PROX-il FUE-ma-rate	oral powder, tablet	300 mg a day	Rx
zidovudine (Retrovir)	zye-DOE-vyoo-deen	capsule, injection, syrup, tablet	PO: 600 mg a day in divided doses IV: 1 mg/kg/dose infused over 1 hr, 5–6 times a day	Rx
Nonnucleoside Reverse Transcriptase Inhibitors (NNRTIs)				
delavirdine (Rescriptor)	de-la-VIR-deen	tablet	400 mg 3 times a day	Rx
doravirine (Pifeltro)	dor-a-VIR-een	tablet	100 mg 1 time a day	Rx
efavirenz (Sustiva)	e-fa-VEER-ens	capsule, tablet	600 mg once a day	Rx
etravirine (Intelence)	e-tra-VEER-een	tablet	200 mg 2 times a day	Rx
Nonnucleoside Reverse Transcriptase Inhibitors (NNRTIs)				
nevirapine (Viramune, Viramune XR)	ne-VYE-ra-peen	oral suspension, tablet	200 mg 1–2 times a day; extended-release: 400 mg 1 time a day	Rx

continues

TABLE 17.2 Commonly Used Antiretroviral Agents—*Continued*

Generic (Brand)	Pronunciation	Dosage Form	Common Dosage	Dispensing Status
rilpivirine (Edurant)	ril-pi-VIR-een	tablet	25 mg 1 time a day	Rx
Protease Inhibitors (PIs)				
atazanavir (Reyataz)	at-a-ZAN-a-veer	capsule, oral packet (powder)	300 mg 1 time a day (must be taken with ritonavir)	Rx
darunavir (Prezista)	da-ROON-a-veer	oral suspension, tablet	600–800 mg 2 times a day (must be taken with ritonavir)	Rx
fosamprenavir (Lexiva)	FOS-am-pren-a-veer	oral suspension, tablet	700–1,400 mg 2 times a day (must be taken with ritonavir)	Rx
lopinavir / ritonavir (Kaletra)	low-PIN-a-veer rye-TON-a-veer	oral solution, tablet	400 mg/100 mg 2 times a day	Rx
nelfinavir (Viracept)	nel-FIN-a-veer	tablet	1,250 mg 2 times a day or 750 mg 3 times a day	Rx
ritonavir (Norvir)	rye-TON-a-veer	capsule, oral solution, tablet	up to 600 mg 2 times a day	Rx
tipranavir (Aptivus)	tip-RAN-a-veer	capsule, oral solution	500 mg 2 times a day (must be taken with ritonavir)	Rx
Fusion Inhibitor				
enfuvirtide (Fuzeon)	en-FOO-vir-tide	injection	SC: 90 mg 2 times a day	Rx
Post-Attachment Inhibitor				
ibalizumab (Trogarzo)	eye-ba-LIZ-ue-mab	IV infusion	2,000 mg 1 time, then 800 mg every 2 weeks	Rx
CCR5 Antagonist				
maraviroc (Selzentry)	ma-RAV-i-rok	oral solution, tablet	150 mg–600 mg 2 times a day	Rx
Integrase Strand Transfer Inhibitors				
bictegravir / emtricitabine / tenofovir alafenamide (Biktarvy)	bik-TEG-ra-vir/em-trye-SYE-ta-bean/te-NO-fo-veer/al-a-FEN-a-mide	tablet	50 mg/200 mg/25 mg 1 time a day	Rx
dolutegravir (Tivicay)	doe-loo-TEG-ra-veer	tablet	50 mg 1–2 times a day	Rx
raltegravir (Isentress)	ral-TEG-ra-veer	oral suspension, tablet	400 mg 2 times a day	Rx

an overview of the NRTIs in current use. Common side effects of NRTIs include GI distress (nausea, diarrhea, abdominal pain), which usually improves within the first two weeks of therapy. More permanent side effects include lactic acidosis with hepatic steatosis (degeneration of the liver). NRTIs contain boxed warnings for liver problems.

The NRTIs commonly used today can be taken with or without food and generally do not interfere with other drugs. These agents are usually administered in two to three doses per day.

Abacavir

Abacavir (Ziagen) is an NRTI and one of the few HIV drugs that penetrate the CNS. This characteristic makes abacavir an invaluable therapeutic weapon because HIV itself is able to penetrate and proliferate within the CNS.

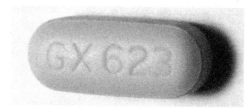

Abacavir has become a key medication in the treatment of HIV because it is able to penetrate the barriers to the CNS.

Dosage Forms and Administration Abacavir is available as a tablet and oral solution. It is usually dosed 300 mg twice a day or 600 mg once a day. Abacavir is also a component of several combination products. Prior to starting treatment with abacavir, patients should be screened for the genetic allele HLA-B*5701.

Side Effects These side effects include rash, nausea, abdominal pain, malaise, or respiratory issues. Patients must be instructed to contact their prescriber if any of these symptoms occur, at which point the prescriber usually stops the medication.

Contraindications Hypersensitivity to a drug contraindicates its use.

Cautions and Considerations The use of alcohol increases abacavir's toxicity, so patients must be instructed to avoid alcohol completely. Patients should also be cautioned about side effects that could signal an adverse and potentially life-threatening reaction to the drug. Abacavir has the potential to cause a severe hypersensitivity syndrome in some individuals, and it carries a boxed warning for this. Symptoms of an abacavir hypersensitivity reaction, which can be fatal, may include fever, malaise, dizziness, headache, nausea, vomiting, and diarrhea. Some patients may also have respiratory symptoms like dyspnea (shortness of breath) and cough. A rash may develop as a late symptom. This hypersensitivity syndrome usually occurs within the first six weeks after starting therapy. Hypersensitivity reactions are more likely to occur in people who test positive for the genetic allele HLA-B*5701; therefore, screening for HLA-B*5701 is recommended before a patient starts abacavir therapy.

Drug Interactions Ganciclovir and valganciclovir may enhance the adverse effects of abacavir. Protease inhibitors may decrease the serum concentration of abacavir. Ribavirin may enhance side effects related to liver toxicity.

Emtricitabine and Lamivudine

Emtricitabine (Emtriva) and **lamivudine (Epivir)** are NRTIs that behave similarly. They can simplify drug regimens because they are often taken one time a day. Both drugs are well tolerated.

Dosage Forms and Administration Emtricitabine is available as a capsule and oral solution, and lamivudine is available as an oral solution and tablet. These medications can be taken without regard to meals.

Side Effects Emtricitabine may discolor the skin (such as by causing hyperpigmentation on the palms or soles). Lamivudine may precipitate pancreatitis.

Contraindications Emtricitabine and lamivudine do not have contraindications.

Cautions and Considerations Lamivudine is indicated to treat HIV and chronic hepatitis B. When used for hepatitis B, lamivudine has several boxed warnings. The first warning is about product selection. The hepatitis B product should not be used to treat HIV. The second warning is about medication discontinuation. After therapy stops, patients should be monitored closely for hepatitis exacerbations. The third warning addresses HIV resistance. Providers must be aware that HIV resistance may emerge when hepatitis B patients with an undiagnosed HIV infection use lamivudine. Lamivudine also has boxed warnings when used in the treatment of HIV, including risks of lactic acidosis and severe hepatomegaly (enlargement of the liver), exacerbation of hepatitis B upon discontinuation of lamivudine, and warnings to use appropriate dosing for HIV.

Emtricitabine has a boxed warning that it should not be used for the treatment of hepatitis. Emtricitabine and lamivudine may cause redistribution of body fat. Both drugs should be used cautiously in patients with renal dysfunction. Emtriciabine and products containing emtricitabine must be dispensed with a Mediation Guide.

Safety Alert

Both lamivudine and emtricia-bine have boxed warnings.

Drug Interactions Emtricitabine and lamivudine should not be used together. Ganciclovir, valganciclovir, and ribavirin may enhance the toxic effects of emtricitabine and lamivudine.

Stavudine

Stavudine (Zerit), an NRTI, is typically well tolerated. Its adverse effects (peripheral neuropathy, pancreatitis, dyslipidemia, hepatic steatosis [fatty liver], and lactic acidosis) generally limit its use. When other options are available, they are used before the patient tries stavudine.

Dosage Forms and Administration Stavudine is available as a capsule and powder for oral solution. It is dosed 30–40 mg every 12 hours and can be taken with or without food.

Side Effects Common side effects include headache, nausea, vomiting, diarrhea, loss of appetite, difficulty falling asleep, and rash.

Contraindications Stavudine does not have contraindications.

Cautions and Considerations Adverse effects of stavudine include peripheral neuropathy, pancreatitis, dyslipidemia, hepatic steatosis (fatty liver), and lactic acidosis. Stavudine has a boxed warning of lactic acidosis and pancreatitis. If a patient taking stavudine develops pancreatitis or it is suspected, they must suspend therapy and discontinue any other agents that may cause pancreatitis. Patients with peripheral neuropathy should use stavudine with caution. Stavudine must be dispensed with a Medication Guide which describes serious side effects including lactic acidosis, liver failure, and neurological problems like peripheral neuropathy.

Drug Interactions Zidovudine may decrease the effectiveness of stavudine.

Tenofovir

Tenofovir (Viread, Vemlidy) is an NRTI available in two different formulations. Tenofovir disoproxil fumarate was the first formulation to market and is available as a single agent and in combination products. Tenofovir alafenamide is only available in combination products. Tenofovir is dosed once daily and can be taken without regard to food.

Side Effects Tenofovir alafenamide has been shown to have reduced long-term renal and bone adverse effects compared to the disoproxil fumarate formulation. Other side effects include dizziness, depression, skin rash, and dyslipidemia.

Contraindications Tenofovir does not have contraindications.

Safety Alert

Tenofovir carries boxed warnings and must be dispensed with a Medication Guide.

Cautions and Considerations Medications containing tenofovir disoproxil fumarate or tenofovir alafenamide contain boxed warnings of posttreatment acute exacerbation of hepatitis B upon discontinuation of therapy. Kidney toxicity is a concern with tenofovir disoproxil fumarate use, so patients should avoid other drugs that are toxic to the kidneys. Use should be discontinued in patients who experience renal function decline. Combination products containing tenofovir must be dispensed with a Medication Guide which describes serious side effects.

Drug Interactions Adefovir may decrease the effectiveness of tenofovir disoproxil fumarate. Tenofovir disoproxil fumarate may increase levels of adefovir. Concomitant use is not recommended.

Zidovudine

Zidovudine (Retrovir), an NRTI, was one of the first drugs developed specifically for the treatment of HIV. With the exception of stavudine, zidovudine can be combined with any of the other NRTIs. The combination of zidovudine with lamivudine, with or without a protease inhibitor, is recommended for the prevention of HIV after a needlestick or sexual exposure.

Dosage Form and Administration Zidovudine is available in capsule, injection, syrup, and tablet form.

Side Effects The most common side effects of zidovudine are headache, anorexia, diarrhea, GI pain, nausea, rash, and anemia.

Contraindications Zidovudine does not have contraindications.

Safety Alert

Zidovudine carries boxed warnings.

Cautions and Considerations Zidovudine has a boxed warning for hematologic toxicity (neutropenia and anemia). It should be used with caution in patients with compromised bone marrow function.

Another boxed warning is present because zidovudine use is associated with myopathy and myositis. Certain combination products such as Trizivir that contain zidovudine must be dispensed with a Medication Guide which describes serious side effects.

Drug Interactions Adverse effects of clozapine may be enhanced by zidovudine use. Zidovudine may decrease the efficacy of stavudine.

Nonnucleoside Reverse Transcriptase Inhibitors

A **nonnucleoside reverse transcriptase inhibitor (NNRTI)** prevents HIV-1 reverse transcriptase from adding new nucleotides to the growing DNA chain. The exact site of action is different from the NRTIs. See Figure 17.2 for an illustration of where NNRTIs work in the HIV life cycle. Table 17.2 includes an overview of the most commonly used NNRTIs.

Delavirdine

Delavirdine (Rescriptor) is not used as much today due to lower efficacy and more complex dosing schedule compared to other NNRTIs.

Dosage Forms and Administration Delavirdine is available in tablet form.

Side Effects Side effects include redistribution or accumulation of body fat, including central obesity (increased abdominal fat), skin rash, headache, nausea, and vomiting. This drug is also associated with rash, but the incidence of rash is lower than it is with nevirapine.

Contraindications Contraindications to delavirdine include concurrent use of alprazolam, astemizole, cisapride, ergot alkaloids, midazolam, pimozide, rifampin, or triazolam.

Cautions and Considerations Delavirdine should not be taken with any antacid. Patients should be instructed to avoid ingesting antacids for one hour before and one hour after the administration of delavirdine.

Drug Interactions Because delavirdine is a cytochrome P450 inhibitor, it has many drug interactions related to cytochrome P450.

Delavirdine inhibits cytochrome P450 3A4 and may increase the serum concentrations of bosutinib, ibrutinib, ivabradine, lomitapide, naloxegol, olaparib, pimozide, simeprevir, suvorexant, tolvaptan, trabectedin, and ulipristal.

Delavirdine also inhibits cytochrome P450 2D6 and may increase the serum concentrations of pimozide and thioridazine.

Delaviridine may enhance the effects of efavirenz and rilpivirine.

Delavirdine may decrease serum concentrations of carbamazepine and etravirine. Fosamprenavir, fosphenytoin, H2 receptor antagonists, proton pump inhibitors (PPIs), rifamycin derivatives, and St. John's wort may decrease the serum concentration of delavirdine.

Doravirine

Doravirine (Pifeltro) is an NNRTI that is generally well tolerated. It is taken one time a day. Doravirine maintains activity in the presence of several common NNRTI drug-resistant mutations, so it may be used in some patients with HIV that have developed resistance to other NNRTIs. In addition, doravirine has fewer drug interactions than other NNRTIs and specifically none with acid-reducing medications. It also has a lower incidence of rash, fewer CNS side effects, and a more favorable lipid profile.

Dosage Forms and Administration Doravirine is available as a once-daily tablet that can be taken with or without food.

Side Effects Side effects include nausea, dizziness, headache, fatigue, diarrhea, abdominal pain, and abnormal dreams.

Contraindications Contraindications to doravirine include coadministration with cytochrome P450 3A4 (CYP3A4) enzyme inducers.

Cautions and Considerations Immune Reconstitution Syndrome (IRIS) may occur in some individuals when beginning therapy. IRIS is an inflammatory response that occurs when the immune system begins to recover and fights residual or opportunistic infections (such as tuberculosis or cytomegalovirus). It may occur in some individuals when beginning therapy.

Drug Interactions Coadministration of doravirine with a CYP3A4 inducer decreases doravirine concentrations and may reduce its efficacy. The following drugs should not be used with doravirine since they may decrease doravirine concentrations: enzalutamide, carbamazepine, oxcarbazepine, phenobarbital, phenytoin, rifampin, rifapentine, rifabutin, mitotane, efavirenz, etravirine, nevirapine, and St. John's wort.

Efavirenz

Efavirenz (Sustiva) has a long duration of action compared to other NNRTIs and is dosed only one time a day, preferably at bedtime. Patients taking efavirenz should be instructed to take it on an empty stomach.

Dosage Forms and Administration Efavirenz is available in a tablet or capsule taken one time a day.

Side Effects Common side effects include dizziness and headache. The drug may also induce vivid dreams, nightmares, and hallucinations. These side effects typically occur between one and three hours after administration and usually subside after two to four weeks on the drug.

Contraindications Efavirenz contraindications include concurrent use of cisapride, ergot alkaloids, midazolam, pimozide, St. John's wort, and triazolam.

Cautions and Considerations CNS side effects are the most common, and dosing at bedtime can help improve tolerability. Hepatic failure has occurred with use. Patients with moderate to severe hepatic dysfunction should avoid efavirenz. Efavirenz may cause false cannabinoid (marijuana) tests. Pregnant individuals should not take efavirenz.

Drug Interactions Efavirenz is a cytochrome P450 mixed inhibitor and inducer and has multiple drug interactions.

Efavirenz is a cytochrome P450 3A4 inducer and may decrease serum concentrations of aripiprazole, axitinib, bedaquiline, bosutinib, enzalutamide, itraconazole, ketoconazole, nisoldipine, olaparib, posaconazole, and simeprevir.

Efavirenz may decrease serum concentrations of atovaquone, carbamazepine, elvitegravir, etravirine, palbociclib, and ulipristal.

Efavirenz may potentiate the toxicities of nevirapine, orphenadrine, and thalidomide.

Efavirenz may decrease the serum concentration of boceprevir; boceprevir may increase the serum concentration of efavirenz.

St. John's wort may decrease the serum concentration of efavirenz.

Etravirine

Etravirine (Intelence) must be taken in combination with other HIV drugs and must never be taken alone. It reduces the HIV level in the blood and increases the levels of WBCs, helping to mitigate the increased risk of infections that occurs with a depressed immune system.

Dosage Forms and Administration Etravirine is available in tablet form.

Side Effects Commonly reported side effects include rash, nausea, hypersensitivity, and redistribution of body fat.

Contraindications Etravirine does not have contraindications.

Cautions and Considerations Etravirine should not be used in treatment-naive patients (patients who have not previously taken antiretroviral drugs). Etravirine should be taken with food.

Drug Interactions Etravirine has many drug interactions. The following drugs should not be used with etravirine.

Etravirine may decrease the serum concentrations of axitinib, bedaquiline, bosutinib, carbamazepine, enzalutamide, nisoldipine, olaparib, palbociclib, ritonavir, and simeprevir.

Etravirine concentrations may be decreased by boceprevir, carbamazepine, efavirenz, fosphenytoin, phenobarbital, phenytoin, primidone, rifamycin derivatives (except rifabutin), St. John's wort, and tipranavir.

Etravirine may increase serum concentrations of efavirenz and fosamprenavir.

Nevirapine

Nevirapine (Viramune, Viramune XR) is associated with a high incidence of rash, especially during the early phases of treatment. To mitigate this effect, the drug is typically administered at a lower dose during the first two weeks of treatment and then increased to the appropriate therapeutic level.

Dosage Forms and Administration Nevirapine is available as an oral suspension or a tablet.

Side Effects Side effects include rash, liver problems, and severe allergic reaction.

Contraindications Nevirapine is contraindicated in patients with moderate to severe liver impairment and should not be used for postexposure prophylaxis.

Safety Alert

Nevirapine has boxed warnings for liver toxicity and for life-threatening skin reactions.

This drug interferes with the effectiveness of oral contraceptives

Cautions and Considerations Nevirapine has two boxed warnings. One addresses liver toxicity that may result in liver failure or death. The greatest risk is within the first six weeks of use, and intensive monitoring is required during the first five months of therapy. The second warns of severe and life-threatening skin reactions. As with liver toxicity, the risk is greatest during the first six weeks of therapy. Nevirapine must be dispensed with a Medication Guide which describes serious side effects including liver problems and severe skin reactions and rashes.

Drug Interactions Nevirapine is a cytochrome P450 inducer. The antibiotic rifampin (a drug used to treat tuberculosis) interferes with the efficacy of nevirapine by reducing its serum concentration in the body. In turn, nevirapine decreases the serum concentration of the protease inhibitor class of antiretrovirals (discussed later in this chapter). As a result, these drugs generally are not prescribed in combination. Nevirapine also decreases the effectiveness of oral contraceptives.

Rilpivirine

Rilpivirine (Edurant) is generally well tolerated compared to older NNRTIs. Rilpivirine is most frequently used in first-time users of antiretroviral medications.

TAKE WITH FOOD

Dosage Forms and Administration Rilpivirine should not be taken with other NNRTIs. It should be taken with food, and it should not be taken by patients requiring a PPI.

Side Effects Side effects include depression, rash, headache, and insomnia.

Contraindications Rilpivirine contraindications include coadministration with anticonvulsants, antimycobacterials, PPIs, systemic dexamethasone, and St. John's wort.

Cautions and Considerations Rilpivirine should be used with caution in patients with a viral load greater than 100,000 copies/mL. A **viral load** is a measurement taken from a blood sample that determines the level of HIV activity and the effectiveness of antiretroviral therapy.

Drug Interactions Dexamethasone, fosphenytoin, oxcarbazepine, phenobarbital, phenytoin, primidone, PPIs, rifamycin derivatives (except rifabutin), and St. John's wort may decrease rilpivirine concentrations. Rilpivirine may increase or decrease serum concentrations of efavirenz and etravirine. Ritonavir may increase serum concentrations of rilpivirine.

Protease Inhibitors

A **protease inhibitor (PI)** inhibits the action of the protease enzyme. Protease cleaves certain HIV protein precursors into smaller proteins so that they can form mature, infectious virions. A protease inhibitor's mechanism results in the production of immature, noninfectious virions instead. PIs are typically combined with other antiretroviral drugs. Their use has led to marked clinical improvement and prolonged survival among HIV-infected patients. Because PIs are metabolized through cytochrome P450, drug interactions are common and can be severe. Statins should not be taken with these drugs.

Side effects associated with all PIs include redistribution of body fat, characterized by a humped back; facial atrophy (a wasting away of facial fat); breast enlargement; hyperglycemia (increased level of glucose in the blood); hyperlipidemia (elevated concentration of lipids in the plasma); and an increase in bleeding episodes in some patients with hemophilia, a hemorrhagic condition caused by a deficiency of a coagulation factor.

PIs are notorious for drug interactions. For this reason, only experienced providers should prescribe PIs. Drug interaction data for PIs is regularly updated. The National Institutes of Health (NIH) publishes data on its AIDSinfo website at http://Pharmacology7e.ParadigmCollege.net/AIDSinfo.

Atazanavir

Atazanavir (Reyataz) is dosed one time a day and should be taken with ritonavir or cobicistat. It does not appear to increase cholesterol or triglyceride levels as most HIV drugs do, but it has similar side effects.

Dosage Forms and Administration Atazanavir should be taken with food and is available as a capsule or oral packet (powder).

Side Effects In addition to the side effects shared by all PIs, one common side effect is jaundice. Patients using atazanavir may notice yellowing of the skin. This yellowing of the skin is benign, but it can be bothersome to patients.

Contraindications Contraindications to atazanavir include concurrent therapy with alfuzosin, cisapride, ergot derivatives, irinotecan, lovastatin, midazolam, nevirapine, pimozide, rifampin, sildenafil, simvastatin, St. John's wort, or triazolam. Atazanavir should not be coadministered with drugs that strongly induce cytochrome P450 3A4 (e.g., phenobarbital, phenytoin), since these drugs lower atazanavir exposure and decrease its efficacy.

Cautions and Considerations Patients using atazanavir may develop diabetes and should be monitored for signs and symptoms of diabetes. Liver and kidney dysfunction may occur with use. Atazanavir has been associated with the development of renal stones and kidney injury.

Drug Interactions PIs have many drug interactions. The most recent interaction information may be obtained at the NIH AIDSinfo website at https://Pharmacology7e.ParadigmEducation.com/AIDSinfo.

Darunavir

Darunavir (Prezista) is a PI that must be administered in combination with ritonavir. This drug received accelerated approval from the FDA so that it could be used in patients resistant to other therapies.

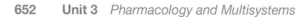

Dosage Forms and Administration Darunavir should be taken with food. It should be stored and dispensed in the original container, tightly closed.

Side Effects In addition to the side effects shared by all PIs, the most common side effects of darunavir are headache, nausea, and diarrhea.

Contraindications Contraindications to darunavir include concurrent therapy with alfuzosin, cisapride, ergot derivatives, irinotecan, lovastatin, midazolam, nevirapine, pimozide, rifampin, sildenafil, simvastatin, St. John's wort, or triazolam. Coadministration with drugs that strongly induce cytochrome P450 3A4 may lead to lower darunavir exposure and loss of efficacy.

Cautions and Considerations Darunavir's chemical structure is related to that of sulfa drugs. Patients with sulfa allergies should use darunavir with caution. Darunavir use may exacerbate kidney and liver toxicities. Darunavir should not be used in children under three years of age.

Drug Interactions PIs have many drug interactions. The most recent interaction information may be obtained at the NIH AIDSinfo website at http://Pharmacology7e .ParadigmCollege.net/AIDSinfo.

Fosamprenavir

Fosamprenavir (Lexiva) is a prodrug of the PI amprenavir. It is better absorbed and tolerated than amprenavir, and it can be taken without regard for meals. Fosamprenavir has largely replaced the use of amprenavir.

Dosage Forms and Administration Fosamprenavir is available as an oral suspension and a tablet.

Side Effects In addition to the side effects shared by PIs, common side effects of fosamprenavir include nausea and diarrhea; however, these effects are reduced compared to those observed with amprenavir use.

Contraindications Contraindications to fosamprenavir include concurrent therapy with alfuzosin, cisapride, ergot derivatives, irinotecan, lovastatin, midazolam, nevirapine, pimozide, rifampin, sildenafil, simvastatin, St. John's wort, or triazolam.

Cautions and Considerations Fosamprenavir's chemical structure is similar to that of sulfa drugs, and caution must be exercised in patients with a sulfa allergy.

Fosamprenavir is associated with hepatic toxicity. Patients with underlying liver disease should use fosamprenavir with caution.

Drug Interactions PIs have many drug interactions. The most recent interaction information may be obtained at the NIH AIDSinfo website at http://Pharmacology7e .ParadigmCollege.net/AIDSinfo.

Lopinavir / Ritonavir

Lopinavir / ritonavir (Kaletra) is a combination product that shares side effects with ritonavir (discussed later in this section).

Dosage Forms and Administration Lopinavir / ritonavir is available as an oral solution and tablet.

Side Effects This combination drug has the side effects shared by all PIs, but because the ritonavir dose is lower when combined with lopinavir, it has fewer intestinal side effects, such as cramping. Other GI side effects, such as diarrhea and nausea, however, are still present. Other side effects include rash, liver dysfunction, and renal dysfunction.

Contraindications Contraindications to lopinavir / ritonavir include concurrent therapy with alfuzosin, cisapride, ergot derivatives, indinavir, irinotecan, lovastatin, midazolam, nevirapine, pimozide, rifampin, sildenafil, simvastatin, St. John's wort, or triazolam. Coadministration with drugs that strongly induce cytochrome P450 3A4 may lead to lower lopinavir / ritonavir exposure and loss of efficacy.

Cautions and Considerations Lopinavir / ritonavir must be dispensed with a Medication Guide which describes serious side effects including drug interactions, inflammation of the pancreas, liver problems, and cardiac rhythm changes.

Lopinavir / ritonavir is available as an oral solution and a tablet. The oral solution contains a high percentage of both alcohol and propylene glycol. Patients taking other drugs that have cautions or contraindications involving alcohol (e.g., metronidazole) should not use the oral solution. Patients should not use other medications that contain propylene glycol while using the oral solution.

Drug Interactions PIs have many drug interactions. The most recent interaction information may be obtained at the NIH AIDSinfo website at http://Pharmacology7e .ParadigmCollege.net/AIDSinfo.

Nelfinavir

Nelfinavir (Viracept) is well tolerated by patients. Although diarrhea is an initial side effect, it generally resolves itself with continued use. Loperamide and calcium carbonate can help control the diarrhea.

Dosage Forms and Administration Nelfinavir is available as a tablet and should be taken with food. If a patient is unable to swallow nelfinavir tablets, they may dissolve a tablet in a small amount of water and consume the solution immediately.

Side Effects In addition to the side effects shared by all PIs, the most common side effect of nelfinavir is diarrhea.

Contraindications Nelfinavir should not be used concurrently with alfuzosin, amiodarone, cisapride, ergot derivatives, lovastatin, midazolam, pimozide, quinidine, rifampin, sildenafil, simvastatin, St. John's wort, or triazolam.

Cautions and Considerations Diarrhea occurs frequently with use of nelfinavir. If a patient uses the method of dissolving a tablet in a small amount of water, then the glass used to dissolve the tablet should be rinsed and the contents ingested to ensure the entire dose is taken. Alternatively, the tablets may be crushed and mixed with a small amount of food. Due to its bitter taste, this drug should not be mixed with acidic beverages or acidic food.

Drug Interactions PIs have many drug interactions. The most recent interaction information may be obtained at the NIH AIDSinfo website at http://Pharmacology7e .ParadigmCollege.net/AIDSinfo.

Ritonavir

Ritonavir (Norvir) is prescribed primarily for its ability to increase the serum concentrations and decrease the dosage frequency of other PIs (an action known as a **boost**). As such, ritonavir is generally prescribed at a low dose in combination with other drugs.

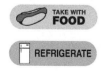

Dosage Forms and Administration Ritonavir, whether in capsule, tablet, or solution form, should be stored in the refrigerator. Ritonavir should be taken with food.

Side Effects In addition to the side effects shared by all PIs, ritonavir has many other side effects, including an altered sense of taste.

Contraindications Ritonavir is contraindicated with the concurrent use of alfuzosin, amiodarone, cisapride, ergot derivatives, flecainide, lovastatin, midazolam, pimozide, propafenone, quinidine, sildenafil, simvastatin, St. John's wort, triazolam, or voriconazole.

Cautions and Considerations Ritonavir has a boxed warning for serious and potentially life-threatening drug interactions. Ritonavir should be used cautiously in patients with cardiac arrhythmias due to the potential for exacerbation of this condition.

Drug Interactions Ritonavir is an extremely potent inhibitor of cytochrome P450 and has many drug interactions. The most recent interaction information may be obtained at the NIH AIDSinfo website at http://Pharmacology7e.ParadigmCollege.net/AIDSinfo.

Tipranavir

Tipranavir (Aptivus) may have some advantages over other PIs. Its structure is more adaptable to protease binding sites than the structure of other PIs. It also has a self-emulsifying drug delivery system (SEDDS) in the form of a soft gelatin capsule. This system improves dissolution and the bioavailability of the drug, which increases systemic circulation and reduces the pill burden.

Dosage Forms and Administration Tipranavir is prescribed with ritonavir (Norvir) as a boost and should be taken with food. Capsules should be stored in the refrigerator but are stable for up to 60 days when not refrigerated. The oral solution should be stored at room temperature.

Side Effects In addition to the side effects shared by all PIs, tipranavir's common side effects are diarrhea, nausea, vomiting, headache, and fatigue.

Contraindications Tipranavir is contraindicated in patients with moderate to severe liver impairment. Tipranavir in combination with ritonavir should not be used with alfuzosin, amiodarone, cisapride, ergot derivatives, flecainide, lovastatin, midazolam, pimozide, propafenone, quinidine, rifampin, sildenafil, simvastatin, St. John's wort, or triazolam.

Cautions and Considerations Tipranavir has a boxed warning because intracranial hemorrhages occurred in participants of clinical studies. It has another boxed warning for hepatotoxicity and may cause hepatitis or exacerbate preexisting hepatitis.

Tipranavir capsules contain dehydrated ethanol and should be avoided in patients taking other drugs that have cautions or contraindications involving ethanol. The oral solution formula contains vitamin E. Individuals using the oral solution should not take additional vitamin E.

Drug Interactions PIs have many drug interactions. The most recent interaction information may be obtained at the NIH AIDSinfo website.

Entry Inhibitors: Fusion Inhibitors, Post-Attachment Inhibitors, and CCR5 Antagonists

Fusion inhibitors, CCR5 antagonists, and post-attachment inhibitors prevent HIV from entering immune cells, which is why these are commonly referred to as **entry inhibitors**. This mechanism of action is a major advancement in HIV treatment because older drugs block replication of the virus only after it has entered the cell.

Enfuvirtide

Enfuvirtide (Fuzeon) is a fusion inhibitor and is administered to HIV patients who are resistant to older drugs.

Dosage Forms and Administration Enfuvirtide is administered subcutaneously. It is distributed as a powder, and sterile water is the diluent. It takes 30 to 45 minutes to dissolve, and reaction at the injection site is common.

Side Effects Side effects include diarrhea, nausea, and fatigue.

Contraindications Enfuvirtide does not have contraindications.

Cautions and Considerations Enfuvirtide may cause hypersensitivity reactions and pneumonia. Enfuvirtide is not appropriate for treatment-naive patients.

Drug Interactions PIs may increase serum concentrations of enfuvirtide.

Ibalizumab

Ibalizumab (Trogarzo) is a humanized IgG4 monoclonal antibody that prevents HIV cell entry by binding a specific spot on of the host CD4 receptor. It is referred to as a **post-attachment inhibitor**. Ibalizumab is used in combination with other antiretroviral medications for the treatment of HIV-1 in heavily treatment-experienced adults with multidrug-resistant infection.

Dosage Forms and Administration Ibalizumab is administered intravenously.

Side Effects Side effects include diarrhea, dizziness, nausea, and rash.

Contraindications Ibalizumab has no contraindications.

Cautions and Considerations Immune reconstitution inflammatory syndrome (IRIS) may occur in some individuals when beginning therapy.

Drug Interactions Ibalizumab has no reported drug interactions.

Maraviroc

Maraviroc (Selzentry) is a chemokine coreceptor (CCR5) antagonist. It blocks the CCR5 coreceptor on the surface of certain immune cells and prevents HIV from entering.

Dosage Forms and Administration Maraviroc must be taken in combination with other antiretroviral drugs. It is taken without regard to food.

Side Effects The most common side effect is a cough. Other side effects include abdominal pain, dizziness, and fever.

Contraindications Maraviroc is contraindicated in patients with severe kidney impairment.

Safety Alert

Maraviroc has a boxed warning for hepatitis.

Cautions and Considerations Maraviroc has a boxed warning for inducing hepatotoxicity with allergic features. While on maraviroc, patients must be monitored closely for infection. Maraviroc must be dispensed with a Medication Guide.

Drug Interactions Maraviroc is a cytochrome P450 substrate and has many drug interactions. Drugs that should be avoided while taking maraviroc include conivaptan, idelalisib, and St. John's wort. Other drug interactions can be found on the NIH AIDSinfo website at http://Pharmacology7e.ParadigmCollege.net/AIDSinfo_2.

Integrase Strand Transfer Inhibitors

Like reverse transcriptase (which is blocked by NRTIs and NNRTIs) and protease (which is blocked by PIs), integrase is an enzyme that HIV needs to reproduce. Figure 17.2 illustrates where **integrase strand transfer inhibitors** (INSTIs) work in the HIV life cycle, and Table 17.2 includes an overview of these drugs. After reverse transcriptase converts HIV RNA into DNA, integrase inserts that DNA into the DNA of the host cell.

Bictegravir

Bictegravir is not available as an individual HIV medication, but it is approved as a component of the fixed-dose combination tablet Biktarvy, which is discussed in the Combining Antiretroviral Medications section.

Dosage Forms and Administration Bictegravir is available as a component of a fixed-dose combination tablet. It is taken one time a day with or without food.

Side effects Side effects include diarrhea, nausea, and headache.

Contraindications Coadministration with rifampin is contraindicated.

Cautions and Considerations Immune reconstitution inflammatory syndrome (IRIS) may occur in some individuals when beginning therapy.

Drug Interactions Bictegravir is a substrate of liver enzymes CYP3A and uridine diphosphate glucuronosyltransferase (UGT1A1). Inducers of these enzymes can decrease the concentrations of bictegravir, which may lead to loss of therapeutic effect. Rifampin, rifapentine, carbamazepine, phenytoin, phenobarbital and St. John's wort are agents that may decrease bictegravir levels. Polyvalent cations like aluminum, calcium, iron, and magnesium that are found in some antacids, laxatives, and mineral supplements can decrease the absorption of bictegravir. Products containing these cations should be taken at least two hours before or two hours after bictegravir. It should be noted that PPIs and H_2 blockers do not affect bictegravir concentrations. Bictegravir can increase concentrations of metformin.

Dolutegravir

Dolutegravir (Tivicay) was approved by the FDA in 2013. Compared with other integrase strand transfer inhibitors, it is well tolerated.

Dosage Forms and Administration Dolutegravir is available as a tablet and as part of a fixed-dose combination tablet.

Side Effects Side effects include elevated serum lipase, insomnia, elevated liver enzymes, and hyperglycemia.

Contraindications Dolutegravir should not be used with dofetilide.

Cautions and Considerations Dolutegravir may cause fat redistribution and hypersensitivity reaction. In patients who have not previously taken antiretrovirals, weight gain may be greater than that observed in patients taking NNRTI or boosted PI regimens.

Drug Interactions Dolutegravir has multiple drug interactions. Drugs that should be avoided when taking dolutegravir include carbamazepine, dofetilide, fosphenytoin, nevirapine, oxcarbazepine, phenobarbital, phenytoin, primidone, and St. John's wort. Polyvalent cations like aluminum, calcium, iron, and magnesium, which are found in some antacids, laxatives, and mineral supplements, can decrease the absorption of dolutegravir. Products containing these cations should be taken at least two hours before or two hours after dolutegravir.

Elvitegravir

Elvitegravir is only available in a combination product. These combination products contain cobicistat, which has many drug interactions.

Dosage Forms and Administration Elvitegravir is available within combination products Genvoya and Stribild, which are available as tablets and taken one time a day.

Side Effects Common side effects include depression, fatigue, insomnia, headache, diarrhea, and abdominal pain.

Contraindications Elvitegravir does not have contraindications.

Work Wise

Raltegravir film-coated tablets, chewable tablets, and oral suspension are not bioequivalent. This means they cannot be substituted on a milligram-to-milligram basis.

Cautions and Considerations Elvitegravir may contribute to lactic acidosis. It should be avoided in patients with severe liver impairment.

Drug Interactions Elvitegravir has many drug interactions. It should be avoided when a patient is using nevirapine, rifabutin, rifampin, or St. John's wort. Elvitegravir may decrease the effectiveness of estrogen-containing contraceptives. Polyvalent cations like aluminum, calcium, iron, and magnesium that are found in some antacids, laxatives, or mineral supplements can decrease the absorption of elvitegravir. Products containing these cations should be taken at least two hours before or two hours after elvitegravir. More information on drug interactions can be found on the NIH AIDSinfo website at http://Pharmacology7e.ParadigmCollege.net/AIDSinfo_3.

Raltegravir

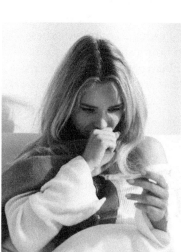

HIV patients are immunocompromised and are vulnerable to illness. Raltegravir increases WBC count and helps fight infections.

Raltegravir (Isentress) is another available integrase strand transfer inhibitor.

Dosage Forms and Administration Raltegravir is available as a chewable tablet, oral suspension, and film-coated tablet.

Side Effects Side effects include nausea, headache, diarrhea, pyrexia (fever), and creatine kinase elevation.

Contraindications Raltegravir does not have contraindications.

Cautions and Considerations Raltegravir is associated with myopathy and rhabdomyolysis (a condition characterized by muscle breakdown). Caution should be exercised in patients with a history of rhabdomyolysis, myopathy, or creatine kinase elevations.

The chewable tablet formulation contains phenylalanine. Patients with phenylalanine sensitivity should avoid this formulation.

Drug Interactions Interactions with aluminum, calcium, iron, and magnesium, which may be found in antacids, laxatives, and mineral supplements can decrease the absorption of raltegravir. These products should be taken at least 2 hours before or 2 hours after raltegravir. Raltegravir may enhance the myopathic effects of fibric acid derivatives and statins (both used for dyslipidemia).

Combining Antiretroviral Medications

None of the antiretroviral medications currently available can eradicate HIV, but when used appropriately, they can decrease viral replication, improve immunologic status, and prolong life. The standard care for the treatment of HIV is to administer several drugs in combination. The regimens are difficult to follow because the drugs must be taken around the clock. Consequently, patient adherence is frequently poor. Clear written instructions for taking the medications, as well as adequate warnings about the potential for drug interactions, may encourage higher patient adherence. Patients who only have to take a single dose per day show higher adherence to therapy than those individuals on a more complex regimen.

To simplify the drug regimen and decrease pill burden, pharmaceutical manufacturers have increasingly developed combination products. There are specific advantages and disadvantages to various combinations. The most obvious advantage is improved patient adherence. A principal disadvantage is that these combination drugs have fixed doses and cannot be used in unstable patients who require frequent dose changes to decrease their viral load.

Efavirenz / emtricitabine / tenofovir (Atripla) is a combination of three different classes of antiretrovirals—an NNRTI (efavirenz), an NRTI (emtricitabine), and tenofovir disoproxil fumarate—in one tablet. The virus can be attacked in three ways simultaneously by the same tablet. The side effects are the same as those of the three individual drugs. The big advantage is that Atripla is dosed one time a day and improves patient adherence. It is recommended as a first-line therapy unless the patient is in the first trimester of pregnancy. It was approved through an accelerated process. It has a boxed warning for lactic acidosis. Atripla must be dispensed in the original unopened container.

Bictegravir / tenofovir / emtricitabine (Biktarvy) contains an INSTI (bictegravir) and two NRTIs (tenofovir and emtricitabine) and is a complete HIV regimen in one tablet. It should not be used in patients with severe renal impairment or severe hepatic impairment. Biktarvy is generally well tolerated. It can be taken with or without food.

Lamivudine / zidovudine (Combivir) comes as a tablet for those individuals who have trouble swallowing a capsule. Its ingredients (Epivir and Retrovir) are both NRTIs. These drugs are synergistic, and the pill burden is decreased. Because Combivir is a fixed dose, it cannot be used in patients requiring dosage adjustments. It also cannot be used in children under 12 years of age.

Abacavir / lamivudine (Epzicom) contains two NRTIs (Ziagen and Epivir) in a fixed combination and a single strength. Epzicom can be taken without regard to food, which improves patient adherence. This point is important because partial adherence can lead to viral resistance, meaning the virus may change or mutate, leading to treatment failure. A card packaged with Epzicom states that if the patient has any two of the following symptoms, the prescriber must be contacted immediately, and the drug must be discontinued:

- fever
- rash
- nausea and vomiting, or diarrhea and cramping
- extreme tiredness or achiness
- shortness of breath, cough, or sore throat

Pharmacy technicians must ensure that patients receive this card when picking up the medication. Technicians should instruct patients to read the card and carry it with them at all times. Providing this patient instruction is *not* considered counseling. In addition, Epzicom must be dispensed with a Medication Guide.

Elvitegravir / cobicistat / emtricitabine / tenofovir disoproxil fumarate (Stribild) is a combination product for the treatment of HIV. It is used as initial treatment for patients new to HIV therapy. As mentioned before, it is similar to Genvoya, with the difference in the two products being the tenofovir component. Elvitegravir / cobicistat / emtricitabine / tenofovir disoproxil fumarate is generally well tolerated but has some limitations, including the risk of bone mineral density loss and renal toxicity due to the tenofovir disoproxil fumarate component. Additionally, patients may experience gastrointestinal side effects like nausea and diarrhea caused by cobicistat. Many drug interactions also exist. The product does contain a boxed warning for an increased risk of posttreatment acute exacerbation of hepatitis B.

Darunavir / cobicistat / emtricitabine / tenofovir alafenamide (Symtuza) is a single-tablet regimen approved to be used in patients who have not received prior HIV treatment or for certain patients with prior treatment where darunavir is still effective. It may have less renal and bone toxicity compared to regimens that use tenofovir disoproxil fumarate. It does have GI side effects and drug interactions due to the cobicistat component.

Emtricitabine / tenofovir (Truvada) has the same drugs as Atripla without efavirenz (Sustiva); that is, this drug is a combination of Emtriva and Viread. Currently, it is a drug recommended for occupational exposure to HIV and as an option for initial treatment. Truvada has also been approved for preexposure prophylaxis (PrEP) to reduce the risk of acquiring HIV. More information on PrEP is presented later in this chapter. It is well tolerated and long acting. Truvada must be dispensed with a Medication Guide.

The most commonly used combinations of antiretroviral drugs are summarized in Table 17.3.

TABLE 17.3 Commonly Used Combination Treatments for HIV

Generic (Brand)	Common Dosage
abacavir / lamivudine (Epzicom)	1 tablet a day
bictegravir / emtricitabine / tenofovir (Biktarvy)	1 tablet a day
darunavir / cobicistat / emtricitabine / tenofovir alafenamide (Symtuza)	1 tablet a day
dolutegravir / lamivudine (Dovato)	1 tablet a day
doravirine / lamivudine / tenofovir (Delstrigo)	1 tablet a day
efavirenz / emtricitabine / tenofovir (Atripla)	1 tablet a day
efavirenz / lamivudine / tenofovir (Symfi, Symfi Lo)	1 tablet a day
Generic (Brand)	**Common Dosage**
elvitegravir / cobicistat / emtricitabine / tenofovir disoproxil fumarate (Stribild)	1 tablet a day
elvitegravir / cobicistat / emtricitabine / tenofovir alafenamide (Genvoya)	1 tablet a day
emtricitabine / tenofovir alafenamide (Descovy)	1 tablet a day
emtricitabine / tenofovir disoproxil fumarate (Truvada)	1 tablet a day
lamivudine / tenofovir (Cimduo)	1 tablet a day
lamivudine / zidovudine (Combivir)	1 tablet 2 times a day

HIV Regimens

The following provides an overview of current recommendations for HIV therapy, specifically the initial regimen recommendations for adults and adolescents.

An antiretroviral regimen for a treatment-naive patient (patient who has not previously taken antiretroviral drugs) generally consists of two nucleoside reverse transcriptase inhibitors (NRTIs) in combination with a third active antiretroviral drug from one of three drug classes: an integrase strand transfer inhibitor (INSTI), a nonnucleoside reverse transcriptase inhibitor (NNRTI), or a protease inhibitor (PI) with a pharmacokinetic enhancer (cobicistat or ritonavir).

The US Department of Health and Human Services Panel on Antiretroviral Guidelines for Adults and Adolescents classifies the following regimens as recommended therapy for treatment-naive patients. Each of these regimens is strongly recommended and supported by evidence and data using randomized controlled trials.

Regimens based on protease inhibitors include darunavir / ritonavir plus tenofovir / emtricitabine.

Regimens based on integrase strand transfer inhibitors include:

- bictegravir / tenofovir alafenamide / emtricitabine
- dolutegravir / abacavir / lamivudine (only for patients who are HLA-B*5701 negative and without chronic hepatitis B virus coinfection)
- dolutegravir plus (emtricitabine or lamivudine) plus (tenofovir alafenamide or tenofovir disoproxil fumarate)
- dolutegravir / lamivudine (except in individuals with HIV RNA > 500,000 copies/mL, with chronic hepatitis B virus [HBV] coinfection, or in whom antiretroviral therapy will be started before the results of HIV genotypic resistance testing for reverse transcriptase or HBV testing are available).

On the basis of individual patient characteristics and needs, an alternate regimen may, in some instances, be the optimal regimen. Given the large number of excellent options for initial therapy, selection of a regimen for a particular patient should be guided by such factors as virologic efficacy, toxicity, pill burden, dosing frequency, drug-drug interaction potential, resistance testing results, comorbid conditions, and cost.

Treatment as Prevention

Treatment as prevention (TasP) is an HIV prevention method in which patients with HIV use effective antiretroviral therapy to suppress viral levels to undetectable levels (<200 copies/mL) to prevent the transmission of HIV to sexual partners. This is also known as *U=U* or *undetectable equals untransmittable*. For people new to antiretroviral treatment, another form of transmittal prevention (such as condoms) should be used for the first six months and until suppression of the viral load to <200 copies/ mL has been confirmed. Patients must be advised that adherence to therapy is critical

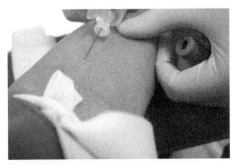

The CDC has developed new guidelines to protect healthcare workers. Healthcare workers who are accidentally exposed to blood with a high virus titer should start PEP immediately.

in maintaining this viral suppression and that it is possible to transmit HIV during treatment interruption. In addition, it is important to remember that this approach does *not* prevent individuals from acquiring other sexually transmitted infections.

Responding to Accidental Exposure

The Centers for Disease Control and Prevention (CDC) have developed guidelines for the management of healthcare worker exposure to HIV. These guidelines include recommendations for the administration of antiretroviral drugs as **postexposure prophylaxis (PEP)**. Healthcare worker risks include exposure to the blood or other body fluids of an HIV-positive patient and needlestick injuries. Following such an exposure, the administration of an appropriate antiretroviral regimen should begin within two hours. Research has shown that prompt treatment can decrease the risk of infection by 80%. Clearly, preventing exposure to HIV through appropriate precautions is the primary means of protection against HIV infection for healthcare workers as well as the public. People accidentally exposed to blood with a high virus titer or to deep needle injury should start PEP immediately (within one to two hours) because they are at a high risk of infection.

Preexposure Prophylaxis (PrEP)

Preexposure prophylaxis (PrEP) is an HIV prevention method via which people who do not have HIV take a specific HIV medicine daily to reduce their risk of acquiring the virus if exposed through sex or injection drug use. Two medications are approved for PrEP: Truvada and Descovy. In patients who are adherent to therapy, these medicines are 90% effective in preventing HIV. Individuals must be advised that adherence to therapy is critical to prevent infection and that this approach does *not* prevent them from acquiring other sexually transmitted infections.

17.4 Immunity and Immunization

Pharm Fact

One way that health professionals can help patients gain immunity is by administering vaccines.

As discussed in Chapter 16, the body responds to pathogens with either the innate immune system or the adaptive immune system. *Immunity* describes resistance to an infectious disease. **Immunization** is the process by which an individual becomes protected against an infectious disease. There are two general ways people acquire immunity: passively and actively. An individual acquires **passive immunity** when preformed antibodies are transferred to them, such as when a fetus receives antibodies during pregnancy (naturally) or a patient receives an injection of immunoglobulins (artificially). Passive immunity provides immediate protection, but the body does not develop immunologic memory.

In contrast to passive immunity, where ready-made antibodies are transferred to an individual, **active immunity** is the process by which a person's body makes its own antibodies to a pathogen. Active immunity acquired naturally occurs when a person is exposed to certain pathogens; active immunity that is acquired artificially typically results from immunization. Vaccination is a tool used for the prevention and elimination of infectious diseases; vaccines prevent an estimated 2 to 3 million deaths worldwide every year.

A vaccine usually contains a component of the virus that causes the infection the vaccine was designed to prevent. Vaccines induce the body to make antibodies, which are proteins that recognize the virus antigen. Anytime these antibodies see the virus, they are able to kill off an infection.

Immunizations

Preventing viral infections by providing immunity is the purpose of immunizations. Immunizations expose a patient to a component of a virus or an altered viral strain that does not produce infection. The exposure of the body to this foreign (though harmless) material promotes the proliferation of B lymphocytes that produce antibodies specific to the introduced virus. Later, if the immunized patient encounters the actual virus, the infection cannot develop, because the patient's defenses are already primed from the vaccine. Because the discovery, testing, production, and implementation of vaccines are very complicated, vaccines are available for only a small number of viruses.

The difficulty of producing effective vaccines is increased by mutations in a virus's genetic material that change the structure and composition of its surface proteins. The patient's defenses are primed against the original virus due to exposure to the vaccine; however, if those defenses do not recognize that the mutated virus is a version of the original virus, they are not primed against it. As a result, the patient's defenses take much longer to mount a strong attack against the mutated virus, and the patient becomes ill in the meantime. Influenza is a virus that mutates this way. Every year, a new influenza vaccine is developed according to which strains (versions) of the virus are predicted to become most prevalent the following year.

Because influenza viruses change from year to year, annual immunizations are needed. The vaccine is only as good as its match to the infecting strain of influenza. This vaccine usually becomes available in September and is administered throughout the flu season. The CDC recommends that everyone six months of age and older receive an annual influenza immunization. The vaccine is made from viral particles that are raised in poultry eggs and then inactivated or killed. For this reason, a healthcare practitioner must confirm that a patient is not allergic to eggs before administering the vaccine. In certain situations, an antiviral medication (oseltamivir) may be prescribed to patients who cannot receive the vaccine or who have recently been exposed to influenza.

Immunizations can reduce and prevent serious diseases, especially among children, when used universally. For example, immunization practices have effectively eliminated smallpox worldwide and have reduced the impact of measles, polio, and influenza.

Various types of vaccines are available (see Table 17.4). A **live attenuated vaccine** uses live but weakened pathogens to induce an immune response. An **inactivated vaccine** uses pathogens that have been killed with chemicals, heat, or radiation.

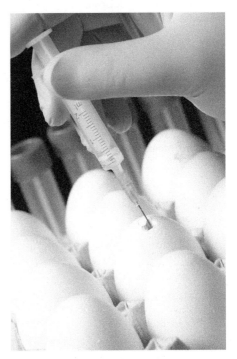

The inactivated form of the influenza vaccine is grown in chicken eggs and should not be administered to patients with egg or chicken allergies.

TABLE 17.4 Common Vaccines

Generic (Brand)	Route of Administration	Prophylactic Use
bacillus Calmette-Guérin (BCG)	injection	patients at high risk of exposure to tuberculosis healthcare workers only in settings where there is high risk of tuberculosis exposure
diphtheria, tetanus, and pertussis (various combinations)	injection	diphtheria, tetanus, and pertussis (whooping cough) in children or adults
Haemophilus influenzae type B, or Hib (ActHIB, HibTITER, PedvaxHIB)	injection	*Haemophilus influenzae* type B in children
hepatitis A (Havrix, Vaqta)	injection	patients at high risk of exposure to hepatitis A
hepatitis B (ENERGIX-B, Recombivax HB)	injection	hepatitis B in children adults at high risk of exposure to hepatitis B healthcare workers
Hib + Hep B (Comvax)	injection	*Haemophilus influenzae* type B and hepatitis B in children
human papillomavirus, or HPV (Gardasil)	injection	children and adults ages 9–26 to prevent genital warts, anal cancer, and cervical cancer
influenza (Afluria, Fluad, Fluarix, Flublok, Flucelvax, FluLaval, Fluzone)	injection	influenza in children and adults
influenza (FluMist)	intranasal	influenza in patients 2–50 years old
Japanese encephalitis (Ixiaro)	injection	recommended for patients at high risk of exposure to Japanese encephalitis
measles, mumps, rubella (MMR II)	injection	measles, mumps, and rubella in adults and children
meningococcal conjugate or Serogroup B meningococcal (Bexsero, Menactra, Menomune)	injection	children ages 11–12 should get a meningococcal conjugate vaccine, with a booster dose at 16 years old patients ages 16–23 may get a serogroup B meningococcal vaccine
pneumococcal, conjugate (Prevnar)	injection	pneumonia and otitis media (ear infections) in children and certain adults
pneumococcal, polyvalent (Pneumovax 23)	injection	pneumonia in patients younger than 2 years or older than 50 years
polio, inactivated, or IPV (IPOL)	injection	poliovirus in children
rotavirus (Rotarix, RotaTeq)	oral	rotavirus in infants and children
typhoid (Typhim VI)	injection	recommended for patients at high risk of exposure to typhoid fever
typhoid (Vivotif)	oral	*Salmonella* Typhi in adults and children
varicella (Varivax)	injection	chicken pox in children
yellow fever (YF-VAX)	injection	recommended for patients at high risk of exposure to yellow fever
zoster (Zostavax)	injection	herpes zoster (shingles) in patients 60 years and older

Immunization Schedule

Several vaccines require multiple doses to produce an adequate immune response and confer upon a patient full immunity to a disease. The CDC publishes a schedule for childhood and adult vaccines. In Canada, the **Public Health Agency** makes immunization recommendations. Certain immunizations are recommended for children, whereas others are more appropriate for adults (see Figures 17.3 and 17.4). In most cases, specific vaccines are required for children entering public school. When the vaccine regimen is complete, most childhood immunizations lead to lifetime immunity. Others—for example, the tetanus and pertussis vaccines—must be readministered periodically as booster shots to continue immunity protection.

Pharmacy technicians should be knowledgeable about immunization schedules and make certain they are personally up to date on their immunizations. Working in the healthcare field without being properly vaccinated increases an individual's risk of exposure to diseases and disease transmission. Certain vaccines are recommended for healthcare workers. These immunizations include the hepatitis B immunization and an annual influenza shot. Many healthcare employers require their employees to get these vaccinations and to keep all others current as part of employment.

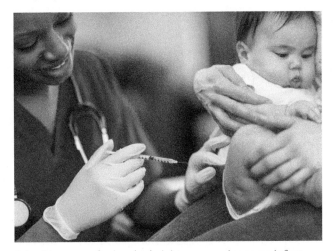

A healthcare professional administers a vaccine to an infant.

Common Vaccines

Work Wise

Yellow fever is a vaccine recommended by the CDC for persons traveling to or living in high-risk areas of South America and Africa. If a patient is traveling to these areas, an opportunity exists to educate them on vaccination best practices.

Many vaccines are administered in physicians' offices, clinics, or inpatient settings. However, a greater number of vaccines is administered in community pharmacies. For example, many patients now receive their annual influenza vaccine at their local pharmacy. In this setting, it is often the pharmacy technician who screens patients, completes the necessary forms, and stocks and stores the vaccines. Some states allow (or are seeking to allow) technicians to administer vaccines. Thus, it is important that the pharmacy technician has a working knowledge of this aspect of practice.

Numerous clinics and pharmacies operate a **travel immunization clinic**, which can help prepare people for travel and provide immunizations and advice about what vaccines are recommended or necessary for global travel. Some diseases are not common enough to warrant mass vaccination in the United States but are found in other parts of the world. When traveling from an area of low rates of infection to areas with high rates, travel vaccines are recommended or required. A **travel vaccine** is a vaccine given in advance of a trip to any location where contact with an infection may occur. Examples of travel vaccines include those for hepatitis and cholera. Travel vaccines must be given well in advance of a trip to allow the immune system enough time to mount the appropriate response and confer full immunity. The time it takes to reach the level of highest immunity differs among vaccines. Many immunizations should be given two or more weeks before travel.

FIGURE 17.3
2020 CDC Immunization Schedule for Adults

The first adult immunization schedule was published by the CDC in 2002 and is updated annually. This figure shows a portion of the 2020 CDC Immunization Schedule for adults. The CDC also publishes an adult immunization schedule based on medical and other indications that is designed for use by healthcare professionals. See https://www.cdc.gov/vaccines/schedules for the complete and most current immunization schedules.

Table 1. Recommended Adult Immunization Schedule for ages 19 years or older, United States, 2020

Always make recommendations by determining needed vaccines based on age (Table 1), assessing for medical conditions and other indications (Table 2), and reviewing special situations (Notes).

Get Email Updates

| Table 1. By age | Table 2. By indications | Schedule Changes & Guidance | Resources for health care providers | Resources for adults | Download schedules app |

- 8.5"x11" print color 📄 [6 pages]
- 8.5"x11" print black and white 📄 [6 pages]
- Compliant version of this schedule

- Vaccines in the Adult Immunization Schedule
- Learn how to display current schedules from your website.
- Hard copies of the schedule are available for free using the CDC-info on Demand order form.

Download Schedules App

Legend

Recommended vaccination for adults who meet age requirement, lack documentation of vaccination, or lack evidence of past infection

Recommended vaccination for adults with an additional risk factor or another indication

Recommended vaccination based on shared clinical decision-making

No recommendation/Not applicable

Vaccine	19-26 years	27-49 years	50-64 years	≥65 years
Influenza inactivated (IIV) or Influenza recombinant (RIV) ❶	1 dose annually			
or Influenza live attenuated (LAIV) ❶	**or** 1 dose annually			
Tetanus, diphtheria, pertussis (Tdap or Td) ❶	1 dose Tdap, then Td or Tdap booster every 10 yrs			
Measles, mumps, rubella (MMR) ❶	1 or 2 doses depending on indication (if born in 1957 or later)			
Varicella (VAR) ❶	2 doses (if born in 1980 or later)		2 doses	
Zoster recombinant (RZV) (preferred) ❶				2 doses
or Zoster live (ZVL) ❶				**or** 1 dose
Human papillomavirus (HPV) ❶	2 or 3 doses depending on age at initial vaccination or condition	27 through 45 years		
Pneumococcal conjugate (PCV13) ❶	1 dose			65 years and older

FIGURE 17.4
2020 CDC Immunization Schedule for Children Ages 0–18

A portion of the immunization schedule for children ages 0 through 18 is shown below. The CDC immunization schedule for children ages 0 through 18 is published annually. See https://www.cdc.gov/vaccines/schedules for the complete and most current immunization schedules.

Table 1. Recommended Child and Adolescent Immunization Schedule for ages 18 years or younger, United States, 2020

Legend

Range of recommended ages for all children	Range of recommended ages for catch-up immunization	Range of recommended ages for certain high-risk groups	Recommended based on shared clinical decision-making or *can be used in this age group	No recommendation/Not applicable

Birth to 15 Months

Vaccine	Birth	1 mo	2 mos	4 mos	6 mos	9 mos	12 mos	15 mos
Hepatitis B ⓘ (HepB)	1st dose	2nd dose			←3rd dose→			
Rotavirus ⓘ (RV) RV1 (2-dose series); RV5 (3-dose series)			1st dose	2nd dose	See notes			
Diphtheria, tetanus, & acellular pertussis ⓘ (DTaP: <7 yrs)			1st dose	2nd dose	3rd dose			←4th dose→
Haemophilus influenzae type b ⓘ (Hib)			1st dose	2nd dose	See notes		←3rd or 4th dose, See notes→	
Pneumococcal conjugate ⓘ (PCV13)			1st dose	2nd dose	3rd dose		←4th dose→	
Inactivated poliovirus ⓘ (IPV: <18 yrs)			1st dose	2nd dose			←3rd dose→	
Influenza (IIV) ⓘ					Annual vaccination 1 or 2 doses			
or Influenza (LAIV) ⓘ								
Measles, mumps, rubella ⓘ (MMR)					See notes		←1st dose→	
Varicella ⓘ (VAR)							←1st dose→	
Hepatitis A ⓘ (HepA)					See notes		←2-dose series, See notes→	
Tetanus, diphtheria, & acellular pertussis ⓘ (Tdap: ≥7 yrs)								
Human papillomavirus ⓘ (HPV)								
Meningococcal ⓘ (MenACWY-D: ≥9 mos; MenACWY-CRM: ≥2 mos)			See notes					
Meningococcal B ⓘ (MenB)								
Pneumococcal polysaccharide ⓘ (PPSV23)								

Range of recommended ages for certain h...

Dosage Forms and Administration Most vaccines require storage in either a refrigerator or freezer. The recommended storage temperature range can differ among vaccines and must be strictly followed. For example, the typhoid vaccine is available in an oral dosage form. The oral vaccine is given as four capsules, one capsule every other day. Oral typhoid capsules must be refrigerated and should be taken with cold or lukewarm water about one hour prior to eating a meal. Most vaccine products cannot be used if frozen. If allowed to warm to room temperature, most vaccines must be used right away (not refrigerated again). In many cases, daily temperature measurement of refrigerators and freezers is required to ensure that stored vaccines are kept at the appropriate temperature and do not spoil. Vaccines that are supplied as powder for injection usually must be used within minutes to hours after reconstitution. Advance mixing and preparation of multiple doses is not recommended. Vaccines should never be mixed in the same syringe with any other medications. If more than one vaccine is administered at the same time, they should be given at different injection sites.

Side Effects Common side effects of vaccines include fever, headache, upset stomach, local injection-site irritation, mild skin rash, and irritability. These symptoms are related to a systemic immune response, which makes a person feel generally tired and achy. It can feel like the onset of the flu, which is why many patients mistakenly believe that the influenza shot gave them the flu. Such symptoms can also occur after injection of other vaccines. All guidelines state specifically that taking acetaminophen for 24 to 48 hours after vaccination usually alleviates these symptoms.

Contraindications The bacillus Calmette-Guérin (BCG) vaccine should not be administered to pregnant patients or to patients who are immunocompromised.

The diphtheria, tetanus, and pertussis vaccine is contraindicated in patients with encephalopathy within seven days of administration of a previous dose of a pertussis vaccine, with or without another identifiable cause. An additional contraindication is progressive neurologic disorder. Certain formulations include latex, and they should not be administered to patients with a latex allergy.

The *Haemophilus influenzae* type B (HIB) vaccine is contraindicated in patients younger than six weeks of age.

The hepatitis A vaccine should not be given to patients with a history of severe reaction to a prior dose of the hepatitis A vaccine or to patients who are highly sensitive to vaccine additives. The hepatitis B vaccine is contraindicated in individuals with a history of hypersensitivity to yeast.

The vaccine for human papillomavirus (HPV) is contraindicated in patients with yeast hypersensitivity.

The influenza vaccine comes in both inactivated and live formulas. The inactivated influenza vaccine is grown in chicken eggs and is contraindicated in patients with egg or chicken allergies. This vaccine should be withheld in children with moderate to severe acute febrile illness and administered only after symptoms resolve. However, minor illness with or without fever is not a contraindication.

Contraindications to the live influenza vaccine include the following: age younger than two years; history of anaphylactic reaction to gelatin or arginine; long-term aspirin or salicylate therapy; history of Guillain-Barré syndrome; asthma in children younger than five years; recurrent wheezing in children ages two through four years; chronic pulmonary, cardiovascular, renal, hepatic, neurologic, hematologic, or metabolic disorders; pregnancy; known or suspected immunodeficiency; or receipt of other live virus vaccine within the previous four weeks.

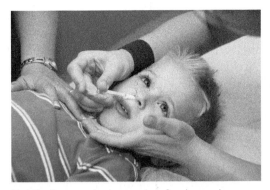

FluMist is a nasal spray option for those who want to get the influenza (flu) vaccine without an injection. This dosage form is only for patients 2 to 50 years of age and contains a live attenuated virus, rather than a deactivated virus. Patients should be made aware of the extra precautions and limitations for the use of FluMist.

The Japanese encephalitis vaccine contains protamine sulfate; therefore, its use should be avoided in patients with protamine hypersensitivity.

Contraindications to the measles, mumps, rubella (MMR) vaccine include anaphylactic reaction to neomycin, pregnancy, and known altered immunodeficiency states. MMR is a live vaccine, and use should be withheld in severe febrile illness until the acute illness has subsided.

The rotavirus vaccine is contraindicated in patients with a history of intussusception (a GI disorder) or severe combined immunodeficiency disease.

The oral typhoid vaccine is contraindicated in immunocompromised patients and patients with an acute febrile illness.

The varicella vaccine is contraindicated in immunocompromised patients because this vaccine contains a live virus.

The yellow fever vaccine should not be given to patients who have a hypersensitivity to egg or chicken protein, children younger than six months, patients who are immunosuppressed (from disorders or use of medications that induce immunosuppression), patients with thymus disorder associated with abnormal immune function, or patients who have undergone organ transplantation.

Contraindications to the herpes zoster vaccine include a history of anaphylactic reaction to gelatin or neomycin, immunosuppression, primary or acquired immunodeficiency states, AIDS or clinical manifestations of HIV, immunosuppressive therapy, and pregnancy.

The meningococcal, pneumococcal, polio (inactivated), and injectable typhoid vaccines do not have contraindications.

Cautions and Considerations Like any drug therapy, vaccinations are not without risk. Patients must receive written information about risks before receiving a vaccination. A **Vaccine Information Statement (VIS)** is available from the CDC for all vaccines on the market. Pharmacy technicians can find samples of these sheets on the CDC website (https://www.cdc.gov/vaccines/hcp/vis/current-vis.html). Prior to vaccination, patients must sign a consent form stating that they are making an informed decision to receive a vaccine and verifying that they have received a VIS for the appropriate vaccine. Quite often, obtaining these signatures and maintaining documentation records are the responsibilities of technicians when vaccines are administered in the pharmacy. These responsibilities should not be taken lightly, because the patient consent form is required by law.

Healthcare personnel giving immunizations must be trained in administering cardiopulmonary resuscitation (CPR) and other necessary treatments in the event of an anaphylactic reaction.

Drug Interactions Patients age 18 or younger receiving the varicella vaccination should avoid taking aspirin or aspirin-containing products for 6 weeks following

Practice Tip

See the CDC website for the most current Vaccine Information Statement (VIS) documents at https://www.cdc.gov/vaccines/hcp/vis/current-vis.html.

administration due to the risk of Reye's syndrome. Following the administration of the varicella vaccine, it is recommended that patients avoid antiviral drugs (such as acyclovir, famciclovir, or valacyclovir) for 14 days. Immune globulins may decrease the response to live vaccines like MMR and varicella vaccines, so it is recommended that these vaccinations be deferred for at least 5 months following administration of immune globulins.

WORKPLACE WISDOM

Some parents choose not to vaccinate their children based on a study that linked autism with the preservatives contained in the measles, mumps, and rubella (MMR) vaccine. This study has since been retracted. Subsequent studies have found no association between the MMR vaccine and autism. The Institute of Medicine and the American Academy of Pediatrics organized panels of independent scientists that concluded there is *no* association between the MMR vaccine and autism. Although subsequent studies did not find a connection, vaccine makers eliminated these preservatives in vaccines for pediatric patients.

17.5 Complementary and Alternative Therapy

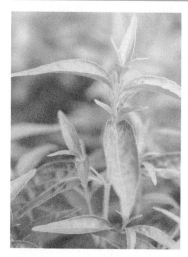

It has been suggested that *Andrographis paniculata* may reduce symptom severity in influenza respiratory infections.

There is some information to suggest that the plant andrographis (*Andrographis paniculata*) may reduce symptom severity and duration of influenza respiratory infections if started quickly (within 36 to 48 hours of symptom onset). Side effects of andrographis include chest discomfort, headache, nausea, and rash. Andrographis may interact with anticoagulants, blood pressure medications, and immunosuppressants.

Colloidal silver is a suspension of submicroscopic silver particles in a colloidal base. Prior to the development of antibiotics, silver-based products were used in the treatment of wounds, bacterial infections, and viral infections. Colloidal silver is used topically (to treat skin infections) and orally (to treat viral, fungal, and bacterial infections). Some individuals use colloidal silver prophylactically for influenza. Total daily silver intake should not exceed 14 mcg/kg. Supplemental silver intake typically exceeds this amount. The risks of silver use are severe and include neurologic deficits and kidney damage. In addition, silver may accumulate in the body and lead to argyria, an irreversible bluish skin discoloration.

Some individuals have used elderberry (*Sambucus nigra*) for influenza. Some evidence suggests it may be effective when initiated within 48 hours of symptom onset. Elderberry extracts may be well tolerated. However, caution should be exercised when using the raw and unripe fruit, seeds, leaves, or other plant parts because they may contain cyanide-like components. Nausea, vomiting, diarrhea, dizziness, numbness, and stupor have been reported with ingestion of unripened fruit and its juice.

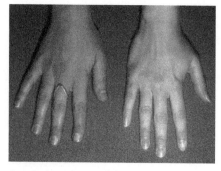

Argyria is an irreversible skin condition that results from silver accumulation.

Review and Assessment

📖 CHAPTER SUMMARY

Viruses and Viral Infections

- Viruses are infectious agents that replicate within a cell by using the host cell's metabolic processes.

- A virus can infect a spectrum of cells, including animal, plant, or bacterial cells.

- All virus-infected cells have some characteristics that are different from those of uninfected cells. These differences offer ways to block viral replication without affecting normal cells.

- Latency is a problem with some viruses. They can lie dormant and then, under certain conditions, reproduce and behave once more like an infectious agent, causing cell damage. Herpesvirus and HIV both have this characteristic.

- Some virus-infected cells produce interferons, which protect neighboring uninfected cells from viral infection.

- Even though the body has defense mechanisms, some viruses can cause normal cells to be transformed into cancer cells.

Antiviral Agents (Nonretroviral)

- A major problem in the development of antivirals is the relationship between host cell and virus. The search for inhibitors of viral activity that are not too toxic to the human host is ongoing.

- Antiherpes agents include acyclovir, famciclovir, valacyclovir, and valganciclovir. Valganciclovir has two boxed warnings: one for hematologic abnormalities and another for reproductive concerns.

- Anti-influenza agents include baloxavir, oseltamivir, peramivir, and zanamivir.

- Ribavirin is another antiviral agent that may be used to treat RSV. Ribavirin has a boxed warning for hemolytic anemia and for teratogenic and embryocidal effects.

HIV/AIDS and Antiretroviral Agents

- Human immunodeficiency virus (HIV) is a retrovirus. It converts its RNA into DNA using the reverse transcriptase enzyme and inserts the DNA into the DNA of the host cell.

- NRTIs work by inhibiting reverse transcriptase. This action prevents the formation of a DNA copy of viral RNA, thus preventing the virus from multiplying or hiding itself within a host cell.

- NNRTIs inhibit HIV reverse transcriptase from adding new nucleotides to the growing DNA chain.

- PIs inhibit the action of the protease enzyme, which cleaves certain HIV protein precursors into smaller proteins, which is necessary for the replication of the virus.

- Fusion inhibitors, also called *entry inhibitors*, prevent HIV from entering immune cells.

- An integrase strand transfer inhibitor blocks the enzyme integrase, which inserts HIV DNA produced by reverse transcriptase into the host cell's DNA.

- Recommended treatment for HIV patients involves a combination of antiretroviral drugs. Because these regimens are often complex and difficult to follow, it is important to encourage proper medication adherence through written instructions and other methods to make taking the regimen easier for patients.

- None of the current drugs can eradicate HIV, but they can improve immunologic status and prolong life.

- An increasing number of manufacturers are combining antiretroviral drugs into one tablet to decrease the pill burden and help improve patient adherence. This innovation is important because partial adherence in patients who have HIV can lead to drug resistance.

Immunity and Immunization

- Immunization can occur naturally, such as in transmission from pregnant parent to fetus and through infection exposure.

- Immunization can also occur artificially, through administration of immunoglobulins or through vaccination.

- The administration of vaccines is the most common form of artificial immunity and is estimated to prevent millions of deaths each year.

- Vaccination recommendations and schedules are released by the CDC in the United States and by the Public Health Agency in Canada.

- Pharmacies are becoming more popular sites of vaccine administration.

- VISs should be given to patients prior to vaccine administration.

- Special attention should be paid to vaccine storage and administration directions.

Complementary and Alternative Therapy

- Patients with HIV and AIDS should discuss any herbal products with a healthcare practitioner prior to use.

- Andrographis, colloidal silver, and elderberry have been used for influenza.

DRUG LIST

Antivirals

Antiherpes Agents
acyclovir (Avaclyr, Sitavig, Zovirax)
famciclovir (Famvir)
valacyclovir (Valtrex)
valganciclovir (Valcyte)

Anti-Influenza Agents
baloxavir marboxil (Xofluza)
oseltamivir (Tamiflu)

peramivir (Rapivab)
zanamivir (Relenza)

Other
ribavirin (Virazole)
palivizumab (Synagis)

Antiretrovirals

NRTIs

abacavir (Ziagen)
palivizumab (Synagis)
abacavir / lamivudine (Epzicom)
abacavir / lamivudine / zidovudine (Trizivir)
efavirenz / emtricitabine / tenofovir (Atripla)
emtricitabine (Emtriva)
emtricitabine / tenofovir disoproxil fumarate (Truvada)
emtricitabine / tenofovir alafenamide (Descovy)
lamivudine (Epivir)
lamivudine / zidovudine (Combivir)
stavudine (Zerit)
tenofovir disoproxil fumarate (Viread)
zidovudine (Retrovir)

NNRTIs

delavirdine (Rescriptor)
doravirine (Pifeltro)
efavirenz (Sustiva)
etravirine (Intelence)
nevirapine (Viramune, Viramune XR)
rilpivirine (Edurant)

PIs

atazanavir (Reyataz)
darunavir (Prezista)
fosamprenavir (Lexiva)
lopinavir / ritonavir (Kaletra)
nelfinavir (Viracept)
ritonavir (Norvir)
tipranavir (Aptivus)

Fusion Inhibitor

enfuvirtide (Fuzeon)

Post-Attachment Inhibitor

ibalizumab (Trogarzo)

CCR5 Antagonist

maraviroc (Selzentry)

Integrase Strand Transfer Inhibitors

bictegravir / emtricitabine / tenofovir alafenamide (Biktarvy)
dolutegravir (Tivicay)
raltegravir (Isentress)

Combinations

abacavir / lamivudine (Epzicom)
abacavir / lamivudine / zidovudine (Trizivir)

bictegravir / tenofovir / emtricitabine (Biktarvy)
doravirine / lamivudine / tenofovir (Delstrigo)
dolutegravir / lamivudine (Dovato)
efavirenz / emtricitabine / tenofovir (Atripla)
efavirenz / lamivudine / tenofovir (Symfi, Symfi Lo)
elvitegravir / cobicistat / emtricitabine / tenofovir alafenamide (Genvoya)
elvitegravir / cobicistat / emtricitabine / tenofovir disoproxil fumarate (Stribild)
emtricitabine / tenofovir (Truvada)
emtricitabine / tenofovir alafenamide (Descovy)
lamivudine / tenofovir (Cimduo)
lamivudine / zidovudine (Combivir)

Boxed Warnings

abacavir / lamivudine (Epzicom)
bictegravir / emtricitabine / tenofovir (Biktarvy)
darunavir / cobicistat / emtricitabine / tenofovir alafenamide (Symtuza)
dolutegravir / lamivudine (Dovato)
doravirine / lamivudine / tenofovir disoproxil fumarate (Delstrigo)
efavirenz / emtricitabine / tenofovir (Atripla)
efavirenz / emtricitabine / tenofovir disoproxil fumarate (Atripla)
efavirenz / lamivudine / tenofovir disoproxil fumarate (Symfi, Symfi Lo)
elvitegravir / cobicistat / emtricitabine / tenofovir alafenamide (Genvoya)
elvitegravir / cobicistat / emtricitabine / tenofovir disoproxil fumarate (Stribild)
emtricitabine (Emtriva)
emtricitabine / tenofovir alafenamide (Descovy)
emtricitabine / tenofovir disoproxil fumarate (Truvada)
lamivudine (Epivir)
lamivudine / tenovovir disoproxil fumarate (Cimduo)
lamivudine / zidovudine (Combivir)
maraviroc (Selzentry)
nevirapine (Viramune)
ribavirin (Virazole)
ritonavir (Norvir)
tenofovir (Viread)
tipranavir (Aptivus)
valacyclovir (Valtrex)
valganciclovir (Valcyte)
zidovudine (Retrovir)

Take a moment to review what you have learned in this chapter and answer the following questions.

1. Which of the following is not treated with acyclovir?
   a chicken pox
   b. genital herpes
   c. influenza
   d. herpes zoster

2. Which drug requires the pharmacy technician to use chemotherapy agent precautions when mixing?
   a. Zovirax
   b. Valcyte
   c. Famvir
   d. Videx

3. Which of the following is administered more than one time a day?
   a. Biktarvy
   b. Truvada
   c. Combivir
   d. Stribild

4. Which medication is used as PrEP?
   a. Truvada
   b. Fortovase
   c. Atripla
   d. Retrovir

5. Which drug is primarily prescribed to boost another drug?
   a. ritonavir (Norvir)
   b. maraviroc (Selzentry)
   c. tenofovir (Viread)
   d. enfuvirtide (Fuzon)

6. Which of the following is an NNRTI?
   a. amantadine
   b. efavirenz
   c. ritonavir
   d. stavudine

7. Stribild is an HIV combination product containing
   a. abacavir and lamivudine.
   b. favirenz, emtricitabine, and tenofovir.
   c. elvitegravir, cobicistat, emtricitabine, and tenofovir.
   d. emtricitabine and tenofovir.

8. Which of the following viral diseases can be prevented with a vaccine?
   a. HSV-1
   b. hepatitis B
   c. hepatitis C
   d. HIV

9. Which of the following brand names refers to an injectable vaccine for influenza?
   a. Pneumovax
   b. FluMist
   c. Fluzone
   d. Varivax

10. What information should be given to patients prior to administering a vaccination?
   a. CDC Immunization Schedule
   b. Vaccine Package Insert
   c. Vaccine Information Statement
   d. Healthcare Directive Form

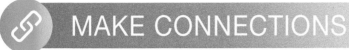

MAKE CONNECTIONS

Take a moment to consider what you have learned in this chapter and respond thoughtfully to the following prompts. Note that some of these activities will require internet access.

1. The drug being dispensed to the patient is Biktarvy. The other technician working with you does not want to wait on the patient for fear of contracting HIV. How will you respond to the technician and the patient?

2. You are on a retreat at a camp in the mountains. An HIV-positive camper forgot to bring an antiseptic. The camp director knows you are in the medical field and asks for your advice. What should you do?

 The online course includes additional review and assessment resources.

18 Pain, Anesthesia, and Drug Therapy

Learning Objectives

1. Describe the major sources of pain. (Section 18.1)

2. Identify the difference between acute and chronic pain. (Section 18.1)

3. Describe the role of opioid analgesics in pain management and the primary hazards of their use. (Section 18.2)

4. Describe the role of nonopioid analgesics in pain management. (Section 18.2)

5. Define opioid use disorder and describe its treatments. (Section 18.3)

6. Explain the purpose of anesthesia and compare the different types of intervention. (Section 18.4)

7. Identify how medications help support sedation and analgesia and the primary risks with use. (Section 18.4)

8. Identify different types of neuromuscular blocking agents and how these agents can be reversed. (Section 18.4)

9. Identify current medications used to manage migraines. (Section 18.5)

ASHP/ACPE Accreditation Standards

To view the *ASHP/ACPE Accreditation Standards* addressed in this chapter, refer to Appendix C.

Many medications are created to control discomfort and minimize pain. Recall that the nervous system is responsible for facilitating signals within the body, and these signals include pain signals. Most drugs commonly used to anesthetize patients, relieve pain, and alleviate migraine headaches interact with the body by influencing the electrical and chemical signaling of the nervous system or its target tissues. This chapter concentrates on these anesthetic agents, opioid and nonopioid analgesics (pain relievers), and agents for migraine headache relief.

18.1 Physiology of Pain

Pain is generally defined as physically or emotionally sensed discomfort that is associated with, or looks like it may be associated with, acute tissue damage or a sensory system malfunction. It is typically categorized and addressed by cause, timing, or how it is experienced.

Pain receptors, also known as *nociceptors*, within the body are activated when a stimulus such as an extreme temperature or a cut could damage tissue. Pain perception arises from the transmission of nerve impulses from these receptors. Serving primarily as a protective signal, pain warns of damage or the presence of disease. It is also a normal part of healing. This process involves inflammation, in which protective cells move into the injured area and release chemical mediators that cause fluids and plasma proteins to leak into the surrounding tissue.

Pain Mechanisms

Pain mechanisms include nociceptive, inflammatory, neuropathic, and centralized pain, and they often overlap. Major sources of pain, their characteristics, and their treatment are listed in Table 18.1.

TABLE 18.1 Major Sources of Pain

Source	Areas Involved	Characteristics	Pain Source Examples	Pharmacologic Management
nociceptive (somatic)	bones, muscles, ligaments	throbbing, stabbing, well localized	osteoarthritis, broken arm, postoperative healing	acetaminophen, NSAIDs, opioids, local anesthetics, antihistamines, dexmedetomidine, low-dose ketamine
nociceptive (visceral)	kidneys, intestines, liver	aching, throbbing, sharp, gnawing, cramping, deep squeezing; associated with sweating, nausea, vomiting	kidney stones, myocardial infarction (heart attack) pain	acetaminophen, NSAIDs, opioid agonists, local anesthetics, antihistamines, dexmedetomidine, low-dose ketamine, antiemetics
neuropathic	nerve damage	burning, tingling, numbing, shooting, viselike, stabbing, constant	diabetic neuropathy, postherpetic neuralgia	antidepressants (duloxetine, venlafaxine, amitriptyline, nortriptyline), anticonvulsants (gabapentin, pregabalin), topicals (lidocaine, capsaicin)
centralized	dysregulated pain processing in the central nervous system	occurring when no pain should be felt	fibromyalgia, sickle cell disease	antidepressants (duloxetine, venlafaxine, amitriptyline, nortriptyline), anticonvulsants (gabapentin, pregabalin)

Nociceptive Pain

Nociceptive pain is perceived when pain receptors sense damage to tissues. This can be either *somatic* nociceptive pain related to skin, muscles, and bones or *visceral* nociceptive pain related to the organs. Pain receptors may be activated via a mechanical injury (such as a cut), a chemical irritation or burn, or a broken bone. The pain signal is then transmitted to the central nervous system (CNS). The CNS messages back to the peripheral nervous system to dampen, or sometimes to amplify, the original pain signal. Pain in this context is primarily a protective signal to warn of damage or the presence of disease and is a normal part of healing. **Inflammatory pain**, a type of nociceptive pain, generally stems from the release of proinflammatory neurotransmitters, such as histamine, prostaglandins, and inflammatory cytokines. During inflammation, protective cells move into the injured area and release chemical mediators that cause fluids and plasma proteins to leak into the surrounding tissue.

Neuropathic Pain

Neuropathic pain is abnormal pain signaling that occurs in the CNS or PNS and occurs when nerve fibers are overactive and send pain signals when pain should be felt. This type of pain is often associated with nerve damage, which usually occurs as a result of trauma to the area caused by disease, lesions, injury, or malfunctions. Examples of conditions predominated by neuropathic pain include diabetic neuropathy, postherpetic neuralgia associated with shingles, stroke or spine injury, and trigeminal neuralgia. Examples that are both nociceptive and neuropathic in nature include arthritis conditions and lower back pain due to spinal nerve compression or injury. Neuropathic pain is traditionally experienced as burning, tingling, numbing, shooting, or stabbing pain that tends to be constant regardless of activity.

Medications often used for this type of pain include:

- pregabalin and gabapentin (see Chapter 7)
- serotonin-norepinephrine reuptake inhibitors (SNRIs): duloxetine, extended-release venlafaxine (see Chapter 8)
- tricyclic antidepressant: amitriptyline (see Chapter 8)
- topical options like OTC capsaicin cream, though that may take a couple of weeks to achieve full effect

Centralized Pain

Centralized pain is a type of pain that happens when the CNS doesn't process pain signals properly. Centralized pain is common in conditions like fibromyalgia, chronic pelvic pain syndromes, and phantom limb pain. It is known to overlap with nociceptive and neuropathic pain. Injuries cause changes in pain receptors and pain processing pathways. These changes include heightening pain receptor sensitivity, activating inflammation, and reducing the body's natural ability to suppress pain signaling. Although these responses occur with a standard injury and usually resolve with healing, sometimes pain amplification is left "on." This reaction may be due to a slow-to-heal nerve injury or chronic inflammation. Rewiring can occur as the changes become semipermanent in the nociceptive or neuropathic pathways, making inflammation and increased sensitivity a chronic problem.

Timing of Pain

Another way to categorize pain is by the timing. The timing of pain is an important element in understanding pain mechanisms and directly managing pain. Pain is typically considered *acute* if it occurs within 6 weeks of a pain-inducing event, while it is thought to have progressed to *chronic* pain if it continues beyond 12 weeks. This type of classification categorizes pain as acute, chronic nonmalignant, or chronic malignant.

Acute pain is associated with trauma or surgery. Acute pain is usually easier to manage by identifying and treating the cause, and it usually disappears once the body has healed. For most individuals, most, if not all, healing is achieved within three months. Acute pain typically consists of nociceptive and inflammatory pain, though there may be elements of neuropathic pain if nerves were affected by the injury.

Chronic nonmalignant pain describes pain that lasts longer than twelve weeks and may or may not have a diagnosed cause. Chronic nonmalignant pain may have one or more pain mechanisms, including nociceptive and inflammatory pathways (like arthritis-related conditions), neuropathic pathways (like diabetic neuropathy), and centralized sensitization (like fibromyalgia).

Chronic malignant pain describes pain that accompanies malignant disease and often increases in severity as the disease progresses. This pain is experienced with cancer; it gets progresively more severe as the disease progresses and near the end of life.

The treatments associated with acute pain and chronic pain differ greatly. Whereas acute pain has a beginning and an end and warns of a problem, chronic pain does not cease when an illness is cured or injury is healed. An individual with chronic pain may also suffer from feelings of helplessness and hopelessness. Chronic pain has the potential to cause additional negative physical, psychological, and social outcomes.

Physiologic responses to pain vary and include the following:

- catabolism (tissues such as muscle are broken down)
- delayed stomach and bowel function
- impaired immune response
- increased autonomic activity (heart rate and blood pressure)
- increased metabolism
- muscle rigidity
- negative emotional response (depression)
- shallow breathing
- water retention

Response to Pain

How pain is experienced is another way of categorizing and addressing pain. **Background pain** is a term used to describe a constant level of pain, while **breakthrough pain** describes when pain of greater intensity occurs intermittently for no particular reason. **Provoked pain** describes pain that is more intense than background pain but has a clear cause, like a wound cleaning.

It is important to note that the experience of pain is incredibly unique to each person, regardless of whether it follows a surgical incision, is persistent lower back pain, or is pain secondary to cancer. Pain is influenced by biological, psychological, and social factors, such as its origin or cause, comorbidities like kidney disease or diabetes, preexisting mood or cognition conditions, personal or family history, psychological coping mechanisms, and familial or community support systems.

Note that studies continue to find that many factors affect an individual's pain threshold. Adequate sleep, mood elevation, diversion, sympathy, and understanding all can raise an individual's pain threshold. Alternatively, fatigue, anxiety, fear, anger, sadness, depression, and isolation can lower the pain threshold.

Because the perception of pain can be subjective, thorough patient assessment and selection of the most successful and cost-effective therapy in pain management is challenging. Goals of pain management include enhancing functionality and productivity to improve the patient's quality of life. Studies have demonstrated that pain is often undertreated, and this deficiency can, in some cases, delay recovery from the condition causing the pain. To adequately control pain, the appropriate medication must sometimes be administered around the clock.

Inadequate treatment of pain can have adverse physiological, psychological, and immunological effects. Good clinical care must be based on the optimization of risk-benefit considerations.

18.2 Opioids and Pain Management

Work Wise

It is worth noting that pain, although a difficult and sometimes traumatic psychological experience, is not innately a deadly medical condition.

A drug that alleviates pain is known as an **analgesic**. In practice, analgesics are typically used to describe drugs addressing nociceptive pain. Most drugs used for neuropathic or centralized pain have other indications, and they are often described as drugs *with analgesic activity*. Opioids are a type of analgesic frequently encountered in pharmacy.

Nociceptive pain often resolves with tissue healing, which should be complete or nearly complete within six weeks. The goal of pain management is to provide enough pain relief using the least amount of drug therapy for the shortest time needed. Pharmacologic therapy for mild nociceptive pain and accompanying inflammation includes acetaminophen, NSAIDs, and antihistamines. In most cases, these nonopioid analgesics are enough to provide adequate pain relief. Options for severe nociceptive pain generally include regional anesthesia (with local anesthetics where possible), opiates, and ketamine.

Nonpharmacologic management should be used when possible and appropriate. It can include psychoeducational interventions like cognitive behavioral therapy and patient education as well as physical interventions like physical therapy, acupuncture, and chiropractic manipulation. Mind-body therapies that mix movement, body awareness, breathing, thought patterns, and emotions can be beneficial. Simpler nonpharmacological methods can include transcutaneous nerve stimulation units, heat, and cold.

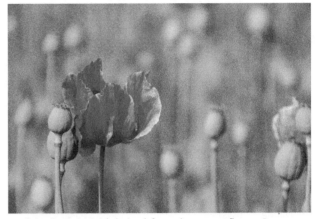

Codeine is an opioid derived from the poppy flower *Papaver somniferum*.

Opioid Analgesics

Members of the **opioid** drug class include naturally occurring opioids, like morphine and codeine from the opium poppy flower *Papaver somniferum*, as well as their semisynthetic derivatives (oxycodone, hydrocodone, hydromorphone, heroin) and synthetic derivatives (methadone, fentanyl). Although *opioid* is a term that can be used to describe all members of this class, the term **opiate** refers only to naturally occurring forms.

Name Exchange

Although narcotic and opioid are often used interchangeably, the term used most often in health care is *opioid*.

These drugs are often referred to as *narcotics*; however, that is a term used more in law enforcement than in pharmacy practice. *Narcotic* stems from the Greek word for "stupor," because these drugs cause a dulling of the senses. In practice, the term *opioid* is more common between prescribers and patients, while the term *narcotic* is used most often when discussing these agents as they relate to the Drug Enforcement Administration (DEA) and regulations.

Opioids and opiates have the ability to reduce pain signals from most sources (analgesia), ease anxiety and cause **sedation** (drowsiness), and produce **euphoria** (feelings of well-being) or **dysphoria** (a state of feeling unwell or unhappy). All opioids have the potential to induce tolerance and dependence.

The brain makes three types of natural opioids in response to pain stimuli; these natural opioids include endorphins, enkephalins, and dynorphins. As pain increases, the levels of these chemicals also increase. When they bind to opioid receptors in the part of the brain that processes pain signals, they provide pain relief. Pain signals originate when nociceptors located in the skin, muscles, bones, organs, joints, and tendons sense stimuli from tissue damage. Opioid medications work by binding and activating the same receptors that these natural substances do. The pain receptors in the CNS are in the limbic system, thalamus, hypothalamus, midbrain, and spinal cord. Additional receptors are found in the adrenal medulla and nerve plexus. The primary opioid receptor target for analgesia is called *mu* (μ; pronounced like "mew"); two others that also provide analgesia are delta (δ) and kappa (κ) receptor targets. Most opioid medications are full mu agonists, and some have mixed opioid receptor activity. Table 18.2 lists products with only one opioid medication, while Table 18.5 addresses combination products.

TABLE 18.2 Commonly Used Opioid Analgesics and Antagonists

Generic (Brand)	Pronunciation	Dosage Form	Common Dosage	Dispensing Status	Controlled Substance Schedule
Mu Opioid Agonists					
codeine (various brands)	KOE-deen	tablet	15–60 mg every 4 hr as needed	Rx	C-II
fentanyl (Abstral, Actiq, Duragesic, Fentora, Lazanda, Subsys)	FEN-ta-nil	buccal tablet, injection, lozenge, nasal spray, sublingual film, sublingual spray, sublingual tablet, transdermal patch	individualized to patient based on dosage form	Rx	C-II
hydrocodone (Hysingla ER, Zohydro ER)	hye-droe-KOE-doan	capsule, tablet	individualized to patient	Rx	C-II
methadone (Dolophine, Methadose)	METH-a-doan	injection, oral solution, suppository, tablet	tablet: 2–4 mg every 4–6 hr as needed; oral solution: 2.5–10 mg every 3–6 hr as needed; IV infusion: 0.2–1 mg every 2–3 hr as needed; IM, SC: 1–2 mg every 2–3 hr	Rx	C-II
morphine (Arymo, Astramorph, Duramorph, Infumorph, Kadian, Mitigo, MS Contin, Oramorph)	MOR-feen	injection, oral dissolving tablet, oral solution, oral tablet	IV: 2.5–10 mg every 8–12 hr; PO: 20–30 mg every 2–4 hr	Rx	C-II
oxycodone (Oxaydo, OxyCONTIN, Roxicodone, Xtampza)	ox-see-KOE-doan	capsule, injection, oral solution, rectal suppository, tablet	PO: 10 mg every 4 hr as needed; IV: 1–4 mg every 4 hr as needed; IM: 5–10 mg every 3–4 hours as needed; rectal: 10 mg every 4 hr as needed	Rx	C-II

continues

TABLE 18.2 Commonly Used Opioid Analgesics and Antagonists—*Continued*

Generic (Brand)	Pronunciation	Dosage Form	Common Dosage	Dispensing Status	Controlled Substance Schedule
tapentadol (Nucynta)	ta-PEN-ta-dol	tablet	50–100 mg every 4–6 hr as needed	Rx	C-II
tramadol (ConZip, Synapryn, Ultram)	TRAM-a-dol	tablet, oral suspension, topical cream, capsule	50–100 mg every 4–6 hr as needed	Rx	C-IV
Mixed Opioid Agents					
buprenorphine (Belbuca, Buprenex, Butrans, Probuphine, Sublocade)	byoo-pre-NOR-feen	buccal film, injection, sublingual tablet, transdermal patch	IV: 0.3 mg every 6–8 hr as needed patch: 5 mcg/hr applied every 7 days sublingual tablet: 2–4 mg per dose, up to 8 mg per day	Rx	C-III
butorphanol	byoo-TOR-fa-nawl	injection, nasal spray	IM: 2 mg every 3–4 hr as needed IV: 1 mg every 3–4 hr as needed spray: 1–2 sprays in each nostril every 3–4 hr as needed	Rx	C-IV
nalbuphine	NAL-byoo-feen	injection	10 mg every 3–6 hr as needed	Rx	
Opioid Antagonists					
naloxone	nal-OX-own	injection, nasal spray	0.4–2 mg every 2–3 min as needed	Rx or directly from pharmacist	
naltrexone (Vivitrol)	nal-TREX-own	injection	PO: 25–100 mg per day IM: 380 mg once every 4 weeks	Rx	

Dosing and Administering Opioids

Progressive increases in opioid-related deaths have led to initiatives to reduce opioid use and overdose. Many opioid products that used to be available have been taken off the market to reduce abuse and overprescribing. Approaches to treating pain have recently evolved to encourage nonopioid pain management whenever possible and to limit use of opioids to short-term therapy.

Morphine is the standard against which all other opioids are measured. Some drugs are more potent (requiring smaller dose for the same effect) than morphine, but doses can be adjusted to provide equivalent effect. An **equianalgesic dose** is a dose that offers an equal amount of analgesia. Equianalgesic doses can be roughly determined using opioid conversion charts; these conversions are also used to determine patients' total daily doses of opioids, defined in morphine milligram equivalents (MME). Table 18.3 lists common opioid analgesics and provides dosage equivalents to 10 mg of morphine.

TABLE 18.3 Conversion Factors for Determining Morphine Milligram Equivalents (MME)

These equivalents will vary slightly, depending on reference. They also do not take individual patient genetics and drug metabolism into account.

Oral Opioid	Multiply by this conversion factor for approximate equivalent dose in MME
codeine (mg/day)	0.15
fentanyl transdermal (mcg/hr)	2.4
hydrocodone (mg/day)	1
hydromorphone (mg/day)	4
methadone 1–20 (mg/day)	4
methadone 21–40 (mg/day)	8
methadone 41–60 (mg/day)	10
methadone ≥ 61 (mg/day)	12
morphine (mg/day)	1
oxycodone (mg/day)	1.5

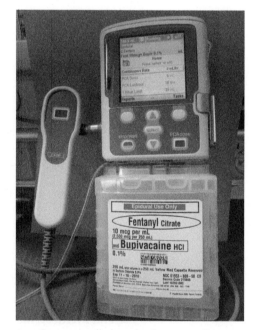

A patient-controlled analgesia pump allows the patient to regulate the amount of pain medication received. This results in better pain control with less drug used.

This PCA pump button should be pushed only BY THE PATIENT

Opioids have no target dose, though with chronic, noncancerous pain, there is little evidence to support significant benefit in increasing doses above 90 MME per day. In contrast, opioid requirements can be significant for cancer-related pain. Nevertheless, just as the pain experience is unique to every patient, so is opioid response. Dosing response can vary due to age, weight, kidney and liver function, genetic differences in drug metabolism, other medications, other medical conditions, the severity of tissue injury or receptor and transmitter dysregulation, and how the patient psychologically processes the pain experience. Since dosing is unique to each patient, opioids should be titrated as needed after other pain medications or nonpharmacological alternatives have been optimized. The best dose is one that allows the patient to complete daily activities and supports quality of life without excessive or intolerable adverse effects. It is worth noting that for the vast majority of patients, it is not possible to achieve complete pain relief.

Opioids can be delivered by several routes. Oral doses of most drugs are essentially equivalent to rectal suppository doses, and intramuscular doses are essentially equivalent to subcutaneous doses. A subcutaneous dose of morphine is two to three times as potent as an oral dose. When patients cannot tolerate oral medications (due to nausea or vomiting, for instance), the rectal suppository route can be considered.

Work Wise

When opioids are dispensed, they must always be counted twice. The number is then circled on either the label of the bottle or the label attached to the back of the prescription. This notation indicates that the correct amount was dispensed and verified, since patients displaying behaviors of substance abuse may say they were shorted.

Another alternative is subcutaneous or IV infusion. Intravenous doses are usually more potent than intramuscular or subcutaneous doses. An effective means of controlling pain in hospitalized patients is the **patient-controlled analgesia (PCA) pump**, given by intravenous infusion. The patient regulates, within prescriber-set limits, the amount of drug received by pushing a button controlled only by the patient. Better pain control can be achieved with lower doses when patients administer the drug at the onset of pain. Once pain has been ongoing for a long time, it is much more difficult to control. Another remarkable development in pain control is the transdermal patch. By providing stable blood levels of drug, the patch seems to control pain more effectively than other forms of delivery while allowing the patient to remain more alert. The route and administration affect both the onset and the duration of action.

Opioid Side Effects

Common effects of opioids include mental clouding or confusion, reduced alertness, nausea, vomiting, dry mouth, constipation, difficulty urinating, flushing, decreased blood pressure, and difficulty breathing (especially in persons with asthma). Most side effects fade within a week or two, except for constipation, which lasts for the duration of opioid therapy. The side effects of opioids should be anticipated and minimized.

Opioids are known to cause constipation or the slowing of movement through the bowels in the days after starting or increasing the dose of an opioid. Opioids inhibit normal peristalsis in the GI system, causing reduced movement. Patients who are prescribed opioids are typically also prescribed laxatives to address this side effect.

Opioid use may also cause urinary retention due to spasmodic activity of the urethra and major sphincter of the bladder. This spasmodic activity can last from 24 to 48 hours and is most pronounced in patients over 55 years of age. Patients can also experience postural hypotension and dizziness.

Nausea is also a common side effect of opioids. Opioids act on an area in the brain identified as the chemoreceptor trigger zone (CTZ), which in turn acts on the vomiting center to produce emesis (the act of vomiting). This can be very dangerous in a patient heavily sedated with opioids, such as in the ICU, because vomit can block the airway. Changing opioids or administering antiemetics may be done to avoid or offset this reaction.

Opioids may stimulate seizures in patients with epileptic disorders, generally when combined with other drugs that can reduce the seizure threshold. Spasms can also be a sign of neurotoxicity and typically are accompanied by slowed cognition and sleepiness.

Most opioids are metabolized by the liver. Serious liver disease may cause the patient to become comatose (a state of profound unconsciousness). Reduced doses must be used in patients with serious liver disease.

Long-term use, particularly of morphine, methadone, or fentanyl, can increase infection risk due to suppression of the immune system.

Opioid Cautions and Considerations

Although opioids and opiates are effective analgesics used for pain, the euphoric effects can cause overuse or misuse. Patients with history of misuse or who are taking opioids for longer than intended can be at risk for developing opioid use disorder. **Opioid use disorder** is characterized by a persistent desire to use opioids. When possible, opioids should be avoided in patients with a history of substance use disorder.

Opioids should be used with caution in patients with liver or kidney disease, as the body will be slower with drug metabolism and elimination. Opioids should also be used with caution in patients with respiratory conditions like COPD, severe asthma, or sleep apnea, since opioids make it harder for the body to obtain sufficient oxygen.

Safety Alert

Two common signs of opioid-caused toxicity or overdose are a low respiratory rate and pinpoint pupils.

Respiratory depression and sedation are dose related. Appropriately prescribed opioids rarely cause clinically significant respiratory depression. Any opioids should be started or increased cautiously in patients with COPD, severe asthma, or sleep apnea. Other CNS depressants, like benzodiazepines, barbiturates, and alcohol, have additive effects, increasing the risk of respiratory depression, profound sedation, coma, and death. These risks are greatest when newly starting, increasing, or adding a CNS depressant.

Symptoms of opioid overdose are respiratory depression, decreased body temperature, decreased blood pressure, tachycardia (abnormally rapid heart rate), and coma. Naloxone and assisted ventilation are used to treat opiate-associated respiratory depression.

Opioids should be used with caution in patients with thyroid dysfunction; with a head injury, as opioids can raise intercranial pressure; or with a mental health disorder, due to increased risk for substance use disorder.

All opioids carry boxed warnings for the following:

Safety Alert

Opioids carry a number of boxed warnings. These include risk of abuse, respiratory depression, and neonatal opioid withdrawal syndrome in exposed infants.

- risk of misuse, abuse, and addiction, which can lead to overdose or death
- risk of life-threatening respiratory depression, particularly with accidental ingestion, a too-high dose at the start of therapy, a dose increase, or a change to a long-acting formulation, or with any drug interaction that causes opioid plasma levels to rise or that further reduces respiratory drive
- risk of neonatal opioid withdrawal syndrome in exposed infants at birth following the pregnant parent's opioid use during pregnancy

Long-term use of opioids can also lead to hypogonadism. Signs in people with testes include decreased testosterone and sperm counts, fatigue, mood effects, and bone loss. There is less literature on presentation in females, but signs may include postmenopausal symptoms, fatigue, mood effects, and bone loss.

An increased risk of overdose can follow interactions with specific drugs that slow opioid metabolism. These drugs can inhibit the liver metabolism enzyme cytochrome P450 3A4, slowing the body's deactivation of opioids.

An increased risk for serotonin syndrome occurs when opioids are taken with antidepressants and other drugs that affect serotonin. Most cases occur within 24 hours of the start or increase of the interacting drug. Signs can include mental status changes (anxiety, disorientation, agitation), sweating, heart palpitations, increase in body temperature, high blood pressure, vomiting, diarrhea, and tremors.

Mu Opioid Agonists

Opioids work by binding and activating the same receptors that the opiates created in the body do. Mu opioid agonists include codeine, fentanyl, hydromorphone, methadone (Dolophine, Methadose), morphine (Arymo, Astramorph, Duramorph, Infumorph, Kadian, Mitigo, MS Contin, Oramorph), oxycodone (Oxaydo, OxyCONTIN, Roxicodone, Xtampza), tapentadol (Nucynta), and tramadol (ConZip, Enovra, Synapryn, Ultram).

Safety Alert

The words *codeine* and *Lodine* (an NSAID) can look alike if written with poor handwriting.

Codeine

Codeine (various brands) is an opioid analgesic indicated, when clinically appropriate, for mild to moderate pain. It is also used off label for short-term cough relief and for restless leg syndrome. It is an alkaloid derived from opium. Codeine is converted to morphine in the liver, is not approved for IV administration, and is most frequently marketed with acetaminophen. While codeine is a Schedule II controlled substance, combinations of codeine with another drug used for mild to moderate pain or diarrhea are Schedule III, Schedule IV, or Schedule V controlled substances. Even in those locales where diluted codeine preparations are available OTC, very few pharmacists will sell them without a prescription. To do so, they must maintain a log. Many states have their own laws regarding these products. Codeine is considered less addictive than other opiates.

Dosage Forms and Administration   Refer to the Dosing and Administering Opioids section.

Side Effects   Refer to the Opioid Side Effects section.

Contraindications   Codeine is contraindicated in patients with a history of hypersensitivity to codeine; patients under 12 years of age; and postoperative, pediatric patients under 18 years of age who received a tonsillectomy or adenoidectomy. Codeine is contraindicated in patients with acute asthma, significant respiratory depression, or hypersensitivity to methadone.

Cautions and Considerations   In addition to standard opioid precautions, further consideration about codeine use should be taken with patients who are older adults. Codeine carries boxed warnings related to addiction, misuse, respiratory depression, neonatal withdrawal syndrome, and combination with benzodiazepines or alcohol. This drug must be dispensed with a Medication Guide.

Drug Interactions   Major drug interactions include concurrent use with other opioid analgesics and CNS depressants, which may result in additive respiratory and cardiovascular depression. Codeine should not be used by patients who have taken an MAOI in the previous fourteen days.

Fentanyl

Fentanyl (Abstral, Actiq, Duragesic, Fentora, Lazanda, Subsys), also discussed in the Anesthesia section, is a potent synthetic analgesic. It comes in a wide variety of forms. Fentanyl also has a variety of formulations used for management of chronic pain, particularly cancer-related pain. Fentanyl should *not* be used for acute pain, because it cannot be titrated quickly in response to patient pain or adverse effects.

Dosage Forms and Administration   One of the most common fentanyl products is Duragesic, a 72-hour transdermal patch. The patch is applied to a dry area on the body and left in place for 72 hours. The patch works by releasing fentanyl into fat tissue, which stores the drug and slowly releases it into the bloodstream. Body temperature, skin type, and placement of the patch all determine how effective the pain control is. Proper disposal of these patches is very important, because used patches still contain some of the drug and must be carefully handled. These patches must not be cut.

Fentanyl buccal lozenges (Actiq) are berry flavored and should be held against the mucosal surfaces inside the mouth and under the tongue. They are most effective when allowed to dissolve over a period of 10 to 15 minutes. The lozenge is less effective if swallowed. A disadvantage to this dosage form is that the dosing is imprecise when a patient doesn't allow the entire lozenge to dissolve before spitting it out.

Abstral is a sublingual form of fentanyl. It is not equivalent to other dosage forms. It comes in a blister pack that must be peeled back. The pill must not be pushed through, as this could damage the pill and alter the dosing. Fentora, the buccal pellet, is effervescent and absorbed through the buccal mucosa. An advantage of this dosage form is quicker absorption into the bloodstream at lower dosage levels. Lazanda is a nasal spray to be used for breakthrough pain. Like Abstral and Subsys, it is not equivalent to other products. Subsys is a sublingual spray. It is not comparable to other fentanyl dosage forms, because there are differences in its pharmacologic profile, and it only has an established conversion process for Actiq.

Side Effects Refer to the Opioid Side Effects section.

Contraindications Intravenous fentanyl is only contraindicated in those with hypersensitivity to fentanyl. Longer-acting products used

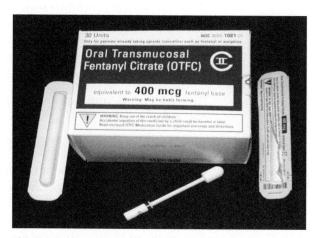

This image shows an example of an oral transmucosal fentanyl lozenge.

for chronic pain are contraindicated in acute or postoperative pain, including headache, migraine, or dental pain. Fentanyl is contraindicated in patients with acute asthma, significant respiratory depression, or hypersensitivity to fentanyl. It also should not be used for acute pain in the emergency room.

Cautions and Considerations General opioid precautions apply to all formulations of fentanyl. Different fentanyl products should not be converted on a microgram-per-microgram basis. Hypoventilation may occur at any dose with transmucosal administration. Proper disposal of patches is important, particularly if children are in the household. Patches must be folded in half, sticky sides together, and flushed down the toilet or returned to a drug take-back program. Subsys is available only through a Risk Evaluation and Mitigation Strategy (REMS), requiring healthcare professionals who want to prescribe or dispense it to enroll in the program.

Fentanyl carries boxed warnings related to addiction, misuse, respiratory depression, neonatal withdrawal syndrome, and combination with benzodiazepines or alcohol. Education programs are available to healthcare providers about opioid use. This drug must be dispensed with a Medication Guide.

Drug Interactions Major drug interactions with fentanyl include other CNS depressants, MAOIs, SSRIs, SNRIs, and dextromethorphan.

Hydrocodone

Hydrocodone (Hysingla ER, Zohydro ER) is an analgesic related to codeine. Hydromorphone is a metabolite of hydrocodone. Because hydrocodone is frequently abused, in 2014, the FDA changed its regulatory status from Schedule III to the more regulated Schedule II.

Dosing Forms and Administration In addition to the information provided in the Dosing and Administering Opioids section, hydrocodone is available as an extended-release, single-drug formulation.

Side Effects Refer to the Opioid Side Effects section.

Contraindications Hydrocodone use is contraindicated in patients with acute asthma, significant respiratory depression, or hypersensitivity or anaphylaxis reactions to opioids.

Cautions and Considerations Hydrocodone carries boxed warnings related to addiction, use, misuse, respiratory depression, neonatal withdrawal syndrome, and combination with benzodiazepines or alcohol. This drug must be dispensed with a Medication Guide. Standard opioid precautions apply to hydrocodone formulations. In addition, in acetaminophen-containing formulations, the total daily dose of acetaminophen, including acetaminophen in both prescription and over-the-counter products, needs to be kept below 4 grams per day. This limit should drop to 3 grams per day in geriatric patients and in those with alcoholism or liver dysfunction.

Drug Interactions Drugs that have major interactions with hydrocodone include drugs with serotonergic activity, such as MAOIs, SSRIs, SNRIs, and dextromethorphan.

Hydromorphone

Safety Alert

To help reduce medication error, technicians should verify both the total dose in milligrams and the total volume in milliliters for hydromorphone and hydromorphone HP, because confusion between the two may result in accidental overdose and death.

Hydromorphone (Dilaudid, Exalgo) is frequently used for pain management. It is preferred over morphine in many cases because of its superior solubility and speed of onset. Hydromorphone has fewer side effects than morphine. Further, patients experience less nausea and vomiting with hydromorphone than with alternatives, and it has no troublesome metabolites. The brand name for the extended-release form is Exalgo, which is for patients who need around-the-clock medication.

Dosage Forms and Administration Refer to the Dosing and Administering Opioids section.

Side Effects Refer to the Opioid Side Effects section.

Contraindications Hydromorphone use is contraindicated in patients with acute asthma, significant respiratory depression, GI obstruction, or hypersensitivity.

Cautions and Considerations Hydromorphone shares the class-wide precautions presented in the Opioid Cautions and Considerations section, including boxed warnings related to addiction, misuse, respiratory depression, and neonatal withdrawal syndrome. This drug must be dispensed with a Medication Guide. It should also be used with care in geriatric patients.

Drug Interactions Drugs that have major interactions with hydromorphone include drugs with serotonergic activity, such as MAOIs, SSRIs, SNRIs, and dextromethorphan.

Methadone

Methadone (Dolophine, Methadose) is used in severe pain management and to prevent withdrawal in patients enrolled in a medication-assisted treatment program for substance use disorder.

Dosage Forms and Administration It is usually prescribed to be taken one time a day if indicated for substance use disorder. For pain management, it is administered every 6 to 12 hours. Methadone dosing and metabolism are unique to every individual, and the dosing cannot be directly converted to and from that of other opioids. Methadone has an analgesic effect that lasts about 4 to 8 hours, while the opioid craving and withdrawal prevention lasts much longer. The craving effect lasts longer because the drug remains in the body for a very long time. Effects on breathing are seen later than pain relief, and they last longer. This means that methadone doses cannot be increased more quickly than every three to five days without risk of a breathing emergency.

The concentrated form of methadone is packaged as a dispersible tablet and as a concentrated solution. Both must be mixed with four ounces of liquid. Patients should ingest the prepared solution immediately after it is mixed. Methadone is a Schedule II controlled substance.

Side Effects Refer to the Opioid Side Effects section.

Contraindications Methadone use is contraindicated in patients with acute asthma, significant respiratory depression, or hypersensitivity to methadone.

Cautions and Considerations Methadone has the standard precautions and boxed warnings common to all the opioids, including addiction, misuse, respiratory depression, neonatal withdrawal syndrome. In addition, it has boxed warnings based upon the dosage form of the drug. In methadone injectable solution, QT interval prolongation and serious cardiac arrhythmias have been observed during treatment, with most cases occurring in individuals receiving higher doses. Methadone oral tablets in suspension have been associated with deaths caused by titration that is too rapid, drug interactions, and cardiac and respiratory side effects. This drug must be dispensed with a Medication Guide.

Methadone should also be used cautiously in older adults and pregnant patients.

Drug Interactions Major drug interactions with methadone include antifungals (such as fluconazole), ziprasidone, dronedarone, linezolid, hydroxychloroquine, additional opioids, donepezil, selective serotonin reuptake inhibitor (SSRI) antidepressants, and ciprofloxacin.

Morphine

Morphine (Arymo ER, Duramorph, Infumorph, Kadian, Mitigo, MS Contin) is the principal alkaloid obtained from opium. It is an extremely versatile drug used in many different settings. Morphine is a strong analgesic used for the relief of severe and chronic pain, for preoperative sedation, and as a supplement to anesthesia. It is the drug of choice for the pain of myocardial infarction (heart attack).

Dosage Forms and Administration Morphine is administered orally, parenterally, intrathecally, epidurally, and rectally. When administered via the intravenous route, it is three to six times more potent than when it is administered orally. Morphine has significant first-pass metabolism. It is readily absorbed from the gut and is absorbed even faster rectally.

Some confusion arises with the morphine sulfate forms of morphine. There are two types of morphine sulfate: immediate release (Duramorph, Infumorph, Mitigo) and extendedrelease (Arymo ER, Kadian, MS Contin). Immediate release allows for quick response to breakthrough pain. As soon as this formulation is administered, the body starts processing the dose. Extended-release formulations have product technology such as special coatings that allow for incremental release of the drug over a period of hours after administration. Immediate-release can generally be given every 4 hours, while extended-release forms are given every 12 to 24 hours.

When a prescriber writes a prescription for morphine, they usually mean the sustained-release form, but if the prescriber does not indicate which form is being prescribed, it is always best to call to make sure.

Side Effects Refer to the Opioid Side Effects section.

Contraindications Morphine use is contraindicated in patients with acute asthma, significant respiratory depression, or hypersensitivity to morphine. Morphine should not be taken by those who are taking an MAOI or have used one in the previous 14 days, or by those with a GI obstruction.

Cautions and Considerations Standard opioid precautions apply when considering morphine use. Infumorph and Mitigo both have formulations available with strengths of 10 mg/mL and 25 mg/mL; these brands should not be confused with Duramorph, which is available in strengths of 0.5 mg/mL and 1 mg/mL. Morphine is the opioid most likely to cause itching. This drug must be dispensed with a Medication Guide.

Drug Interactions Drugs that have major interactions with morphine include other CNS depressants like benzodiazepines and Z-drugs for insomnia (such as eszopiclone, zaleplon, and zolpidem).

Oxycodone

Oxycodone (Oxaydo, OxyCONTIN, Roxicodone, Xtampza) is generally used in moderate to severe pain.

Dosage Forms and Administration When a prescriber writes an order for OxyCONTIN, verification is prudent, as OxyCONTIN is only available as a 12-hour extended-release tablet, and it is not interchangeable with generic, immediate-release oxycodone.

Since oxycodone is one of the most frequently abused opioids, the pharmaceutical industry has started making abuse-deterrent formulations to reduce tampering. A recent formulation of OxyCONTIN forms a viscous hydrogel when mixed with aqueous liquid for dissolution.

Side Effects Refer to the Opioid Side Effects section.

Contraindications Oxycodone is contraindicated in patients with acute asthma, significant respiratory depression, hypersensitivity to oxycodone, or elevated levels of carbon dioxide.

Cautions and Considerations Standard opioid precautions apply to oxycodone. Oxycodone carries boxed warnings related to addiction, misuse, respiratory depression, neonatal withdrawal syndrome, and combination with benzodiazepines or alcohol. This drug must be dispensed with a Medication Guide. With oral solutions, care should be taken to ensure that milligrams and milliliters are not confused, as that can cause dosing errors. If an acetaminophen combination product is being used, the patient should keep their total daily dose of acetaminophen, including OTC products, under 4 grams daily to prevent liver toxicity. If the patient has liver disease, high alcohol intake, or is geriatric, this limit should be reduced to 3 grams daily.

Drug Interactions Drug interactions include drugs with serotonergic activity, such as MAOIs, SSRIs, SNRIs, and dextromethorphan. Caution should be used when adding or increasing any antifungals, calcium channel blockers, macrolide antibiotics, paroxetine, fluoxetine, or bupropion.

Tapentadol

Tapentadol (Nucynta) is a derivative of tramadol that has two analgesic mechanisms. It is indicated for use in adults for moderate to severe pain as well as for pain associated with diabetic neuropathy. It may be less constipating than other opioid alternatives. There is also an extended-release form of this drug that should not be mixed with alcohol, whether the alcohol is taken as a beverage or as an additive in another product like a cough syrup or mouthwash.

Dosage Forms and Administration Refer to the Dosing and Administering Opioids section.

Side Effects Refer to the Opioid Side Effects section.

Contraindications Tapentadol is contraindicated in patients with documented anaphylactic reactions to tapentadol, in those insufficiently monitored with respiratory insufficiency or with significant asthma, in those who are taking an MAOI or have used one in the previous 14 days, and in those with a GI obstruction.

Cautions and Considerations Standard opioid precautions apply to tapentadol. Tapentadol carries boxed warnings related to addiction, misuse, respiratory depression, neonatal withdrawal syndrome, and combination with benzodiazepines or alcohol. This drug must be dispensed with a Medication Guide. Caution should be taken regarding use in patients with a history of alcohol use or with severe liver disease.

Drug Interactions Drug interactions include concurrent use of opioid analgesics, because this may result in additive CNS and respiratory depression.

Tramadol

Safety Alert

Tramadol, trazodone (an antidepressant), and Toradol (an NSAID) could be confused.

Tramadol (ConZip, Synapryn, Ultram) is a weak synthetic mu agonist that is notable for its additional serotonin and norephinephrine reuptake inhibition (like the SNRIs duloxetine and venlafaxine).

Dosage Forms and Administration When given in combination with Tylenol, it has a high success rate in treating pain. Because the drug has a slow onset, it was originally promoted as a nonaddictive substance. However, due to evidence of addictive properties, it was classified as a Schedule IV controlled substance in 2014.

Side Effects The most common side effects include dizziness, vertigo, nausea, constipation, and headache.

Contraindications Use is contraindicated in patients with a history of hypersensitivity to tramadol; patients under 12 years of age; postoperative pediatric patients who received a tonsillectomy or adenoidectomy; inadequately monitored patients with acute or severe asthma; patients experiencing significant respiratory depression; patients with GI obstruction, such as a known or suspected paralytic ileus; and patients currently on an MAOI who have taken an MAOI in the previous 14 days.

Cautions and Considerations Standard opioid precautions apply to tramadol. Tramadol carries boxed warnings related to addiction, misuse, respiratory depression, neonatal withdrawal syndrome, and combination with benzodiazepines or alcohol. This drug must be dispensed with a Medication Guide. Additionally, tramadol has some significant CYP3A4 and CYP2D6 drug interactions, so starting or stopping other medications must include tramadol dosing reconsideration. Patients with diabetes should be aware of increased hypoglycemia risk in the first 30 days of tramadol use.

Drug Interactions Drug interactions include drugs with serotonergic activity (such as MAOIs, SSRIs, SNRIs, and dextromethorphan), CYP3A4 inhibitors, and CYP2D6 inhibitors.

Mixed Opioid Agonists

Certain opioids are considered mixed agonists, meaning they may fully activate receptors in certain conditions but not all. These agents include buprenorphine (Belbuca, Buprenex, Butrans, Probuphine, Sublocade), butorphanol, and nalbuphine.

Buprenorphine

Buprenorphine (Belbuca, Buprenex, Butrans, Probuphine, Sublocade) is used to manage moderate to severe chronic pain and to prevent opioid withdrawal. Buprenorphine is indicated for acute and chronic pain. Generally, if it is formulated by itself, it is indicated for pain management. Exceptions are Sublocade (an extended-release subcutaneous injection) and Probuphine (a subdermal implant), which are used for substance use disorder. If buprenorphine is paired with naloxone, as in Suboxone, the formulation is indicated for substance use disorder, though it can be written off label for chronic pain. Buprenorphine / naloxone prescriptions for substance use disorder require the prescriber to have a buprenorphine waiver (referred to as an XDEA number).

Contraindications Buprenorphine use is contraindicated in patients with a history of hypersensitivity to buprenorphine. It is also contraindicated in patients with respiratory depression, severe asthma, or gastrointestinal obstruction if they cannot be closely monitored.

Cautions and Considerations Buprenorphine should not be swallowed. Buprenorphine carries boxed warnings related to addiction, misuse, respiratory depression, neonatal withdrawal syndrome, and combination with benzodiazepines or alcohol. This drug must be dispensed with a Medication Guide. Healthcare professionals who want to prescribe or dispense buprenorphine must enroll in the REMS program.

Drug Interactions Major drug interactions with buprenorphine include naltrexone, phenobarbital, opioids, carbamazepine, benzodiazepines, and other CNS depressants. Each of these may increase toxicity and result in CNS depression or respiratory depression. Buprenorphine is sometimes stopped in advance of surgery so that it does not interfere with pain management.

Butorphanol

Butorphanol is an analgesic that is more potent than morphine, yet it has less of a negative effect on cardiovascular and respiratory systems. It is used for acute, severe pain, often relating to an operation or during childbirth. It is unlikely to be used for chronic pain, and while it has been used historically to treat acute migraines, many preferred agents now exist for migraine management.

Contraindications Butorphanol use is contraindicated in patients with a history of hypersensitivity to butorphanol or benzethonium chloride; in inadequately monitored patients with acute or severe asthma; in those experiencing significant respiratory depression; and in patients with GI obstruction, such as a known or suspected paralytic ileus. Butorphanol is contraindicated in patients with acute asthma, significant respiratory depression, or hypersensitivity to methadone.

Cautions and Considerations Butorphanol has the standard cautions and considerations common to the opioid class.

Drug Interactions Major drug interactions with butorphanol include other CNS depressants, like benzodiazepines and Z-drugs for insomnia (such as eszopiclone, zaleplon, and zolpidem).

Nalbuphine

Nalbuphine is the only opioid agonist that is not a controlled substance. It is able to provide analgesia, though the relief experience may not feel the same to patients, as it has no euphoric effect like what often occurs with mu receptor agonism. In fact, the patient may feel a "heaviness." Nalbuphine routes of administration are subcutaneous, intramuscular, and intravenous. This agent is also used for morphine-induced itching.

Contraindications Contraindications to nalbuphine include documented anaphylactic reactions to nalbuphine, respiratory depression, severe asthma, and GI obstruction.

Cautions and Considerations Standard opioid precautions apply to nalbuphine.

Drug Interactions Drug interactions include other CNS depressants, like benzodiazepines and Z-drugs for insomnia (such as eszopiclone, zaleplon, and zolpidem). Nalbuphine could reduce full analgesia efficacy if given with other opioids.

18.3 Opioid Use Disorder and Treatments

When used chronically, opioid analgesics can produce physical dependence, meaning withdrawal symptoms occur when decreasing or discontinuing use. Recall that opioid use disorder (OUD) is a condition that can occur with long-term, or chronic, use of an opioid analgesic and is characterized by a persistent desire to use opioids. Overuse of prescription opioids can be problematic and can lead to illegal opioid use (heroin). Signs of opioid use disorder include:

- continued use that interferes with interpersonal relationships or work
- persistent desire or unsuccessful effort to reduce use
- excessive time spent seeking opioid use or recovering from it
- elimination or reduction in important activities due to use
- use of opioid while driving or engaging in other hazardous activities
- need for increased doses to receive the same effects
- withdrawal symptoms when opioid is decreased

Patients exhibiting these signs should be referred to a healthcare provider for evaluation. Treatment for opioid use disorder involves both medical treatment for withdrawal and behavioral approaches. Medications can be used to decrease physical symptoms of withdrawal during treatment. Methadone is often used in this manner because it has fewer euphoric effects and can be used to slowly wean a patient from use. Risk of relapse will persist.

Pharm Fact

In March 2018, the CDC released a guideline for prescribing opioids for chronic pain. The guideline provides recommendations for primary care clinicians and addresses (1) when to initiate or continue opioids for chronic pain, (2) opioid selection, and (3) assessing risk and addressing harms of opioids.

Although patients undergoing chronic opioid therapy do become physically dependent, opioid use disorder must not be confused with dependence. Dependence is a physical and emotional reliance on a drug. Patients who are dependent will experience an abstinence syndrome (withdrawal) when drug therapy is discontinued or when the dose is reduced substantially.

In contrast, opioid use disorder is a compulsive disorder that leads to continued use of the drug despite harm to the user. Symptoms of opioid use disorder include preoccupation with drugs, refusal to taper off medication, a strong preference for a specific opioid, and a general decrease in ability to function. A patient with opioid use disorder usually does not take the medication as prescribed. People with opioid use disorder have a tendency to rely on multiple prescribers and pharmacies to conceal their behavior. Pharmacy technicians must be alert to these signs of addiction when dispensing opioids, because it is their legal and moral responsibility to notify the pharmacist, the prescribing physician, or both if drug-seeking behavior is suspected. Technicians should always watch for signs of abuse of these drugs, without prejudging patients.

Pharmacy technicians should be alert to the following signs of opioid use disorder:

- forged prescriptions
- frequent prescription loss
- changes made to the prescription: for example, adding a zero to the number 10
- unsanctioned dose escalation
- patient repeatedly saying they were shorted when medication was dispensed
- patient demands a specific brand name/generic manufacturer
- patient wants to pay cash despite having insurance

One of the most difficult tasks for the pharmacy team is to assess opioid use in patients. The pharmacy team commonly does not know what illness is being treated. Technicians should never hesitate to call the prescribing physician to verify and clarify a prescription for pain. Although the intention is certainly not to cause patients to feel uncomfortable or embarrassed, the pharmacy team must always be on the alert for those who abuse these medications, because opioid use disorder itself is an illness.

Patients are generally more successful at addressing addiction if the symptoms of withdrawal are medically treated. Table 18.4 lists drugs commonly used to treat addiction.

Pharm Fact

Methadone is used as an opioid for analgesia, but it can also be used in opioid use disorder to assist a patient to slowly decrease the dose and use of opioids.

It is very important that the pharmacy team acknowledge the value of opioids in the treatment of pain as well as the potential for drug diversion. The federal regulation pertinent to controlled substances states that prescriptions can be "issued for a legitimate medical purpose by an individual practitioner acting in the usual course of . . . professional practice." It is imperative that documentation of the medical purpose be in the medical records. The pharmacy team must serve as both gatekeeper and advocate for patients who are in pain.

TABLE 18.4 Medications Used to Treat Substance Use Disorder

Generic (Brand)	Pronunciation	Dosage Form	Common Dosage	Dispensing Status	Controlled Substance Schedule
buprenorphine (Probuphine, Sublocade)	byoo-pre-NOR-feen	implant, injection	SC: 0.3 mg every 6–8 hr implant: 4 implants inserted every 6 months for 1 year	Rx	C-III
buprenorphine / naloxone (Bunavail, Suboxone, Zubsolv)	byoo-pre-NOR-feen nal-OX-oan	buccal film, sublingual film, sublingual tablet	PO: 2.1 mg/0.3 mg to 16 mg/4 mg a day	Rx	C-III
methadone (Dolophine, Methadose)	METH-a-doan	injection, oral dissolving tablet, oral solution, oral tablet	IV: 2.5–10 mg every 8–12 hr PO: 30–120 mg a day	Rx	C-II
naltrexone (Vivitrol)	nal-TREKS-oan	injection, oral tablet	IM: 380 mg every 4 weeks PO: 25–50 mg a day	Rx	

Opioid Antagonists

Opioid antagonists work by binding to opioid receptors and blocking the effects of opioids. These include naloxone and naltrexone (Vivitrol). Opioid antagonist agents are useful when the effects of an opioid need to be reversed.

Naloxone

Naloxone (Narcan) is an opioid antagonist with deep attraction to the mu receptor. It is used in respiratory emergencies following known or suspected **opioid toxicity**. Opioid toxicity can result in slow breathing, absence of breathing, deep sedation, lack of response to voice or physical touch, pinpoint pupils when the eyelid is raised, or a combination of these effects. When naloxone is administered, it replaces opioids that were binding and activating the mu receptor. As an antagonist, naloxone does not activate the receptor and essentially turns the receptor off, reversing the toxicity and sedation and allowing normal breathing patterns to restart. The FDA has recommended that healthcare providers discuss the availability of naloxone with all patients who are prescribed opioid analgesics and consider prescribing it to patients who are at increased risk of opioid overdose. These include patients who are also taking benzodiazepines or other CNS depressants, currently have opioid use disorder or a history of it, or have experienced an opioid overdose.

Pharmacists may consider prescribing naloxone to patients prescribed medications to treat opioid use disorder (such as methadone or buprenorphine), patients at risk of opioid overdose, and patients taking opioids. Pharmacists may also dispense naloxone to household members of such patients to use in case of overdose or ingestion of opioids by children.

Dosage Forms and Administration Naloxone can be given intramuscularly or intravenously. In a community setting, it is more likely to be an intranasal spray formulation. When given intranasally, its effect is usually seen within 2 minutes. After the first dose is given, it is critical that the patient is brought to emergency services or that emergency services are called. This is because most opioids have a longer duration of action than naloxone's 30 minutes, and the patient's difficulty breathing will likely restart as the naloxone fades. Repeated doses of naloxone can be given if they are available, as often as every 2 to 3 minutes, with a fresh unit used each time.

Side Effects The patient will likely experience headache and nasal symptoms after administration. If a patient takes opioids regularly and is physically dependent, expect them to wake up agitated, in pain, and possibly aggressive.

Contraindications Naloxone is contraindicated in patients who have anaphylactic reactions to naloxone.

Cautions and Considerations Withdrawal will occur if the patient is physically dependent on opioids. This can include pain, tachycardia, hypertension, sweating, abdominal cramps and diarrhea, nausea, and agitation. Respiratory and central nervous system depression may restart after naloxone fades. Emergency services should be seen or called as soon as possible after the first dose is given.

Drug Interactions If a patient is taking a peripherally acting mu opioid antagonist for opioid-caused constipation, naloxone will have an additive effect. This could increase GI opioid withdrawal symptoms, like abdominal cramps and diarrhea.

Pharm Fact

Pharmacists can prescribe naloxone to family members of a patient with opioid use disorder to have on hand in the case of overdose.

Naltrexone

Naltrexone (Vivitrol) is an opioid antagonist that binds opioid receptors, particularly the mu subtype. When binding to a receptor, naltrexone prevents activation of the opioid receptors by the body's endogenous (naturally made) opioids as well as exogenous (taken or administered) opioid agonists. Naltrexone is related to naloxone but has a longer half-life and is indicated for use to treat alcohol dependence and opioid use disorder. The mechanism through which naltrexone is able to reduce alcohol consumption is not understood, though it seems to involve the endogenous opioid system. The use of low-dose naltrexone (about a tenth of current dosing standards) for central sensitization and neuropathic pain conditions, like fibromyalgia and Crohn's disease, is an area of ongoing research.

Dosage Forms and Administration Naltrexone can be taken orally but is more often administered as a monthly injection intramuscularly into the upper, outer quadrant of the gluteal area (buttock). Vivitrol administration is a service increasingly available in community pharmacy settings.

Side Effects Common side effects include headache, dizziness, nausea, vomiting, stomach pain, diarrhea, anxiety, drowsiness, dry mouth, sore throat, skin rash, fainting, and pain at the injection site. Naltrexone can also affect liver function. Patients must be monitored for all these effects.

Contraindications Contraindications include current opioid dependence or use of opioid analgesics, acute withdrawal, and hypersensitivity to naltrexone or other formulation components.

Cautions and Considerations Injection site reactions are normal, typically presenting as pain, tenderness, swelling, bruising, redness, and itching. Liver function should be monitored, partially because this patient population is already at risk of hepatitis and liver dysfunction. There may be a risk of eosinophilic pneumonia, which would present as difficulty breathing and shortness of breath and lack of response to antibiotics. The patient must have abstained from opioid use for the previous one to two weeks before receiving naltrexone to prevent acute withdrawal effects. If the patient restarts opioids within four weeks after a naltrexone dose, they will be at increased risk of respiratory emergency, as their body will have lost some tolerance during that time and the previous daily opioid intake might now be too high. It is also possible for a patient to take high quantities of opioids at any time after a Vivitrol administration, overwhelming naltrexone's blocking effect. Naltrexone does not prevent or reduce alcohol withdrawal symptoms; it only reduces consumption.

Drug Interactions Opioid agonists should be avoided due to reduced or prevented effect. Additionally, peripherally acting mu opioid agonists should be avoided due to increased effect.

18.4 Anesthesia

Anesthesia is an intervention used for intentional loss of feeling in a person's body or part of the body when pain relief, anxiety relief, or muscle relaxation is required for patient care. Pain is a general sense of the body that detects tissue damage. Pain receptors send impulses through sensory neurons to the CNS. Anesthetics work by manipulating the nervous system so that pain or the conscious perception of pain is inhibited.

Pharm Fact

Anesthesia was first used in 1846 by a dentist and a surgeon at Massachusetts General Hospital to remove a tumor from a patient's neck.

Particular types of anesthesia are selected depending on the situation. The types of anesthesia available include general anesthesia, neuraxial anesthesia, and local anesthesia. **General anesthesia** causes reversible unconsciousness and absence of response to otherwise painful stimuli. During general anesthesia, the patient is unconscious, and usually airway support or intubation is required. General anesthesia is used for more complex operations. **Neuraxial anesthesia** blocks sensation through the injection of an anesthetic agent into a nerve in the central nervous system without making the patient unconscious. An example of neuraxial anesthesia is an epidural during childbirth. **Local anesthesia** (a reversible loss of sensation in a defined area of the body) is used with nerve blocks for significant local pain reduction, such as for a procedure on an arm or a leg.

Table 18.5 identifies commonly used anesthetic agents. Common dosages for many of these agents vary based on patient needs and are administered in an inpatient setting.

TABLE 18.5 Commonly Used Anesthetics

Generic (Brand)	Pronunciation	Dosage Form	Common Dosage	Dispensing Status	Controlled Substance Schedule
Inhaled Agents					
desflurane (Suprane)	des-FLOO-rayn	gas	dosage varies by patient	Rx	
isoflurane (Forane)	eye-soe-FLOO-rayn	gas	dosage varies by patient	Rx	
nitrous oxide	NYE-trus OX-ide	gas	dosage varies by patient	Rx	
sevoflurane (Ultane)	see-voe-FLOO-rane	gas	dosage varies by patient	Rx	
Injectable Agents					
alfentanil (Alfenta)	al-FEN-ta-nil	intravenous, injection	dosage varies by patient	Rx	C-II
dexmedetomidine (Precedex)	deks-MED-e-toe-mi-deen	intravenous	dosage varies by patient	Rx	
etomidate (Amidate)	e-TOM-i-date	intravenous, injection	dosage varies by patient	Rx	
fentanyl	FEN-ta-nil	intravenous, injection, prefilled syringe	dosage varies by patient	Rx	C-II
ketamine (Ketalar)	KET-a-meen	intravenous, injection, prefilled syringe	dosage varies by patient	Rx	C-III
morphine (various brands)	MOR-feen	intravenous, IM injection, prefilled syringe, oral liquid, capsule, tablet, suppository	dosage varies by patient	Rx	C-II
propofol (Diprivan)	PRO-po-fawl	intravenous, injection, prefilled syringe	dosage varies by patient	Rx	

continues

TABLE 18.5 Commonly Used Anesthetics—*Continued*

Generic (Brand)	Pronunciation	Dosage Form	Common Dosage	Dispensing Status	Controlled Substance Schedule
remifentanil (Ultiva)	rem-i-FEN-ta-nil	intravenous, injection, prefilled syringe	dosage varies by patient	Rx	C-II
sufentanil (Sufenta)	soo-FEN-ta-nil	intravenous, injection	dosage varies by patient	Rx	C-II
Induction Agents					
Barbiturates					
methohexital (Brevital)	meth-oh-HEKS-i-tal	intravenous, injection, prefilled syringe	dosage varies by patient	Rx	C-IV
Benzodiazepines					
diazepam (Valium)	dye-AZ-e-pam	intravenous, injection, intramuscular, rectal gel, nasal spray, oral liquid, tablet	dosage varies by patient	Rx	C-IV
lorazepam (Ativan)	lor-AZ-e-pam	intravenous, injection, intramuscular, prefilled syringe, oral liquid, nasal solution	dosage varies by patient	Rx	C-IV
midazolam	mid-AZ-oh-lam	intravenous, injection, intramuscular	dosage varies by patient	Rx	C-IV
Neuromuscular Blocking Agents					
Short Duration					
succinylcholine (Anectine, Quelicin)	sux-in-il-KOE-leen	intravenous, intramuscular, prefilled syringe, nasal spray	dosage varies by patient	Rx	
Intermediate Duration					
atracurium	a-tra-KYOO-ree-um	intravenous	dosage varies by patient	Rx	
cisatracurium (Nimbex)	sis-a-tra-KYOO-ree-um	intravenous	dosage varies by patient	Rx	
rocuronium (Zemuron)	roe-kyoor-OH-nee-um	intravenous, prefilled syringe	dosage varies by patient	Rx	
vecuronium (Norcuron)	vek-ue-ROE-nee-um	intravenous, prefilled syringe	dosage varies by patient	Rx	
Extended Duration					
pancuronium (Pavulon)	pan-kyoo-ROE-nee-um	intravenous	dosage varies by patient	Rx	

continues

TABLE 18.5 Commonly Used Anesthetics—*Continued*

Generic (Brand)	Pronunciation	Dosage Form	Common Dosage	Dispensing Status	Controlled Substance Schedule
Agents for Malignant Hyperthermia					
dantrolene (Dantrium, Revonto, Ryanodex)	DAN-troe-leen	capsule, injection	2.5–10 mg/kg	Rx	
Local Anesthetics					
Esters					
benzocaine (various brands)	BEN-zoe-kayn	cream, ear drops, gel, lozenge, ointment, oral liquid, oral paste, spray	dosage varies by patient	OTC	
chloroprocaine (Nesacaine)	klor-oh-PROE-kayn	injection	dosage varies by patient	Rx	
dyclonine (Sucrets)	DYE-kloe-neen	liquid spray, lozenge/troche, solution	dosage varies by patient	OTC	
tetracaine (Cepacol Viractin, Pontocaine)	TET-ra-kayn	gel, injection, ophthalmic solution, oral liquid	dosage varies by patient	OTC, Rx	
Amides					
bupivacaine	byoo-PIV-a-kayn	injection	dosage varies by patient	Rx	
lidocaine (various brands)	LYE-doe-kayn	cream, gel, injection, lotion, ointment, oral, patch, solution (external and mouth/throat), topical	dosage varies by patient	OTC, Rx	
lidocaine / epinephrine (Xylocaine with epinephrine)	LYE-doe-kayn ep-i-NEF-rin	injection	dosage varies by patient	Rx	
lidocaine / prilocaine (various brands)	LYE-doe-kayn PRIL-oh-kayn	cream	dosage varies by patient	Rx	
mepivacaine (Carbocaine, Polocaine)	me-PIV-a-kayn	injection	dosage varies by patient	Rx	
ropivacaine (Naropin)	roe-PIV-a-kane	injection	dosage varies by patient	Rx	

A physician who oversees administration of anesthesia during surgery is known as an **anesthesiologist**. The care team can also include certified registered nurse anesthetists (CRNAs) or anesthesia assistants (AAs). The physiologic effects of general anesthesia involve many systems, as described in Table 18.6. In contrast, local and neuraxil anesthetics block the transmission of pain signals to the CNS from a specific anatomic site; however, they cause no changes in awareness or sensory perception in other areas.

TABLE 18.6 Physiologic Effects of General Anesthesia

Body System	Effects
nervous system	All nerve tissue function in the peripheral system is depressed.
respiratory system	Function is depressed, and the anesthesiologist controls oxygen concentration and ventilation (exchange of air between the lungs and ambient air). Inhaled anesthetics, which are drawn into the lungs, generally irritate the respiratory tract and salivary glands, causing increased mucus secretion, coughing, and spasm.
endocrine system	Some anesthetics cause pituitary secretion of antidiuretic hormone, which may cause postoperative urinary retention. The adrenal medulla may release epinephrine and norepinephrine, which can counter depression caused by inhibited nerves.
cardiovascular system	The activity of cardiac muscle in the myocardium is reduced, and the resultant loss of tone reduces blood pressure. Vagus nerve inhibition increases the heart rate. Some drugs make the heart sensitive, which may cause arrhythmias (variations from the normal rhythm of the heart).
skeletal muscular system	Anesthesia depresses systems within the brain and spinal reflexes, causing some muscle relaxation.
GI system	Common GI effects are nausea and vomiting.
hepatic system	Some medications are suspected of causing liver damage.

General anesthesia is characterized by four reversible conditions:

- unconsciousness (unawareness)
- analgesia (relief of pain)
- paralysis (skeletal muscle relaxation)
- amnesia upon recovery

There are three phases of general anesthesia: *induction*, or "putting the patient under"; *maintenance* of the general anesthesia; and *emergence*. To maintain anesthesia appropriately, indicators are used to assess the patient's status. These indicators include:

- oxygenation (inhaled oxygen and blood oxygen content)
- ventilation (exhaled carbon dioxide, lung volume and pressures, and ventilator feedback if intubated)
- circulation (cardiac activity and blood pressure)
- temperature

General anesthetics can be administered in different ways, and several factors must be considered before, during, and after their administration. Some of these considerations are briefly discussed in the following section.

General Anesthetics: Inhaled Agents

Inhaled anesthetics are stored under high pressure and are provided by the manufacturer in steel cylinders. Though informally referred to as "compressed gas," some of these chemicals are in liquid form in the cylinders and transform into a gas when released. During surgery, anesthesiologists administer inhaled anesthetics through a face mask. Interestingly, the respiratory system excretes 80%-90% of the inhaled anesthetics. Common side effects associated with inhaled anesthetics include a reduction in blood pressure; **hypervolemia**, or excessive blood volume in the body; a reduction in renal function; and nausea and vomiting. The most commonly used inhaled anesthetics are listed in Table 18.5.

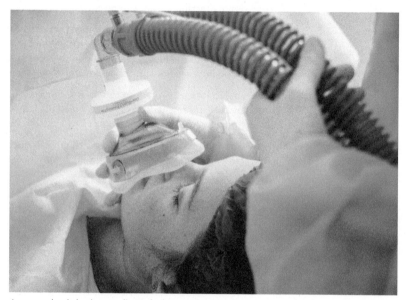

An anesthesiologist applies inhalant anesthetics during surgery.

Nitrous Oxide

Nitrous oxide (N₂O) is not a potent anesthetic, and it usually is used with other agents. Its effects are limited to reducing blood pressure and providing analgesia; it does not induce amnesia or relax skeletal muscle. It has the tremendous advantage of being rapidly eliminated; its disadvantage is that it may cause hypoxia, a reduction in the oxygen supplied to a tissue, despite adequate perfusion by blood. In balanced anesthesia, nitrous oxide is supplemented with a hypnotic (a barbiturate or a benzodiazepine), analgesics (intravenous narcotics), and muscle relaxants. It is administered with more powerful anesthetics to hasten the uptake of the more powerful agents.

Dosage Forms and Administration Nitrous oxide may be used alone, particularly in dental procedures, which is the most common use of this drug.

Side Effects Nitrous oxide is generally well tolerated. Side effects of nitrous oxide include memory loss and mildly slowed breathing.

Contraindications Nitrous oxide should not be administered with oxygen. No patient should receive more than two hours of continuously inhaled nitrous oxide.

Cautions and Considerations Nitrous oxide should not be administered to patients with hypovolemia, shock, pneumothorax, or cardiac disease (severe hypotension), as it may cause arrhythmias, cardiac depression, pulmonary hypertension, or systemic hypotension.

Drug Interactions The use of nitrous oxide with other CNS depressants, such as opioid analgesics, benzodiazepines, and alcohol may result in increased or additive CNS depressant effects.

Isoflurane

Isoflurane (Forane) produces rapid induction and recovery, with no excessive tracheal or salivary secretions. The disadvantages are progressive respiratory and blood pressure depression, with possible malignant hyperthermia. Isoflurane may cause less renal and hepatic toxicity than any other commonly employed anesthetic. Isoflurane's chemical structure is similar to that of enflurane, an inhaled anesthetic that is no longer available in the United States.

Contraindications Contraindications include hypersensitivity to isoflurane or other halogenated agents as well as known or suspected genetic susceptibility to malignant hyperthermia.

Cautions and Considerations Isoflurane should not be used with carbon dioxide absorbents. Deep anesthesia with isoflurane may cause dose-related hypotension and respiratory depression, and it may cause increases in cerebrospinal fluid pressure. Isoflurane is not recommended for individuals with coronary artery disease, as it may increase the risk of myocardial ischemia.

Drug Interactions The use of isoflurane with neuromuscular blocking agents may result in respiratory depression and apnea. Concurrent use of isoflurane and St. John's wort may increase the risk of cardiovascular collapse, delayed emergence from anesthesia, or both.

Desflurane

Desflurane (Suprane) is an easily controlled anesthetic used in both inpatient and outpatient practice due to its rapid onset and a patient's rapid recovery from it. It reduces the required dose of neuromuscular blocking agents. However, desflurane also produces a high incidence of moderate to severe upper respiratory irritation in children and is therefore not recommended for use in the pediatric population when inducing anesthesia. It can be used for maintenance of general anesthesia.

Dosage Forms and Administration Desflurane is inhaled.

Side Effects Common side effects of desflurane include nausea, vomiting, and cough. Serious effects can include difficulty breathing, changes in heart rhythm, and elevated potassium.

Contraindications Contraindications include hypersensitivity to desflurane or other halogenated agents as well as known or suspected genetic susceptibility to malignant hyperthermia. Desflurane should not be used in individuals who have a history of moderate to severe hepatic dysfunction following halogenated agent use. It should not be used to induce anesthesia in pediatric patients.

Cautions and Considerations Desflurane is not recommended as a sole agent for anesthetic induction in individuals with coronary artery disease or other conditions for which increases in heart rate or blood pressure are undesirable.

As the dose of desflurane increases, there is a corresponding increase in hypotension and respiratory depression, and increases in cerebrospinal fluid pressure may occur.

Drug Interactions The use of desflurane with nitrous oxide may result in a decrease in the minimum alveolar concentration of desflurane. When used together, desflurane may excessively prolong the neuromuscular blocking effects of cisatracurium.

Sevoflurane

Sevoflurane (Ultane) is used for induction and maintenance of general anesthesia. It can be used for mask induction before switching to desflurane for maintenance, as it is less irritating to mucous membranes.

Dosage Forms and Administration Sevoflurane is administered via inhalation for general anesthesia.

Side Effects Common side effects of sevoflurane include nausea, vomiting, drowsiness, agitation, cough, and shivering. Serious effects can include heart arrhythmias, liver failure, elevated potassium, seizure, and difficulty breathing.

Contraindications Sevoflurane is contraindicated in patients with hypersensitivity to sevoflurane or other halogenated agents as well as known or suspected genetic susceptibility to malignant hyperthermia.

Cautions and Considerations Sevoflurane should not be used with carbon dioxide absorbents because the combination may form carbon monoxide. QT prolongation is a concern with sevoflurane use, particularly in combination with antiarrhythmic agents, in older patients, or in patients with congenital QT prolongation. Dose-related hypotension or respiratory depression may occur. Prior exposure to halogenated hydrocarbon anesthetics may increase risk of hepatic injury. Increased risk of preoperative seizures may occur with administration of sevoflurane, primarily in young adults and children aged two months and older.

Drug Interactions Use of a number of QT-prolonging agents like dronedarone, ziprasidone, and cisapride raise the risk of arrythmias and torsades de pointes when used concurrently with sevoflurane. Use with St. John's wort may increase the risk of cardiovascular collapse and delayed emergence from anesthesia.

General Anesthetics: Injectable Agents

The injectable anesthetics include the ultrashort-acting barbiturates and benzodiazepines. A **barbiturate** is a depressant for the central nervous system that also acts as an antianxiety, hypnotic, and anticonvulsant agent. A **benzodiazepine** is one of a class of drugs that act as a sedative, hypnotic, antianxiety, and anticonvulsant agent. The IV products are very lipid soluble. They are distributed initially to the brain, liver (where they are metabolized), kidneys, and other organs with high-volume blood flow and later to fat and muscle. Body distribution away from the central nervous system lowers concentrations at sites of activity where anesthesia is maintained. Most of the injectable anesthetics are administered by an IV drip, but some have other dosage forms. Table 18.5 lists the most commonly used injectable anesthesia agents. Almost all the injectable anesthetics are controlled substances.

Etomidate

Etomidate (Amidate) is a hypnotic with ultrashort-acting properties that is used to supplement a weak anesthetic (such as nitrous oxide) and for short outpatient procedures, such as gynecologic procedures (like dilation and curettage). It is also used for sedation in rapid sequence intubation. It may cause transient involuntary muscle contractions.

Dosage Forms and Administration Like most other general anesthetics, etomidate is most commonly administered via IV drip.

Side Effects Side effects for etomidate include nausea and vomiting during the recovery period.

Contraindications Contraindications include hypersensitivity to etomidate.

Cautions and Considerations Etomidate may induce cardiac depression in older patients, especially those with hypertension, or an acute episode in those with heart failure. It can also induce adrenal insufficiency by reducing plasma aldosterone and cortisol, leading to loss of blood pressure and perfusion of tissues. Individuals with renal impairment may also be at risk of drug toxicity.

Drug Interactions Taking oxycodone and etomidate may worsen CNS depression, respiratory depression, or both. St. John's wort interacts with anesthetics in general but not with etomidate.

Fentanyl

Fentanyl is an opioid analgesic that is used as an adjunct medication in anesthesia procedures, as most anesthesia agents do not provide pain relief when they sedate the patient. It can be used as a preoperative medication and is a preferred analgesic for open-heart surgery, because it lacks some of the cardiac depressant (diminishing heart function) actions of other anesthetics. Fentanyl is frequently administered intrathecally as part of spinal anesthesia. The IV form of this drug is used most often in the operating room.

The potency of fentanyl is much greater than that of morphine. It has several analogs that are used exclusively in the operating room. **Alfentanil (Alfenta)** is an ultrashort-acting (30 to 60 minutes) analgesic. **Sufentanil (Sufenta)** is 5 to 10 times more potent than fentanyl. **Remifentanyl (Ultiva)** is the shortest-acting opioid, with a duration of effect lasting 3 to 10 minutes. It has the benefit of rapid offset, even after prolonged infusions during surgeries. Anesthesiologists prefer anesthetics that promote rapid patient recovery.

Dosage Forms and Administration Like most other general anesthetics, fentanyl is most commonly administered via IV drip. While the intravenous infusion or injection is most often used for acute or anesthesia purposes, other fentanyl formulations include transdermal patches, buccal (dissolves in cheek pouch) tablets, buccal lozenges, sublingual tablets, sublingual spray, and intranasal delivery.

Side Effects Side effects for fentanyl include confusion, dizziness, drowsiness, nausea, vomiting, constipation, blurred vision, rash (with transdermal patch), muscle weakness, and slowed or difficult breathing. Fentanyl can also alter heart rhythm, cause chest pain, and alter kidney or liver function. Monitoring is needed for patients with a history of heart, kidney, or liver disease using fentanyl.

Contraindications Contraindications for fentanyl include intolerance to fentanyl products. Though not used for anesthesia, it is worth noting that nonintravenous formulations have other contraindications: transdermal patches, which last three to seven days, are contraindicated for acute or operation-related pain since they cannot be adjusted quickly while pain is resolving with healing or if a breathing emergency occurs. Some other long-acting formulations are contraindicated in patients with severe asthma or a known or suspected gastrointestinal obstruction. These long-acting formulations should not be used in opioid-naive patients.

Cautions and Considerations Fentanyl has multiple boxed warnings common to all opioids. Life-threatening respiratory depression can occur when a dose that is too high is used at the start of therapy, during a dose increase, when changing to a long-acting formulation, when starting a medication that inhibits liver enzymes so opioid plasma levels rise, or when stopping a medication that increases liver enzymes so opioid plasma levels rise. There is a risk of misuse, abuse, and addiction that can lead to overdose or death. Use of benzodiazepines or other CNS depressants can increase the risk of respiratory depression or sedation. Use of multimodal analgesia helps reduce the risk of both.

Older adults or debilitated patients are at a higher risk of respiratory depression and other adverse events when using fentanyl.

Drug Interactions When fentanyl is taken with CNS depressants (including alcohol), there may be additive respiratory and CNS depressant effects as well as increased sedation and dizziness. Serotonin syndrome may occur in patients taking fentanyl with monoamine oxidase inhibitors (MAOIs) or other serotonergic agents. Taking fentanyl with amphetamines may increase the analgesic effects of fentanyl.

Ketamine

Ketamine (Ketalar) produces a type of anesthesia known as *dissociative amnesia*, in which the patient appears to be awake but neither responds to pain nor remembers the procedure. This agent enhances muscle tone and increases blood pressure, heart rate, and respiratory secretions. Onset is quick (within 30 seconds), and effects last 5 to 10 minutes. Ketamine is a preferred agent for anesthesia in pediatric patients because it has some pain-relieving properties. Ketamine can also be used to reduce opioid use.

Dosage Forms and Administration Like most other general anesthetics, ketamine is most commonly administered via IV drip.

Side Effects Side effects for ketamine include an extended emergence from anesthesia that can consist of a dreamlike state, confusion, and hallucinations. Other common side effects can include rash, nausea, vomiting, increased urination, and double vision. Serious side effects include slowed breathing or heart rate, increased blood pressure, and seizure.

Contraindications Contraindications for ketamine include conditions in which a significant increase in blood pressure would be dangerous to the patient and hypersensitivity to ketamine or any other product component. Ketamine is also contraindicated in patients with known or suspected schizophrenia.

Cautions and Considerations Ketamine should not be taken with alcohol or given to patients with a history of alcohol abuse. Emergence reactions can occur with ketamine. These reactions (for example, vivid dreams, hallucinations, or delirium) can occur in addition to confusion or irrational behavior for up to 24 hours following the procedure. Rapid administration or overdose of ketamine may increase the risk of respiratory depression and apnea. Ketamine can increase blood pressure as well as raise pressure inside the CNS and eyes. Cardiac decompensation can also occur, so monitoring is recommended.

Safety Alert

Diprivan and Diflucan might be confused. This could be life threatening if an ICU patient who needs Diflucan for an infection receives Diprivan instead.

Drug Interactions Taking St. John's wort and ketamine may increase the risk of cardiovascular collapse and delayed emergence from anesthesia. Combined use of ketamine and other CNS depressants may increase the risk of additive CNS depressant effects.

Propofol

Propofol (Diprivan) is used to maintain anesthesia and sedation or to treat agitation in patients in the intensive care unit (ICU). It has demonstrated antiemetic and antiepileptic properties. Any unused drug must be discarded after 12 hours. Propofol should be mixed only with 5% dextrose. It is a white emulsion, stable in glass containers, and should be stored at room temperature. When drawn up, propofol must be labeled immediately, as it can be confused with liposomal bupivacaine, another white-appearing local anesthetic frequently used in anesthesia procedures. Bupivacane can lead to cardiac complications if given mistakenly.

Dosage Forms and Administration Like most other general anesthetics, propofol is most commonly administered via IV drip.

Side Effects The side effects of propofol are drowsiness, respiratory depression, motor restlessness, and decreased blood pressure. Propofol changes urine color to green, pink, or rust.

Contraindications Contraindications include moderate to severe allergies to eggs, egg products, soybeans, soy products, or peanuts as well as hypersensitivity to propofol or any other product component.

Cautions and Considerations Cardiorespiratory effects, including hypotension and cardiovascular depression, may occur in vulnerable populations. Due to the oil-in-water formulation, continuous propofol can also raise serum triglycerides, causing hyperlipidemia.

Drug Interactions Taking St. John's wort and ketamine may increase the risk of cardiovascular collapse and delayed emergence from anesthesia. Combined use of other anesthetics (such as lidocaine and bupivacaine) may increase the hypnotic effect of propofol.

Dexmedetomidine

Dexmedetomidine (Precedex) is an agent that sees frequent use as a sedative agent in less invasive procedures and as a temporary dosage for patients who are being weaned off of propofol. While dexmedetomidine cannot sedate a patient as deeply as propofol, it does have some analgesic properties that are useful for reducing anxiety and opioid use as well. Unlike opioids and propofol, it does not compromise a patient's ability to breathe.

Dosage Forms and Administration Dexmedetomidine is given as an infusion (usually in the intensive care unit) or intranasally for specific types of surgery.

Side Effects Common side effects can include increases in blood pressure, nausea, and fever.

Contraindications Dexmedetomidine has no known contraindications.

Cautions and Considerations Caution should be used when prescribing this agent for patients with cardiac dysfunction, such as advanced heart block or low blood pressure. Heart arrythmias and drops in blood pressure can occur, which are rare but serious side effects. Tolerance and dose-related adverse effects become more likely when use of this agent continues beyond 24 hours.

Drug Interactions Though dexmedetomidine does not affect respiratory drive, it is still categorized as a CNS depressant and primarily interacts with other CNS depressants. This combination is commonly coadministered in general practice, so monitoring is necessary.

Anesthesia Induction Agents

Medication is sometimes used preoperatively to control sedation, reduce postoperative pain, cause amnesia, and decrease anxiety. This preanesthesia is called *induction*. These medications can also provide mild anesthesia for short and less invasive

> ▲ **Name Exchange**
> Dexmedetomidine is frequently referred to as *dex* and by its brand name Precedex.

procedures than surgery, such as a colonoscopy or dental procedure. They work quickly and wear off relatively quickly as compared to other general anesthetics. Review of an individual patient's medication history is important in determining which medications to use.

Methohexital

The barbiturate **methohexital (Brevital)** is used primarily for induction in short procedures. Methohexital can be used to induce anesthesia prior to administration of another agent or alone for short procedures. The big advantages of the barbiturates are rapid induction, fast recovery, and little postanesthetic excitement and vomiting.

Dosage Forms and Administration Like most other general anesthetics, methohexital is most commonly administered via IV drip.

Side Effects In patients who are awake, these agents may cause excitement or delirium in the presence of pain. Common side effects can include nausea, vomiting, allergic reaction, headache, hiccups, and abdominal pain. Respiratory depression or laryngospasm may occur. Serious side effects can include difficulty breathing, low blood pressure, and cardiac arrest.

Contraindications Methohexital is contraindicated in the absence of suitable veins for IV administration, in acute intermittent porphyria, and in patients with a hypersensitivity to barbiturates.

Cautions and Considerations Methohexital should be used with caution in patients with severe cardiovascular disease, hypotension/shock, liver or kidney disease, respiratory impairment or obstruction, or severe anemia.

Drug Interactions Methohexital's major drug interaction is with other CNS depressants, such as benzodiazepines and opiates.

Benzodiazepines

The benzodiazepines, **diazepam (Valium)**, **lorazepam (Ativan)**, and **midazolam**, are used for induction, short procedures, and dental procedures. They are metabolized to active products, so they work longer than barbiturates. Midazolam has the fastest onset of action, greatest potency, and most rapid elimination and is thus the preferred agent. Similar to ketamine, it produces dissociative amnesia; patients do not remember the procedure. It is used even though sometimes patients carry on a strange conversation during the procedure. Benzodiazepines are also useful for controlling and preventing seizures.

Dosage Forms and Administration Like most other general anesthetics, benzodiazepines are most commonly administered by injection for short-term sedation and relaxation ahead of anesthesia. They are most used for short-duration procedures.

Side Effects Some patients can experience unexpected reactions from benzodiazepines, exhibiting behavior more aggressive or hyperactive than sedative in nature. Others can experience sleep-related effects, like driving, cooking, or making phone calls without awareness that they are doing so.

Contraindications Boxed warnings for benzodiazepines include the risk of respiratory depression. Doses must be monitored closely. Depending on the specific benzodiazepine used, they are sometimes contraindicated in patients with glaucoma, sleep apnea, or severe respiratory impairment. Patients who have experienced Stevens-Johnson syndrome or severe allergic reaction to a benzodiazepine, such as angioedema (swelling of the tongue or throat), should not use benzodiazepines.

Cautions and Considerations Because benzodiazepines can cause unexpected and severe adverse reactions, patients should be monitored and must be informed of the risks. Because they can cause respiratory depression, they should be used with caution in patients with respiratory disease.

Drug Interactions Major drug interactions occur with CNS depressants.

When conducting anesthesia, it is critical that reversal agents are available. They are necessary to respond to an overdose emergency. Antagonist drugs, substances that interfere with or inhibit the physiologic action of another, are used to reverse the effects of benzodiazepine and opioid overdoses; antagonists commonly used for this purpose are listed in Table 18.7. All operating rooms and emergency rooms maintain an adequate, quickly accessible supply of these drugs.

Neuromuscular Blocking Agents

Safety Alert

Most neuromuscular blocking agents must be refrigerated and are expensive. Failure to store them correctly could be very costly.

Neuromuscular blocking agents paralyze the patient's skeletal muscles, which enables a surgeon to operate with greater accuracy and safety. Neuromuscular blocking is often used as an adjunct to general anesthesia to enable **endotracheal intubation**, the insertion of a tube into the trachea to maintain an open airway and deliver oxygen and general anesthesia directly to the lungs. Neuromuscular blocking agents are some of the most dangerous drugs, because their administration results in immediate skeletal muscle paralysis. When stocking neuromuscular blocking agents, technicians should always flag this type of drug with a label to alert everyone explicitly that the drug will paralyze whoever receives it. Every effort should be made to make sure these agents are not stored close to a look-alike drug. Table 18.5 gives an overview of the most commonly used neuromuscular blocking agents, many of which must be stored in a refrigerator.

Succinylcholine

There are two mechanisms for achieving neuromuscular blockade. **Succinylcholine (Anectine, Quelicin)**, often referred to as *sux*, is the only agent that works via a depolarizing (neutralizing) mechanism. Succinylcholine works as an agonist of the nicotinic cholinergic receptors. These receptors briefly allow ions to pass through when acetylcholine binds to them, producing a pulse of electrical current that causes the muscle to contract. Succinylcholine holds the ion channels open, causing a persistent depolarization at the motor endplate—in other words, it shorts out the electrical signal.

The result is a brief period of skeletal muscle paralysis.

Dosage Forms and Administration Like most other general anesthetics, neuromuscular blocking agents are administrered via IV drip.

Side Effects Bradycardia (irregular and slow heartbeats) may occur; if they do, they are reversed with atropine.

Contraindications Succinylcholine use is contraindicated in the acute phase of injury after trauma, as it may result in hyperkalemia (high blood potassium levels) and cardiac arrest. It is also contraindicated for patients with a history of malignant hyperthermia, skeletal muscle myopathies, or hypersensitivity to succinylcholine.

Cautions and Considerations Succinylcholine carries a boxed warning associated with rare reports of healthy children with previously undiagnosed skeletal muscle myopathy developing acute rhabdomyolysis with hyperkalemia after succinylcholine was administered. This was followed by ventricular dysrhythmias, cardiac arrest, and death. Use of this medication in children is restricted to emergency intubation and situations when the airway must be immediately secured. This medication should also be used with caution in patients with an abdominal infection, bradycardia, digoxin toxicity, hyperkalemia, other electrolyte abnormalities, or subarachnoid hemorrhage or with a history of repeated use.

Drug Interactions Major drug interactions with succinylcholine include St. John's wort, systemic lidocaine, digoxin, quinine, aminoglycoside antibiotics (such as tobramycin and gentamicin), and donepezil. Concurrent use of these with succinylcholine may result in respiratory depression, cardiovascular distress, or prolongation of the neuromuscular blockade.

Intermediate and Extended Duration Neuromuscular Blockers

The second mechanism for achieving neuromuscular blockade is through nondepolarizing agents that are competitive antagonists to acetylcholine at the nicotinic cholinergic receptors. They prevent acetylcholine from binding to the receptors to start the electrical signal, paralyzing the skeletal muscles. Nondepolarizing agents have a longer duration of action than succinylcholine and are categorized accordingly in Table 18.5.

Dosage Forms and Administration Intermediate and long-acting neuromuscular blockers are used as adjunct to anesthesia to relax muscles for surgery. They are administered by IV injection. Dosing is individualized to the patient, and therapy during anesthesia is monitored closely by an anesthesiologist.

Side Effects The most common side effect is extended action beyond the time period needed. This can result in muscle weakness, apnea, and slowed (or even absence of) respiration. For this reason, these agents are considered high-risk medications.

Contraindications Contraindications include hypersensitivity to nondepolarizing neuromuscular blocking agents. Vials of these agents sometimes contain benzyl alcohol. When used in newborns, these agents can cause potentially fatal gasping syndrome. These agents should not be used in neonates or newborn babies.

Cautions and Considerations Patients should be constantly monitored during administration by individuals specifically trained on these medications. Blood pressure, heart rate, peripheral nerve stimulation, blood gases, and ventilation must all be monitored. Nondepolarizing neuromuscular blocking agents should be used with caution in individuals with a history of allergic reactions to these agents, as severe anaphylactic reactions have occurred. Nondepolarizing neuromuscular blocking agents should only be used along with appropriate amounts of anesthesia, as these products have not been shown to influence consciousness, thought processes, or pain thresholds.

Vecuronium and pancuronium have boxed warnings and should be administered by trained individuals familiar with their actions, characteristics, and hazards.

Drug Interactions When nondepolarizing neuromuscular blocking agents are given with other anesthetics, it can cause prolongation of the neuromuscular blocking effects. The combination of bactericidal antibiotics may also cause prolonged neuromuscular blockade, which may lead to respiratory depression and paralysis.

Phenytoin, when used with rocuronium, may reduce the efficacy of the neuromuscular blockade. In addition, the administration of rocuronium with epinephrine may put the patient at increased risk of postoperative reparalysis.

Drugs Used to Reverse Anesthesia or Overdose

When a patient is oversedated with anesthesia or has taken too much of a benzodiazepine or opioid, medications can be used to reverse those effects. Flumazenil and

Pharm Fact

Nondepolarizing agents have a longer duration of action than succinylcholine and are categorized accordingly in Table 18.5.

Pharm Fact

Neuromuscular blockers are high-alert medications. With the exception of vecuronium (Norcuron), which is stable at room temperature, most neuromuscular blocking agents are stored under refrigeration. Once removed from the refrigerator, the expiration date for storage at room temperature will depend on the drug and should be noted as the discard by date.

naloxone are used by healthcare professionals when needed. Naloxone can also be used by a caregiver when someone is unconscious from an opioid overdose.

Anticholinesterase agents, such as neostigmine and pyridostigmine, are used to reverse nondepolarizing neuromuscular blocking agents. They work by inhibiting the enzyme that breaks down acetylcholine, thereby restoring transmission of impulses across the neuromuscular junction. These agents are also useful in treating myasthenia gravis. See table 18.7 for a list of commonly used antagonists for overdose reversal.

TABLE 18.7 **Commonly Used Antagonists to Reverse Anesthesia or Overdose**

Generic (Brand)	Pronunciation	Dosage Form	Common Dosage	Dispensing Status
flumazenil (Romazicon)	floo-MAZ-eh-nil	injection	0.2 mg	Rx
naloxone (Narcan)	nal-OX-oan	injection, nasal spray, prefilled syringe	0.4–2 mg	Rx
neostigmine (Bloxiverz)	nee-oh-STIG-meen	injection, prefilled syringe	individualized to patient	Rx
pyridostigmine (Mestinon, Regonol)	peer-id-oh-STIG-meen	injection, oral syrup, tablet	individualized to patient	Rx

Flumazenil

Flumazenil (Romazicon) antagonizes benzodiazepines by competing at the same receptor sites, which blocks sedative effects and improves respiratory function. It is used for complete or partial reversal of the effects of benzodiazepines used as general anesthesia or to reverse the effects of a benzodiazepine overdose.

Dosage Forms and Administration Like most other general anesthetics, flumazenil is most commonly administered via IV drip.

Side Effects Adverse reactions include headache, nausea, vomiting, dizziness, and agitation.

Contraindications Use of flumazenil is contraindicated with hypersensitivity to flumazenil or benzodiazepines, signs of serious tricyclic antidepressant overdose, or use of a benzodiazepine for control of a life-threatening condition.

Cautions and Considerations Flumazenil carries a boxed warning for increased risk of seizures, specifically in association with concurrent major sedative-hypnotic drug withdrawal, recent therapy with repeated doses of parenteral benzodiazepines, myoclonic jerking or seizure activity prior to flumazenil administration in overdose cases, or concurrent serious tricyclic antidepressant overdose. Flumazenil should be used with caution in an ICU setting and with patients who have head injuries, respiratory distress, epilepsy, or drug or alcohol dependence. Patients should continue to be monitored following administration, as depending on the dose, the flumazenil might wear off sooner than the benzodiazepine, leading to resedation.

Drug Interactions Major drug interactions occur with concurrent use of other benzodiazepines, which may facilitate seizures, and with concurrent use of selected benzodiazepine receptor agonists, which can decrease the effectiveness of the receptor agonist.

Naloxone

Naloxone (Narcan) is an antagonist that competes for opiate receptor sites. Although this drug has a greater affinity for the receptor, its action is much shorter than that of the competing narcotic. Thus, when the naloxone wears off, the opioid reattaches to the receptor. Consequently, naloxone must be given repeatedly until the opioid is cleared from the patient's system. Naloxone must be stored in a dark space. Due to the increase in opioid overdoses in the United States, there is a growing movement for naloxone to be carried widely.

Dosage Forms and Administration Like most other general anesthetics, naloxone is commonly administered intranasally or with an autoinjector if overdose is experienced at home. It is given by injection when experienced in the hospital or emergency department.

Side Effects Side effects of naloxone can include flushing, sweating, increased blood pressure, agitation, confusion, dizziness, headache, irritability, outbursts, nausea, vomiting, and yawning. Serious side effects can include seizure, difficulty breathing, and fever.

Contraindication Naloxone use is contraindicated in individuals with hypersensitivity to naloxone.

Cautions and Considerations Naloxone should be used with caution in abrupt postoperative reversal of opioids, during labor, in neonates, and in patients with agitation, physical dependence on opioids, liver disease, kidney disease, respiratory depression caused by nonopioid drugs, or septic shock. It is common for the shock of acute withdrawal and return of pain to cause agitated behavior in the rescued patient.

Drug Interactions Major drug interactions with naloxone include opioids and clonidine.

Neostigmine and Pyridostimine

To reverse the effects of a nondepolarizing neuromuscular blocking drug requires the administration of an anticholinesterase agent, such as **neostigmine (Bloxiverz)** or **pyridostigmine (Mestinon, Regonol)**. These drugs potentiate the action of acetylcholine by inhibiting its destruction by the enzyme acetylcholinesterase, thereby restoring the transmission of impulses across the neuromuscular junctions.

Dosage Forms and Administration When used to reverse the effects of neuromuscular blocking agents, neostigmine and pyridostigmine are used as intravenous injection. The oral dosage forms of anticholinesterase agents are also used in the treatment of myasthenia gravis, a neuromuscular disease that is characterized by weakness of the skeletal muscles of the body.

Side Effects Common side effects for anticholinesterase agents include stomachache, diarrhea, muscle aches, twitching, dry skin, and nose bleeds.

Contraindications Contraindications for anticholinesterase drugs include hypersensitivity to anticholinesterase drugs, intestinal or urinary tract obstruction, and peritonitis.

Cautions and Considerations Anticholinesterase drugs should be used with caution in patients with cardiovascular disease, renal impairment, or hepatic impairment. Vulnerable populations (such as infants and small children) may be at an increased risk for complications. Older adult patients given either of these agents during anesthesia will have to be monitored longer than normal. This may involve keeping the patient longer in the recovery suite after anesthesia.

Drug Interactions Taking anticholinesterase drugs with succinylcholine may result in increasing the neuromuscular blockade. Also, concurrent use with corticosteroids may decrease the effectiveness of anticholinesterase drugs. Finally, neostigmine can have an additive effect when combined with other seizure threshold–lowering drugs.

General Anesthetics and Malignant Hyperthermia

Malignant hyperthermia is a rare but serious side effect of anesthesia. It is a sudden and rapid rise in body temperature with accompanying irregularities in heart rhythm and breathing. Body temperature can increase to 110°F or more, and this is accompanied by other symptoms that include increased body metabolism and muscle rigidity (inflexibility or stiffness). Malignant hyperthermia is potentially life threatening and must be treated immediately. If left untreated, death may result from cardiac arrest, brain damage, internal hemorrhaging, or failure of other body systems.

Treatment of malignant hyperthermia involves the IV infusion of the drug **dantrolene (Dantrium, Revonto, Ryanodex)**, a skeletal muscle relaxant also used to treat multiple sclerosis, stroke, cerebral palsy, and spinal cord injury (see Chapter 6 for more information). Dantrolene is thought to reduce muscle tone and metabolism. Hospitals require that a specialized drug kit for the treatment of malignant hyperthermia be immediately accessible wherever anesthesia is administered. It is usually the responsibility of the pharmacy technician to maintain these kits and to make sure that the drugs are up to date, because dantrolene has a very short shelf life and must be replenished frequently.

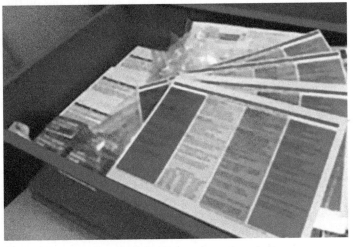

This image is an example of a malignant hyperthermia kit.

A malignant hyperthermia kit generally contains the following components:

- dantrolene (Dantrium, Revonto, Ryanodex)
- sterile water for injection
- sodium bicarbonate, 8.4%
- dextrose, 50%
- calcium chloride, 10%
- regular insulin (refrigerated)
- lidocaine* for injection, 2% (amiodarone is also acceptable)
- refrigerated saline solution

*Lidocaine or procainamide should not be given if a wide QRS complex arrhythmia is likely due to hyperkalemia; this may result in asystole.

Local Anesthetics

Local anesthesia produces a transient and reversible loss of sensation in a defined area of the body without altering alertness or mental function. The introduction of cocaine as a topical ophthalmologic anesthetic in 1884 opened the first era of local anesthesia, and cocaine is still used today for procedures on the eye and nasal passages. Lidocaine, introduced in the 1940s, is now the most widely used local anesthetic. Local anesthetics decrease the neuronal membrane's permeability to ions. This inhibits depolarization, which results in blockade of conduction. Local anesthesia is advantageous because it affects both types of nervous tissue: sensory and motor. The action is reversible, and there is no residual nerve damage. Nerve fibers (cells) determine the degree and speed with which a local anesthetic acts. In response to the activity of the anesthetic, function is lost in the following order:

1. pain perception
2. temperature sensation
3. touch sensation
4. proprioception (recognition of body position, posture, and joint positions)
5. skeletal muscle tone

Local anesthetics depress small, uninsulated fibers first and larger, insulated nerve fibers last. For smaller fibers, the onset of action is much shorter. As a result, the concentration of the drug required to depress sensory signaling is smaller as well. The systemic action that the local anesthetic has on the nervous tissue depends on the time the drug is in contact with that tissue. The action of a local anesthetic can also depend on other factors. For example, inflammation in the tissue and dilation of the blood vessels in the area has the potential to reduce drug activity and duration of action. On the other hand, adding a vasoconstrictor (such as epinephrine) slows the absorption of a drug into the bloodstream, allowing for a longer duration of action. Dentists commonly employ epinephrine to keep the local anesthetic drug at the injection site so that the numbness from the local anesthetic will last longer.

Local anesthetics are classified by their chemical structures into esters and amides. An **ester** is relatively easily broken down, so local anesthetics that are esters are short acting and are metabolized in plasma and tissue fluids. Esters include **benzocaine (various brands)**, **chloroprocaine (Nesacaine)**, **dyclonine (Sucrets)**, and **tetracaine (Cepacol Viractin, Pontocaine)**. An **amide** is more difficult to break down, so amide-containing local anesthetics are longer acting and are metabolized by liver enzymes. Amides include lidocaine, **bupivacaine, lidocaine / epinephrine (Xylocaine with epinephrine)**, **lidocaine / prilocaine (various brands)**, **mepivacaine (Carbocaine, Polocaine)**, and **ropivacaine (Naropin)**. Metabolites of both classes are excreted in urine. Table 18.5 lists the most commonly used local anesthetics in these two classes.

All local anesthetics, except cocaine (used for eye and nose surgery), cause relaxation of vascular smooth muscles and can lead to vascular collapse. Hypersensitivity or an allergy to a particular local agent can cause histamine release at the injection site. The most common reactions to the ester class of local anesthetics are skin rashes, edema, and asthma. This hypersensitivity usually develops when the agent is used frequently or for prolonged periods. An amide can usually be substituted for an ester to prevent these hypersensitivity reactions.

Local anesthetics are commonly combined with other drugs. They are available in a variety of dosage forms for use in a range of conditions. These dosage forms and applications are as follows:

Safety Alert

Epinephrine should not be used as a vasoconstrictor in numbed areas of the fingers, toes, ears, nose, or external genitals, because cutting blood flow at these extremities may result in ischemia and subsequent gangrene.

- epidural (injection into the space outside the dura mater membrane of the vertebral canal)—to block afferent-pain nerve impulses to provide regional anesthesia
- infiltration (superficial injection)—to suture (stitch) cuts, perform dental procedures, and block small nerves
- injection (nerve block via an injection or continuous infusion)—to prevent transmission of pain impulses, particularly in the extremities (arms and legs) and sometimes on the torso
- IV—for reasons other than anesthesia
- spinal (subarachnoid or intrathecal injection into the innermost space of the spinal cord)—to block afferent pain nerve impulses from the lower part of the body
- topical—to treat sunburn, insect bites, and hemorrhoids

Although local anesthetics are administered to produce a pharmacologic response in a well-defined area of the body, occasionally, an anesthetic is absorbed into the blood from the administration site. It can then affect organs along the way, the most serious effects being those on the blood vessels, heart, and brain.

Lidocaine (various brands) can be administered with a patch, an adhesive strip that should be placed directly onto dry, clean skin at the site of pain.

Dosage Forms and Administration A patch should be applied only to intact skin and may be cut with scissors to fit a smaller area. As many as three patches may be applied in one area if the patch size is too small to cover the painful area. A patch is worn for 12 hours and then must be completely removed for 12 hours. Hands should be washed immediately after applying a patch. Patches are especially useful to treat pain caused by shingles.

Side Effects Side effects of lidocaine include low blood pressure, swelling, skin irritation, nausea, and vomiting.

Contraindications Lidocaine use is contraindicated in patients with a history of hypersensitivity to local amide anesthetics.

Cautions and Considerations Lidocaine topical solutions carry a boxed warning for risk of seizures, cardiopulmonary arrest, and death when not administered according to dosing and administration instructions in patients under three years of age. It should be avoided for teething pain. Lidocaine should be used with caution in patients with severe shock, bradycardia, impaired cardiovascular function, acute porphyria, severe liver disease, or epilepsy, and with geriatric and pediatric patients. Excessive dosing can lead to toxicity, which can include headaches, dizziness, drowsiness, numbness, tingling, seizures, cardiac arrythmias, and even heart attack.

Drug Interactions Major drug interactions with lidocaine include antiarrhythmic drugs, metoprolol, St. John's wort, phenytoin, propofol, and propranolol, because potentially toxic side effects may lead to cardiovascular collapse, seizures, and respiratory depression.

18.5 Migraine Headaches and Drug Treatments

Migraine is a neurological disorder most commonly associated with an episodic and painful headache. This headache is moderate or severe in pain intensity, seems to pulse or throb, and is generally centered behind one eye and temple. It can be accompanied by sensory and GI disturbances that can severely affect quality of life and daily function. Vomiting and anorexia are common during the episode, and approximately 90% of all migraine sufferers report nausea. Photophobia (sensitivity to light), phonophobia (sensitivity to sound), and hyperesthesia (increased sensitivity to stimulation) are also common.

A classic migraine has four phases: premonitory (before headache), aura (may or may not occur; arrives immediately before or with headache), headache, and postdrome (after headache has faded). The duration and overlap of these phases can vary. Premonitory symptoms can start hours before the migraine headache phase and may include yawning, fatigue, difficulty concentrating, increased urinary frequency, mood changes or irritability, light or sound sensitivity, and neck pain or stiffness.

About 30% of migraine attacks are preceded by a subjective sensation or motor phenomenon known as an **aura**, which entails visual or sensory disturbances such as flashing lights; shimmering heat waves; bright lights; dark holes in the visual field; blurred, cloudy vision; or transient loss of vision. Aura seems to be induced by a wave of depolarization spreading through the cerebral cortex after starting in the visual cortex. It is unclear if aura triggers the headache or if aura itself is painful. Reasons for the headache's occurrence remain unclear, and research is ongoing. Evidence does suggest that migraine pain is related to nociceptive pain pathways in the trigeminal ganglion (which connects to the trigeminal cranial nerve). Many other parts of the brain and brain stem also affect these pathways and are responsible for other migraine symptoms. The headache usually dissipates in six hours but sometimes lasts one to two days.

The pain of migraine headaches seems to be primarily managed by two neurotransmitters: serotonin (also known as 5-HT) and calcitonin gene-related peptide (CGRP). When 5-HT receptors in the trigeminal ganglion are activated by serotonin or serotonin agonists (ergots and triptans), they inhibit CGRP release. CGRP is a vasodilator and activates trigeminal pain pathways.

Diet, stress, sleep habits, certain medications, hormonal fluctuations, depression, atmospheric changes, and environmental irritants have all been implicated as causative factors that lower the threshold for neural transmission in the trigeminal nerve system, which is implicated in migraine pain. Medication overuse can worsen migraines. This overuse can occur when a patient uses migraine medication or analgesics 10 days or more a month, uses opioids daily for at least 3 months, or uses NSAIDs or acetaminophen at least 15 days a month for at least 3 months. Even relatively low use of barbiturates and opioids is a risk factor for the worsening of acute migraines to chronic migraines. Other medications that can worsen migraines include estrogen-containing products, decongestants, SSRIs, and proton pump inhibitors.

The initial treatment for a migraine should focus primarily on nondrug interventions. Identifying and eliminating trigger factors may be effective for many patients. For example, a quiet environment and sleep may help as many as 25% of patients during an acute attack. Lying down in a dark room often helps. When symptoms are severe or debilitating and attacks are frequent, drug therapy may be indicated. Sedative, antiemetic, and opioid agents are helpful.

The medications used in migraine therapy can be divided into two classes: preventative therapy and acute therapy.

Preventative or *prophylactic therapy* is aimed at preventing or reducing recurrence. Prophylaxis is indicated if migraines occur more than twice a month, occur in predictable patterns, or become refractory (stop responding) to acute therapy. Propranolol (Inderal), a beta-blocker (Chapter 10), is the drug used most often for prophylaxis of migraines. Prophylactic therapies for migraines include the following classes of drugs:

- antihypertensives (beta-blockers, calcium channel blockers, ACE inhibitors, and ARBs)
- antidepressants

- anticonvulsants (gabapentin, topiramate, valproate)
- CGRP antagonist monoclonal antibodies (eptinezumab, erenumab, fremanezumab, galcanezumab)
- NSAIDs
- SSRIs

Acute or *abortive therapy* for migraine headaches treats acute migraine headaches after they begin. The abortive drugs should be taken at the first sign of a headache. Patients must be educated about the importance of treating an attack as soon as possible—long before it develops into a full migraine, when treatments are much less effective. Abortive therapy is most effective when it begins at the first sign of aura or headache. The traditional therapies for acute migraine include simple analgesics (acetaminophen, NSAIDs), triptans, combinations of triptans with NSAIDs, antiemetics for nausea, lasmiditan, CGRP antagonists, and ergots. Uncommon therapies include ergots such as dihydroergotamine and ergotamine.

Research has shown that combination regimens are more effective at treating migraine headaches and have lower recurrence rates than monotherapy. These advantages are especially true for combinations of a triptan and an NSAID. Table 18.8 gives an overview of commonly used agents for migraine headaches.

TABLE 18.8 Commonly Used Agents to Treat Migraines

Generic (Brand)	Pronunciation	Dosage Form	Common Dosage	Dispensing Status
5HT Agonists: Selective Serotonin Receptor Agonists				
almotriptan (Axert)	al-moe-TRIP-tan	tablet	25 mg	Rx
eletriptan (Relpax)	el-e-TRIP-tan	tablet	20–40 mg	Rx
frovatriptan (Frova)	froe-va-TRIP-tan	tablet	2.5–7.5 mg	Rx
naratriptan (Amerge)	NAR-a-trip-tan	tablet	1–2.5 mg	Rx
rizatriptan (Maxalt, Maxalt-MLT)	rye-za-TRIP-tan	sublingual tablet, tablet	5–10 mg	Rx
sumatriptan (Imitrex, Onzetra Xsail, Sumavel DosePro, Tosymra, Zembrace SymTouch)	soo-ma-TRIP-tan	nasal spray, nasal powder, subcutaneous injection, tablet	nasal: 30 mg PO: 50–100 mg SC: 6 mg	Rx
sumatriptan / naproxen (Treximet)	soo-ma-TRIP-tan na-PROX-en	tablet	nasal: 2.5–5 mg PO: 1.25–2.5 mg	Rx
zolmitriptan (Zomig, Zomig ZMT)	zohl-mi-TRIP-tan	nasal spray, sublingual tablet, tablet	nasal 2.5–5 mg PO: 1.25–2.5 mg	Rx
Ergot Derivatives				
dihydroergotamine (D.H.E. 45, Migranal)	dye-hye-droe-er-GOT-a-meen	injection (IM, IV, SC), nasal spray	injection: 1 mg nasal: 2 mg	Rx
ergotamine (Ergomar)	er-GOT-a-meen	sublingual tablet	2 mg	Rx
Calcitonin Gene-Related Peptide (CGRP) Receptor Antagonists				
rimegepant (Nurtec)	rih-ME-jeh-pant	sublingual tablet	75 mg a day	Rx
ubrogepant (Ubrelvy)	ue-BROE-jeh-pant	tablet	200 mg a day	Rx

continues

TABLE 18.8 Commonly Used Agents to Treat Migraines—*Continued*

Generic (Brand)	Pronunciation	Dosage Form	Common Dosage	Dispensing Status
Antiemetic Agents				
chlorpromazine	klor-PROE-ma-zeen	intramuscular injection, intravenous injection, tablet	10–25 mg	Rx
metoclopramide (Reglan)	met-oh-KLOE-pra-mide	injection (IV), oral solution, oral disintegrating tablet, tablet	10 mg	Rx
prochlorperazine (Compro)	proe-klor-PER-a-zeen	injection (IM, IV), rectal suppository, tablet	40 mg	Rx
Combinations				
acetaminophen / aspirin / caffeine (Excedrin)	a-seet-a-MIN-oh-fen AS-pir-in KAF-een	tablet	250 mg/250 mg/ 65 mg	OTC
butalbital / acetaminophen / caffeine (Capacet, Esgic, Fioricet, Vanatol LQ, Zebutal)	byoo-TAL-bi-tal a-seet-a-MIN-oh-fen KAF-een	capsule, oral solution, tablet	varies based on dosage form and brand	Rx
butalbital / aspirin / caffeine (Fiorinal)	byoo-TAL-bi-tal AS-pir-in KAF-een	capsule, tablet	50 mg/325 mg/ 40 mg; 1–2 capsules or tablets (max 6 a day)	Rx

5HT Agonists

Migraine-specific products called *5HT agonists* or *triptans* offer good efficacy and rapid onset of action. **5HT agonists** bind to serotonin receptors, causing dilated blood vessels in the dura mater to constrict and acting on nerves in the trigeminal system, preventing inflammation and reducing pain signal transmission. They are available in various dosage forms. If a patient does not respond to one, they may respond well to another. There is some variation in activity between the triptans.

Almotriptan (Axert) is available as a tablet and has effect onset about 45 to 60 minutes after administration. It generally is consistent in providing relief. It is also better tolerated than some of the other migraine medications.

Eletriptan (Relpax) is available as a tablet; onset of effect is about 30 minutes. It is most effective at doses of 80 mg. However, since the highest dose available in the United States is 40 mg, patients may find more success with other options. In addition, eletriptan is more likely than other triptans to have drug interactions. The maximum is two 40 mg doses in 24 hours, but the effects seem to last longer than with most migraine treatments.

Frovatriptan (Frova) has a slow onset to effect, about four hours, but it has a relatively long half-life. It is available as a tablet in one strength.

Naratriptan (Amerge) is the gentlest triptan because it has slow onset, approximately four hours, and a favorable safety profile. It has a long half-life, which is generally associated with a low likelihood of migraine recurrence.

Rizatriptan (Maxalt, Maxalt-MLT) tablets are quickly absorbed and have the most rapid onset of action of all the oral migraine therapies. Many patients experience relief as soon as 30 minutes after taking this drug. The tablet is placed on the tongue and allowed to quickly dissolve. Maxalt is not absorbed as rapidly as Maxalt-MLT.

Sumatriptan (Imitrex, Onzetra Xsail, Sumavel DosePro, Tosymra, Zembrace SymTouch) first entered the market as a subcutaneous injection and now is also available in tablet form and as a nasal spray and an inhaled nasal powder. When injected, sumatriptan is effective in approximately 15 minutes, the fastest onset of action available among the triptans. If sumatriptan is taken orally, onset slows to 45 to 60 minutes until effect after administration. The subcutaneous administration route is especially beneficial to patients with diminished gastric absorption or nausea and vomiting. The patient should receive an injection at the first sign of a headache. **Sumatriptan / naproxen (Treximet)** is also available as a combination product. It is more effective than sumatriptan alone.

Zolmitriptan (Zomig, Zomig ZMT) takes about 45 to 60 minutes for onset of action when taken orally. Intranasal zolmitriptan is faster than oral tablets.

Dosage Forms and Administration Oral disintegrating tablets can be taken without water. The tablet should be removed from the blister pack and placed on the tongue. To use the nasal spray, the patient should blow their nose prior to use and then insert the spray tip into a nostril, pinch the other nostril closed, and apply one spray. They should breathe gently through the mouth for 5 to 10 seconds. The injection product is injected subcutaneously into the abdomen or thigh. It should not be injected into the arm. This product is one-time use only—discard after use.

Side Effects The most common side effect of triptans is an unpleasant taste in the mouth, but patients can also experience dizziness, drowsiness, flushing, sweating, headache, and nausea. Serious effects can include chest pain, allergic reaction, and facial swelling.

Contraindications Contraindications to triptans include cerebrovascular syndromes, ischemic cardiac syndromes, uncontrolled hypertension, and hepatic impairment. Use of a triptan is contraindicated within 24 hours of taking an ergotamine-containing or ergot-type medication or within 24 hours of taking a different triptan.

Cautions and Considerations Triptans should be administered with caution in patients with coronary artery disease or hepatic impairment. The use of triptans should be limited to nine administrations a month. This is due to the medications' ability to cause medication-overuse headaches. Patients needing to use zomitriptan more often than nine times in a month should talk with their prescriber about taking prophylaxis therapy to prevent migraines rather than treating them once they occur. Sumatriptan / naproxen combination products must be dispensed with a Medication Guide.

Drug Interactions Drug interactions include MAOIs; concurrent use may increase the risk of serotonin syndrome. Other serotonergic agents, such as SSRIs, are generally safe, as their primary serotonin receptor targets differ. Concurrent use of ketoconazole, itraconazole, and amiodarone may increase toxicity.

Ergot Derivatives

Ergotamine, an alkaloid derived from the **ergot** group of fungi, which live parasitically on grasses such as rye, is used in the treatment of migraine headaches. These medications bind to the same receptors that triptans target, addressing migraines through the same mechanism. This is why triptans and ergot derivatives cannot be taken together. To be effective, ergotamine therapy should be initiated early in a migraine attack.

Dosage Forms and Administration **Dihydroergotamine (D.H.E. 45, Migranal)** is an alpha-adrenergic blocker in addition to having its primary migraine activity at the serotonin receptors. It is available as a nasal spray or as a solution for subcutaneous, intramuscular, or intravenous administration. It is often given with an antiemetic like metoclopramide, which is also known to have some antimigraine effect. This drug does not work as quickly as sumatriptan, but its effect lasts longer.

Ergotamine (Ergomar) is a direct vasoconstrictor of smooth muscle in cranial blood vessels and is used to treat migraines. It is unclear if the drug is truly effective at relieving migraines, and its benefits are questionable when compared to the side effects of nausea and vomiting.

Side Effects Ergotamine has significant adverse effects that limit its usefulness. The most common, regardless of the administration route, are nausea and vomiting. These effects may be exacerbated if a rectal suppository is used, because absorption is enhanced. Ergotism (a syndrome of progressive vasoconstriction and ischemia of vital organs) and ergot headache (a medication-headache cycle occurring with daily use of ergotamine) have been reported. To avoid these adverse effects, patients should be told the maximum daily and weekly dosages and the importance of avoiding ergotamine use on consecutive days or more than twice a week.

Contraindications Ergot derivatives are contraindicated in patients who have myocardial infarction and in those who are pregnant or lactating.

Cautions and Considerations Ergot derivatives carry a risk for serious or life-threatening peripheral ischemia with the concurrent use of CYP3A4 inhibitors. Derivatives should also be used with caution in patients at risk for cardiovascular or cerebrovascular events.

Drug Interactions Concurrent use of ergot derivative drugs with CYP3A4 inhibitors like ketoconazole, voriconazole, or macrolide antibiotics may increase the risk of nausea and vomiting.

Calcitonin Gene-Related Peptide (CGRP) Receptor Antagonists

CGRP receptor antagonists are a new class of drugs used for migraine. Two tablet options are currently available for acute migraine management. A **CGRP receptor antagonist** works by blocking activation of the trigeminal pain pathways. This drug class can be a useful alternative to triptans and ergots since it works similarly but does not have the same vasoconstriction, which may be preferred in patients with cardiovascular conditions. In addition, four monoclonal antibody CGRP receptor antagonists are available via monthly injections for migraine prevention (not for acute migraine). **Ubrogepant (Ubrelvy)** was the first agent in this drug class, gaining FDA approval in December 2019.

Dosage Forms and Administration Ubrogepant is a tablet that can be taken with or without food, though its effect can be delayed if taken with a high-fat meal. **Rimegepant (Nurtec)** is available as an orally disintegrating tablet that cannot be swallowed.

Side Effects The most common side effect of ubrogepant and rimegepant is nausea.

Contraindications Ubrogepant cannot be used with CYP3A4 inhibitors (antifungals, diltiazem, and verapamil). Rimegepant cannot be used if there is any history of hypersensitivity to the formulation.

Cautions and Considerations Ubrogepant and rimegepant should not be used in patients with end-stage kidney disease or with severe liver disease.

Drug Interactions Ubrogepant and rimegepant interact with antifungals, diltiazem, verapamil, rifampin, carbamazepine, St. John's wort, and phenytoin. Close monitoring is needed to determine appropriate dosing if either drug is taken with one of these medications.

Antiemetic Agents

Antiemetics are commonly prescribed to treat nausea and vomiting as well as dizziness. A number of agents can be used as antiemetic treatments. Most of these agents work by blocking specific neurotransmitters. These can include serotonin, dopamine, acetylcholine, and histamine antagonists. Antimetic agents can alleviate nausea and vomiting associated with migraine headaches.

Chlorpromazine is effective in some migraines that are unresponsive to ergotamines. It has antiemetic properties and is also used to treat hiccups.

Metoclopramide (Reglan) is available as an IV injection, oral solution, oral disintegrating tablet, and tablet. It can be used to reduce nausea and vomiting and to enhance the absorption of other antimigraine products by reducing gastritis (inflammation of the stomach). It is comparable to sumatriptan and is reasonable to use for migraine relief before starting triptan therapy.

Prochlorperazine (Compro) is also an antiemetic with antimigraine activity. It is comparable to IV metoclopramide and subcutaneous sumatriptan for acute migraine treatment.

Dosage Forms and Administration Prochlorperazine and chlorpromazine have formulations allowing for intramuscular, intravenous, oral tablet, and rectal suppository administration. Prochlorperazine is also frequently used with diphenhydramine due to movement reactions (risk of extrapyramidal side effects and tardive dyskinesia).

Side Effects Side effects of chlorpromazine include drowsiness, extrapyramidal side effects, and orthostatic hypotension. Metoclopramide also tends to cause drowsiness and is frequently given with diphenhydramine to prevent restlessness and movement-related side effects. Frequent side effects of prochlorperazine include drowsiness and hypotension.

Contraindications Antiemetic agents are contraindicated in patients with epilepsy or gastrointestinal hemorrhage who are concurrently taking large doses of CNS depressants or who have hypersensitivity to antiemetic medications.

Cautions and Considerations Antiemetic agents should be administered with caution in patients with liver disease or congestive heart failure. Concomitant use with alcohol should be avoided. Chlorpromazine, metoclopromide, and prochlorperazine carry boxed warnings. Metoclopramide treatment is associated with an increased risk of tardive dyskinesia, a serious movement disorder. Chlorpromazine treatment is not approved for patients with dementia-related psychosis, because it is associated with an increased risk of death. These agents must be dispensed with a Medication Guide.

Drug Interactions Drugs that may interact with chlorpromazine include tricyclic antidepressants and trazodone, because they may increase the risk for extrapyramidal reactions and neuroleptic malignant syndrome. Amitriptyline should not be used with chlorpromazine because it may increase the risk of fatal heart arrhythmia.

Combination Agents

OTC and prescription products that combine multiple agents into one product are also used to treat migraine headache. The most used combination product, **acetaminophen / aspirin / caffeine (Excedrin)**, is available OTC. It is recommended to treat most types of headache as well as migraines that are mild and occur only occasionally.

Butalbital / acetaminophen / caffeine (Fioricet) and **butalbital / aspirin / caffeine (Fiorinal)** are combination drugs often used to treat migraine and tension headaches. The butalbital / aspirin combination is regulated as a Schedule III controlled substance, whereas the acetaminophen combination is not.

Contraindications Acetaminophen / aspirin / caffeine does not have contraindications. Contraindications to butalbital combination drugs include hemorrhagic medical conditions, peptic ulcer (or other serious gastrointestinal lesions), porphyria, and hypersensitivity to any component of the medication.

Cautions and Considerations Acetaminophen / aspirin / caffeine should be used with caution in patients with liver disease. Rarely, severe skin reactions to acetaminophen can occur. The product should be immediately discontinued if skin reaction occurs. Butalbital combination drugs should be used with caution in pediatric patients and in patients with severe hepatic impairment. Fioricet carries a boxed warning for liver failure associated with acetaminophen use greater than 4 g a day.

Drug Interactions Acetaminophen / aspirin / caffeine should not be used with other medications that affect anticoagulation or platelets, such as warfarin, bemiparin, or ginkgo biloba. It also should not be used with theophylline or medications that cause liver toxicity. Drug interactions include the concurrent use of SSRIs and NSAIDs, as these may result in an increased risk of bleeding. Concurrent use with benzodiazepines or opioid analgesics may result in additive respiratory depression.

18.6 Complementary and Alternative Therapies

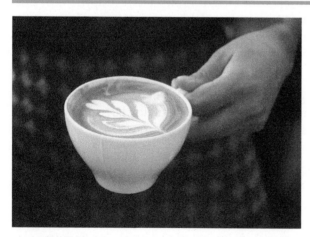

The caffeine in coffee can sometimes be used to treat headaches, fatigue, and drowsiness.

Caffeine is a CNS stimulant used in combination with other analgesics to treat headache. It is sometimes used to treat fatigue and drowsiness in doses of 100–200 mg. It should not be used more than every three to four hours. Caffeine is available in tablets, capsules, gum, and lozenges. Side effects include rapid heartbeat, palpitations, insomnia, restlessness, ringing in the ears, tremors, light-headedness, nausea, vomiting, stomach pain, and an itchy skin rash. Taking caffeine with food can help with these effects, and typically doses should be decreased if such effects occur.

Capsaicin is a chemical derived from cayenne peppers that is used as a topical treatment for pain. It has been found to be effective in diabetic neuropathy, arthritis, and headache pain. It works by exhausting the supply of substance P, a substrate in pain nerve endings in the skin. At first, burning, itching, and tingling occur, and then analgesic effects take hold once substance P is depleted. It may be about a week before some relief starts taking effect. Capsaicin should not be taken orally, be inhaled, or be applied to the eye because severe burning can occur.

Patients should wear gloves during application and wash their hands thoroughly afterward to avoid these effects.

Feverfew is a plant product used orally for migraine pain. It is occasionally used to treat other pain conditions, including menstrual cramps and arthritis. It has been found to improve nausea, vomiting, and light sensitivity experienced during a migraine. Feverfew is generally well tolerated, but side effects include heartburn, nausea, diarrhea, constipation, abdominal pain, and gas. Chewing on feverfew leaves has caused mouth ulceration. Feverfew is dosed at 50–100 mg a day to prevent migraine rather than being used to treat migraine once it has already started.

Cannabis sativa, commonly known as *marijuana*, is a plant that is used for medical and recreational purposes. Cannabinoid, including cannabidiol (CBD), compounds in the plant are associated with pain relief and are distinct from tetrahydrocannabinol, or THC, which is associated with psychological effects. Synthetic and natural CBD extracts may be used to provide relief of chronic or neuropathic pain. CBD can be administered via oral, sublingual, and intramuscular routes. To receive effects of CBD via inhalation, medical marijuana is used. Side effects of CBD include dizziness, weight gain, and heart disease. Inhaled marijuana may increase the risk of lung cancer.

Butterbur is an herbal product that is sometimes taken to prevent migraines. Taken twice a day, over time it has been found to reduce the frequency and severity as well as to shorten the length of migraine headaches. Some butterbur products contain pyrrolizidine alkaloids (PAs), which are harmful and unsafe. Patients should seek out only those butterbur products that are PA free. Side effects can include diarrhea, upset stomach, drowsiness, and itchy eyes. Patients who are allergic to ragweed, marigolds, or daisies should not use butterbur.

Review and Assessment

CHAPTER SUMMARY

Physiology of Pain

- Neuropathic pain is frequently managed with gabapentinoids, SNRIs, tricyclic antidepressants, and topical medications.

- Pain is classified as acute, chronic nonmalignant, or chronic malignant.

Opioids and Pain Management

- Morphine is the standard against which all other opioids are measured.

- Opiates are naturally occurring substances, while opioids are semi-synthetic derivatives and synthetic substances.

- Opioids and opiates have similar side effects, which include constipation, urinary retention, and nausea.

- Dosing is unique to each patient and should support general quality of life and the ability to complete daily activities. For the vast majority of patients, complete pain relief may not be possible.

- The patient-controlled analgesia (PCA) pump is an effective means of controlling pain; the pump allows the patient to regulate, within certain limits, the amount of drug received. Better pain control is achieved with less drug.

- The transdermal patch controls pain and allows the patient to remain more alert than with most other methods.

- Most opioid side effects fade within a week or two, except for constipation, which lasts for the duration of opioid therapy.

- Opioids act on the chemoreceptor trigger zone (CTZ) of the brain, which in turn stimulates the vomiting center.

- Opioid use disorder is a condition that can occur with long-term use of an opioid analgesic; it is characterized by a persistent desire to use opioids, interference with relationships and other life activities, and the need to increase doses to receive the same effects.

- Fentanyl is manufactured as a buccal tablet, injection, lozenge, nasal spray, sublingual film, sublingual spray, sublingual tablet, and transdermal patch.

- Naloxone is an opioid antagonist used in respiratory emergencies following known or suspected opioid toxicity events.

- Nociceptive pharmacologic therapy options include regional anesthesia with local anesthetics, opioid agonists, ketamine, acetaminophen, NSAIDs, and antihistamines.

- Combination opioid and nonopioid analgesics can result in superior pain relief at lower doses than either alone.

Opioid Use Disorder and Treatments

- Various agents are used to treat opioid use disorder and assist patients with withdrawal symptoms.

- Methadone (Dolophine, Methadose), naltrexone (Vivitrol), buprenorphine (Probuphine, Sublocade), and buprenorphine / naloxone (Suboxone) are used to treat opioid use disorder.

Anesthesia

- General anesthesia causes reversible unconsciousness and absence of response to stimulation. It is characterized by four actions: unconsciousness, analgesia, paralysis (skeletal muscle relaxation), and amnesia upon recovery.

- The advantage of nitrous oxide is that it is rapidly eliminated.

- Naloxone and flumazenil (Romazicon) are given to reverse overdoses of specific drugs.

- Neuromuscular blocking is important as an adjunct to general anesthesia to facilitate endotracheal intubation and to ensure that the patient does not move during surgery.

- Neuromuscular blocking agents act via a depolarizing mechanism or as antagonists to acetylcholine at the nicotinic cholinergic receptors.

- Medication is sometimes used preoperatively to control sedation, reduce postoperative pain, cause amnesia, and decrease anxiety.

- Anticholinesterase agents reverse the effects of neuromuscular blockers.

- Local anesthetics are advantageous because they affect all types of nervous tissue. They relieve pain without decreasing the level of alertness or mental function.

Migraine Headaches and Drug Treatments

- Drug treatments for migraine headaches are divided into two groups: acute and prophylactic therapies.

- Prophylactic drugs include anticonvulsants, beta-blockers, calcium channel blockers, feverfew, NSAIDs, SSRIs, and tricyclic antidepressants.

- Patients who are using acute drug therapy for migraine headaches should initiate therapy at the first sign of a headache.

- Triptans are used for the relief of migraine headaches. They are used at the first sign of headache.

- CGRP receptor antagonists can be used as an alternative to triptans for acute migraine management, and they may be better for patients with cardiovascular medical conditions.

- Butalbital is combined with other drugs to treat migraine and tension headaches.

Complementary and Alternative Therapies

- Caffeine is a CNS stimulant and is used in combination with other agents to treat headaches.

- Capsaicin (derived from cayenne peppers) may be used as a topical treatment for pain.

- Feverfew and butterbur are plant products that are used for migraine pain.

- Cannabinoid, including cannabidiol (CBD), compounds derived from the *Cannabis sativa* plant are associated with pain relief.

DRUG LIST

Opioid Analgesics
codeine (various brands)
fentanyl (Abstral, Actiq, Duragesic, Fentora, Lazanda, Subsys)
hydromorphone (Dilaudid, Exalgo)
methadone (Dolophine, Methadose)
morphine (Arymo, Astramorph, Dura-morph, Infumorph, Kadian, Mitigo, MS Contin, Oramorph)
oxycodone (Oxaydo, OxyCONTIN, Roxico-done, Xtampza)
tapentadol (Nucynta)
tramadol (ConZip, Synapryn, Ultram)

Mixed Opioid Agonists
buprenorphine (Belbuca, Buprenex, Butrans, Probuphine, Sublocade)
butorphanol
nalbuphine

Opioid Antagonists
naloxone (Narcan)
naltrexone (Vivitrol)

Drugs Used to Treat Substance Use Disorder
buprenorphine (Probuphine, Sublocade)
buprenorphine / naloxone (Bunavail, Subox-one, Zubsolv)
methadone (Dolophine, Methadose)
naltrexone (Vivitrol)

Inhaled Anesthetics
desflurane (Suprane)
isoflurane (Forane)
nitrous oxide
sevoflurane (Ultane)

Injectable Anesthetics
alfentanil (Alfenta)
dexmedetomidine (Precedex)
etomidate (Amidate)
fentanyl
ketamine (Ketalar)
morphine (various brands)
propofol (Diprivan)

remifentanyl (Ultiva)
sufentanil (Sufenta)

Barbiturates
methohexital (Brevital)

Benzodiazepines
diazepam (Valium)
lorazepam (Ativan)
midazolam

Agent for Malignant Hyperthermia
dantrolene (Dantrium, Revonto, Ryanodex)

Neuromuscular Blocking Agents
atracurium
cisatracurium (Nimbex)
pancuronium (Pavulon)
rocuronium (Zemuron)
succinylcholine (Anectine, Quelicin)
vecuronium (Norcuron)

Antagonists to Reverse Overdoses
flumazenil (Romazicon)
naloxone (Narcan)
neostigmine (Bloxiverz)
pyridostigmine (Mestinon, Regonol)

Local Anesthetics

Esters
benzocaine (various brands)
chloroprocaine (Nesacaine)
dyclonine (Sucrets)
tetracaine (Cepacol Viractin, Pontocaine)

Amides
bupivacaine
lidocaine (various brands)
lidocaine / epinephrine (Xylocaine with epinephrine)
lidocaine / prilocaine (various brands)
mepivacaine (Carbocaine, Polocaine)
ropivacaine (Naropin)

Migraine Headaches

5HT Agonists
almotriptan (Axert)
eletriptan (Relpax)

frovatriptan (Frova)
naratriptan (Amerge)
rizatriptan (Maxalt, Maxalt-MLT)
sumatriptan (Imitrex, Onzetra Xsail,
    Sumavel DosePro, Tosymra, Zembrace
    SymTouch)
sumatriptan / naproxen (Treximet)
zolmitriptan (Zomig, Zomig ZMT)

Ergot Derivatives
dihydroergotamine (D.H.E. 45, Migranal)
ergotamine (Ergomar)

Calcitonin Gene-Related Peptide (CGRP)
    Receptor Antagonists
rimegepant (Nurtec)
ubrogepant (Ubrelvy)

Antiemetic Agents
chlorpromazine
metoclopramide (Reglan)
prochlorperazine (Compro)

Combinations
acetaminophen / aspirin / caffeine (Excedrin)
butalbital / acetaminophen / caffeine
    (Capacet, Esgic, Fioricet, Vanatol LQ,
    Zebutal)
butalbital / aspirin / caffeine (Fiorinal)

Boxed Warnings
Note that only certain forms of the drugs in
    this list have boxed warnings.
bupivacaine
buprenorphine (Belbuca, Buprenex, Butrans,
    Probuphine, Sublocade)
buprenorphine / naloxone (Bunavail, Subox-
    one, Zubsolv)
butalbital / acetaminophen / caffeine
    (Fioricet)
butorphanol (Stadol)
chlorpromazine
codeine (various brands)
dantrolene (Dantrium, Revonto, Ryanodex)
diazepam (Valium)
fentanyl (Abstral, Actiq, Duragesic, Fentora,
    Lazanda, Subsys)
flumazenil (Romazicon)
hydrocodone
hydromorphone (Dilaudid, Exalgo)
ketamine (Ketalar)

lidocaine (topical solution)
lorazepam (Ativan)
methadone (Dolophine, Methadose)
metoclopramide (Metozolv, Reglan)
midazolam
morphine (Arymo, Astramorph, Dura-
    morph, Infumorph, Kadian, Mitigo, MS
    Contin, Oramorph)
nalbuphine (Nubain)
oxycodone (Oxaydo, OxyCONTIN, Roxico-
    done, Xtampza)
pancuronium (Pavulon)
pentazocine (Talwin)
prochlorperazine (Compazine, Compro)
rocuronium (Zemuron)
succinylcholine (Anectine, Quelicin)
tapentadol (Nuycynta)
tramadol (ConZip, Enovra, Synapryn,
    Ultram)
vecuronium (Norcuron)

Medication Guides
buprenorphine (Belbuca, Buprenex, Butrans,
    Probuphine, Sublocade)
buprenorphine / naloxone (Bunavail, Subox-
    one, Zubsolv)
codeine (various brands)
fentanyl (Abstral, Actiq, Duragesic, Fentora,
    Lazanda, Subsys)
hydromorphone (Dilaudid, Exalgo)
methadone (Dolophine, Methadose)
metoclopramide (Metozolv, Reglan)
morphine (Arymo, Astramorph, Dura-
    morph, Infumorph, Kadian, Mitigo, MS
    Contin, Oramorph)
oxycodone (Oxaydo, OxyCONTIN, Roxico-
    done, Xtampza)
oxycodone / ibuprofen (Combunox)
oxymorphone (Opana)
sumatriptan / naproxen (Treximet)
tapentadol (Nuycynta)
tramadol (ConZip, Enovra, Synapryn,
    Ultram)

Take a moment to review what you have learned in this chapter and answer the following questions.

1. Which one of these medications is used for local anesthesia?
   a. desflurane
   b. propofol
   c. midazolam
   d. lidocaine

2. The weakest general anesthetic is
   a. sevoflurane.
   b. nitrous oxide.
   c. midazolam.
   d. propofol.

3. Which agent has a side effect of high blood pressure?
   a. propofol
   b. fentanyl
   c. ketamine
   d. midazolam

4. Which of these neuromuscular blocking agents will have the shortest duration of action?
   a. rocuronium
   b. succinylcholine
   c. pancuronium
   d. vecuronium

5. Which of the following is required for a valid Suboxone prescription, written for substance use disorder?
   a. days supply
   b. patient's opioid MME prior to starting Suboxone
   c. prescriber's XDEA number
   d. ICD-10 code

6. Which medication can reverse opioid-induced emergencies?
   a. fentanyl
   b. buprenorphine
   c. naloxone
   d. codeine

7. Which of the following opioid side effects makes opioid toxicity deadly?
   a. sedation
   b. slowed breathing
   c. hypotension
   d. constipation

8. Which of the following side effects never fades while on long-term opioid therapy?
   a. sedation
   b. hypotension
   c. nausea
   d. constipation

9. What medication should not be taken within 24 hours of a triptan?
   a. ergot
   b. NSAID
   c. metoclopramide
   d. butalbital / acetaminophen / caffeine

10. Which neurotransmitter activates the trigeminal pain pathways during a migraine?
    a. 5HT
    b. CGRP
    c. histamine
    d. prostaglandins

MAKE CONNECTIONS

Take a moment to consider what you have learned in this chapter and respond thoughtfully to the following prompts. Note that some of these activities will require internet access.

1. How do nociceptive pain, neuropathic pain, and centralized sensitization pain differ? Compare and contrast how they are managed.

2. Why should any patient getting an opioid analgesic be offered naloxone?

 The online course includes additional review and assessment resources.

Nutrition, Fluids, Electrolytes, and Drug Therapy

19

Learning Objectives

1 Describe how the body uses vitamins and the common signs and symptoms of vitamin deficiency. (Section 19.1)

2 Explain how fluids and electrolytes are used in the body. (Section 19.2)

3 Describe how electrolyte replacement products are used. (Section 19.2)

4 Define obesity. (Section 19.3)

5 Describe the prescription treatments for obesity. (Section 19.3)

6 Compare and contrast enteral and parenteral nutrition, including their purposes, ingredients, stability, and complications. (Section 19.4)

ASHP/ACPE Accreditation Standards

To view the *ASHP/ACPE Accreditation Standards* addressed in this chapter, refer to Appendix C.

Consumption of food and other nondrug substances has far-reaching effects on the health of the human body. Food contains vitamins, minerals, and other nutrients that maintain body function and aid in disease prevention and treatment. Electrolytes such as sodium, potassium, and calcium regulate electrical activity in the body and need to be kept in balance with bodily fluids. Plant substances such as herbs can affect the body, and many of them have medicinal applications. Nutrition is an important component of health and wellness. When an individual receives too much or too little of the daily caloric, protein, or micronutrient needs for their age and size, overnutrition (obesity) or undernutrition (malnutrition) can result. Both obesity and malnutrition can have negative health effects and can increase morbidity and mortality. According to the World Health Organization, global obesity has more than tripled since 1975, and more than 1.9 billion adults were overweight in 2016. Once a problem associated with high-income countries, obesity is now on the rise in low- and middle-income countries. In fact, most of the world's population lives in countries where being overweight kills more people than being underweight. Malnutrition, however, is still a major concern. It is estimated that malnutrition contributes to more than one-third of child deaths worldwide.

19.1 Vitamins

A **vitamin** is an organic substance that is necessary for normal metabolic functioning. With the exception of vitamin D, vitamins are not synthesized in the body in sufficient amounts. Usually a vitamin is a **coenzyme** (a chemical other than a protein that an enzyme needs for assistance in performing a metabolic function) or is converted to a coenzyme in the body. Vitamins are naturally present in many foods and can be added to foods as supplements. If dietary intake of any of these substances is inadequate, a deficiency results and can lead to serious illness.

Vitamins are classified as either fat soluble or water soluble and serve a variety of purposes throughout the body. Table 19.1 lists the main vitamins needed to maintain a baseline of health.

TABLE 19.1 Commonly Used Vitamins

Vitamin	Function in Human Body
Fat Soluble	
A (carotenoid, retinol)	bones, skin, eyes, reproduction
D (calciferol)	bones
E (tocopherol)	eyes, immunity, dementia
K (phylloquinone, phytonadione)	blood clotting
Water Soluble	
B_1 (thiamine)	metabolism, mental, cardiac
B_2 (riboflavin)	hair, skin, nails
B_3 (niacin)	cholesterol levels, brain cells, skin, bowel
B_5 (pantothenic acid)	growth, normal physiological functions, energy production
B_6 (pyridoxine)	nerves
B_7 (biotin)	hair, energy production, growth
B_9 (folate / folic acid)	red blood cells, depression
B_{12} (cobalamin)	red blood cells
C (ascorbic acid)	immunity

Fat-Soluble Vitamins

A **fat-soluble vitamin** is a vitamin the body absorbs along with dietary fat and maintains in large stores, mainly in the liver. Due to the body's ability to store vitamins, deficiency develops only after several months of restricted intake. It is possible to ingest too much of a fat-soluble vitamin, which can result in toxic levels in the body. The fat-soluble vitamins are vitamins A, D, E, and K.

Vitamin A

Vitamin A is a family of compounds referred to as *retinoic acids* and can be found in two forms: provitamin A carotenoids such as beta-carotene and preformed vitamin A retinoids such as retinol, retinal, retinoic acid, and retinyl esters. Vitamin A is needed for vision, growth, bone formation, reproduction, immune system function, and skin health.

Provitamin A carotenoids must be metabolized into active vitamin A via a highly regulated process. Provitamin A carotenoids can be found in green leafy vegetables,

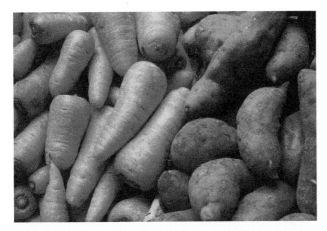

Carrots and sweet potatoes are rich sources of beta-carotene. In fact, the compound beta-carotene gives these vegetables their orange color.

sweet potatoes, and carrots. Because the body regulates conversion to active vitamin A on an as-needed basis, excessive intake of provitamin A is unlikely to cause toxicity.

Preformed vitamin A is a more active form and is found mostly in animal sources and supplements. Butter, egg yolk, kidney, and liver are common food sources of preformed vitamin A. Absorption and storage of preformed vitamin A are efficient, but toxicity can occur if excessive quantities are ingested.

Vitamin A supplements are used primarily to treat deficiency. Vitamin A deficiency is rarely seen in the United States, but it is the third most common nutritional deficiency in the world. It may result in **keratomalacia**, a softening and ulceration of the cornea of the eye.

Signs and symptoms of keratomalacia include skin rash, corneal degeneration, night blindness, and dry eyes. Other manifestations of vitamin A deficiency include poor bone growth, dermatologic problems, and weakened immune system.

Vitamin A is also used to treat cataracts and to reduce postpartum complications and complications of human immunodeficiency virus (HIV), measles, malaria, and ulcerative colitis.

Excessive intake of vitamin A, usually from ingestion of preformed vitamin A, may cause toxicity. Signs and symptoms of vitamin A toxicity include nausea, vomiting, vertigo, blurry vision, hair loss, headache, irritability, skin peeling, and bone and liver problems.

Excessive vitamin A can be highly teratogenic, especially in the first trimester of pregnancy, and can lead to spontaneous abortions and fetal malformations.

The US Department of Agriculture (USDA) suggests a recommended daily allowance of 750 mcg (as retinol activity equivalents) of vitamin A during pregnancy. Doses in excess of this allowance are contraindicated in pregnant individuals.

Vitamin D

The D vitamins are collectively known as **calciferol**. **Vitamin D** was first identified as a vitamin in the early 20th century and is now also recognized as a hormone. Vitamin D and its metabolites play an important role in maintaining calcium and phosphate levels in the body. There is evidence to suggest that vitamin D plays a role in insulin resistance, obesity, metabolic syndrome, and various cancers.

Vitamin D has two major forms: ergocalciferol (vitamin D_2) and cholecalciferol (vitamin D_3). Both forms of vitamin D are converted in the body to the active metabolite, calcitriol. **Ergocalciferol** is largely human made and added to foods. **Cholecalciferol** is synthesized in the skin in response to sunlight and can be consumed in the diet through the intake of certain animal-based foods. Sunlight usually provides 80%–90% of the body's vitamin D stores. Both forms of vitamin D are made commercially and can be found in dietary supplements and fortified foods.

There are few naturally occurring food sources of vitamin D. These sources include fatty fish, fish liver oil, and egg yolks.

Vitamin D is used to treat **rickets**, a childhood disease in which a lack of vitamin D results in bone softening and muscle weakness. A hallmark of rickets is bowlegs. Vitamin D can also be used to treat **osteomalacia**, a bone disorder that presents as bone pain, muscle weakness, difficulty walking, and bone fractures. The National Osteoporosis Foundation recommends that adults over 50 years old take 800 to 1,000 IU of vitamin D per day along with calcium to prevent osteoporosis.

Excessive intake of vitamin D can lead to toxicity. Signs and symptoms of vitamin D toxicity include high blood calcium levels, kidney stones, nausea, vomiting, thirst, increased urination, muscle weakness, and bone pain.

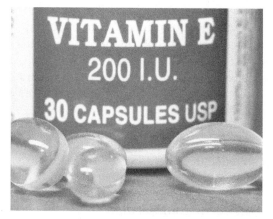

Vitamin E supplements are typically in capsule form.

Vitamin E

The physiologic role of **vitamin E**, or **tocopherol**, is still being defined, but it is thought to work as an antioxidant. Vitamin E is found in a variety of food products, including oils, meat, eggs, and green leafy vegetables. Abundant in olive oil and sunflower oil, alpha-tocopherol is the form of vitamin E best known for its role in human health. Gamma-tocopherol can be found in soybean oil and corn oil.

Vitamin E deficiency rarely occurs except in cases of specific genetic or malabsorption disorders. Vitamin E deficiency can cause neuromuscular disorders, fragile red blood cells (RBCs), and hemolysis, and it may be treated with supplementation.

Laboratory studies support the use of vitamin E in the treatment of macular degeneration and Alzheimer's disease. Vitamin E also has been shown to reduce the risk of some cancers and dementia and to improve immune system function. Other indications for the use of vitamin E include diabetic retinopathy, cardiovascular disease, and prevention of chemotherapy-induced side effects. Topical use of vitamin E can improve skin health, healing, and hydration.

Very high doses of vitamin E may result in bleeding or stroke.

Safety Alert

Patients who are taking warfarin, a common anticoagulant, need to monitor their intake of foods rich in vitamin K.

Vitamin K

Vitamin K functions as a coenzyme for the hepatic production of blood clotting factors and for bone metabolism. Dietary forms of vitamin K (**phylloquinone** and **phytonadione**) are found in green leafy vegetables such as spinach, broccoli, and brussels sprouts and in fats such as plant oils and margarine.

Vitamin K deficiency is rare in otherwise healthy adults. Signs and symptoms of vitamin K deficiency usually are associated with impaired coagulation (such as easy bruising, mucosal bleeding, or blood in the urine or stool). Therefore, vitamin K is administered in situations where blood clotting is desired. One of these situations is the reversal of warfarin, a common anticoagulant.

Another indication for the administration of vitamin K is deficiency caused by drug therapy (for example, salicylates, sulfonamides, quinine, quinidine, and broad-spectrum antibiotics). Vitamin K injection may also be administered to neonates suffering from a deficiency.

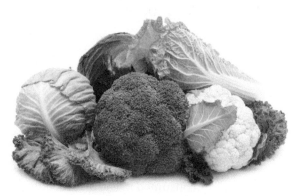

Vitamin K can be found naturally in many commonly consumed vegetables, including broccoli, cabbage, and kale.

Vitamin K can interact with anticoagulants, tetracycline, and retinoids (such as retinol, isotretoin, and acetretin). Patients should not take vitamin K supplements if they take these other prescription medications.

Vitamin K toxicity is rare. Signs of toxicity include anemia and jaundice. Patients who are taking warfarin, a common anticoagulant, need to monitor their intake of foods rich in vitamin K. These foods include green leafy vegetables, green onions, and avocados. Most patients can consume these foods as long as they keep their intake consistent.

Water-Soluble Vitamins

Safety Alert

Pharmacy technicians should be aware that one B vitamin is not interchangeable with another. For example, B_3 (or niacin) may be used for cholesterol, whereas B_{12} (cobalamin) may be used for anemia.

Water-soluble vitamins (the B vitamins and vitamin C) are present in extracellular fluids, which are readily excreted by the kidneys. Because these vitamins are not stored in the body and the kidneys rapidly remove any excess, a deficiency quickly becomes apparent if dietary sources are inadequate, but an overdose is unlikely to be as serious as with fat-soluble vitamins. The B vitamins include vitamins B_1, B_2, B_3, B_5, B_6, B_7, B_9, and B_{12}. Each of these B vitamins has their own unique properties.

Vitamin B_1

Vitamin B_1, or **thiamine**, is an important coenzyme involved in carbohydrate metabolism. It also plays a role in nerve impulse propagation. Thiamine is found in food products such as yeast, legumes, pork, rice, and cereals. However, thiamine is denatured at high temperatures, and cooking, baking, canning, and pasteurization can destroy it.

Thiamine supplements are used to treat vitamin B_1 deficiency. Signs and symptoms of vitamin B_1 deficiency include impaired memory, lactic acidosis, visual disturbances, and mental status changes. Thiamine deficiency is most common during pregnancy and in **Wernicke-Korsakoff syndrome**, which can occur in patients with alcohol use disorder. Patients with known alcohol use disorder may be given thiamine supplements when hospitalized to combat symptoms of alcohol withdrawal. In addition, thiamine supplements are used to treat patients who have **beriberi**, a disease that results from a diet low in vitamin B_1. Beriberi presents with numbness and tingling, edema, and heart failure.

Vitamin B_2

Vitamin B_2, or **riboflavin**, is a coenzyme involved in tissue respiration and normal cell metabolism. Riboflavin is found in many foods, including cereal, green vegetables, milk, and some meats. It is also made in the intestines by bacteria.

Riboflavin is typically used to treat vitamin B_2 deficiency, but it can also be used in doses of 400 mg a day to decrease migraine headaches. Signs of vitamin B_2 deficiency include mucositis, skin rash, cracked lips, photophobia, tearing, poor vision, poor wound healing, and anemia.

Vitamin B_3

Vitamin B_3, or **niacin**, is essential for reactions in the body that produce **adenosine triphosphate (ATP)**, a critical molecule in cellular energy production. The two most common forms of niacin are nicotinic acid and nicotinamide. Niacin also helps regulate the production and activity of cholesterol molecules in the blood. Vitamin B_3 is found in yeast, peanuts, peas, beans, whole grains, potatoes, and lean meats.

Niacin may be used to treat patients with dyslipidemia, a condition signified by elevated total or low-density lipoprotein (LDL) cholesterol levels or low levels of high-density lipoprotein (HDL) cholesterol. Niacin lowers triglycerides and LDL levels and raises HDL levels but may not have significant effects on cardiovascular outcomes such as preventing heart attack. The dose required for these effects is at least 1,200 mg a day.

In addition, niacin supplements are used to treat vitamin B_3 deficiency. This deficiency may result from the use of certain medications, such as 5-fluorouracil, isoniazid, phenobarbital, azathioprine, and chloramphenicol.

A deficiency of vitamin B_3 may result in **pellagra**, a disease that presents with hyperpigmented rash in areas of exposed skin, red tongue, swelling of the mouth and tongue, diarrhea, sensitivity to light, and neurologic symptoms such as insomnia, anxiety, and disorientation. Pellagra often develops in patients who have certain gastrointestinal (GI) diseases or alcohol use disorder.

Vitamin B_5

Vitamin B_5, or pantothenic acid, is a precursor to coenzyme A. Coenzyme A has an important role in the synthesis of many molecules, such as vitamins A and D, cholesterol, steroids, heme, fatty acids, amino acids, and proteins. Vitamin B_5 is found in whole grains, potatoes, chicken, beef, egg yolk, liver, kidney, broccoli, and milk. Pantothenic acid can also be produced by bacteria in the colon.

Pantothenic acid supplements are usually used to treat vitamin B_5 deficiency. Signs of deficiency include paresthesia, dysesthesia, fatigue, malaise, headache, insomnia, vomiting, and abdominal cramps.

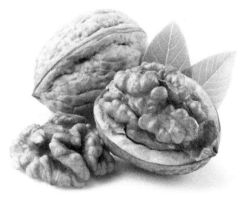

Walnuts are a rich source of pantothenic acid.

Vitamin B_6

Vitamin B_6 is converted in the body to the coenzymes responsible for amino acid metabolism. Common forms include **pyridoxine**, which vitamin B_6 is often called, as well as pyridoxal and pyridoxamine. Pyridoxine and pyridoxamine are predominantly found in plant-based foods such as vegetables, whole grains, and nuts. Pyridoxal is most commonly derived from foods with animal sources. Cooking, processing, and storage can reduce vitamin B_6 levels by up to 50%.

Pyridoxine is used to treat and prevent vitamin B_6 deficiency. Dermatitis may be present in patients with pyridoxine deficiency. Other side effects include neuropathy, weakness, dizziness, and anemia.

Vitamin B_7

Vitamin B_7, or biotin, a coenzyme involved in metabolism, plays an essential role in many processes, including cell replication. Biotin can be found in a variety of plants (particularly peanuts and green leafy vegetables), liver, egg yolk, soybeans, and yeast.

Biotin supplements are taken for vitamin B_7 deficiency. Signs of deficiency include skin rash, hair loss, change in hair color, depression, tiredness, hallucinations, and numbness and tingling. Biotin deficiency is typically associated with pregnancy, long-term parenteral nutrition, and malnutrition that may be due to impaired absorption in patients with short bowel syndrome. Consumption of large quantities of raw egg whites can also lead to biotin deficiency.

Vitamin B$_9$

Vitamin B$_9$, also known as **folic acid** and **folate**, plays a major role in intracellular metabolism and the breakdown of **homocysteine**, an amino acid associated with cardiovascular disease. It is also involved in the production of the neurotransmitter serotonin. Folic acid is frequently added to foods but is naturally found in green leafy vegetables, fruits, cereals, grains, and red meat.

Folic acid supplements are used to treat vitamin B$_9$ deficiency. Signs of deficiency include anemia, diarrhea, and a swollen or painful tongue. A lack of vitamin B$_9$ also has a deleterious effect on the cardiovascular system and is associated with a heightened risk of coronary heart disease, stroke, and peripheral vascular disease.

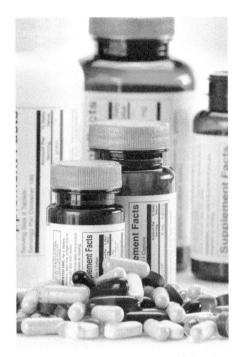

Self-medicating with large doses of vitamins can cause problems. A well-balanced diet is the best way to ensure good health.

Deficiencies in folic acid cause anemia and neural tube defects in developing fetuses. Consequently, folic acid supplements are highly recommended for all individuals who are pregnant or planning to become pregnant. Taking folic acid can greatly reduce the incidence of some birth defects.

Vitamin B$_9$ supplements are also used to reduce homocysteine levels in patients with end-stage kidney disease. Other uses include treatment for chronic fatigue syndrome, depression, and vitiligo.

Vitamin B$_{12}$

Vitamin B$_{12}$, or **cobalamin**, is a coenzyme necessary for cell reproduction, normal growth, and RBC production. It is found in fish, milk, bread, and meat. Intestinal absorption of vitamin B$_{12}$ requires intrinsic factor, which is produced in the stomach. Patients who have undergone a gastrectomy need to take lifelong vitamin B$_{12}$ injections because they are unable to produce intrinsic factor.

Vitamin B$_{12}$ deficiency takes a long time to develop and is easily treated with supplements. It is most common in older adults and strict vegetarians. Signs of B$_{12}$ deficiency include anemia, swollen or painful tongue, and nerve pain and degeneration.

Other indications for cobalamin supplements are pernicious anemia and end-stage renal disease. Vitamin B$_{12}$ can be applied topically for psoriasis and atopic dermatitis.

Vitamin C

Vitamin C, or **ascorbic acid**, is best known for its role in immune system function and as an antioxidant. An **antioxidant** is one of a number of substances believed to help prevent cell damage caused by free radicals. Vitamin C is found in citrus fruits, tomatoes, potatoes, brussels sprouts, cauliflower, broccoli, strawberries, blueberries, cabbage, and spinach.

Small doses (100–250 mg a day) of vitamin C supplements are used to treat deficiency. Signs of deficiency include poor wound healing, fatigue, and depression. Vitamin C is most effective for treating a severe deficiency known as **scurvy**, a disease rarely seen in the United States. Scurvy presents with fatigue, anemia, hemorrhage, nosebleeds, spongy gums, and enlargement of hair follicles. Other indications for vitamin C supplements are macular degeneration, seasonal allergies, and poor iron absorption. They are also used for the reduction of tyrosinemia in premature infants on high-protein diets.

Many individuals also take large doses of vitamin C supplements (1–3 g a day) because they believe it helps prevent illnesses such as the common cold, cancer, atherosclerosis, and sunburn. The FDA has approved a health claim for the use of vitamin C in the prevention of cancer. However, patients should be aware that high doses of supplemental vitamin C may increase their risk for kidney stones and may cause undesirable side effects such as diarrhea and gastrointestinal upset.

19.2 Fluids, Electrolytes, and Acid-Base Balance

Fluids and electrolytes are highly related and dependent on each other within the body. A change in one component usually causes subsequent changes to the other. An **electrolyte** is a substance that dissociates (separates) into ions within a solution or solvent (usually water) and is thus capable of conducting electricity. Water moves from areas of low solute (dissolved substance) concentration to areas of high solute concentration in an attempt to maintain equilibrium. Thus, fluids and electrolytes move around the body in relation to each other. A loss of fluids in one area of the body prompts a shift in fluids from another area to replace what was lost. During this shift, electrolytes are exchanged in an effort to balance the concentration of solutes between fluid compartments of the body.

Fluids

The human body consists of about 60% water and varies between the average male body and the average female body. (Figure 19.1 shows the percentage of body weight that is made up of water in the average adult man and the average adult woman.) The difference is due to skeletal weight and the inverse relation of water to adipose (fat) tissue. The percentage of body water (that is, fluid levels), often referred to as **total body water (TBW)**, varies according to weight, sex, and age and is influenced by any accompanying medical conditions.

Fatty tissue holds little water. Therefore, the proportion of water in people with more fatty tissue may be as little as 55%, whereas in people who are lean it may be as much as 70%. Women generally have more fat than men; therefore, they have proportionally less body water. As an individual's body ages, the body retains less and less water. Newborns may have as much as 75% or more water by weight; older adults may have 60% or less.

Water deficits are caused by loss of bodily fluids as a result of such conditions as vomiting, diarrhea, edema, and excessive sweating from fever; large urine output; and acute weight loss (more than 5% of body weight). A water deficit can cause dry skin and mucous membranes, longitudinal wrinkling of the tongue, hypotension, tachycardia, and lowered body temperature. A loss of 25% of body water can lead to death.

To maintain the overall equilibrium in concentration of total molecules on the inside and outside of a cell, water moves passively across cellular membranes in a process known as **osmosis**. If a solute (for example, an ion) is added to one side of the membrane, water moves to that side to keep the concentration constant on both sides. Often, the concentration of intracellular and extracellular fluid remains constant.

FIGURE 19.1
Water as
Percentage of
Body Weight
in Average
Adult Men and
Women

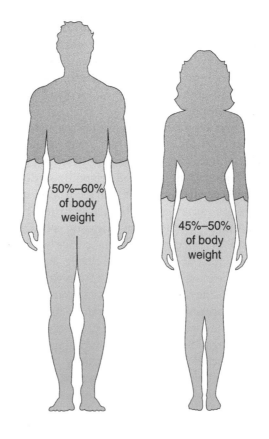

50%–60%
of body
weight

45%–50%
of body
weight

Bodily fluids are divided into two categories: **intracellular** (inside cells) and **extracellular** (outside cells). Intracellular fluid makes up about two-thirds of the body's fluids and is found *inside* cells. Extracellular fluid is found *outside* cells, in the spaces between cells or inside the vasculature in lymph fluid and plasma. Bodily fluids are in equilibrium across the capillary walls. The chemical and physical processes that occur to maintain equilibrium are some of the most important processes in the human body.

Fluids and Solutions

IV fluid products are used to replace fluids and electrolytes lost through dehydration. Parenteral nutrition solutions discussed later in this chapter are primarily used to supply essential trace minerals and daily caloric needs along with providing daily fluid and electrolyte needs. IV fluids can be categorized by tonicity or content (for instance, IV fluid content might consist of colloids or crystalloids).

Tonicity refers to the concentration of a solute in a solvent (liquid vehicle, such as water) and how that concentration affects the movement of water across membranes. The concept of tonicity refers only to molecules, such as ions and electrolytes, that do not move easily across membranes. Fluid and electrolyte products have labeled concentrations in grams of solute per 100 mL of solvent, which is displayed as percent concentration.

A related concept that affects tonicity is **osmolarity**. Osmolarity refers to the concentration of all molecules, both those that move across membranes and those that do not, in a set volume of fluid. Osmolarity is measured in milliosmoles (mOsm) per liter (L). The osmolarity of plasma is approximately 275–300 mOsm/L.

An **isotonic solution** describes a solution with the same level of particles, and thus the same tonicity, as bodily fluids. That means that isotonic solutions have a concentration similar to that of blood plasma. Isotonic fluid products replace daily fluid and electrolyte loss and prevent dehydration. When administered by IV solution, an isotonic solution maintains the normal balance between the vascular volume and interstitial spaces. Isotonic solutions are sometimes referred to as *maintenance solutions*. The most common isotonic IV solution used is normal saline (0.9% NaCl). Figure 19.2 shows what can happen when cells in the blood or body are exposed to solutions that are not isotonic.

A **hypertonic solution** contains a higher concentration of solute than bodily fluids contain. Cells placed in a hypertonic solution shrivel and shrink as water passes out through the cell membrane (see Figure 19.2). The osmolarity of these products is usually over 350 mOsm/L. Hypertonic solutions are used when urgent sodium replenishment is needed as part of hydration. They are indicated for severe sodium depletion from excess sweating, vomiting, or diarrhea. They are also used to treat excessive water intake, overuse of enemas or irrigating solutions (during surgery), and when sodium-free fluids and electrolyte products have been used for fluid replacement. Hypertonic solutions must be administered slowly and monitored closely. If they are given too quickly, the mass exodus of fluid from vital tissues can cause damage. Resulting fluid overload inside the blood vessels can cause heart failure.

A **hypotonic solution** contains a lower concentration of solute than bodily fluids contain. The osmolarity of these products is usually less than 280 mOsm/L. Hypotonic solutions treat dehydration by diluting the concentration of particles within the bloodstream, which decreases the osmolarity. Water leaves the blood and enters interstitial and intracellular spaces. Cells placed in a hypotonic solution swell and burst as water rushes into the cell. Hypotonic solutions are commonly referred to as *hydrating solutions*, because they are used to correct dehydration. Hypotonic solutions must be used with caution. If they are administered too quickly, fluid shifts into the cerebral compartment and causes increased intracranial pressure and brain damage.

FIGURE 19.2
Tonicity Effects on Cells in Solution

Hypertonic solutions cause water to flow out of cells, while hypotonic solutions cause a net flow of water into cells.

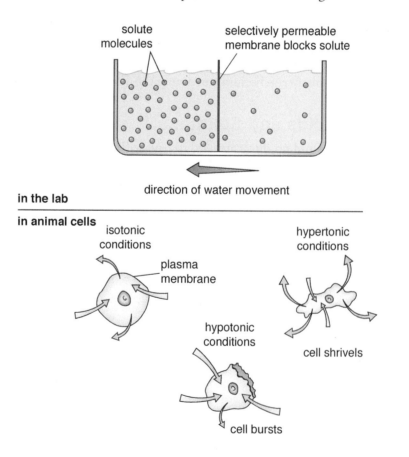

1,000 ml

Lactated Ringer's and 5% Dextrose®

Injection

Lactated Ringer's is a crystalloid solution that is often used in combination with 5% dextrose.

A **crystalloid solution** contains small ions and molecules (electrolytes). Crystalloid solutions are used to replace lost fluid and treat dehydration. They are used on a daily basis as a liquid vehicle for administering IV drugs. Both normal saline and dextrose in water are crystalloid solutions. Dextrose is desirable when a patient has a need for caloric energy (such as in malnutrition) or when glucose levels are low. Table 19.2 contains examples of common crystalloid solutions along with their associated osmolarity.

A **colloid solution** is a solution that contains proteins and other large molecules (such as fats). Molecules in colloid products are so large that they do not quickly or easily move from the bloodstream to surrounding tissues. In that way, colloids act similarly to hypertonic solutions. They increase the osmolarity of blood plasma, which pulls fluid from interstitial spaces. Colloid solutions are commonly referred to as *blood volume expanders*. Examples of colloid solutions include albumin, dextran, and blood itself.

TABLE 19.2 Common Electrolyte Solutions

Tonicity	Solution	Osmolarity (mOsm/L)
hypotonic (hydrating) solutions	0.45% NaCl (½ NS)	154
	dextrose 2.5% in sterile water ($D_{2.5}W$)	140
isotonic solutions	dextrose 5% in sterile water (D_5W)	252
	0.9% NaCl (normal saline [NS])	308
	lactated Ringer's solution (LR)	273
hypertonic solutions	dextrose 5% in 0.45% NaCl (D_5W in ½ NS)	406
	dextrose 5% in 0.9% NaCl (D_5W in NS)	560
	dextrose 10% in sterile water ($D_{10}W$)	505
	3, 5, 14.6, and 23.4% NaCl concentrates	varies

WORKPLACE WISDOM

Hypertonic solutions can be quite irritating and corrosive to tissues and blood vessels. They must be administered via a central IV line (an IV line surgically inserted into a port in a central vein), not a peripheral IV line placed in the arm or hand.

Sterile water for injection is a product available in the pharmacy. It is used for diluting other IV drugs or fluids and should never be administered by itself. Injecting or administering pure water through an IV line causes mass hemolysis as water rushes from the plasma into red blood cells, quickly bursting them. Hemolysis destroys the blood and releases intracellular material in mass amounts, resulting in death.

Electrolytes, Electrolyte Deficiency, and Electrolyte Replacement

Electrolytes are molecular compounds that form ions when dissolved in water. Because water forms the majority of bodily fluid, electrolytes exist throughout the body as positively or negatively charged ions. For example, sodium chloride (table salt) dissociates into sodium (Na^+) and chloride (Cl^-) when dissolved in water. A positively charged ion is called a **cation**, and a negatively charged ion is called an **anion**. Important cations in the body are sodium (Na^+), potassium (K^+), calcium (Ca^{2+}), and magnesium (Mg^{2+}). Important anions include chloride (Cl^-), bicarbonate (HCO_3^-), and, at times, phosphate (PO_4^-). The concentration of electrolytes is measured in **milliequivalents (mEq)** per liter (L). Electrolytes are present in both intracellular and extracellular fluid, though in differing concentrations, depending on the ion. Specific ion pumps (such as sodium-potassium ion pumps) and channels (such as chloride channels) in cellular membranes maintain these concentrations. See Tables 19.3 and 19.4 for common electrolyte products used in pediatrics and adults. Note that electrolyte doses are individualized to patients according to their lab results.

TABLE 19.3 Common Oral Liquid Electrolyte Mixtures

Product	Electrolyte Content	Other Content
Infalyte	Na, K, Cl	rice syrup
Naturalyte	Na, K, Cl	dextrose
Pedialyte (solution, freezer pops, gelatin)	Na, K, Cl	dextrose
Rehydrate	Na, K, Cl	dextrose

TABLE 19.4 Common Electrolyte Replacement Products

Generic (Brand)	Pronunciation	Dosage Form	Dispensing Status
Sodium			
sodium acetate	SOE-dee-um AS-e-tate	injection	Rx
sodium chloride (Slo-Salt, Sustain)	SOE-dee-um KLOR-ide	injection, nasal solution, ophthalmic solution, tablet	Rx
sodium phosphate* (Fleet Enema, Fleet Enema Extra, Fleet Pedia-Lax Enema, OsmoPrep)	SOE-dee-um FOS-fate	concentrate for oral solution, injection, rectal enema	OTC, Rx
Potassium			
potassium acetate	poe-TASS-ee-um AS-e-tate	IV additive (diluted to 40–80 mEq/L)	Rx
potassium chloride (Effer-K, K-Dur, Klor-Con, K-Sol, K-Tab, K-99, Micro-K)	poe-TASS-ee-um KLOR-ide	IV additive, liquid, tablet	Rx
potassium phosphate*	poe-TASS-ee-um FOS-fate	IV additive	Rx

continues

TABLE 19.4 Common Electrolyte Replacement Products—*Continued*

Generic (Brand)	Pronunciation	Dosage Form	Dispensing Status
Calcium			
calcium acetate (Eliphos, PhosLo, Phoslyra)	KAL-see-um AS-e-tate	capsule, oral solution, tablet	Rx, OTC
calcium carbonate (Cal-Gest, Caltrate, Florical, Os Cal, Maalox, Oysco 500, Titralac, Tums)	KAL-see-um KAR-bo-nate	capsule, chewable tablet, oral suspension, tablet	OTC
calcium chloride	KAL-see-um KLOR-ide	injection	Rx
calcium citrate (Cal-Cee, Calcitrate, Citracal)	KAL-see-um SI-trate	tablet	OTC
calcium gluconate	KAL-see-um GLOO-koh-nate	capsule, injection, tablet	Rx, OTC
calcium lactate (Cal-Lac)	KAL-see-um LAK-tate	capsule, tablet	OTC
Magnesium			
magnesium gluconate (Mag-G, Magtrate, Magonate)	mag-NEE-zee-um GLOO-koh-nate	oral suspension, tablet	OTC
magnesium lactate (Mag-Tab)	mag-NEE-zee-um LAK-tate	tablet	OTC
magnesium oxide (Elite Magnesium, Mag-200, Mag-Cap, Mag-Ox, Maox, Uro-Mag)	mag-NEE-zee-um OX-side	capsule, tablet	OTC
magnesium sulfate (Mag-200)	mag-NEE-zee-um SUL-fate	capsule, injection	Rx, OTC
Phosphate			

*Phosphate-containing products are listed by salt.

Sodium (Na⁺)

Sodium, which comes in multiple salts (**sodium acetate**, **sodium chloride**, and **sodium phosphate**), is the primary cation of extracellular fluid. Sodium has a variety of crucial functions, including retaining fluid in the body, generating and transmitting nerve impulses, maintaining acid-base balance, regulating enzyme activities, and regulating the osmolarity and electroneutrality of cells. The kidneys are responsible for maintaining normal sodium concentrations in plasma and other body fluids. The average diet provides sufficient sodium to meet the body's requirements.

Hyponatremia is low sodium concentration relative to the normal range. Hyponatremia is related to sodium loss or a relative excess of water in the extracellular space. It can be caused by excessive water intake, overuse of salt-wasting diuretics, adrenal gland insufficiency, kidney failure, or liver failure. Low sodium concentrations can also occur with fluid loss caused by excessive sweating or vomiting. **Hypernatremia** is high sodium concentration relative to the normal range. Hypernatremia can be caused by dehydration from lack of fluid intake, diarrhea, or deficiency of antidiuretic hormone. Heart disease and kidney failure can also cause hypernatremia.

Dosage Forms and Administration Dosing of sodium chloride replacements must be individualized depending on the reason for the imbalance and on the fluid status of the patient.

Side Effects Side effects of sodium products are rare and mostly involve instances when sodium supplementation has exceeded the need. Administering more sodium-containing fluid than needed can result in fluid overload, which can cause swelling, cardiac dysfunction, and accumulation of fluid in the lungs.

Contraindications Contraindications to sodium chloride include hypertonic uterus, hypernatremia, and fluid retention.

Cautions and Considerations Monitoring is required when sodium supplements are used to treat patients with kidney failure or kidney impairment. Patients with kidney problems should notify their healthcare providers before taking an electrolyte supplement.

Drug Interactions Sodium supplements do not have drug interactions.

Safety Alert

The Institute for Safe Medication Practices publishes a list of high-alert medications that may cause significant patient harm when used in error. Potassium chloride for injection is included on this list. Errors in injectable potassium chloride administration can cause heart abnormalities and even death.

Potassium (K⁺)

Potassium, which comes in multiple salts (**potassium acetate**, **potassium chloride**, **potassium phosphate**), is the primary cation of intracellular fluid. Potassium is important in the regulation of the acid-base balance and water balance of the body, in protein synthesis and carbohydrate metabolism, in muscle building, and in the function of the nervous system.

Hypokalemia is a condition of lower-than-normal potassium concentration. Potassium can be lost through overuse of potassium-wasting diuretics, vomiting or gastric suctioning, or excessive urine output. Signs of hypokalemia include reduced muscle tone (decreased reflexes), weakness, confusion, drowsiness, depression, low blood pressure, and cardiac arrhythmias. Hyperkalemia results from an increase in potassium levels. High potassium is a dangerous condition because cardiac function and contractility are greatly affected. Cardiac arrest can occur when potassium levels are too high. Hyperkalemia can be caused by kidney failure, diarrhea, excessive use of potassium-sparing diuretics, Cushing's syndrome, severe burns, and septic shock (severe systemic infection). Signs and symptoms include depressed breathing, diarrhea, nausea, vomiting, irritability, confusion, anxiety, intestinal upset, and cardiac arrhythmias.

Oral potassium supplements are typically used to replace potassium lost from diuresis. Some diuretics deplete potassium, so patients must take a potassium supplement while on those drug therapies.

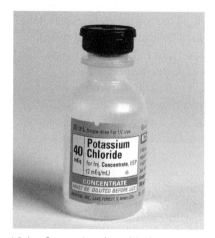

Vials of potassium have black tops to help alert healthcare providers to dilute their contents prior to administration.

Dosage Forms and Administration Doses are individualized to patients. Intravenous potassium solutions should be diluted to a concentration no greater than 100 mEq/L. More concentrated solutions may cause phlebitis (inflammation of the vein), and rapid infusions can result in lethal cardiac arrhythmias. Klor-Con is a brand name for oral potassium and is commonly used by patients who take diuretics.

Side Effects Common side effects of high potassium levels include nausea, vomiting, diarrhea, and abdominal pain. In some cases, potassium supplements have been associated with GI ulceration. At minimum, they can be irritating to the GI tract. Patients should take oral potassium products with a full glass of water to reduce these effects. Taking potassium supplements with food may also decrease stomach upset.

Contraindications Potassium replacements are contraindicated in hyperkalemia and diseases in which high potassium levels may be encountered. Solid potassium dosage forms are contraindicated in patients who may have delay or arrest in passage through the gastrointestinal tract.

Cautions and Considerations Injectable potassium products must be diluted before administration. Potassium is diluted and added to a large-volume IV solution, then mixed well before administration. Such infusions must also be administered slowly because they can be irritating to the veins and painful for the patient. Usually, 40 mEq of potassium are added to 1 L IV fluid. The maximum safe concentration is 100 mEq/L.

Administering too much potassium can be fatal because it interferes with heart function and causes cardiac arrest. For this reason, vials of potassium concentrate have black tops. Injectable potassium products must be mixed well, so that the entire IV bag has a consistent concentration. Fully agitating the IV bag once potassium is added helps ensure consistent mixing.

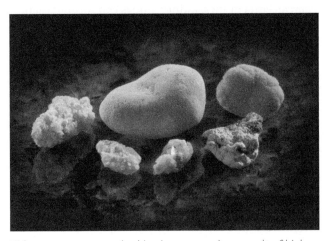

Kidney stones, as seen in this picture, may be a result of high calcium levels.

Calcium (Ca^{2+})

Calcium is important in bone formation, muscle contraction, and blood coagulation. When a patient's blood test shows low calcium, their albumin levels should be checked. Low albumin often results in low calcium levels, because calcium is highly bound to this protein.

Recall that hypocalcemia is a depletion in calcium levels in the body. Low calcium can be caused by insufficient calcium intake or parathyroid disease. Signs and symptoms of hypocalcemia include hyperexcitability of nerves and muscle contraction (tetany). Muscle spasms, seizures, and even death can occur. **Hypercalcemia** is an excess of calcium in the blood. It can be caused by excessive intake of calcium supplements and by some cancerous tumors. When calcium levels are high, crystals form in the urine and cause kidney stones.

Oral calcium products are used to prevent and treat bone loss from osteoporosis, rickets (which may be caused by calcium deficiency or vitamin D deficiency), and osteomalacia. They are also used for tetany. They are absorbed more efficiently when taken with vitamin D. Various calcium salts are used for different purposes. Six calcium salts currently in use are calcium chloride, calcium carbonate, calcium citrate, calcium acetate, calcium gluconate, and calcium lactate.

Calcium chloride moderates nerve and muscle performance through regulation of the action potential excitation threshold. **Calcium carbonate (Caltrate, Os-Cal, Tums)** is typically used as an antacid and is sold under many brand names, such as Tums. It is also used as a dietary supplement to prevent a negative calcium balance. **Calcium citrate (Calcitrate)** is better absorbed than other calcium products. It should be given in combination with vitamin D to build bones.

Calcium acetate (Eliphos, PhosLo, Phoslyra) is used to control hyperphosphatemia in end-stage renal failure. It binds to the phosphorus in the GI tract more efficiently than other calcium salts. This efficient binding is due to its lower solubility and subsequent reduced absorption and increased formation of calcium phosphate. **Calcium gluconate** is used to prevent negative calcium balances. It moderates muscle and nerve performance and allows normal cardiac function. **Calcium lactate (Cal-Lac)** is used to prevent and treat calcium deficiencies.

Dosage Forms and Administration Calcium chloride is only available as an injection product. It is the fastest of the calcium salts to diffuse into the bloodstream, so it is the salt primarily used in cardiac emergencies. If infused directly into an IV line or mixed in too high a concentration with phosphate, calcium precipitates. Calcium carbonate is taken only by mouth. Calcium cannot penetrate bone without the aid of vitamin D, so most of these supplements have vitamin D added to them. Calcium citrate should be taken in two or three doses separated by six hours. Calcium acetate can be administered as a capsule, tablet, or injection. Calcium gluconate is used in total parenteral nutrition and can be taken orally or parenterally.

Side Effects A common side effect of calcium supplementation is constipation. Taking calcium supplements with food and drinking plenty of water may diminish occurrences of constipation. If hypercalcemia occurs, kidney stones can form. Patients should seek medical attention if they have back or flank pain or difficult or painful urination, especially if associated with nausea and vomiting. These can be signs of kidney stone formation.

Contraindications Calcium chloride is contraindicated in digoxin toxicity. The gluconate form of calcium should not be used in patients with ventricular fibrillation or hypercalcemia, and it should not be used concomitantly with ceftriaxone in neonates. Calcium lactate is contraindicated in hypercalcemia and ventricular fibrillation. Calcium carbonate and citrate do not have contraindications.

Cautions and Considerations Most electrolyte products cannot be used in patients with kidney failure or kidney impairment. If they are used in these cases, they must be monitored closely. Patients with kidney problems should notify their healthcare providers before taking an electrolyte supplement.

Drug Interactions Calcium and phosphate salts cannot always be mixed in the same IV bags. They can chelate, or bond chemically to form an insoluble precipitate. The precipitate appears as small white specks or lumps of material within the bag. If infused through an IV, the precipitate clogs capillaries and has severe adverse effects for the patient.

Magnesium (Mg^{2+})

Magnesium, which comes in multiple salts (**magnesium gluconate, magnesium lactate, magnesium oxide,** and **magnesium sulfate**), is the second most abundant cation in intracellular fluids. Most magnesium is found in bones and within cells. Many body enzymes and enzyme systems need magnesium for activation. Magnesium helps transmit impulses across neuromuscular junctions, maintain normal nerve and muscular function, and steady heart rhythms.

Hypomagnesemia is a depletion of magnesium in the body. Magnesium can be lost through alcohol abuse, pregnancy-induced hypertension, or drug therapy that causes increased magnesium excretion. Digoxin, estrogen, and diuretics can deplete magnesium. Signs and symptoms of hypomagnesemia include muscle cramps, confusion, hypertension, tachycardia, arrhythmias, tremors, hyperactive reflexes, hallucinations, and seizures. **Hypermagnesemia** is an excess of magnesium in the body.

It can be caused by renal failure, an overdose of IV magnesium infusion, or use of enemas containing magnesium. Symptoms of hypermagnesemia may not immediately be apparent to patients. Signs include reduced deep tendon reflexes and changes in cardiac function.

Other than for treating a deficiency, oral magnesium products have been used with some controversy in people with heart disease and diabetes. Magnesium sulfate is commonly used to treat preeclampsia and eclampsia.

Dosage Forms and Administration Although oral magnesium is available, magnesium sulfate is administered intravenously for acute prevention of uterine contractions in preterm labor.

Side Effects Common side effects of magnesium supplements include diarrhea. Taking magnesium supplements with food can decrease this effect. Over time, this effect usually decreases.

Contraindications Magnesium products have no contraindications.

Cautions and Considerations Most electrolyte products cannot be used in patients with kidney failure or kidney impairment. If they are used in these cases, they must be monitored closely. Patients with kidney problems should notify their healthcare providers before taking an electrolyte supplement.

Drug Interactions Magnesium can reduce the effects of some antibiotics (see Chapter 16) and bisphosphonates (see Chapter 6). Patients should take magnesium at least two hours before or after taking these other medications.

Chloride (Cl⁻)

In the body, **chloride** functions to transport carbon dioxide, form hydrochloric acid in the stomach, retain potassium, and maintain the osmolarity of the cells. An excess or deficiency of chloride mainly effects the acid-base balance in the body.

Hypochloremia is a depletion of chloride in the body caused by loss of fluid from diuretic use, excessive production of urine or sweat, or from gastric suctioning. **Hyperchloremia** is an excess of chloride within the body, typically caused by diarrhea, kidney disease, or diabetes insipidus.

Phosphate (PO_4^{3-})

Phosphate is an anion that plays an important role in energy production within cells. Without sufficient phosphate, normal cell function is not possible. Phosphate is commonly counterbalanced with calcium in the bloodstream. Excessive intake of phosphate can deplete calcium levels and affect bone health.

Hypophosphatemia is a drop in phosphate in the bloodstream. It can be caused by anorexia or severe malnutrition. Signs and symptoms include weakness, respiratory failure, heart failure, hemolysis, and rhabdomyolysis (mass muscle tissue breakdown). **Hyperphosphatemia**, or excess phosphate in the blood, can be caused by tumor lysis syndrome (a condition that can occur when receiving chemotherapy drugs for large cancer tumors), rhabdomyolysis, lactic acidosis, or diabetic ketoacidosis. Taking bisphosphonates or too much vitamin D, or overusing bowel prep products containing phosphate can also cause hyperphosphatemia. Symptoms of hyperphosphatemia are not always apparent to patients but often include kidney damage or failure. Phosphate products are used primarily in cases of malnourishment. Some patients do not acquire sufficient phosphate because they have GI absorption abnormalities.

Dosage Forms and Administration Phosphate comes in various forms in combination with other minerals and in multivitamins. Dosing is individualized.

Side Effects Common side effects of phosphate-containing supplements include stomach upset and diarrhea. Over time, these effects usually subside. Phosphate supplements have also been associated with kidney stones. Patients should seek medical attention if they have back or flank pain or difficult or painful urination, especially if associated with nausea and vomiting. These can be signs of kidney stone formation.

Contraindications Phosphate replacements are contraindicated in hyperphosphatemia and hypocalcemia. Potassium phosphate is contraindicated in hyperkalemia.

Cautions and Considerations Most electrolyte products cannot be used in patients with kidney failure or kidney impairment. If they are used in these cases, they must be monitored closely. Patients with kidney problems should notify their healthcare providers before taking an electrolyte supplement.

Drug Interactions Calcium and phosphate salts cannot always be mixed in the same IV bags. They can chelate, or bond chemically to form an insoluble precipitate. The precipitate appears as small white specks or lumps of material within the bag. If infused through an IV, the precipitate clogs capillaries and has severe adverse effects for the patient. To prevent this interaction in a TPN, items are mixed in a specific order. Phosphates are added first, followed by micronutrients with chloride and acetate, and then magnesium is added. All of these are added prior to calcium.

Acidifying and Alkalinizing Agents

Acidosis occurs when the pH of blood and/or extracellular fluid drops below the normal range, less than 7.35. **Metabolic acidosis** occurs when excess acid is produced, bicarbonate is lost (such as with diarrhea), or the kidneys do not excrete enough acid. **Respiratory acidosis** results from slow breathing and retention of carbon dioxide in the blood.

Alkalosis occurs when there is a relative excess of bicarbonate in the blood and/or extracellular fluid and the pH rises above the normal range, more than 7.45. Hydrogen ions can be lost from the GI tract (such as by vomiting) or in urine. **Metabolic alkalosis** takes place when excess acid is excreted via the kidneys (such as in overdiuresis) or acid is lost from the stomach (from vomiting or gastric suction). **Respiratory alkalosis** occurs when breathing becomes more rapid and more carbon dioxide is exhaled and eliminated from the blood.

When a metabolic or respiratory process is contributing to an acid-base imbalance, the other pathway makes adjustments for it. Correction in pH can occur quickly with respiratory changes, but metabolic correction takes time. In either case, drug therapy may be needed to address the imbalance if it is severe or urgent.

Some electrolyte products are used primarily for their acidic or basic properties in alkalosis or acidosis rather than for electrolyte deficiencies. Acidic electrolyte products are used to treat alkalosis, and basic products are used to treat acidosis (see Table 19.5).

Dosage Forms and Administration **Ammonium chloride** is an acidic substance used for hypochloremia and metabolic alkalosis. It is typically administered in doses of 100–200 mEq mixed with 500–1,000 mL normal saline and then infused slowly over approximately three hours. This infusion prompts the kidneys to use ammonium in place of sodium in excretion processes. Less sodium is then available to combine to make sodium bicarbonate.

Sodium bicarbonate is a basic substance used as an antacid for heartburn and acid indigestion, a systemic alkalinizer for treating metabolic acidosis, and a urinary

Pharm Fact

Sodium bicarbonate (baking soda), sometimes used to correct acid-base imbalances, can be found in the pharmacy and at the grocery store. When combined with moisture and an acidic ingredient in baking, sodium bicarbonate produces bubbles of carbon dioxide. This helps baked goods to rise.

TABLE 19.5 Common Acidifying and Alkalinizing Products

Generic Drug	Pronunciation	Dosage Form	Dispensing Status
Acidifying Agent			
ammonium chloride	a-MONE-ee-yum KLOR-ide	injection	Rx
Alkalinizing Agent			
sodium bicarbonate (Alka-Seltzer)	SOE-dee-um bye-KAR-bo-nate	injection, powder, tablet	Rx, OTC

alkalinizer when treating hemolytic emergencies or overdoses of salicylates or lithium. When sodium bicarbonate is used as an antacid, adult patients take 325–2,000 mg one to four times a day. The oral powder is taken by mixing a half teaspoon in half a glass (120 mL) of water and drinking as often as every two hours. As an oral systemic alkalinizer, 1,000–2,000 mg of sodium bicarbonate are dissolved in 1–2 L of water and consumed within one hour. When using the IV form for systemic alkalinization, 2–5 mEq/kg are given over four to eight hours, which allows blood pH to be adjusted upward gently. As a urinary alkalinizer, the dose is six 650 mg tablets initially and then two to four tablets every four hours under the supervision of a physician.

Side Effects Close supervision and monitoring must accompany use of any acidifying or alkalinizing agent to prevent overcorrections in pH. Most side effects are related to overshooting pH goals. Excess ammonium chloride can result in ammonium toxicity. Patients must be watched for pallor, sweating, retching, irregular breathing, changes in heart rate, twitching, and convulsions. If these effects are left untreated, coma and death could occur. Excess sodium bicarbonate can result in sodium toxicity, which causes fluid overload. Renal function and cardiac function are impaired when sodium and water retention occur.

Sodium bicarbonate is a hypertonic solution that can cause extravasation (ulceration of local tissue at the injection site). As with chemical burns, this causes tissue necrosis (death) and skin sloughing. To prevent extravasation, any pain experienced during infusion should be given prompt attention and treatment.

Contraindications Ammonium chloride is contraindicated in severe liver or kidney dysfunction. Contraindications to sodium bicarbonate include alkalosis, hypernatremia, severe pulmonary edema, hypocalcemia, and abdominal pain of unknown origin.

Cautions and Considerations The concentrations and rates of infusion must be precise to prevent adverse effects. For instance, the maximum concentration of ammonium chloride when mixed should be 1%–2%. The maximum infusion rate of ammonium chloride is 5 mL/min to prevent venous irritation and ammonium toxicity. For the same reason, sodium bicarbonate is also typically given slowly. In these cases, healthcare providers must be very attentive to signs of extravasation. Controlled infusion rates and frequent laboratory tests are necessary to prevent dramatic swings in pH and allow for gradual, safe correction of acidosis or alkalosis.

Drug Interactions Ammonium chloride interacts with alpha and beta agonists, amantadine, amphetamines, diuretics, and salicylates. Sodium bicarbonate interacts with alpha and beta agonists, amantadine, amphetamines, methylphenidate, flecanide, fosinopril, iron supplements, lithium, and several antiviral medications. Patients should be monitored when taking any of these medications together.

19.3 Obesity and Drug Therapy

Work Wise

Pharmacy technicians encounter patients of a wide variety of sizes. It is important to treat all patients with empathy and understanding and to avoid giving the impression of being judgmental about a person's appearance.

Obesity is a condition characterized by the excessive accumulation and storage of fat in the body. Obesity is recognized as a disease by many health-related organizations such as the World Health Organization and the American Medical Association and is considered a global health challenge. The CDC estimates that in 2015, nearly 40% of adults and 19% of children in the United States had obesity. This statistic has climbed over the past few decades. Figure 19.3 illustrates obesity prevalence throughout the United States. Body weight regulation is complex and it involves the influences of the environment, genetics, and physiology.

Environmental factors that contribute to obesity include leading a sedentary lifestyle, having a readily available food supply, and consuming increased amounts of fats and refined sugars and decreased amounts of fruits and vegetables. These specific environmental factors are prevalent in the United States. Food portions are larger than those in other industrialized countries, and the lifestyle of many individuals has become sedentary, as technology has made many manual labor tasks less necessary.

Genetics is a major factor in obesity and the distribution of body fat. For instance, obesity among first-degree relatives (parents and siblings) is a strong predictor of obesity in adulthood.

FIGURE 19.3 CDC Obesity Prevalence Map

According to the CDC, the prevalence of obesity in the United States varies from state to state. The causes of obesity are multifactorial and not fully understood. Environmental, genetic, physiologic, and psychological factors all contribute in different ways to the development of obesity.

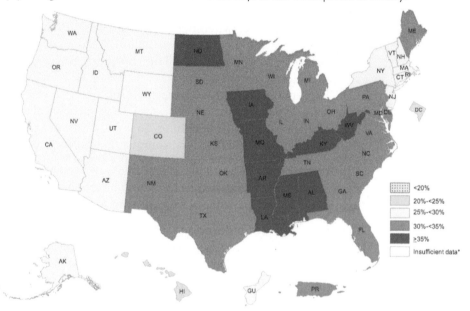

Physiologic factors affect appetite control. Peptides such as leptin and incretins as well as neurotransmitters such as serotonin, norepinephrine, and dopamine are involved in satiety, the sensation of feeling full and satisfied. As weight and adipose (fat) tissue accumulate, it is thought that the normal release and sensitivity to these hormones and neurotransmitters are affected. Other physiologic contributors include medical conditions such as hypothyroidism and Cushing's syndrome. Certain drugs, such as corticosteroids, also cause fat redistribution and appetite changes that foster weight gain.

Obesity is associated with serious health risks and mortality (see Table 19.6). **Centrally distributed fat** is adipose tissue that accumulates in the abdominal area, rather than in the hips, thighs, or buttocks. This kind of fat distribution is linked to heart disease and diabetes. People with obesity also have greater rates of depression, psychological disturbances, and certain types of cancer. Consequently, preventing and treating obesity is an important effort within health care. Reducing body weight has been shown to reduce morbidity and mortality in patients with obesity.

TABLE 19.6 Comorbid Conditions of Obesity

breast and colon cancer	hypertension
congestive heart failure	inflammatory disorders
coronary artery disease	obstructive airway disease
degenerative bone and joint disease	osteoarthritis
depression	polycystic ovarian syndrome
eating disorders	pulmonary hypertension
gallbladder inflammation	skin tags, stretch marks, and other dermatologic problems
gastroesophageal reflux disorder	sleep apnea
hiatal hernia	stroke
high cholesterol	type 2 diabetes

Clinical guidelines recommend progressive treatment dependent on the severity of obesity. First line treatment for obesity is lifestyle intervention—a combination of diet and exercise—and behavior modification. Initial treatment should create a caloric deficit by reducing caloric intake, increasing caloric expenditure, or both. Patients who restrict caloric intake and also perform physical activity will lose weight. Some individuals find these interventions difficult. Lifestyle changes must be permanent to keep off lost weight. Consequently, providing products and services for weight loss and physical fitness is a billion-dollar industry.

Many diets tend to restrict specific components of nutrition to achieve weight loss. Popular weight-loss programs include those that restrict the intake of carbohydrates, fats, or both. These programs are often unsustainable because they do not represent a balanced way to eat that ensures adequate nutrition in the long term. The most successful and healthy diets are those that restrict caloric intake while maintaining a proper balance of nutrients.

Based on the patient's level of obesity and the risk of obesity-associated disease, some patients require medication and surgical interventions to help achieve weight loss needed to improve comorbid conditions. Drug therapy is available to some patients. Drug therapy for weight loss includes lipase inhibitors, sympathomimetic agents, glucagon-like peptide-1 (GLP-1) receptor agonists, opioid agonist, and buproprion. These agents are identified in Table 19.7. Some patients are candidates for more aggressive therapy options. Medications and surgical intervention can achieve significant weight loss. Surgical options are collectively referred to as **bariatric surgery** and include (1) restrictive procedures (**laparoscopic gastric banding**) that effectively make the stomach smaller and prevent excess food intake, and (2) malabsorptive techniques (**gastric bypass** or gastric sleeve surgery) that bypass parts of the intestine, thus preventing nutrients from being fully absorbed. Surgical patients must meet specific criteria prior to surgery. Usually, surgical methods are limited to patients with a body mass index (BMI) of 40 or higher. Some patients with a BMI of 30 or higher will be considered candidates for surgery if they have comorbid health conditions (see Table 19.6).

TABLE 19.7 Common Agents Used to Treat Obesity

Generic (Brand)	Pronunciation	Dosage Form	Common Doages	Dispensing Status	Controlled Substance Schedule
Lipase Inhibitor					
orlistat (Alli, Xenical)	OR-li-stat	capsule	180 mg a day; 360 mg a day	OTC, Rx	
Sympathomimetic Agents					
diethylpropion	dye-eth-ill-PROE-pee-on	tablet	25–75 mg a day	Rx	C-IV
phendimetrazine (Bontril PDM)	fen-di-MEH-tra-zeen	capsule, tablet	210 mg a day	Rx	C-III
phentermine (Adipex, Adipex-P, Lomaira)	FEN-ter-meen	capsule, tablet	15–37.5 mg a day	Rx	C-IV
Combination Product					
phentermine / topiramate (Qsymia)	FEN-ter-meen toe-PEER-i-mate	capsule	3.75 mg/23 mg a day	Rx	C-IV
Glucagon-Like Peptide 1 (GLP-1) Receptor Agonist					
liraglutide (Saxenda)	lir-a-GLOO-tide	injection	SC: 0.6–3 mg 1 time a week	Rx	
Opioid Agonist and Bupropion					
naltrexone / bupropion (Contrave)	nal-TREK-sown byoo-PROW-pee-aan	tablet	90 mg/8 mg	Rx	

Lipase Inhibitor

Lipase inhibitors are medications commonly used to treat obesity. As the name suggests, a **lipase inhibitor** works by binding to gastric and pancreatic lipase enzymes in the intestines, thereby preventing the enzymes from breaking down fats into a form that can be absorbed. Fat then passes through the intestines, where it is excreted in stool. **Orlistat (Alli, Xenical)**, a commercially available lipase inhibitor, is available over the counter and by prescription.

Dosage Forms and Administration Orlistat is taken three times a day with each meal that contains fat.

Side Effects Common side effects of orlistat include fatty or oily stools, fecal incontinence or urgency, gas, and diarrhea. These effects may decrease over time. Patients can reduce or prevent these effects by limiting fat intake to less than 30% of total calories. Patients who do not may find that the side effects become intolerable.

Contraindications Orlistat is contraindicated in chronic malabsorption syndrome, cholestasis, and pregnancy.

Cautions and Considerations Because orlistat interferes with the absorption of fat, it can also prevent absorption of fat-soluble vitamins. Patients should take multivitamin supplements to combat potential vitamin deficiencies.

Drug Interactions Orlistat may decrease concentrations of amiodarone, anticonvulsants, cyclosporine, levothyroxine, multivitamins, and vitamin D analogs. Warfarin levels may be increased by orlistat.

Sympathomimetic Drugs

One class of drugs used to treat obesity, **sympathomimetics**, stimulates the central nervous system (CNS), much as amphetamines do. These medications should only be used short term. Sympathomimetics are used with exercise, behavior modification, and reduced caloric intake to produce weight loss in patients with a BMI of 30 or higher (or over 27 with the presence of other risk factors, such as high blood pressure, diabetes, or high cholesterol). The sympathomimetic agents used for weight loss include **diethylpropion, phendimetrazine (Bontril PDM), phentermine (Adipex, Adipex-P, Lomaira)** and **phentermine / topiramate (Qysmia)**. The sympathomimetics stimulate dopamine and norepinephrine and prevent the reuptake of serotonin. Increased neurotransmitter levels signal a sense of satiety. In effect, patients do not feel as hungry.

Dosage Forms and Administration Fast-acting dosage forms are taken 30 minutes to 1 hour prior to eating, and long-acting forms are taken once a day.

Side Effects Common side effects of sympathomimetics are headache, stomachache, insomnia, nervousness, tachycardia, and irritability. Taking these medications in the morning may help reduce insomnia, but other effects can be limiting if they are bothersome. Sympathomimetics can also cause dry mouth, difficulty urinating, and constipation. Patients with urinary problems should not take these medications, and drinking plenty of water can help with these effects. Sympathomimetics can cause impotence. Patients should discuss the risks and benefits of sympathomimetics with their healthcare practitioners.

A less common side effect of sympathomimetics is serotonin syndrome, which causes a dangerous rise in blood pressure and heart rate. Other symptoms include agitation, confusion, twitching, and shivering. Serotonin syndrome is a serious health condition and can even result in death.

Contraindications Sympathomimetics are contraindicated in patients with coronary heart disease, high blood pressure, or hyperthyroidism and in patients with a history of drug abuse. In addition, phendimetrazine and phentermine are contraindicated in pregnancy.

Cautions and Considerations All CNS stimulants are controlled substances and have addiction and abuse potential. State laws and regulations governing pharmacy practice and procedures for dispensing these agents should be consulted. Phentermine / topiramate can only be dispensed through an REMS program and must include a Medication Guide.

Drug Interactions Sympathomimetics may enhance the analgesic effect of opioids. They may decrease the sedative effects of antihistamines and drugs for insomnia. Sympathomimetics may increase blood pressure and may enhance the hypertensive effects of other drugs, such as linezolid and monoamine oxidase inhibitors (MAOIs). Lithium may decrease the stimulatory effects of sympathomimetics.

Glucagon-Like Peptide 1 (GLP-1) Receptor Agonists

Glucagon-like peptide is a gastric hormone that stimulates glucose-dependent insulin secretion and inhibits glucagon release and gastric emptying. It acts as a regulator of appetite and caloric intake. **Glucagon-like peptide 1 (GLP-1) receptor agonists** act similarly to endogenous glucagon-like peptide, and there is evidence to suggest these medications decrease body weight through decreased caloric intake. **Liraglutide (Saxenda)**, a glucagon-like peptide 1 (GLP-1) receptor agonist, is indicated as an adjunct therapy to a reduced-calorie diet and increased physical activity for long-term weight management in adults with a BMI of 30 or higher (or 27 or higher with the presence of other risk factors, such as high blood pressure, diabetes, or high cholesterol).

Dosage Forms and Administration Liraglutide is available as a solution for subcutaneous injection.

Side Effects Liraglutide may cause nausea, hypoglycemia, diarrhea, constipation, vomiting, headache, decreased appetite, dyspepsia, fatigue, dizziness, abdominal pain, and increased lipase activity.

Contraindications Liraglutide is contraindicated in patients with a personal or family history of medullary thyroid carcinoma or multiple endocrine neoplasia type 2. Liraglutide should not be used by pregnant patients.

Cautions and Considerations Because liraglutide can cause insulin secretion, it should be used cautiously with other drugs that cause insulin secretion such as sulfonylureas or meglitinides. Due to possible increased risk of thyroid tumors with use, patients should be counseled about the symptoms of thyroid tumors. Liraglutide has been associated with acute pancreatitis and gallbladder disease. Patients should discontinue use if either of these conditions is suspected or confirmed. Liraglutide has a boxed warning related to thyroid cancer. Patients with a family history of medullary thyroid carcinoma should not use liraglutide. Liraglutide must be dispensed with a Medication Guide.

Opioid Antagonist and Bupropion

Naltrexone / bupropion (Contrave) is an opioid antagonist and dopamine and norepinephrine reuptake inhibitor combination drug. It is used for weight loss as an adjunct to dietary and lifestyle modifications. Candidates for this drug include patients with a BMI of 30 or higher or of 27 or higher if they have at least one weight-related comorbidity such as type 2 diabetes mellitus, hyperlipidemia, or hypertension.

Dosage Forms and Administration Naltrexone / bupropion is taken two times a day and should not be taken with high-fat meals.

Side Effects Common side effects include nausea, constipation, headache, vomiting, dizziness, insomnia, and dry mouth.

Contraindications Naltrexone / bupropion is contraindicated in pregnancy and in patients with uncontrolled hypertension, seizure disorder, or chronic opioid use.

Cautions and Considerations Naltrexone / bupropion may increase the risk of suicidal thinking and behavior in children, adolescents, and young adults between the ages of 18 and 24 with major depressive disorder or other psychiatric disorders. For this reason, naltrexone / bupropion carries a boxed warning that states it may increase risk of suicidal ideation and must be dispensed with a Medication Guide.

Special precautions should be taken when naltrexone / bupropion is taken in combination with digoxin, dopaminergic drugs, or drugs that lower the seizure threshold.

Drug Interactions Naltrexone / bupropion inhibits a liver metabolizing enzyme, which can increase concentrations of certain antidepressants, antipsychotics, beta-blockers, and antiarrhythmics. It should not be used within 14 days of taking another product containing bupropion or an MAOI inhibitor.

19.4 Malnutrition and Drug Therapy

Malnutrition is a lack of adequate nutrient intake to supply basic metabolic needs. It can be related to an overall lack of calorie or protein consumption, or it may be associated with a deficiency in a specific micronutrient (for example, a vitamin or mineral). Malnutrition is most prevalent in underdeveloped countries. Children living in these poorer nations are especially vulnerable to malnutrition. They often develop **marasmus**, a chronic condition caused by inadequate caloric and protein intake over a prolonged period. Wasting of muscle and fat tissue is observed, a condition known as **cachexia**. Individuals in these underdeveloped countries are also at risk for **kwashiorkor**, a condition in which caloric intake is adequate but protein intake is deficient. These patients, paradoxically, usually appear well nourished because heightened metabolic rates break down protein stores but leave adipose tissue intact. However, patients may accumulate fluid in the abdomen, hands, face, and feet.

In the United States, malnutrition is most often encountered in the inpatient setting, where it is associated with disease states, acute illness, and even drug therapy. Some causes for malnutrition include the following:

- anorexia nervosa
- food allergies or intolerance
- chronic infection or inflammatory conditions
- cancer
- endocrine disorders
- pulmonary disease
- cirrhosis of the liver
- renal failure
- nausea, vomiting, or diarrhea
- trauma, burns, or sepsis
- inflammatory bowel disease, Crohn's disease, or short bowel syndrome
- inadequate parenteral or enteral nutrition
- psychiatric or psychological conditions

Signs of malnutrition include weight loss, skin changes (too dry, shiny, or scaly), hair loss, fatigue, poor wound healing, pallor (pale skin), sunken eyes, dry mouth and eyes, visible loss of muscle mass, and fluid accumulation in the abdomen or around the ankles and tailbone.

An individual cannot go longer than 7 to 10 days without food or nutrition; malnutrition will ensue and negatively affect health outcomes. When a patient cannot be fed normally, nutrition must be supplied by alternative methods. Enteral nutrition and parenteral nutrition are artificial ways to feed patients that do not involve swallowing.

Enteral Nutrition

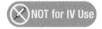

Pharm Fact

An NG tube, also known as a *Levin tube*, is made from lightweight polyurethane material.

Enteral nutrition is a method of feeding a patient liquid nutrients through a tube inserted into the GI tract. The tube can be inserted manually or surgically. A nasogastric (NG) tube is manually inserted. A gastrostomy (G) tube and a jejunostomy (J) tube are placed surgically in the stomach and jejunum, respectively (see Figure 19.4). A liquid nutrient formula is injected through the tube, either in bolus doses to mimic eating a meal or continuously with an enteral pump.

Indications for enteral feeding include bowel obstruction, short bowel syndrome, and Crohn's disease. Patients in long-term care who are unable to swallow foods voluntarily because of a severe stroke or prolonged coma may have an enteral feeding tube to maintain their hydration status.

FIGURE 19.4
**Enteral
Feeding Tube
Sites**

NG tubes are
uncomfortable
for patients, so
such tubes are
suitable only for
short-term use. If
enteral feeding is
necessary for more
than a few days, a
G tube or J tube is
placed surgically.

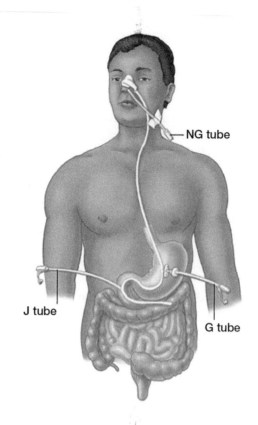

— NG tube

J tube

G tube

Specialized enteral feeding products are available for specific conditions, so patients must be matched with appropriate formulas. Healthcare personnel should never administer enteral nutrition through an intravenous (IV) line. These preparations are neither sterile nor formulated for that use. Enteral feeding is preferred to parenteral feeding because it keeps the GI tract functional and prevents abdominal infections. Various enteral feeding products are highlighted in Table 19.8.

TABLE 19.8 **Commonly Used Enteral Nutrition Formulations**

Enteral Feeding Product	Population Receiving
Fibersource HN, Jevity Plus	patients with high protein needs, noninjured patients, patients in long-term care
Fibersource, Jevity	patients with an intact GI tract who are unable to eat for any of various reasons
Isosource VHN, Promote	patients with very high protein needs, trauma victims, burn victims
Nepro, Novasource Renal	renal patients on dialysis
Impact, Perative	immunocompromised patients, abdomen trauma victims, seriously ill patients
Glucerna	patients with diabetes

Parenteral Nutrition

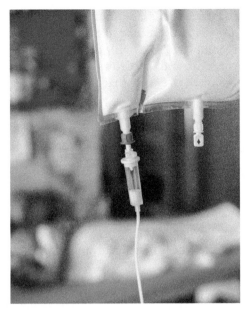

Parenteral nutrition is administered intravenously.

Parenteral nutrition (PN), often referred to as **total parenteral nutrition (TPN)**, is provided by feeding a patient through an IV line. PN is used when the digestive tract cannot be used for nutrient absorption. Indications for PN include severe burns, intolerance to enteral feeding, anorexia nervosa (refusal to eat), pancreatitis, severe gallbladder disease, inflammatory bowel disease, and severe diarrhea. PN may also be necessary in pregnancy, acquired immunodeficiency syndrome (AIDS), and cancer.

PN carries risks for complications. It is complex in that it supplies all the fluids, electrolytes, nutrients (carbohydrates, proteins, and fats), vitamins, and minerals that a patient needs intravenously. If an essential nutrient or trace element is not included, a patient can easily become nutritionally deficient or imbalanced. Regular laboratory monitoring is necessary to guide PN therapy and protect against infection. Special care must be taken when adding trace minerals to a PN formula because of the heightened risk of underdosing or overdosing these elements.

Complications of Parenteral Nutrition

Patients may experience various complications as a result of PN, including the following:

- acid-base imbalance
- dehydration
- elevated serum triglycerides
- failure to induce anabolism
- high serum lipid concentrations
- hyperammonemia
- hyperglycemia or hypoglycemia
- hypoalbuminemia
- imbalance of electrolytes
- liver toxicity

Even patients without diabetes may show increased blood sugar levels when on PN; therefore, insulin may be added to the solution for these patients.

Infections are frequently a problem for patients receiving parenteral nutrition. PN solutions are rich in nutrients and therefore capable of hosting many types of bacteria and fungi. Aseptic technique should be used in the preparation of parenteral products, and the solution should be tested for microbial growth. The area around the central line should be inspected for infection often; the line may need to be removed and replaced in the case of infection. PN may be discontinued in the case of line infection and may be reformulated when restarted.

Preparing Parenteral Nutrition Solutions

PN solutions are formulated to ensure adequate absorption of nutrients from circulation, providing fluids, carbohydrates, and protein while maintaining osmolarity.

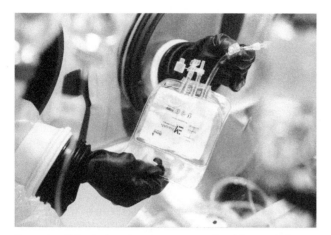

Preparing PN solutions is a process completed by specially trained pharmacy technicians.

Preparing PN solutions is a process completed by specially trained pharmacy technicians. This process is completed in a sterile compounding environment, and strict rules and methods must be followed to ensure that PN solutions are formulated correctly.

Two types of PN solutions are available: (1) a **total nutrient admixture (TNA)**, or **three-in-one**, a solution that contains lipids in addition to amino acids and dextrose, and (2) a **two-in-one**, a solution that includes amino acids and dextrose but does not contain lipids. Both three-in-one and two-in-one solutions have electrolytes added. The three-in-one formulations offer the following advantages:

- lower cost of preparation and delivery
- less nursing time needed for administration
- potentially reduced risk of sepsis

The three-in-one formulations also have two disadvantages. First, the risk of IV line occlusion is greater, and larger filters must be used. Larger filters lead to less microbial elimination. Second, if precipitation of the electrolytes occurs, it cannot be seen because of the opacity of lipid formulations.

With either type of PN solution, the electrolytes are added to the mixture during initial preparation, but the vitamins are always added just before administration. PN solutions are only stable for 24 hours after the addition of vitamins. Both types of PN solution may remain at room temperature for 24 hours (usually a parenteral bag is hung this long). Otherwise, the solution is always stored in the refrigerator.

When mixing a three-in-one PN, electrolytes should be added carefully. A preparation method called **pooling** saves considerable time, but this method is controversial because precipitation is more common when it is used. In pooling, all the electrolytes except phosphate are put into a small-volume parenteral bag and then transferred into each batch. Cysteine is sometimes added to prevent precipitation of the electrolytes. If pooling is used, the phosphates must be separate from the calcium and magnesium. The phosphates should be injected into the bag first; next, the amino acids, dextrose, lipids, and water should be added; and then, the pooled electrolytes are added. When the PN is mixed in this way, precipitation is very unlikely to occur.

Solutions that contain lipids should be carefully inspected in the pharmacy and before infusion for **cracking**, or separation. Cracking can be demonstrated by adding hydrochloric acid to the PN solution. The result is a distinct separation of the oil that is easily visible.

Another way to mix three-in-one and two-in-one PN solutions while preventing both precipitation of electrolytes and cracking is to use a **compounder**. A compounder is an automated pumping system that compounds multiple ingredients into a finished solution in a single patient bag. Pharmacies that use automated compounders are able to increase the accuracy of patient-specific PN formulas and reduce the time it takes to make a single patient PN bag. Many compounder machines have safety checks in place, such as a bar-code scanning verification process; a daily setup priming and verification process; and calibration for accuracy.

To provide all nutrients intravenously, PN solutions must contain a large number of components in a relatively small volume of fluid. The possibility of

REFRIGERATE

component interactions and microprecipitation is quite high and must be considered when mixing each batch. Solutions that do not contain lipids should be inspected during preparation against both black and white backgrounds with proper lighting. It is advantageous to look for particulate matter before adding insulin or other additives. All bags with precipitates should be discarded.

Calcium and phosphorus are the electrolytes that cause the most problems with precipitation. The phosphate ion should always be added to the bag first and mixed thoroughly with other ingredients. After the PN solution is mixed, the calcium ion is added with constant swirling. Calcium chloride should not be used; calcium gluconate is preferred. The sulfate salt is the preferred form for magnesium. The actual concentration of magnesium depends on the amount of calcium, because both destabilize the lipid emulsion.

Table 19.9 lists the recommended multivitamin and trace element additions for PN. These come in one bottle and are added to the PN as close to the time of administration as possible because vitamins degrade more rapidly than other components. Table 19.10 lists other additions, which may vary according to the product and patient needs.

After the PN solution is mixed and given a final inspection, each batch should be clearly labeled with the patient's name, address or hospital unit, solution name, concentration and volume, and additives. Instructions for the additives, such as vitamins,

TABLE 19.9 Recommended Additions for PN

Additives	Pronunciation	Daily Adult Dose
Multivitamins		
ascorbic acid (vitamin C)	a-SKOR-bik AS-id	60 mg
biotin (vitamin B_7)	BYE-oh-tin	150 mcg
cobalamin (vitamin B_{12})	koe-BAL-a-min	2 mcg
dexpanthenol (vitamin B_5) as d-pantothenyl alcohol	deks-PAN-the-nole	15 mg
ergocalciferol (vitamin D_2)	er-goe-kal-SIF-e-rawl	200 mg
folic acid (vitamin B_9)	FOE-lik AS-id	180 mcg
niacin (vitamin B_3)	NYE-a-sin	15 mg
phytonadione (vitamin K)	fye-toe-na-DYE-one	150 mcg
pyridoxine (vitamin B_6)	peer-i-DOX-een	1.6 mg
retinol (vitamin A)	RE-tin-awl	800 mg
riboflavin (vitamin B_2)	RYE-boe-flay-vin	1.3 mg
thiamine (vitamin B_1)	THYE-a-min	1.1 mg
tocopherol (vitamin E)	to-KOF-er-awl	12 mg
Trace Elements		
chromium	CROW-mee-um	10–15 mcg
copper	COP-ur	0.5–1.5 mg
manganese	MAN-gah-knees	0.15–0.80 mg
multitrace-4 formulation (chromium, copper, manganese, zinc)		1 mL (4 mcg, 400 mcg, 100 mcg, 1 mg)

continues

TABLE 19.9 Recommended Additions for PN—*Continued*

Additives	Pronunciation	Daily Adult Dose
multitrace-5 formulation (chromium, copper, manganese, selenium, zinc)		1 mL (4 mcg, 400 mcg, 100 mcg, 20 mcg, 1 mg)
selenium	suh-LEE-nee-um	20–60 mcg
zinc	ZINK	2.5–4 mg

should be given on the label, and a beyond-use date must be included on any IV product. In many practice settings, it is the pharmacy technician who mixes PN solutions, which are then checked by the pharmacist and sent out to the patient.

TABLE 19.10 Other Additives and Medications in PN

Additive	Amount per Day
acetate	variable (as needed to maintain acid-base balance)
calcium	10–15 mEq
chloride	variable (as needed to maintain acid-base balance)
magnesium	8–20 mEq
phosphate	20–40 mmol
potassium	1–2 mEq/kg
sodium	12 mEq/kg
insulin, regular	variable (dependent on blood glucose)

19.5 Complementary and Alternative Therapies

While bacteria and other microorganisms are often thought of as harmful, many microorganisms are needed to help the body function. For example, the normal bacteria of the intestinal tract help digest food, destroy harmful microorganisms, and even produce vitamins. When normal bacteria levels are altered, patients may experience health consequences. Sometimes **probiotics**, which are live microorganisms ingested for health benefits, are used to maintain or restore normal bacteria in the body. Various probiotic formulations are available (see Table 19.11 for more information).

Researchers are studying the efficacy of probiotics for various health disorders. Probiotics are commonly used for gastrointestinal disorders such as irritable bowel syndrome and diarrhea. They may also be used for dermatologic conditions such as eczema, genitourinary disorders such as vaginal infections, and allergies.

Probiotics are generally safe for individuals. However, as they contain live microorganisms, probiotics should not be used in patients with compromised immune systems. Common side effects include stomach upset, abdominal cramping, soft stools, and flatulence.

TABLE 19.11 Common Probiotic Products

Probiotic	Species	Form	Use
acidophilus (generic)	*Lactobacillus acidophilus*	capsule, liquid, powder	diarrhea, vaginitis
Activia	*Bifidobacterium animalis*	yogurt	constipation
Align	*Bifidobacterium infantis*	capsule	irritable bowel syndrome
Culturelle	*Lactobacillus rhamnosus* GG	capsule, chewable tablet	diarrhea
Flora-Q	*Lactobacillus acidophilus, Bifidobacterium, L. paracasei, Streptococcus thermophilus*	capsule	irritable bowel syndrome
Florastor	*Saccharomyces boulardii*	capsule, powder (packet)	diarrhea
Lactinex	*Lactobacillus acidophilus, L. helveticus*	granules, tablet	diarrhea
VSL#3	*Bifidobacterium breve, B. lactis, Lactobacillus acidophilus, L. plantarum, L. paracasei, L. helveticus, Streptococcus thermophilus*	capsule, powder (packet)	ulcerative colitis

Review and Assessment

CHAPTER SUMMARY

Vitamins

- Vitamins are classified as water soluble or fat soluble. The B vitamins and vitamin C are water soluble; vitamins A, D, E, and K are fat soluble.

- Vitamin supplementation may be necessary to treat or prevent certain medical conditions.

- It is possible to ingest too much of a fat-soluble vitamin; an overdose is less likely to be serious with a water-soluble vitamin.

Fluids, Electrolytes, and Acid-Base Balance

- Water is the major component of living cells. Bodily fluids are divided into two categories: intracellular and extracellular.

- Water deficits are caused by loss of bodily fluids as a result of such conditions as vomiting, diarrhea, edema, and excessive sweating from fever; high urine output; and acute weight loss of more than 5% of body weight. Water loss can cause dryness of skin and mucous membranes, longitudinal wrinkling of the tongue, hypotension, tachycardia, and lowered body temperature. A loss of 25% of body water can result in death.

- An isotonic solution has the same level of particles, and thus the same tonicity, as bodily fluids.

- Sodium is the primary cation of extracellular fluid.

- Potassium is the primary cation of intracellular fluid.

- Calcium is important in bone formation, muscle contraction, and blood coagulation.

- Calcium comes in multiple salt forms, including calcium chloride, calcium carbonate, calcium citrate, calcium acetate, and calcium gluconate.

- Hydrogen ions regulate the acidity or alkalinity of bodily fluids.

Obesity and Drug Treatments

- Obesity, a major health concern, is characterized by excessive accumulation and storage of fat in the body.

- Lipase inhibitors, sympathomimetic agents, naltrexone / bupropion, and glucagon-like peptide 1 (GLP-1) receptor agonists may be used in appropriate patients for obesity.

Malnutrition and Drug Treatments

- Malnutrition is a lack of adequate nutrient intake to supply basic metabolic needs.

- Enteral formulas, which are introduced through a tube directly into the GI tract, are preferred to feeding by vein (parenteral nutrition) because they keep the GI tract functional and prevent abdominal infections. Technicians should always label enteral preparations so that they are not confused with intravenous preparations.

- The advantages of three-in-one formulations are lower costs of preparation and delivery, less nursing time needed for administration, and potentially reduced risk of sepsis.

- Two disadvantages of three-in-ones are their greater risk of IV line occlusion and the difficulty of seeing precipitates in them due to their opacity.

Complementary and Alternative Therapies

- Probiotics are live microorganisms ingested for health benefits.

- Probiotics are used to maintain or restore normal bacteria in the body.

DRUG LIST

Vitamins
A (carotenoid, retinol)
B_1 (thiamine)
B_2 (riboflavin)
B_3 (niacin)
B_5 (pantothenic acid)
B_6 (pyridoxine)
B_7 (biotin)
B_9 (folate, folic acid)
B_{12} (cobalamin)
C (ascorbic acid)
D (calciferol)
E (tocopherol)
K (phylloquinone, phytonadione)

Electrolytes
calcium, Ca^{2+}
chloride, Cl^-
magnesium, Mg^{2+}
phosphate, PO_4^{3-}
potassium, K^+ (Klor-Con)
sodium, Na^+

Lipase Inhibitor
orlistat (Alli, Xenical)

Sympathomimetic Agents
diethylpropion
phendimetrazine (Bontril PDM)
phentermine (Adipex-P, Lomaira)
phentermine / topiramate (Qsymia)

Glucagon-Like Peptide 1 (GLP-1) Receptor Agonist
liraglutide (Saxenda)

Opioid Agonist and Bupropion
naltrexone / bupropion (Contrave)

Enteral Nutrition Formulations
Fibersource
Fibersource HN
Glucerna
Impact
Isosource VHN
Jevity
Jevity Plus
Nepro
Novasource Renal
Perative
Promote

Probiotics
acidophilus
Activia
Align
Culturelle
Flora-Q
Florastor
Lactinex
VSL#3

Boxed Warnings
bupropion
liraglutide

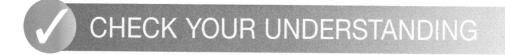
Take a moment to review what you have learned in this chapter and answer the following questions.

1. Which of the following is a fat-soluble vitamin?
   a. vitamin A
   b. vitamin B
   c. vitamin C
   d. niacin

2. Patients who are taking warfarin should monitor their intake of which vitamin?
   a. vitamin A
   b. vitamin D
   c. vitamin E
   d. vitamin K

3. Which electrolyte is found primarily in intracellular fluid (inside the cell)?
   a. sodium
   b. chloride
   c. potassium
   d. calcium

4. Which of the following is an isotonic solution used as an IV fluid?
   a. dextrose 10% in sterile water
   b. dextrose 5% in 0.9% NaCl
   c. 0.45% NaCl
   d. lactated Ringer's solution

5. Which of the following is *not* a comorbid condition of obesity?
   a. congestive heart failure
   b. depression
   c. type 2 diabetes
   d. anemia

6. Which of the following medications for weight loss may cause nutritional deficiencies?
   a. phentermine
   b. liraglutide
   c. orlistat
   d. naltrexone / bupropion

7. Which two electrolytes need to be added to a parenteral nutrition bag separately to prevent precipitation?
   a. magnesium, chloride
   b. phosphate, calcium
   c. potassium, phosphate
   d. sodium, chloride

8. Which of the following electrolytes must be diluted prior to administration?
   a. sodium
   b. potassium
   c. calcium
   d. magnesium

9. Which of the following is an indication for enteral feeding?
   a. Crohn's disease
   b. severe burns
   c. anorexia nervosa
   d. pancreatitis

10. Parenteral nutrition can be given through which of the following tubes?
   a. nasogastric
   b. gastrostomy
   c. jejunostomy
   d. intravenous

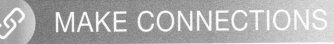

MAKE CONNECTIONS

Take a moment to consider what you have learned in this chapter and respond thoughtfully to the following prompts. Note that some of these activities will require internet access.

1. Peter walks into the pharmacy with a prescription for a medication to help him reach his weight-loss goals. He recently started making dietary and lifestyle adjustments, and his doctor recommended and prescribed orlistat. What is the OTC product that contains orlistat, and how does it work? How should Peter take this medication, and what side effects might be common? When filling the prescription, you notice he also takes amiodarone and warfarin. What should you alert the pharmacist about?

2. Stacey brings in a prescription for amoxicillin and mentions that her prescriber suggested that she take a probiotic along with it. Describe the benefits she may experience when taking a probiotic product, especially in combination with an antibiotic.

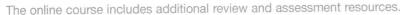

The online course includes additional review and assessment resources.

20

Cancer and Drug Therapy

Nelly G. Adel, PharmD, BCOP, BCPS

Learning Objectives

1 Describe the basic physiology of cancer and the growth of tumor cells. (Section 20.1)

2 Provide examples of traditional chemotherapy drugs, hormonal anticancer therapies, and targeted anticancer drug therapies. (Sections 20.3 to 20.5)

3 Identify the generic names, brand names, indications, dosage ranges, side effects, and considerations associated with drugs commonly used to treat cancer. (Sections 20.3 to 20.5)

4 Justify the development of immunotherapy as a viable treatment option. (Section 20.6)

5 Explain strategies that help prevent chemotherapy-related errors. (Section 20.7)

ASHP/ACPE Accreditation Standards
To view the *ASHP/ACPE Accreditation Standards* addressed in this chapter, refer to Appendix C.

ancer is the second leading cause of death in United States. According to *Cancer Facts & Figures*, published by the American Cancer Society, 1.8 million new cancer diagnoses are expected to occur in 2020, with approximately 606,520 cancer deaths. These grim statistics are a reminder of the overwhelming impact cancer can have on individuals, their families and caregivers, and the healthcare system. As part of this system, most pharmacy technicians will be involved in caring for patients with cancer.

This chapter provides an overview of cancer and methods used to treat it. These methods include surgery, radiation, chemotherapy, and immunotherapy. Of these methods, chemotherapy and immunotherapy require the most knowledge of drugs and their effects in the body. Chemotherapy drugs are a complicated group of medications with a narrow therapeutic index and the potential for severe toxicity. These medications are traditionally administered in a hospital or an outpatient chemotherapy infusion center by the intravenous (IV) route. Most IV chemotherapy drugs are prepared by pharmacists or pharmacy technicians in these settings. However, the availability of orally administered chemotherapy agents has increased over the last decade. As a result, the care of patients with cancer has been shifting into outpatient and community practice settings. In addition to understanding chemotherapy medications, pharmacy technicians must be aware of the necessary safety measures required during the preparation and handling of these medications.

Improvements have been made not only to chemotherapy drugs but also to other anticancer drug treatments, including immunotherapy. This chapter discusses what pharmacy technicians need to know about these drugs and how they affect cancer patients.

20.1 Cancer and Its Development

Cancer is a group of diseases characterized by the uncontrolled growth (also known as uncontrolled *proliferation* or *multiplication*) and spread of abnormal cells. It can result in death if the spread is not controlled. The real causes of cancer are not fully understood; however, cancer has numerous known risk factors. These include modifiable risk factors (such as tobacco use and inactivity) and unmodifiable risk factors (such as inherited genetic mutations). Various risk factors may act together to initiate and promote cancer growth.

Normally, cells multiply until they have met the body's needs and then stop multiplying. For example, epidermal cells multiply to replace skin cells lost due to damage or aging and then stop multiplying when those lost cells have been replaced. In some cases, however, multiplying cells avoid the normal process of stopping or dying. This results in the abnormal cell proliferation that characterizes cancer. Cells originating from a single cell are called **monoclonal**. Cancer is thought to be composed of monoclonal cells originating from a single cell that has lost the ability to control its proliferation.

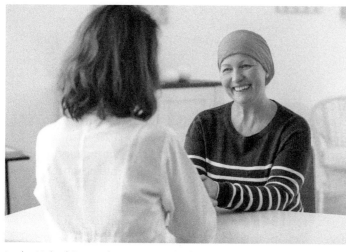

In the United States, breast cancer is the most common cancer among women.

This abnormal cell growth is caused by genetic changes within a cell that can result from external or internal factors. External factors include certain lifestyle choices such as tobacco or heavy alcohol use, sun exposure, diet, and physical inactivity; they also include some infectious disease processes and exposure to environmental carcinogens (such as pesticides or asbestos). Internal factors that can cause genetic changes within a cell include immune disorders, hormones, and genetic mutations. Although some cancers are hereditary, many more cancers result from some combination of lifestyle, environmental, and genetic factors.

Pathophysiology of Cancer

Scientists have discovered the role of genes in cancer development. Their research has established correlations between certain genetic mutations and the development of particular cancers. Identifying these correlations has been instrumental in the development of early cancer screening methods (such as colonoscopy, mammography, and Pap smears) as well as targeting drug therapy for specific cancers. Both strategies continue to improve the early diagnosis and treatment of patients with cancer.

The two major classes of genes that play a role in cancer development are *oncogenes* and *tumor suppressor genes*. Scientists have identified changes to these genes as the **drivers of cancer**: genetic alterations that promote cancer progression.

Oncogenes

An **oncogene** is a gene that promotes cancer formation. An oncogene is a gene that develops from a **proto-oncogene**, a gene that codes for growth factors or their receptors (see Figure 20.1). Growth factors are substances that promote cellular growth. All cells possess proto-oncogenes for normal function. Alterations to a proto-oncogene from exposure to chemicals, viruses, radiation, or hereditary factors can activate an oncogene that promotes abnormal cell growth. One example of an oncogene is the *ERBB2* gene (also called the *HER2/neu* gene), which codes for a growth-factor receptor found in some forms of breast cancer and gastric cancer.

FIGURE 20.1 Oncogenes and Cancer Formation

The activation of an oncogene converts a normal cell to a cancer cell.

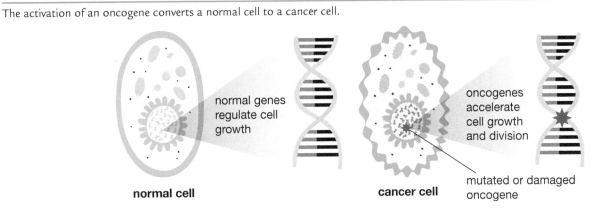

normal cell   normal genes regulate cell growth   **cancer cell**   oncogenes accelerate cell growth and division   mutated or damaged oncogene

Tumor Suppressor Genes

A **tumor suppressor gene** downregulates (decreases the quantity of) or turns off the production of cancer cells (see Figure 20.2). Tumor suppressor genes are the brakes that inhibit inappropriate cell growth. Mutations or deletions of tumor suppressor genes can result in uncontrolled cell growth. One of the most common tumor suppressor genes is *TP53*, which codes for the protein p53. In abnormal or aging cells, p53 halts cell division and induces **apoptosis**, or programmed cell death. Mutations of *TP53* are linked to resistance to many chemotherapy drugs.

FIGURE 20.2 Tumor Suppressor Gene

A mutated gene can lead to cancer development, as the duplicated, damaged gene leads to more damaged genes.

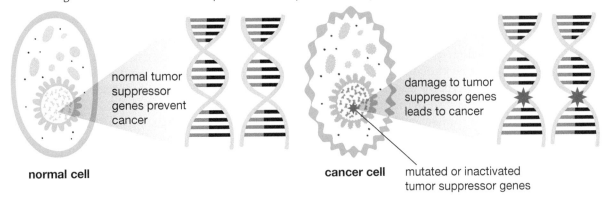

normal cell   normal tumor suppressor genes prevent cancer   **cancer cell**   damage to tumor suppressor genes leads to cancer   mutated or inactivated tumor suppressor genes

Tumor Cell Proliferation and Tumor Burden

Tumor cells usually grow and divide rapidly. The increase in the number of tumor cells is known as **tumor cell proliferation** (see Figure 20.3). Tumor cells exhibit different stages and rates of growth. The exponential phase, which is where the most rapid growth rate occurs, is where the tumor is most sensitive to chemotherapy agents that will attack and destroy rapidly reproducing cells. After a tumor has reached a certain size, its growth slows.

The term **tumor burden** refers to the number of cancer cells in a tumor or the size of the tumor tissue. This measurement is a determining factor in the effectiveness of chemotherapy. The smaller the tumor burden, the more effective chemotherapy is.

Dose-dense chemotherapy, the practice of administering chemotherapy doses more frequently than in standard treatment to allow fewer cells to regrow between doses, is based on the cell kill hypothesis. The **cell kill hypothesis** is a theory that chemotherapy will only kill a certain percentage of cancer cells and not *all* cancer cells but can reduce the number of cancer cells low enough that the normal defense mechanism typically takes over to eradicate the remaining cancer cells.

FIGURE 20.3 Tumor Cell Proliferation Model

A tumor must reach a certain size before it can be detected. Unfortunately, chemotherapy drugs can kill only a percentage of cancer cells in the tumor after this point, instead of completely eradicating it.

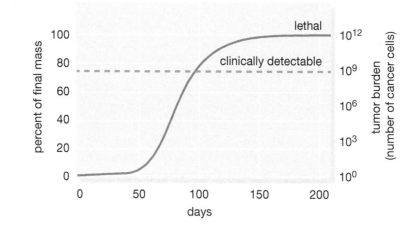

20.2 Cancer Stages and Treatments

Four major modalities (methods) are used to treat cancer. These methods—surgery, radiation therapy, immunotherapy, and chemotherapy—may be used alone or combined. Treatments of different cancers vary based on the tumor type; tumor location; and extent, or stage, of the disease. Most cancers are considered to have four stages (see Table 20.1), and the stage of the disease is important to identify when determining the best treatment. Tumors at stage I or II are **localized** (confined to one location in the body, called the *primary site*) and are usually easier to treat than tumors that have spread to other parts of the body. The spreading of a tumor from its primary site to other parts of the body is known as **metastasis**. Cancer is considered stage IV when a tumor has metastasized.

TABLE 20.1 Stages of Cancer

Stage	Description
I	The tumor is relatively small and has not grown outside the organ in which it began growing.
II	The tumor is larger than in stage I but has not spread to nearby tissues.
III	The tumor is large and has spread to nearby tissues and lymph nodes.
IV	The tumor has spread to another site in the body (via the blood or lymphatic system).

Surgery

The most curable types of cancer are localized tumors that can be surgically **resected** (removed). Ideally, a tumor can be removed without leaving any cancer cells at the site of the resection. The surgeon typically removes a little bit of normal tissue around the site of the tumor, an area known as the **margin**. Once the tumor is completely resected, the surgeon assesses the site of removal for residual tumor cells. The absence of tumor cells there, a condition known as a **negative margin**, lowers the risk of tumor regrowth.

Pharm Fact

The earliest known recorded description of cancer that survives today is in the Edwin Smith Papyrus, which dates from about 1600 BCE. It describes what appears to be breast cancer. The author wrote, "There is no treatment."

Radiation Therapy

Some tumors occur in locations that are difficult to reach with surgery (e.g., brain tumors). Other tumors may be too extensive to remove without damaging normal tissue or structures. In these situations, radiation therapy may be a better option. **Radiation therapy** involves the use of external beam radiation delivered from a machine outside the body to the site of a tumor. Radiation therapy may be used to rapidly shrink the mass of a tumor that is causing pain or growing too close to vital organs or structures, such as the spinal cord. Sometimes, radiation therapy is used after surgery to "clean up" areas of residual tumor that might have been left behind. This type of radiation therapy is called **adjuvant radiation therapy**.

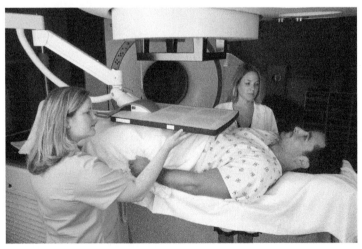

Almost half of all patients who have cancer undergo radiation therapy.

Immunotherapy

Immunotherapy is a type of cancer treatment that uses medications to stimulate the immune system to stop or slow the growth of cancer cells. Two common immunotherapy drugs are interferons and interleukins, which are used to treat melanoma (an often-fatal skin cancer) and renal cell carcinoma (an aggressive kidney cancer).

Immune checkpoint inhibitors, another type of immunotherapy, prevent cancer cells from "turning off" immune cells (cells that help the body fight infections and some diseases). Immune checkpoint inhibitors are a broad category of antineoplastic agents approved for several tumor types. Additional information on immunotherapy is covered later in this chapter.

Chemotherapy

Chemotherapy is defined as the administration of drugs to treat cancer by killing or stopping the growth of cancer cells. Chemotherapy drugs are also known as *chemotherapeutics, cytotoxic drugs,* and *anticancer drugs.* This treatment method provides systemic exposure to anticancer therapy as a mean of affecting the primary tumor as well as any migrating tumor cells. Chemotherapy may be described as primary, neoadjuvant, adjuvant, or palliative, depending on the goals of therapy.

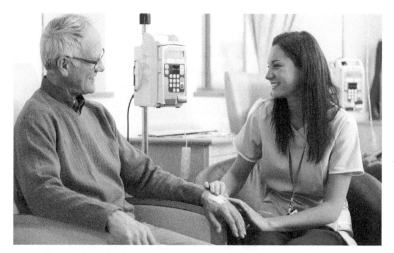

According to the American Cancer Society, prostate cancer is the most common cancer among men.

Primary Chemotherapy

Primary chemotherapy refers to the initial treatment of cancer with chemotherapy with curative intent. A **curative** act or treatment is one administered with the intent to cure an illness. Some cancers that can be cured with primary chemotherapy are Hodgkin's disease, lymphoma, leukemia, and testicular cancer.

Neoadjuvant Chemotherapy

Neoadjuvant chemotherapy is the administration of therapeutic agents *before* surgery. The main aim of neoadjuvant chemotherapy is to minimize or shrink a tumor so that surgery is easier to perform and more successful. For example, breast cancer patients may opt for neoadjuvant chemotherapy prior to breast surgery. This prereduction of cancer cells may allow for the removal of a limited amount of breast tissue (a lumpectomy) instead of the whole breast (a mastectomy). Administering neoadjuvant chemotherapy can give the patient the option of preserving the breast and avoiding major surgery.

Adjuvant Chemotherapy

Adjuvant chemotherapy refers to the treatment of residual cancer cells *after* removal or reduction of a tumor by surgery. An example of adjuvant therapy is the administration of chemotherapy, hormone therapy, or both following a lumpectomy or mastectomy for breast cancer. The patient receives adjuvant chemotherapy and radiation after surgery to ensure that any remaining cancer cells are eradicated. Both adjuvant and neoadjuvant chemotherapy can be curative if the tumor is effectively removed.

Palliative Chemotherapy

Palliative chemotherapy is given for cancer that is not curable. The usual goals of palliative chemotherapy are to prolong a patient's life and to improve the patient's quality of life by decreasing the tumor size and reducing the symptoms caused by the tumor. In this phase, it is important for patients to understand that the tumor will not disappear; rather, palliative chemotherapy minimizes the tumor's growth and the disease's progression.

20.3 Chemotherapy Drugs

Pharm Fact

In 1908, Paul Ehrlich won a Nobel Prize for his pioneering work. Today, he is considered to be the father of chemotherapy.

In the late 19th century, German bacteriologist Paul Ehrlich used methylene blue stain to demonstrate cell pathology. His research in the use of chemical compounds to identify and treat diseases paved the way for genetic studies in cancer research and the development of drugs that interfere with the cell cycle. A drug that is toxic to or kills the cell is referred to as a **cytotoxic drug**. The therapeutic use of these drugs became known as *chemotherapy*, a term Ehrlich coined from the words *chemical* and *therapy*. Multiple factors affect tumor response to chemotherapy drugs. These factors include the size of the tumor (tumor burden), cell resistance to the chemotherapy agent, amount of chemotherapy administered, and condition of the patient prior to chemotherapy.

Cell Cycle and Mechanism of Action

Grasping how chemotherapy drugs work requires an understanding of the cell cycle. The **cell cycle** is the process by which both normal cells and cancer cells divide. Because most cancer cells have lost their checks and balances on the rate of cellular replication, chemotherapy drugs are designed to interfere with the cell cycle at specific points.

The cell cycle is a series of phases that all cells, both normal and cancerous, go through to form new cells. The cycle begins with the cell in a resting phase (G_0). In the G_1 phase, the cell grows larger and begins to make proteins. During the S phase, chromosomes are copied so the two new cells being created will have identical DNA. In the G_2 phase, the cell begins to divide. Finally, in the M phase, the cell splits into two cells. This last phase is also known as *mitosis*. Figure 20.4 identifies the phases of the cell cycle and some of the activities that occur during those phases. Chemotherapy agents each target one or more phases of the cell cycle.

Cell Cycle–Specific Drugs

A **cell cycle–specific drug** exerts its effects on rapidly dividing cancer cells, which are the most sensitive to the effects of chemotherapy. Drugs of this class target cancer cells as they move into a specific nonresting phase of the cell cycle: when the cell prepares to divide, when the cell divides, or when the cell enlarges and makes new proteins. As a result, they minimize exposure to normal cells that may be in the resting

FIGURE 20.4
Cell Cycle and Cell Phase Chemotherapy Agents

This image depicts the phases of the cell cycle and identifies the sites of action of various chemotherapy agents. For example, mitotic inhibitors affect a cell during the M (or mitosis) phase.

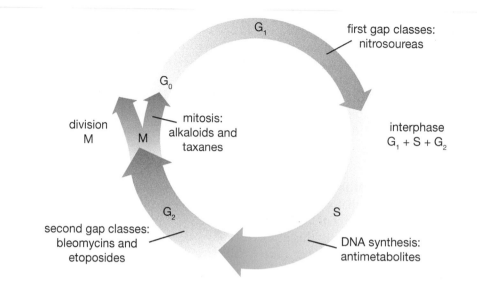

phase of the cell cycle (see Figure 20.4). For this reason, these drugs are considered schedule dependent and are administered as continuous infusions (e.g., fluorouracil and cytarabine) or in repeated bolus doses (e.g., weekly bleomycin).

Cell Cycle–Nonspecific Drugs

Cell cycle-nonspecific agents act on all phases of the cell cycle, including the resting phase. As a result, these drugs have little control over which cells they affect. They are especially valuable for treating slow-growing cancers. Unlike cell cycle-specific drugs, cell cycle-nonspecific drugs are given in large doses. These bolus doses are given over a short period of time so that they can kill the largest possible number of cells.

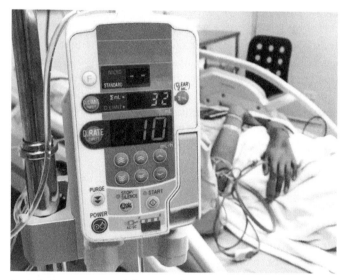

An infusion pump set delivers IV chemotherapy to a patient. The pump delivers medication at a controlled IV flow rate specified by the prescriber or pharmacist.

Cytotoxic Drugs and Side Effects

Cancer may be treated with chemotherapy, hormonal therapies, immunotherapy drugs, or one of the newer targeted anticancer therapies. Recall that a cytotoxic drug works by interrupting the normal process of cell function or proliferation. Table 20.2 lists common chemotherapy agents. It offers examples of chemotherapy drugs within each cytotoxic drug class along with those drugs' dosage forms and common indications. The table also lists the primary side effects for each class. Chemotherapy drugs of all types are available only by prescription, and common dosages vary significantly.

TABLE 20.2 Common Chemotherapy Agents and Their Indications and Side Effects

Generic (Brand)	Pronunciation	Dosage Form	Common Indications	Main Side Effects
Alkylating Agents				
bendamustine (Treanda)	ben-da-MUSS-teen	injection	chronic lymphocytic leukemia, lymphoma	bone marrow suppression, alopecia, nausea and vomiting, infertility, secondary cancers
busulfan (Myleran)	byoo-SUL-fan	tablet	leukemia, bone marrow transplant	
carboplatin (Paraplatin)	kar-boe-PLA-tin	injection	breast cancer, lung cancer, ovarian cancer	
chlorambucil (Leukeran)	klor-AM-byoo-sill	tablet	chronic lymphocytic leukemia	
cisplatin (Platinol)	sis-PLA-tin	injection	bladder cancer, bone cancer, cervical cancer, ovarian cancer, sarcoma, testicular cancer	
cyclophosphamide (Cytoxan)	sye-kloe-FOS-fa-mide	injection, tablet	breast cancer, immune system diseases (e.g., arthritis, lupus), leukemia, lymphoma	
dacarbazine (DTIC-Dome)	da-CAR-ba-zeen	injection	brain tumor	
ifosfamide (Ifex)	eye-FOSS-fam-ide	injection	lymphoma, sarcoma, testicular cancer	
mechlorethamine (Mustargen)	me-klor-ETH-a-meen	injectable	Hodgkin's disease, lymphoma	
melphalan (Alkeran)	MEL-fa-lan	injection, tablet	multiple myeloma	
oxaliplatin (Eloxatin)	ox-A-li-pla-tin	injection	colon cancer	
procarbazine (Matulane)	proe-KAR-ba-zeen	capsule	brain tumor, Hodgkin's disease	
temozolomide (Temodar)	te-mo-ZOLE-oh-mide	capsule	brain tumor, melanoma	
Nitrosoureas				
carmustine (BiCNU)	kar-MUS-teen	injection	brain tumor, bone marrow suppression, alopecia, nausea, vomiting, infertility, secondary cancers	
lomustine (Gleostine)	loe-MUS-teen	capsule	brain tumor	
Antimetabolites				
capecitabine (Xeloda)	kap-pe-SITE-a-been	tablet	breast cancer, colon cancer	bone marrow suppression, immune system suppression, mucositis
cladribine (Leustatin)	KLA-dra-been	injection	leukemia	
clofarabine (Clolar)	cloh-FAR-a-been	injection	pediatric leukemia	
cytarabine (Cytosar-U)	sye-TARE-a-been	injection	leukemia, lymphoma	

continues

TABLE 20.2 Common Chemotherapy Agents and Their Indications and Side Effects—*Continued*

Generic (Brand)	Pronunciation	Dosage Form	Common Indications	Main Side Effects
decitabine (Dacogen)	deh-SEE-tah-been	injection	adult leukemia	
fludarabine (Fludara)	floo-DARE-a-been	injection	leukemia, lymphoma	
fluorouracil (Adrucil)	flure-oh-YOOR-a-sill	injection, topical solution	breast cancer, colon cancer, premalignant skin conditions (some), skin cancers (some)	
gemcitabine (Gemzar)	jem-SIT-a-been	injection	bladder cancer, breast cancer, lung cancer, ovarian cancer, pancreatic cancer	
hydroxyurea (Hydrea)	hye-drox-ee-yoor-EE-a	capsule, tablet	leukemia, sickle cell anemia	
mercaptopurine (Purinethol)	mer-kap-toe-PYOOR-een	oral suspension, tablet	leukemia	
methotrexate (various brands)	meth-o-TREX-ate	injection (IM, IT, IV, SC), tablet	breast cancer, bone cancer, immune system diseases, leukemia, lymphoma, psoriasis, rheumatoid arthritis, systemic lupus erythematosus	
nelarabine (Arranon)	ne-LA-ra-been	injection	acute lymphoblastic leukemia	
pemetrexed (Alimta)	pe-me-TREX-ed	injection	lung cancer	
thioguanine (Tabloid)	thye-oh-GWAH-neen	tablet	pediatric leukemia	
Topoisomerase Inhibitors				
doxorubicin (Adriamycin)	dox-oh-ROO-bi-sin	injection	bone cancer, breast cancer, leukemia, lymphoma, multiple myeloma, sarcoma	
doxorubicin lipid complex (Doxil)	dox-oh-ROO-bi-sin LIP-id COM-plex	injection	bone cancer, breast cancer, leukemia, lymphoma, multiple myeloma, sarcoma	
epirubicin (Ellence)	ep-i-ROO-bi-sin	injection	breast cancer, esophageal cancer, stomach cancer	
etoposide (VePesid)	e-toe-POE-side	capsule, injection	leukemia, lung cancer, lymphoma, testicular cancer	
idarubicin (Idamycin)	eye-da-ROO-bi-sin	injection	acute leukemia	

continues

TABLE 20.2 Common Chemotherapy Agents and Their Indications and Side Effects—*Continued*

Generic (Brand)	Pronunciation	Dosage Form	Common Indications	Main Side Effects
Anthracyclines				
daunorubicin (Cerubidine, Daunomycin)	daw-noe-ROO-bi-sin	injection	leukemia	bone marrow suppression, nausea and vomiting, mucositis, alopecia, diarrhea
mitoxantrone (Novantrone)	mye-toe-ZAN-trone	injection	breast cancer, leukemia, lymphoma	
Campothecins				
irinotecan (Camptosar)	eye-ri-noe-TEE-kan	injection	colon cancer, lung cancer	
irinotecan liposomal (Onivyde)	eye-ri-noe-TEE-kan ly-po-SO-mal	injection	colon cancer, lung cancer	
topotecan (Hycamtin)	toe-poe-TEE-kan	capsule, injection	lung cancer, ovarian cancer	
Antimicrotubule Agents				
Taxanes				
docetaxel (Taxotere)	doe-se-TAX-el	injection	breast cancer, lung cancer, prostate cancer	bone marrow suppression, mucositis, alopecia, nerve toxicity
eribulin (Halaven)	er-i-BU-lin	injection	breast cancer, leukemia	
paclitaxel (Taxol)	pak-li-TAX-el	injection	breast cancer, lung cancer, ovarian cancer	
paclitaxel albumin bound (Abraxane)	pak-li-TAX-el al-BYOO-min bound	injection	breast cancer, lung cancer, ovarian cancer	
Vinca Alkaloids				
vinblastine (Velban)	vin-BLASS-teen	injection	lymphoma, testicular cancer	
vincristine (Oncovin)	vin-KRISS-teen	injection	leukemia, lymphoma	
vincristine liposomal (Marqibo)	vin-KRISS-teen ly-po-SO-mal	injection	leukemia, lymphoma	
vinorelbine (Navelbine)	vine-oh-REL-been	injection	breast cancer, lung cancer	
Miscellaneous Agents				
asparaginase	asp-air-ah-gen-AYZE	injection	acute lymphocytic leukemia	allergic reaction
bleomycin	blee-O-my-sin	injection	testicular cancer, Hodgkin's disease	pulmonary fibrosis

Although chemotherapy drugs exert the majority of their effects on cancer cells, these agents do not target tumor cells specifically. As a result, chemotherapy drugs cause numerous side effects related to normal cell function. Side effects from traditional chemotherapy drugs include **bone marrow suppression** (decreased production of blood cells, increased risks of infections and bleeding), **alopecia** (hair loss), nausea and vomiting, and **mucositis** (inflammation and ulceration of the mucous membranes lining the mouth and gastrointestinal tract). Major side effects of chemotherapy can be overwhelming. The Chemo Man in Figure 20.5 was created to help healthcare workers associate the side effects of chemotherapy with various body organs.

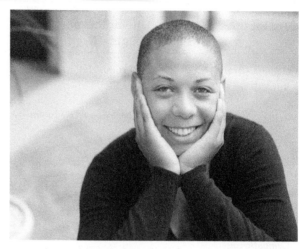

For patients with cancer, alopecia typically begins within the first two weeks of chemotherapy treatment and progressively worsens over the following two months.

FIGURE 20.5
Chemo Man

Chemo Man illustrates where various chemotherapy agents (listed in the key) affect the body. This illustration can be used for memorizing side effects of chemotherapy agents.

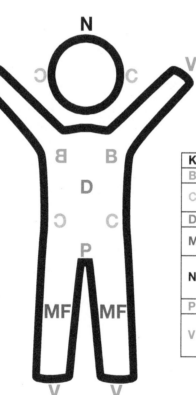

Key	Agent(s)	Side Effects
B	bleomycin, busulfan	pulmonary fibrosis
C	cisplatin, carboplatin	nephrotoxicity, ototoxicity
D	doxorubicin	cardiotoxicity
MF	methotrexate and 5-fluorouracil	myelosuppression
N	nitrosoureas (lomustine, carmustine)	neurotoxicity (cross the blood-brain barrier)
P	cyclophosphamide	hemorrhagic cystitis
V	vinca alkaloids (vincristine, vinblastine)	peripheral neuropathy

Among the many chemotherapy drug classes are alkylating agents, antimetabolites, topoisomerase inhibitors, and antimicrotubule agents. Each chemotherapy drug in these classes has one or more specific toxicities that must be addressed with preventive measures. Table 20.3 identifies some of the unique side effects of specific chemotherapy drugs and the measures taken to prevent those drugs' toxicities. Although many risks are associated with traditional chemotherapy agents, the use of these powerful drugs continues to cure many patients of cancer or to slow the progression of their disease, which prolongs their lives. Chemotherapy drugs remain a critical component of cancer treatment.

TABLE 20.3 Unique Toxicities of Chemotherapy Agents

Drug	Toxicity	Preventive
Alkylating Agents		
cisplatin	kidney damage	Aggressively administer IV fluids before and after each dose.
	potassium and magnesium loss	Provide potassium and magnesium supplements.
	nerve pain, nerve damage, or both	Assess level of nerve damage with each treatment. Stop treatment at onset of symptoms. Limit doses to ≤100 mg/m² for a cycle of treatment.
ifosfamide	hemorrhagic cystitis and CNS toxicity	Administer IV fluids during and after treatment. Give mesna (a bladder protectant) during and after treatment.
oxaliplatin	nerve pain, nerve damage, or both (hands, feet, throat)	Caution patients to avoid cold temperatures. Advise patients to avoid cold beverages. Limit doses or stop treatment if symptoms do not reverse.
Antimetabolites		
capecitabine	hand-foot syndrome	Advise patients to use emollients on hands and feet.
	diarrhea	Limit doses or stop therapy if symptoms develop.
cytarabine	conjunctivitis	Administer steroid eye drops during treatment whenever patients receive doses >1,000 mg/m².
methotrexate	kidney damage	Aggressively administer IV fluids. Provide urinary alkalinization using sodium bicarbonate.
	severe bone marrow suppression and mucosal toxicity	Maintain leucovorin rescue during the administration of methotrexate.
pemetrexed	severe bone marrow suppression	Administer folic acid and vitamin B supplements, starting 5–7 days before treatment.
	skin rash	Give dexamethasone, starting 1 day before treatment.
Topoisomerase Inhibitors		
Anthracyclines		
daunorubicin, doxorubicin, epirubicin, idarubicin	cardiac toxicity: cardiomyopathy, congestive heart failure	Track and limit cumulative doses. Monitor heart function. Stop treatment if symptoms develop.
irinotecan	severe diarrhea	Before irinotecan administration, administer atropine for diarrhea. Educate patients about how and when to take antidiarrheal agents (e.g., loperamide [Imodium], atropine / diphenoxylate [Lomotil]) after treatment.

continues

TABLE 20.3 Unique Toxicities of Chemotherapy Agents—*Continued*

Drug	Toxicity	Preventive
Antimicrotubule Agents		
paclitaxel	allergic reaction	Premedicate patients with diphenhydramine, famotidine, or another H_2 blocker or with dexamethasone.
	nerve pain, nerve damage, or both	Decrease dose or stop treatment if symptoms occur.
vincristine	nerve damage	Cap individual doses at 2 mg.
		Stop treatment if symptoms develop.
Miscellaneous Agent		
bleomycin	lung damage	Track cumulative dose and limit it to <400 units.
		Limit individual doses to ≤30 units.
		Avoid giving to patients with kidney dysfunction.

One of the most serious side effects of methotrexate (MTX), an antimetabolite, is kidney damage. When methotrexate is administered in doses above 1,000 mg, it can accumulate in the kidneys and form damaging renal crystals. To prevent such accumulation, patients are given IV fluids containing sodium bicarbonate or sodium acetate to alkalinize (increase the pH of) the urine. Increasing the urine pH makes methotrexate more soluble and prevents renal crystals from forming.

In high doses, methotrexate can also cause severe bone marrow suppression and mucosal injury in the GI tract. These side effects occur because methotrexate interferes with an enzyme, dihydrofolate reductase, that is important in normal bone marrow and mucosal cell development. **Leucovorin**, also called *folinic acid*, is a by-product of this enzyme. The administration of leucovorin to patients who have received high-dose methotrexate rescues normal cells from a leucovorin shortage and allows them to resume their normal proliferation.

This process, known as **leucovorin rescue**, is usually initiated 19 to 36 hours after the start of the methotrexate infusion, thus allowing the methotrexate to exert its action on cancer cells. Timing is essential for leucovorin rescue because leucovorin cannot rescue cells that have been exposed to high levels of methotrexate for more than 48 hours. In pediatric patients who are having delayed methotrexate clearance, the use of the orphan drug carboxypeptidase is a must.

Combination Chemotherapy

To reduce a cancer's potential resistance to treatment, **combination chemotherapy** is usually administered. This type of regimen is designed to include two or more drugs that have:

- proven efficacy against the tumor being treated
- nonoverlapping toxicities
- different mechanisms of action

Some drug combinations elicit an enhanced response because the agents work together to amplify the individual effects of each. This is called a **synergistic effect**. The most important thing to know about combinations of anticancer drugs is that a combination's benefits and effects cannot always be accurately predicted prior to comprehensive testing on human subjects. Combination chemotherapy regimens must be selected based on the proven—not hypothetical—safety and efficacy of the combination. One chemotherapeutic agent is not always effective in killing the intended tumor cells. Combination chemotherapy allows for additional benefit when the chemotherapeutic agents have different mechanisms of action.

Alkylating Agents

The oldest category of traditional chemotherapy drugs is the alkylating agents. **Alkylating agents** work by binding to and damaging deoxyribonucleic acid (DNA) during the cell division process, ultimately preventing cell replication. The first drug identified as having anticancer activity in this category was **mechlorethamine (Mustargen)**, or nitrogen mustard, a derivative of mustard gas. The release of mustard gas during World War I was discovered to play a role in decreasing lymphocyte activity within soldiers who were exposed to the gas. The discovery of this reaction led to the development of this agent as a treatment for lymphoma, a cancer of the lymphatic system. Alkylating agents have a broad spectrum of anticancer activity and are used to treat a variety of cancer types. Refer to Table 20.2 for examples of specific alkylating agents, their indications, and their dosage forms.

Cisplatin (Platinol) is used to treat many diseases, including lung, ovarian, and bone cancers. It is a critical component of the chemotherapy regimens for testicular cancer.

Cyclophosphamide (Cytoxan) plays an important role in treating lymphoma, leukemia, and breast cancer.

Carmustine (BiCNU) and **lomustine (Gleostine)** are in the **nitrosourea** category of alkylating agents. Nitrosoureas have the ability to penetrate the central nervous system (CNS) and are frequently used in the treatment of brain tumors.

Dosage Forms and Administration Alkylating agents are available in either oral or injectable dosage forms. The unique toxicities associated with specific alkylating agents (see Table 20.3) require monitoring of the patient and use of preventive measures. For example, maximum limits are placed on the dosing of cisplatin to avoid overdoses and severe toxicities, and IV fluids are recommended before and after cisplatin administration.

Side Effects The most common side effect of alkylating agents is bone marrow suppression. Alkylating agents also cause nausea, vomiting, and alopecia. As noted in Table 20.3, many alkylating agents have unique toxicities. Cisplatin, for example, causes **peripheral neuropathy** (extremely painful damage to the peripheral nervous system, especially affecting the hands and feet) and **ototoxicity** (damage to the nerves that affect hearing). Patients must be carefully assessed for these side effects between cycles of treatment, and doses should be decreased or stopped when symptoms develop.

Because alkylating agents damage DNA, they are also considered **mutagenic**, meaning they can cause changes in genetic material. As mutagens, these drugs have the potential to cause certain types of **secondary cancers**, also called *secondary malignancy*, in patients who have received them. The potential to cause secondary cancers is a rare but very serious side effect.

Alkylating agents are also known to damage reproductive tissue, and patients who receive these medications may become infertile.

Contraindications Although alkylating agents are associated with several potential toxicities, there are very few absolute contraindications to the use of these agents in cancer treatment. A history of allergic reaction is one contraindication to the use of specific alkylating agents. Some alkylating agents, such as cisplatin, **carboplatin**

(Paraplatin), and **oxaliplatin (Eloxatin)**, are associated with a higher risk of allergic or hypersensitivity reaction. Patients who have exhibited an allergy to one of these agents may need to avoid treatment with another agent in the platin category. Skin tests to assess the risk of an allergic reaction, a protocol for administering sequentially escalating doses in a "desensitization" regimen, or both can be ordered as a means of managing patients who do not have other treatment options. Certain alkylating agents may be contraindicated for some patients due to those agents' particular toxicities. For example, patients with kidney dysfunction may not be good candidates for cisplatin therapy, which could worsen their kidney function, or for ifosfamide therapy, which can cause serious CNS toxicity (causing an altered mental status) when given to patients with kidney dysfunction.

Cautions and Considerations These agents carry numerous boxed warnings and should be dispensed with Medication Guides. Cisplatin has a boxed warning for nephrotoxicity, myelosuppression, nausea, vomiting, and ototoxicity. Proper hydration and an antiemetic regimen should be administered to the patient prior to starting the infusion of this chemotherapy agent.

Busulfan has a boxed warning for severe myelosuppression. Blood count should be monitored.

Dacarbazine has a boxed warning for myelosuppression and hepatic necrosis and is a carcinogenic and teratogenic.

Melphalan has a boxed warning for bone marrow suppression.

Carmustine has a boxed warning for bone marrow suppression and pulmonary toxicity.

Ifosfamide can lead to several toxicities, including CNS toxicity and bladder toxicity, referred to as *hemorrhagic cystitis* (bleeding of the bladder). A drug called mercaptoethane sulfonate can protect against hemorrhagic cystitis.

Alkylating agents are hazardous drugs and require special precautions for personnel who prepare or handle them. Some alkylating agents are absorbed through the skin, so extreme caution must be used.

Drug Interactions Alkylating agents may increase the adverse effects of immunosuppressants (such as steroids and other cancer therapies). Caution should be exercised with concurrent use of alkylating agents and other immunosuppressants. Drug interactions for this class of drug are numerous and should be confirmed when prescribed.

Antimetabolites

Another class of chemotherapy drugs is the antimetabolites. An **antimetabolite** works during the synthesis phase, or S phase, of the cell cycle. These medications have differing mechanisms of action. Some antimetabolites inhibit enzyme production or activity that is needed for DNA or ribonucleic acid (RNA) synthesis. Methotrexate, cytarabine, and **fluorouracil (Adrucil)** interefere with enzymes that are essential for tumor cell proliferation. Antimetabolites may also act as false nucleotides (a **nucleotide** is the basic structural component of DNA and RNA). Because they resemble DNA nucleotides, these antimetabolites become incorporated into DNA during synthesis, which inhibits the synthesis of normal DNA. Their incorporation inhibits synthesis of normal DNA. **Mercaptopurine (Purinethol)** and **thioguanine (Tabloid)** are antimetabolite drugs that interfere with cell synthesis by replacing normal nucleotides in DNA and RNA production.

Antimetabolite drugs are used to treat a variety of cancers (see Table 20.2). For example, fluorouracil and its oral counterpart, **capecitabine (Xeloda)**, are commonly used to treat colon cancer. A topical form of fluorouracil is used to treat some low-grade skin cancers and precancerous skin lesions. **Gemcitabine (Gemzar)** is used to treat lung

Practice Tip

Methylene blue and thiamine are two agents that can be administered to patients with CNS-related ifosfamide toxicity.

Safety Alert

Ifosfamide can cause severe hemorrhagic cystitis and is always prescribed with the bladder protective agent mesna. Orders for the administration of ifosfamide without mesna should always be questioned.

and pancreatic cancers, and **pemetrexed (Alimta)** is critical in the treatment of certain types of lung cancer. **Cytarabine (Cytosar-U)** and **fludarabine (Fludara)** are primarily used to treat different types of leukemia and lymphoma. Uniquely, cytarabine can be safely introduced by **intrathecal (IT) administration** (administered directly into the CNS via a lumbar puncture or spinal tap) in patients who have leukemia cells in their cerebrospinal fluid. **Hydroxyurea (Hydrea)** is an oral antimetabolite commonly used to rapidly lower white blood cell counts in patients who have leukemia. Hydroxyurea is also used to help decrease painful crisis episodes in individuals with sickle cell anemia.

Methotrexate is commonly used to treat leukemia, bone cancer, breast cancer, lymphoma, and a variety of nonmalignant immunologic conditions, such as psoriasis, rheumatoid arthritis, and systemic lupus erythematosus. Methotrexate suppresses immune system function and is one of the most complicated antimetabolites to administer.

Safety Alert

Even in very low doses, methotrexate can be extremely toxic, especially if it is administered incorrectly. Methotrexate is never administered daily for extended periods. Daily orders for even very low doses (e.g., 2.5 mg PO once a day) should always be questioned.

Pharm Fact

Treatment decisions are always based on a risk-benefit assessment.

Dosage Forms and Administration Administration of antimetabolite drugs includes various preventive measures for avoiding toxicities associated with each drug. See Tables 20.2 and 20.3 as well as the following section on side effects. Because antimetabolites are cell cycle–specific drugs, their cytotoxic effects (effects on the cell) and side effects may change depending on how they are administered. For example, if administered incorrectly, methotrexate can result in serious and sometimes fatal toxicities. Methotrexate may be prepared for administration by different routes, including oral, IV, intrathecal (IT), intramuscular, and subcutaneous. It is given in a wide range of doses, from 5 mg once a week for rheumatoid arthritis to 20 g once or twice a month when used for bone cancer (osteosarcoma or lymphoma).

Sometimes, the administration of an antimetabolite is manipulated to provide the best therapeutic effect. For example, for newly diagnosed patients with acute leukemia, cytarabine is typically administered as a 24-hour continuous infusion for seven days. Administering this cell cycle–specific agent continuously ensures that it is present during the synthesis phase of the cell cycle, when cells are most susceptible to its toxic effects. In contrast, gemcitabine is a cell cycle–specific drug typically administered as a 30-minute infusion. Extending the duration to 60 minutes might seriously increase the toxicity of this drug. Dosage schedules for antimetabolite drugs must be carefully followed to prevent excessive toxicity from these agents.

Side Effects The main side effects the various antimetabolites have in common are bone marrow suppression, immune system suppression, and mucositis. Higher doses of methotrexate may require the administration of leucovorin rescue to address these toxicities.

The oral antimetabolite capecitabine can cause a debilitating reaction called **hand-foot syndrome**, also know as *palmar-plantar erythrodysesthesia*. In hand-foot syndrome, patients experience painful sloughing and peeling of the skin on the palms of the hands and soles of the feet. The appearance of this condition in patients taking oral capecitabine necessitates a pause in treatment as well as a reduction in subsequent doses.

Cytarabine is used in a wide range of doses. High doses may result in **conjunctivitis**. To prevent this side effect, patients receiving high-dose cytarabine must also receive steroid eye drops (e.g., dexamethasone, prednisolone) during therapy and for 24 to 48 hours after completion of therapy.

Contraindications Like alkylating agents, antimetabolite drugs have very few absolute contraindications.

For individuals who have a deficiency or lack of an enzyme called *dihydropyrimidine dehydrogenase* (which helps to break down and eliminate fluorouracil and capecitabine), a significant reduction in doses or a selection of alternative agents may be necessary. These individuals are extremely susceptible to the side effects of fluorouracil and capecitabine.

Methotrexate should not be administered as part of an anticancer treatment regimen to individuals who are pregnant. Due to its unique toxicity profile, methotrexate also should not be administered to patients with severe kidney dysfunction. Furthermore, because methotrexate accumulates in interstitial spaces (a condition known as *third-space fluid shift*), this medication should be avoided or administered with extreme caution in patients who have ascites or pleural effusions.

Cautions and Considerations Antimetabolites are hazardous drugs and require special precautions for all personnel who prepare or handle them. Cytarabine and methotrexate carry a boxed warning for bone marrow suppression. Methotrexate also carries boxed warnings for liver, kidney, and lung toxicity; diarrhea; and ulcerative stomatitis. Careful monitoring of methotrexate drug level is recommended to determine clearance and when to administer leucovorin rescue.

Drug Interactions Antimetabolites may increase the adverse effects of other immunosuppressants. Caution should be exercised with concurrent use of antimetabolites and other immunosuppressants. Antimetabolites may increase the adverse effects and decrease the efficacy of live vaccines. Live vaccines should not be administered until at least three months after immunosuppressants have been discontinued. As with other cytotoxic drugs, drug interactions for this class of drug are numerous and should be confirmed when prescribed.

Topoisomerase Inhibitors

Topoisomerases are enzymes required for DNA synthesis and cell replication. DNA has a tightly coiled structure and must be unwound during the replication process. Topoisomerases make temporary breaks and repairs in DNA strands, which helps unwind the DNA and allows the transcription process to occur. There are two types of topoisomerase enzymes: a **topoisomerase I enzyme** causes single-strand DNA breaks, and a **topoisomerase II enzyme** causes double-strand DNA breaks. Topoisomerase inhibitors interfere with the DNA repair function of topoisomerases (I and II) and disrupt the cell replication process. (See Table 20.2 for more information on topoisomerase inhibitors.)

A **topoisomerase I inhibitor** is a member of the subset of drugs that inhibit topoisomerase I enzymes. These include topotecan and irinotecan, both derived from a tree, *Camptotheca acuminata*, that is native to China. **Topotecan (Hycamtin)** is commonly used to treat ovarian cancer and lung cancer. **Irinotecan (Camptosar)** is most frequently used to treat lung cancer and colon cancer. Both of these agents are also used to treat brain tumors or brain metastases because of their ability to penetrate the CNS.

An **anthracycline** is a member of a large category of commonly used topoisomerase II inhibitors. A **topoisomerase II inhibitor** is a member of the subset of drugs that inhibit topoisomerase II enzymes. Anthracyclines, also known as *DNA intercalating agents*, inhibit topoisomerase activity by inserting themselves (or intercalating) into strands of DNA. These agents include daunorubicin, doxorubicin, epirubicin, and idarubicin. They are derived from *Streptomyces* bacteria, which are found in soil and produce a red pigment.

Doxorubicin (Adriamycin) is part of curative chemotherapy regimens for breast cancer and lymphoma. It is also used in many other types of cancers. **Daunorubicin** and **idarubicin (Idamycin)** are primarily used to treat leukemia. **Epirubicin (Ellence)** is most frequently used to treat breast, esophageal, and stomach cancers. Pharmacy technicians who work with chemotherapy patients may hear the term **R-CHOP** used in the workplace (see Table 20.4). This is an acronym that refers to a combination of

TABLE 20.4 A Typical Regimen of Rituximab with Cyclophosphamide, Doxorubicin, Vincristine, and Prednisone (R-CHOP)

Drug	Dose
rituximab	intravenous infusion (375 mg/m²) on day 1
cyclophosphamide	intravenous bolus (750 mg/m²) on day 1
doxorubicin	intravenous bolus (50 mg/m²) on day 1
vincristine	intravenous bolus (1.4 mg/m²) on day 1
prednisone	oral administration (100 mg) on days 1–5

various chemotherapy agents to a monoclonal antibody: **r**ituximab (Rituxan), **c**yclophosphamide (Cytoxan), **h**ydroxydaunorubicin (better known as *doxyrubicin*), **O**ncovin (brand name of vincristine), and **p**rednisone.

Etoposide and mitoxantrone are two other topoisomerase II inhibitors. **Etoposide (VePesid)** is derived from the American mayapple plant and is commonly used to treat leukemia, lung cancer, lymphoma, and testicular cancer. **Mitoxantrone (Novantrone)** is similar in activity to the anthracyclines but has an inky blue color. This medication is frequently used to treat breast cancer, leukemia, and lymphoma.

Dosage Forms and Administration Some topoisomerase inhibitors are prepared in a lipid formulation, known as a **liposomal product**, to help decrease toxicity. The drugs doxorubicin (Doxil) and irinotecan (Onivyde) have liposomal formulations. Paclitaxel is available in an albumin bound formulation called Abraxane.

Side Effects Side effects common to most topoisomerase inhibitors include bone marrow suppression, nausea and vomiting, mucositis, alopecia, and diarrhea. Because topoisomerase inhibitors interfere with DNA synthesis, these agents also have the ability to cause secondary cancers such as acute leukemia. Although the potential to cause secondary cancers is rare, it is a serious side effect of topoisomerase inhibitors.

Another serious toxicity of anthracyclines is **cardiac toxicity**, the ability to cause heart damage, although such damage typically occurs many years after patients have received the drug. The risk of cardiac toxicity with anthracyclines is cumulative, increasing with each dose the patient receives. The best way to limit the risk of cardiac toxicity with these drugs is to track the patient's cumulative exposure and stop treatment after they have reached a **threshold dose**. The threshold dose is different for each anthracycline drug. For example, the lifetime cumulative dose limit for doxorubicin is approximately 450 mg/m², whereas the cumulative dose limit for idarubicin is approximately 225 mg/m² (Table 20.5).

TABLE 20.5 Relative Cardiotoxicity of Anthracycline Agents

Agent	Conversion Factor	Cumulative Dose Limit
daunorubicin	0.5	900 mg/m²
doxorubicin	1	450 mg/m²
epirubicin	0.5	935 mg/m²
idarubicin	2	225 mg/m²

Unlike other topoisomerase inhibitors, irinotecan has severe diarrhea as a side effect. If not managed quickly, diarrhea from irinotecan can lead to serious complications. Patients who experience this type of diarrhea are treated with atropine, an injectable anticholinergic drug. The most serious form of diarrhea occurs in the days following administration of irinotecan. Patients must be adequately warned about the potential for this side effect and educated on how to appropriately administer antidiarrheal agents, such as loperamide, at the onset of symptoms.

Contraindications Topoisomerase inhibitors have few absolute contraindications. However, patients with a history of cardiac disease, evidence of congestive heart failure, or cardiac dysfunction may not be good candidates for any of the anthracycline agents.

Many of the topoisomerase drugs are eliminated from the body through the liver and the biliary systems. Therefore, patients with significant liver dysfunction may not be able to tolerate drugs such as anthracyclines or irinotecan.

Topotecan is eliminated by the kidneys, so patients with significant kidney dysfunction are not good candidates for this agent.

Cautions and Considerations Irinotecan has a boxed warning for severe diarrhea, acute diarrhea within 24 hours of administration, and late diarrhea occurring more than 24 hours post infusion. Patients should be monitored for fluid imbalance. Topotecan has a boxed warning for bone marrow suppression.

Daunorubicin has a boxed warning for bone marrow suppression and cardiac toxicity. Doxorubicin has a boxed warning for myelosuppression, secondary malignancy, and cardiotoxicity.

Patients with a mutation of the *UGT1A* gene (which encodes an enzyme responsible for breaking down irinotecan in the liver) are susceptible to increased toxicity when irinotecan is administered in high doses. A commercial test is available to identify patients who have this genetic mutation. However, the clinical utility of this test is not widely established; therefore, it is not recommended for routine use.

Anthracyclines, such as daunorubicin, doxorubicin, epirubicin, and idarubicin, cause severe tissue damage if an infusion leaks under the skin during administration. This leaking and the related damage is called **extravasation**. A drug that causes extravasation injury is referred to as a **vesicant** (see Table 20.6).

TABLE 20.6 Chemotherapy Vesicant Drugs

daunorubicin	idarubicin	vinblastine
doxorubicin	mechlorethamine	vincristine
epirubicin	mitomycin	vinorelbine

Drug Interactions Topoisomerase inhibitors may increase the adverse effects of other immunosuppressants. Caution should be exercised with concurrent use of topoisomerase inhibitors and other immunosuppressants. Topoisomerase inhibitors may increase the adverse effects and decrease the efficacy of live vaccines. Live vaccines should not be administered until at least three months after immunosuppressants have been discontinued. As with other cytotoxic drugs, drug interactions for this class of drug are numerous and should be confirmed when prescribed.

Antimicrotubule Agents

A **microtubule** is any of the minute tubules in a cell's cytoskeleton. Important to cell function, microtubules play a role in maintaining cell shape and structure and are critical elements in the process of cell division, or mitosis. An **antimicrotubule agent** is an agent that interferes with the formation and function of microtubules, ultimately preventing cell growth and division.

Most antimicrotubule drugs are derived from plant sources. **Paclitaxel (Taxol)** and **docetaxel (Taxotere)** are taxanes. A **taxane** is a member of a class of antimicrotubule drugs derived from the bark and needles of yew trees. **Vincristine (Oncovin)**, **vinblastine (Velban)**, and **vinorelbine (Navelbine)** are vinca alkaloids. A **vinca alkaloid** is a member of a class of antimicrotubule drugs derived from periwinkle plants. Antimicrotubule agents are important components in the treatment of lung, breast, ovarian, prostate, and testicular cancers, as well as for some types of leukemia and lymphoma.

Dosage Forms and Administration Vincristine and vinblastine must never be administered by the intrathecal (IT) route. Fatalities have occurred with the inadvertent administration of vincristine as an IT agent. The ISMP recommends dispensing vincristine in a small minibag infusion instead of in a syringe.

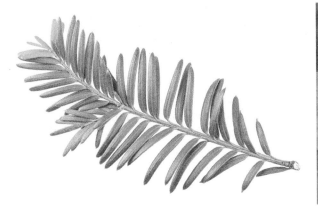
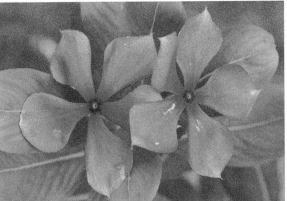

Yew needles (left) and periwinkle (right) are the plant sources for several antimicrotubule agents used in chemotherapy. The study of natural cancer-fighting sources is ongoing; for instance, scientists recently discovered that a berry from the blushwood tree (a species found only in North Queensland, Australia) holds promise for treating head and neck tumors and melanomas.

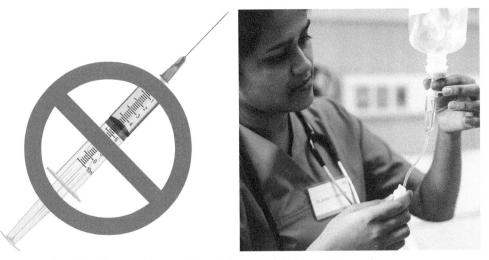

Vincristine should be dispensed in a minibag with proper labeling, not in a syringe.

Side Effects Like other traditional cytotoxic drugs, antimicrotubule agents cause bone marrow suppression, mucositis, and alopecia. The degree of alopecia varies. For example, patients receiving paclitaxel may experience total body alopecia, including loss of eyelashes, eyebrows, and pubic hair. Nausea and vomiting with antimicrotubule agents may occur but is generally mild.

Because microtubules also play an important role in nerve function, many antimicrotubule agents cause peripheral neuropathy. Vincristine, in particular, can cause neurotoxicity to the GI tract. While on therapy with vincristine, patients must be closely monitored to make sure they do not develop **ileus**, a condition in which GI motility is severely reduced.

Side effects of taxanes (such as paclitaxel and docetaxel) that are not shared with other antimicrotubule agents include bone and muscle aches (myalgia), which can occur for several days after an infusion. These side effects are typically managed with an OTC pain reliever such as acetaminophen or ibuprofen. **Paclitaxel albumin bound (Abraxane)** was developed to decrease infusion-related reactions.

Contraindications The antimicrotubule agents paclitaxel and docetaxel are contraindicated in patients who have a history of hypersensitivity reaction.

Vincristine should not be administered to patients who have a history of peripheral neuropathy. This medication may worsen the neuropathy.

Paclitaxel, docetaxel, vincristine, and vinblastine are contraindicated for patients with significant liver dysfunction because these agents are eliminated by the hepatic and biliary system.

Cautions and Considerations Because they are yew tree derivatives, paclitaxel and docetaxel are commonly associated with allergic reactions during drug administration. Patients typically require premedication with antihistamines and corticosteroids to prevent severe allergic reactions to these drugs. Patients who have had allergic reactions to one or both of these agents may require additional premedication with corticosteroids or may not be able to tolerate reexposure to the agent, depending on the severity of the reaction. Paclitaxel and docetaxel have boxed warnings for anaphylaxis and severe hypersensitivity reaction. All patients should receive corticosteroids, diphenhydramine, and H2 antagonists prior to administration of each dose.

Docetaxel also carries boxed warnings for liver toxicity, edema, and myelosuppression.

Vincristine and vinblastine carry boxed warnings related to administration, noting they are fatal if given intrathecally.

Drug Interactions Antimicrotubule agents may increase the adverse effects of other immunosuppressants. Caution should be exercised with concurrent use of antimicrotubule agents and other immunosuppressants. Antimicrotubule agents may increase the adverse effects and decrease the efficacy of live vaccines. Live vaccines should not be administered until at least three months after immunosuppressants have been discontinued. As with other cytotoxic drugs, drug interactions for this class of drug are numerous and should be confirmed when prescribed.

Miscellaneous Chemotherapy Drugs

Two commonly used chemotherapy drugs that do not fit into the other cytotoxic drug categories are bleomycin and asparaginase.

Bleomycin works by cutting or breaking DNA strands, preventing the process of cell proliferation. It is part of the curative chemotherapy regimens used to treat testicular cancer and Hodgkin's disease (a type of lymphoma).

Asparaginase is a drug with a very narrow spectrum of activity. Asparaginase is used to treat acute lymphocytic leukemia, a common and often curable type of leukemia in children. Leukemia cells require a large amount of the amino acid **asparagine** to proliferate. Unlike normal cells, leukemia cells are not able to make asparagine. Asparaginase is an enzyme that breaks down asparagine, depriving leukemia cells of this essential amino acid. Consequently, these leukemia cells will not be able to survive and will die.

Dosage Forms and Administration Unlike many other cytotoxic drugs, one advantage of bleomycin is that it does not cause bone marrow suppression. However, this medication can cause a deadly type of lung toxicity known as **pulmonary fibrosis**. This condition occurs when the delicate tissue of the lung is damaged or scarred. It is important to track and limit cumulative doses of bleomycin to decrease the risk of pulmonary fibrosis.

Side Effects Allergic reaction is one of the most common side effects of asparaginase therapy. Because asparaginase products are made from two different bacterial sources, patients who develop an allergic reaction to one product can often safely switch to the other product. Asparaginase can also interfere with normal protein synthesis in patients who are receiving it. Patients receiving asparaginase therapy must be closely monitored for effects on clotting factors and might be at a higher risk for bleeding or clotting.

A common side effect of bleomycin is pulmonary fibrosis.

Pharm Fact

Pulmonary fibrosis is the most severe toxicity associated with bleomycin. Its occurrence is higher in patients over 60 and in those receiving a total dose greater than 400 units.

Contraindications Because of the risk of lung toxicity, patients older than 60 years of age may not be good candidates for treatment with bleomycin. Younger patients who are athletes may also choose to limit their exposure to bleomycin in an effort to preserve their lung function. Asparaginase is contraindicated in patients with liver toxicity. Proper liver enzyme monitoring is advised.

Cautions and Considerations Patients who have received bleomycin may be at a higher risk for respiratory problems during surgery with general anesthesia. Asparaginase has boxed warnings for allergic reactions and liver toxicity.

Drug Interactions These cytotoxic drugs may increase the adverse effects of other immunosuppressants. Caution should be exercised with concurrent use of cytotoxic drugs and other immunosuppressants. Cytotoxic drugs may increase the adverse effects and decrease the efficacy of live vaccines. Live vaccines should not be administered until at least three months after immunosuppressants have been discontinued. Drug interactions related to specific agents are numerous and should be confirmed when prescribed.

20.4 Hormonal Drug Therapies

Although the treatment of certain tumors requires the administration of cytotoxic drugs to interrupt cell proliferation, other tumors can be affected by altering hormone levels within the body. These types of cancer depend on naturally occurring hormones for growth. In tumors that are known to be dependent on specific hormones for proliferation, one treatment strategy is to block the activity of those hormones. Hormonal drug therapies, also called *endocrine drug therapies*, target the hormone that is contributing to the growth of a specific type of tumor. For example, estrogen and progesterone are hormones that frequently stimulate breast tumors. Prostate cancer is often dependent on androgens, such as testosterone, for growth. Hormonal drug therapies work by stopping the production of or access to those hormones to prevent the continued growth of these tumors. Drug classes associated with hormonal drug therapies include antiestrogens, antiandrogens, and luteinizing hormone–releasing hormone agonists. A newer class given in combination with hormonal therapy is the cyclin-dependent kinase 4/6 inhibitors (CDK 4/6 inhibitors). Cyclin-dependent kinases (CDKs) play a role in regulating the cell cycle.

TABLE 20.7 **Commonly Used Hormonal Therapy Agents**

Generic (Brand)	Pronunciation	Dosage Form	Common Dosage	Common Indications
Antiestrogens				
tamoxifen (Nolvadex)	ta-MOX-eh-fen	tablet	20 mg daily	breast cancer
anastrozole (Arimidex)	ah-NA-stro-zole	tablet	1 mg daily	breast cancer
letrozole (Femara)	LET-ro-zole	tablet	2.5 mg daily	breast cancer
exemestane (Aromasin)	EX-ah-mess-tine	tablet	25 mg daily	breast cancer
Antiandrogens				
abiraterone (Zytiga)	ab-er-RAT-eh-ron	tablet	1,000 mg daily	prostate cancer
bicalutamide (Casodex)	bye-ca-LOO-ta-myde	tablet	50 mg daily	prostate cancer
enzalutamide (Xtandi)	en-zah-LOO-ta-myde	tablet	160 mg daily	prostate cancer
flutamide (Eulexin)	FLOO-ta-myde	tablet	250 mg every 8 hr	prostate cancer
apalutamide (Erleada),	ah-pa-LOO-ta-myde	tablet	240 mg daily	prostate cancer
darolutamide (Nubeqa)	dah-ro-LOO-ta-myde	tablet	600 mg 2 times a day	prostate cancer
nilutamide (Nilandron)	nigh-LOO-ta-myde	tablet	300 mg for 30 days, then 150 mg a day	prostate cancer
Luteinizing hormone–releasing hormone (LHRH)				
leuprolide (Lupron)	LOO-pro-lyde	injection	IM: 7.5 mg per month 22.5 mg every 3 months	breast cancer, prostate cancer
goserelin (Zoladex)	GO-seh-rell-in	implant injection	SC: 3.6mg every 28 days	breast cancer, prostate cancer
Cyclin-Dependent Kinase 4/6 Inhibitors				
abemaciclib (verzenio)	uh-BEH-ma-sye-klib	tablet	200 mg 2 times a day	breast cancer
palbociclib (Ibrance)	pal-boe-SYE-klib	tablet	125 mg daily	breast cancer
ribociclib (Kisqali)	RYE-boe-sye-klib	tablet	600 mg daily	breast cancer

Antiestrogens

Members of the **antiestrogen** drug class work by interfering with estrogen production or by blocking estrogen receptors on tumor cells, inhibiting estrogen's ability to enhance tumor growth. Drugs within this class, such as anastrozole, exemestane, letrozole, and tamoxifen, are commonly used to treat breast cancer. **Tamoxifen (Nolvadex)** works by blocking estrogen receptors and can be used in the treatment of breast cancer in patients of any age.

Anastrozole (Arimidex), **letrozole (Femara)**, and **exemestane (Aromasin)** are aromatase inhibitors. An **aromatase inhibitor** blocks the effects of estrogen by preventing synthesis of estrogen in the body. However, aromatase inhibitors only work in individuals who have experienced menopause. Aromatase inhibitors do not adequately inhibit ovarian production of estrogen in younger patients who have not undergone menopause; this counteracts the effects of these agents in these patients.

Dosage Forms and Administration These agents are administered orally. They are all available as tablets and administered once or twice a day. Both anastrozole and letrozole can be taken with or without food.

Side Effects Side effects of antiestrogen therapy are very similar to menopausal symptoms, such as hot flashes, mood swings, and depression. In addition, the use of these agents can increase a patient's risk for blood clots and endometrial cancer.

Contraindications Antiestrogen agents should be avoided in patients who are pregnant or trying to become pregnant. A history of blood clots may also be a contra-indication for therapy with an antiestrogen agent. However, physicians and patients may decide that the potential benefits of therapy outweigh the risks and choose to initiate therapy with enhanced monitoring for signs and symptoms of blood clots.

Cautions and Considerations Tamoxifen has a boxed warning for uterine malig-nancies, thromboembolic events, strokes, and pulmonary embolism. Careful consid-eration is required for patients who have coagulation abnormalities. Although it is associated with an increased risk of endometrial cancer, tamoxifen is approved for the prevention of breast cancer in patients who are at very high risk for developing the disease. Patients using tamoxifen for breast cancer prevention must be closely moni-tored for endometrial changes that are early indicators of cancer.

Drug Interactions Tamoxifen decreases levels of anastrozole and letrozole by an unspecified interaction mechanism. Letrozole should not be given concurrently with other estrogens or estrogen-containing products. In addition to these interactions, other interactions exist and should be confirmed when these agents are prescribed.

Antiandrogens

Members of the **antiandrogen** drug class work by blocking the activity of testoster-one at the receptor level or by interfering with the production of testosterone. These medications include **abiraterone (Zytiga)**, **bicalutamide (Casodex)**, **enzalutamide (Xtandi)**, and **flutamide (Eulexin)** and are used to treat prostate cancer. Newly approved agents for prostate cancer are **apalutamide (Erleada)**, **darolutamide (Nubeqa)**, and **nilutamide (Nilandron)**.

Dosage Forms and Administration Bicalutamide, flutamide, and nilutamide are considered older agents. All are given orally with various dosages and frequency. Abiraterone has fewer side effects compared to the older agents. It is given as a 1,000 mg tablet once daily.

Side Effects Side effects of antiandrogen agents include hot flashes, breast tender-ness, **gynecomastia** (enlargement of the breasts), and decreased libido. Many antian-drogen agents also cause toxicity to the liver.

Contraindications Antiandrogen agents do not have contraindications.

Cautions and Considerations Patients taking antiandrogen agents must be educated by the pharmacist about the potential for these agents to interact with other drugs. For example, both bicalutamide and flutamide can increase the anticoagulant effects of warfarin. For this reason, patients must be instructed not to add new drugs to their regimen without consulting a healthcare professional who is aware of all of their medications.

Drug Interactions Drug interactions related to these agents are numerous and should be confirmed when prescribed.

Luteinizing Hormone–Releasing Hormone Agonists

Luteinizing hormone–releasing hormone (LHRH), also known as *gonadotropin-releasing hormone*, stimulates the production of reproductive hormones in people of all genders. LHRH initially stimulates the production of sex hormones; however, over time, continuous exposure to LHRH ultimately shuts down the production of sex hormones through a negative feedback loop. **Leuprolide (Lupron)** and **goserelin (Zoladex)** are analogs of naturally occurring LHRH. Members of the **luteinizing hormone–releasing hormone (LHRH) agonist** drug class are frequently given to patients with hormone-sensitive tumors, such as breast and prostate cancers, to eliminate the source of endogenous estrogen, progesterone, and testosterone production.

Dosage Forms and Administration These medications are usually administered as intramuscular injections (IM). Proper dosing and frequency may vary depending on patient preference—whether they prefer to come on a monthly basis or every three months.

Side Effects LHRH agonists cause many of the same side effects that are seen with antiandrogens. These side effects include hot flashes, gynecomastia, breast tenderness, decreased libido, and liver abnormalities. In addition, these agents can also cause local reactions or pain at the injection site.

Contraindications Individuals who are breast-feeding or pregnant should not be exposed to these drugs.

Cautions and Considerations Because LHRH analogs initially *stimulate* the production of testosterone, patients with prostate cancer may experience a flare of symptoms at the onset of therapy. This reaction can be significant if the tumor is close to vital structures (e.g., the spinal cord) or is associated with pain. To prevent this type of flare reaction, patients are commonly prescribed an antiandrogen such as bicalutamide to overlap with the first few weeks of LHRH agonist therapy.

LHRH agonists have a variety of dosage forms and durations. For example, these medications are prepared as injections that are effective for days, weeks, or months. Pharmacy technicians who handle LHRH agonists must be aware of the different formulations of these agents.

Drug Interactions Goserelin and leuprolide have an additive effect when combined with other drugs that prolong the QT interval (such as amiodarone, disopyramide, dolasetron, moxifloxacin, quinidine, and ziprasidone). Goserelin and leuprolide may decrease the effectiveness of drugs that are used to treat diabetes.

Cyclin-Dependent Kinase (CDK 4/6) Inhibitors

Members of the **cyclin-dependent kinase 4/6 (CDK 4/6) inhibitor** drug class target the enzymes CDK4 and CDK6. Cyclin-dependent kinases, or CDKs, are enzymes that are important for cell division. CDK 4/6 inhibitors interrupt signals that stimulate the proliferation of malignant cells. Certain cancers, such as hormone receptor–positive breast cancer, are more likely to have disturbances in CDK4 and CDK6. Accordingly, CDK 4/6 inhibitors play an essential role in the treatment of those cancers.

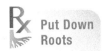
Currently there are three FDA-approved CDK 4/6 inhibitors, **palbociclib (Ibrance), ribociclib (Kisqali)**, and **abemaciclib (Verzenio)**, for the treatment of patients with hormone receptor–positive, human epidermal growth factor (*HER2*)–negative advanced or metastatic breast cancer. Most often, CDK 4/6 inhibitors are administered with other hormonal therapies. The CDK 4/6 inhibitor abemaciclib may be used alone to treat hormone receptor–positive, *HER2*-negative metastatic breast cancer in pretreated patients.

Dosage Forms and Administration The CDK 4/6 inhibitors are administered orally. Special dose modifications should be considered when side effects are encountered.

Side Effects The most common side effects of CDK 4/6 inhibitors are fatigue and GI disturbances, including nausea, diarrhea, and vomiting. Bone marrow suppression resulting in neutropenia and leukopenia is common with this class, although anemia and thrombocytopenia are less common. The side effects of CDK 4/6 inhibitor therapy are typically less severe than those of chemotherapy.

Contraindications CDK 4/6 inhibitors have no contraindications.

Cautions and Considerations The most common adverse event associated with palbociclib and ribociclib is neutropenia; however, febrile neutropenia is rare, and the neutropenia is typically easily reversible when the drug is held (temporarily discontinued). Ribociclib is associated with hepatobiliary toxicity and QT prolongation, requiring additional monitoring and dose modification. GI toxicity and fatigue are more prevalent with abemaciclib than with the other CDK 4/6 inhibitors.

Drug Interactions Drug interactions related to these agents are numerous and should be confirmed when prescribed.

20.5 Targeted Anticancer Therapies

As scientists have learned more about the biology of cancer, they have identified features of certain types of cancer that are critical for tumor cell growth. These critical components have become targets for more sophisticated cancer treatments. A **targeted anticancer therapy**, for example, is directed at specific molecules that are required for tumor cell development, proliferation, or growth. By targeting specific features of tumor cells, a targeted anticancer therapy exerts fewer effects on normal cells and is usually better tolerated than a traditional cytotoxic drug.

Because targeted anticancer therapies are relatively new agents in the arsenal of cancer-fighting drugs, oncologists are still learning about them. Although these therapies have some serious and unusual side effects, they typically offer patients much more direct cancer treatment with fewer side effects than those of traditional cytotoxic drugs. Many believe targeted anticancer therapies are the future of anticancer treatment. Table 20.8 provides an overview of these therapies, which include angiogenesis inhibitors, monoclonal antibodies, signal transduction inhibitors, Bruton's tyrosine kinase inhibitors, and PI3K/Akt/mTOR pathway agents. Note that dosage varies per indication and individual.

TABLE 20.8 Common Targeted Anticancer Therapy Agents

Generic (Brand)	Pronunciation	Dosage Forms	Common Indications
Angiogenesis Inhibitors			
lenalidomide (Revlimid)	leh-nuh-LIH-doh-mide	capsule	multiple myeloma
thalidomide (Thalomid)	thuh-LIH-doh-mide	capsule	multiple myeloma
pomalidomide (Pomalyst)	pom-uh-LIH-doh-mide	capsule	multiple myeloma
Tyrosine Kinase Inhibitors			
afatinib (Gilotrif)	ah-FA-ti-nib	tablet	lung cancer
axitinib (Inlyta)	ak-sih-TIH-nib	tablet	kidney cancer
cabozantinib (Cabometyx)	ca-boh-zan-TIH-nib	capsule, tablet	kidney cancer, thyroid cancer
dacomitinib (Vizimpro)	da-KOH-mi-ti-nib	tablet	lung cancer
erlotinib (Tarceva)	er-LO-ti-nib	tablet	lung cancer
gefitinib (Iressa)	GEH-fih-ti-nib	tablet	lung cancer
lapatinib (Tykerb)	LAP-ah-ti-nib	tablet	breast cancer
lenvatinib (Lenvima)	len-vah-TIH-nib	capsule	kidney cancer
neratinib (Nerlynx)	ner-RAT-in-ib	tablet	breast cancer
osimertinib (Tagrisso)	OH-seh-mer-ti-nib	tablet	lung cancer
pazopanib (Votrient)	paz-OH-peh-nib	tablet	kidney cancer
regorafenib (Stivarga)	reg-OH-raff-ih-nib	tablet	colon cancer
sorafenib (Nexavar)	so-ra-FEN-ib	tablet	liver cancer
sunitinib (Sutent)	soo-NIT-in-ib	capsule	kidney cancer
vandetanib (Caprelsa)	van-DEBT-ah-nib	tablet	lung cancer, thyroid cancer
Monoclonal Antibodies			
Anti-VEGF			
bevacizumab (Avastin)	be-va-KIZ-oo-mab	injection	colon cancer
ramucirumab (Cyramza)	rah-mu-SUR-u-mab	injection	colon cancer
ziv-aflibercept (Zaltrap)	ZIV-af-LIB-er-sept	injection	colon cancer
Anti-HER2			
ado-trastuzumab emtansine (Kadcyla)	a-DOE tras-tu-zu-MAB em-TAN-syn	injection	breast cancer
fam-trastuzumab deruxtecan (Enhertu)	FAM tras-tu-zu-MAB de-ruks-tee-can	injection	breast cancer
pertuzumab (Perjeta)	per-TOO-zoo-mab	injection	breast cancer
trastuzumab (Herceptin)	traz-TOO-zoo-mab	injection	breast cancer
Anti-EGFR			
cetuximab (Erbitux)	se-TUX-i-mab	injection	colon cancer

continues

TABLE 20.8 Common Targeted Anticancer Therapy Agents—*Continued*

Generic (Brand)	Pronunciation	Dosage Forms	Common Indications
necitumumab (Portrazza)	neh-see-tu-MYOO-mab	injection	lung cancer
panitumumab (Vectibix)	pan-i-TU-mu-mab	injection	colon cancer
Anti-CD20			
rituximab (Rituxan)	ri-TUX-i-mab	injection	lymphoma
Signal Transduction Inhibitors			
bosutinib (Bosulif)	boe-SUE-ti-nib	tablet	chronic myelogenous leukemia
dasatinib (Sprycel)	da-SAT-in-ib	tablet	chronic myelogenous leukemia
imatinib (Gleevec)	i-MAT-i-nib	tablet	chronic myelogenous leukemia
nilotinib (Tasigna)	ni-LO-ti-nib	capsule	chronic myelogenous leukemia
ponatinib (Iclusig)	pon-AT-ah-nib	tablet	chronic myelogenous leukemia
Bruton's Tyrosine Kinase Inhibitors			
acalabrutinib (Calquence)	AYE-kahl-ah-brew-ti-nib	capsule	mantle cell lymphoma
ibrutinib (Imbruvica)	AYE-brew-ti-nib	capsule, tablet	chronic myelogenous leukemia
zanubrutinib (Brukinsa)	ZAN-ib-brew-ti-nib	capsule	mantle cell lymphoma
PI3K/AKT/mTOR Pathway Agents			
alpelisib (Piqray)	al-peh-LIH-sib	tablet	chronic lymphocytic leukemia, metastatic breast cancer
idelalisib (Zydelig)	eye-DEL-eh-lih-sib	tablet	chronic lymphocytic leukemia

Angiogenesis Inhibitors

Although some targeted anticancer therapies have narrow therapeutic applications, many agents have been developed to target a wider variety of cancers. An **angiogenesis inhibitor**, commonly referred to as a *vascular endothelial growth factor (VEGF) inhibitor*, works by preventing tumor cells from building blood vessels that would supply the tumor with vital nutrients. By inhibiting new blood vessel formation at the site of the tumor, it causes the tumor cells to eventually die.

Put Down Roots

Recognizing common drug stems (such as *-lidomide* and *-nib*) will help you recognize agents in the same drug class.

Lenalidomide (Revlimid), **thalidomide (Thalomid)**, and **pomalidomide (Pomalyst)** are oral agents primarily used to treat a type of blood cancer called *multiple myeloma*. These drugs are usually used in combination with dexamethasone for the treatment of multiple myeloma.

Bevacizumab (Avastin), **ramucirumab (Cyramza)**, and **ziv-aflibercept (Zaltrap)** are monoclonal antibodies, which are a type of angiogenesis inhibitors given intravenously. They have significant anticancer activity in various solid tumors. These medications also seem to enhance the effects of cytotoxic drugs when dispensed with them.

Axitinib (Inlyta), **cabozantinib (Cabometyx)**, **lenvatinib (Lenvima)**, **pazopanib (Votrient)**, **regorafenib (Stivarga)**, **sorafenib (Nexavar)**, **sunitinib (sutent)**, and **vandetanib (Caprelsa)** are oral tyrosine kinase inhibitors, a type of angiogenesis inhibitor targeting the intracellular domain of the vascular endothelial growth factor (VEGF) receptor. They play a major role in the treatment of various solid tumors.

Dosage Forms and Administration Bevacizumab, ramucirumab, and ziv-aflibercept are monoclonal antibodies given as intravenous infusion. Other small-molecule tyrosine kinases inhibitors (sorafenib and others) are given orally.

Side Effects Although most side effects associated with targeted anticancer therapies are less severe and more manageable than those seen with cytotoxic drugs, some of these drugs can cause very serious reactions. Bevacizumab has the potential to interfere with wound healing and normal blood vessel formation. It may also cause bleeding in the GI tract, nose, and CNS. Further, it can give rise to hypertension and kidney damage, so blood pressure measurements and urine samples must be evaluated prior to treatment.

Contraindications Bevacizumab is contraindicated in patients who have active bleeding (such as nosebleeds or blood in sputum) and in patients who have a significant risk of bleeding. Lenalidomide and thalidomide both have severe teratogenic effects, and these medications are contraindicated in patients who are pregnant.

Pharm Fact

Lenalidomide and thalidomide are agents that require a Risk Evaluation and Mitigation Strategy (REMS) to ensure the benefits of the medication outweigh the risks.

Cautions and Considerations Because bevacizumab interferes with normal wound healing, this medication must not be given to patients within four weeks of a surgical procedure.

Lenalidomide and thalidomide carry boxed warnings for their severe teratogenic effects. Lenalidomide and thalidomide are reproductive toxins and should not be handled by healthcare personnel who are pregnant, possibly pregnant, or trying to conceive. Because of the high risk for reproductive toxicity, the prescribing and dispensing of these agents is strictly regulated. Prescribers, patients, and pharmacies must be registered with the manufacturers of these agents with REMS in order to access these drugs.

Drug Interactions Angiogenesis inhibitors may decrease the effectiveness of live vaccines; coadministration is not recommended. Drug interactions related to these agents are numerous and should be confirmed when prescribed.

Monoclonal Antibodies

A **monoclonal antibody** is an antibody that has been developed from a single type of immune cell that was cloned from a parent cell. These antibodies are directed against a specific marker or antigen on target cells. Monoclonal antibodies are developed from a variety of sources, including mouse, bacterial, and human cell lines. Some of these medications designed to target specific markers on tumor cells have a limited range of activity.

Monoclonal antibodies include *HER2* inhibitors, CD20 targeting agents, and EGFR inhibitors.

Put Down Roots

The suffix *-mab* is common for monoclonal antibodies.

Trastuzumab (Herceptin) is a monoclonal antibody that targets the *HER2/neu* receptor commonly found on breast cancer cells. **Pertuzumab (Perjeta)**, **ado-trastuzumab emtansine (Kadcyla)**, and **fam-trastuzumab deruxetcan (Enhertu)** are all newer *HER2* receptor inhibitors used in various stages of breast cancer treatment. **Lapatinib (Tykerb)** and neratinib are the two oral agents that block the intracellular domain of *HER2* and the epidermal growth factor receptor (EGFR) pathway and, as such, have shown effectiveness in the treatment of breast cancer.

Rituximab (Rituxan), developed to treat non-Hodgkin's lymphoma, targets a specific marker (CD20) on B lymphocytes. Because lymphocytes are active in various immunologic diseases, such as rheumatoid arthritis, rituximab has become a mainstay treatment of many nonmalignant conditions through the same mechanism of action: the targeting of CD20. **Ofatumumab (Arzerra)** and **obinutuzumab (Gazyva)** are newer CD20 inhibitors used in various combinations to treat lymphoma.

Cetuximab (Erbitux), panitumumab (Vectibix), and **necitumumab (Portrazza)** are monoclonal antibodies that target EGFR, a growth factor receptor present on many types of cancer cells. Cetuximab has shown potential in treating head, neck, colon, lung, and pancreatic cancers. Panitumumab is used to treat colon and rectal cancers. Necitumumab has shown efficacy in squamous non–small cell lung cancer. They are all administered as intravenous infusions. **Dacomitinib (Vizimpro), erlotinib (Tarceva), gefitinib (Iressa), osimertinib (Tagrisso), neratinib (Nerlynx),** and **vandatinib (Caprelsa)** are all oral tyrosine kinase inhibitors targeting EGFR receptors approved for the treatment of a wide variety of cancers. Figure 20.6 shows the EGFR pathway and the various agents that target the EGFR receptor (both intracellularly and extracellularly). Cetuximab and others act on the extracellular domain of the receptors and initiate the blocking of cell growth through the PI3K/AKT/mTOR pathway. Note that there are other pathways that are potentially affected.

FIGURE 20.6
EGFR Pathway

Various agents inhibit the cell growth, proliferation, and survival of a cancer cell. This figure illustrates how the EGFR receptor sends signals via the PI3K / AKT / mTOR pathway or via the RS, RAF, MEK, ERK pathway. It also demonstrates the inhibition of these pathways with various agents.

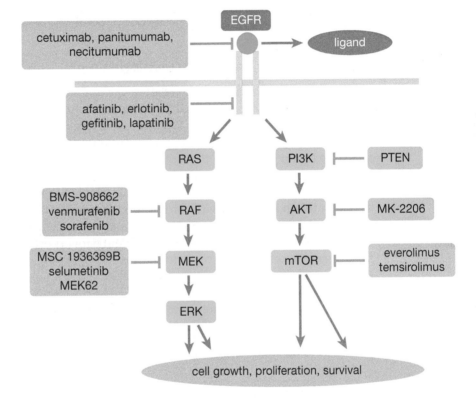

Dosage Forms and Administration Monoclonal antibodies are large molecules that are given intravenously. Because these agents are approved in various cancers, they are given at various doses and frequencies. Special care should be taken to check the patient's disease state, the drug's indications, and the prescribed dosage.

Safety Alert

Many monoclonal antibodies and some chemotherapy drugs pose a high risk of causing anaphylaxis.

Side Effects Because monoclonal antibodies are frequently derived from animal sources, these medications can cause allergic reactions, such as fever, chills, and flushing. Infusion reactions with rituximab and cetuximab can be prevented by premedicating patients with acetaminophen, diphenhydramine, or possibly corticosteroids. More serious allergic reactions, such as anaphylaxis, necessitate a change in therapy.

Contraindications Specific contraindications to monoclonal antibodies have not been determined.

Cautions and Considerations Trastuzumab has a boxed warning for cardiotoxicity, pulmonary toxicity, and infusion-related reaction. Patients should be monitored while receiving this agent.

Rituximab carries a boxed warning for tumor lysis syndrome, hepatitis B virus reactivation, severe mucocutaneous reaction, and fatal infusion reactions. Patients should be carefully monitored while the medication is infused.

Many targeted anticancer therapies cause acne-like skin reactions. Sometimes, such a rash is a sign that the treatment is working. For example, patients who develop a rash while receiving cetuximab generally have a better response to treatment than those who do not develop a rash. These rashes can usually be managed with topical creams and antibiotic gels. On some occasions, a rash may be so severe that treatment must be stopped.

Drug Interactions Trastuzumab can intensify the adverse cardiac side effects of anthracyclines. It may increase the adverse effects of other immunosuppressants. Drug interactions related to monoclonal antibodies are numerous and should be confirmed when prescribed.

Signal Transduction Inhibitors

Certain targeted anticancer therapies affect the molecular abnormalities associated with specific tumor types. A **signal transduction inhibitor** is a drug of this type that targets tumor cell receptors. Typically, signal transduction inhibitors are small-molecule oral agents that block or prevent communication and intracellular functions related to tumor growth and proliferation.

Many types of signal transduction inhibitors have been developed for cancer treatment. **Imatinib (Gleevec)** and **dasatinib (Sprycel)** target a specific chromosomal mutation associated with chronic myelogenous leukemia (CML). This type of cancer can be fatal if it is not managed in the early stage of the disease. These drugs have revolutionized the way CML is treated, and patients on oral therapy can maintain their disease state for many years without the risk of disease progression. However, because imatinib and dasatinib work against the specific abnormality associated with CML, these drugs have not been very useful in the treatment of other types of cancer. Newer agents in this same category of drugs include **bosutinib (Bosulif)**, **nilotinib (Tasigna)**, and **ponatinib (Iclusig)**.

Dosage Forms and Administration These agents are administered orally. Dosages vary depending on whether the disease is newly diagnosed or recurrent.

Side Effects Targeted anticancer therapies are generally better tolerated than traditional chemotherapy drugs. The side effects associated with signal transduction inhibitors vary greatly, depending on the specific target of the agent.

Edema, or the swelling of tissues caused by excessive fluid retention, is one side effect of some of these agents. In addition, many signal transduction inhibitors can cause hypertension and changes in normal cardiac conduction. Medications used to treat CML can cause mild bone marrow suppression.

Contraindications Signal transduction inhibitors have no specific contraindications. Patients who become pregnant while taking a signal transduction inhibitor must consult with their obstetrics and gynecology practitioner and their medical oncologist to discuss the potential risks and benefits of continuing the agent during pregnancy.

Cautions and Considerations Patients who are taking oral signal transduction inhibitors to treat CML must continue their therapy without interruption to avoid progression to the accelerated phase of this disease.

Practice Tip

In the United States, 5,000 patients are diagnosed with chronic myelogenous leukemia (CML) every year. Prior to the approval of imatinib and the other tyrosine kinase inhibitors for CML treatment, the best chance for long-term survival with CML required bone marrow transplantation (BMT), an intensive procedure associated with a mortality rate as high as 25%. Now patients with CML are treated with oral signal transduction inhibitors and have long-term survival rates as high as 90% without needing to undergo BMT.

Practice Tip

Ponatinib may cause heart or blood vessel problems. It was withdrawn from the market but later allowed for patients who are responding to the treatment of CML with this agent.

Drug Interactions Pharmacy technicians should have a heightened awareness of the potential for drug interactions during signal transduction inhibitor therapy. Prescription drugs as well as OTC and herbal or supplemental therapies have been shown to decrease the effectiveness of these agents. For example, histamine blockers and proton pump inhibitors used for stomach acid suppression, such as famotidine or omeprazole, can decrease the absorption of dasatinib. Certain herbal therapies, such as St. John's wort, can decrease the efficacy of imatinib. Agents that interfere with the activity of these signal transduction inhibitors put patients at risk for disease progression. Other drug interactions can result in toxicity of these targeted anticancer therapies. Therefore, when pharmacy technicians are updating a patient's medical profile, they should inquire about the use of herbal therapies.

Drug interactions related to these agents are numerous and should be confirmed when prescribed.

Bruton's Tyrosine Kinase Inhibitors

A **Bruton's tyrosine kinase (BTK) inhibitor** blocks the enzyme BTK, which is a crucial part of the B cell receptor signaling pathway. Certain B cells in leukemia and lymphoma use B cell receptor signaling for growth and survival. The rationale for using BTK inhibitors in cancer is to block this signaling and trigger cell death. This class of medications shows activity in the treatment of chronic lymphocytic leukemia (CLL), follicular lymphoma, mantle cell lymphoma, and marginal zone lymphoma. Three FDA-approved agents are used in the treatment of these diseases: **ibrutinib (Imbruvica)**, **zanubrutinib (Brukinsa)**, and **acalabrutinib (Calquence)**.

Dosage Forms and Administration BTK inhibitors are administered orally.

Side Effects Common side effects include pneumonia, upper respiratory tract infection, sinusitis, skin infection, low neutrophil counts, low platelet counts, headache, bleeding, bruising, diarrhea, and vomiting.

Contraindications BTK inhibitors have no contraindications.

Cautions and Considerations Atrial fibrillation (AF) is a significant side effect. The intersection between BTK inhibitor therapy for B-cell malignancies and AF represents a complex area of management with scant evidence for guidance. The interplay between increased bleeding risk and the thromboembolic complications of AF must be carefully considered.

Drug Interactions Ibrutinib has many drug interactions with anticoagulants, antiarrhythmic agents, and other agents.

Strong CYP3A4 inhibitors, such as ketoconazole, itraconazole, ritonavir, and grapefruit juice, can increase serum concentrations of ibrutinib by more than tenfold. Strong CYP3A4 inducers, such as phenobarbital, phenytoin, glucocorticoids, and St. John's Wort, can significantly decrease serum concentrations of ibrutinib. Both strong CYP3A4 inducers and inhibitors should be avoided, or ibrutinib should be held (stopped for a short time) if a strong CYP3A4 inhibitor must be given. If moderate CYP3A4 inducers or inhibitors must be given, it is recommended that the dose of ibrutinib be decreased to 140 mg daily until the inhibitor or inducer is discontinued.

PI3K/AKT/mTOR Pathway Agents

The PI3K/AKT/mTOR pathway is a significant signaling pathway within cells. This pathway is responsible for regulating cellular processes, including cell survival, proliferation, and growth. Increased activity of this pathway is often associated with tumor progression and resistance to cancer therapies. The activation of the PI3K/AKT/mTOR pathway has been implicated in treatment resistance to targeted therapies in multiple tumor types.

Two FDA-approved medications that target the PI3K/AKT/mTOR pathway are primarily used in treatment modalities. **Idelalisib (Zydelig)** is approved in combination with rituximab for the treatment of chronic lymphocytic leukemia. **Alpelisib (Piqray)** is approved for the treatment of metastatic breast cancer in postmenopausal patients whose tumors have the *PIK3A* mutation and are hormone receptor positive and *HER2* negative.

Dosage Forms and Administration These agents are administered orally.

Side Effects Alpelisib and idelalisib can cause similar side effects, including high blood sugar levels; signs of kidney, liver, or pancreatic problems; diarrhea; rash; low blood counts; nausea and vomiting; fatigue; decreased appetite; mouth sores; weight loss; low calcium levels; blood clotting problems; and hair loss.

Contraindications Patients with a history of severe skin reactions should tell their doctor before taking PI3K/AKT/mTOR pathway agents.

Cautions and Considerations Very severe skin reactions, such as rashes with peeling and blistering, are known to occur in patients using alpelisib and idelalisib. Patients should be monitored for these reactions. Idelalisib can cause liver damage and has a boxed warning for this toxicity. Other idelalisib boxed warnings include severe diarrhea or colitis, pneumonitis, infection, and intestinal perforation. Idelalisib must be dispensed with a Medication Guide.

Drug Interactions Drug interactions with other agents are a concern, especially when those other agents are taken orally.

20.6 Immunotherapy

 Pharm Fact

Another type of immunotherapy involves treatment with CAR T cells. This work is completed in a laboratory, not in a pharmacy, so pharmacy personnel are not involved in the preparation or handling of CAR T-cell therapy.

The immune system plays important roles in protecting patients from microbes (such as viruses and bacteria) and in clearing the body's own unhealthy and ailing cells. The T cells of the immune system have the capacity to selectively recognize and kill pathogens or unhealthy cells, including cancer cells. See Chapters 16 and 17 for additional information on the immune system. The purpose of immunotherapy, as it relates to cancer, is to help the body find and attack cancer cells that would otherwise evade the body's natural immune system.

Immune Checkpoints

In most cases, T cells and other immune system components can locate pathogens, unhealthy cells, and dying cells and effectively attack and remove them from the body. Cancer cells, however, are complex and have the ability to exploit the immune system's processes.

Checkpoints within these processes ensure that immune system cells do not mistakenly destroy healthy cells during an immune response (known as an *autoimmune reaction*). Cancer cells can exploit these immune checkpoints to evade immune detection and elimination. Immune checkpoint inhibitors are the type of immuno-therapy that pharmacy personnel encounter most often. These agents are CTLA-4 inhibitors, PD-1 inhibitors, and PD-L1 inhibitors. An example of an immune check-point inhibitor interaction is shown in Figure 20.7.

FIGURE 20.7 Mechanism of Action of Immunotherapy

In some cases, a tumor's presence creates a microenvironment that does not allow T cells to recognize the tumor. In such an environment, the tumor is allowed to grow and survive. The discovery of programmed cell death protein 1 (PD-1) on T cells and programmed death ligand-1 (PD-L1) on tumor cells prompted the development of immunotherapy. Immunotherapy agents activate T cells and allow them to fight cancers.

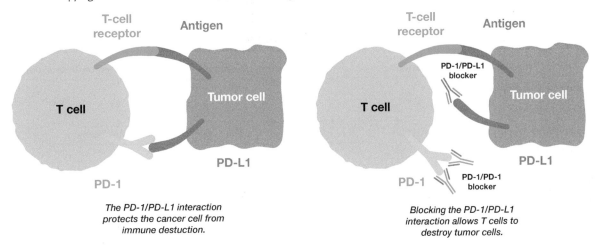

The PD-1/PD-L1 interaction protects the cancer cell from immune destuction.

Blocking the PD-1/PD-L1 interaction allows T cells to destroy tumor cells.

By blocking immune checkpoint proteins and protein receptors, including PD-1, PD-L1, and CTLA-4, with monoclonal antibodies, the immune system can overcome cancer's ability to resist immune responses and can stimulate the body's own mecha-nisms to remain effective in their defenses against cancer.

Cytotoxic T-Lymphocyte-Associated Protein 4 (CTLA-4)

Cytotoxic T-lymphocyte-associated protein 4 (CTLA-4) is a protein receptor that functions as an immune checkpoint within T cells. CTLA-4 downregulates immune responses. CTLA-4 is expressed in regulatory T cells, making the T cells unable to identify and fight cancer cells.

Programmed Death Pathway

The PD-1 (programmed cell death-1) receptor is expressed on the surface of activated T cells. Its ligands, PD-L1 and PD-L2, are expressed on the surface of dendritic cells or macrophages. PD-1, PD-L1, and PD-L2 belong to the family of immune checkpoint proteins that can halt or limit the development of the T-cell response. The PD-1/PD-L1 interaction ensures that the immune system is activated only at the appropriate time in order to minimize the possibility of chronic autoimmune inflammation.

Under normal conditions, the immune system performs a series of steps, known as the **cancer immunity cycle**, that leads to an anticancer immune response and cancer cell death. These steps include:

1. Tumor cells produce mutated antigens that are captured by dendritic cells.
2. The dendritic cells prime T cells with tumor antigen and stimulate the activa-tion of cytotoxic T cells.

3. Activated T cells then travel to the tumor and infiltrate the tumor environment.

4. The activated T cells recognize and bind to the cancer cells.

5. The bound effector T cells release cytotoxins, which induce apoptosis (cell self-destruction) in their target cancer cells.

The PD-1/PD-L1 pathway is an adaptive immune resistance mechanism used by tumor cells in response to antitumor activity. PD-L1 is overexpressed on tumor cells or on nontransformed cells in the tumor environment. Excess PD-L1 on the tumor cells binds to PD-1 receptors on the activated T cells, which inhibits or stops the cytotoxic T cells. These deactivated T cells remain inhibited in the tumor environment.

TABLE 20.9 Common Agents Used for Immunotherapy

Generic (Brand)	Pronunciation	Dosage Form	Common Dosage	Common Indications
Immune Checkpoint Inhibitors				
CTLA4 inhibitor				
ipilimumab (Yervoy)	ip-i-LI-mu-mab	injection	3 mg/kg or 10 mg/kg	melanoma
PD-1 Inhibitors				
cemiplimab (Libtayo)	SEM-ip-li-mab	injection	350 mg	cutaneous squamous cell carcinoma (CSCC)
nivolumab (Opdivo)	ni-VO-lu-mab	injection	480 mg	melanoma
pembrolizumab (Keytruda)	pen-bro-LI-zu-mab	injection	200 mg flat dose	melanoma
PD-L1 Inhibitors				
atezolizumab (Tecentriq)	a-te-zo-LI-zu-mab	injection	1,200 mg	urothelial carcinoma, non–small cell lung cancer
avelumab (Bavencio)	a-VE-lu-mab	injection	800 mg	Merkel cell carcinoma
durvalumab (Imfinzi)	dur-VA-lu-mab	injection	1,500 mg	bladder cancer, lung cancer

Practice Tip

Not all patients respond to PD-1 and PD-L1 inhibitors. The FDA has approved several assays to measure the level of PD-L1 expressed by tumor cells in order to predict the likelihood of response to an inhibitor. A higher mutation burden is also predictive of response to anti-PD-1 and anti-PD-L1 agents.

Immune Checkpoint Inhibitors

The interaction of the programmed death ligand-1 present on tumor cells and the programed cell death protein 1 (PD-1) present on T cells reduces the T cells' ability to function appropriately, which prevents the immune system from attacking the tumor cells. Use of an inhibitor that blocks the interaction of PD-L1 with the PD-1 receptor can prevent the cancer from evading the immune system this way. Several PD-1 and PD-L1 inhibitors are approved for use in advanced melanoma, non–small cell lung cancer, renal cell carcinoma, bladder cancer, and Hodgkin's lymphoma, among other cancer types. These inhibitors are used in many outpatient cancer clinics.

Using immune checkpoint inhibitors with other therapies can shrink tumors in a higher number of patients across a wider range of tumor types than traditional treatment can. Such treatments are also associated with lower toxicity levels than other immunotherapies, with long-term response to therapy. Ipilimumab (Yervoy), a human CTLA-4-blocking monoclonal antibody, was the first FDA-approved checkpoint inhibitor. Like PD-1, CTLA-4 is a protein receptor found on T cells that acts as a negative regulator of T-cell activation.

Current PD-1 inhibitors include pembrolizumab, nivolumab, and cemiplimab. **Pembrolizumab (Keytruda)** was the first immunotherapy drug approved for the treatment of melanoma. **Nivolumab (Opdivo)** was the second immunotherapy drug approved for melanoma and consequently received approval for the treatment of various solid tumors and lymphoma. **Cemiplimab (Libtayo)** was recently approved for the treatment of cutaneous squamous cell carcinoma (CSCC) and in patients with locally advanced CSCC who are not candidates for curative surgery or curative radiation.

PD-L1 inhibitors include atezolizumab, avelumab, and durvalumab. **Atezolizumab (Tecentriq)** is a fully human monoclonal antibody approved for urothelial carcinoma and non–small cell lung cancer.

Avelumab (Bavencio) is a fully human monoclonal antibody approved for the treatment of metastatic Merkel cell carcinoma. **Durvalumab (Imfinzi)** is a fully human monoclonal antibody approved for the treatment of urothelial carcinoma and unresectable non–small cell lung cancer after chemoradiation.

All of these agents are being studied in various clinical trials in combination with chemotherapy and have been tested in upfront, neoadjuvant, adjuvant, and metastatic settings. The roles of these agents are expanding rapidly. Monitoring the data is advised for staying current regarding approvals.

Dosage Form and Administration All of these agents are administered intravenously.

Side Effects The most common side effects of these agents include diarrhea, pneumonitis, rash, changes in hormonal levels, problems with kidney function, and GI disturbances (colitis), which could be severe. The side effects of these agents are referred to as *immune-related adverse events (irAEs)* or *immune-mediated adverse events (imAEs)*. Checkpoint inhibitors commonly affect the skin, GI, endocrine, pulmonary, and renal systems. Patients should be educated about these side effects and be instructed when to call the physician and when the onset of the side effects would occur. Table 20.10 includes a list of possible laboratory tests and qualitative monitoring that could be used to monitor the effects of checkpoint inhibitors.

TABLE 20.10 Monitoring Options for Checkpoint Inhibitors

Laboratory Monitoring	Qualitative Monitoring
• complete blood count (CBC) with differential	• neurologic changes
• comprehensive metabolic panel (CMP): liver, renal, glucose	• mood
	• libido
	• diarrhea
• hemoglobin A1c (HbA1c)	• rash
• adrenocorticotropic hormone (ACTH)	• fatigue
• thyroid-stimulating hormone (TSH), free T4	• pulmonary dysfunction

Contraindications Currently these agents cannot be administered to pregnant patients or to patients who have an autoimmune disease.

Cautions and Considerations All immunotherapy or checkpoint inhibitors have boxed warnings for severe and fatal immune mediated adverse reactions, which affect various organs in the body. They also carry boxed warnings for infusion-related reactions, some of which are life threatening. Close monitoring during the infusion is advised. All require Medication Guides. Since these medications have serious reactions, patient counseling and education are crucial in managing side effects.

Drug Interactions These agents have many side effects. Reading the package insert and checking for potential drug interactions is important prior to the start of therapy.

TABLE 20.11 Onset of Common imAEs of Checkpoint Inhibitors

imAE	Onset	Incidence (Any Grade)
adrenal insufficiency	10–17 weeks	0.7%
colitis	5–10 weeks	8%-27%
dermatologic reactions	4–6 weeks (1–2 cycles)	30%-50%
hepatitis	6–12 weeks	2%-10%
hyperthyroidism	6–7 weeks (2–68 months)	2.5%
hypophysitis	10 weeks	1.2%
hypothyroidism	10 weeks (4–68 months)	6.5%
insulin-deficient diabetes	varies widely	0.2%
nephritis	13 weeks (3–35 months)	1%-2%
pneumonitis	12 weeks (2–24 months)	0%-10%

20.7 Handling Hazardous Agents

Many pharmacy technicians, especially those working in a hospital setting, occasionally handle hazardous drugs (HDs), especially in compounding nonsterile and sterile medications. Others specialize in hazardous or nuclear compounding. Anticancer agents are considered hazardous drugs. Handling chemotherapy agents poses a risk of accidental exposure to these hazardous drugs and a risk of experiencing long-term effects as a result. Common means of accidental exposure include inhalation, ingestion, injection, and topical absorption. Table 20.12 identifies when these types of accidental exposures are most likely to occur.

TABLE 20.12 Hazardous Drug Exposure Examples

Means of Exposure	Common Circumstances
inhalation	capsules or tablets are opened, broken, or crushed
	hazardous drugs are prepared without adequate respiratory protection
ingestion	eating or drinking in areas where hazardous drugs are stored or prepared
	placing food on contaminated surfaces
	touching food or mouth with contaminated hands
injection	needlestick injury during the preparation of hazardous drugs
topical absorption	handling oral or injectable hazardous agents without donning personal protective equipment (PPE)
	accidental powder or liquid spillage from broken vials or leaky IV bags

Toxic agents and other hazardous drugs are considered hazardous materials. A **hazardous material (hazmat)** is any material that can be dangerous to life or to the environment and usually requires a special procedure for cleanup. Studies have shown that personnel handling hazardous drugs during reception and delivery of ingredients and final products experience more exposure than previously known.

USP Chapter <800> outlines the requirements for the receipt, storage, mixing, preparation, compounding, dispensing, and administration of hazardous drugs to protect patients, healthcare personnel, and the environment.

According to *USP* <800>, personnel in a hospital or compounding facility who come into any level of contact with HDs require specialized equipment, training, protective clothing, and knowledge of procedures for the handling, preparation, and disposal of these substances. Hospitals are required to develop written policies and procedures for each aspect of HD use to be in compliance with the United States Pharmacopeia (USP) and The Joint Commission, as well as with state and federal regulations.

Personal Protective Equipment

Pharmacy personnel must protect themselves when handling any hazardous materials. **Personal protective equipment (PPE)** is used to protect the handler from exposure to hazardous drugs or their residue (from the outsides of vials, bottles, or IV bags). PPE should be used at all times when handling hazardous drugs in any dosage form. PPE also protects products by keeping contaminants on the handler's skin, such as lint or bacteria, away from the product. PPE includes the following garments:

- a disposable gown made of material that is impermeable to fluid
- sterile chemotherapy gloves
- chemotherapy safety glasses
- hair and shoe covers
- a disposable respirator

Hazardous drug compounding has additional PPE requirements to meet standards set by the National Institute for Occupational Safety and Health. These requirements include:

- a nonpermeable sterile gown
- hair and shoe covers
- eye and face protection (goggles and shield)
- a special hazardous face mask with respiratory protection (a surgical mask is insufficient)
- two pairs of sterile chemotherapy gloves

Hazardous compounding PPE should be worn by pharmacy technicians when handling HDs, receiving or transporting intact or broken supplies, stocking or working on inventory control for the compounding area, engaging in nonsterile or sterile compounding, collecting or disposing of compounding waste, completing routine cleaning, or managing spills.

Before personnel leave the hazardous drug preparation area, all disposable protective garb must be discarded in a sealable bag in a specially marked container.

Spill Kit

In addition to wearing PPE, individuals working with hazardous drugs should be trained to clean up small accidental spills in ways that reduce potential exposure to hazardous drugs. To help with this task, healthcare personnel should have access to a **spill kit** in every area where hazardous drugs are prepared, administered, or transported. All cleanup supplies used must be placed in sealed plastic bags and disposed of in appropriately labeled chemotherapy waste containers. Large spills may need to be cleaned up by a hazardous materials (hazmat) team.

Hazardous Drug Communication Program

Every institution that prepares, dispenses, or administers hazardous medications is required to have a hazardous drugs communication program to identify drugs that require special handling and to outline the protocol for managing spills and other accidental exposures. Pharmacy technicians should consult the Policy and Procedures (P&P) manual of their facility to learn these hazardous drug handling requirements. If an accidental spill occurs, personnel should refer to the appropriate **Safety Data Sheet (SDS)**—formerly referred to as a *Material Safety Data Sheet*—to guide the cleanup process (see Figure 20.8). SDSs are available from manufacturers for all potentially hazardous drugs and chemical products. These sheets identify a drug or chemical and list its potential hazards, handling and storage requirements, first-aid measures for accidental exposure, and other critical information. SDSs for pharmaceutical products may be obtained from a variety of internet resources. Workplaces that handle hazardous drugs, such as chemotherapy agents, should keep copies of SDSs on file or have an established internet link for each product they carry for easy reference when needed.

FIGURE 20.8 Safety Data Sheet

The Occupational Safety and Health Administration requires chemical manufacturers to provide SDSs for all hazardous chemical products.

spectrum®

SAFETY DATA SHEET

Preparation Date: 3/6/2013 **Revision Date:** 4/4/2016 **Revision Number:** G3

1. IDENTIFICATION

Product identifier

Product code: M1435
Product Name: METHOTREXATE, USP

Other means of identification

Synonyms: Amethopterin; (+)-Amethopterin; Amethopterine; 4-Amino-4-deoxy-N-methylpteroylglutamate; 4-Amino-4-deoxy-N-methylpteroylglutamic acid; 4-Amino-10-methylfolic acid; 4-Amino-N-methylpteroylglutamic acid; Antifolan; L-(+)-N-(p-(((2,4-Diamino-6-pteridinyl)methyl)methylamino)benzoyl)glutamic acid; N-(p-(((2,4-Diamino-6-pteridinyl)methyl)methylamino)benzoyl)-L-(+)-glutamic acid; N-(p-(((2,4-Diamino-6-pteridyl)methyl)methylamino)benzoyl)glutamic acid; N-Bismethylpteroylglutamic acid; Ledertrexate; Methylaminopterin; Methylaminopterinum; L-Glutamic acid, N-(4-(((2,4-diamino-6 pteridinyl)methyl)methylamino)benzoyl)-; Glutamic acid, N-(p-(((2,4-diamino-6-pteridinyl)methyl)methylamino)benzoyl)-, L-(+)-
CAS #: 59-05-2
RTECS # MA1225000
CI#: Not available

Recommended use of the chemical and restrictions on use
Recommended use: Medication.
Uses advised against No information available

Supplier: Spectrum Chemical Mfg. Corp
14422 South San Pedro St.
Gardena, CA 90248
(310) 516-8000
Order Online At: https://www.spectrumchemical.com

Emergency telephone number Chemtrec 1-800-424-9300
Contact Person: Martin LaBenz (West Coast)
Contact Person: Ibad Tirmiz (East Coast)

2. HAZARDS IDENTIFICATION

Classification

This chemical is considered hazardous according to the 2012 OSHA Hazard Communication Standard (29 CFR 1910.1200)

Considered a dangerous substance or mixture according to the Globally Harmonized System (GHS)

Acute toxicity - Oral	Category 3
Reproductive toxicity	Category 1B

Product code: M1435 **Product name:** METHOTREXATE, USP 1 / 13

Preventing Chemotherapy-Related Medication Errors

Medication errors can occur at any step in processing an order. The risks associated with chemotherapy medication errors are severe, and steps should be taken to avoid these errors. A **prescribing error** occurs when a prescriber makes an error in the order for a chemotherapy agent. A **transcription error** occurs when a written chemotherapy order is incorrectly transcribed into the dispensing or computer system. (Transcription errors are virtually eliminated by the use of computerized provider order entry systems.) A **preparation error** occurs when a chemotherapy agent is prepared incorrectly.

Pharmacy technicians can help prevent multiple types of errors, including:

Safety Alert

Everyone on the healthcare team plays a role in preventing medication errors with chemotherapy drugs. Pharmacy technicians should be deliberate and methodical and should implement checks and balances to ensure the safety of patients and of themselves.

- **errors in calculations:** by double-checking every calculation and verifying that the correct concentration of the drug on hand was chosen
- **errors in pharmacist order entry:** by comparing the final product label to the original physician order for verification of drug, dose, administration schedule, route, and duration of therapy
- **errors in dosing:** by ensuring adherence to specific manufacturer-provided drug warnings
- **errors in administration route:** by using a syringe overwrap (provided by the manufacturer) for vincristine and vinblastine to draw attention to the fact that giving these drugs by the IT route is lethal for the patient

Several chemotherapy drugs have look-alike, sound-alike names or have similar packaging. To prevent inadvertent chemotherapy product mix-ups, healthcare personnel must implement storage and handling measures such as:

- not storing look-alike, sound-alike drugs next to each other
- affixing look-alike, sound-alike labels to certain medication containers
- using color-coded or labeled storage bins
- following manufacturers' warnings on hazardous drug products
- noticing tall man lettering on medication labels (e.g., CISplatin versus CARBOplatin, vinCRIStine versus vinBLAStine). In tall man lettering, the differing parts of two similar words are emphasized using capital letters (see Figure 20.9).

FIGURE 20.9 Carboplatin Medication Label

The medication label for carboplatin uses tall man lettering to prevent confusion with cisplatin, another chemotherapy drug with a similar name.

20.8 Complementary and Alternative Therapies

Many patients feel a loss of control when they are diagnosed with cancer or when their disease progresses. Consequently, some patients seek nontraditional or alternative approaches for treatment of their disease. Others simply prefer nontraditional therapies because of their holistic lifestyle or fundamental belief system. Although many herbal, supplemental, and complementary therapies are harmless, some are associated with significant toxicity or have the potential to negatively interact with traditional cancer treatments. In general, there is little scientific evidence to support many of the claims that are made for the curative potential of supplemental and herbal therapies for cancer; however, some of these therapies may provide effective symptom relief. Pharmacy technicians should encourage patients to discuss these therapies with their oncology health professionals to determine if these therapies are safe to use with their current cancer medications.

Alternative techniques that may improve quality of life for patients with cancer include meditation and guided imagery. These techniques may improve mood, sleep quality, and stress related to cancer treatment. Neither should be used as a sole treatment; they should be used in addition to other therapies.

Review and Assessment

CHAPTER SUMMARY

Cancer and Its Development

- Cancer is a group of diseases characterized by the uncontrolled growth of abnormal cells.

- Oncogenes (promoters of cancer formation) and tumor suppressor genes (down-regulators of cancer cells) play a major role in cancer.

- Tumor cells proliferate rapidly. During the exponential phase, a tumor is most sensitive to chemotherapy agents.

- A tumor burden is the number of cells in a tumor or the size of the tumor tissue. The smaller the tumor burden, the more effective chemotherapy will be.

Cancer Stages and Treatments

- Four major modalities are used to treat cancer: surgery, radiation therapy, immunotherapy, and chemotherapy. These treatments may be used alone or combined.

- Chemotherapy may be described as primary, neoadjuvant, adjuvant, or palliative.

Chemotherapy Drugs

- Many factors affect tumor response to chemotherapy drugs.

- Chemotherapy drugs are designed to interfere with the cell cycle at different points and have a narrow window between safe, therapeutic use and the potential for great toxicity.

- A cell cycle–specific drug works on a specific phase of the cell cycle: when the cell prepares to divide, when the cell divides, or when the cell enlarges and makes new proteins.

- Cytotoxic drugs work by interfering with the normal processes of cell function or proliferation.

- To decrease the potential for treatment resistance, combination chemotherapy is usually administered.

- Alkylating agents, antimetabolites, topoisomerase inhibitors, and antimicrotubule agents are the main categories of cytotoxic drugs.

- Cytotoxic drugs cause numerous side effects related to normal cell function, including bone marrow suppression, alopecia, nausea, vomiting, and mucositis.

Hormonal Drug Therapies

- Some tumors can be affected by altering hormone levels within the body.

- These types of cancer depend on naturally occurring hormones for growth.

- Hormonal drugs target the hormonal agent that is contributing to the growth of a specific type of tumor. These therapies block the activity of that hormone.

- Hormonal drug therapies include anti-estrogens, antiandrogens, and LHRH agonists.

Targeted Anticancer Therapies

- Targeted anticancer therapies (angiogenesis inhibitors, monoclonal antibodies, signal transduction inhibitors, Bruton's tyrosine kinase inhibitors, and PI3K/AKT/mTOR pathway agents) are relatively new agents in the arsenal of cancer-fighting drugs.

- These therapies are directed at specific molecules that are required for tumor cell development, proliferation, and growth.

- Although targeted anticancer therapies have some serious and unusual side effects, they typically offer patients much more direct cancer treatment.

Immunotherapy

- The purpose of immunotherapy, as it relates to cancer, is to help the body find and attack cancer cells that would otherwise evade the body's natural immune system.

- Immune checkpoint inhibitors are the most common type of immunotherapy.

Handling Hazardous Agents

- Per *USP* <800>, personnel who come into any kind of contact with hazardous drugs (HDs) require specialized equipment, training, protective clothing, and procedures.

- All individuals who handle or administer chemotherapy medications must don PPE and have access to spill kits and SDSs.

- Safety measures for storing and handling HDs must include measures such as separate storage areas for look-alike, sound-alike drugs; the application of labels to call attention to look-alike, sound-alike medications; and the use of color-coded storage bins.

- Pharmacy technicians should be alert to tall man lettering and to manufacturers' warnings on hazardous drug products.

Complementary and Alternative Therapies

- Meditation and guided imagery may improve the quality of life of patients with cancer.

- These techniques may improve mood, sleep quality, and stress related to cancer treatment. Neither should be used as a sole treatment; they should be used in addition to other therapies

DRUG LIST

Chemotherapy Drugs

Alkylating Agents
bendamustine (Treanda)
busulfan (Myleran)
carboplatin (Paraplatin)
carmustine (BiCNU)
chlorambucil (Leukeran)
cisplatin (Platinol)
cyclophosphamide (Cytoxan)
dacarbazine (DTIC-Dome)
ifosfamide (Ifex)
lomustine (CCNU) (Gleostine)

mechlorethamine (Mustargen)
melphalan (Alkeran)
oxaliplatin (Eloxatin)
procarbazine (Matulane)
temozolomide (Temodar)

Antimetabolites
capecitabine (Xeloda)
cladribine (Leustatin)
clofarabine (Clolar)
cytarabine (Cytosar-U)
decitabine (Dacogen)
fludarabine (Fludara)

fluorouracil (Adrucil)
gemcitabine (Gemzar)
hydroxyurea (Hydrea)
mercaptopurine (Purinethol)
methotrexate (various brands)
nelarabine (Arranon)
pemetrexed (Alimta)
thioguanine (Tabloid)

Topoisomerase Inhibitors
daunorubicin (Cerubidine)
daunorubicin liposomal (DaunoXome)
doxorubicin (Adriamycin)
doxorubicin lipid complex (Doxil)
epirubicin (Ellence)
etoposide (VePesid)
idarubicin (Idamycin)
irinotecan (Camptosar)
mitoxantrone (Novantrone)
topotecan (Hycamtin)

Antimicrotubule Agents
docetaxel (Taxotere)
eribulin (Halaven)
paclitaxel (Taxol)
vinblastine (Velban)
vincristine (Oncovin)
vinorelbine (Navelbine)

Chemotherapy Vesicant Drugs
daunorubicin (Cerubidine, Daunomycin)
doxorubicin (Adriamycin)
epirubicin (Ellence)
idarubicin (Idamycin)
mechlorethamine (Mustargen)
mitomycin
vinblastine (Velban)
vincristine (Oncovin)
vinorelbine (Navelbine)

Miscellaneous Cytotoxic Drugs
asparaginase
bleomycin

Hormonal Drug Therapies

Antiestrogens
anastrozole (Arimidex)
exemestane (Aromasin)
letrozole (Femara)
tamoxifen (Nolvadex)

Antiandrogens
abiraterone (Zytiga)
apalutamide (Erleada)
bicalutamide (Casodex)
darolutamide (Nubeqa)
enzalutamide (Xtandi)
flutamide
nilutamide (Nilandron)

*Luteinizing Hormone–Releasing Hormone
Agonists*
goserelin (Zoladex)
leuprolide (Lupron)

Cyclin-Dependent Kinase 4/6 Inhibitors
abemaciclib (Verzenio)
palbociclib (Ibrance)
ribociclib (Kisqali)

Targeted Anticancer Therapies

Angiogenesis Inhibitors
lenalidomide (Revlimid)
thalidomide (Thalomid)
pomalidomide (Pomalyst)

Tyrosine Kinase Inhibitors
afatinib (Gilotrif)
axitinib (Inlyta)
cabozantinib (Cabometyx, Cometriq)
dacomitinib (Vizimpro)
erlotinib (Tarceva)
gefitinib (Iressa)
lapatinib (Tykerb)
lenvatinib (Lenvima)
neratinib (Nerlynx)
osimertinib (Tagrisso)
pazopanib (Votrient)
regorafenib (Stivarga)
sorafenib (Nexavar)
sunitinib (Sutent)
vandetanib (Caprelsa)

Monoclonal Antibodies

Anti-CD20
obinutuzumab (Gazyva)
ofatumumab (Arzerra)
rituximab (Rituxan)

Anti-EGFR
cetuximab (Erbitux)
necitumumab (Portrazza)
panitumumab (Vectibix)

Anti-HER2
ado-trastuzumab emtansine (Kadcyla)
fam-trastuzumab deruxetcan (Enhertu)
pertuzumab (Perjeta)
trastuzumab (Herceptin)

Anti-VEGF
bevacizumab (Avastin)
ramucirumab (Cyramza)
ziv-aflibercept (Zaltrap)

Signal Transduction Inhibitors
bosutinib (Bosulif)
dasatinib (Sprycel)

imatinib (Gleevec)
nilotinib (Tasigna)
ponatinib (Iclusig)

Bruton's Tyrosine Kinase Inhibitors
acalabrutinib (Calquence)
ibrutinib (Imbruvica)
zanubrutinib (Brukinsa)

PI3K/Akt/mTOR Pathway Inhibitors
alpelisib (Piqray)
idelalisib (Zydelig)

✓ CHECK YOUR UNDERSTANDING

Take a moment to review what you have learned in this chapter and answer the following questions.

1. Which chemotherapy drug has heart failure as a serious toxicity?
   a. vincristine
   b. doxorubicin
   c. bleomycin
   d. etoposide

2. What is the name of the process in which tumors spread from the primary site to other parts of the body?
   a. metastasis
   b. alkalinization
   c. extravasation
   d. angiogenesis

3. Which chemotherapy drug must never be administered by the IT route?
   a. methotrexate
   b. vincristine
   c. cytarabine
   d. hydrocortisone

4. Which chemotherapy drug does not cause bone marrow suppression as a common side effect?
   a. cyclophosphamide
   b. doxorubicin
   c. bleomycin
   d. topotecan

5. Which medication is an example of an antimetabolite drug?
   a. cytarabine
   b. irinotecan
   c. paclitaxel
   d. vincristine

6. Which chemotherapy agent is available in an oral dosage form?
   a. capecitabine
   b. cytarabine
   c. vincristine
   d. leuprolide

7. Which statement best describes the relationship between cancer and oncogenes?
   a. Tumors are formed by a collection of oncogenes.
   b. Oncogenes promote cancer formation.
   c. Oncogenes suppress tumor formation.
   d. Oncogenes kill cancer cells.

8. Which description most accurately reflects adjuvant therapy?
   a. Chemotherapy administered to a patient with leukemia with the intent to cure the disease
   b. Radiation therapy administered to treat a new brain tumor
   c. Radiation administered before surgery to reduce the size of the tumor for resection
   d. Radiation therapy administered after surgery to kill any residual disease

9. Which drug is commonly given as a rescue medication to prevent bone marrow suppression and mucosal toxicity from high-dose methotrexate?
   a. folic acid
   b. leucovorin
   c. mesna
   d. sodium bicarbonate

10. Which statement best describes the anticancer effects of tamoxifen?
    a. Tamoxifen is a monoclonal antibody that targets the estrogen receptor.
    b. Tamoxifen is an antiestrogen agent.
    c. Tamoxifen is a topoisomerase I inhibitor.
    d. Tamoxifen is an antimicrotubule agent.

MAKE CONNECTIONS

Take a moment to consider what you have learned in this chapter and respond thoughtfully to the following prompts. Note that some of these activities will require internet access.

1. Orders have arrived for rituximab (Rituxan). There are no orders for premedications for this patient. What should you do?

2. Tatyana Reichova is a 36-year-old woman with advanced cervical cancer. She is scheduled to receive her fourth treatment of cisplatin and radiation therapy. The treatment typically requires her to be in the infusion room for six to eight hours. Ms. Reichova has two young children at home and wants to know if there is any way to eliminate the IV fluids that she always receives before and after each dose of her cisplatin, to shorten her time away from home. Should the IV fluids be eliminated from her treatment regimen? Explain your reasoning.

 The online course includes additional review and assessment resources.

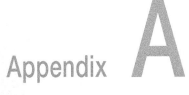

Common Pharmacy Abbreviations and Acronyms

The abbreviations with red lines through them are ones that are still in use but are discouraged by Institute for Safe Medication Practices (ISMP). The ISMP recommends the use of the correct words instead. Many of these discouraged abbreviations are also on the Joint Commission's Official "Do Not Use" List of Abbreviations.

Abbreviation	Meaning
A-B-C	
aaa	apply to affected area
ACA	Affordable Care Act (Patient Protection and Affordable Care Act)
~~ac; a.c.; AC~~	before meals
ACE	angiotensin-converting enzyme inhibitors
ad; a.d.; AD	right ear
ADD	attention-deficit disorder
ADH	antidiuretic hormone
ADHD	attention-deficit hyperactivity disorder
ADME	absorption, distribution, metabolism, and elimination
ADR	adverse drug reaction
AIDS	acquired immune deficiency syndrome
AM; a.m.	morning
ANDA	Abbreviated New Drug Application
APAP	acetaminophen; Tylenol
AphA	American Pharmacy Association
ARBs	angiotensin receptor blockers
~~as; a.s.; AS~~	left ear
ASA	aspirin
~~au; a.u.; AU~~	both ears; each ear
b.i.d.; BID	twice daily
BMI	Body Mass Index
BP	blood pressure
BUD	beyond-use date
°C	degrees centigrade; temperature in degrees centigrade
Ca^{++}	calcium

Abbreviation	Meaning
Cap, cap	capsule
CDC	Centers for Disease Control and Prevention
CF	cystic fibrosis
CHF	congestive heart failure
CNS	Central Nervous System
COPD	chronic obstructive pulmonary disease
CPR	cardio pulminary resuscitation
CSP	compounded sterile preparation
CV	cardiovascular
D-E-F	
D$_5$; D$_5$W; D5W	dextrose 5% in water
D$_5$ ¼; D5 1/4	dextrose 5% in ¼ normal saline; dextrose 5% in 0.225% sodium chloride
D$_5$ ⅓; D5 1/3	dextrose 5% in ⅓ normal saline; dextrose 5% in 0.33% sodium chloride
D$_5$ ½; D5 1/2	dextrose 5% in ½ normal saline; dextrose 5% in 0.45% sodium chloride
D$_5$LR; D5LR	dextrose 5% in lactated Ringer's solution
D$_5$NS; D5NS	dextrose 5% in normal saline; dextrose 5% in 0.9% sodium chloride
DAW	dispense as written
DC; d/c	discontinue
D/C	discharge
DCA	direct compounding area
Dig	digoxin
disp	dispense
EC	enteric-coated
Elix	elixir
eMAR	electronic medication administration record
EPO	epoetin alfa; erythropoietin
ER; XR; XL	extended-release
°F	degrees Fahrenheit; temperature in degrees Fahrenheit
FeSO$_4$	ferrous sulfate; iron
G-H-I	
g, G	gram
gr	grain
GI	gastrointestinal
GMP	good manufacturing practice
gtt; gtts	drop; drops
h; hr	hour
HC	hydrocortisone
HCTZ	hydrochlorothiazide
HIPAA	Health Insurance Portability and Accountability Act
HIV	human immunodeficiency virus
HMO	Health Maintenance Organization
HRT	hormone replacement therapy

Abbreviation	Meaning
h.s.; HS	bedtime
IBU	ibuprofen; Motrin
ICU	intensive care unit
IM	intramuscular
IND	Investigational New Drug Application
Inj	injection
IPA	isopropyl alcohol
ISDN	isosorbide dinitrate
ISMO	isosorbide mononitrate
ISMP	Institute for Safe Medication Practices
IV	intravenous
IVF	intravenous fluid
IVP	intravenous push
IVPB	intravenous piggyback
J-K-L	
K; K+	potassium
KCl	potassium chloride
kg	kilogram
L	liter
LAFW	laminar airflow workbench; hood
lb	pound
LD	loading dose
LVP	large-volume parenteral
JCAHO	Joint Commission on the Accreditation of Healthcare Organizations
M-N-O	
Mag; Mg; MAG	magnesium
MAR	medication administration record
mcg	microgram
MDI	metered-dose inhaler
MDV	multiple-dose vial
mEq	milliequivalent
mg	milligram
MgSO$_4$	magnesium sulfate; magnesium
mL	milliliter
mL/hr	milliliters per hour
mL/min	milliliters per minute

Abbreviation	Meaning
MMR	measles, mumps, and rubella vaccine
MRSA	methiciliin-resistant S. aureaus
MOM; M.O.M.	milk of magnesia
~~M.S.~~	morphine sulfate (save MS for multiple sclerosis)
~~MU†~~; ~~mu~~	million units
MVI; MVI-12	multiple vitamin injection; multivitamins for parenteral administration
Na⁺	sodium
NABP	National Association of Boards of Pharmacy
NaCl	sodium chloride; salt
NDA	New Drug App
NDC	National Drug Code
NF; non-form	nonformulary
NKA	no known allergies
NKDA	no known drug allergies
NPO, npo	nothing by mouth
NR; d.n.r.	no refills; do not repeat
NS	normal saline; 0.9% sodium chloride
½ NS	one-half normal saline; 0.45% sodium chloride
¼ NS	one-quarter normal saline; 0.225% sodium chloride
NSAID	nonsteroidal anti-inflammatory drug
NTG	nitroglycerin
OC	oral contraceptive
~~od~~; ~~o.d.~~; ~~OD~~	right eye
ODT	orally disintegrating tablet
OPTH; OPHTH; Opth	ophthalmic
~~os~~; ~~o.s.~~; ~~OS~~	left eye
OTC	over the counter; no prescription required
~~ou~~; ~~o.u.~~; ~~OU~~	both eyes; each eye
oz	ounce
P-Q-R	
p.c.; PC	after meals
PCA	patient-controlled anesthesia
PCN	penicillin
pH	acid-base balance
PHI	protected health information
PM; p.m.	afternoon; evening
PN	paternal nutrition

Abbreviation	Meaning
PNS	peripheral nervous system
PO; po	orally; by mouth
PPE	personal protective equipment
PPI	proton pump inhibitor
PR	per rectum; rectally
PRN; p.r.n.	as needed; as occasion requires
PTSD	Post Traumatic Stress Disorder
PV	per vagina; vaginally
PVC	polyvinyl chloride
q	every
q.h.; qhour	every hour
q2h	every 2 hours
q4h	every 4 hours
q6h	every 6 hours
q8h	every 8 hours
q12h	every 12 hours
q24h	every 24 hours
q48h	every 48 hours
QA	quality assurance
QAM; qam	every morning
qDay; QD	every day
q.i.d.; QID	four times daily
QOD; Q other day; Q.O. Day	every other day
QPM; qpm	every evening
qs; qsad	quantity sufficient; a sufficient quantity to make
QTY; qty	quantity
qwk; qweek	every week
RA	rheumatoid arthritis
RDA	recommended daily allowance
Rx	prescription; pharmacy; medication; drug; recipe; take
S-T	
sig	write on label; signa; directions
SL; sub-L	sublingual
SMZ-TMP	sulfamethoxazole and trimethoprim; Bactrim
SNRI	serotonin nonrepinephrine reuptake inhibitor
SPF	sunburn protection factor

Abbreviation	Meaning
SR	sustained-release
~~SS~~; ~~ss~~	one-half
SSRI	selective serotonin reuptake inhibitor (don't use for sliding scale insulins)
STAT, Stat	immediately; now
STD	sexually transmitted disease
~~Sub-Q~~; ~~SC~~; ~~SQ~~; ~~sq~~, subcut, SUBCUT	subcutaneous
SUPP; Supp	suppository
susp	suspension
SVP	small-volume parenteral
SW	sterile water
SWFI	sterile water for injection
Tab; tab	tablet
TB	tuberculosis
TBSP; tbsp	tablespoon; tablespoonful; 15 mL
TDS	transdermal delivery system
~~t.i.d.~~; ~~TID~~	three times daily
~~t.i.w.~~; ~~TIW~~	three times a week
TKO; TKVO; KO; KVO	to keep open; to keep vein open; keep open; keep vein open (a slow IV flow rate)
TNA	Total Nutrition Admixture
TPN	total parenteral nutrition
TSP; tsp	teaspoon; teaspoonful; 5 mL
U-V-W	
~~U or u~~	unit
~~u-d, UD, ut dictum~~	as directed
ung	ointment
USP	U.S. Pharmacopoeial Convention
USP-NF	U.S. Pharmacopoeia-National Forumulary <italics>
UTI	urinary tract infection
UV	ultraviolet light
VAG; vag	vagina; vaginally
Vanco	vancomycin
VO; V.O.; V/O	verbal order
w/o	without
X-Y-Z	
Zn	zinc
Z-Pak	azithromycin; Zithromax

Common Look-Alike and Sound-Alike Medications

While manufacturers have an obligation to review new trademarks for error potential before use, there are some actions that prescribers, pharmacists, and pharmacy technicians can do to help prevent errors with products that have look- or sound-alike names. The Institute for Safe Medication Practices (ISMP) provides several types of tools that are designed to prevent dispensing errors. These include the following recommended actions as well as a list of look-alike and sound-alike drugs.

- **Use electronic prescribing** to prevent confusion with handwritten drug names.

- **Encourage physicians to write prescriptions that clearly specify the dosage form, drug strength, and complete directions.** They should include the product's indication on all outpatient prescriptions and on inpatient *prn* orders. With name pairs known to be problematic, reduce the potential for confusion by writing prescriptions using both the brand and generic name. Listing both names on medication administration records and automated dispensing cabinet computer screens also may be helpful.

- **Whenever possible, determine the purpose of the medication** before dispensing or administering it. Many products with look-alike or sound-alike names are used for different purposes.

- **Accept verbal or telephone orders only when truly necessary.** Require staff to read back all orders, spell the product name, and state its indication. Like medication names, numbers can sound alike, so staff should read the dosage back in numerals (eg. "one five" for 15 milligrams) to ensure clear interpretation of dose.

- **When feasible, use magnifying lenses and copyholders** under good lighting to keep prescriptions and orders at eye level during transcription to improve the likelihood of proper interpretation of look-alike product names.

- **Change the appearance of look-alike product names** on computer screens, pharmacy and nursing unit shelf labels, and bins (including automated dispensing cabinets), pharmacy product labels, and medication administration records by highlighting, through bold face, color, and/or capital letters, the parts of the names that are different (e.g., hydrOXYzine, hydrALAzine). These are called "tall man" letters.

- **Install a computerized reminder** (also placed on automated dispensing cabinet screens) for the most serious confusing name pairs so that an alert is generated when entering prescriptions for either drug. If possible, make the reminder auditory as well as visual.

- **Affix "name alert" stickers** in areas where look-alike or sound-alike products are stored (available from pharmacy label manufacturers).

- **Store products with look-alike or sound-alike names in different locations.** Avoid storing both products in the fast-mover area. Use a shelf sticker to help locate the product that is moved.

- **Continue to employ an independent check in the dispensing process** (one person interprets and enters the prescription into the computer and another reviews the printed label against the original prescription and the product).

- **Open the prescription bottle or the unit dose package in front of the patient** to confirm the expected product appearance and review the indication. Caution patients about error potential when taking products that have a look-alike or sound-alike counterpart. Take the time to fully investigate the situation if a patient states he or she is taking an unknown medication.

- **Monitor reported errors caused by look-alike and sound-alike medication names** and alert staff to mistakes.

- **Look for the possibility of name confusion when a new product is added to the formulary.** Have a few clinicians handwrite the product name and directions, as they would appear in a typical order. Ask frontline nurses, pharmacists, technicians, unit secretaries, and physicians to view the samples of the written product name as well as pronounce it to determine if it looks or sounds like any other drug product or medical term. It may be helpful to have clinicians first look at the scripted product name to determine how they would interpret it before the actual product name is provided to them for pronunciation. Once the product name is known, clinicians may be less likely to see more familiar product names in the written samples. If the potential for confusion with other products is identified, take steps to avoid errors as listed below.

- **Encourage reporting of errors** and potentially hazardous conditions with look-alike and sound-alike product names and use the information to establish priorities for error reduction. Also maintain awareness of problematic product names and error prevention recommendations provided by ISMP (www.ismp.org and also listed on the quarterly *Action Agenda*), FDA (www.fda.gov), and United States Pharmacopoeia (USP; www.usp.org).

- **Review any look-alike and sound-alike drug name pairs in use at your practice location.** Go to ISMP's website to review these medications, available at https://www.ismp.org/recommendations/confused-drug-names-list. Decide what actions might be warranted to prevent medication errors. Stay current with alerts from ISMP, FDA, and USP in case new problematic name pairs emerge.

ASHP/ACPE
Accreditation Standards

The following identifies the *ASHP/ACPE Accreditation Standards* addressed in each chapter of Paradigm's *Pharmacology for Technicians*, Seventh Edition. This appendix identifies the *ASHP/ACPE Standards* associated with the chapter content. This list is meant for guidance purposes only and was compiled by the authors and editor. Neither ASHP nor ACPE has participated in or had any role in creating the list of standards or any other content that is included in this book.

Units 1: Introduction to Pharmacology

Chapter 1: Introduction to Pharmacology and Medications in the Body
1.8, 1.10, 2.3, 2.5, 2.7, 4.2

Chapter 2: Pharmaceutical Development
1.8, 1.10, 2.1, 2.3, 2.5, 2.7, 2.9, 3.3, 3.5, 3.6, 3.8, 3.10–3.12, 3.18, 3.19, 3.28, 3.30, 3.31, 4.1, 4.2, 4.7, 4.11, 4.12, 5.1, 5.2, 5.3, 5.4, 5.5, 5.10

Chapter 3: Pharmacology Study for the Pharmacy Technician
1.6, 1.8, 1.10, 2.1, 2.5, 4.2

Chapter 4: Medication Safety and Prescription Orders
1.4, 1.8, 1.9, 1.10, 2.2, 2.3, 2.5, 2.7, 2.10, 3.3, 3.6, 3.7, 3.11, 3.12, 3.13, 3.22, 4.1, 4.2, 4.5, 4.7, 4.9, 4.11, 4.12, 5.1, 5.2, 5.3, 5.5, 5.10

Unit 2: Body Systems and Corresponding Drug Therapies

Chapter 5 The Integumentary System and Drug Therapy
1.1, 1.8, 1.10, 2.4, 2.5, 2.7, 3.1, 3.2, 3.3, 3.4, 3.6, 3.11, 4.2

Chapter 6: The Musculoskeletal System and Drug Therapy
1.8, 1.10, 2.3, 2.4, 2.5, 2.7, 3.1, 3.2, 3.3, 3.4, 3.6, 3.11, 4.2f

Chapter 7: The Nervous System, Central Nervous System Disorders, and Drug Therapy
1.8, 1.10, 2.5, 2.7, 3.1, 3.2, 3.3, 3.4, 3.6, 3.11, 4.2

Chapter 8: The Nervous System, Mental Health, and Drug Therapy
1.8, 1.10, 2.5, 2.7, 3.1, 3.2, 3.3, 3.4, 3.6, 3.11, 4.2

Chapter 9: The Sensory System and Drug Therapy
1.8, 1.10, 2.4, 2.5, 2.7, 3.1, 3.2, 3.3, 3.4, 3.6, 3.11, 3.26, 4.2

Chapter 10: The Cardiovascular System and Drug Therapy
1.8, 1.10, 2.4, 2.5, 2.7, 2.9, 2.11, 3.1, 3.2, 3.3, 3.4, 3.6, 3.11, 4.2

Chapter 11: The Respiratory System and Drug Therapy
1.8, 1.10, 2.5, 2.7, 3.1, 3.2, 3.3, 3.4, 3.6, 3.11, 4.2

Chapter 12: The Gastrointestinal System and Drug Therapy
1.8, 1.9, 1.10, 1.12, 2.1, 2.3, 2.4, 2.5, 2.6, 2.7, 3.1, 3.2, 3.3, 3.4, 3.6, 3.11, 4.2

Chapter 13: The Endocrine System and Drug Therapy
1.8, 1.10, 2.5, 2.7, 3.1, 3.2, 3.3, 3.4, 3.6, 3.11, 4.2

Chapter 14: The Reproductive System and Drug Therapy
1.8, 1.10, 2.5, 2.7, 2.9, 3.1, 3.2, 3.3, 3.4, 3.6, 3.11, 3.30, 4.2, 5.10

Chapter 15: The Renal System and Drug Therapy
1.8, 1.10, 2.1, 2.3, 2.4, 2.5, 2.7, 3.1, 3.2, 3.3, 3.4, 3.6, 3.11, 4.2

Unit 3: Pharmacology and Multisystems

Chapter 16: The Immune System, Bacterial Infections, Fungal Infections, and Drug Therapy
1.8, 1.10, 2.5, 2.7, 3.1, 3.2, 3.3, 3.4, 3.6, 3.11, 3.16, 4.2

Chapter 17: The Immune System, Viral Infections, and Drug Therapy
1.1, 1.2, 1.3, 1.5, 1.7, 1.8, 1.10, 2.5, 2.7, 2.11, 3.1, 3.2, 3.3, 3.4, 3.6, 3.11, 3.29, 4.2

Chapter 18: Pain, Anesthesia, and Drug Therapy
1.8, 1.10, 2.5, 2.7, 3.1, 3.2, 3.3, 3.4, 3.6, 3.11, 4.2, 5.1, 5.2, 5.10

Chapter 19: Nutrition, Fluids, Electrolytes, and Drug Therapy
1.8, 1.10, 2.5, 2.7, 2.11, 3.1, 3.2, 3.3, 3.4, 3.6, 3.11, 3.23, 4.2

Chapter 20: Cancer and Drug Therapy
1.8, 1.10, 2.5, 2.7, 3.1, 3.2, 3.3, 3.4, 3.6, 3.9, 3.11, 3.15, 3.22, 3.25, 3.29, 4.2, 4.4, 4.9, 5.6

GLOSSARY

5-alpha-reductase inhibitor   a drug used to treat BPH and male-pattern hair loss

5HT agonist   describes a drug that binds to serotonin receptors and causes dilatation of blood vessels in the dura mater, preventing inflammation, and reducing pain signal transmission; also known as *triptans*

5-hydroxytryptophan   the chemical precursor to serotonin; a complementary or alternative therapy that can improve motor symptoms in patients with Parkinson's disease

abbreviated new drug application   the application drug companies send to the FDA to market a generic product

absence seizure   a type of generalized seizure characterized by a sudden, momentary break in consciousness; formerly known as a petit mal seizure

absorption   the uptake of essential nutrients and drugs into the bloodstream

acetylcholine (ACh)   a neurotransmitter that binds to ACh receptors on the membranes of muscle cells, beginning a process that ultimately results in muscle contraction

acidosis   a condition that occurs when the pH of blood and/or extracellular fluid drops below the normal range, less than 7.35

acne   an inflammation of the skin, usually on the face and neck, that is caused by increased activity of the sebaceous glands at puberty

acne vulgaris   formation of comedones, papules, pimples, and/or cysts in the skin of the face and upper trunk; these lesions occur when hair follicles and sebaceous glands are blocked and become inflamed

acquired immunodeficiency syndrome (AIDS)   the advanced and severe form of HIV

actinic keratosis   a precancerous skin condition resulting from overexposure to sunlight

action potential   the electrical signal that causes a muscle to contract

active immunity   the process by which a person's body makes its own antibodies to a pathogen

acupuncture   a process that involves penetrating the skin with thin needles in specific areas to manage pain

acute   short, severe course

acute coronary syndrome   a situation in which the blood supplied to the heart is suddenly blocked

acute kidney disease   the rapid reduction in kidney function, which may be caused by renal ischemia, trauma, pregnancy, extracellular volume depletion, hemorrhage, surgery, or shock

acute kidney failure   a decrease in kidney function that occurs over hours, days, or weeks; also known as *acute renal failure* and *acute kidney injury*

acute pain   associated with trauma or surgery; usually treatable

acute viral infection   an infection that quickly resolves with no latent infection

adaptive immune system   system within the body that learns and remembers specific pathogens it has encountered and provides long-lasting protection and defense against recurring infections; also known as the *acquired immune system*

Addison's disease   a life-threatening deficiency of glucocorticoids and mineralocorticoids that is treated with daily administration of corticosteroids

addition   the combined effect of two drugs

adenosine triphosphate   a critical molecule in cellular energy production

adenosine triphosphate–citrate lyase (ACL) inhibitor   an agent that lowers LDL by inhibiting cholesterol synthesis in the liver

adherence   taking a medication correctly or as prescribed

adipose tissue the layer of skin consisting of fat cells

adjunct therapy a drug used in combination with a primary drug for improved effect

adjuvant chemotherapy the treatment of residual cancer cells after removal or reduction of the tumor by surgery

adjuvant radiation therapy radiation therapy used in conjunction with surgery to "clean up" areas of residual tumor

ADME absorption, distribution, metabolism, and elimination; see pharmacokinetics

adsorbents a class of antidiarrheals

adverse drug reaction an unexpected negative consequence from taking a drug

adverse effect a secondary response to a drug other than the primary therapeutic effect that the drug was intended to produce, also known as *side effect*

aerobic needing oxygen in order to survive

afferent system the sensory division of the nervous system, carrying information from sensory receptors to the central nervous system

affinity the strength by which a particular chemical messenger binds to its receptor site on a cell

agonist a drug that binds to a particular receptor site and triggers the cell's response in a manner similar to the action of the body's own chemical messenger

agranulocytosis a reduction in white blood cells

alcohol dependence a pattern of alcohol use that involves problems controlling drinking and preoccupation with alcohol; also known as *alcoholism*

aldosterone antagonist agent that works byinhibiting a hormone that promotes fluid retention

aldosterone a hormone that promotes sodium and water reabsorption in the distal convoluted tubule and collecting duct of the nephron

alimentary tract the GI tract, made up of the mouth, esophagus, stomach, small intestine, colon, and rectum

alkalosis a condition that occurs when there is a relative excess of bicarbonate in the blood and/or extracellular fluid and the pH rises above the normal range, more than 7.45

alkylating agent a member of a class of cytotoxic drugs that bind to and damage DNA during cell division, preventing cell replication

allergen a substance that produces an allergic response

allergic asthma asthma exacerbated by airborne allergens

allergic response an instance in which the immune system overreacts to an otherwise harmless substance

allergy a state of heightened sensitivity as a result of exposure to a particular substance

alopecia hair loss

alpha receptor an adrenergic receptor that binds the neurotransmitters epinephrine and norepinephrine, facilitating constriction of blood vessels

alpha-blocker a drug used to treat patients who have BPH; it inhibits alpha-1 receptors in the prostate gland and bladder (and in blood vessels in the rest of the body), improving urine flow

alternative medicine medical products and practices that are not part of standard care

Alzheimer's disease a degenerative disorder of the brain that leads to progressive dementia and changes in personality and behavior

amide a longer-acting local anesthetic that is metabolized by liver enzymes

aminoglycoside a member of a class of antibiotics that inhibits bacterial protein synthesis by binding to ribosomal subunits; commonly used to treat serious infections

aminosalicylates drugs used for both induction and maintenance of remission in patients with Crohn's disease and ulcerative colitis

ammonium chloride a salt of ammonium

amylase a pancreatic enzyme necessary to help digest carbohydrates

amylin a hormone coproduced with insulin that reduces glucagon production, slows gastric emptying, and produces satiety

amyotrophic lateral sclerosis (ALS) a degenerative disease of the motor nerves; also known as *Lou Gehrig's disease*

anaerobic capable of surviving in the absence of oxygen

analgesic a drug that alleviates or reduces pain

anaphylactic reaction a severe allergic response resulting in immediate life-threatening respiratory distress, usually followed by vascular collapse and shock and accompanied by hives

anaphylaxis a serious or life-threatening allergic response often involving hives, swelling, and lowered blood pressure

androgen any of a group of hormones that promote the development and maintenance of typically masculine physical characteristics

anemia a below-normal concentration of red blood cells or hemoglobin in the blood

anesthesia an intervention that causes loss of feeling in all or part of the body by manipulating the nervous system to inhibit pain or the conscious perception of pain

anesthesiologist a physician who oversees administration of anesthesia during surgery

angina pectoris chest pain caused by inadequate blood flow to a portion of the heart

angioedema swelling under the skin that can be a life-threatening allergic reaction, manifested by a swelling of the tongue, lips, or eyes

angiogenesis inhibitor a drug that prevents tumor cells from building blood vessels that would supply the tumor with vital nutrients

angiotensin a hormone that causes vasoconstriction and an increase in blood pressure

angiotensin receptor blocker (ARB) a drug that blocks the action of angiotensin II

angiotensin-converting enzyme the enzyme that converts angiotensin I to angiotensin II

angiotensin-converting enzyme (ACE) inhibitors a commonly used drug class that blocks the action of angiotensin-converting enzyme

anion a negatively charged ion

anorexia a loss of appetite for food (as a medical condition)

antacids medications preventing or correcting acidity, especially in the stomach

antagonist a drug that binds to a receptor site and blocks the action of the endogenous messenger or other drugs

anterior chamber the container behind the cornea that holds the aqueous humor of the eye

anthracycline a member of a large category of topoisomerase II inhibitors; also known as a *DNA intercalating agent*

antiandrogen a member of a class of drugs that block the activity of testosterone at the receptor level

antibiotic a chemical substance with the ability to kill or inhibit the growth of bacteria by interfering with bacteria biological processes

antibiotic resistance the development by bacteria of defense mechanisms that resist or inactivate antibiotics used on those bacteria

antibody a Y-shaped protein that recognizes and then binds to a specific type of antigen after the immune system has been exposed to that antigen

anticholinergic agent agent that inhibits acetylcholine, a neurotransmitter that stimulates smooth muscle in the lungs to constrict

anticholinesterase one of a class of drugs that potentiate the action of acetylcholine by inhibiting the enzyme acetylcholinesterase, which breaks down acetylcholine

anticoagulant a drug that prevents clot formation by inhibiting clotting factors

anticonvulsant a drug used to control seizures

antidiarrheals drugs that prevent or alleviate diarrhea symptoms

antiemetic a drug that prevents or controls nausea and vomiting

antiestrogen a member of a class of drugs commonly used to treat breast cancer

antigen a molecule or molecular structure, often found on the surfaces of pathogens such as bacteria or viruses; elicits an immune response and can bind with an antibody, T cell, or other product of that response

antihistamine drug that blocks the H_1 receptors

antimetabolite a member of a class of drugs that work during the synthesis phase of the cell cycle

antimicrotubule agent a drug that interferes with the formation and function of microtubules

antimuscarinic a drug that works by inhibiting acetylcholine in the nerves that control involuntary bladder contraction and emptying

antioxidant one of a number of substances believed to help prevent cell damage caused by free radicals

antiplatelet agent a drug that interferes with the chemical reactions that cause platelets to be sticky and aggregate

antiplatelet a drug that reduces the risk of clot formation by inhibiting platelet aggregation

antipsychotic drug a drug that is used to treat schizophrenia and that reduces symptoms such as hallucinations, delusions, and thought disorders; also known as a *neuroleptic drug*

antipyretic fever reducing

antiretroviral a drug that limits the progression of HIV or other retrovirus infections

antiseptic a substance that kills or inhibits the growth of microorganisms on the outside of the body

antitussive drug that blocks or suppresses a cough

antiviral drug an agent that prevents virus replication in a host cell without interfering with the host's normal function

anuria an inability to produce urine

anxiety a state of uneasiness characterized by apprehension and worry about possible events

apoptosis programmed cell death

apothecary forerunner of the modern pharmacists; a shop where medicines are gathered, stored, and compounded by skilled artisans using herbs and other natural ingredients

aqueous humor the fluid in the anterior chamber that lubricates and protects the lens of the eye

aromatase inhibitor a member of a class of drugs that block the effects of estrogen by preventing synthesis of estrogen in the body

arrhythmia a variation in heartbeat; irregular heartbeat

artery a vessel that carries oxygen-enriched blood from the heart to other parts of the body

arthritis disorder characterized by persistent pain due to functional problems of the joints

ascites abnormal buildup of fluid in the abdomen, usually caused by cirrhosis of the liver

asparagine an amino acid that is needed for leukemia cells to proliferate

aspiration inhalation of fluids from the mouth and throat

asthma inflammatory disorder of the airways; causes coughing, wheezing, breathlessness, and chest tightness; occurs in intermittent attacks that involve a reversible airway obstruction; precipitated by specific triggering events that vary in severity from patient to patient

asthma attack an acute difficulty with breathing

atherosclerosis accumulation of cholesterol and fats on the inner surfaces of arteries, eventually clogging the arteries and leading to MI or stroke

atonic seizure a type of generalized seizure characterized by sudden loss of both muscle tone and consciousness

atopic dermatitis a chronic itchy eruption of unknown origin, although allergic, hereditary, and psychogenic factors may be involved; also known as *eczema*

atrioventricular (AV) node the part of the heart's conduction system that carries the action potential from the atria to the ventricles with a delay

attention deficit hyperactivity disorder (ADHD) a disorder that manifests as difficulty focusing and concentrating overactivity, and difficulty in impulse control

atypical antipsychotic a first-line drug therapy for schizophrenia and other psychoses

aura an unusual sensation, such as one of light, sound, or taste, occurring at the onset of a seizure or other neurological condition, such as a migraine

automated dispensing process a computerized drug storage device that automatically tracks drug distribution

autonomic nervous system the part of the nervous system's efferent (motor) system that regulates involuntary motor activity such as that of cardiac muscle

azole a member of a family of fungi that interfere with fungal cytochrome P450 and inhibit the formation of the fungal cell wall

background pain a term used to describe a constant level of pain

bacteria single-celled microorganisms that exist in three primary forms: spherical (cocci), rod shaped (bacilli), and spiral (spirilla)

bacterial infection   a condition in which bacteria grow in body tissues and cause tissue damage to the host either by their presence or by toxins they produce

bactericidal agent   a drug that kills bacteria

bacteriostatic agent   a drug that inhibits the growth or multiplication of bacteria

barbiturate   one of a class of central nervous system depressants that also act as antianxiety, hypnotic, and anticonvulsant agents

bariatric surgery   any of several surgical options for achieving significant weight loss

basal cell carcinoma   a slow-growing skin cancer that rarely metastasizes

basal insulin   insulin released throughout the day and night to allow energy for basic cellular function

basal nuclei   symmetric, subcortical masses of gray matter embedded in the lower portions of the cerebral hemisphere; part of the extrapyramidal system; also known as *basal ganglia*

Beers Criteria   a list of drugs for which monitoring is especially important in older adult patients; also known as *Beers List*

benign prostatic hyperplasia (BPH)   an abnormal enlargement of the prostate gland, usually associated with aging

benzamides   drugs that cause dopamine antagonism and, at higher doses, 5-HT3 antagonism

benzodiazepine   one of a class of drugs that act as sedative, hypnotic, antianxiety, and anticonvulsant agents

beriberi   a condition associated with a diet low in vitamin B_1 that presents with numbness, tingling, edema, and heart failure

beta-1 receptor (ß1)   an adrenergic receptor that binds the neurotransmitters epinephrine and norepinephrine, increasing the heart rate and contractive force of the heart; found primarily in the heart and kidneys

beta-2 receptor (ß2)   an adrenergic receptor that binds the neurotransmitters epinephrine and norepinephrine, influencing dilation of bronchial tubes and blood vessels; found primarily in the lungs

beta-3 adrenoceptor agonist   a drug that works by relaxing the detrusor muscles during urine storage, increasing bladder capacity

beta-blocker   a class II antiarrhythmic drug that competitively blocks response to beta-adrenergic stimulation and therefore lowers heart rate

beta-carotene   a pigment in plants that is converted to vitamin A, an essential vitamin

beta-lactamase   an enzyme that destroys the beta-lactam ring present in the molecular structure of all penicillins

beta-lactamase inhibitor   an agent that inhibits beta-lactamase

bifidobacteria   not yet thoroughly studied agents that may be effective for diarrhea management

bile   an alkaline fluid produced by the liver; assists in the digestion and absorption of fat and cholesterol

bile acid sequestrant   an agent that forms a non-absorbable complex with bile acids in the intestines, which is eliminated in the feces

bioavailability   the fraction of drug made available at the site of physiological activity

biologic drugs   complex, large molecules that are created in a laboratory and derived from various living organisms such as bacteria, mammals, plants, insects, and birds

biologic response modifiers   drugs that target the part of the immune system responsible for inflammation and joint damage

biosimilar drug   highly similar to the reference or originator drug, with no clinically meaningful differences between that product and the reference product regarding safety, purity, and potency (safety and effectiveness)

bipolar disorder   a condition in which a patient presents with mood swings that alternate between periods of depression and periods of mania

black box warning   information printed on a drug package insert to alert prescribers to potential problems; also known as *boxed warning*

blocking (study method)   a study method involving practicing one skill at a time before moving on to the next

blood pressure (BP)   the force of blood in the circulatory system

blood urea nitrogen (BUN)   a blood test used to diagnose and monitor kidney function

blood-brain barrier   a barrier that prevents many substances from entering the cerebrospinal fluid from the blood; formed by glial cells that envelope the capillaries in the central nervous system, presenting a barrier to many water-soluble compounds, although they are permeable to lipid soluble substances

bolus insulin   insulin released at mealtimes to react with glucose entering the body from food intake

bone marrow suppression   a decrease in production of blood cells and increased risks of infections and bleeding

bone marrow   the spongy material inside bones that is responsible for white blood cells, red blood cells, and platelets

bone mineral density   the amount of mineral content for a particular volume of bone; can help indicate a patient's risk of osteoporosis

bone remodeling   the continual process of bone buildup and breakdown to maintain mineral balance in the body

boost   a drug given to increase the serum concentration of another drug

bowel evacuant   an agent used to empty the colon prior to GI examination or after ingestion of toxic substances

boxed warning   warning alert placed on a package insert inside a black box, identifies known problems associated with the use of the drug; also known as *black box warning*

bradycardia   abnormally slow heart rate

brand name   the name under which the manufacturer markets a drug; also known as the *trade name* or *proprietary name*

breakthrough pain   describes pain of great intensity that appears intermittently

broad-spectrum antibiotic   an antibiotic that is effective against multiple organisms

bronchitis   a condition in which the lining of the bronchial airways becomes inflamed, which obstructs exhalation

bronchodilator   an agent that relaxes smooth muscle cells of the bronchioles, thereby increasing airway diameter and improving the movement of gases into and out of the lungs

bronchospasm   spasmodic contraction of the smooth muscles of the bronchioles

Bruton's tyrosine kinase (BTK) inhibitor   a member of a drug class that blocks the enzyme BTK, a crucial part of the B-cell receptor signaling pathway

buccal   administration route via the mucous membrane between the cheek and the gums

bulk-forming agent   medication used to treat constipation; a type of laxative

bundle of His   the part of the heart's conduction system between the atrioventricular node and the Purkinje fibers

butterbur   herbal product; thought to prevent migraines

cachexia   a condition in which muscle and fat tissue waste away

calciferol   the collective name of the D vitamins

calcimimetic   a drug that lowers parathyroid hormone and calcium levels by increasing the parathyroid gland's sensitivity to calcium in the blood

calcineurin inhibitors   used to treat severe eczema

calcium channel blocker   a class IV antiarrhythmic drug that impedes the movement of calcium ions into cardiac muscle cells, reducing cell contractility, lowering the cell's need for energy and oxygen, and relaxing coronary vascular smooth muscle, which allows coronary arteries and arterioles to dilate and increases oxygen delivery

cancer immunity cycle   a series of steps that the immune system performs to elicit an anticancer immune response and cancer cell death

cancer   a group of diseases characterized by the uncontrolled growth of abnormal (or dysfunctional) cells

Candida   a common fungus that causes vaginal yeast infections and oral thrush

capacitance   the amount of blood held in the circulatory system

capillary   a tiny blood vessel in which fluids, gases, and nutrients are exchanged between the blood and body tissues

capsaicin chemical derived from cayenne peppers; used as a topical treatment for pain

capsid a protein shell that surrounds and protects the nucleic acid within a virus particle

carbapenem a member of a class of drugs used for mixed infections that have both Gram-positive and Gram-negative bacteria

carbonic anhydrase inhibitor a diuretic that acts in the nephrons to increase excretion of bicarbonate ions, increase urine volume, and change urine pH from acidic to alkaline

carbuncle a coalescent mass of infected hair follicles that is deeper than a furuncle

cardiac muscle heart muscle; responsible for the involuntary contraction of the heart

cardiac output the force and volume of blood coming from the heart

cardiac toxicity the ability to cause heart damage

cardiovascular system the body system that includes the heart and blood vessels and circulates blood throughout the body; also known as the *circulatory system*

cataplexy short periods of muscle weakness and loss of muscle tone associated with sudden emotions such as joy, fear, or anger; a symptom of narcolepsy

cation a positively charged ion

CD4 cell an infection-fighting cell that is important in the body's immune response

ceiling effect a point at which no clinical response occurs with increased dosage of a drug

cell cycle the process by which both normal cells and cancer cells divide

cell cycle–specific drug a drug that exerts its effects on rapidly dividing cancer cells

cell kill hypothesis the predominant hypothesis applied in cancer treatment; presumes that each cycle of chemotherapy kills a certain percentage of cancer cells

Centers for Disease Control and Prevention a governmental organization aimed to protect Americans from health, safety, and security threats

central nervous system (CNS) the brain and spinal cord; processes incoming information, determines responses, and coordinates other body systems

centralized pain pain that occurs when the central nervous system does not process pain signals properly

centrally distributed fat adipose tissue that accumulates in the abdominal area rather than in the hips, thighs, or buttocks

cephalosporin a member of a class of antibiotics that has a mechanism of action similar to that of penicillins but differs in antibacterial spectrum, resistance to beta-lactamase, and pharmacokinetics; divided into first-, second-, third-, fourth-, and fifth-generation agents

cerebrovascular accident (CVA) an event that interrupts oxygen supply to an area of the brain; medical term for stroke

cerumen earwax

cervical cap a contraceptive device inserted inside the vagina that fits over the cervix to prevent sperm from entering the uterus

CGRP receptor antagonist a member of the drug class that works by blocking activation of the trigeminal pain pathways

chancre a painless ulcer at the site of an infection

chemical dependence a person's inability to control their use of some chemical substance

chemoreceptor trigger zone (CTZ) an area below the floor of the fourth ventricle of the brain that can trigger nausea and vomiting when certain signals are received

chemotherapy the administration of drugs to treat cancer by killing or stopping the growth of cancer cells

cholecalciferol another name for vitamin D_3; synthesized in the skin in response to sunlight

cholescystectomy surgical removal of the gallbladder

cholesterol an odorless, white, waxlike, powdery substance that is present in all foods of animal origin but not in foods of plant origin

choline a nutrient related to B vitamins; may be effective for asthma management

chronic persisting for a long time

chronic kidney disease (CKD) a disease that involves progressive damage to kidney tissue, resulting in tissue death over time

chronic malignant pain pain that accompanies malignant disease and often increases in severity as the disease progresses

chronic nonmalignant pain pain that lasts for more than twelve weeks and may or may not have a diagnosed cause

chronic obstructive pulmonary disease (COPD) a chronic lung disease that impedes airflow and causes breathing difficulty; two types are chronic bronchitis and emphysema

chronic viral infection an infection that has a protracted course with long periods of remission interspersed with recurrence

C-I schedule I controlled substance; a drug with the highest potential for abuse, which may be used only for research under a special license

C-II schedule II controlled substance; a drug with a high potential for abuse, for which dispensing is severely restricted and prescriptions may not be refilled

C-III schedule III controlled substance; a drug with a moderate potential for abuse that can be refilled no more than five times in six months and only if authorized by the physician for this time period

C-IV schedule IV controlled substance; a drug dispensed under the same restrictions as schedule III but having less potential for abuse

ciliary muscle the part of the eye that holds the lens in place

circadian regularly recurring on a cycle of 24 hours

clearance the rate at which a drug is eliminated from a specific volume of blood per unit of time

clinical trial drug testing on humans; used to determine drug safety and efficacy

clotting cascade a series of events that initiates blood clotting, or coagulation

CNS stimulant a drug that affects the levels of certain chemicals in the brain, temporarily boosting mental and physical processes

coating agent an agent used to treat ulcers by forming a protective coat or layer over the ulcer

cobalamin a coenzyme necessary for cell reproduction, normal growth, and RBC production; also known as *vitamin B12*

cochlea the part of the ear that produces pressure waves

Cockcroft and Gault equation a formula commonly used to calculate creatinine clearance

cocktail a combination of drugs used in conjunction with each other to take advantage of the effects of synergistic drug therapy

codeine a morphine derivative with antitussive and analgesic properties; the traditional agent used to treat a cough related to bronchitis

coenzyme a chemical other than a protein that an enzyme needs for assistance in performing a metabolic function

colloid solution an IV solution that contains proteins and other large molecules, such as fats

colon part of the lower GI system; also known as the *large intestine*

colonic segmentation when the colon acts as if it is divided into small parts that move independently of each other rather than contributing to an integrated overall motion

color blindness a condition in which cone cells do not differentiate certain colors

combination chemotherapy a regimen of two or more chemotherapy drugs combined to reduce a cancer's potential resistance to treatment; the agents should have proven efficacy, nonoverlapping toxicities, and different mechanisms of action

combination therapy the use of two or more drugs from different classes; also known as *polytherapy*

common cold a mild, self-limited viral infection

community acquired contracted outside of a hospital or nursing home

community-acquired pneumonia pneumonia infection that results from exposure outside of an inpatient facility

competitive inhibition a process whereby a drug blocks enzyme activity and impairs the metabolism of another drug; can usually be overcome by increasing the dosage of the drug

complement system a collection of proteins that trigger one another in a chain reaction to enhance the immune system by attracting inflammatory cells, marking some bacteria for destruction by phagocytes, killing other pathogenic microbes directly, and clearing immune complexes from the body

complementary and alternative medicine medicine practices that are not part of standard care but are sometimes used in conjunction with standard practices

complete inhibition a state in which a drug cannot be metabolized by a person's body, regardless of the dosage

complex focal seizure a type of focal seizure in which the patient experiences impaired consciousness, often with confusion, a blank stare, and postseizure amnesia

compounder an automated pumping system that compounds multiple ingredients into a finished solution in a single patient bag of parenteral nutrition solution

computerized physician order entry a database entry for prescriptions records

concomitant accompanying

conduction system a system consisting of cardiac muscle cells and conducting fibers that coordinate contraction of the heart

cone cells photoreceptor cells in the retina of the eye which are responsible for color vision

conjunctiva the mucous membrane of the socket that holds the eye in place

conjunctivitis inflammation of the mucous membranes surrounding the eye; also known as *pink eye*

constipation a condition in which an individual has difficulty emptying their bowels; characterized by infrequent bowel movements, small stool size, or hard stools

constriction narrowing

contact dermatitis an inflammatory reaction produced by contact with an irritating agent

contemporary pharmacy a science based on systematic research to determine the origin, nature, chemistry, effects, and uses of drugs.

contiguity principle a study method that aligns words to corresponding graphics

contraception any practice that serves to prevent pregnancy during sexual activity

contraindication a disease, condition, or symptom for which a drug will not be beneficial and may do harm

controlled substance a drug with potential for abuse; organized into five categories or schedules that specify the way the drug must be stored, dispensed, recorded, and inventoried

convulsion involuntary contraction or series of contractions of the voluntary muscles

cornea the protective cover for the anterior chamber, iris, and pupil of the eye

corticosteroid any of several steroid hormones produced by the adrenal cortex

corticosteroid class of drug that acts as an anti-inflammatory agent to suppress the immune responses; resembles certain chemicals naturally produced by the adrenal gland and inhibits inflammatory cells by stimulating adenylate cylase

cotinine a major metabolite of nicotine

cough reflex a coordinated series of events, initiated by stimulation of receptors in the lungs and airways, that results in a cough

cracking a separation of lipid from a parenteral nutrition solution

cradle cap colloquial term for seborrheic dermatitis

cranberry juice liquid extracted from cranberries that may be used to prevent urinary tract infections

creatinine clearance (CrCl) a value used to assess kidney health

Crohn's disease an inflammatory bowel disease that causes chronic diarrhea and may affect the entire GI tract from mouth to anus

crystalloid solution an IV solution containing electrolytes

culture and sensitivity (C&S) test a laboratory test that helps determine which antibiotics have the best effect on a pathogen culture

curative an act or treatment administered with the intent to cure an illness

Cushing's syndrome a disease caused by overproduction of steroids, excessive administration of corticosteroids over an extended period, or adrenal gland tumors

cyclic lipopeptide   a member of a class of drugs that bind to bacterial membranes, causing cell membrane depolarization

cyclin-dependent kinase 4/6 (CDK 4/6) inhibitor   a member of a drug class that targets CDK4 and CDK6, enzymes important to cell division

cyclooxygenase-1   an enzyme that promotes the production of prostaglandins and causes pain and inflammation; also produces prostaglandins that protect the stomach lining

cyclooxygenase-2   an enzyme that is associated with the pain and inflammation of arthritis

cystic duct   connection between the gallbladder and the common bile duct and common hepatic duct

cystic fibrosis (CF)   a hereditary disorder that involves widespread dysfunction of the gastrointestinal and pulmonary systems

cystitis   a lower urinary tract infection

cytochrome P-450   a system of enzymes that plays a key role in metabolizing drugs and other substances

cytotoxic drug   a drug that interrupts the normal process of cell function or proliferation

cytotoxic T-lymphocyte-associated protein 4 (CTLA-4)   a protein receptor that functions as an immune checkpoint within T cells

dandruff   a malfunction of the oil-producing glands around hair follicles on the scalp

DEA Form 222   the form used to order C-II substances

decongestant   an agent that causes the mucous membranes to shrink, thereby allowing the sinus cavities to drain

deep vein thrombosis (DVT)   a condition caused by a blood clot that forms in a vein deep in the body

delirium tremens   a condition caused by cessation of alcohol consumption in which coarse, irregular tremors are accompanied by vivid hallucinations

dendrite   a branchlike extension from a neuron's cell body

depolarization   reversal of the negative voltage across a heart or nerve cell membrane, caused by an inflow of positive ions

depression   a condition characterized by pessimism, worry, intense sadness, loss of concentration, slowing of mental processes, dysphoric mood, loss of interest in usual activities, and problems with eating and sleeping

dermatitis   a condition of inflamed skin

dermatophyte   a type of fungus that can cause infection of the skin

dermis   layer of skin below the epidermis

detrusor muscles   muscles that cause the bladder to contract

diabetes   a disease characterized by high blood glucose due to insufficient levels of insulin

diabetic neuropathy   a lack of blood flow to nerves that leaves them unable to function

diabetic retinopathy   damage to the blood vessels in the retina due to diabetes; rupture of these vessels can cause loss of sight

dialysate   a fluid used in dialysis that draws toxins from the body into itself

dialysis   an artificial method of filtering blood and correcting the electrolyte imbalances caused by kidney failure

diaper rash   common in infants, when skin remains wet for long periods and bacteria growing on the skin turns into a rash

diaphragm   a contraceptive device inserted inside the vagina to prevent sperm from entering the uterus

diarrhea   excessive, soft, or watery stool

diastole   the period when the heart muscle relaxes, allowing blood to passively flow into the heart and fill its chambers

diastolic blood pressure   a measurement of the blood pressure when the heart relaxes and fills with blood (diastole)

dietary supplement   a category of nonprescription drugs that includes vitamins, minerals, and herbs, which is not regulated by the FDA

digestion   breakdown of large food molecules to smaller ones

dihydropyridine calcium channel blocker   a first-line therapy for hypertension that reduces blood pressure by dilating the arterioles; used to treat most supraventricular tachyarrhythmias

dilation widening

dipeptidyl peptidase-4 inhibitor one of a class of agents for treating diabetes that slow the inactivation of incretin hormones, allowing them to persist longer and produce beneficial effects

diplopia the perception of two images of a single object

disease-modifying antirheumatic drugs agents that can potentially modify the progression of rheumatoid arthritis

disinfectant an agent that destroys infectious organisms on nonliving objects

dispense as written instruction in a prescription to prevent substitution of a generic drug for a branded drug

distribution the process by which a drug moves from the blood into other body fluids and tissues to its sites of action

disulfiram-like reaction an adverse reaction to a substance leading to nausea, vomiting, flushing, dizziness, throbbing headache, chest and abdominal discomfort, and general hangover-like symptoms

diuretic a substance that rids the body of excess fluid and electrolytes by increasing urine output

diverticular disease formation and inflammation of an outpocketing from the colon wall

dopamine-norepinephrine reuptake inhibitor (DNRI) a class of drugs that works by blocking the reuptake of dopamine and norephinephrine, increasing the levels of both neurotransmitters

dosage the specific amount, dose, number, and dose frequency of an administered drug

dose the quantity of a drug administered at one time

dose-dense chemotherapy the practice of administering chemotherapy doses more frequently than in standard treatment to allow fewer cells to regrow between doses

dose-response curve the visual chart of how a drug reaches a point where a larger dose reaches its ceiling effect

double-blind study a clinical trial in which neither the trial participants nor the study staff know whether a particular participant is in the control group or the experimental group

drivers of cancer genetic alterations that promote cancer progression

drug a medicinal substance or remedy used to change the way a living organism functions; also called a medication

drug abuse the use of a drug for purposes other than those prescribed and/or in amounts that were not directed

drug addiction a dependence characterized by a perceived need to take a drug to attain the psychological and physical effects of mood-altering substances

drug class a category of drugs; includes drugs that share similar characteristics

drug dependence a state in which a person's body has adapted physiologically and psychologically to a drug and cannot function without it

Drug Enforcement Administration (DEA) the branch of the US Justice Department that is responsible for regulating the sale and use of drugs with abuse potential

drug interaction a change in the action of a drug caused by another drug, a food, or a substance such as alcohol or nicotine

drug sponsor the entity, usually a pharmaceutical company, responsible for testing the efficacy and safety of a drug and proposing the drug for approval

drug stem a group of letters in the drug's generic name that helps identify the drug class

dry powder inhaler (DPI) a type of inhaler used to deliver medications (such as inhaled corticosteroids); activated by taking a deep breath through the device

drying agent used for treatment or prevention of otitis externa; also known as *swimmer's ear*

duodenal ulcer a peptic lesion situated in the duodenum

duration of action the length of time a drug gives the desired response or is at the therapeutic level

Durham-Humphrey Amendment legislation that established distinctions between prescription drugs and nonprescription drugs

dysarthria imperfect articulation of speech

dyskinesia impairment of the power of voluntary movement

dyslipidemia   an abnormal amount of lipids in the blood

dyspareunia   painful intercourse

dysphagia   difficulty in swallowing

dysphoria   a state of feeling unwell or unhappy

dyspnea   labored or difficult breathing; shortness of breath

ear canal   the part of the ear that sound travels through to reach the eardrum; also known as *auditory canal*

eardrop   topical otic preparation

earwax dissolver   used to loosen and dissolve cerumen in patients with cerumen impaction

echinacea (Echinacea purpurea)   an herb some patients use to treat the common cold, respiratory tract infections, or vaginal yeast infections

echinocandin   a member of a class of antifungals that work by inhibiting the synthesis of D-glucan, an integral component of the fungal cell wall

eczema   a dry, flaky, red, itchy skin inflammation; also known as *atopic dermatitis*

educational research   the scientific field of study that examines learning and education

efferent system   the motor division of the nervous system, carrying information from the central nervous system to parts of the body to produce a response

electrolyte   a substance that dissociates into ions within a solution or solvent and is thus capable of conducting electricity

elimination   removal of a drug or its metabolites from the body by excretion; the process of filtering waste products

embolus   an abnormal particle, such as a blood clot or air bubble, that circulates in the blood

emergency contraceptive   a drug taken within 120 hours of having sex that stops the release of an egg from the ovary to prevent fertilization by sperm; if the patient is already pregnant, the drug has no effect

emesis   vomiting

emetic   a substance that induces vomiting

emphysema   an irreversible lung disease characterized by destruction of the alveoli in the lungs, which allows air to accumulate in tissues and organs

empirical treatment   use of a medication to treat a patient before the specific microorganism causing their infection is identified

emulsify   enable mixing with water

endocrine system   a collection of ductless glands and other structures that secrete hormones directly into the bloodstream

endogenous anxiety   anxiety caused by factors within the person's body

endogenous chemical messengers   chemical messengers that originate within the body

endometrium   the inner membrane of the uterus

endotracheal intubation   the insertion of a tube into the trachea to keep it open and deliver oxygen and general anesthesia directly to the lungs

enema   procedure in which liquid or gas is introduced into the rectum

enteral nutrition   a method of feeding a patient liquid nutrients through a tube inserted into the gastrointestinal tract

entry inhibitor   see *fusion inhibitor*

envelope   the membrane surrounding the capsid of some viruses; carries surface proteins that attach to the host cell's receptors

enzyme   biological molecule that catalyzes chemical reactions in the body

eosinophilic asthma   asthma that produces an increase in eosinophils (a type of white blood cell), which are thought to cause inflammation

epidermis   the top layer of the skin

epigastric area   the region of the upper abdomen immediately below the ribs

epilepsy   a neurologic disorder involving sudden and recurring seizures

e-prescription   an electronic prescription transmitted directly from prescriber to pharmacy

equianalgesic dose   a dose that offers an equal amount of analgesia

erectile dysfunction   a chronic inability to achieve a penile erection or to maintain one until ejaculation

ergosterol   a lipid unique to fungi

ergot   a group of fungi from which is derived the alkaloid ergotamine, which is used in the treatment of migraines

erysipelas   a skin infection characterized by redness and warmth, local pain, swollen plaques with sharply established borders, chills, malaise, and fever; a form of cellulitis

erythropoiesis   the process of making red blood cells

erythropoietin   a hormone secreted by the kidneys that stimulates the production of red blood cells

erythropoietin-stimulating agent (ESA)   a drug that induces red blood cell production by activating the release of reticulocytes (immature red blood cells)

Escherichia coli (E. coli)   a bacterial cause of diarrhea

esophageal hiatus   the opening in the diaphragm through which normally only the esophagus passes

esophagitis   inflammation of the esophagus

esophagus   part of the upper GI system

ester   one of a class of short-acting local anesthetics metabolized in plasma and tissue fluids

estrogen   any of the group of hormones produced primarily in the ovaries that regulate the reproductive system and produce typically feminine secondary sex characteristics

ethanol   the intoxicating agent in liquors and an anesthetic; also known as *alcohol*

eukaryotic   having a defined nucleus

euphoria   a state of feeling of well-being

eustachian tube   the part of the ear that connects to the throat to allow fluid to drain

exogenous anxiety   anxiety caused by factors outside person's body

exophthalmos   a condition in which fat collects behind the eyeball

expectorant   an agent that decreases the thickness and stickiness of mucus, enabling the patient to rid the lungs and airway of mucus by coughing

external condom   a condom placed over the erect penis before sexual activity to form a physical barrier (previously known as a male condom)

external ear   the part of the ear that captures sound waves

external ear infection (otitis externa)   an infection of the ear canal usually caused by bacteria or fungi that thrive in moist environments

external urethral sphincter   a voluntary muscle that holds urine in the bladder before it exits the body; also known as *external urinary sphincter*

extracellular   outside of cells

extrapyramidal symptom (EPS)   a symptom involving loss of control of muscle movements, caused by the blocking of dopamine receptors in the basal ganglia; also known as *EPS effect*

extravasation   an infusion leak under the skin during administration

fat-soluble vitamin   a vitamin the body absorbs along with dietary fat and maintains in large stores; the fat-soluble vitamins are vitamins A, D, E, and K

feedback mechanism   continuous feedback from the body that causes increases or decreases in the production of various hormones

feminizing hormone therapy   a reduction of androgen activity and use of hormone therapy to induce the development of typically secondary sex characteristics in a person who was assigned male at birth

feverfew   plant product used orally for migraine pain

fiber   the undigested residue of fruits, vegetables, and other foods of plant origin that remains after digestion by the human GI enzymes; characterized by fermentability and may be either water soluble or insoluble

fibrate   see fibric acid derivative

fibric acid derivative   a drug used to lower high cholesterol, especially high triglycerides

fibrillation   an abnormal rhythm that occurs when large portions of the heart beat out of sequence

fibrin   a protein that arranges into threads and ultimately leads to the formation of a blood clot

fibrinogen   a protein produced in the liver that reacts with thrombin to create fibrin

fibromyalgia   a condition characterized by long-term pain throughout the entire body

fight-or-flight response   the body's physical preparation to either escape or do battle when faced with danger

filtrate   fluids and by-products filtered from the blood in the glomerulus and other parts of a nephron

filtration   the removal of substances from the blood as part of the formation of urine by the glomerulus and renal tubules of the nephrons; also known as *elimination*

first order   depending directly on the concentration of the drug; elimination of most drugs is a first-order process in which a constant fraction of the drug is eliminated per unit of time

first-dose effect   a sudden or severe blood pressure decrease from the first dose of a medication; causes dizziness or fainting

first-pass effect   the extent to which a drug is metabolized by the liver before reaching the target sites or systemic circulation

first-phase insulin response   the immediate burst of insulin that occurs with or slightly before the first bite of food

fixed mindset   the belief that intelligence, character, and drive are static and will never change

flatulence   gas from the GI system

fluoroquinolone   a member of a class of drugs that kill bacteria by inhibiting the enzyme that helps DNA coil; also known as a *quinolone*

flutter   an abnormal rhythm that occurs when select portions of the heart beat slightly out of sync with the rest of the heart

focal seizure   an abnormal electrical discharge centered in a specific area of the brain; usually caused by trauma

folate-deficiency anemia   anemia caused by a lack of folic acid in the blood

folic acid   a vitamin that helps the body produce and maintain RBCs; also known as *folate* and *vitamin B$_9$*

folliculitis   a hair follicle inflammation presenting as a minute, red, pustulated nodule without involvement of the surrounding tissue

Food and Drug Administration (FDA)   the agency of the federal government that is responsible for ensuring the safety of drugs and food prepared for the market

fungus   a single-celled organism that is similar to an animal cell and to a green plant cell

furuncle   a staphylococcal infection of a sebaceous gland and the associated hair follicle; also known as a *boil*

fusion inhibitor   a drug that prevents HIV from entering the immune cells; also known as *entry inhibitor*

gallbladder   a pear-shaped organ located below the liver in the upper right abdomen that stores bile

gallstone dissolution agent   drug that assists in removing gallstones from the GI and urinary tracts

gastric bypass   a malabsorptive bariatric surgery that bypasses parts of the intestine to prevent the full absorption of nutrients from foods

gastric stasis   lack of stomach motility

gastric ulcer   a local excavation in the gastric mucosa

gastritis   irritation or inflammation of the stomach lining

gastroesophageal reflux disease (GERD)   a GI disease characterized by radiating burning or pain in the chest and an acid taste; caused by backflow of acidic stomach contents through an incompetent lower esophageal sphincter; also known as *heartburn*

gastrointestinal (GI) system   the system of organs that processes foods and liquids

gender transition   a process that is social, physical, or both that seeks to align a person's gender identity with their outward appearance; it may include hormone therapy and other medical interventions

gene therapy   the process of adding new genes to help the body fight or treat disease, replacing defective genes with healthy ones, or deactivating specific genes

general anesthesia   anesthesia that causes reversible unconsciousness and absence of response to otherwise painful stimuli; during general anesthesia, the patient is unconscious

generalized seizure a seizure that involves both hemispheres of the brain simultaneously and has no local origin; types include tonic-clonic (formerly known as grand mal), absence (formerly known as petit mal), myoclonic, and atonic seizures

generalized viral infection an infection that has or is spreading to other tissues by way of the bloodstream or the CNS

generation one of five numbered groups into which cephalosporins are organized

generic name a name that identifies a drug independently of its manufacturer; sometimes denotes a drug that is not protected by a trademark

genital herpes a sexually transmitted disease caused by the herpes simplex virus; characterized by lesions that cause a burning sensation

gestational diabetes diabetes that occurs during pregnancy due to insulin resistance caused by elevated hormones

ghost tablet the empty shell of an osmotic controlled-release oral delivery system tablet; excreted in the stool after the drug has dissolved

GI bleed condition in which ulceration erodes into a blood vessel

GI tract a continuous tube that begins in the mouth and extends through the pharynx, esophagus, stomach, small intestine, and large intestine to end at the anus

GI transit time the time it takes for material to pass from the mouth to the anus; the slower the GI transit time, the greater the amounts of nutrients and water absorbed; also known as *bowel transit time*

glaucoma a chronic eye disorder characterized by abnormally high internal eye pressure that damages the optic nerve and causes partial or complete loss of vision

glitazone see thiazolidinedione

glomerular filtration the process of filtering excess fluid and waste products out of the blood into the urine-collecting tubules of a kidney; the first step in making urine

glomerular filtration rate a value used to assess kidney health

glomerulus a network of capillaries contained in a nephron

GLP-1 an endogenous incretin hormone that GLP-1 agonists mimic

glucagon-like peptide a gastric hormone that stimulates glucose-dependent insulin secretion and inhibits glucagon release and gastric emptying; acts as a regulator of appetite and caloric intake

glucagon-like peptide 1 (GLP-1) receptor agonist an agent that treats diabetes by mimicking the endogenous incretin hormones GLP-1 and glucose-dependent insulinotropic polypeptide

glucocorticoid a corticosteroid involved in cholesterol, fat, and protein metabolism

gluconeogenesis the conversion of fatty acids and proteins to glucose

glucose-dependent insulinotropic polypeptide an endogenous incretin hormone that GLP-1 agonists mimic

glycoprotein antagonist an antiplatelet agent that binds to receptors on platelets, preventing platelet aggregation as well as the binding of fibrinogen and other adhesive molecules

glycosylated hemoglobin (A1c) an average of the sugar measured in blood glucose over a period of time

gouty arthritis a disease resulting from the improper excretion of uric acid; also called gout

Gram-negative bacteria bacteria with a thin cell wall that does not absorb Gram stain

Gram-positive bacteria bacteria with a thick cell wall that absorbs Gram stain and appears purple

grand mal seizure *see* tonic-clonic seizure

Graves' disease a condition in which the production of thyroid hormones is increased

growth hormone deficiency a condition in which the pituitary gland doesn't produce enough growth hormone, which leads to stunted height, stunted muscle development, or both

growth hormone a fundamental hormone that affects metabolism, skeletal growth, and somatic growth; a deficiency in this hormone causes growth retardation

growth hormone–releasing factor a neuropeptide secreted by the hypothalamus that stimulates the secretion of growth hormone by the pituitary

growth mindset the belief that intelligence, character, and drive as evolving characteristics can be changed

gynecomastia an enlargement of the breasts

gynecomastia excessive development of mammary glands, with or without tenderness

half-life the time necessary for the body to eliminate half of the drug in the body at any time; written as $t_{1/2}$

hand-foot syndrome a painful sloughing and peeling of the skin on the palms of the hands and soles of the feet; also known as *palmar-plantar erythema*

hazardous material (hazmat) a material that can be dangerous to life or the environment; usually requires a special procedure for cleanup

heart failure (HF) a condition in which the heart can no longer pump adequate blood to the body's tissues

heart rate the rate at which the sinoatrial node fires and the heart beats, typically 60 to 100 times per minute

Helicobacter pylori (H. pylori) a bacterium that contributes to the development of many gastric ulcers

hemodialysis the process of diverting blood flow through a machine that mechanically filters blood and returns the blood to the body

hemorrhagic stroke a rupture in a blood vessel that supplies an area of the brain

hemorrhoids a condition marked by engorgement of the vascular cushions situated within the anal sphincter muscles; result from pressure exerted on anal veins while straining to pass a stool

heparin a naturally occurring circulatory anticoagulant produced in mast cells

heparin-induced thrombocytopenia a low platelet count caused by heparin or an LMWH; can be life-threatening

hepatitis a disease of the liver that causes inflammation, can be acute or chronic, and has several forms, A through G

hepatitis A a viral form of hepatitis that is usually mild and transient and can be spread from one person to another

hepatitis B a viral form of hepatitis that can be acute or chronic; transmitted parenterally, through body fluids, from sexual contact, and perinatally

hepatitis C an infection of the liver that cannot be spread from one person to another by contact; most commonly transmitted by blood transfusions or illicit drug use

herniation a protrusion through a weakened muscular wall

hiatal hernia a protrusion through the esophageal hiatus of the diaphragm

high-density lipoprotein (HDL) a lipoprotein that absorbs cholesterol and transports it to the liver to be excreted from the body; also known as *good cholesterol*

hip fracture a break in the upper quarter of the femur (thigh) bone often caused by osteoporosis

hirsutism abnormal hairiness

histamine H_2 receptor antagonist an agent that blocks acid and pepsin secretion in response to histamine, gastrin, foods, abdominal distension, caffeine, or cholinergic stimulation; used to treat GERD and H. pylori

histamine a chemical produced by the body that evokes the symptoms of an allergic reaction

histoplasmosis a pulmonary disease caused by a fungus, usually from accumulated bat or bird droppings; also known as the *summer flu*

HMG-CoA reductase inhibitor a drug that inhibits the rate-limiting step in cholesterol formation

homeostasis stability of the organism

homocysteine an amino acid associated with cardiovascular disease

hormone therapy treatment to relieve symptoms of a deficiency in sex hormones, to augment sexual characteristics, or to support gender identity and transition; also known as *hormone replacement therapy*

hormone a secretion released by an endocrine gland into the circulatory system that has a specific regulatory effect on organs and other tissues

human chorionic gonadotropin a glycoprotein produced by trophoblastic cells and their descendants in the placenta

human immunodeficiency virus (HIV)   a retrovirus transmitted in body fluids that causes AIDS by attacking T lymphocytes

Huntington's disease   a neurodegenerative disorder characterized by brief, repetitive, involuntary movements; also known as *Huntington's chorea*

hydrocortisone   the pharmaceutical term for cortisol

hyperaldosteronism   a condition in which the body produces too much aldosterone

hypercalcemia   an excess of calcium in the blood

hypercapnia   icreased carbon dioxide in the blood

hyperchloremia   an excess of chloride in the body

hypercholesterolemia   a disorder characterized by excessive cholesterol

hyperglycemia   an elevated blood sugar level

hyperkalemia   an elevated potassium level

hyperlipidemia   an elevation of the levels of one or more of the lipoproteins in the blood

hypermagnesemia   an excess of magnesium in the body

hypernatremia   an elevated sodium concentration relative to the normal range

hyperphosphatemia   an excess of phosphate in the blood that can be caused by tumor lysis syndrome, rhabdomyolysis, lactic acidosis, or diabetic ketoacidosis

hyperpnea   abnormal increase in the depth of breathing

hypertension   elevated blood pressure

hyperthyroidism   a condition caused by excessive thyroid hormone; also known as *thyrotoxicosis*

hypertonic solution   a solution with a higher concentration of solute than bodily fluids contain

hypervolemia   excessive blood volume in the body

hypnotic   a drug that induces sleep

hypocalcemia   a condition in which the calcium level in the blood is below normal

hypochloremia   a depletion of chloride in the body caused by loss of fluid

hypoglycemia   a low blood glucose level (less than 70 mg/dL)

hypogonadism   a condition in which the body's sex glands produce few or no hormones

hypokalemia   a condition of potassium concentration that is lower than normal

hypomagnesemia   a depletion of magnesium in the body

hyponatremia   a low sodium concentration relative to the normal range

hypophosphatemia   a drop in phosphate in the bloodstream

hypothalamic-pituitary-adrenal axis suppression   a condition that causes appetite changes, weight gain, fat redistribution, fluid retention, and insomnia

hypothyroidism   a deficiency of thyroid activity that results in tiredness, lethargy, hair loss, weight gain, changes in sleep, depressed mood, and increased appetite

hypotonic solution   a solution with a lower concentration of solute than bodily fluids contain

hypoxia   reduction of oxygen in the blood

idiosyncratic reaction   an unusual or unexpected response to a drug that is unrelated to the dose given

ileus   a condition in which gastrointestinal motility is severely reduced

immune checkpoint inhibitor   an agent used in therapies to prevent cancer cells from "turning off" immune cells

immune system   a complex system made up of specialized organs, ducts, cells, and proteins; responsible for fighting infections and protecting the body

immunization   the process whereby a person acquires resistance to an infectious disease

immunocompromised   having a deficiency in the immune system response

immunoglobulin   an antibody that reacts to a specific foreign substance or organism and may prevent its antigen from attaching to a cell receptor or may destroy the substance or organism

immunosuppressant   a drug that strategically suppresses the body's immune system

immunosuppressive agent   drug that interferes with nucleic acid synthesis in both normal and precancerous cells; the overall action is suppression of the immune system

immunotherapy a type of cancer treatment that stimulates the immune system to stop or slow the growth of cancer cells

impetigo a superficial, highly contagious skin infection; characterized by small red spots that evolve into vesicles, break, and become encrusted and surrounded by a zone of erythema

inactivated vaccine a vaccine that uses pathogens that have been killed with chemicals, heat, or radiation

incontinence the inability to retain urine in the bladder

indication the common intended use of a drug to treat a specific disease, symptom, or condition

induction the process whereby a drug increases the concentration of certain enzymes that affect the pharmacologic response to another drug

induration a circular area of hardened tissue that indicates a positive reaction to a skin test in people who have been exposed to or have the disease that the test is for (e.g., tuberculosis)

infix letters within a word that have a specific meaning

inflammation the body's response to tissue injury or infection, commonly including heat, redness, and swelling

inflammatory pain a type of nociceptive pain; stems from the release of proinflammatory neurotransmitters (histamine, prostaglandins, etc.)

influenza the flu; a common viral infection

inhalation route method of administering a medication through the respiratory system

inhibition the process whereby a drug blocks enzyme activity and impairs the metabolism of another drug

innate immune system the immune system a person is born with, which orchestrates the body's automatic response to pathogens and provides nonspecific immunity

inner ear the part of the ear that includes the semicircular canals and the cochlea

insomnia difficulty falling asleep or staying asleep, or not feeling refreshed upon awakening

instillation administration of a medication drop by drop

institutional setting facility that assumes total care of patients

insulin a hormone that helps cells burn glucose for energy

insulin pump a device that delivers insulin through a tiny tube inserted just under the skin

insulin secretagogue an agent that stimulates insulin production from the pancreas to directly lower blood glucose levels

integrase strand transfer inhibitor a drug that prevents DNA produced by the reverse transcriptase of HIV from becoming incorporated into the patient's DNA

integrase an enzyme that integrates HIV DNA into the DNA of the host CD4 cell

integumentary system describes the system of tissue that protects and covers the body, including skin, nails, and hair

interchangeable products biosimilar products that meet additional requirements from more evaluations and tests; expected to produce the same clinical results as the reference drug

interferon a substance that exerts virus-nonspecific but host-specific antiviral activity by inducing the production of antiviral proteins that disrupt the synthesis of viral RNA

interleaving a study method of mixing (interleaving) practice on several related skills together

intermediate-acting insulin insulin that begins to be effective in 30 to 60 minutes and lasts 6 to 8 hours in most cases

internal condom a condom inserted into the vagina before sexual activity to form a physical barrier between the penis and vagina (previously known as a female condom)

internal urethral sphincter an involuntary muscle that prevents urine leakage; also known as *internal urinary sphincter*

international normalized ratio (INR) a blood test that measures how long it takes blood to clot

intracellular within a cell

intradermal injected into the skin

intramuscular injected into a muscle

intraocular pressure the buildup of force inside the eye

intraspinal injected into the spinal column

intrathecal (IT) administration the administration of drugs directly into the CNS via a lumbar puncture or spinal tap

intrauterine device a contraceptive device placed into the uterus by a healthcare practitioner; it stays in place for up to 10 years

intravenous administration of a medication through a vein, thereby avoiding the first-pass effect

investigational drug a chemical or biological substance that the FDA has approved for testing on humans in clinical trials; also known as an *experimental drug*

iris the coloring around the pupil of the eye

iron supplementation the process of replacing iron in the blood

irritable bowel syndrome (IBS) a functional disorder in which the lower GI tract does not have appropriate tone or spasticity to regulate bowel activity

irritant receptor a nerve cell in the lungs and airways that responds to coarse particles and chemicals to trigger a cough

ischemia an inadequate blood supply to an organ, usually due to blockage in the coronary arteries

ischemic stroke a stroke resulting from an obstruction of blood flow to part of the brain

isomer one of two or more compounds that contain the same number and type of atoms but have different molecular structures

isotonic solution a solution with the same level of particles, and thus the same tonicity, as body fluids

IV fluid a fluid used to replace fluids and electrolytes lost through dehydration

IVIG the notation for immune globulin that is given intravenously

jaundice a yellowing of the skin and eyes

joint place of union or junction between two or more bones of the skeleton

kava an extract derived from a Piper methysticum plant, may be used to treat anxiety and insomnia

keratolytic an agent that breaks down and peels off dead skin cells to keep them from clogging pores

keratomalacia a softening and ulceration of the cornea of the eye

kidney one of two bean-shaped organs that filter excess minerals and water from the body to the bladder

kidney transplantation the process of surgically implanting a kidney from a living or deceased donor into a recipient

kwashiorkor a condition in which caloric intake is adequate but protein intake is deficient

lactic acidosis a potentially fatal condition that can be a side effect of metformin and requires medical care and hospitalization

lactobacilli Gram-positive bacteria that are normally found in the GI tract

laparoscopic gastric banding a restrictive type of bariatric surgery that effectively makes the stomach smaller to prevent excess food intake

large molecules proteins that have a therapeutic effect; also called biologics

latency the ability of a virus to lie dormant and then, under certain conditions, reproduce and again behave like an infectious agent, causing cell damage

laxatives drugs that relieve constipation

legend drug a drug that requires a prescription; labeled "Rx only" on a medication stock bottle

lens the part of the eye that focuses light onto the back of the eye, much like the lens of a camera

leucovorin a by-product of dihydrofolate reductase that helps prevent harmful effects of certain chemotherapy drugs; also known as *folinic acid*

leucovorin rescue the administration of leucovorin to patients who have received high-dose methotrexate; this action rescues normal cells from a leucovorin shortage and allows them to resume their normal proliferation

leukotriene inhibitor an agent that blocks the body's inflammatory responses to leukotrienes or blocks their synthesis

lice wingless insects that live parasitically on various animals, including most mammals

lincosamide a member of a class of drugs that block bacteria's ability to produce proteins for survival

lipase a pancreatic enzyme to help digest fat

lipase inhibitor an agent that binds to gastric and pancreatic lipase enzymes in the intestines, preventing enzymes from breaking down fats to be absorbed

lipid a fatty molecule that is an important constituent of cell membranes; includes natural oils, waxes, and steroids

lipoprotein a spherical particle containing a core of triglycerides and cholesterol, in varying proportions, surrounded by a surface coat of phospholipids

liposomal product a drug prepared in a lipid formulation

live attenuated vaccine a vaccine that uses live but weakened pathogens to produce an immune response

liver an organ that produces bile and removes harmful substances before they reach general circulation

loading dose the amount of a drug that will bring its blood concentration rapidly to a therapeutic level

local affecting only a small area of the body

local anesthesia the production of transient and reversible loss of sensation in a defined area of the body without altering alertness or mental function

local effect an action of a drug that is confined to a specific part of the body

local infection an infection restricted to or pertaining to one area of the body

local viral infection a viral infection affecting tissues of a single system, such as the respiratory tract, the skin, or an eye

localized confined to one location in the body

long QT syndrome (or QT prolongation) a heart rhythm disorder

long-acting beta-2 agonist (LABA) drug that is similar to short-acting beta agonists but does not have to be administered as frequently

long-acting insulin insulin that works for approximately 24 hours and is injected one time a day

long-term persistent medication a drug used regularly to prevent asthma symptoms or attacks

loop diuretic a drug that inhibits the reabsorption of sodium, chloride, and water in the ascending loop of Henle, thereby causing increased urinary output

loop of Henle a long, U-shaped portion of a nephron from which water and salts are reabsorbed into the blood

low-density lipoprotein (LDL) a lipoprotein that at high levels causes plaque buildup in the vasculature and can lead to heart disease or stroke; also known as *bad cholesterol*

low-molecular-weight heparin (LMWH) an anticoagulant derived from heparin

luteinizing hormone–releasing hormone (LHRH) a hormone that stimulates the production of reproductive hormones in all genders; also known as *gonadotropin-releasing hormone*

luteinizing hormone–releasing hormone (LHRH) agonist a member of a class of drugs given to patients with hormone-sensitive tumors

lymphatic system the network of tubes and lymph nodes throughout the body

macrolide a member of a class of drugs that block bacteria's ability to produce proteins for survival

macula a spot near the center of the retina containing the focal point where light is concentrated for vision

maintenance dose amount of a drug administered at regular intervals to keep the blood concentration at a therapeutic level

malabsorption imperfect absorption of food material by the small intestine

malignant hyperthermia a sudden and rapid rise in body temperature, irregularities in heart rhythm and breathing; a serious side effect of anesthesia

malignant melanoma a highly malignant skin cancer formed from pigment-producing skin cells

malleus incus and stapes the bones of the middle ear that vibrate in response to sound waves

malnutrition a lack of adequate nutrient intake to supply basic metabolic needs

mania a state of overly high energy, excitement, hyperactivity, optimism, and increased psychomotor activity

marasmus a chronic condition caused by inadequate caloric and protein intake over a prolonged time

margin the area of normal tissue around the site of a tumor

masculinizing hormone therapy the use of hormone therapy to induce the development of typically masculine secondary sex characteristics in a person who was assigned female at birth

massing a study method that entails studying just once or twice in a short period of time; also known as *cramming*

mast cell stabilizer an agent that stabilizes mast cell membranes against rupture caused by antigenic substances and thereby reduces the amount of histamine and other inflammatory substances released in airway tissues

medical dictionary resource that defines commonly used terms in the healthcare field

medication error any preventable event that may cause or lead to inappropriate medication use or patient harm

Medication Guide a drug- or drug class–specific guide that the FDA mandates be issued with certain drugs to help prevent adverse events

medication reconciliation the process of obtaining a complete and accurate drug profile for a patient at each transition of care

medication use process the steps needed to provide a medication to a patient; includes the manufacturing, procurement, prescribing, filling or dispensing, administering, and monitoring of a medication

MedlinePlus a health information website published by the US National Library of Medicine

MedWatch a program run by the FDA for reporting serious adverse events, product problems, or medication errors after a drug has been approved and gone to market; serves as a clearinghouse to provide information on safety alerts for drugs, biologics, dietary supplements, and medical devices, as well as drug recalls

meglitinide one of a class of diabetes medications that increase the secretion of insulin from the pancreas; drugs in this class act within 10 minutes and last around 2 hours

melasma patches of darkened skin on the face

melatonin a naturally produced hormone that helps regulate circadian rhythms

membrane-stabilizing agent a class I anti-arrhythmic drug that slows the movement of ions into cardiac cells, reducing the action potential and damping abnormal rhythms and heartbeats

menopause describes the time when the menstrual cycle stops for one year, usually marking the end of reproductive years

metabolic acidosis a form of acidosis occurring when excess acid is produced, bicarbonate is lost, or the kidneys do not excrete enough acid

metabolic alkalosis a form of alkalosis occurring when excess acid is excreted via the kidneys or acid is lost from the stomach

metabolic pathway the sequence of chemical steps that convert a drug into a metabolite

metabolism the process by which drugs are chemically converted to other compounds

metabolite a substance into which a drug is chemically converted in the body

metastasis the spreading of a tumor from its primary site to other parts of the body

metered-dose inhaler (MDI) a device that delivers a specific amount of medication (as for asthma) in a fine spray in order to reach the innermost parts of the lungs

methemoglobinemia a disorder in which an abnormal form of hemoglobin is produced

methicillin-resistant Staphylococcus aureus (MRSA) a bacteria that causes infections and is resistant to certain drugs

methotrexate a drug used to treat leukemia, bone cancer, breast cancer, and lymphoma

microtubule a part of a cell that helps maintain its structure and is critical to mitosis

micturition the urination process in which detrusor muscles relax the external urinary sphincter, which pushes out urine from the body

middle ear the part of the ear beyond the eardrum

middle ear infection (otitis media) condition in which fluid from the middle ear does not drain well, allowing bacteria and viruses to flourish

migraine a moderate to severe, throbbing, unilateral headache, often accompanied by nausea, photophobia, phonophobia, or hyperesthesia

milliequivalent a unit commonly used to measure electrolytes

mineralocorticoid a corticosteroid involved in regulating electrolyte and water balance

minimum inhibitory concentration the lowest concentration of an antibiotic needed to inhibit the growth of a bacteria

mnemonic device a learning technique that uses a pattern of letters, ideas, or associations to assist in information retention or retrieval

monoamine oxidase inhibitor a drug that inhibits the activity of the enzymes that break down catecholamines (such as norepinephrine)

monobactam a member of a class of drugs used for Gram-negative bacterial infections

monoclonal originating from a single cell

monoclonal antibody an antibody produced in a laboratory from an isolated specific lymphocyte that produces a pure antibody against a known, specific antigen

monotherapy the use of a single drug to treat a disorder or disease

motor end plate a complex branching at the end of a motor neuron's axon where it meets a muscle fiber; part of a neuromuscular junction

mucolytic an agent that destroys or dissolves mucus

mucositis inflammation and ulceration of the mucous membranes

multidrug-resistant tuberculosis a strain of tuberculosis that is highly resistant to many currently used drugs

multiple sclerosis (MS) an autoimmune disease in which the myelin sheaths around nerves degenerate

multitasking the act of trying to complete multiple tasks at the same time

muscle an organ that produces movement by contracting (shortening itself)

muscle fasciculation a small, local, involuntary muscular contraction visible under the skin

muscle relaxant a drug that provides skeletal muscle relaxation or relief from muscle spasms as well as pain relief

muscle spasm an involuntary contraction of muscle fibers; also called a cramp

mutagenic having the ability to cause changes in genetic material

myasthenia gravis an autoimmune disorder of the neuromuscular junction in which the acetylcholine receptors are destroyed at the motor end plate, preventing muscles from responding to nerve signals to move them

myocardial infarction (MI) a heart attack; occurs when a region of the cardiac muscle is deprived of oxygen

myoclonic seizure a type of generalized seizure characterized by sudden muscle contractions with no loss of consciousness

naked virus a virus without an envelope covering the capsid

narcolepsy a sleep disorder in which inappropriate attacks of sleep occur during the daytime hours

narrow therapeutic index describes when a small difference in dose or blood concentration of a drug may lead to serious therapeutic failures or adverse drug reactions

narrow-angle glaucoma an acute eye condition that comes on quickly and is resolved with surgery followed by drugs

nasal corticosteroid a type of steroid sprayed or inhaled into the nose to treat allergies

nasal irrigation a flushing of the nasal cavity to remove excess mucus and debris from the nose and sinuses

nasal route administration of medication via the nose

National Institutes of Health a governmental medical research agency of the United States

national waiting list the list of candidates who are eligible for kidney transplantation; a person's place on the list depends on factors such as type of kidney problem, disease severity, and likelihood of transplant success

nebulizer a device that creates a mist from air flowing over a liquid and is used in the administration of inhaled medications

negative feedback a feedback process that occurs when the level of hormone in the blood or the level of a chemical it affects moves above or below a desired range; when this occurs, hormone production is lowered or raised in the opposite direction to bring the blood level of the hormone or the chemical it affects back into the appropriate range

negative margin an absence of tumor cells bordering the site of a tumor removal

neoadjuvant chemotherapy chemotherapy used to shrink a tumor so it can be safely and completely removed with surgery

nephron the functional filtering unit of the kidney

nephrotoxicity toxicity that causes damage to the kidneys

neuraxial anesthesia a type of anesthesia that blocks sensation through the injection of an agent into a nerve in the central nervous system without making the patient unconscious

neuroleptic drug see antipsychotic drug

neuromuscular blockade the blocking of neuromuscular transmission; skeletal muscle paralysis

neuromuscular blocking skeletal muscle paralysis

neuromuscular blocking agent an agent that paralyzes the patient's skeletal muscle

neuron a type of cell that transmits information through electrical and chemical signals

neuropathic pain abnormal pain signaling due to overactive nerve fibers

neurotransmitter a substance that controls ion channel molecules in a neuron's cell membrane, allowing or inhibiting transmission of nerve impulses across synapses

new drug application the vehicle through which drug sponsors formally propose that the FDA approve a new pharmaceutical for sale and marketing in the United States

nicotine the addictive component of tobacco

nicotine supplement agent that is used to reduce absorbed nicotine slowly over time

nitrate a drug that dilates coronary vessels, allowing more oxygen and nutrients to reach cardiac muscle cells thereby relieving chest pain and ischemia

nitroimidazole a member of a class of drugs effective against fungi, protozoa, and bacteria

nitrosourea a type of alkylating agent with the ability to penetrate the CNS; used in the treatment of brain tumors

nociceptive pain pain perceived when tissue is damaged

nocturia excessive nighttime urination

nodular acne formation of comedones, papules, pimples, and/or cysts in the skin of the face and upper trunk; these lesions occur when hair follicles and

nonadherence the failure to take a medication as prescribed

noncompetitive inhibition a process whereby a drug blocks enzyme activity and impairs the metabolism of another drug, leading to complete inhibition

noninstitutional setting facility such as a clinic or community pharmacy that offers same-day patient care

nonnucleoside reverse transcriptase inhibitor (NNRTI) a drug that prevents HIV-1 reverse transcriptase from adding new nucleotides to the growing DNA chain

nonpathologic not related to disease

nonproprietary name identifies the drug without regard to who is manufacturing and marketing the drug, also known as *generic name*

nonspecific immunity the type of immunity provided by the innate immune system, which responds similarly to all pathogens; also known as *innate immunity*

nonsteroid hormone a hormone that does not have the ability to penetrate cells but binds to receptors on a cell membrane to activate secondary messengers within the cell

nonsteroidal anti-inflammatory drugs a class of drugs that provides reduction of pain, swelling, inflammation, and fever

nonvirilized lacking typically male secondary sex characteristics despite having been born with testes

normal saline   a sterile IV or irrigation solution containing a concentration of 0.9% sodium chloride in water

Norwalk virus   viral infection that causes diarrhea

nosocomial infection   an infection acquired by a patient in a hospital or nursing home

nosocomial pneumonia   pneumonia acquired while a patient is hospitalized or living in a long-term care facility

nucleoside reverse transcriptase inhibitor (NRTI)   a drug that inhibits HIV reverse transcriptase by competing with natural nucleic acid building blocks, causing termination of the DNA chain

nucleotide   the basic structural component of DNA and RNA

obesity   a condition characterized by excessive accumulation and storage of fat in the body

obsessive-compulsive disorder   a disorder characterized by recurrent, persistent thoughts or behaviors, such as urges to perform repetitive acts like handwashing

off-label use   the use of a medication for an unapproved indication

olive oil   oil extracted from olives

oncogene   a gene that promotes cancer formation

on-off phenomenon   a wide fluctuation between abnormally increased and abnormally diminished motor function, present in many patients with Parkinson's disease after about five years of levodopa / carbidopa therapy

open-angle glaucoma   a slowly progressing chronic eye condition managed with medication alone

ophthalmic glaucoma agent   topical medication that reduces production of aqueous humor or its drainage from the anterior chamber

ophthalmic ointment   eye ointment

ophthalmic route   method of administering medication through the eye

opiate   any of the naturally occurring opioid analgesics, such as morphine or codeine, from the poppy flower Papaver somniferum

opioid   a substance, whether a drug or a chemical naturally produced by the body, that acts on

opioid receptors to reduce the sensation of pain; also known as a *narcotic*

opioid toxicity   results in slow breathing, absence of breathing, deep sedation, lack of response, or combination of these effects

opioid use disorder   a condition that can occur with long-term use of an opioid analgesic; characterized by persistent desire to use opioids, interference with relationships and other life activities, and the need to increase doses to receive the same effects

optic nerve   the nerve connecting the eye to the brain

oral candidiasis   an infection in the mouth caused by yeast-like fungi of the genus Candida

oral contraceptive   one or more hormonal compounds taken orally to prevent the occurrence of pregnancy

oral herpes   painful, fluid-filled lesions most commonly located around the mouth, chin, and upper lip; also known as *cold sores* or *fever blisters*

oral iron supplement   an iron supplement that is taken by mouth

oral thyroid supplementation   the administration of an agent to artificially provide adequate hormone levels

oral   administration of a medication by mouth in either solid form (as a tablet or capsule) or in liquid form (as a solution or syrup); also known as *peroral (po)*

order   a prescription issued in an institutional setting; also known as a *medication order*

organ of Corti   the sensory hairs lining the surface of the cochlea

orthostatic hypotension   a drop in blood pressure upon positional change that causes dizziness

osmolarity   the concentration of all molecules in a set volume of fluid

osmosis   the movement of fluid molecules across a semipermeable membrane from a higher concentration to a lower concentration

osmotic laxative   an organic substance that draws water into the colon and thereby stimulates evacuation

osteoarthritis   a degenerative joint disease resulting in loss of cartilage, cartilage elasticity, and bone thickness

osteoblast a cell that takes calcium from the blood and uses it to build bone tissue

osteoclast a cell that breaks down bone and releases calcium into the bloodstream

osteomalacia a bone disorder that presents as bone pain, muscle weakness, difficulty walking, and bone fractures and can be treated with vitamin D

osteoporosis a condition in which the patient experiences reduced bone mineral density, disrupted microarchitecture of bone structure, and increased likelihood of fracture

otic route method of administering medication in the ear

ototoxicity the ability to damage the organs of hearing

ototoxicity damage to the nerves that affect hearing

oval window the entrance to the inner ear

overflow incontinence the involuntary release of urine when the bladder becomes overly full, even if the individual feels no urge to urinate

over-the-counter drug a drug that may be sold without a prescription

oxazolidinone a member of a class of drugs that inhibit bacterial protein synthesis

oxytocic agent a drug that promotes contraction of uterine smooth muscle at term of pregnancy

package insert a document that accompanies the stock sent from the wholesaler; also known as *patient package insert*

pain physically or emotionally sensed discomfort that is or may be associated with acute tissue damage or a sensory system malfunction

palliative chemotherapy chemotherapy given for cancer that is not curable

pancreas a glandular organ of the GI system that makes enzymes to help digest carbohydrates, fats and proteins and that produces hormones such as insulin and glucagon to help maintain appropriate blood sugar levels in the body

pancreatic enzyme supplements pancreatic enzymes given to patients with cystic fibrosis to help prevent ductal obstructions and steatorrhea

panic disorder a disorder characterized by involuntary, intense, overwhelming, and uncontrollable anxiety

parasympathetic nervous system the part of the autonomic nervous system that controls rest, digestion, and homeostasis (maintenance of stable physiological conditions)

parenteral administered by injection rather than by way of the alimentary canal

parenteral iron supplement an iron supplement that is administered intravenously

parenteral nutrition nutrition provided by feeding a patient through an IV line; also known as *total parenteral nutrition*

Parkinson's disease (PD) a neurologic disorder characterized by akinesia, resting tremors, and muscular rigidity

paroxysmal sudden and recurring

passive immunity immunization that occurs when antibodies are transferred to the fetus during pregnancy

patent a government protection that gives a drug company the exclusive right to manufacture a drug for a certain number of years; protects the company's investment in developing the drug

pathogen a microorganism, such as a bacteria or virus, capable of causing an infection or disease

pathogenic causing or capable of causing disease or infection

pathologic manifestations of disease

patient-controlled analgesia pump a means of pain control whereby the patient can regulate, within certain limits, the amount of drug received

peak expiratory flow rate (PEFR) the maximum flow rate generated during a forced expiration, measured in liters per minute

peak flow meter a device used to measure peak expiratory flow rate as an indication of respiratory status; usually used by patients who have asthma

pediculosis an infestation of lice

pellagra a disease that presents with hyperpigmented rash in areas of exposed skin, swelling of the mouth and tongue, diarrhea, and anxiety; often develops in patients with gastrointestinal diseases or alcohol use disorder

penicillin a member of a class of antibiotics obtained from Penicillium chrysogenum; kills bacteria by preventing them from forming a rigid cell wall, thereby allowing an excessive amount of water to enter through osmosis and cause lysis of the bacterium cell

peptic disease disorder of the upper GI tract caused by the action of acid and pepsin; includes mucosal injury, erythema, erosions, and frank ulceration

peptic ulcer an ulcer formed at any part of the GI tract exposed to acid and pepsin

percussion a tapping movement to induce cough and expectoration of sputum from the lungs

percutaneous coronary intervention (PCI) a nonsurgical procedure in which a catheter is used to place a stent to open blood vessels in the heart

perimenopause a period of time prior to menopause, characterized by a gradual loss of ovarian function and irregular bleeding

peripheral nervous system (PNS) the nerves and sensory receptors located outside the central nervous system, transmitting neural signals between the body and the central nervous system

peripheral neuropathy extremely painful damage to the peripheral nervous system, especially affecting the hands and feet

peripheral vascular resistance (PVR) the degree to which the blood vessels are constricted or relaxed

peristalsis muscle contractions that propel fecal matter along the colon

peritoneal dialysis a procedure that puts dialysate into the abdominal cavity for a certain period

peroral comes from the Latin per os, meaning, "by opening"; commonly known as the oral route

personal protective equipment (PPE) equipment that must be worn at all times when handling hazardous drugs

petit mal seizure *see* absence seizure

pH a measurement of acidity or alkalinity

phagocystosis the process by which phagocytes engulf and usually destroy pathogens and other particulate matter

pharmacist an individual who is licensed to prepare and sell or dispense drugs and compounds and to fill prescriptions

pharmacodynamics the study of how a drug affects the body

pharmacognosy the study and identification of natural sources for drugs

pharmacokinetic modeling a method of mathematically describing the process of absorption, distribution, metabolism, and elimination of a drug within the body

pharmacokinetics individualized doses of drugs based on absorption, distribution, metabolism, and elimination of drugs from the body; the study of how the body affects drugs

pharmacologic effect the action of a drug on a living system

pharmacology the science of drugs and their interactions with the systems of living animals

pharmacopoeia an official listing of medic-inal preparations

Pharmacy Technician Certification Board (PTCB) a national organization that develops pharmacy technician standards and serves as a credentialing agency for pharmacy technicians

Pharmacy Technician Educators Council (PTEC) an organization of instructors dedicated to developing and sharing pharmacy technician program curriculums, educational materials, and instructional materials, advocating for greater education, training, certification, and responsibilities for technicians across the states

pharmacy technician an individual working in a pharmacy who, under the supervision of a licensed pharmacist, assists in activities not requiring the professional judgment of a pharmacist

pharmakon a Greek word meaning a "magic spell," "remedy," or "poison" that was used in early records to represent the concept of a drug

phenothiazine a drug that controls vomiting by inhibiting the CTZ

phlebitis inflammation of a vein

phosphate an anion that plays a role in energy production within cells

phosphate binder a medication that prevents phosphate absorption

phosphodiesterase-4 inhibitor a type of drug that prevents leukocytes and neutrophils from infiltrating the lungs

phosphodiesterase-5 inhibitor any of the class of drugs most frequently used to treat erectile dysfunction

photosensitivity an abnormal response of the skin or eye to sunlight

phytoestrogen a plant source of protein and fiber used in complementary and alternative medicine for conditions including hot flashes; also known as *isoflavone* and *soy*

phytonadione a dietary form of vitamin K

pimples a pore or follicle clogged with oil, dirt, or dead skin cells; can either be an open clogged pore, known as a *blackhead*, or a closed clogged pore, known as a *whitehead*

placebo an inactive substance with no treatment value

pneumonia a common lung infection caused by microorganisms that gain access to the lower respiratory tract

polyene a member of a class of drugs that interfere with cell-wall permeability

polypharmacy the concurrent use of multiple medications

pooling a time-saving process used in the preparation of a three-in-one parenteral nutrition in which all electrolytes except phosphate are put into a small-volume parenteral bag and then transferred into each batch

positive feedback feedback from the body's systems that promotes continued production of hormone or of a chemical the hormone affects without keeping blood levels within a particular range

post-attachment inhibitor a drug that inhibits HIV from entering the immune cells

postexposure prophylaxis (PEP) the administration of antiretrovirals after exposure to HIV

posttraumatic stress disorder (PTSD) a disorder characterized by persistent agitation or persistent, recurrent fear after the end of a traumatic event and lasting for over a month or impairing work or relationships

potassium-sparing diuretic drug that promotes excretion of water and sodium but inhibits the exchange of potassium for sodium in the nephrons

potentiation when one drug increases or prolongs the effect of another drug

prandial mealtime

precaution a disease, symptom, or condition for which the drug will not be beneficial and may do harm

preexposure prophylaxis (PrEP) an HIV prevention method in which people without HIV take an HIV medicine daily to reduce their risk of acquiring the virus if exposed through sex or injection drug use

prefix a group of letters occurring at the beginning of a word, base, or phrase

premenstrual dysphoric disorder a severe form of premenstrual syndrome

preparation error when an agent is prepared incorrectly

presbycusis hearing loss due to damage to the organ of Corti

prescribing error an error that occurs when a prescriber makes an incorrect order for a drug

prescription a direction for medication to be dispensed to a patient, written by a physician or a qualified licensed practitioner and filled by a pharmacist; known as an order when the medication is requested in a hospital setting

priapism a prolonged penile erection

primary chemotherapy the initial treatment of cancer with chemotherapy with curative intent

priming the act of pumping a nasal sprayer or inhaler a few times until an even amount of medication exits the applicator

probiotic a live microorganism ingested for health benefits

prodrug a compound that must be metabolized in the body to form an active pharmacologic agent

progesterone the hormone that prepares the uterus for a fertilized ovum

progestin any of a group of synthetic hormones that emulate the effects of progesterone

prokaryotic lacking a defined nucleus

prophylactic drug a drug that prevents or decreases the severity of a disease

prophylaxis effect of a drug in preventing infection or disease

prostaglandin E1 analog drug used in the treatment of ulcers

protease a pancreatic enzyme necessary to break down proteins

protease inhibitor (PI) a drug that prevents protease from cleaving certain HIV protein precursors into the smaller proteins needed for the formation of new infectious virions

proton pump inhibitor (PPI) a class of drugs that works to stop stomach acid; blocks acid secretion by inhibiting the enzyme that pumps hydrogen ions into the stomach

proto-oncogene a gene that codes for growth factors or their receptors

protozoan a single-celled organism that inhabits water and soil

provoked pain pain with a clear cause; more intense than background pain

pruritic itchy

pruritus itching sensation

psoriasis a skin disorder characterized by well-defined patches of raised, silvery or white, flaky, and pruritic skin; can affect any part of the body

ptosis paralytic drooping of the upper eyelid

Public Health Agency Canada's agency for public health and emergency preparedness against infections and chronic disease

pulmonary embolism (PE) a sudden blocking of the pulmonary artery by a blood clot

pulmonary fibrosis a type of lung toxicity

pulmonary function test a test done to assess asthma severity

pulse dosing dosing that produces escalating antibiotic levels early in the dosing interval followed by a prolonged dose-free period

pupil the black center of the eye

purified protein derivative (PPD) an agent used in a tuberculin skin test

Purkinje fiber one of the conduction system's fibers that stretches from the bundle of His through the ventricles to contract the lower part of the heart

pyelonephritis an infection of the upper urinary tract

QT interval the time between depolarization and repolarization of the ventricles of the heart during a heartbeat, as shown on an electrocardiogram

quick-relief medication drug used intermittently to provide rapid relief as needed

quinolone a member of a class of antibiotics that kill bacteria by inhibiting the enzyme that helps DNA to coil

radiation therapy the use of external beam radiation delivered from a machine outside the body to the site of a tumor

radioiodine the removal or reduction of the thyroid via radioactive iodine

rapid-acting insulin insulin that begins to work in 10 minutes and lasts as long as 2 hours

R-CHOP an acronym for a combination chemotherapy regimen: **r**ituximab (Rituxan), **c**yclophosphamide (Cytoxan), **h**ydroxydaunorubicin (better known as doxorubicin), **O**ncovin (brand name of vincristine), and **p**rednisone

rDNA type of DNA that has been formed in a laboratory by combining two or more different strands of DNA from different organisms

reabsorption the process by which substances are pulled back into the blood after waste products have been removed during the formation of urine

receptor a protein molecule on the surface of or within a cell that recognizes and binds with specific molecules, thereby producing some effect within the cell

rectal route administration of medication via the rectum

rectum the final portion of the large intestine where solid waste is stored until it passes through the anus

reflux backflow; specifically in GERD, the backflow of acidic stomach contents through an incompetent lower esophageal sphincter

regurgitation the action when swallowed food goes back up through one's throat

renal artery a branch of the abdominal aorta that brings blood into the kidneys

renal cortex the outer layer of a kidney; it and the renal medulla are responsible for filtration

renal medulla a structure in the body of each kidney that performs filtration

renal system   the body system composed of the kidneys, ureters, bladder, and urethra; also known as the *urinary system*

renal transplant drug   a medication that assists the body in accepting a transplanted kidney

renal vein   a vein that transfers filtered blood from the kidneys back into the bloodstream

renin-angiotensin system   the feedback mechanism that is regulated by the kidneys and balances fluid volume and vessel constriction in the circulatory system

repolarization   restoration of the negative voltage across a heart or nerve cell membrane, caused by an outflow of positive ions

resected   removed surgically

respiratory acidosis   a form of acidosis resulting from slow breathing and retention of carbon dioxide in the blood

respiratory alkalosis   a form of alkalosis occurring when breathing becomes more rapid and more carbon dioxide is exhaled and eliminated from the blood

respiratory distress syndrome (RDS)   a syndrome occurring in neonates that is characterized by acute asphyxia with hypoxia and acidosis

respiratory system   a system of organs responsible for obtaining oxygen from the air, supplying it to cells in the body, and removing carbon dioxide from the body

restless legs syndrome (RLS)   an overpowering sensation causing the urge to move the legs, especially while at rest

reticulocyte   an immature red blood cell

retina   the membrane containing the photoreceptor cells that detect light and color in the eye

retinoid   compound related to vitamin A that helps increase cell turnover in follicles

retrovirus   a virus that can copy its RNA genetic information into the host's DNA

reverse transcriptase   a retroviral enzyme that makes a DNA copy from an RNA original

rheumatoid arthritis   an autoimmune disorder in which the immune system destroys the synovial membrane of the joint, producing inflammation

rhinitis medicamentosa   a condition of decreased response that results when nasal decongestants are used over prolonged periods; also known as *rebound congestion*

rickets   a childhood disease in which a lack of vitamin D results in bone softening and muscle weakness

ringworm   a fungus that infects the horny (scaly) layer of skin or the nails; also known as *tinea*

Risk Evaluation and Mitigation Strategy   FDA-mandated programs for prescribing, dispensing, or taking certain drugs to manage associated risks

rod cell   a type of cell in the retina responsible for night vision

rosacea   chronic dermatologic disorder involving inflammation of the skin of the face; also known as *acne rosacea*

rotavirus   a viral infection that causes diarrhea

Rx   the symbol for a drug prescription

Saccharomyces boulardii (S. boulardii)   yeast organism that lives in the human GI tract

Safety Data Sheet (SDS)   the guide for a drug cleanup process

salicylates   a class of nonnarcotic analgesics that have pain-relieving, antipyretic (fever-reducing), and anti-inflammatory properties

saline nasal spray   a salt-water nasal spray that can also be used to help relieve nasal congestion by helping to loosen secretions

saliva   lubrication for food

salivary glands   small glands responsible for producing saliva

salmonella   infectious cause of diarrhea

satiety   a sensation of fullness and satisfaction

saw palmetto   a plant that may provide treatment for BPH symptoms

scabies   intense itching and threadlike lesions caused by mites

schizophrenia   a chronic mental health disorder characterized by delusions, disorganized speech and behavior, decrease in emotional range, and neurocognitive deficits

sclera the outer coating of the eyeball; also known as *the white of the eye*

scurvy a disease rarely seen in the United States, indicative of severe lack of vitamin C

seasonal affective disorder a form of depression that recurs in the fall and winter and remits in the spring and summer

sebaceous gland secretes sebum, a substance that oils the skin and hair

seborrheic dermatitis greasy, scaly area on the skin that sometimes appears red, brown, or yellow; also known as *cradle cap*

sebum an oil, produced by sebaceous glands around hair follicles, that when overproduced creates acne

secondary cancer an additional cancer in conjunction with the first cancer the patient was trying to cure

secondary diabetes diabetes caused by drugs

second-phase insulin secretion the continued but somewhat slower release of insulin in the hours after eating

secretion the release of cell products, such as hydrogen ions, potassium ions, and acids and bases, into urine

sedation a state of eased anxiety and drowsiness that can typically be induced by opioids

seizure an overfiring of the neurons of the brain and nervous system, resulting in a change in behavior or function; can result in convulsions, loss of control over movements, loss of consciousness, or distortion of senses

seizure threshold describes a person's likelihood to have a seizure

selective estrogen receptor modulators drugs for treating osteoporosis that work as estrogen receptors by mimicking the beneficial effects of estrogen on bone mineral density

selective serotonin reuptake inhibitor an antidepressant drug that blocks the reabsorption of serotonin, with little effect on norepinephrine and fewer side effects than other antidepressant drugs

self-injector pen a syringe that only needs to pierce the skin to pump medicine into the body

self-testing a study method that uses self-assessment to retain information; also known as *retrieval practice*

semicircular canals canals in the inner ear that are full of fluid and maintain the body's balance and orientation

sepsis a life-threatening systemic inflammatory response to an infection

serotonin (5-HT) receptor antagonist antiemetic used to prevent and treat severe nausea and vomiting associated with chemotherapeutic medications

serotonin syndrome a potentially fatal condition caused by combining antidepressants that increase serotonin levels with other medications that also stimulate serotonin receptors

serotonin-norepinephrine reuptake inhibitor an antidepressant drug that blocks the reabsorption of serotonin and norepinephrine, increasing the levels of both neurotransmitters

serum creatinine a blood test used to diagnose and monitor kidney function

sexual dysfunction persistent, recurrent problems with sexual response, including decreased desire, reduced arousal, inability to achieve orgasm, and pain during sexual intercourse

shiatsu acupressure the application of pressure to the discrete points on the body in order to provide therapeutic effects

short-acting beta-2 agonist (SABA) a bronchodilator that relieves acute asthma symptoms

short-acting insulin insulin that begins to work in around 30 minutes and lasts up to 4 hours

side effect a secondary response to a drug other than the primary therapeutic effect for which the drug was intended

signal transduction inhibitor a member of a drug class designed to target tumor cell receptors

simple focal seizure a type of focal seizure in which the patient does not lose consciousness and may have some muscular activity manifested as twitching as well as sensory hallucinations

sinoatrial (SA) node area of the heart that generates heartbeats, known as the heart's natural pacemaker

skeletal muscle   striated muscle in which contraction is voluntary, or under direct control; also known as *voluntary muscle*

slow viral infection   an infection that maintains a progressive course over months or years, inflicting cumulative damage to body tissues, ultimately ending in the host's death

small intestine   part of the lower GI system; the site where most digestion and nutrient absorption occur

small molecules   drugs produced synthetically from chemical substances and have a low molecular weight

smooth muscle   muscle in which contraction is involuntary; often found in organs (such as the stomach); also known as *involuntary muscle*

sodium bicarbonate   a basic substance used as an antacid for heartburn and acid indigestion, a systemic alkalinizer for treating metabolic acidosis, and a urinary alkalinizer when treating hemolytic emergencies and drug overdoses

sodium channel blocker   a drug that makes neurons less likely to fire by blocking the flow of positively charged sodium ions

sodium-glucose linked transporter-2 inhibitor   one of a class of diabetes medications that work by blocking the reabsorption of glucose that the kidneys filter out of the bloodstream

solubility   a drug's ability to dissolve in body fluids

solution   an active drug that is dissolved in liquid

somatic nervous system   the part of the nervous system's efferent (motor) system that regulates voluntary motor activity such as that of skeletal muscles

somatic sensory system   comprised of nerves that sense touch, pressure, temperature, and painful stimuli on the surface of the body

spacer   a device used with a metered-dose inhaler to decrease the amount of spray deposited on the back of the throat and swallowed

spacing   a study method involving multiple small study sessions spread across a long period of time

specificity   the property of a receptor site that enables it to bind only with a specific chemical messenger; to bind with a specific cell type, the messenger must have a chemical structure that is complementary to the structure of that cell's receptors

spectrum of activity   the range of bacteria against which an agent is effective

spermicide   an agent that kills sperm cells on contact

spill kit   a kit used in the cleanup of hazardous drug spills; must be available where hazardous drugs are prepared, administered, or transported

spleen   an organ that filters blood and removes microbes and damaged red blood cells

squamous cell carcinoma   a skin cancer that grows more rapidly than basal cell carcinoma but in which metastasis is uncommon

St. John's wort   a type of plant that may be taken orally for mild depression, the active ingredient is hypericin, which has activity similar to that of SSRIs

stable angina   a type of angina characterized by effort-induced chest pain from physical activity or emotional stress; usually predictable and reproducible

Staphylococcus aureus   a bacteria that causes infections on the skin and requires antibiotics to treat

status asthmaticus   a medical emergency that begins as an asthma attack but does not respond to normal management; can result in loss of consciousness and death

status epilepticus   a serious disorder involving tonic-clonic convulsions that last at least 30 minutes

steatorrhea   fatty, foul-smelling diarrhea that occurs when dietary fat is not properly absorbed in the gastrointestinal tract

steroid hormone   a messenger hormone that passes directly into the cells of the target organ

Stevens-Johnson syndrome   a sometimes-fatal allergic reaction marked by red blotches on the skin

stimulant laxative   a laxative used to treat acute constipation by stimulating neurons that control bowel muscles, enhancing peristalis and GI motility

stomach organ composed of layers of smooth muscle and lined with glands that secrete gastric juice; part of the upper GI system

stress ulcer a peptic ulcer, usually gastric, that occurs in a clinical setting; caused by a breakdown of natural mucosal resistance

stretch receptor a nerve cell in the lungs and airways that responds to elongation of muscle to trigger a cough

striated striped

stroke see cerebrovascular accident (CVA)

subcutaneous (SC, SQ, or subcut) injected into the tissue just beneath the skin

subcutaneous tissue the innermost layer of skin connecting the dermis to underlying organs and tissues

sublingual administration route via mucous membrane under the tongue

substantia nigra dark-gray matter in the midbrain containing neurons that release dopamine to help control movement; PD involves destruction of these neurons

suffix a group of letters occurring at the end of a word, base, or phrase that has the ability to add to or change the meaning of the word

sulfonamide a sulfa drug; a member of a class of bacteriostatic antibiotics that work by blocking bacteria from making folic acid, which is essential to their survival

sulfonylurea one of a class of diabetes medications that increase secretion of insulin from the pancreas; drugs in this class can take 30 minutes or more to start working and can last for 8 hours or longer

sun protection factor a measurement of the effectiveness of a sunscreen

suppository soft, rounded pieces of cocoa butter, glycerin, or a synthetic base containing medication; administration via the rectum

suppuration formation or discharge of pus

surfactant a fluid that reduces surface tension between the air in the alveoli and the inner surfaces of the alveoli, allowing gas to be exchanged between the lung and the air

surfactant laxative a stool softener that has a detergent activity that facilitates mixing of fat and water, making the stool soft and mushy

suspension active drug particles that are mixed, but not dissolved, in liquid

sweat gland a type of gland in the skin that produces water and salts; also known as an *eccrine sweat gland*

sympathetic nervous system the part of the autonomic nervous system that controls fight-or-flight functions such as heart rate increase and pupil dilation

sympathomimetic one of a class of drugs that treat obesity by stimulating the central nervous system, much as amphetamines do

synapse the connection between neurons that allows signal, or impulse to travel

synergism the combined effect of two drugs is more intense or greater than the sum of their individual effects systemic effect the distribution of a drug that has a generalized, all-inclusive effect on the body

synergistic drug therapy drug therapy using two or more drugs together because they employ different mechanisms of action that work better together than either drug works alone

synergistic effect the result of a drug combination that elicits an enhanced response because the agents work together to amplify the individual effects of each

systemic pertaining to or affecting the body as a whole

systemic absorption absorption into the bloodstream

systole the period during which the heart is contracting and actively pumping blood

systolic blood pressure a measurement of the pressure when the heart contracts, ejecting blood (systole)

tachycardia an excessively fast heart rate

tachypnea very rapid respiration causing a flushed appearance; a characteristic of emphysema

tardive dyskinesia a neurological disorder characterized by involuntary movements of the mouth, lips, and tongue

target a cell, tissue, or organ that is affected by a particular hormone

targeted anticancer therapy a drug therapy directed at specific molecular entities required for tumor cell development, proliferation, and growth

taxane a member of a class of antimicrotubule drugs derived from the bark and needles of yew trees

testosterone an androgen that is responsible for sperm production, sexual potency, and the maintenance of muscle mass and strength, among other functions

tetracycline a member of a class of broad-spectrum bacteriostatic antibiotics that inhibit protein synthesis within bacterial cells

therapeutic agent a drug that can be used to treat a disease or relieve symptoms of a disease or condition

therapeutic effect the desired action of a drug in the treatment of a particular disease state or symptom

therapeutic level the amount of drug in a patient's blood at which beneficial effects occur

therapeutic range the optimum dosage, providing the best chance for successful therapy; dosing below this range has little effect on the healing process, while overdosing can lead to toxicity and death

thiazide and thiazide-related diuretics diuretics that work by blocking a molecular pump that pulls sodium and chloride back into the blood from the distal convoluted tubule

thiazolidinedione a member of a class of drugs that directly increase insulin sensitivity in cells by stimulating the production of more insulin receptors; also known as *glitazone*

three-in-one see total nutrient admixture

threshold dose the lifetime cumulative dose limit for a drug

thrombin an enzyme in blood plasma that causes blood clotting by reacting with fibrinogen to form fibrin

thrombocytopenia low platelet count

thrombolytic agent an agent that dissolves clots by binding to the clot protein formed by fibrin

thrombus a blood clot that stays attached to its point of origin

thyroid gland a gland that produces hormones that stimulate various body tissues to increase their metabolic activity

thyroid storm a life-threatening medical emergency with the symptoms of hyperthyroidism, but more exaggerated

thyroxine (T_4) a hormone produced by the thyroid gland that can increase metabolic activity; tends to be less active than triiodothyronine (T_3)

tinnitus a ringing in the ears

tocolytic agent a drug that slows labor in pregnancy; used to treat premature labor

tolerance a decrease in response to the effects of a drug as it continues to be administered

tonic-clonic seizure a type of generalized seizure characterized by body rigidity followed by muscle jerks; formerly known as a grand mal seizure

tonicity the concentration of a solute (dissolved substance) in a solvent (liquid vehicle, such as water) and how that concentration affects the movement of water across membranes within the body

tophus a deposit of sodium urate around a joint, which is a symptom of gout

topical corticosteroids anti-inflammatory agents that treat contact dermatitis, eczema, psoriasis, and allergic reactions

topical applied to the surface of the skin or mucous membranes

topoisomerase I enzyme an enzyme that causes single-strand DNA breaks

topoisomerase I inhibitor a member of the subset of drugs that inhibit topoisomerase I enzymes

topoisomerase II enzyme an enzyme that causes double-strand DNA breaks

topoisomerase II inhibitor a member of the subset of drugs that inhibit topoisomerase II enzymes

total body water the amount of water in the body including intracellular and extracellular fluids

total cholesterol a measure of the total amount of cholesterol in the body based on HDL, LDL, and triglyceride levels

total nutrient admixture an amino acid–dextrose–lipid formulation used for parenteral nutrition; also known as a *three-in-one*

total parenteral nutrition   nutrition provided by feeding a patient through an IV line; also known as *parenteral nutrition*

transcription error   an error that occurs when a written order for a drug is incorrectly transcribed into the dispensing or computer system

transdermal contraceptive   a stick-on patch that delivers a combination of estrogen and progesterone in a steady supply through the skin

transgender   having a gender identity that differs from the sex a person was assigned at birth, which is typically limited to male or female

transient ischemic attack (TIA)   a temporary neurologic change that occurs when part of the brain lacks sufficient blood supply over a brief period of time; it may be a warning sign and predictor of imminent stroke

travel immunization clinic   a clinical site that provides immunizations and advice about what vaccines are needed

travel vaccine   a vaccine given prior to travel to allow the immune system time to confer full immunity

traveler's diarrhea   diarrhea caused by ingesting contaminated food or water; so called because it is often contracted by travelers in countries where the water supply is contaminated

treatment as prevention (TasP)   an HIV prevention method in which patients with HIV use antiretroviral therapy to suppress viral levels to undetectable levels in order to prevent the transmission of HIV to sexual partners

tricyclic antidepressant   one of a class of antidepressant drugs, developed earlier than the SSRIs and SNRIs, that prevents neuron reuptake of norepinephrine, serotonin, or both

triglyceride   a neutral fat stored in adipose tissue that releases free fatty acids into the blood

triiodothyronine (T$_3$)   a hormone produced by the thyroid gland that can increase metabolic activity; tends to be more active than thyroxine (T$_4$)

T-score   the result of a bone mineral density screening, which helps determine a patient's risk of osteoporosis

tuberculosis (TB)   a disease of the lungs and other body tissues and organs caused by Mycobacterium tuberculosis

tumor burden   the number of cancer cells in a tumor or the size of the tumor tissue

tumor cell proliferation   the exponential rate of growth early on in tumor development

tumor suppressor gene   a gene that turns off or downregulates the proliferation of cancer cells

two-in-one   a formulation for parenteral nutrition that contains amino acids and dextrose but no lipids

tympanic membrane   eardrum

type 1 diabetes   insulin-dependent diabetes in which the patient has no ability to produce insulin

type 2 diabetes   a type of diabetes characterized by insulin insufficiency or by the resistance of the target tissues to the insulin produced

ulcer   a local defect or excavation of the surface of an organ or tissue

ulcerative colitis   irritation and inflammation of the large bowel or colon, causing it to look scraped; characterized by bloody mucus and leading to watery diarrhea containing blood, mucus, and pus

uncoating   a virion's shedding of its capsid before presenting its RNA or DNA to the host cell's nucleus

unstable angina   a type of angina characterized by chest pain that occurs with increasing frequency, diminishes the patient's ability to work, and has a decreasing response to treatment; it may signal an oncoming MI

uremia   the clinical syndrome resulting from renal dysfunction in which excessive products of protein metabolism, such as urea, are retained in the blood

ureter   one of two pairedmuscular ducts that extend from the kidneys to the bladder

urge incontinence   a type of incontinence in which patients experience a sudden need to urinate that is difficult to delay; also known as *overactive bladder*

urinary analgesic   a pain reliever used for relieving discomfort caused by UTIs

urinary bladder   an organ that collects and holds urine until the fluid exits the body during urination

urinary incontinence   an involuntary loss or leakage of urine from the bladder

urinary retention   a condition in which the kidneys produce urine, but the micturition process does not function properly, and consequently, urine accumulates in the bladder

urinary retention   the inability to partially or completely empty the bladder, may result from prostate hypertrophy, malignancies, kidney stones, anticholinergic drug intake, or urinary tract infections

urinary tract infection   an infection caused by bacteria, usually E. coli, that enter via the urethra and progress up the urinary tract; characterized by the presence of bacteria in the urine with localized symptoms

urine   a modified filtrate of plasma created from filtration of waste substances in the kidneys

urticaria   hives

US Pharmacopeia   the independent, scientific organization responsible for setting official quality standards for all drugs sold in the United States, as well as standards for practice

Vaccine Information Statement (VIS)   a list of risks associated with a vaccination

vaginal ring   a combination contraceptive that is inserted into the vagina; contains synthetic estrogen and progesterone

vaginal route   administration of medication via the vagina

variant angina   a type of angina characterized by chest pain due to coronary artery spasm; usually not stress induced

vasodilator   a drug that relaxes smooth muscle and causes blood vessels to dilate

vasomotor   affecting constriction and dilation of blood vessels

vein   a vessel that carries oxygen-depleted blood toward the heart

vertigo   a malfunction of the semicircular canals resulting in balance problems and dizziness

vesicant   a drug that can cause an extravasation injury

vial   a container that holds medicine

vinca alkaloid   a member of a class of antimicrotubule drugs derived from periwinkle plants

viral load   a measurement taken from a blood sample that determines the level of HIV activity and the effectiveness of antiretroviral therapy

virilization   the development of typically masculine secondary sex characteristics

virion   an individual virus particle capable of infecting a living cell; consists of nucleic acid surrounded by a capsid (protein shell) and sometimes an envelope

virus   a minute infectious agent that does not have all the components of a cell and thus can replicate only within a living host cell

visceral sensory system   comprised of nerves that sense pain or reflex signals in the internal organs and blood vessels

vitamin   an organic substance that the body needs for normal metabolic functioning but does not synthesize, so the body must obtain it from food

vitamin A   a vitamin essential to photoreceptor cell growth and regeneration

vitamin B$_{12}$ a vitamin naturally occurring in many animal products such as meat, fish, poultry, eggs, and milk; also known as *cobalamin*

vitamin D analog   a treatment for psoriasis

vitamin D   a vitamin with many responsibilities in the body, including regulating calcium, phosphorus, and parathyroid hormone levels

vitreous humor   the fluid inside the eye, behind the lens

wart   a virally caused epidermal tumor

washout period   the period of time a patient must wait between discontinuing one drug therapy and starting another so that the first drug is out of the patient's system before the new drug takes effect

water-soluble vitamin   a vitamin that is excreted in the urine and is not stored in the body; includes vitamin C and the B vitamins

Wernicke-Korsakoff syndrome   a syndrome in which thiamine deficiency is present; occurs in patients with alcohol use disorder

wheals   slightly elevated, red areas on the body surface

wheezing   a whistling respiratory sound

wrinkle   a line or crease in the skin

xanthine derivative a drug that causes relaxation of airway smooth muscle, thus causing airway dilation and better air movement

yoga an ascetic discipline in which breath control, simple meditation, and the adoption of bodily postures is practiced for health and relaxation

zero order not depending on the concentration of the drug in the body; elimination of alcohol is a zero-order process in which a constant quantity of the drug is removed per unit of time

GENERIC AND BRAND NAME DRUG INDEX

Note: Locators followed by the letters *f* and *t* refers to figures and tables.

A

abacavir, 644*t*, 646, 659, 660*t*, 661
abciximab, 324*t*, 332
Abelcet, 374*t*, 617*t*, 620
abemaciclib, 790*t*, 793
abiglutide, 484
Abilify, 230*t*, 233–234
abiraterone, 790*t*, 791
A/B Otic Drops, 275*t*
Abraxane, 777*t*, 785, 788
Abreva, 103*t*, 107
Absorica, 93*t*, 94
Abstral, 682*t*, 687
acalabrutinib, 795*t*, 799
acamprosate, 253–254, 253*t*
Accolate, 78*t*, 350*t*, 354
Accuneb, 349*t*, 351
Accupril, 289*t*
acebutolol, 290*t*, 296
Aceon, 289*t*
Acetadote, 126
acetaminophen, 5, 123, 125–126, 569,
    621, 681, 689, 716, 718*t*, 722, 797
Acetasol, 275*t*
acetazolamide, 90*t*, 266*t*, 553*t*, 554
acetic acid, 275*t*
acetylcysteine, 126
acetylsalicylic acid, 152
Achromycin V, 614*t*
acidophilus, 761*t*
Aciphex, 412*t*, 414, 418*t*
acitretin, 521, 522
aclidinium, 359*t*, 361
aclidinium-formoterol, 360*t*, 365
Aclovate, 98*t*
Actigall, 424–425
Actiq, 682*t*, 687
Activase, 324*t*
Activella, 500*t*, 505, 506
Activia, 761*t*
Actonel, 142, 142*t*
Actoplus Met, 478*t*
Actos, 478*t*, 488
acyclovir, 103*t*, 107, 635*t*, 636*t*, 637, 670
Aczone, 92, 93*t*
Adalat CC, 289*t*
adalimumab, 4, 5*t*, 98, 132, 132*t*, 133,
    134*t*, 136*t*
adapalene, 93*t*, 94
Adasuve, 230*t*

Adcirca, 508, 508*t*
Adderall, 199*t*
additional opioids, 690
Addyi, 508*t*, 510
adefovir, 78*t*
Adhansia XR, 199*t*
Adipex-P, 752*t*, 753
Adlyxin, 477*t*, 484
Admelog, 476*t*, 481*t*, 482
ado-trastuzumab, 796
ado-trastuzumab emtansine, 794*t*
Adoxa, 592*t*, 604
Adriamycin, 776*t*, 784
Adrucil, 776*t*, 782
Advair Diskus, 350*t*, 360*t*, 365
Advair HFA, 350*t*, 360*t*, 365
Advil, 124*t*, 127–128, 379*t*
Adzenys, 199*t*
aemifentanyl, 705
afatinib, 794*t*
Afeditab, 289*t*
Afeditab CR, 289*t*
Afinitor, 78*t*
Afirmelle, 514*t*, 516
Afluria, 664*t*
Afrezza, 475*t*, 481*t*, 482
Aftera, 515*t*, 518
Aggrastat, 324*t*, 332
Aggrenox, 78*t*
A-Hydrocort, 419*t*
AirDuo Respiclick, 350*t*, 360*t*, 365
AK-Pred, 269*t*
Ala-Cort, 98*t*
Alavert, 379*t*, 380*t*, 388
albiglutide, 477*t*
albuterol, 50*t*, 349*t*, 351
alcium carbonate, 745
alclometasone, 98*t*
Aldactone, 501*t*, 507, 553*t*, 557
Aldex, 379*t*
aldosterone, 557
alendronate, 142, 142*t*
Alevazol, 103*t*, 106
Aleve, 125*t*, 127
Aleve-D, 379*t*
Alfenta, 698*t*, 705
alfentanil, 698*t*, 705
alfuzosin, 548*t*, 549, 653, 655
Align, 761*t*
Alimta, 776*t*, 783

Alinia, 426*t*, 430
aliskiren, 78*t*, 290*t*, 296, 570
Alka-Seltzer, 749*t*
Alkeran, 775*t*
Allegra, 380*t*, 388
Allegra-D, 379*t*
Alleroff, 380*t*, 388
Aller-Tec, 380*t*, 388
Alli, 752, 752*t*
allopurinol, 138, 138*t*, 139
almotriptan, 717*t*, 718
aloe gel, 113
alogliptin/metformin, 477*t*, 485
Aloprim, 138*t*, 139
Alora, 500*t*, 501*t*, 504
Aloxi, 444*t*, 446
alpelisib, 795*t*, 800
Alphagan P, 267*t*
5-alpha-reductase inhibitor, 550
AlphaTrex, 99*t*
alprazolam, 241*t*, 243, 518*t*, 619, 649
alprostadil, 508*t*, 510
Alrex, 269*t*
Altabax, 103*t*, 105
Altace, 289*t*
Altavera, 514*t*, 516
alteplase, 324*t*
AlternaGel, 411*t*
Altoprev, 314*t*
Altreno, 93*t*, 95
aluminum hydroxide, 411*t*, 434*t*
Alvesco, 349*t*, 352
Alyacen, 514*t*, 516
Alyq, 508, 508*t*
Amabelz, 500*t*, 505
amantadine, 186*t*, 191
Amaryl, 478*t*, 487
Ambien, 245*t*, 247
AmBisome, 374*t*, 617*t*, 620
amcinonide, 99*t*
Amerge, 717*t*, 718
A-MethaPred, 419*t*
Amethia, 514*t*, 516
Amethyst, 514*t*, 516
Amidate, 698*t*, 704
amikacin, 592*t*
amiloride, 553*t*, 556, 557
aminoglycosides, 543, 555, 587, 602, 603
aminosalicylates, 421
amioarone, 455

amiodarone, 90t, 300t, 302, 303t, 316, 329t, 595, 655, 719, 792
Amitiza, 434t, 438
amitriptyline, 72t, 214t, 220t, 518t, 679, 721
amlodipine, 289t
amlodipine-atorvastatin, 315
ammonium chloride, 748, 749, 749t
Amnesteem, 93t, 94
amoxicillin, 544, 589t, 590t, 596, 609t
amoxicillin-clavulanate, 78t
Amoxil, 589t, 596, 609t
amphetamine, 199t, 753
amphotericin B, 374t, 543, 617t, 620
amphotericin B lipid complex, 617t, 620
amphotericin B liposomal, 617t, 620
ampicillin, 589t, 590t, 609t
Amrix, 147t, 148t, 149t
amylin, 484
anabolic steroids, 35t
Anacaine, 90, 90t, 111t, 113
Anafranil, 214t
anakinra, 132, 132t, 133, 134t, 136t
Anaprox, 125t, 127
Anaprox DS, 125t, 127
anastrozole, 505, 790, 790t, 791
Ancef, 590t, 597
Ancobon, 617t, 621
andexanet alfa, 323t, 328
Andexxa, 323t, 328
Androderm, 500t, 501t, 502
AndroGel, 500t, 501t, 502
androgen, 473, 550
Anectine, 699t, 709
Angeliq, 500t, 505
Angiomax, 322t, 324
Anoro Ellipta, 359t, 360t, 366
Antabuse, 253t, 254
Antara, 314t
anthracycline, 784
antiandrogen, 507, 791
anticholinergic antiemetics, 445
anticholinergics, 545t
anticholinesterase, 712
anticoagulants, 505
antiestrogen, 790
antihistamine, 445, 621
antimetabolite, 782
antimuscarinics, 545t, 547
antineoplastic drugs, 543
antipyrine-benzocaine, 275t
antiretroviral, 642
Antistaphylococcal Penicillins, 589t
Antivert, 444t
antiviral drug, 635
Anusol HC, 442t
Anzemet, 444t, 446
apalutamide, 790t, 791
Apexicon, 99t
Apidra, 476t, 481t, 482
apixaban, 323t, 327, 327t
Aplenzin, 214t, 224–225, 393t, 394–395
Aplicare, 111t, 112
Apokyn, 185t, 186–187

apomorphine, 185t, 186–187
apraclonidine, 267t
aprepitant, 445t, 448–449, 473, 521, 522
Apri, 514t, 516
Apriso, 420t, 421
Aptensio XR, 199t
Aptiom, 170t, 171t, 173
Aptivus, 645t
Aquanil, 98t
Aralast NP, 366
Aranelle, 514t, 516
Aranesp, 560, 560t
Arava, 132t, 133, 134t, 135t
arformoterol, 360t, 364
Aricept, 196, 196t
Aricept ODT, 196, 196t
Arimidex, 790, 790t
aripiprazole, 230t, 233–234, 568
aripiprazole lauroxil, 230t, 233–234
Aristada, 230t, 233–234
Arixtra, 323t, 327
armodafinil, 245t, 249
Armour Thyroid, 467t, 469
Arnuity Ellipta, 349t, 352
Aromasin, 790, 790t
Arranon, 776t
arsphenamine, 25
Arthrotec, 125t, 128
Arymo, 682t, 696
Arymo ER, 690
Arzerra, 796
Asacol, 420t, 421
ascorbic acid, 759t
Ascriptin, 152t
asenapine, 230t, 234
Ashlyna, 514t, 516
Asmanex, 349t, 352
asparaginase, 777t, 789
asparagine, 789
aspirin, 4, 78t, 152, 152t, 157t, 268t, 323t, 330, 417, 417t, 718t, 722
Astagraf XL, 569, 569t
Astelin, 380t, 389
astemizole, 602, 649
Astepro, 380t, 389
Astramorph, 682t, 696
Atacand, 289t, 292, 292t
atazanavir, 521, 522, 645t, 652
Atelvia, 142, 142t
atenolol, 290t, 295, 296, 553t, 558
atezolizumab, 802t, 803
Ativan, 241t, 243, 699t, 708
atomoxetine, 199t, 200, 568
atorvastatin, 4, 314t, 316, 570, 619
atracurium, 699t
Atralin, 93t, 95
Atripla, 78t, 643, 644t, 659, 660t
atropine, 300t, 304, 305t
Atrovent, 359t, 361
Aubagio, 192t, 194, 194t
Aubra, 514t, 516
Augmentin, 78t, 544, 590t, 596, 609t
Augmentin XR, 590t, 609t
Auralgan, 275t

auranofin, 132t, 133, 134t, 135t
Aurodex, 275t
AuroDri, 275t
Avaclyr, 635t, 636t, 637
Avage, 93t, 94
avanafil, 508, 508t
Avandia, 478t, 488
Avapro, 289t, 292t
Avar Cleanser, 93t, 96
Avar-E Emollient, 93t, 96
Avastin, 794t, 795, 796
Aveed, 500t, 501t, 502
Avelox, 593t
avelumab, 802t, 803
Aventyl, 214t
Aviane, 514t, 516
Avita, 93t, 95
Avodart, 548t, 550
Avonex, 192, 192t
Axert, 717t, 718
Axid, 411t, 412
Axid AR, 411t, 412
Axiron, 500t, 501t, 502
axitinib, 794t, 795
Ayuna, 514t, 516
Azactam, 591t, 599
Azasan, 132, 132t, 135t, 202, 202t
AzaSite, 271t, 272
azathioprine, 98, 132, 132t, 134t, 135t, 202, 202t, 420t, 423, 622
azelaic acid, 92, 93t
azelastine, 380t, 389, 511
Azelex, 92, 93t
Azilect, 185t, 189
azilsartan, 78t, 289t, 292, 292t
azithromycin, 271t, 272, 368t, 592t, 596, 601, 602, 610t, 612, 613, 614t
azithromycin Z-Pak, 601
Azopt, 266t
Azo Urinary Pain Relief, 544t, 545
aztreonam, 368t, 369, 591t, 599, 600
Azulfidine, 132, 132t, 134t, 136t, 420t, 421–422
Azulfidine EN-tabs, 132, 132t, 136t
Azurette, 514t, 516

B

bacillus Calmette-Guérin (BCG), 664t, 668
bacitracin, 103t, 104, 610t
bacitracin-neomycin-polymyxin B, 103t, 104
baclofen, 147t, 148t, 149t
Bactrim, 544, 589t, 593, 610t
Bactrim DS, 544, 589t, 593
baloxavir marboxil, 636t, 639
Balziva, 514t, 516
Banzel, 170t, 172t, 174
Baraclude, 450–451, 450t
barbiturates, 519, 521, 522, 686, 704
Basaglar KwikPen, 476, 481t, 482
Bavencio, 802t, 803
becaplermin, 478t, 489

beclomethasone, 349t, 352, 380t, 390
Beconase AQ, 380t, 390
Bekyree, 514t, 516
Belbuca, 683t, 692, 693
Belviq, 33, 33f
bempedoic acid, 315t, 318
bempedoic acid-ezetimibe, 315
Benadryl, 232, 232t, 380t, 387, 444t
benazepril, 289t
bendamustine, 775t
Benefiber, 433t, 435
Benicar, 289t, 292, 292t
benralizumab, 350t, 355
Benzac, 92, 93t
benzalkonium chloride, 111t, 112
benzamides, 447
benzocaine, 90, 90t, 111t, 113, 700t, 714
benzodiazepine, 35t, 242–243, 245t,
    250–251, 619, 686, 689, 691, 693,
    694, 704
benzonatate, 378t, 382
benzoyl peroxide, 92, 93t
benztropine, 185t, 188, 232, 232t
benzyl alcohol, 563
beractant, 371, 373t
besifloxacin, 271t, 273
Besivance, 271t, 273
beta-3 adrenergic agonist, 547
Betadine, 111t, 112
Betagan, 265t
betamethasone, 471t, 616t
betamethasone dipropionate, 99t
betamethasone valerate, 99t
Betapace, 290t, 295
Betaseron, 192, 192t
beta-sitosterol, 333
betaxolol, 265t, 290t, 296
Bethkis, 368t, 369
Betimol, 265t
Betoptic-S, 265t
bevacizumab, 794t, 795, 796
Bevespi Aerosphere, 360t, 365
Beyaz, 514t, 516
Biaxin, 592t, 601, 610t
Biaxin Filmtab, 592t
Biaxin XL Filmtab, 592t
Biaxin XL Pac, 592t
bicalutamide, 790t, 791
bicarbonate, 411t
Bicillin L-A, 614t
BiCNU, 775t, 781
bictegravir, 645t, 657, 659, 660t
biguanide, 485–486
Bijuva, 500t, 505
Biktarvy, 643, 645t, 659, 660t
bile acid sequestrants, 521, 522
bimatoprost, 265t
Binostro, 142, 142t
Biopatch, 111t, 113
biotin, 732t, 736, 759t
bisacodyl, 434t, 438
bismuth subcitrate potassium/metroni-
    dazole/tetracycline, 417–418
bismuth subsalicylate, 426–427, 426t

bisoprolol, 290t, 296, 553t, 558
bisphosphonates, 142–143, 142t
bivalirudin, 322t, 324
bleomycin, 777t, 780t, 788, 789
Bleph-10, 271t, 272, 611t
Bleph-30, 271t
Blephamide, 272t
Bloxiverz, 711t, 712
boceprevir, 650
Boniva, 142, 142t
boric acid, 275t
bosentan, 519
Bosulif, 795t, 798
bosutinib, 511, 570, 649, 795t, 798
Breo Ellipta, 350t, 360t, 365
Brevibloc, 290t, 295
Brevital, 699t, 708
Brevoxyl, 92, 93t
brexpiprazole, 230t, 234–235, 568
Briellyn, 514t, 516
Brilinta, 323t, 331
brimonidine, 92, 93t, 95, 267t
brinzolamide, 266t
brivaracetam, 171t, 182, 183t
Briviact, 171t, 182, 183t
Bromfed DM, 378t
bromocriptine, 185t, 187
Brovana, 360t, 364
Brukinsa, 795t, 799
budesonide, 349t, 352, 380t, 390,
    419t, 471t
budesonide-formoterol, 350t, 360t
Bufferin, 152t
bumetanide, 553t, 554, 555, 556
Bumex, 553t, 554
Bunavail, 695t
bupivacaine, 700t, 714
Buprenex, 683t, 692, 693
buprenorphine, 683t, 692, 693, 695t
bupropion, 214t, 220t, 224–225, 393t,
    394–395, 752t, 754
Burrows, 275t
buspirone, 241t, 244
busulfan, 775t, 782
butaconazole, 618
butalbital, 718t, 722
butenafine, 103t, 105, 617t, 621, 622
butoconazole, 616t
butorphanol, 683t, 692, 693
Butrans, 683t, 692, 693
Bydureon, 477t, 484
Byetta, 477t, 484
Bystolic, 290t, 296

C

Cabometyx, 794t, 795
cabozantinib, 794t, 795
Caduet, 315
caffeine, 606, 718t, 722
calamine, 98t, 101–102
Calan, 290t
calciferol, 732t, 733

calcipotriene, 98t, 101
Calcitrate, 745
Calcitrene, 98t, 101
calcitriol, 565t, 566, 567
calcium acetate, 745
calcium carbonate, 411t
calcium carbonate/famotidine-
    magnesium hydroxide, 411t, 412
calcium carbonate/magnesium
    hydroxide, 411t
calcium carbonate/simethicone, 434t
calcium chloride, 745
calcium citrate, 745
calcium gluconate, 746
calcium lactate, 746
calfactant, 372, 373t
Cal-Lac, 746
Cambia, 124t, 127
Camila, 514t, 516
Campral, 253–254, 253t
Camptosar, 777t, 784
Camrese, 514t, 516
canagliflozin/metformin, 477t, 478t, 487
Canasa, 420t, 421
Cancidas, 617t, 619
candesartan, 289t, 292, 292t
cannabinoid test, 650
Capacet, 718t
capecitabine, 775t, 779t, 782, 783
Capex, 99t
Caplyta, 230t, 236–237
Capoten, 289t
Caprelsa, 794t, 795, 797
capsaicin, 722
captopril, 289t
Carafate, 412t, 415
carbamazepine, 9, 170t, 171t, 173, 227t,
    228, 329t, 455, 469, 473, 487,
    518t, 521, 522, 551, 650, 657, 693
carbamide peroxide, 111t, 113, 275t
carbapenems, 599, 600
Carbatrol, 170t, 171t, 173, 227t, 228
Carbocaine, 700t, 714
carboplatin, 775t, 781–782, 807
Cardene, 289t
Cardizem, 290t
Cardizem CD, 290t
Cardizem LA, 290t
Cardura, 548t
Cardura XL, 548t
cariprazine, 230t, 235
carisoprodol, 147t, 148t, 149t
carmustine, 775t, 781, 782
CaroSpir, 501t, 507, 553t, 557
carotenoid, 732t
carteolol, 265t
Cartia XT, 290t
carvedilol, 290t, 295
Casodex, 790t, 791
caspofungin, 49t, 617t, 619
Casporyn HC Otic Suspension, 275t
Catapres, 200
Caverject, 508t, 509
Cayston, 368t, 369, 591t, 599

Caziant, 514t, 516
CCR5 antagonists, 643
Cedax, 591t, 597
cefaclor, 590t, 610t
cefazolin, 590t, 597, 598
cefdinir, 591t, 597, 610t
cefditoren, 591t, 597, 598
cefepime, 591t, 597
cefiderocol, 591t
cefixime, 591t, 597, 610t
cefotaxime, 591t, 597
cefotetan, 590t, 598
cefoxitin, 590t, 598
cefpodoxime, 591t, 597, 598
ceftaroline, 591t, 597
ceftazidime, 591t, 597
ceftibuten, 591t, 597
Ceftin, 590t, 597
ceftriaxone, 591t, 597, 599, 612,
    613, 614t
cefuroxime, 590t, 597
Celebrex, 125t, 129–130
celecoxib, 125t, 129–130
Celestone, 471t
Celexa, 4, 213t, 215–216, 241t
CellCept, 569, 569t
cemiplimab, 802t, 803
Centany, 103t, 104
Cepacol Viractin, 700t, 714
cephalexin, 590t, 596, 610t
cephalosporin, 587, 596, 597, 598,
    599, 602
Cerebyx, 170t, 171t, 176
CereVe, 93t, 95
Cerubidine, 777t
Cervidil, 524t, 526
Cetamide, 271t
cetirizine, 267t, 380t, 388
cetirizine-pseudoephedrine, 379t
Cetraxal, 275t, 593t
cetuximab, 794t, 797
Chantix, 393t, 395
Chateal, 514t, 516
Cheratussin AC, 379t
chlorambucil, 775t
chloramphenicol, 564
chlordiazepoxide, 72t, 241t, 243,
    518t, 619
chlorhexidine gluconate, 111t, 113
chloride, 747
chloroprocaine, 700t, 714
chloroquine, 50t
chlorothiazide, 553t, 558
chlorpheniramine, 267t, 380t, 387
chlorpheniramine-hydrocodone,
    380t, 387
chlorpromazine, 49t, 72t, 267t, 595,
    718t, 721
chlorthalidone, 553t, 558
Chlor-Trimeton, 380t, 387
chlorzoxazone, 147t, 148t, 149t
cholecalciferol, 733
cholestyramine, 314t, 317, 570
cholic acid, 570

choline magnesium trisalicylate, 152,
    152t, 157t
chronic opioid therapy, 694
Cialis, 508, 508t
ciclesonide, 349t, 352, 381t, 390
Ciclodan, 103t, 105
ciclopirox, 103t, 105, 617t, 621
cilastatin, 591t, 599
Ciloxan, 271t, 273, 593t, 610t
Cimduo, 660t
cimetidine, 316, 329t, 411t, 412, 413, 551
cinacalcet, 565t, 567
Cinqair, 350t, 355
Cipro, 544, 593t, 610t
Ciprodex, 275t
ciprofloxacin, 271t, 273, 275t, 469, 544,
    593t, 610t, 690
ciprofloxacin-dexamethasone, 275t
ciprofloxacin-hydrocortisone, 275t
Cipro HC, 275t
cisapride, 455, 595, 602, 619, 649, 653,
    655, 704
cisatracurium, 699t
cisplatin, 775t, 779t, 781, 782
citalopram, 4, 213t, 215–216, 220t, 241t
Citrucel, 433t, 435
cladribine, 192t, 193, 194t, 775t
Claforan, 591t, 597
Claravis, 93t, 94
Clarinex, 380t, 388
Clarinex Reditabs, 388
clarithromycin, 551, 557, 592t, 596, 601,
    602, 610t
Claritin, 380t, 388
Claritin D, 379t
clavulanate, 544, 590t, 596, 609t
Clearasil, 92, 93t, 95
clemastine, 380t, 387
Cleocin, 592t, 601, 610t
Cleocin T, 92, 93t
Climara, 500t, 501t, 504
Climara Pro, 500t, 506
Clindagel, 92, 93t
clindamycin, 92, 93t, 592t, 596, 601,
    602, 610t
Clindesse, 92, 93t
Clindets, 92, 93t
clobetasol propionate, 99t
Clobex, 99t
clocortolone, 99t
Clodan, 99t
Cloderm, 99t
clofarabine, 775t
Clofibrate, 425
Clolar, 775t
clomifene, 49t
clomipramine, 90t, 214t, 221t
clonazepam, 241t, 243, 619
clonidine, 200
clopidogrel, 323t, 330
clorazepate, 72t, 241t
Clorox, 111t, 112
clotrimazole, 103t, 106, 616t, 618
clove oil, 113

clozapine, 230t, 235–236, 471, 570
Clozaril, 230t, 235–236
cobalamin, 732t, 737, 759t
cobicistat, 660, 660t
codeine, 35t, 268t, 378t, 381, 568, 682t,
    684t, 686, 696
coenzyme, 736
Colace, 433t, 436
colchicine, 138, 138t, 139, 505, 506,
    564, 619
Colcrys, 138t, 139
colesevelam, 315t, 317
Colestid, 315t
colestipol, 315t, 317
Colyte, 434t, 439–440
CombiPatch, 500t, 506
Combivent Respimat, 359t, 360t, 365
Combivir, 644t, 659, 660t
Compazine, 444t, 447
Compro, 230t, 718t, 721
Comtan, 185t, 189
Concerta, 199t
conivaptan, 455, 511, 570
conjugate, 664t
Contrave, 752t, 754
ConZip, 683t, 686, 692
Copaxone, 192t, 193, 194t
Copegus, 450t, 452
Cordarone, 300t
Coreg, 290t, 295
Coreg CR, 290t
Corgard, 290t, 295
Cortaid, 90t, 91, 98t
Cortane, 275t
Cortef, 98t, 419t, 471t
corticosteroids, 420–421, 472, 473, 559
Cortifoam, 442t
cortisol, 527
cortisone, 471t
Cortisporin Otic Solution, 275t
Cortifoam, 442t
Cortizone, 90t, 91
Cotempla XR, 199t
Cozaar, 289t, 292t
Creon, 78t
Crestor, 314t
Crinone, 500t, 501t, 505
Crixivan, 78t
crizotinib, 570
cromolyn sodium, 350t
Cubicin, 593t, 607
Culturelle, 761t
curare, 24
Curosurf, 372, 373t
Cutivate, 99t
cyanocobalamin, 560t, 563, 564
Cyclafem, 514t, 516
cyclic antidepressants, 214t,
    220–223, 220t
cyclobenzaprine, 147t, 148t, 149t
cyclooxygenase-1 (COX-1), 129
cyclooxygenase-2 (COX-2), 129
cyclophosphamide, 202, 202t, 775t, 781,
    785, 785t
Cycloset, 185t, 187

Cyclosporine, 569
cyclosporine, 78t, 98, 269, 269t, 316, 423, 430, 455, 566, 569, 569t, 570, 619
Cymbalta, 213t, 219, 241t
CYP3A4 inhibitors, 692
CYP2D6 inhibitors, 692
cyproheptadine, 90t
Cyramza, 794t, 795
Cyred, 514t, 516
Cyred EQ, 514t, 516
Cysteine, 758
cytarabine, 775t, 779t, 782, 783, 784
cytochrome P450, 557, 649
cytochrome P450 3A4, 649
cytochrome P450 inhibitor, 649
cytokines, 569
Cytomel, 467t, 468
Cytosar-U, 775t, 783
Cytotec, 412t, 415, 524t, 526
Cytoxan, 202, 202t, 775t, 781, 785

D

dabigatran, 78t, 322t, 324
dacarbazine, 90t, 775t, 782
Dacogen, 776t
dacomitinib, 794t, 797
Daliresp, 366
dalteparin, 323t, 326
Dantrium, 147t, 148t, 150t, 700t, 713
dantrolene, 147t, 148t, 150t, 700t, 713
dapagliflozin, 477t, 478t, 487
dapsone, 92, 93t
daptomycin, 587, 593t, 607, 608
darbepoetin alfa, 560, 560t
darifenacin, 545t, 546
darolutamide, 790t, 791
darunavir, 521, 522, 645t, 652, 660, 660t, 661
dasabuvir, 450t, 454–455
dasatinib, 413, 795t, 798, 799
Dasetta, 514t, 516
Daunomycin, 777t
daunorubicin, 777t, 779t, 784, 785t, 786, 786t
Dayhist Allergy, 380t, 387
Daysee, 514t, 516
Daytrana, 199t
Deblitane, 514t, 516
Debrox, 275t
Decadron, 471, 471t
decitabine, 776t
delavirdine, 413, 644t, 648, 649
Delestrogen, 501t
Delstrigo, 660t
Delsym, 378t, 382–383
Delyla, 514t, 516
Delzicol, 420t, 421
Demadex, 553t, 554
Denorex Everyday Dandruff Shampoo, 99t, 102
denosumab, 142t, 144
Depakene, 170t, 177, 178t, 227t, 228
Depakote, 170t, 177, 178t, 227t, 228

Depakote ER, 170t, 177
Depakote Sprinkle, 170t, 177
Depo- Estradiol, 501t
Depo-Medrol, 419t, 471, 471t
Depo-Provera, 515t, 521
Depo-SubQ Provera 104, 515t, 521
Depo-Testosterone, 500t, 501t, 502
DermaFungal, 103t
Dermarest, 98t
Dermatop, 99t
Dermoplast, 90, 90t, 111t, 113
Descovy, 644t, 660t
Desenex, 103t, 106, 616t, 618
desflurane, 698t, 703
desipramine, 49t, 214t, 221t
Desitin Maximum Strength Original, 111t, 112
desloratadine, 380t, 388
desogestrel, 514t
desonide, 99t
DesOwen, 99t
desoximetasone, 99t
Desquam-X, 92, 93t
desvenlafaxine, 213t, 218
Detrol, 546, 546t
Dexabliss, 471, 471t
dexamethasone, 268, 269t, 471, 471t, 472, 651
Dexilant, 411t, 414
dexlansoprazole, 411t, 414
dexmedetomidine, 698t, 707
dexmethylphenidate, 199t
DexPak, 471, 471t
dexpanthenol, 759t
dextroamphetamine-amphetamine, 199t
dextromethorphan, 378t, 382–383
dextromethorphan-pseudoephedrine-brompheniramine, 378t
DiaBeta, 478t, 487
Diamox, 266t
Diamox Sequels, 553t, 554
Diastat, 147t, 148t, 150t, 241t
diazepam, 72t, 147t, 148t, 150t, 241t, 243, 518t, 619, 699t, 708
dichlorphenamide, 266t
diclofenac, 124t, 127
diclofenac-misoprostol, 125t
dicloxacillin, 589t
dienogest, 523t
diethylpropion, 752t, 753
difenoxin/atropine, 426t, 428
difenozin/atropine, 427–428
Differin, 93t, 94
Diflucan, 616t, 618
DigiFab, 300t, 304
Digitek, 300t, 304, 305t
Digox, 300t, 304, 305t
digoxin, 4, 5t, 50t, 300t, 304, 305t, 425t
digoxin immune Fab, 300t, 304
dihydroergotamine, 602, 717t, 720
dihydrotestosterone (DHT), 550
Dilacor XR, 290t
Dilantin, 170t, 172t, 174–176
Dilatrate-SR, 307t, 308

Dilaudid, 689
diltiazem, 90t, 290t, 602
Dilt-XR, 290t
dimenhydrinate, 444t
dimethyl fumarate, 192t, 193, 194t
dinoprostone, 524t, 526, 527
Diovan, 289t, 292t
dipeptidyl peptidase-4 (DPP-4) inhibitor, 485
diphenhydramine, 90t, 232, 232t, 267t, 380t, 387, 444t, 797
diphenoxylate/atropine, 426t, 427–428, 428
diphtheria, 664t, 668
Diprivan, 698t, 706
Diprolene, 99t
dipyridamole, 72t, 78t
diroximel fumarate, 192t, 193, 194t
Disalcid, 152, 152t, 157t
disopyramide, 300t, 300t, 301t, 595, 619, 792
disulfiram, 253t, 254
Ditropan, 546, 546t
Diuril, 553t, 558
divalproex, 227t, 228
divalproex sodium, 177
docetaxel, 777t, 787, 788
docosanol, 103t, 107
docusate, 433t, 436
docusate senna, 433t, 436
docusate sodium, 277
dofetilide, 300t, 302, 303t, 413, 595, 619, 657
dolasetron, 444t, 446, 595, 792
Dolophine, 682t, 689, 695t, 696
dolutegravir, 645t, 657, 660t, 661
donepezil, 196, 196t, 690
dopamine, 510
Doral, 245t, 250–251
doravirine, 644t, 649, 660t
Doribax, 591t, 599
doripenem, 591t, 599, 600
dornase alfa, 367, 368t, 369
Doryx, 613
dorzolamide, 266t
Dotti, 500t, 501t, 504
DoubleDex, 471, 471t
Dovato, 643, 660t
Dovonex, 98t, 101
doxazosin, 548t, 549
doxepin, 214t, 221–222, 221t
Doxil, 776t, 785
doxorubicin, 505, 506, 568, 776t, 779t, 784, 785, 785t, 786, 786t
doxorubicin lipid complex, 776t
Doxy, 613
doxycline, 604
doxycycline, 49t, 563, 592t, 604, 610t, 614t
d-pantothenyl alcohol, 759t
Dramamine, 444t
dronedarone, 300t, 302, 303t, 316, 570, 619, 690, 704

droperidol, 595
Drospirenone, 500*t*, 505, 514*t*, 517
DTIC-Dome, 775*t*
Duaklir Pressair, 360*t*, 365
Duexis, 128
dulaglutide, 477*t*, 484
Dulcolax, 434*t*, 438
Dulera, 350*t*, 360*t*, 365
duloxetine, 213*t*, 219, 221*t*, 241*t*
DuoNeb, 359*t*, 360*t*, 365
Duopa, 185*t*, 186
dupilumab, 350*t*, 355
Dupixent, 350*t*, 355
Duragesic, 682*t*, 687
Duramorph, 682*t*, 690, 691, 696
Durlaza, 152*t*, 157*t*
durvalumab, 802*t*, 803
dutasteride, 548*t*, 550, 551
dxycycline, 613
Dyanavel, 199*t*
Dyazide, 553*t*, 558
dyclonine, 700*t*, 714
Dyna-Hex, 111*t*, 113
dynorphins, 681
Dyrenium, 553*t*, 556
Dyspnea, 438

E

EarDry, 275*t*
echinocandin, 619
EC-Naprosyn, 125*t*, 127
EContra One-Step, 515*t*, 518
EC-RX Progesterone, 501*t*
Edarbi, 78*t*, 289*t*, 292, 292*t*
Edecrin, 553*t*, 554
Edex, 508*t*, 509
Edluar, 245*t*, 247
edoxaban, 323*t*, 327, 327*t*
Edurant, 651
efavirenz, 78*t*, 487, 519, 521, 522, 602,
    644*t*, 649, 650, 651, 659, 660*t*
efavirenze, 455
Effexor, 214*t*, 220, 241*t*
Effient, 78*t*, 323*t*, 331
Elavil, 72*t*
elbasvir/grazoprevier, 450*t*, 453–454
Eldepryl, 185*t*, 189, 214*t*, 223
Elepsia XR, 171*t*, 182, 183*t*
Elestrin, 500*t*, 501*t*, 504
eletriptan, 717*t*, 718
elexacaftor-ivacaftor-tezacaftor,
    368*t*, 370
Elidel, 98*t*, 100
eliglustat, 568
Elimite, 108*t*, 110
Eliphos, 745
Eliquis, 323*t*, 327
Elixophyllin, 351*t*, 356
Ella, 78*t*, 515*t*
Ellence, 776*t*, 784
Elocon, 99*t*
Eloxatin, 775*t*, 781–782
EluRyng, 515*t*, 520

eluxadoline, 510
elvitegravir, 658, 660, 660*t*
Emend, 445*t*, 448–449, 473
Emoquette, 514*t*, 516
empagliflozin, 477*t*, 478*t*, 487
Emsam, 185*t*, 189, 214*t*, 223
emtansine, 796
emtricitabine, 78*t*, 644*t*, 645*t*, 646, 647,
    659, 660, 660*t*, 661
Emtriva, 644*t*, 646
Enablex, 545*t*, 546
enalapril, 47, 289*t*
enalaprilat, 289*t*
Enbrel, 4, 98, 132, 132*t*, 135*t*, 136*t*
Endometrin, 500*t*, 501*t*, 505
endorphins, 681
enfuvirtide, 645*t*, 656
Engerix-B, 449
Enhertu, 794*t*, 796
enkephalins, 681
EnovaRx, 147*t*, 148*t*, 149*t*
Enova RX-Baclofen, 147*t*, 148*t*, 149*t*
Enovra, 686
enoxaparin, 323*t*, 326
Enpresse, 514*t*, 516
Enskyce, 514*t*, 516
entacapone, 185*t*, 189
entecavir, 450–451, 450*t*
Entocort EC, 419*t*, 471*t*
Entresto, 311, 311*t*
Entyvio, 420*t*, 422
Enulose, 433*t*, 436–437
Envarsus XR, 569, 569*t*
enzalutamide, 790*t*, 791
Epaned, 289*t*
Epanova, 315*t*, 319
Epclusa, 450*t*, 455
ephalosporin, 612
epinephrine, 73, 700*t*, 714
epirubicin, 413, 776*t*, 779*t*, 784, 785*t*,
    786, 786*t*
Epitol, 170*t*, 171*t*, 173, 227*t*, 228
Epivir, 450*t*, 451, 644*t*, 646
Epivir-HBV, 450*t*, 451
eplerenone, 553*t*, 556, 557, 570, 619
epoetin alfa, 560, 560*t*
Epogen, 560, 560*t*
eprosartan, 289*t*, 292*t*
Epsom salts, 433*t*
eptifibatide, 324*t*, 332
Epzicom, 644*t*, 659, 660*t*
Equalactin, 433*t*, 435
Equetro, 170*t*, 171*t*, 173, 227*t*, 228
equianalgesic dose, 683
Erbitux, 794*t*, 797
ergocalciferol, 733, 759*t*
Ergomar, 4, 717*t*, 720
ergot alkaloids, 619, 649
ergotamine, 4, 602, 619, 717*t*, 720
ergot derivatives, 653, 655
eribulin, 777*t*
Erleada, 790*t*, 791
erlotinib, 794*t*, 797
Errin, 514*t*, 516

Ertaczo, 103*t*, 106
ertapenem, 591*t*, 599
ertugliflozin, 477*t*, 478*t*, 487
Ery, 92, 93*t*
EryC, 592*t*, 613, 614*t*
Erygel, 92, 93*t*
EryPed, 592*t*, 610*t*
Ery-Tab, 592*t*, 613, 614*t*
Erythrocin, 592*t*, 613, 614*t*
erythromycin, 92, 93*t*, 271*t*, 272, 455,
    518*t*, 551, 592*t*, 600, 610*t*, 611*t*,
    613, 614*t*
erythropoiesis, 559
erythropoietin, 539, 559
erythropoietin stimulating
    agent (ESA), 560
escitalopram, 213*t*, 215–216, 221*t*, 241*t*
Esgic, 718*t*
eslicarbazepine, 170*t*, 171*t*, 173
esmolol, 290*t*, 295, 296
esomeprazole, 411*t*, 414, 418*t*
esomeprazole-naproxen, 125*t*
Estarylla, 514*t*, 516
estazolam, 245*t*, 250–251
Estrace, 500*t*, 501*t*, 504
estradiol, 523, 524
estradiol plus levonorgestrel, 519
estradiol valerate, 523*t*, 524
Estring, 500*t*, 504
EstroGel, 500*t*, 504
Estrogel, 501*t*
estrogen, 519
eszopiclone, 245*t*, 247, 691, 693, 694
etanercept, 4, 98, 132, 132*t*, 133, 135*t*, 136*t*
ethacrynic acid, 553*t*, 554, 555
ethambutol, 373*t*, 374
ethinyl estradiol, 514*t*, 517, 519, 520
ethosuximide, 170*t*, 177, 178*t*
etodolac, 124*t*, 127, 128
etomidate, 698*t*, 704
etonogestrel, 520, 521, 522
etoposide, 50*t*, 776*t*, 785
etravirine, 78*t*, 602, 644*t*, 650, 651
Eulexin, 790*t*, 791
Euthyrox, 467*t*, 468
Evamist, 500*t*, 501*t*, 504
Evekeo, 199*t*
Evenity, 142*t*, 144
everolimus, 78*t*
evirapine, 653
Evista, 142*t*, 143
Evoclin, 92, 93*t*
Exalgo, 689
Excedrin, 718*t*, 722
Exelon, 196, 196*t*
exemestane, 790, 790*t*
exenatide, 477*t*, 484
exenatide ER, 477*t*
ex-lax, 433*t*, 434*t*, 436, 438
Extavia, 192, 192*t*
Extina, 103*t*, 106, 616*t*, 618
Ezallor, 314*t*
ezetimibe, 315*t*, 318, 333
ezetimibe-simvastatin, 315

F

Fabior, 93t, 94
FaLessa, 514t, 516
Falmina, 514t, 516
famciclovir, 636t, 637, 638, 670
famotidine, 411t, 412, 413
fam-trastuzumab deruxtecan, 794t, 796
Famvir, 636t, 637
Fanapt, 230t, 236
Farxiga, 478t, 487
Fasenra, 350t, 355
Fayosim, 514t, 516
FazaClo ODT, 230t, 235–236
febuxostat, 138, 138t, 140, 423
felbamate, 170t, 181, 182t, 518t, 519
Felbatol, 170t, 181, 182t
Feldene, 125t, 127, 128
felodipine, 289t, 619
Femara, 790, 790t
Femhrt, 500t, 505
Femiron, 560t, 561
Femring, 500t, 504
Femynor, 514t, 516
fenofibrate, 314t, 317, 329t
fenofibric acid, 314t, 317
fentanyl, 35t, 268t, 682t, 685, 687, 688,
        696, 698t, 705
fentanyl buccal lozenges, 687
fentanyl transdermal, 684t
Fentora, 682t, 687
Feraheme, 560t, 561, 561t
Ferate, 560t, 561
Fergon, 560t, 561
Ferosol, 560t, 561
FeroSul, 560t, 561
Ferrlecit, 560t, 561, 561t
Ferrocite, 560t, 561
ferrous fumarate, 560t, 561
ferrous gluconate, 560t, 561
ferrous sulfate, 560t, 561
ferumoxytol, 560t, 561, 561t, 562
fesoterodine, 545t, 546, 619
Fetroja, 591t
Fetzima, 213t, 219
Fexmid, 147t, 148t, 149t
fexofenadine, 380t, 388
fexofenadine-pseudoephedrine, 379t
fexophenadine, 267t
Fiasp, 476t, 481t, 482
Fiberall, 433t, 435
FiberCon, 433t, 435
Fiber-Lax, 433t, 435
Fibricor, 314t
Filgrastim, 49t
Finacea, 92, 93t
finasteride, 548t, 550
fingolimod, 192t, 193, 194t
Fioricet, 718t, 722
Fiorinal, 718t, 722
First-Baclofen, 147t, 148t, 149t
First-Progesterone, 500t, 505
Flagyl, 593t, 606, 613, 614t
Flagyl ER, 613, 614t

Flanax, 125t, 127
Flarex, 269t
Flatulence, 439
flecainide, 300, 300t, 301t, 655
Flector Patch, 127
Fleet Glycerin Suppositories, 433t
Fletcher's Laxatives, 434t, 438
flibanserin, 508t, 510
Flolipid, 314t
Flomax, 548t, 549
Flonase Allergy Relief, 381t, 390
Flonase Sensimist, 381t, 390
Flora-Q, 761t
Florastor, 761t
Floxin Otic, 275t
Flovent, 349t, 352
fluconazole, 329t, 518t, 616t, 618
flucytosine, 617t, 621, 622
Fludara, 776t, 783
fludarabine, 776t, 783
FluLaval, 664t
flumazenil, 710, 711, 711t
fluocinolone acetonide, 99t
fluocinonide, 99t
fluoromethalone (FML), 268, 269t
fluoroquinolone, 563
fluorouracil (5-FU), 90t, 776t, 782, 783
fluoxetine, 49t, 213t, 216, 329t
fluphenazine, 230t, 267t
flurazepam, 245t, 250–251, 518t
flutamide, 790t, 791
fluticasone, 99t, 349t, 352, 390
fluticasone furoate, 381t
fluticasone propionate, 381t
fluticasone-salmeterol, 350t, 360t, 365
fluticasone-umeclidinium-vilanterol,
        360t, 365
fluticasone-vilanterol, 350t, 360t, 365
fluvastatin, 314t, 316, 329t
fluvoxamine, 213t, 216–217
Fluzone, 664t
FML, 269t
FML-S, 271t
Focalin, 199t
Focalin XR, 199t
Folate, 737
folic acid, 560t, 563, 564, 759t
fondaparinux, 323t, 327, 327t
Forane, 698t, 703
Forfivo, 224–225, 393t, 394–395
Forfivo XL, 214t
formoterol, 360t, 364
Fortamet, 477t, 485
Fortaz, 591t, 597
Forteo, 142t, 144
Fortesta, 500t, 501t, 502
Fosamax, 142, 142t
fosamprenavir, 645t, 653
fosaprepitant, 445t
foscarnet, 570

fosfomycin, 544
fosinopril, 289t
fosphenytoin, 170t, 171t, 176, 469, 487,
        521, 522, 564, 650, 651, 657
Fostex, 93t, 95
Fragmin, 323t, 326
Frova, 717t, 718
frovatriptan, 717t, 718
fungal cytochrome P450, 615
Fungi-Guard, 103t, 106
Furadantin, 544
furosemide, 11f, 90t, 268t, 553t, 554, 556
FusePaq, 147t
fusidic acid, 455, 511
Fuzeon, 645t, 656
Fyavolv, 500t, 505
Fycompa, 170t, 181, 182t

G

gabapentin, 78t, 170t, 178, 180t, 204
Gabitril, 170t, 179, 180t
Gablofen, 147t, 148t, 149t
galantamine, 196, 196t
ganciclovir, 638, 646, 647
gancilovir interferon, 622
Garamycin, 592t
Garamycin Ophthalmic, 271t
Gardasil, 664t
Gas-X, 434t, 439
gatifloxacin, 271t, 273, 611t
GaviLyte-C, 434t, 439–440
GaviLyte-G, 434t, 439–440
GaviLyte-N, 434t, 439–440
Gaviscon, 37, 411t
Gazyva, 796
gefitinib, 794t, 797
Gelnique, 546, 546t
gemcitabine, 776t, 782
gemfibrozil, 314t, 329t
Gemzar, 776t, 782
Generess FE, 514t, 516
Gengraf, 78t, 569, 569t
Genoptic, 271t, 272, 611t
Genotropin, 528, 528t
Gentak, 271t, 272, 592t, 611t
gentamicin, 271t, 272, 592t, 611t
gentamicin-prednisolone, 271t
Gentasol, 271t, 592t
Gentopic, 592t
Genvoya, 660t
Geodon, 231t, 239–240
Gianvi, 514t, 516
Gilenya, 192t, 193, 194t
Glassia, 366
glatiramer acetate, 192t, 193, 194t
Glatopa, 192t, 193
glecaprevir/pibrentasvir, 450t, 454
Gleevec, 795t, 798
Gleostine, 775t, 781
glimepiride, 478t, 487
glipizide, 477t, 478t, 487
glitazone, 488
Gloperba, 138t, 139

glucocorticoids, 528
glucosamine, 155
Glucotrol, 478t, 487
Glucotrol XL, 478t, 487
Glumetza, 477t, 485
glyburide, 477t, 478t, 487
glycerin, 433t, 436
glycopyrrolate, 359t, 361–362
glycopyrrolate-formoterol, 360t, 365
Glynase, 478t, 487
Gly-Oxide Oral, 111t, 113
Gocovri, 186t, 191
golimumab, 132, 132t, 133, 135t, 137t
GoLYTELY, 434t, 439–440
GoNitro, 307t, 308
goserelin, 790t, 792
granisetron, 444t, 446
Grifulvin V, 617t, 621
griseofulvin, 90t, 518t, 519, 521, 522,
    617t, 621
Gris-PEG, 617t, 621
guaifenesin, 378t, 383
guaifenesin-codeine, 378t
guaifenesin-dextromethorphan, 378t
guaifenesin-pseudoephedrine, 379t
guanfacine, 200
Gynazole-1, 616t, 618
gynecomastia, 550, 557, 791
Gynecort, 98t
Gyne-Lotrimin, 103t, 106

H

Haemophilus influenzae type B (HIB), 668
Halaven, 777t
halcinonide, 99t
Halcion, 245t, 250–251
Haldol, 230t
HalfLYTELY, 439–440
halobetasol propionate, 99t
Halog, 99t
haloperidol, 90t, 230t, 267t
Halothane, 49t
Harvoni, 450t, 452–453
Havrix, 664t
H2 blockers, 73
HCTZ, 553t, 558
Heather, 514t, 516
Hemocyte, 560t, 561
heparin, 67, 323t, 325–326, 583
hepatitis A, 664t, 668
Hepsera, 78t
Herceptin, 794t, 796
heroin, 35t, 681, 694
herpes zoster, 669
Hibiclens, 111t, 113
histamine, 583, 678
Horizant, 78t
Humalog, 476t, 481t, 482
Humalog 50/50, 477t, 481t
Humalog 75/25, 476t, 481t
Humatrope, 528, 528t
Humira, 4, 5t, 98, 132, 132t, 134t, 136t
Humulin 70/30, 476t, 481t

Humulin 70/30 Kwikpen, 476t, 481t
Humulin N, 481t, 482
Humulin R, 476t, 481t, 482
Humulin R U-500, 476t, 481t, 482
Humulin R U-500 Kwikpen, 476t,
    481t, 482
HurriCaine, 90, 90t, 111t, 113
Hycamtin, 777t, 784
Hydrea, 776t, 783
hydrcortisone, 90t, 91
hydrochlorothiazide, 268t, 553t,
    556, 558
hydrocodone, 35t, 681, 682t, 684t, 688
hydrocodone-chlorpheniramine,
    378t, 382
hydrocortisone, 98t, 419t, 420, 442t,
    471t, 518t
hydrocortisone acetate, 98t
hydrocortisone butyrate, 99t
hydrocortisone probutate, 99t
hydrocortisone valerate, 99t
hydrogen peroxide, 111t, 112
hydromorphone, 35t, 268t, 681, 684t,
    689, 696
hydroxide, 412
hydroxychloroquine, 132, 132t, 134t,
    135t, 690
5-hydroxytryptophan, 204
hydroxyurea, 776t, 783
hydroxyzine, 241t, 244
hyperaldosteronism, 557
hyperuricemia, 558
hypoparathyroidism, 567
Hysingla ER, 682t, 688
Hyzaar, 553t, 558

I

ibalizumab, 645t, 656
ibandronate, 142, 142t
Ibrance, 790t, 793
ibrutinib, 649, 795t, 799
ibuprofen, 124t, 127–128, 268t, 417, 417t
ibuprofen-famotidine, 125t, 128
ibuprofen-pseudoephedrine, 379t
ibuprofen-pseudoephedrine chlorpheni-
    ramine, 379t
Iclusig, 795t, 798
Idamycin, 776t, 784
idarubicin, 776t, 779t, 784, 785t, 786
idarucizumab, 323t, 325
idelalisib, 455, 511, 570, 795t, 800
Ifex, 775t
ifosfamide, 775t, 779t, 782
iloperidone, 230t, 236, 568
Ilotycin, 272, 611t
imatinib, 795t, 798, 799
Imbruvica, 795t, 799
Imfinzi, 802t, 803
imipenem, 591t, 599
imipramine, 214t, 221–222, 518t
Imitrex, 717t, 719
Imodium, 426t, 429
Imodium A-D, 426t, 429

Imuran, 132, 132t, 134t, 135t, 202, 202t,
    420t, 423
Incassia, 514t, 516
Incruse Ellipta, 362–363
indapamide, 553t, 558
Inderal, 290t
Inderal LA, 290t, 295
Inderal XL, 290t, 295
indinavir, 78t, 653
Indocin, 72t, 127, 524t, 526
indomethacin, 72t, 127, 129, 524t, 526
Infasurf, 372, 373t
INFeD, 561t
Infed, 560t, 561
inflammatory cytokines, 678
infliximab, 132, 132t, 133, 135t, 137t
Infumorph, 682t, 690, 691, 696
inhaled insulin, 475t
Inlyta, 794t, 795
InnoPran XL, 290t, 295
Inspra, 553t, 557
Instacort, 98t, 99t
insulin, 25, 67, 480, 481t, 483, 527
insulin aspart, 476t, 481t, 482
insulin aspart protamine, 477t, 481t
insulin degludec, 476t, 481t, 483
insulin degludec/liraglutide, 481t
insulin detemir, 476t, 481t, 483
insulin glargine, 481t, 482
insulin glulisine, 476t, 481t, 482
insulin human inhalation, 481t, 482
insulin lispro, 476t, 481t, 482
insulin lispro protamine/lispro 50/50,
    477t, 481t
insulin lispro protamine/lispro 75/25,
    476t, 481t
insulin NPH/regular 70/30, 476t, 481t
insulin secretagogue, 487
integrase strand transfer inhibitors
    (INSTIs), 643, 657
Integrilin, 324t, 332
Intelence, 78t, 644t, 650
interferon beta-1a, 192, 192t
interferon beta-1b, 192, 192t
Intermezzo, 245t, 247
intrathecal (IT), 783
Introvale, 514t, 516
Intuniv, 200
Invanz, 591t, 599
Invega, 231t, 239
Invega Sustenna, 231t
Invega Trinza, 231t
Inveltys, 269t
Invokamet, 477t
Invokamet XR, 477t
Invokana, 478t, 487
ipecac, 24
ipilimumab, 802t
ipratropium, 359t, 361, 547
ipratropium-albuterol, 359t, 360t, 365
Iquix, 271t, 273
irbesartan, 289t, 292t
Iressa, 794t, 797
irinotecan, 619, 653, 777t, 779t, 784, 785

irinotecan liposomal, 777t
iron dextran, 560t, 561, 561t, 562
iron sucrose, 560t, 561, 561t, 562
Isentress, 645t, 658
Isibloom, 514t, 516
isoflurane, 698t, 703
isoniazid, 49, 373t, 374–375, 551
isopropyl alcohol, 111t, 112
isopropyl alcohol-glycerin, 275t
isoproterenol, 300t, 304, 305t
Isordil, 307t, 308
isosorbide dinitrate, 307t, 308, 508, 509
isosorbide mononitrate, 307t, 308, 508, 509
isotretinoin, 93t, 94, 268t
isradipine, 289t
istradefylline, 186t, 191
Isuprel, 304, 305t
itraconazole, 374t, 518t, 549, 551, 557, 616t, 618, 619, 719
ivabradine, 649
ivacaftor, 368t, 370
ivermectin, 108t, 110
Ixiaro, 664t

J

Jaimiesse, 514t, 516
Jalyn, 548t, 550
Janumet, 478t
Januvia, 477t, 485
Japanese encephalitis, 664t
Jardiance, 478t, 487
Jasmiel, 514t, 516
Jencycla, 514t, 516
Jentadueto, 477t
Jentadueto XR, 477t
Jinteli, 500t, 505
Jolessa, 514t, 516
Jornay PM, 199t
Juleber, 514t, 516

K

Kadcyla, 796
Kadian, 682t, 690, 696
Kaitlib Fe, 514t, 516
Kaletra, 645t, 653
Kalliga, 514t, 516
Kalydeco, 368t, 370
Kaopectate, 426–427, 426t
Kapvay, 200
Kariva, 514t, 516
Kaspargo, 290t, 295
Katerzia, 289t
kava, 255
Kazano, 477t
Keflex, 590t, 610t
Kefzol, 590t, 597
Kelnor, 514t, 516
Kenalog, 99t
Keppra, 171t, 182, 183t
Keppra XR, 171t, 182, 183t
keratolytic agent, 95

Kericort, 98t
Ketalar, 698t, 706
ketamine, 681, 698t, 706
ketoconazole, 49t, 103t, 106, 415, 518t, 549, 551, 557, 568, 616t, 618, 719, 720
Ketodan Kit, 103t
ketoprofen, 124t, 127
ketorolac, 124t, 127, 129, 417t
Keveyis, 266t
Keytruda, 802t, 803
Kineret, 132, 132t, 134t, 136t
Kisqali, 790t, 793
Kitabis Pak, 368t, 369
Klarity-A, 271t, 272
Klonopin, 241t, 243
Kombiglyze XR, 478t
Konsyl Fiber, 433t, 435
Kurvelo, 514t, 516
Kuvan, 78t
Kwikpen, 481t
Kyleena, 515t, 522
Kytril, 444t, 446

L

labetalol, 290t, 295
lacosamide, 170t, 172t, 174
lactate, 746
Lactinex, 761t
lactulose, 433t, 436–437
Lamictal, 170t, 180, 182t
Lamictal CD, 170t, 180, 182t
Lamictal ODT, 170t, 180, 182t
Lamictal XR, 170t, 180, 182t
Lamisil, 103t
Lamisil AF Defense, 103t, 106
Lamisil AT, 103t, 105, 617t, 621
lamivudine, 450t, 451, 644t, 646, 647, 648, 659, 660t, 661
lamotrigine, 170t, 180, 182t, 521, 522
Lanacane, 90, 90t, 111t, 113
Lanacort, 98t
Lanoxin, 4, 300t, 304, 305t
lansoprazole, 411t, 414, 418t
lansoprazole-amoxicillin-clarithromycin, 418
Lantus, 481t, 482
Lantus SoloStar, 481t, 482
lapatinib, 794t, 796
Larissia, 514t, 516
Lasix, 553t, 554
latanoprost, 265t
latanoprostene bumod, 265t
Latuda, 230t, 237
Layolis FE, 514t, 516
Lazanda, 682t, 687
ledipasvir, 450t, 452–453, 455
Leena, 514t, 516
leflunomide, 132t, 133, 134t, 135t
lenalidomide, 561, 794t, 795, 796
lenvatinib, 794t, 795
Lenvima, 794t, 795
Lescol, 314t
Lessina, 514t, 516

letrozole, 790, 790t, 791
Leucovorin, 780
Leukeran, 775t
leuprolide, 790t, 792
Leustatin, 192t, 193, 194t, 775t
levalbuterol, 349t, 351
Levemir, 476t, 481t, 483
levetiracetam, 171t, 182, 183t
Levitra, 508, 508t
levobunolol, 265t
levodopa-carbidopa, 185t, 186
levodopa-carbidopa-entacapone, 185t
levofloxacin, 49t, 271t, 273, 544, 593t
levomilnacipran, 213t, 219
Levonest, 514t, 516
levonorgestrel, 518, 519, 520, 522
Levora, 514t, 516
Levo-T, 467t, 468
Levothyroid, 467t, 468
levothyroxine, 329t, 467t, 468, 469, 566
Levoxyl, 467t, 468
Lexapro, 213t, 215–216, 241t
Lexette, 99t
Lexiva, 645t, 653
Lialda, 420t, 421
Librium, 72t, 241t, 243
Libtayo, 802t, 803
Licide, 108t, 110
Lidex, 99t
lidocaine, 49t, 90, 90t, 300, 300t, 301t, 700t, 714, 715
Lidoderm, 90, 90t
Lidopin, 90, 90t
lifitegrast, 269, 269t
Liletta, 515t, 522
Lillow, 514t, 516
linagliptin, 477t, 478t, 485
lincosamide, 601
linezolid, 593t, 607, 610t, 690
Lioresal, 147t, 148t, 149t
liothyronine, 467t, 468, 469
Lipitor, 4, 314t
Lipofen, 314t
liraglutide, 477t, 484, 752t, 753, 754
lisdexamfetamine, 199t
lisinopril, 50t, 289t, 553t, 558
lithium, 227–228, 227t
Lithobid, 227–228, 227t
Livalo, 314t
lixisenatide, 477t, 484
Locoid, 99t
Lodine, 124t, 127, 128
LoJaimiesse, 514t, 516
Lomaira, 752t, 753
Lomotil, 426t, 427–428, 428
lomustine, 775t, 781
Lonhala Magnair, 359t, 361–362
loperamide, 426t, 429
Lopid, 314t
Lopidine, 267t
lopinavir, 645t, 653, 654
Lopreeza, 500t, 505
Lopressor, 290t, 295

Loprox, 103*t*, 105, 617*t*, 621
loratadine, 380*t*, 388
loratadine-pseudoephedrine, 379*t*
loratidine, 267*t*
lorazepam, 49*t*, 241*t*, 243, 699*t*, 708
lorcaserin, 33, 33*f*
Loryna, 514*t*, 516
Lorzone, 147*t*, 148*t*, 149*t*
losartan, 49*t*, 289*t*, 292*t*, 553*t*, 558
LoSeasonique, 514*t*, 516
Lotamox, 268
Lotensin, 289*t*
lotepredninol, 268, 269*t*
Lotrimin, 616*t*, 618
Lotrimin AF, 103*t*, 106, 616*t*
Lotrimin Ultra, 103*t*, 105, 617*t*, 621
Lotrisone, 616*t*
lovastatin, 314*t*, 316, 329*t*, 570, 602, 619, 653, 655
Lovaza, 315*t*, 319
Lovenox, 323*t*, 326
loxapine, 230*t*
Lo-Zumandimine, 514*t*, 516
lubiprostone, 434*t*, 438
lumacaftor-ivacaftor, 368*t*, 370
lumateperone, 230*t*, 236–237
Lumify, 267*t*
Lumigan, 265*t*
Luminal, 179, 180*t*
Lunesta, 245*t*, 247
luoroquinolone, 605
Lupron, 790*t*, 792
lurasidone, 230*t*, 237, 619
Lutera, 514*t*, 516
Luvox, 213*t*, 216–217
Luxiq, 99*t*
Lyrica, 170*t*, 179, 180*t*
lysergic acid diethylamide (LSD), 35*t*
Lysteda, 523, 523*t*
Lyumjev, 476*t*, 481*t*, 482
Lyza, 514*t*, 516

M

Maalox, 411*t*, 434*t*
Macrobid, 65*f*, 544, 589*t*, 594
Macrodantin, 544, 589*t*, 594
macrolides, 587, 601, 602, 612, 720
magnesium, 746, 747
magnesium carbonate, 411*t*
magnesium gluconate, 746
magnesium hydroxide, 411*t*, 433*t*, 434*t*, 437
magnesium oxide, 746
magnesium sulfate, 433*t*, 524*t*, 526, 746
Maltsupex, 433*t*, 435
maprotiline, 90*t*
maraviroc, 645*t*, 656
marijuana, 35*t*
Marlissa, 514*t*, 516
Marqibo, 777*t*
Matulane, 775*t*
Matzim LA, 290*t*
Mavenclad, 192*t*, 193, 194*t*

Mavik, 289*t*
Mavyret, 450*t*, 454
Maxalt, 717*t*, 718
Maxalt-MLT, 717*t*, 718
MAX Care-Pak, 471, 471*t*
Maxipime, 591*t*, 597
Maxitrol, 271*t*
Maxzide, 553*t*, 558
Mayzent, 192*t*, 194, 194*t*
measles, mumps, rubella (MMR), 669
mechlorethamine, 775*t*, 781
meclizine, 444*t*
Medrol, 419*t*, 471, 471*t*
Medrol DosePak, 471*t*
medroxyprogesterone, 500*t*, 521
mefloquine, 595
Mefoxin, 590*t*
meglitinides, 487, 488
melatonin, 255
Mellaril, 72*t*
meloxicam, 125*t*, 127
melphalan, 775*t*, 782
memantine, 196*t*, 197
Menostar, 500*t*, 501*t*, 504
Mentax, 103*t*, 105, 617*t*, 621
meperidine, 35*t*, 268*t*
Mephyton, 78*t*, 323*t*, 329
mepivacaine, 700*t*, 714
mepolizumab, 350*t*, 355
meprobamate, 35*t*
mercaptopurine, 423, 776*t*, 782
meropenem, 591*t*, 599
Merrem, 591*t*, 599
mesalamine, 420*t*, 421
Mestinon, 202, 202*t*, 711*t*, 712
Metadate CD, 199*t*
Metamucil, 433*t*, 435
metaproterenol, 349*t*, 351
Metaxall, 147*t*, 148*t*, 150*t*
metaxalone, 147*t*, 148*t*, 150*t*
metformin, 477*t*, 478*t*, 485–486, 486
methadone, 438, 602, 619, 682*t*, 684*t*, 685, 689, 690, 694, 695*t*, 696
Methadose, 682*t*, 689, 695*t*, 696
methazolamide, 266*t*
methicillin, 596
methimazole, 467*t*, 470, 471
methocarbamol, 147*t*, 148*t*, 150*t*
methohexital, 699*t*, 708
methotrexate, 90*t*, 98, 132, 132*t*, 133, 134*t*, 136*t*, 563, 776*t*, 779*t*, 780, 782, 783, 784
methoxyflurane, 418
methylcellulose, 433*t*, 435
methylergometrine, 619
Methylin, 199*t*
methylnaltrexone, 434*t*
methylphenidate extended release, 199*t*
methylphenidate immediate release, 199*t*
methylprednisolone, 419*t*, 420, 471, 471*t*, 518*t*
metipranolol, 265*t*
metoclopramide, 445*t*, 448, 718*t*, 721

metoclopromide, 721
metolazone, 90*t*, 268*t*, 553*t*, 558
metoprolol, 290*t*, 295, 296, 568
MetroCream, 92, 93*t*, 593*t*, 606, 613, 614*t*
MetroGel, 92, 93*t*, 593*t*, 606, 613, 614*t*
MetroGel Vaginal, 613, 614*t*
MetroLotion, 92, 93*t*, 593*t*, 606
metronidazole, 92, 93*t*, 329*t*, 587, 593*t*, 606, 614*t*, 654
Mevacor, 314*t*
mexiletine, 300, 300*t*, 301*t*
Mexitil, 300*t*
Micaderm, 103*t*, 106
micafungin, 617*t*, 619
Micardis, 289*t*, 292, 292*t*
Micatin, 103*t*, 106, 616*t*, 618
miconazole, 103*t*, 106, 616*t*
miconozole, 618
midazolam, 49*t*, 649, 653, 654, 655, 699*t*, 708
mifepristone, 521, 522, 570
Migranal, 717*t*, 719, 720
Mili, 514*t*, 516
milnacipran, 214*t*, 219–220
Mimvey, 500*t*, 505
Minitran, 307*t*, 308
Minivelle, 500*t*, 501*t*, 504
Minocin, 592*t*
minocycline, 592*t*, 604
mirabegron, 546*t*, 547
MiraLax, 433*t*, 437
Mirapex, 185*t*, 187, 204
Mirapex ER, 185*t*, 187, 204
Mircette, 514*t*, 516
Mirena, 515*t*, 522
mirtazapine, 214*t*, 222–223
Mirvaso, 93*t*, 95
misoprostol, 412*t*, 415, 524*t*, 526, 527
Mitigare, 138*t*, 139
Mitigo, 682*t*, 690, 691, 696
mitoxantrone, 192*t*, 193, 194*t*, 777*t*, 785
Mobic, 125*t*, 127
modafinil, 245*t*, 248
Moderiba, 450*t*, 452
moexipril, 289*t*
molidone, 230*t*
mometasone, 349*t*, 352, 381*t*, 390
mometasone-formoterol, 350*t*, 360*t*, 365
mometasone furoate, 99*t*
Monistat, 616*t*, 618
monobactam, 599
Mono-Linyah, 514*t*, 516
montelukast, 50*t*, 350*t*, 354
Monurol, 544
morphine, 4, 33*f*, 35*t*, 268*t*, 682*t*, 683, 684*t*, 685, 690, 691, 696, 698*t*
morphine milligram equivalents (MME), 683
Motofen, 426*t*, 428
Motrin, 124*t*, 127–128
MoviPrep, 434*t*, 439–440
Moxatag, 589*t*, 596
Moxeza, 271*t*, 273, 593*t*, 611*t*

moxifloxacin, 271*t*, 273, 593*t*, 595, 611*t*, 792
MS Contin, 682*t*, 690, 696
mtronidazole, 613
Mucinex, 378*t*, 383
Mucinex D, 379*t*
Mucinex DM, 378*t*378*t*
Mucomyst, 126, 367
Multaq, 300*t*, 302, 303*t*
mupirocin, 103*t*, 104
Murine, 275*t*
Muse, 508*t*, 509
Mustargen, 775*t*, 781
Mycamine, 617*t*, 619
My Choice, 515*t*, 518
Mycitracin Triple Antibiotic, 103*t*, 104
mycophenolate, 521, 522, 566, 569, 570
mycophenolate mofetil, 569, 569*t*
mycophenolic acid, 569, 569*t*, 570
Mydayis, 199*t*
Myfortic, 569, 569*t*
Mylanta, 411*t*, 434*t*
Mylanta Maximum Strength, 434*t*
Myleran, 775*t*
Myorisan, 93*t*, 94
Myrbetriq, 546*t*, 547
Mysoline, 170*t*, 179, 180*t*
My Way, 515*t*, 518
Myxredlin, 476*t*, 481*t*, 482

N

nabumetone, 125*t*, 127
N-acetylcysteine, 367
nadolol, 290*t*, 295
nafcillin, 589*t*
nalbuphine, 683*t*, 692, 693
naloxone, 683*t*, 695*t*, 696, 711, 711*t*
naltrexone, 253*t*, 255, 683*t*, 693, 695*t*, 697, 752*t*, 754
Namenda, 196*t*, 197
Namzaric, 196, 196*t*
Naprelan, 125*t*, 127
Naprosyn, 125*t*, 127
naproxen, 78*t*, 125*t*, 127, 417*t*, 717*t*, 719
naproxen-esomeprazole, 128
naproxen-pseudoephedrine, 379*t*
naratriptan, 717*t*, 718
Narcan, 696, 711*t*, 712
Nardil, 214*t*, 223
Naropin, 700*t*, 714
Nasacort Allergy 24 HR, 381*t*, 390
Nasonex, 381*t*, 390
natalizumab, 192*t*, 193, 194*t*, 423, 570
Natazia, 501*t*, 523, 523*t*
nateglinide, 478*t*, 487
Nature-Throid, 467*t*, 469
Navelbine, 777*t*, 787
nebivolol, 290*t*, 296
necitumumab, 795*t*, 797
Necon, 514*t*, 516
nefazodone, 316, 551
nelarabine, 776*t*
nelfinavir, 645*t*, 654

neomycin-polymyxin B-dexamethasone, 271*t*
neomycin-polymyxin B-hydrocortisone, 275*t*
Neoral, 78*t*, 569, 569*t*
Neosporin, 103*t*, 104
Neosporin AF, 103*t*, 106
neostigmine, 711*t*, 712
Neo-Synephrine, 379*t*, 386
nephrotoxic drugs, 543
neratinib, 794*t*, 797
Nerlynx, 794*t*, 797
Nesacaine, 700*t*, 714
Neupro, 185*t*, 187, 204
Neurontin, 170*t*, 178, 180*t*, 204
neutral protamine hagedorn (NPH) insulin, 481*t*, 482
Neutrogena, 93*t*, 95
nevirapine, 644*t*, 651, 654, 657
New Day, 515*t*, 518
Nexavar, 794*t*, 795
Nexium, 411*t*, 414, 418*t*
Nexletol, 315*t*, 318
Nexlizet, 315
Nexplanon, 515*t*, 521
Nexterone, 300*t*, 302, 303*t*
niacin, 732*t*, 735, 736, 759*t*
nicardipine, 289*t*, 294
Nicoderm CQ, 393*t*
Nicorette, 393*t*
nicotine, 393*t*
Nicotrol, 393*t*
Nifediac, 289*t*
nifedipine, 49*t*, 78*t*, 289*t*, 294, 524*t*, 526
Nikki, 514*t*, 516
Nilandron, 790*t*, 791
nilotinib, 795*t*, 798
nilutamide, 790*t*, 791
Nimbex, 699*t*
nisoldipine, 289*t*, 619
nitazoxanide, 426*t*, 430
Nitro-Bid, 307*t*, 308
Nitro-Dur, 307*t*, 308
nitrofurantoin, 544, 589*t*, 594
nitrofurantoin monohydrate, 65*f*
nitroglycerin, 67*f*, 78*t*, 142–143, 307*t*, 308, 442*t*, 443., 508, 509
nitroimidazole, 606
Nitrolingual, 307*t*, 308
NitroMist, 307*t*, 308
nitrosourea, 781
Nitrostat, 78*t*, 307*t*, 308
Nitro-Time, 307*t*, 308
nitrous oxide, 698*t*
nivolumab, 802*t*, 803
Nix, 108*t*, 110
nizatidine, 411*t*, 412, 413
Nizoral, 103*t*, 106, 616*t*, 618
Nolvadex, 790, 790*t*
nonnucleoside reverse transcriptase inhibitors (NNRTIs), 643, 648
nonsteroidal anti-inflammatory drugs (NSAIDs), 124*t*–125*t*, 126–129, 543, 603

Nora-Be, 514*t*, 516
Norcuron, 699*t*
norelgestromin, 519
norepinephrine, 510
norfloxacin, 595
Noritate, 92, 93*t*
Noritate Cream, 593*t*, 606
Norlyda, 514*t*, 516
Norlyroc, 514*t*, 516
normal saline (NS), 620
Norpace, 300, 300*t*, 301*t*
Norpramin, 214*t*
Nortrel, 514*t*, 516
nortriptyline, 214*t*
Norvasc, 289*t*
Norvir, 78*t*, 645*t*, 654
Nourianz, 186*t*, 191
Novantron, 192*t*, 193, 194*t*
Novantrone, 777*t*, 785
Novolin 70/30, 476*t*, 481*t*
Novolin 70/30 Flexpen, 476*t*, 481*t*
Novolin N, 481*t*
Novolin R, 476*t*, 481*t*, 482
Novolin 70/30 Relion, 476*t*, 481*t*
Novolin R Flexpen, 476*t*, 481*t*, 482
Novolin R Relion, 476*t*, 481*t*, 482
NovoLog, 476*t*, 481*t*, 482
Novolog 70/30, 477*t*, 481*t*
NovoLog Mix 70/30, 476*t*, 481*t*, 482
Noxafil, 617*t*, 618
Nubeqa, 790*t*, 791
Nucala, 350*t*, 355
nucleotide, 782
NuCort, 98*t*
Nucynta, 683*t*, 686, 691
NuLYTELY, 434*t*, 439–440
Nuplazid, 231*t*, 238
NuPrep, 111*t*, 112
Nurtec, 717*t*, 720
NuvaRing, 515*t*, 520
Nuvessa, 593*t*, 606, 613, 614*t*
Nuvigil, 245*t*, 249
Nyamyc, 617*t*
nystatin, 617*t*, 620, 621
Nystop, 617*t*

O

obinutuzumab, 796
Ocella, 514*t*, 516
Ocuflox, 271*t*, 273, 611*t*
Ocuvite, 277
ofatumumab, 796
ofloxacin, 271*t*, 273, 275*t*, 611*t*
olanzapine, 230*t*, 237–238, 267*t*
olaparib, 649
olmesartan, 289*t*, 292, 292*t*
olodaterol, 360*t*, 364
olopatadine, 380*t*, 389
Olux, 99*t*
Olysio, 450*t*, 455
omalizumab, 350*t*, 355
ombitasvir-paritaprevir, 450*t*, 454–455
omega-3 fatty acid, 315*t*, 319

omeprazole, 5t, 411t, 413, 414, 418t
omeprazole/sodium, 411t
omeprazole/sodium bicarbonate, 414
Omnaris, 381t, 390
Omnitrope, 528, 528t
Oncovin, 777t, 785, 787
ondansetron, 444t, 446
Onglyza, 477t, 485
Onivyde, 777t, 785
Onmel, 616t
Onzetra Xsail, 717t, 719
Opcicon One-Step, 515t, 518
Opdivo, 802t, 803
opiates, 681
opioids, 684, 693
OptiPranolol, 265t
Oracea, 592t, 604
oral midazolam, 619
oral typhoid, 669
Oramorph, 682t, 696
Orap, 230t
Orapred ODT, 471t
Oravig, 616t, 618
Orkambi, 368t, 370
orlistat, 469, 752, 752t
orphenadrine, 147t, 148t, 150t, 511
Orsythia, 514t, 516
Ortho- Micronor, 514t, 516
oseltamivir, 636t, 639, 640
osimertinib, 794t, 797
Osmolex ER, 186t, 191
osteomalacia, 733
Otiprio, 275t, 593t
oxacillin, 590t
oxaliplatin, 775t, 779t, 781–782
Oxaydo, 682t, 686, 691
oxazepam, 241t, 243
oxazolidinone, 607
oxcarbazepine, 170t, 172t, 173, 519, 651, 657
oxcarbazine, 78t
Oxtellar XR, 170t, 172t, 173
Oxy, 93t, 95
Oxy 10, 92, 93t
oxybutynin, 546, 546t
oxycodone, 35t, 268t, 681, 682t, 684t, 686, 691
OxyCONTIN, 682t, 686, 691
oxymorphone, 268t
oxytocin, 524t, 527
Oxytrol, 546, 546t
Ozempic, 477t, 484

P

Pacerone, 300t, 302, 303t
paclitaxel, 777t, 780t, 787, 788
paclitaxel albumin bound, 777t, 788
palbociclib, 790t, 793
paliperidone, 231t, 239
palivizumab, 636t, 641
palonosetron, 444t, 446
Pamelor, 214t
pancrealipase, 78t

Pancreaze, 78t
pancuronium, 699t
Pandel, 99t
panitumumab, 795t, 797
PanOxyl, 92, 93t
pantoprazole, 5, 411t, 414, 418t
pantothenic acid, 732t, 736
Paragard, 515t
paraldehyde, 511
Paraplatin, 775t, 781–782
parathyroid carcinomas, 567
Parlodel, 185t, 187
Parnate, 214t, 223
paroxetine, 213t, 217, 241t
Pataday, 380t, 389
Patanase, 380t, 389
Patanol, 380t, 389
pathogens, 587, 595
Pavulon, 699t
Paxil, 213t, 217, 241t
pazopanib, 413, 455, 505, 506, 511, 570, 794t, 795
Pediapred, 471t
Pediazole, 592t
Pegasys, 450t, 451–452
peginterferon, 452
peginterferon alfa-2a, 450t, 451–452
pellagra, 736
pembrolizumab, 802t, 803
pemetrexed, 776t, 783
pemetrexedv, 779t
penicillin, 25, 518t, 587, 588, 595, 602, 610t, 612
penicillin G, 589t
penicillin G benzathine, 596, 614t
penicillin V potassium, 589t
Penlac, 103t, 105, 617t, 621
Pennsaid, 124t, 127
Pentasa, 420t, 421
Pepcid, 411t, 412
Pepcid AC, 411t, 412
Pepcid Complete, 411t, 412
Pepto-Bismol, 426–427, 426t
peramivir, 636t, 640
perampanel, 170t, 181, 182t
Perforomist, 360t, 364
perindopril, 289t
Perjeta, 794t, 796
permethrin, 108, 108t, 110
perphenazine, 230t
Persantine, 72t
pertussis, 664t
pertussis vaccine, 668
pertuzumab, 794t, 796
Pexeva, 217, 241t
Pfizerpen, 589t
P-glycoprotine, 455
phenazopyridine, 544t, 545
phendimetrazine, 752t, 753
phenelzine, 214t, 223
Phenergan, 444t, 447–448
Phenobarbital, 49t
phenobarbital, 35t, 170t, 179, 180t, 455, 487, 518t, 564, 650, 651, 657, 693

phenothiazines, 90t, 447
phentermine, 752t, 753
phenylephrine, 379t, 386
Phenytek, 170t
phenytoin, 170t, 172t, 174–176, 329t, 455, 469, 473, 487, 518t, 521, 522, 564, 568, 650, 651, 657
Philith, 514t, 516
Phillips' Milk of Magnesia, 411t, 433t, 437
PhosLo, 745
Phoslyra, 745
phosphate, 747
phosphodiesterase inhibitors, 509
phylloquinone, 732t, 734
phytoestrogen, 529
phytonadione, 323t, 329, 732t, 734, 759t
phytondione, 78t
Pifeltro, 644t, 649
pimavanserin, 231t, 238
pimecrolimus, 98t, 100, 570
pimozide, 230t, 413, 568, 570, 602, 619, 649, 653, 654, 655
Pimtrea, 514t, 516
pioglitazone, 478t, 488
piperacillin, 590t
Piqray, 795t, 800
Pirmella, 514t, 516
piroxicam, 125t, 127, 128
pitavastatin, 314t, 316, 570
Pitocin, 524t
pitolisant, 245t, 249
Plan B One-Step, 518
Plaquenil, 132, 132t, 134t, 135t
Platinol, 775t, 781
Plavix, 323t
Plendil, 289t
Plexion, 93t, 96
Plexion Cleanser, 93t, 96
pneumococcal, 664t
Pneumovax 23, 664t
Podactin, 103t, 106
Polocaine, 700t, 714
polycarbophil, 433t, 435
polyethylene glycol 3350, 433t, 434t, 437, 439–440
polyvalent, 664t
pomalidomide, 794t, 795
Pomalyst, 794t, 795
ponatinib, 795t, 798
Pontocaine, 700t, 714
poractant alfa, 372, 373t
Portia, 514t, 516
Portrazza, 795t, 797
posaconazole, 617t, 618
post-attachment inhibitors (PAIs), 643
potassium acetate, 744
potassium chloride, 744
potassium phosphate, 744
potassium-sparing diuretics, 570
povidone-iodine, 111t, 112
PPIs, 651
Pradaxa, 78t, 322t, 324
pramipexole, 185t, 187, 204

pramlintide, 477t, 484
prasugrel, 78t, 323t, 331
Pravachol, 314t
pravastatin, 314t, 316
pravastatin-buffered aspirin, 315
Pravigard PAC, 315
Pravix, 330
Praxbind, 323t, 325
Precedex, 698t, 707
Pred Forte, 268, 269t
Pred-G, 271t
Pred Mild, 269t
prednicarbate, 99t
prednisolone, 268, 269t, 471t, 518t
prednisone, 138, 420, 471, 471t, 518t,
    785, 785t
Prednisone Intensol, 471, 471t
Prefest, 500t, 505, 506
pregabalin, 170t, 179, 180t
Premphase, 500t, 505
Prempro, 500t, 505
Prepidil, 524t, 526
Prevacid, 411t, 414, 418t
Prevalite, 314t
Preventeza, 515t, 518
Previfem, 514t, 516
Prevnar, 664t
Prevpac, 418
Prezista, 645t, 652
Priftin, 373t, 375
prilocaine, 700t, 714
Prilosec, 5t, 411t, 414, 418t
Prilosec OTC, 411t, 414
Primaxin, 591t, 599
primidone, 170t, 179, 180t, 487, 518t,
    564, 650, 651, 657
Prinivil, 289t
Prinzide, 553t, 558
Pristiq, 213t, 218
ProAir, 349t, 351
probenecid, 138t, 140
Probuphine, 683t, 692, 693, 695t
procainamide, 300t, 301t, 595
procarbazine, 90t, 775t
Procardia, 78t, 289t, 524t, 526
Procardia XL, 289t
prochlorperazine, 230t, 444t, 447,
    718t, 721
Procrit, 560, 560t
Pro-Ex, 103t, 106
progesterone, 519, 528
Prograf, 569, 569t
Prolastin-C, 366
Prolia, 142t, 144
Promethazien DM, 378t
promethazine, 444t, 447–448
promethazine-codeine, 378t
promethazine-dextromethorphan, 378t
Prometh DM, 378t
Prometrium, 500t, 501t, 505
Prontosil, 25
propafenone, 300, 300t, 301t, 655
Propecia, 548t, 550
propofol, 698t, 706

propranolol, 50t, 290t, 295
propylene glycol, 268
propylthiouracil (PTU), 467t, 470, 471
Proscar, 548t, 550
Prostaglandin E1 analogs, 415
prostaglandins, 678
Prostin E2, 524t, 526
protamine sulfate, 323t, 327
protease inhibitors (PIs), 643, 651
Protonix, 5, 411t, 414, 418t
Protopic, 98t, 100
protozoan, 429
Proventil, 349t, 351
Provera, 515t, 521
Provigil, 245t, 248
Prozac, 213t, 216
Pseudodine, 379t
pseudoephedrine, 379t, 385
pseudohypoparathyroidism, 567
Psorion, 99t
psyllium, 433t, 435
Pulmicort, 349t, 352
Pulmozyme, 367, 368t, 369
Purinethol, 776t, 782
Pylera, 417–418, 418
pyrazinamide, 373t, 375
pyrethrin, 108t, 110
Pyridium, 544t, 545
pyridostigmine, 202, 202t, 711t, 712
pyridoxamine, 736
pyridoxine, 732t, 736, 759t
pyrithione zinc, 99t, 102

Q

Qbrelis, 289t
Qternmet XR, 478t
QT prolongation, 595
Quartette, 514t, 516
quazepam, 245t, 250–251
Qudexy XR, 171t, 181, 182t
Quelicin, 699t, 709
Questran, 314t
Questran Light, 314t
quetiapine, 231t, 238
Quillichew ER, 199t
Quillivant XR, 199t
quinapril, 289t
quinidine, 90t, 300t, 301t, 595, 619,
    655, 792
quinolones, 90t, 566, 605, 606
Quixin, 271t, 273
Quoliana, 267t
QVAR, 349t, 352
Qysmia, 752t, 753

R

rabeprazole, 412t, 414, 418t
raloxifene, 142t, 143, 469
raltegravir, 645t, 658
ramelteon, 245t, 250
ramipril, 289t
ramucirumab, 794t, 795, 796

Ranexa, 307t, 309–310
Ranitidine, 50t
ranolazine, 290t, 307t, 309–310, 619
Rapivab, 636t, 640
rasagiline, 185t, 189
Rayos, 471, 471t
Razadyne, 196, 196t
Razadyne ER, 196, 196t
R-CHOP, 784
React, 515t, 518
Rebetol, 450t, 452
Rebif, 192, 192t
Reclast, 142, 142t
Reclipsen, 514t, 516
Recombivax HB, 449
Rectiv, 142–143, 307t, 308, 442t
refapentine, 455
Refissa, 93t, 95
Refresh, 268, 269t
Reglan, 445t, 448, 718t, 721
Regonol, 711t, 712
regorafenib, 794t
Regranex, 478t, 489
regular insulin, 476t
regular insulin U-100, 481t, 482
regular insulin U-500, 476t, 481t, 482
Relafen, 125t, 127
Relenza, 636t, 640
Relistor, 434t
Relpax, 717t, 718
Remeron, 214t, 222–223
Remicade, 132, 132t, 135t, 137t
remifentanil, 699t
Renagel, 565t, 566
renin, 539
Renova, 93t, 95
Renvela, 565t, 566
ReoPro, 324t, 332
Requip, 185t, 187, 204
Requip XL, 185t, 187, 204
Rescriptor, 644t, 648
Rescula, 265t
reserpine, 72t
reslizumab, 350t, 355
Restasis, 269, 269t
Restoril, 245t, 250–251
Retacrit, 560, 560t
retapamulin, 103t, 105
Retavase, 324t
reticulocyte, 560
Retin-A, 93t, 95
retinol, 732t, 759t
Retrovir, 644t, 648
Revatio, 508, 508t
revefenacin, 359t, 362
ReVia, 253t, 255
Revlimid, 794t, 795
Revonto, 147t, 148t, 150t, 700t, 713
Rexulti, 230t, 234–235
Reyataz, 645t, 652
Rheumatrex, 132, 132t, 134t, 136t
Rhinocort Aqua, 380t, 390
Ribasphere, 450t, 452
Ribasphere RibaPak, 450t, 452

ribavirin, 450t, 452, 636t, 641, 642, 647
ribociclib, 790t, 793
riboflavin, 732t, 735, 759t
RID, 108t, 110
Ridaura, 132t, 134t, 135t
rifabutin, 455
Rifadin, 373t, 375
rifampin, 329t, 373t, 375, 455, 469,
    473, 487, 518t, 619, 649, 653,
    654, 655
rifamycin, 551, 570, 649, 650, 651
rifapentine, 373t, 375
rifaximin, 426t, 430
rilpivirine, 645t, 649, 651
Rilutek, 203
riluzole, 203
Rimactane, 373t, 375
rimegepant, 717t, 720
Rinvoq, 132t, 133, 135t, 137t
Riomet, 477t, 485
Riomet ER, 477t, 485
risedronate, 142, 142t, 413
Risk Evaluation and Mitigation Strategy
    (REMS), 688
RisperDAL, 231t, 239
risperidone, 231t, 239, 267t
Ritalin, 199t
Ritalin LA, 199t
ritonavir, 78t, 450t, 454–455, 455, 549,
    557, 645t, 653, 654, 655
ritonavir plus tenofovir, 661
Rituxan, 785, 795t, 796
rituximab, 785, 785t, 795t, 796,
    797, 798
rivaroxaban, 323t, 327, 327t, 505, 506
rivastigmine, 196, 196t
Rivelsa, 514t, 516
rizatriptan, 717t, 718
Robaxin, 147t, 148t, 150t
Robitussin, 378t
Rocaltrol, 565t, 567
Rocephin, 591t, 597, 613, 614t
rocuronium, 699t
Roflumilast, 366
Rolaids, 411t
Romazicon, 711t, 711t
romosozumab, 142t, 144
Romycin Ophthalmic, 271t
ropinirole, 185t, 187, 204
ropivacaine, 700t, 714
Rosadan, 92, 93t
rosiglitazone, 478t, 488
rosuvastatin, 314t, 329t
Rotarix, 664t
rotavirus, 664t
rotigotine, 185t, 187, 204
Roweepra, 171t, 182, 183t
Roxicodone, 682t, 686, 691
Rozerem, 245t, 250
rufinamide, 170t, 172t, 174
Ryanodex, 147t, 148t, 150t, 700t, 713
Rybelsus, 477t, 484
Rytary, 185t, 186
Rythmol, 300, 300t, 301t

S

Sabril, 170t, 172t, 176–177
sacubitril-valsartan, 311, 311t
safinamide, 185t, 190
Safyral, 516
Saint-John′s-wort, 455
Saizen, 528, 528t
salicylates, 151–154, 152t, 154t
salicylic acid, 93t, 95
Salix alba, 155
salmeterol, 360t, 364
salsalate, 152, 152t, 157t
Salvarsan, 25
Sanctura, 546, 546t
Sandimmune, 78t, 569, 569t
Saphris, 230t, 234
sapropterin, 78t
Saquinavir, 50t
Sarafem, 213t, 216
sargramostim, 49t
Savaysa, 323t, 327
Savella, 214t, 219–220
saxagliptin, 477t, 478t, 485
Saxenda, 752t, 753
Scopace, 444t
scopolamine, 444t, 547
Seasonique, 514t, 516
Sectral, 290t, 296
Segluromet, 477t
selective serotonin reuptake inhibitor
    (SSRI), 690
selegiline, 185t, 189, 214t, 223
selenium sulfide, 99t, 102
SelRex, 99t
Selsun Blue, 99t, 102
Selzentry, 645t, 656
semaglutide, 477t, 484
Semglee, 481t, 482
senna, 434t, 438
Senokot-S, 433t, 436
Sensipar, 565t, 567
Septra, 589t, 593, 610t
Septra DS, 589t, 593
Serevent, 360t, 364
Sernivo, 99t
Seroquel, 231t, 238
Seroquel XR, 231t, 238
Serostim, 528, 528t
serotonin, 510, 686
sertaconazole, 103t, 106
sertraline, 90t, 213t, 217–218, 241t
Setlakin, 514t, 516
sevelamer, 469, 565t, 566
sevelamer hydrochloride, 566
sevoflurane, 698t, 704
Sharobel, 514t, 516
sildenafil, 49t, 508, 508t, 653, 654, 655
Silenor, 214t, 221–222
silodosin, 505, 506, 511, 570
Silvadene, 90t, 91
silver nitrate, 4, 5t
silver sulfadiazine, 90t, 91
simeprevir, 450t, 455, 506, 570, 649

simethicone, 49, 411t, 434t, 439
Similiya, 516
Simpesse, 514t, 516
Simponi, 132, 132t, 135t, 137t
Simponi Aria, 132, 132t, 137t
simvastatin, 50t, 90t, 314t, 316, 329t,
    570, 602, 619, 653, 654, 655
Sinemet, 185t, 186
Singulair, 350t, 354
siponimod, 192t, 194, 194t
sirolimus, 570
sitagliptin, 477t, 478t, 485
Sitavig, 103t, 107, 635t, 636t, 637
Skelaxin, 147t, 148t, 150t
Sklice, 108t, 110
Skyla, 515t, 522
Slow Iron, 561
sodium bicarbonate, 748, 749, 749t
Sodium Diuril, 553t, 558
Sodium Edecrin, 553t, 554
sodium ferric gluconate, 560t, 561, 561t,
    562, 563
sodium hypochlorite, 111t, 112
sodium phosphate, 434t
Sodium Sulamyd, 271t
sodium sulfacetamide / sulfur, 93t, 96
sofosbuvir, 450t, 452–453, 455
Solaraze, 127
solifenacin, 546, 546t, 619
Solodyn, 592t
SoloStar, 476t
solriamfetol, 245t, 250
Solu-Cortef, 419t, 471t
Solu-Medrol, 419t, 471, 471t
Soma, 147t, 148t, 149t
somatotropin, 50t, 505, 528
somatropin, 528, 529
Sonata, 245t, 247
Soolantra, 108t, 110
Soothe, 268, 269t
sorafenib, 794t, 795
Sorilux, 98t, 101
Sorine, 290t, 295
sotalol, 90t, 290t, 295, 595
Sotylize, 290t, 295
Sovaldi, 450t, 452–453
Spectracef, 591t, 597
Spiriva HandiHaler, 359t, 363
Spiriva Respimat, 359t
spironolactone, 553t, 556, 557
Sporanox, 374t, 616t, 618
Sprintec, 514t, 516
Spritam, 171t, 182, 183t
Sprycel, 795t, 798
Sronyx, 514t, 516
SSD, 90t, 91
Stalevo, 185t
Starlix, 478t, 487
statins, 652
stavudine, 644t, 647, 648
Staxyn, 508, 508t
Steglatro, 478t, 487
Stelara, 420t, 422–423
Stendra, 508, 508t

Sterapred, 420
Stiolto Respimat, 360t, 366
Stivarga, 794t
St. John's wort, 256
Strattera, 199t, 200
Stribild, 643, 660, 660t
Stridex, 93t, 95
Striverdi Respimat, 360t, 364
Styrofoam, 569
Sublocade, 683t, 692, 693, 695t
Suboxone, 695t
Subsys, 682t, 687
succinylcholine, 699t, 709
sucralfate, 412t, 415
Sucrets, 700t, 714
Sudafed, 379t, 385
Sudafed 12 Hour Pressure/Pain, 379t
Sudafed PE, 379t, 386
Sufenta, 699t, 705
sufentanil, 699t, 705
Sular, 289t
sulbactam, 590t
sulfacetamide, 271t, 272, 611t
sulfacetamide-fluorometholone, 271t
sulfacetamide-prednisolone, 272t
Sulfacleanse, 93t, 96
sulfadoxine, 564
sulfa drugs, 588
sulfamethoxazole, 329t, 544, 589t, 593, 594, 610t
Sulfamez Wash, 93t, 96
sulfas, 25, 90t
sulfasalazine, 132, 132t, 133, 134t, 136t, 420t, 421–422, 564
Sulfatrim, 544, 610t
Sulfazine, 420t, 421–422
sulfonamides, 587
sulfonylurea, 487
sulfonylureas, 90t, 487, 488
Sumadan, 93t, 96
Sumadan Wash, 93t, 96
sumatriptan, 50t, 78t, 717t, 719
Sumavel DosePro, 717t, 719
Sumaxin, 93t, 96
Sumaxin CP, 93t, 96
sunitinib, 795
Sunosi, 245t, 250
Suprane, 698t, 703
Suprax, 591t, 597, 610t
Surfak, 433t, 436
Survanta, 371, 373t
Sustiva, 644t, 649
sutent, 795
suvorexant, 649
Syeda, 514t, 516
Symbicort, 350t, 360t
Symdeko, 368t, 370
Symfi, 660t
Symfi Lo, 660t
SymlinPen, 477t, 484
Symmetrel, 186t, 191
Symtuza, 660, 660t
Synagis, 636t, 641
Synalar, 99t

Synapryn, 683t, 686, 692
Synjardy, 477t
Synjardy XR, 477t
Synthroid, 467t, 468
Systane, 268, 269t

T
Tabloid, 776t, 782
tacrolimus, 98t, 100, 566, 569, 569t, 570, 595
tadalafil, 508, 508t
tafluprost, 265t
Tagamet, 411t, 412
Tagamet HB, 411t, 412
Tagrisso, 794t, 797
Take Action, 515t, 518
Tambocor, 300, 300t, 301t
Tamiflu, 636t, 639
tamoxifen, 49t, 329t, 568, 790, 790t, 791
tamsulosin, 548t, 549, 550, 551
Tapazole, 467t, 470
tapentadol, 683t, 686, 691, 692
TaperDex, 471, 471t
Tarceva, 794t, 797
Tasigna, 795t, 798
Tasmar, 185t, 189
Tatzia XT, 290t
Tavist, 380t, 387
Tavist Allergy, 387
taxanes, 787, 788
Taxol, 777t, 787
Taxotere, 777t, 787
tazarotene, 93t, 94
Tazicef, 591t, 597
tazobactam, 590t
Tazorac, 93t, 94
Tears, 268, 269t
Tecentriq, 802t, 803
Tecfidera, 192t, 193, 194t
Teflaro, 591t, 597
Tegretol, 9, 170t, 171t, 173, 227t, 228
Tekturna, 78t, 296
telbuvidine, 78t
telithromycin, 619
telmisartan, 289t, 292, 292t
temazepam, 245t, 250–251
Temodar, 775t
Temovate, 99t
temozolomide, 775t
temsirolimus, 570
tenecteplase, 324t
Tenex, 200
tenofovir, 78t, 453, 644t, 647, 659, 660, 660t
tenofovir alafenamide, 450t, 644t, 645t, 647, 660, 660t
tenofovir disoproxil fumarate, 450t, 644t, 660, 660t
Tenoretic, 553t, 558
Tenormin, 290t, 295
terazosin, 50t, 548t, 549
Terbinafine, 50t
terbinafine, 103t, 105, 106, 617t, 621, 622

teriflunomide, 192t, 194, 194t
teriparatide, 142t, 144
Tessalon, 378t, 382
Testopel, 500t, 501t, 502
testosterone, 550
tetanus, 664t, 668
tetrabenazine, 203–204
tetracaine, 700t, 714
tetracyclic antidepressants, 214t, 222–223
tetracyclines, 90t, 518t, 587, 592t, 604, 610t, 614t
tetracyclines chelate, 604
Teveten, 289t, 292t
Texacort, 98t
tezacaftor-ivacaftor, 368t, 370
T/Gel Daily Control, 99t, 102
thalidomide, 511, 794t, 795, 796
Thalomid, 794t, 795
Theo-24, 351t, 356
Theochron, 351t, 356
theophylline, 50t, 351t, 356, 469, 518t, 606
thiamine, 732t, 759t
thiazides, 90t, 556, 558, 559
thiazolidinediones (TZDs), 475, 488
thioguanine, 776t, 782
thioridazine, 72t, 230t, 413, 568
Thorazine, 72t
thyroid desiccated, 467t, 469
thyroxine, 527
Tiadylt ER, 290t
tiagabine, 170t, 179, 180t
Tiazac, 290t
ticagrelor, 323t, 331, 619
ticarcillin, 49t, 590t
tigecycline, 604
Tiglutik, 203
Tikosyn, 300t, 302, 303t
timolol, 265t, 290t, 295
Timoptic, 265t
Timoptic GFS, 265t
Timoptic XE, 265t
Tinactin, 103t, 106
tioconazole, 617t
tiotropium, 359t, 363
tiotropium-olodaterol, 360t, 366
tipranavir, 455, 645t, 655
tirofiban, 324t, 332
Tirosint, 467t, 468
Tivicay, 645t, 657
Tivorbex, 127, 524t, 526
tizanidine, 147t, 148t, 150t
Tobi, 368t, 369
Tobi Podhaler, 368t, 369
TobraDex, 272t
Tobradol, 147t
Tobradol FusePaq, 148t, 149t
Tobradol RapidPaq, 147t, 148t, 149t
tobramycin, 271t, 272, 368t, 369, 592t, 611t
tobramycin-dexamethasone, 272t
Tobrex, 271t, 272, 592t, 611t
tocolytic agent, 526

tocopherol, 732t, 734, 759t
tofacitinib, 423, 570
Tofranil, 214t, 221–222
tolcapone, 185t, 189
tolnaftate, 103t, 106
Tolsura, 374t
tolterodine, 546, 546t
tolvaptan, 50t, 649
Topamax, 171t, 181, 182t
Topicaine, 90, 90t
Topicort, 99t
TopiDex, 471, 471t
topiramate, 171t, 181, 182t, 752t, 753
topotecan, 50t, 455, 505, 506, 511, 570, 777t, 784, 786
Toprol-XL, 290t, 295
Toradol, 124t, 127
torsemide, 553t, 554, 555
Tosymra, 717t, 719
Toujeo Max SoloStar, 481t, 482
Toujeo SoloStar, 481t
Tovet, 99t
Toviaz, 545t, 546
trabectedin, 649
Tradjenta, 477t, 485
tramadol, 683t, 686, 692
trandolapril, 289t
tranexamic acid, 523, 523t
transcriptase inhibitors (NRTIs), 643
Transderm Scop, 444t
Tranxene, 72t, 241t
tranylcypromine, 214t, 223
trastuzumab, 794t, 796, 798
Travatan-Z, 265t
travoprost, 265t
trazodone, 214t, 225–226
Treanda, 775t
Trelegy Ellipta, 360t, 365
Tresiba, 476t, 481t, 483
Tresiba FlexTouch, 476t, 481t, 483
tretinoin, 93t, 95
Tretin-X, 93t, 95
Trexall, 132
Treximet, 78t, 717t, 719
Triacin, 379t
triamcinolone, 99t, 138, 381t, 390
Triaminic, 378t
triamterene, 553t, 556, 557, 558
triamterine, 268t
triazolam, 245t, 250–251, 518t, 619, 649, 653
TriCor, 314t
tricyclic antidepressants, 568
Triderm, 99t
Tridesilon, 99t
Tri-Estarylla, 514t, 516
Tri Femynor, 514t, 516
trifluoperazine, 230t
trihexyphenidyl, 185t, 188
Trijardy XR, 478t
Trikafta, 368t, 370
Trileptal, 78t, 170t, 172t, 173
Tri-Linyah, 514t, 516
Trilipix, 314t

Trilisate, 152, 152t, 157t
Tri-Lo-Estarylla, 514t, 516
Tri-Lo-Marzia, 514t, 516
Tri-Lo-Mili, 514t, 516
Tri-Lo-Sprintec, 514t, 516
TriLyte, 434t, 439–440
trimethoprim, 544, 589t, 593, 594, 610t
Tri-Mili, 514t, 516
TriNessa, 514t
Triostat, 467t, 468
Triple Antibiotic Ointment, 103t, 104
Tri-Previfem, 514t, 516
triprolidine-pseudoephedrine, 379t
Tri-Sprintec, 514t, 516
Triumeq, 643
Trivagizole 3, 616t
Trivora, 514t, 516
Tri-VyLibra, 514t, 516
Trizivir, 644t
Trogarzo, 645t, 656
Trokendi XR, 171t, 181, 182t
trospium, 546, 546t
Trulicity, 477t, 484
Trusopt, 266t
Trusopt Ocumeter Plus, 266t
Truvada, 78t, 643, 644t, 660, 660t
Tucks, 98t
Tudorza Pressair, 359t, 361
Tulana, 514t, 516
Tums, 411t
TussiCaps, 378t, 380t, 382, 387
Tussionex, 378t, 380t, 382, 387
Twirla, 515t, 519
Tydemy, 514t, 516
Tygacil, 604
Tykerb, 794t, 796
Tylenol, 5, 123, 125–126
Typhim VI, 664t
Tysabri, 192t, 193, 194t
Tyzeka, 78t

U

Ubrelvy, 717t, 720
ubrogepant, 717t, 720
Uceris, 471t
ulipristal, 78t, 506, 518, 519, 521, 522, 649
Uloric, 138t, 140
Ultane, 698t, 704
Ultiva, 699t, 705
Ultram, 683t, 686, 692
Ultravate, 99t
umeclidinium-vilanterol, 359t, 360t, 362–363, 366
Unasyn, 590t
Unifiber, 433t, 435
Unithroid, 467t, 468
unoprostone, 265t
upadacitinib, 132t, 133, 135t, 137t
Uroxatral, 548t, 549
ursodiol, 424–425
ustekinumab, 420t, 422–423
uterine, 527

V

Vabomere, 599
vaborbactam, 591t, 599
Vabormere, 591t
Vagifem, 500t, 504
vaginal ring, 520
Vagistat-1, 617t
valacyclovir, 636t, 638, 670
Valcyte, 636t, 638
valganciclovir, 636t, 638, 639, 646, 647
Valium, 72t, 147t, 148t, 150t, 241t, 243, 699t, 708
valproate, 170t, 177
valproic acid, 177, 178t, 227t, 228
valsartan, 289t, 292t
Valtoco, 241t
Valtrex, 636t, 638
Vanatol LQ, 718t
Vancocin, 593t, 608, 608f, 609
vancomycin, 593t, 608
vandatinib, 797
Vandazole, 593t, 606
vandetanib, 794t, 795
Vanos, 99t
Vaqta, 664t
vardenafil, 508, 508t
varenicline, 393t, 395
varicella vaccine, 669
Varivax, 664t
Vasaotec, 47
Vascepa, 315t, 319
Vasocidin, 272t
Vasotec, 289t
Vectibix, 795t, 797
vecuronium, 699t
vedolizumab, 420t, 422
Velban, 777t, 787
Velivet, 514t, 516
velpatasvir, 450t, 455
Veltin, 92, 93t
Vemlidy, 450t, 453, 647
venlafaxine, 214t, 220, 241t
Venofer, 560t, 561, 561t
Ventolin, 349t, 351
VePesid, 776t, 785
verapamil, 290t
Verdeso, 99t
Verelan, 290t
Veripred, 471t
Versacloz, 230t, 235–236
Vertigo, 444
Vesicare, 546, 546t
Vfend, 618
Viagra, 508, 508t
Vibramycin, 592t, 604, 610t, 613, 614t
Victoza, 477t, 484
Viekira Pak, 450t, 454–455
Vienva, 514t, 516
vigabatrin, 170t, 172t, 176–177
Vigamox, 271t, 273, 593t, 611t
Vimovo, 125t, 128
Vimpat, 170t, 172t, 174
Vimpat IV, 170t, 172t, 174

vinblastine, 90t, 777t, 787, 788
vinca alkaloid, 787
vincristine, 455, 505, 506, 511, 570, 777t, 780t, 785t, 787, 788
vincristine liposomal, 777t
vinorelbine, 777t, 787
Viokase, 78t
Viorele, 514t, 516
Viracept, 645t, 654
Viramune, 644t, 651
Viramune XR, 644t, 651
Virazole, 450t, 452, 636t, 641
Viread, 78t, 450t, 453, 644t, 647
Viroxyn, 111t, 112
Visicol, 434t
Vistaril, 241t, 244
vitamin B9, 560t
vitamin B12, 560t
Vitrasert, 638
Vitus, 382
Vivelle-Dot, 500t, 501t, 504
Vivitrol, 253t, 255, 683t, 695t, 697
Vivotif, 664t
Vizimpro, 794t, 797
Volnea, 514t, 516
Voltaren Gel, 124t, 127
voriconazole, 329t, 618, 720
vortioxetine, 568
Votrient, 794t, 795
Vraylar, 230t, 235
VSL#3, 761t
Vumerity, 192t, 193, 194t
Vyfemla, 514t, 516
VyLibra, 514t, 516
Vytorin, 315
Vyvanse, 199t
Vyzulta, 265t

W

Wakix, 245t, 249
warfarin, 323t, 328–329, 423
Welchol, 315t
Wellbutrin, 214t, 224–225
Wellbutrin SR, 214t, 393t, 394–395
Wellbutrin XL, 214t
Wera, 514t, 516
wheat dextrin, 433t, 435
Willow bark, 155
Wymza Fe, 514t, 516

X

Xadago, 185t, 190
Xalatan, 265t
Xanax, 241t, 243
Xarelto, 323t, 327

Xeloda, 775t, 782
Xenazine, 203–204
Xenical, 752, 752t
Xgeva, 142t, 144
Xifaxan, 426t, 430
Xigduo XR, 477t
Xiidra, 269, 269t
Xofluza, 636t, 639
Xolair, 350t, 355
Xolegel, 103t, 106
Xolido, 90, 90t
Xopenex, 349t, 351
Xtampza, 682t, 686, 691
Xtandi, 790t, 791
Xulane, 515t, 519
Xultophy, 481t
Xylocaine, 90, 90t, 300t, 700t, 714
Xyosted, 501t

Y

Yasmin 28, 514t, 516
Yaz, 514t, 516
ydroxydaunorubicin, 785
yellow fever, 669
Yervoy, 802t
YF-VAX, 664t
Yupelri, 359t, 362

Z

zafirlukast, 78t, 350t, 354
zaleplon, 245t, 247, 691, 693, 694
Zaltrap, 794t, 795
Zanaflex, 147t, 148t, 150t
zanamivir, 636t, 640
zanubrutinib, 795t, 799
Zarah, 514t, 516
Zarontin, 170t, 177, 178t
Zaroxolyn, 553t, 558
Z-drugs, 691
Zebeta, 290t, 296
Zebutal, 718t
Zegerid, 411t, 414
Zelapar, 185t, 189, 214t, 223
Zemaira, 366
Zembrace SymTouch, 717t, 719
Zemuron, 699t
Zenatane, 93t, 94
Zenpep, 78t
Zeosorb, 103t, 106
Zepatier, 450t, 453–454
Zerit, 644t, 647
Zestoretic, 553t, 558
Zestril, 289t
Zetia, 315t, 318, 333
Zetonna, 381t, 390

Ziac, 553t, 558
Ziagen, 644t, 646
Ziana, 92, 93t
zidovudine, 644t, 648, 659, 660t
zileuton, 350t, 354
Zinacef, 590t, 597
zinc oxide, 111t, 112
Zioptan, 265t
ziprasidone, 231t, 239–240, 595, 690, 704, 792
Zipsor, 124t, 127
Zithromax, 368t, 592t, 601, 610t, 613, 614t
Zithromax Tri-Pak, 592t, 610t, 613, 614t
Zithromax Z-Pak, 610t, 613, 614t
zivaflibercept, 796
ziv-aflibercept, 794t, 795
Zmax, 592t
Zocor, 314t
zodiazepine, 711
Zofran, 444t, 446
Zohydro ER, 682t, 688
Zoladex, 790t, 792
zoledronic acid, 142, 142t
Zolegel, 616t, 618
zolmitriptan, 717t, 719
Zoloft, 213t, 217–218, 241t
zolpidem, 245t, 247, 691, 693, 694
Zolpimist, 245t, 247
Zomacton, 528, 528t
Zomig, 717t, 719
Zomig ZMT, 717t, 719
Zonatuss, 378t, 382
Zonegran, 170t, 177, 178t
zonisamide, 170t, 177, 178t
Zorbtive, 528, 528t
Zorvolex, 124t, 127
Zostavax, 664t
Zosyn, 590t
Zovia, 514t, 516
Zovirax, 103t, 107, 635t, 636t, 637
Zoxyn, 590t
Z-Pak, 592t
Zubsolv, 695t
Zumandimine, 514t, 516
Zyban, 214t, 224–225
Zydelig, 795t, 800
Zyflo, 350t, 354
Zylet, 269t
Zyloprim, 138t, 139
Zymaxid, 271t, 273, 611t
Zypitamag, 314t
Zyprexa, 237–238
Zyprexa Relprevv, 230t, 237–238
Zyrexa, 230t
Zyrtec, 380t, 388
Zyrtec-D, 379t
Zyvox, 593t, 607, 610t

SUBJECT INDEX

Note: Locators followed by the letters *f* and *t* refers to figures and tables.

A

Abbreviated New Drug Application
(ANDA), 36
abbreviations, used on prescriptions, 62,
62t, 63t
absence seizure, 168–169
absorption, 405
absorption, distribution, metabolism,
and elimination (ADME), 65
absorption, of drug, 8–9
ACE inhibitors, 310, 311
CAPTOPRIL mnemonic, 51, 51t
photosensitivity and, 90t
acetylcholine (ACh), 123, 164, 165t
myasthenia gravis and, 201
acidifying and alkalinizing agents,
748–749, 749t
acidosis, 748
acne vulgaris, 91–96
ACPE (Accreditation Counsel of
Pharmacy Education), 28
acquired immunodeficiency syndrome
(AIDS), 642
acronym mnemonic method, 50
acrostics mnemonic method, 50
actinic keratosis, 89
action potential, 286, 286f
active immunity, 662
acupuncture, 154
acute coronary syndrome, 331
acute cough, 345
acute kidney disease, 542
acute pain, 679
acute viral infection, 634
adaptive immune system, 583
addiction, 14, 15t
alcohol dependence, 251–255
Addison's disease, 472
adenosine triphosphate (ATP), 735
adenosine triphosphate-citrate lyase
(ACL) inhibitor, 315–316, 315t
adherence, 65
adipose tissue, 88
adjunct therapy, 552
adjuvant chemotherapy, 773
adjuvant radiation therapy, 771
ADME, 7–10, 8f
adrenal glands and corticosteroids,
466–467
Addison's disease, 472
corticosteroid therapy, 472–473
Cushing's syndrome, 472

adsorbents, 426–427
advanced chronic kidney disease, 564–568
calcimimetic, 567–568
phosphate binders, 566
vitamin D supplements, 566–567
adverse drug reactions (ADRs), 71–72, 71t
adverse effect, defined, 13
aerobic, 584
afferent system, 162, 162f
affinity, 6
agonist, 6–7, 7f
agranulocytosis, 235
airway clearance therapy (ACT), 367
akathisia, 231
albumin, 70
alcohol
dependence and withdrawal from,
252–253, 252t, 253t
effects on metabolism, 252
alcohol antagonists, 253–255, 253t
alcohol dependence, 251–255
alcoholism, 251
aldosterone, 70
aldosterone antagonists, 312
alimentary tract, 405
alkalosis, 748
alkylating agents, 781–782
allergen, 14, 73
allergic response, 14
allergy
allergic response, 73
asthma and, 355
defined, 73
drug therapy, 376–390
histamine and, 73
aloe gel, 113
alopecia, 470, 778
alpha-blockers, 297, 549
alpha receptors, 165, 265t
alpha tocopherol (vitamin E), 334
ALS. *See* amyotrophic lateral sclerosis (ALS)
alternative medicine, 15
alveolus, 358, 358f
Alzheimer, Alois, 195
Alzheimer's disease, 195–197
American Association of Pharmacy
Technician (AAPT), 28, 80
American Pharmaceutical Association, 24
American Pharmacists Association
(APhA), 24, 28
American Society of Health-System
Pharmacists (ASHP), 28

aminoglycosides, 271t, 602
aminosalicylates, 421–422
ammonium chloride, 748
amylase, 369
amyotrophic lateral sclerosis (ALS), 203
anaerobic, 584
analgesics, 123, 268t, 681
defined, 123
nonnarcotic, 123–126
anaphylactic reaction, 14
anaphylaxis, 386–387
androgen, 498–499
anemia, renal system and, 559–564
B vitamins, 563–564
erythropoietin-stimulating agents,
560–561
oral and parenteral iron supplements,
561–563
anesthesia, 697–715, 698–701t
drugs used to reverse, 710–713, 711t
induction agents, 707–709
inhaled agents, 702–704
injectable agents, 704–707
local anesthetics, 714–715
malignant hyperthermia and, 713
neuromuscular blocking agents,
709–710
anesthesiologist, 701
angina pectoris, 305–310
metabolic modifier, 307t, 309–304
nitrates, 307t, 308–309
overview of drug therapy for, 307t
symptoms and risk factors of, 306
types of, 305–306
angioedema, 14
angiogenesis inhibitors, 795–796
angiotensin-converting enzyme, 291, 311
inhibitor, 289t, 291–292
angiotensin receptor blocker (ARB),
289t, 292–293, 292t
angiotensin receptor-neprilysin
inhibitors (ARNIs), 311–312, 311t
anion, 742
anorexia, 216
antacids, 410
antagonists, 7, 7f, 15t
anterior chamber, 264, 264f
antiandrogen drug, 791
antiandrogens, 791–792
antibiotic drugs, 589–593t, 589–609
aminoglycosides, 602–603
carbapenems, 599–600

antibiotic drugs (continued)
  cephalosporins, 597–599
  daptomycin, 607–608
  fluoroquinolones, 605–606
  lincosamides, 600–602
  linezolid, 607
  macrolides, 600–602
  metronidazole, 606–607
  monobactams, 599–600
  nitrofurantoin, 593–595
  penicillins, 595–596
  storage of, 609–610t
  sulfonamide, 593–595
  tetracyclines, 604–605
  vancomycin, 608–609
antibiotic resistance, 588
antibiotics
  for bacterial infections, 586
  for cystic fibrosis, 368–369
  ear infections, 275–276, 275t
  eye infections, 270–273, 271–272t
  photosensitivity and, 90t
  for urinary tract infection, 544
antibody, 583
anticancer therapies, 793–880, 794–795t
anticholinergics, 185t, 188, 359t,
    360–363, 445, 546
anticholinesterase agents, 711
anticoagulant agents, 322–323t, 322–329
  direct thrombin inhibitors, 322t,
    324–325
  Factor Xa inhibitors, 323t, 327–328
  heparin, 323t, 325–327
  low-molecular-weight heparins, 323t,
    326
  vitamin K antagonists, 323t, 328–330
anticoagulants, 310
anticonvulsant drugs
  calcium channel blockers, 170t,
    177–178, 178t
  GABA enhancers, 170t, 178–179, 180t
  glutamate inhibitors, 170–171t,
    180–183, 182t
  overview of, 169–170
  sodium channel blockers, 170–172t,
    173–177
  synaptic vesicle protein binder, 171t,
    182–183, 183t
antidepressants, 267t
  cyclic antidepressants, 214t, 220–223
  Medication Guides and, 212
  monoamine oxidase inhibitor (MAOI),
    214t, 223–224
  overview, 212
  photosensitivity and, 90t
  selective serotonin reuptake inhibitor
    (SSRI), 213–218, 213t
  serotonin-norepinephrine reuptake
    inhibitor (SNRI), 213–214t,
    218–220
  serotonin syndrome, 213
antidiarrheals, 426
antiemetic, 444
antiemetic agents, 721

antiepileptic drugs, 169–183, 170–172t
antiestrogen drug, 790
antiestrogens, 790–791
antiflatulent agents, 439
antigen, 14, 583
  defined, 386
antiherpes agents, 637–639
antihistamines, 73, 267t, 445
  first-generation, 387–388
  most commonly used, 380t
  overview of, 386–387
  photosensitivity and, 90t
  second-generation, 388–389
  therapeutic uses of, 387
anti-influenza agents, 639–641
antimetabolites, 782–784
antimicrotubule agents, 786–788
antimotility drugs, 427–429
antioxidant, 737
antiplatelet agents, 322–323t, 330–332
  general, 323t, 330–332
  glycoprotein antagonists, 324t, 332
antipsychotic drugs, 229, 267t
  atypical, 230–231t, 232–240
  photosensitivity and, 90t
  side effects of, 229–232
  typical, 229–232, 230–231t
antipyretic analgesic, 123
antiretroviral, 642
antiretroviral agents, 642–662, 644–645t
  combining antiretroviral medications,
    659–661
  entry inhibitors, 655–656
  integrase strand transfer inhibitors,
    657–658
  nonnucleoside reverse transcriptase
    inhibitors, 648–651
  nucleoside reverse transcriptase
    inhibitors, 643–648
  protease inhibitors, 651–655
antiseptics, 111–113, 111t, 112t, 589
antitussives, 377, 378t, 381–383
antiviral agents, 635–636t, 635–642
  antiherpes agents, 637–639
  anti-influenza agents, 639–641
  therapeutic uses of, 635
antiviral drug, 635
anuria, 542
anxiety
  antianxiety drugs, 241t, 242–244
  complementary and alternative
    therapies for, 255
  endogenous, 240
  exogenous, 240
  panic disorders, 241–242
  symptoms of, 240
apocrine sweat glands, 88
apoptosis, 769
apothecary, 24
aqueous humor, 264
arachidonic acid, 151, 151f
Aristotle, 22
arrhythmia, 297–305, 595
  beta-blocker, 302

calcium channel blocker, 304
calcium channel blockers, 293
defined, 293
ECG and conduction system of,
    297–299, 298–299f
membrane-stabilizing agent
    (Class I), 300–301t, 300–302
potassium channel blockers, 300t,
    302–303, 303t
artery, 283, 284f
arthritis, 70
  analgesics, 123–126
  COX-2 inhibitors, 125t, 129–130
  defined, 123
  disease-modifying antirheumatic
    drugs (DMARDs), 131–137
  gouty arthritis, 137–140, 138f
  nonsteroidal anti-inflammatory
    drugs (NSAIDs), 124–125t,
    126–129
  osteoarthritis, 123–130, 124f
  rheumatoid arthritis, 130–137, 130f
ascorbic acid, 737
asparaginase, 789
aspiration, 371
aspirin, 323t, 330
asthma, 345–356, 345f, 349–351t
  allergic, 355
  anatomy and physiology of,
    345–346, 345f
  asthmatic response, 345–346, 345f
  characteristics of, 345
  drug therapy for, 347–356
  management of, 346–349
  status asthmaticus, 347
  triggers, 346
asthma attack, 345–346, 345f
atherosclerosis, 313
athlete's foot, 106
atonic seizure, 169
atopic dermatitis, 97
atrial fibrillation, 298, 299t
atrial flutter, 297–298, 299t
atrioventricular (AV) node, 286, 286f,
    297–299, 298–299f
attention deficit hyperactivity disorder
    (ADHD), 197–200, 199t
atypical antipsychotics, 232–240
aura, 169, 716
autoimmune disease, 130
automated dispensing process, 27
autonomic nervous system, 162, 162f
azoles, 618

B

background pain, 680
bacteria, 587
bacterial infections, 584–588,
    585–586t, 585f
  antibiotic selection, 586–587
  antibiotic side effects
    and dispensing issues, 588
  antimicrobial resistance, 588

skin, 103t, 104–105
   types of bacteria, 584–586, 585f
bactericidal agent, 587
bacteriostatic agent, 587
Ballington, Don, 28
Banting, Frederick, 25
barbiturate, 704
bariatric surgery, 751
basal cell carcinoma, 89
basal insulin, 478
basal nuclei, 184, 185f
basal rate, 478
Beers List, 71–72
Bencao Gangmu (Compendium of Materia Medica), 22
benign prostatic hyperplasia (BPH), 548–551, 548t
   alpha-blockers, 549–550
   5-alpha-reductase inhibitor, 550–551
benzodiazepines, 704, 708
beriberi, 735
Bernard, Claude, 24, 24f
Best, Charles, 25
beta-3 adrenergic agonist, 547
beta-blocker, 290t, 265t, 268t, 294–296, 302, 310, 312
beta-carotene, 277
beta-lactamase, 595
   inhibitor, 595
beta-1 receptors, 165, 294–295
beta-2 receptors, 165, 294–295
bifidobacteria, 456
bile, 407
   acid sequestrants, 314–315t, 317–318
bioavailability, 10
biologic drugs, 36
biologic response modifiers, 131
biologic therapy, 422–423
biosimilar drug, 37
biotin, 736
bipolar disorders
   drug therapy for, 226–228
   overview of, 226–227
   signs of, 226–227
bismuth subcitrate potassium / metronidazole / tetracycline, 417
bismuth subsalicylate, 426
bisphosphonates, 142–143, 142t
Black Box warning, 33, 33f
bleomycin, 788
blocking study method, 44–45
blood
   binding of blood to plasma proteins, 9
   lab values for blood counts, 26t
blood-brain barrier, 9
blood clots
   anticoagulant agents, 322–329
   antiplatelet agents, 322, 330–332
   deep vein thrombosis (DVT), 319–320
   direct thrombin inhibitors, 322t, 324–325

Factor Xa inhibitors, 323t, 327–328
glycoprotein antagonists, 324t, 332
heparin, 323t, 325–327
low-molecular-weight heparins, 323t, 326
overview of, 319
pulmonary embolism, 319
thrombolytic agents, 324t, 333
vitamin K antagonists, 323t, 328–330
blood pressure
   defined, 287
   diastolic, 288
   factors affecting, 287–288
   hypertension, 288–297
   mechanism for maintaining, 287, 287f
   systolic, 287–288
blood urea nitrogen (BUN), 542
boil, 104
bolus insulin, 478
bolus rate, 478
bone marrow, 582
bone marrow suppression, 778
bone mineral density (BMD), 141
bone remodeling, 122, 122f
bones
   aging and, 70
   anatomy and physiology of, 120–122f, 120–123
   osteoporosis, 140–145
Boswellia serrata, 396
bowel evacuants, 439–440
bowel transit time, 407
boxed warning, 33, 33f
bradycardia, 299t
   defined, 293
bradykinin, 6
brain
   anatomy of, 184–185f
   Parkinson's Disease and, 183–184, 184f, 185f
   stroke, 321–322
brand name, 5
breakthrough pain, 680
broad-spectrum antibiotic, 587
bronchitis, 357–359
bronchodilators, 349t, 351–352
bronchospasm, 346
Bruton's tyrosine kinase (BTK) inhibitor, 799
buccal route, 67
bulk-forming agents, 435
buprenorphine, 693
butorphanol, 693

C

cachexia, 755
calamine, 101–102
calciferol, 733
calcimimetics, 567
calcineurin inhibitors, 100–101
calcium acetate, 745

calcium (Ca²⁺), 745–746
calcium carbonate, 745
calcium channel blockers, 289–290t, 293–294, 304, 310
   as antiepileptic drug therapy, 170t, 177–178, 178t
calcium chloride, 745
calcium citrate, 745
calcium gluconate, 746
calcium lactate, 746
callus, 87
cancer, 767–812
   chemotherapy drugs, 773–789, 775–777t
      alkylating agents, 781–782
      antimetabolites, 782–784
      antimicrotubule agents, 786–788
      asparaginase, 789
      bleomycin, 788
      cell cycle and mechanism of action, 773–774
      combination chemotherapy, 780–781
      cytotoxic drugs and side effects, 774–780, 775–777t, 779–780t
      topoisomerase inhibitors, 784–786
   complementary and alternative therapies, 808
   defined, 768
   development of, 768–770
   handling hazardous agents, 804–807, 804t
      hazardous drug communication program, 806
      personal protective equipment, 805
      prevention of chemotherapy-related medication errors, 807
      spill kit, 806
   hormonal drug therapies, 789–793, 790t
      antiandrogens, 791–792
      antiestrogens, 790–791
      cyclin-dependent kinase 4/6 (CDK 4/6) inhibitor, 792–793
      luteinizing hormone–releasing hormone (lhrh), 792
   immunotherapy, 800–804, 802–804t
      cytotoxic t-lymphocyte-associated protein 4 (CTLA-4), 801
      immune checkpoint inhibitors, 802–804
      immune checkpoints, 800–801
      programmed death pathway, 801–802
   pathophysiology of, 768–769
      oncogenes, 769, 769f
      tumor suppressor gene, 769, 769f
   skin, 89
   stages, treatment and, 770–773, 771t
      chemotherapy, 772–773
      immunotherapy, 772
      radiation therapy, 771
      surgery, 771

cancer (*continued*)
  targeted anticancer therapies, 793–880, 794–795t
    angiogenesis inhibitors, 795–796
    Bruton's tyrosine kinase (BTK) inhibitor, 799
    monoclonal antibodies, 796–798
    PI3K/AKT/mTOR pathway agents, 800
    signal transduction inhibitors, 798–799
  tumor burden, 770
  tumor cell proliferation, 770
Candida, 615
Candida infection, 105, 389
capacitance, 287
capsid, 632
CAPTOPRIL Mnemonic, 51, 51t
carbapenem, 599
carbonic anhydrase inhibitors, 266t, 554
carbuncle, 104
cardiac muscle, 121, 121f
cardiac output (CO), 287
cardiac toxicity, 785
cardiovascular diseases
  angina, 305–310
  arrhythmia, 297–305
  clotting disorders, 319–333
  complementary and alternative therapies, 333–334
  heart anatomy and physiology, 283–284, 284–285f
  heart failure, 310–312, 311t
  high cholesterol and related diseases, 313–319
  hypertension, 288–297, 289–290t
  myocardial infarction (heart attack), 306–307
  photosensitivity and drugs treating, 90t
  stroke, 321–333
cardiovascular system
  blood pressure, 287–288, 287f
  cardiac contractility, 286, 286f
  heart anatomy and physiology, 283–284, 284–285f
cataplexy, 248
catecholamines, 223
Catechol-O-Methyl Transferase (COMT) inhibitors, 185t, 188–189
cation, 742
CD4 cell, 642
ceiling effect, 10, 11f
cell cycle, 773
  and mechanism of action, 773–774
cell cycle–nonspecific agents, 774
cell cycle–specific drug, 773
cell kill hypothesis, 770
cells, drug binding to cellular constituents, 9
Centers for Disease Control and Prevention (CDC), 54
centralized pain, 679
centrally distributed fat, 750
central nervous system, 162

cephalosporins, 597
cerebral hemorrhage, 321–322
cerebrovascular accidents (CVAs), 321
cerumen, 273
cervical cap, 512
CFTR modulators, 370
CGRP receptor antagonist, 720–721
Chain, Ernst, 25
chancre, 612
chemical dependence, 252, 252t
chemoreceptor trigger zone (CTZ), 443
chemotherapeutic agents, 268t
  photosensitivity and drugs treating, 90t
chemotherapy, 772–773
  drugs, 773–789, 775–777t
    alkylating agents, 781–782
    antimetabolites, 782–784
    antimicrotubule agents, 786–788
    asparaginase, 789
    bleomycin, 788
    cell cycle and mechanism of action, 773–774
    combination chemotherapy, 780–781
    cytotoxic drugs and side effects, 774–780, 775–777t, 779–780t
    topoisomerase inhibitors, 784–786
children
  aspirin and Reye's syndrome, 154
  dosage considerations, 73
  drug action considerations, 72–73
  OTC and, 73
Chinese medicine, 22
chiropractic care, 155
chlamydia, 611
chloride (Cl⁻), 747
chlorofluorocarbons (CFCs), 347
cholecalciferol, 733
cholecystectomy, 424
cholesterol
  defined, 313
  HDL, 313
  high
    adenosine triphosphate-citrate lyase (ACL) inhibitor, 315–316, 315t
    bile acid sequestrants, 314–315t, 317–318
    fibric acid derivatives, 314t, 317
    HMG-CoA reductase inhibitors, 314t, 315–316
    lipid-lowering agents, 314–315t, 314–319
    omega-3 fatty acids, 319
    overview of, 313–315
    statins, 314t, 315–316
  lab values, 26t
  LDL, 313
  total, 313
  triglycerides, 313
choline, 396
chondroitin, 155
chronic cough, 345
chronic dry eye, 267–269t, 267–270
chronic kidney disease, 551–559, 551t

carbonic anhydrase inhibitors, 554
  loop diuretic, 554–556
  potassium-sparing diuretic, 556–557
  thiazide and thiazide-related diuretics, 558–559
chronic malignant pain, 680
chronic nonmalignant pain, 679
chronic obstructive pulmonary disease (COPD), 70, 356–367, 359–360t
  anatomy and physiology of, 356–359, 357f, 358f
chronic viral infection, 634
ciliary muscle, 264, 264f
circadian rhythm, 467
circulatory system. *See* cardiovascular system
clearance, 10
clinical trials, 30–32
clotting cascade, 320, 320f
clotting disorders and stroke, 319–333
clove oil, 113, 277
CNS stimulants, 198–200, 199t
coagulation cascade, 320
coating agents, 415
cobalamin, 737
cochlea, 273–274, 274f
Cockcroft and Gault equation, 543
cocktail, 642
codeine, 686–687
colloid solution, 741
colon, 406
colonic segmentation, 441
color blindness, 263–264
combination agents, migraine headaches, 722
combination chemotherapy, 780–781
combination therapy, 169
common cold, drug therapy for, 376–390
community-acquired infections, 597
community-acquired pneumonia (CAP), 371
competitive inhibition, 10
Complementary and Alternative Medicine (CAM), 16
complementary and alternative therapies
  acupuncture, 154
  aloe gel, 113
  alpha tocopherol (vitamin E), 334
  for anxiety, 5
  beta-carotene, 277
  Boswellia serrata, 396
  for cancer, 808
  cardiovascular diseases, 333–334
  chiropractic care, 155
  choline, 396
  chondroitin, 155
  clove oil, 113, 277
  for depression, 256
  for endocrine diseases, 490
  garlic, 334
  for gastrointestinal diseases, 456
  for gastrointestinal disorders, 760, 760t
  ginkgo biloba, 205

5-hydroxytryptophan, 204
  for immune system, 622
  for insomnia, 255–256
  kava, 255
  melatonin, 255
  for musculoskeletal system, 154–155
  nasal irrigation, 396
  for nervous system, 204–205
  olive oil, 277
  for pain, 722–723
  plant sterol esters, 333
  red yeast rice, 333
  for renal diseases, 571
  for reproductive diseases, 529–530
  respiratory system, 396
  for skin, 111
  St. John's wort, 256
  for viral infections, 670
  Vitamin A, 277
  Willow bark (*Salix alba*), 155
  yoga, 204, 396
complementary medicine, 16
complement system, 583
complete inhibition, 10
complex focal seizure, 167
compliance, reasons for noncompliance, 75–76
compounder, 758
computerized physician order entry (CPOE), 77
concomitant, 126
conduction system, 284
cone cells color blindness, 263
conjugated estrogen, 504
conjunctiva, 264, 264f
conjunctivitis, 270–273, 271–272t, 783
constipation and flatulence, 70, 430–440
  antiflatulent agents, 439
  bowel evacuants, 439–440
  bulk-forming laxatives, 435
  fiber and fiber supplementation, 432–433, 433–434t
  osmotic laxatives, 436–437
  other agents, 438
  stimulant laxatives, 437–438
  stool softeners/surfactant laxatives, 436
contact dermatitis, 96, 96f
contiguity principle, 45
contraception, 511–524
  barrier contraception, 511–513
    diaphragms and cervical caps, 512–513
    external condoms, 511–512
    internal condoms, 512
  heavy menstrual bleeding, 523–524
  hormonal contraceptives, 513–522, 514–515t
    emergency contraceptives, 518–519
    implantable contraceptives, 521–522
    injectable contraceptives, 521
    intrauterine devices, 522
    oral contraceptives, 516–518
    transdermal contraceptives, 519–520
    vaginal contraceptives, 520
contraindication, 13

controlled substances
  defined, 34
  drug label, 35f
  drug regulation for, 34, 35t
  institutional procedures for, 64
  schedules, 35f
Controlled Substances Act, 34
  schedules for, 34, 35t
convulsion, 166
Cordus, Valerius, 23
cornea, 264, 264f
coronary artery disease, 70
corticosteroids, 97, 349–350t, 352–353, 420–421, 466
  nasal, 380–381t, 389–390
  side effects of, 352–353
  topical for skin, 98–99t, 100
cotinine, 392
cough reflex, 377
coughs, drug therapy for, 376–390
COX-2 inhibitors, 125t, 129–130
cracking, 758
cradle cap, 96
cramming study method, 44
cranberry juice, 571
creatinine clearance (CrCl), 543
Crohn's disease and ulcerative colitis, 419–423
  aminosalicylates, 421–422
  biologic therapies, 422–423
  corticosteroids, 420–421
  immunosuppressants, 423
cromolyn sodium, 355
crystalloid solution, 741
culture and sensitivity (C&S) test, 587
curative act, 772
Cushing's syndrome, 472
cyclic antidepressants, 214t, 220–223
cyclic lipopeptide, 607
cyclin-dependent kinase 4/6 (CDK 4/6) inhibitor, 792–793
cyclooxygenase, 129, 151, 151f
cyclooxygenase-1 (COX-1), 129
cyclooxygenase-2 (COX-2), 129
cystic duct, 424
cystic fibrosis, 367–370
cystitis, 543
cytochrome P-450, 9
  drug interactions and, 14
cytotoxic drug, 773
  and side effects, 774–780, 775–777t, 779–780t
cytotoxic t-lymphocyte-associated protein 4 (CTLA-4), 801

D

dandruff, 97, 102, 102f
DEA Form 222, 34
decongestants
  most commonly used, 379t, 385–386
  overview of, 383–384
  side effects and dispensing issues of, 384, 385t

deep vein thrombosis (DVT), 319–320
delirium tremens (DTs), 253
De Materia Medica (Dioscorides), 22
dendrite, 163, 164f
dependence, drug, 14
  alcohol, 251–255
depolarization, 286, 286f
depression
  complementary and alternative therapies for, 256
  cyclic antidepressants, 214t, 220–223
  drug therapy for, 213–226
  monoamine oxidase inhibitor (MAOI), 214t, 223–224
  overview of, 212
  selective serotonin reuptake inhibitor (SSRI), 213–218, 213t
  serotonin-norepinephrine reuptake inhibitor (SNRI), 213–214t, 218–220
  serotonin syndrome, 213
dermatitis, 96–102, 98–99t
dermatophyte fungi, 615
dermis, 88, 88f
desflurane, 703
detrusor muscle, 542
dexmedetomidine, 707
diabetes, 473–489, 474f, 475–478t
  agents, photosensitivity and drugs treating, 90t
  defined, 473
  dipeptidyl peptidase-4 (DPP-4) inhibitor, 485
  glucagon, 489
  glucagon-like peptide 1 (GLP-1) receptor agonist, 484–485
  insulin, 478–484, 479–480f, 481t
  insulin secretagogue, 487–488
  metformin, 485–486
  sodium-glucose linked transporter-2 (SGLT-2) inhibitor, 487
  thiazolidinediones, 488–489
  treatment of, 475–478t
  types of, 474–478
diabetic neuropathy, 219, 474
diabetic retinopathy, 474
dialysate, 564
dialysis, 564–568, 565f, 565t
  calcimimetic, 567–568
  phosphate binders, 566
  vitamin D supplements, 566–567
diaper rash, 96–97
diaphragm, 512
diarrhea, 425–430
  adsorbents, 426–427
  antimotility drugs, 427–429
  drugs for infectious, 429–430
diastole, 284
diastolic blood pressure, 288
dietary supplement, 16–17
Dietary Supplement Health and Education Act (DSHEA), 16
difenoxin/atropine, 428
digestion, 405
dihydropyridine calcium channel blocker, 293

Dioscorides, 22
dipeptidyl peptidase-4 (DPP-4)
    inhibitor, 484
diphenoxylate/atropine, 427–428
diplopia, 201
direct renin inhibitors, 290t, 296–297
direct thrombin inhibitors, 322t, 324–325
disease-modifying antirheumatic drugs
    (DMARDs), 131–137, 132t
disinfectants, 111–113, 111t, 112t, 589
disk inhaler, 640
Dispensatorium, 23
dispense as written (DAW), 468
dissociative amnesia, 706
distribution, of drug, 9
diuretics, 70, 268t, 552
    loop, 312
    photosensitivity and drugs
        treating, 90t
    thiazide, 297
diverticular disease, 440–441
docusate, 436
docusate senna, 436
Domagk, Gerhardt, 25
dopamine, 164, 165t
    antipyschotic drugs and, 229–231,
        232–250
    Parkinson's disease and, 183–188
    schizophrenia and, 229
dopamine agonists, 185t, 186–188
dopamine receptor antagonists, 447–448
dosage forms, 65, 66t
dosage routes, 65–68, 66t
    buccal, 67
    children and, 73
    defined, 10
    inhalation, 68
    loading dose, 12
    maintenance dose, 12
    ophthalmic, 68
    oral, 66–67, 66t
    otic, 68
    parenteral, 66t, 67
    peroral, 66
    rectal, 68
    sublingual, 67
    topical, 66t, 68
    vaginal, 68
dose-dense chemotherapy, 770
dose-response curve, 10–11, 11f
double blind study, 30
drivers of cancer, 768
drug abuse, 14
drug action
    absorption, 8–9
    agonists and antagonists, 6–7, 7f
    distribution, 9
    elderly patient considerations, 69–72
    elimination, 10
    induction and inhibition, 9–10
    mechanisms of, 6–7, 7f
    messengers, 6
    metabolism, 9–10
    parameters for, 10–12

pediatric considerations, 72–73
pharmacodynamics, 6–7
receptors, 6
specificity and affinity, 6
drug approval process
    Abbreviated New Drug Application
        (ANDA), 36
    clinical trial phases, 31
    FDA approval process, 31–32
    postmarketing surveillance, 32
drug class
    defined, 47
    learning drugs by, 47–48, 48f
Drug Enforcement Administration
    (DEA)
    regulating controlled substances,
        34, 35t
    number, on prescription, 60, 61f
drug regulation, 29–38
    biosimilar medication, 37
    Black Box warning, 33, 33f
    controlled substances, 34, 35t
    drug approval process, 29–32
    by FDA, 29–33
    medication guides, 32–33
    over-the-counter (OTC) drug, 37–38
    removing drug from market, 32, 33
drug(s)
    action of, 6–10
    allergic response, 14
    approval process, 29–32
    beneficial effects of, 13
    biologic, 36
    biosimilar, 37
    brand or trade name, 5
    defined, 3
    generic, 36
    generic name, 5
    half-life, 13
    history of medicinal drugs, 21–25
    indication and contraindication, 13
    interactions, 14–15
    label, 35f
    legend, 29
    names, 5
    origins and sources, 4, 5t
    over-the-counter, 29, 37–38
    pharmacologic effect, 4
    regulation of, 29–38
    resource apps for, 53–54
    side effects of, 13–14
    sponsor, 29
drug stems, identifying drugs utilizing
    generic drug stems, 48–49, 48f,
        49–50t
drying agents, 275t, 277
dry-powder inhaler, 347
duodenal ulcer, 416
duration of action, 12, 12f
Durham-Humphrey Amendment, 29
dysarthria, 201
dyskinesia, 186
dyslipidemia
    causes of, 313

drug therapy for, 314–319
dyspareunia, 503
dysphagia, 201
dysphoria, 681
dyspnea, 345, 438
dystonia, 232

E

eardrops, 276, 277f
ears
    anatomy and physiology, 273–274,
        274f
    external ear infection (otitis externa),
        275–277, 275t
    middle ear infection (otitis media),
        274–277, 275t
earwax removers, 275t, 277
Ebers Papyrus, 22
eccrine sweat glands, 88
echinacea (echinacea purpurea), 622
echinocandins, 619
eczema, 96–102, 97f, 98–99t
efferent system, 162, 162f
Ehrlich, Paul, 25
elderly patients
    adverse drug reactions (ADRs), 71, 71t
    altered drug responses, 71–72
    Beers List, 71–72
    changes in physiologic function, 69–70
    cognitive abilities and, 72
    drug action considerations, 69–72
    polypharmacy, 72
electrocardiogram (ECG), 297–299,
    298–299f
electrolyte replacement, 742–743t
electrolytes, 738, 741–743t, 742–748
    calcium (Ca2+), 745–746
    chloride (Cl-), 747
    magnesium (Mg2+), 746–747
    phosphate (PO4 3-), 747–748
    potassium (K+), 744–745
    sodium (Na+), 743–744
elimination, of drug, 10
    first-order, 12
    zero-order, 12
emboli, 319
emergency contraceptive, 518–519
emesis, 443
emetic (vomit-inducing) action, 252
emphysema, 357–359
empirical learning, 22
empirical treatment, 587
endocrine system, 463–494
    adrenal glands, 471–473
    anatomy and physiology,
        463–467, 464f
        adrenal glands and corticosteroids,
            466–467
        pancreas, 467
        thyroid gland, 465–466, 466f
    complementary and alternative
        therapies, 490

defined, 463
diabetes, 473–489, 474f, 475–478t
thyroid disorders, 467–471
endocytosis, 632
endogenous anxiety, 240
endogenous chemical messengers, 6
endometrium, 499
endotracheal intubation, 709
end-stage chronic kidney disease, 568–571
immunosuppressants, 569–570, 569t
enema, 68, 431
enteral nutrition, 755–756, 756t
entry inhibitors, 655–656
envelope, 632
enzymes, seizures and, 167
eosinophilic asthma, 355
epidermis, 87, 88f
epigastric area, 408
epilepsy, 166–183, 170–172t
epinephrine, 164, 464
Epocrates, 53
e-prescribing, 77
e-prescription
defined, 60
elements of, 60, 61f
EPS effects, 229
equianalgesic dose, 683
erectile dysfunction (ED), 508–510
ergocalciferol, 733
ergosterol, 615
ergot derivatives, 719–720
erysipelas, 104
erythromycin, 600
erythropoiesis, 559
erythropoietin, 559
erythropoietinstimulating agent (ESA), 560
Escherichia coli (E. coli), 425
esophageal hiatus, 441
esophagitis, 408
ester, 714
estrogen, 499
estrogen-only hormone therapy products, 504–505
ethanol (alcohol), 252
etomidate, 704
eukaryotic, 614
euphoria, 681
eustachian tube, 273, 274f
evidence-based study methods, 43–47
contiguity principle, 45
eliminating distractions, 46
growth mindset, 46–47
interleaving vs. blocking, 44–45
self-testing, 45
spacing, 44
Exam for the Certification of Pharmacy Technicians (ExCPT), 28
exogenous anxiety, 240
exophthalmos, 470
expectorants, 378– 379t, 383–384
external condom, 511
external ear, 273, 274f
external ear infection (otitis externa),
275–277, 275t
extracellular (outside cells), 739
extrapyramidal symptoms (EPS), 229
extravasation, 786
eyes
aging and, 70
anatomy and physiology, 263–264, 264f
chronic dry eye, 267–269t, 267–270
conjunctivitis, 270–273, 271–272t
dispensing opthalmic products, 270f
glaucoma, 265–266t, 265–267

F
Factor Xa inhibitors, 323t, 327–328
fascia, 88
fat-soluble vitamins, 732–734
vitamin A, 732–733
vitamin D, 733–734
vitamin E, 734
vitamin K, 734–735
Federal Food and Drug Act, 29
feedback mechanism, 464
feminizing hormone therapy, 507
fentanyl, 687–688, 705
fever, 123
fiber, 432
fibric acid derivatives, 314t, 317
fibrillation, 298, 299t
fibrin, 319
fibrinogen, 319
fibrinolytic agents, 322–323t
fibromyalgia, 204
fight-or-flight response, 464
filtrate, 541
first-order elimination, 12
first-pass effect, 11, 67, 407, 408f
first-phase insulin secretion, 484
5-alpha-reductase inhibitor, 550
5HT agonists, 718–719
5-hydroxytryptamine, 164, 165t
5-hydroxytryptophan, 204
fixed mindset, 46
flatulence and constipation, 430–440
antiflatulent agents, 439
bowel evacuants, 439–440
bulk-forming laxatives, 435
fiber and fiber supplementation, 432–433, 433–434t
osmotic laxatives, 436–437
other agents, 438
stimulant laxatives, 437–438
stool softeners/surfactant laxatives, 436
Fleming, Alexander, 25
Florey, Howard, 25
fluids, 738–739
and solutions, 739–741
flumazenil, 711
fluoroquinolones, 605
flutter, 297–298, 299t
focal (partial) seizures, 167–168, 168f
folate, 737
folate-deficiency anemia, 563
folic acid, 563, 737
folliculitis, 104
food
absorption process and, 66
drug interactions and, 15
Food, Drug and Cosmetic Act, 29
Food and Drug Administration (FDA)
dietary supplements and, 16–17
drug approval process, 29–32
formation of, 29
medication guides, 32–33
Orange, Purple and Green Books, 52–53
postmarketing surveillance, 32
pregnancy categories, 32
removing drugs from market, 32, 33
website as health information resource, 54
fungi and fungal diseases, 614–622, 615–617t
azoles, 618–619
echinocandins, 619–620
polyenes, 620–621
skin infections, 103t, 105–107
fungus, 614
furuncle, 104

G
GABA enhancers, 170t, 178–179, 180t
Galen, 22
gallbladder, 407
gallstones, 424–425
dissolution agents, 424–425
gamma-aminobutyric acid (GABA), 164, 165t, 167
garlic, 334
gastric bypass, 751
gastric ulcer, 416
gastritis, 417
gastroesophageal reflux disease (GERD), 408–416
antacids, 410–412, 411–412t
coating agents, 415
histamine H2-receptor antagonist, 412–413
prostaglandin E1 analogs, 415–416
proton pump inhibitors, 413–415
gastrointestinal (GI) system, 405–460
anatomy and physiology, 405–408, 406f
complementary and alternative therapies, 456
constipation, 430–440
Crohn's disease, 419–423
defined, 405
diarrhea, 425–430
diverticular disease, 440–441
flatulence, 430–440
gallstones, 424–425
gastroesophageal reflux disease, 408–416
hemorrhoids, 442–443

gastrointestinal (*continued*)
  hepatitis, 449–455
  hiatal hernia, 441
  irritable bowel syndrome, 441
  nausea and vomiting, 443–449
  peptic disease, 416–419
  ulcerative colitis, 419–423
gastrointestinal (GI) tract, aging and, 405, 70
gender transition, 507
general anesthesia, 698
generalized seizure, 168–169, 168*f*
generalized viral infection, 634
generation, 597
generic drugs, 36
  identifying drugs utilizing generic drug stems, 48–49, 48*f*, 49–50*t*
generic name, 5
gene therapy, 370
genital herpes, 637
gestational diabetes, 474
ghost tablet, 239
GI bleed, 417
ginger, 456
gingival hyperplasia, 175*f*
ginkgo biloba, 205
GI transit time, 407
glaucoma, 265–266*t*, 265–267
glitazone, 488
glomerular filtration, 540
glomerular filtration rate (GFR), 542
glomerulus, 540
glucagon, 489
glucagon-like peptide 1 (GLP-1) receptor agonist, 484
glucocorticoid, 466
gluconeogenesis, 466
glucosamine, 155
glucose-dependent insulinotropic polypeptide, 484
glutamate, 164, 165*t*, 167
glutamate inhibitors, 170–171*t*, 180–183, 182*t*
glycerin, 436
glycoprotein antagonists, 324*t*, 332
glycosylated hemoglobin (A1c), 475
gonorrhea, 612
gouty arthritis, 137–140, 138*f*
governement healthcare websites, 54–55
gram-negative bacteria, 586
gram-positive bacteria, 586
grand mal seizure, 168
Graves' disease, 470
Greek alphabet, 22, 23*t*
Green Book, as study aid, 53
growth disorders, 527–529
growth hormone, 528–529
  deficiency, 528
growth hormone–releasing factor (GHRF), 528
growth mindset, 46–47
gynecomastia, 502, 791

H
half-life, 13
handfoot syndrome, 783
handling hazardous agents, cancer and, 804–807, 804*t*
  hazardous drug communication program, 806
  personal protective equipment, 805
  prevention of chemotherapy-related medication errors, 807
hand washing, 377
hazardous drug communication program, 806
hazardous material (hazmat), 805
H2 blockers, 73
Health Canada, 29
Health Insurance Portability and Accountability Act (HIPAA), 79
hearing, aging and, 70
heart. *See also* cardiovascular diseases
  aging and, 70
  anatomy and physiology, 283–284, 284–285*f*
  cardiac contractility, 286, 286*f*
  ECG and conduction system of, 297–299, 298–299*f*
  heart failure, 310–312, 311*t*
  myocardial infarction (heart attack), 306–307
heartburn. *See* gastroesophageal reflux disease (GERD)
heart disease. *See* cardiovascular diseases
heart failure
  drug therapy for, 311–312, 311*t*
  overview of, 310
heart rate (HR), 286
heavy menstrual bleeding, 523–524
hemodialysis, 564, 565*f*
hemorrhagic stroke, 321–322, 321*f*
hemorrhoids, 442–443
heparin, 323*t*, 325–327
heparin antidote, 323*t*, 327
heparin-induced thrombocytopenia (HIT), 326
hepatitis, 449–455, 633
  hepatitis B and hepatitis C agents, 449–455, 450*t*
Hepatitis A, 449
Hepatitis B, 449
Hepatitis C, 449
herpes simplex virus (HSV), 107
high-density lipoproteins (HDL), 313
hip fracture, 141
Hippocrates, 22, 22*f*
hirsutism, 502
histamine, 6
  in allergic response, 73
histamine H2-receptor antagonist, 412
histoplasmosis, 376
HIV/AIDS agents, 642–662, 660*t*.
  See also antiretroviral agents
  preexposure prophylaxis, 662

regimens, 661
responding to accidental exposure, 662
treatment as prevention, 661
HMG-CoA reductase inhibitors, 314*t*, 315–316
homeopathy, 17
homeostasis, 5
homocysteine, 737
hormonal drug therapies, 789–793, 790*t*
  antiandrogens, 791–792
  antiestrogens, 790–791
  cyclin-dependent kinase 4/6 (CDK 4/6) inhibitor, 792–793
  luteinizing hormone–releasing hormone (lhrh), 792
  for treating osteoporosis, 141
hormone replacement therapy, 499–507, 500–501*t*
  female hypogonadism and menopause, 503–506
  gender-affirming hormone therapy, 506–507
  male hypogonadism, 501–503
hormones, 463
  aging and, 70
hormone therapy, 141, 268*t*, 499
hot flashes, 503
human chorionic gonadotropic (hCG), 525
human immunodeficiency virus (HIV), 642
humors, 22
Huntington's disease (Huntington's chorea), 203–204
hydrocodone, 688–689
hydrofluoroalkane (HFA), 347
hydromorphone, 689
hypercalcemia, 745
hypercapnia, 70
hyperchloremia, 747
hypercholesterolemia, 313
hyperglycemia, 473
hyperkalemia, 291
hyperlipidemia, 313
hypermagnesemia, 746
hypernatremia, 743
hyperphosphatemia, 747
hyperpnea, 153
hypertension, 70, 288–297
  alpha-blockers, 297
  angiotensin-converting enzyme (ACE) inhibitor, 289*t*, 291–292
  angiotensin receptor blocker (ARB), 289*t*, 292–293, 292*t*
  beta-blocker, 290*t*, 294–296
  calcium channel blocker, 289–290*t*, 293–294
  defined, 288
  direct renin inhibitors, 290*t*, 296–297
  overview of drug therapy for, 288, 289–290*t*
  thiazide diuretics, 297
hyperthyroidism, 470

hypertonic solution, 739
hypervolemia, 702
hypnotics, 244–247, 245*t*, 250
hypocalcemia, 568
hypochloremia, 747
hypoglycemia, 474
hypogonadism, 501
hypokalemia, 744
hypomagnesemia, 746
hyponatremia, 743
hypophosphatemia, 747
hypothalamic-pituitary-adrenal (HPA)
    axis suppression, 98
hypothalamic-pituitary axis, 465
hypothalmus releasing factors, 465
hypothyroidism, 468
hypotonic solution, 739
hypoxia, 70

I

idiosyncratic reaction, 14
Illinois Council of Health-System
    Pharmacists (ICHP), 28
immune checkpoint inhibitors, 772,
    802–804
immune checkpoints, 800–801
immune system
    allergic response, 14
    anatomy and physiology, 582–584
    antibiotic drugs, 589–593*t*, 589–609
        storage of, 609–610*t*
    autoimmune disease, 130
    bacterial infections, 584–588,
        585–586*t*, 585*f*
    complementary and alternative
        therapies, 622
    defined, 582
    description of, 581
    fungal diseases, 614–622, 615–617*t*
    ophthalmic antibiotics, 610–611*t*
    sexually transmitted infections,
        611–613, 614*t*
    viral infections, 631–674, 635–636*t*,
        644–645*t*, 660*t*
immunizations, 662–664
    common vaccines, 664*t*, 665–670
    schedule, 665
immunocompromised patients, 633
immunoglobulin, 634
immunosuppressants, 423
    for Crohn's disease and ulcerative
        colitis, 423
    for kidney transplantation, 569–570
immunotherapy, 772, 800–804,
    802–804*t*
    cytotoxic t-lymphocyte-associated
        protein 4 (CTLA-4), 801
    immune checkpoints, 800–801
    inhibitors, 802–804
    programmed death pathway, 801–802
impetigo, 104, 104*f*
implantable contraceptives, 521

inactivated vaccine, 663
incontinence, 70
incretin mimetic, 484
incus, 273, 274*f*
Indian medicine, 22
indication, 13
induction, 9
    agents, 707–709
induration, 373
infection local, 68
infections. *See also* bacterial infection;
    fungi and fungal diseases; viral
    infections
    bacterial, 103*t*, 104–105
    ear, 275–277, 275*t*
    eye, 270–273, 271–272*t*
    fungal, 103*t*, 105–107
    of skin, 102–107
    viral, 107
inflammation
    defined, 151
    drug therapy for, 151–154
    salicylates, 151–153, 152*t*, 154*t*
inflammatory pain, 678
influenza, 632
inhalation route, 68
inhaled agents, 702–704
inhaler
    CFC, 347
    dry-powder, 347
    HFA, 347
    steps for using, 348
inhibition, 10
injectable agents, 704–707
injectable contraceptives, 521
injection
    as dosage route, 67
    needle size, 67
innate immune system, 583
inner ear, 273, 274*f*
inscription, 60*t*
insomnia, 244–245, 255–256
instillation, 68
Institute for Safe Medication Practices
    (ISMP), 37, 62
institutional setting, 59
insulin, 467
insulin aspart, 482
insulin degludec, 482
insulin detemir, 482
    insulin glargine, 482
insulin glulisine, 482
insulin human inhalation, 482
insulin lispro, 482
insulin pump, 479
insulin secretagogue, 487
integrase, 642
integrase strand transfer inhibitors
    (INSTIs), 657–658
integrative medicine, 16
integumentary system, 87–88.
    See also skin
interaction, 14–15
interchangeable products, 37

interferon, 635
    for multiple sclerosis, 191–192
interleaving study method, 44–45
intermediate-acting insulin, 479
internal condom, 512
international normalized ratio (INR), 329
intracellular (inside cells), 739
intradermal injection, 67
intramuscular (IM) injection, 67
intraocular pressure, 265
intraspinal injection, 67
intrathecal injection, 67
intrauterine device (IUD), 522
intravenous (IV) injection, 67
investigational drug, defined, 30
Investigational New Drug (IND)
    Application, 5
iris, 263, 264*f*
iron supplementation, 561
    oral, 561
    parenteral, 561
irritable bowel syndrome (IBS), 441
irritant receptor, 377
ischemia, 305
ischemic stroke, 321, 321*f*
islets of Langerhans, 467, 473
isoflurane, 703
isomer, 198
isotonic solution, 739
IV fluid, 739

J

jaundice, 602
jock itch, 106
joints
    anatomy and physiology of, 120–122*f*,
        120–123
    gouty arthritis, 137–140, 138*f*
    inflammation and swelling,
        151–154, 151*f*
    osteoarthritis, 123–130, 124*f*
    rheumatoid arthritis, 130–137, 130*f*
    types of, and function, 120, 121*f*

K

K-BANK Mnemonic, 51, 51*t*
keratolytic agent, 95
keratomalacia, 733
ketamine, 706
kidneys, 539–540*f*, 539–541
    aging and, 70, 71
kidney transplantation, 568–571
Koch, Robert, 111
kwashiorkor, 755

L

labels, medication, 74, 74*f*, 75*f*
    controlled substances, 35*f*
    right drug and, 64, 65*f*

laboratory values, 25, 26t
lactic acidosis, 486
lactobacilli, 456
lactulose, 436–437
lansoprazole-amoxicillin-
    clarithromycin, 418
laparoscopic gastric banding, 751
latency, 634
laxatives, 431
legend drug, 29
lens, 263, 264f
leucovorin rescue, 780
leukotriene inhibitor, 350t, 353–354
Lexicomp, 53
lice, 108–110, 110f
lidocaine, 715
lincosamide, 601
lipase, 369
    inhibitors, 752
lipid-lowering agents, 314–315t, 314–319
lipids, 7
lipoprotein, 313
liposomal product, 785
Li Shizhen, 22
Lister, Joseph, 25, 111
live attenuated vaccine, 663
liver, 407
    enzyme lab values, 26t
loading dose, 12, 601
local anesthesia, 698
local anesthetics, 714–715
local effect, 13, 68
local infection, 68
local viral infection, 634
long-acting beta agonists (LABAs),
    359t, 363–364
long-acting insulin, 479
long QT syndrome, 595
long-term persistent medications, 347
loop diuretics, 312, 554
loop of Henle, 541
loperamide, 429
Lou Gehrig's disease, 203
low-density lipoproteins (LDL), 313
low-molecular-weight heparins, 323t, 326
lubiprostone, 438
lungs. See also respiratory system
    aging and, 70
    exchange of oxygen/carbon dioxide in
        lungs, 343–344, 344f
    natural defense system, 358, 358f
lymphatic system, 582

M

macrolides, 271t, 272, 601
macula, 264, 264f
magnesium hydroxide, 437
magnesium (Mg²⁺), 746–747
maintenance dose, 12
malabsorption, 369
malignant hyperthermia, 713
malleus, 273, 274f
malnutrition, 754–759, 759–760t

enteral nutrition, 755–756, 756t
parenteral nutrition, 757–760,
    759–760t
mania, 226
marasmus, 755
margin, 771
marijuana, 723
masculinizing hormone therapy, 507
massing study method, 44
mast cells, 346
    stabilizers, 350t, 355
mechlorethamine, 781
medical dictionaries, 55
Medical Dictionary (Stedman), 55
medication errors, reporting systems
    for, 79
medication guide, 32–33
medication management
    instructions for, 74, 75
    labels, 74, 74f, 75f
    noncompliance and, 75–76
    OTC drugs and, 74–75
    patient's history and, 74
medication order, 59
    institutional setting, 63–64
medication reconciliation, 79
medication safety
    e-prescribing, 77
    medication error reporting
        systems, 79
    medication reconciliation, 79
    medications dispensed in original
        container, 78, 78t
    physical order entry, 77
    potential errors, 76, 77t
    prescription abbreviations, 62, 63t
    removing drugs from market, 32, 33
    rights of medication administration,
        64, 65f
    tamper-resistant pads, 79
    technician's role in, 77
medication use process, 76, 77t
medicinal drug history, 21–25
MedlinePlus, 54
MedWatch, 32, 37
meglitinide, 487
melanoma, 89
melasma, 504
membrane-stabilizing agent (Class I),
    300–301t, 300–302
menopause, 503
Merriam-Webster Medical Dictionary, 55
mesalamine, 421
messengers, 6
metabolic acidosis, 748
metabolic alkalosis, 748
metabolic modifier, 307t, 309–304
metabolic pathway, 9
metabolism, of drug, 9–10
metabolite, 9
metastasis, 771
metered dose inhaler (MDI), 347–348
metformin, 484
methadone, 689–690
methemoglobinemia, 91

methicillin-resistant *Staphylococcus aureus*
    (MRSA) infections, 596
methohexital, 708
methylcellulose, 435
Michigan Pharmacists Association
    (MPA), 28
Micromedex, 53
microtubule, 786
micturition, 542
Middle Ages, 23
middle ear, 273, 274f
middle ear infection (otitis media),
    274–277, 275t
migraine headaches, 715–722, 717–718t
    antiemetic agents, 721
    CGRP receptor antagonist, 720–721
    combination agents, 722
    ergot derivatives, 719–720
    5HT agonists, 718–719
milliequivalents (mEq), 742
mineralocorticoid, 466
minimum inhibitory concentration
    (MIC), 587
mites, 108, 108f, 109f
mixed opioid agonists, 692–694
mnemonic devices
    acronym and acrostic method, 50
    defined, 50
    in pharmacology, 51, 51t
    songs, stories and rhymes, 51
monoamine oxidase inhibitor (MAOI)
    for depression, 214t, 223–224
    for Parkinson's Disease, 185t, 189–190
monobactam, 599
monoclonal antibodies, 350t, 355–356,
    768, 796–798
monotherapy, 169
mood disorders, 212–226
morphine, 690–691
motor end plate, 201, 201f
mucolytics, 367
mucositis, 778
multidrug-resistant tuberculosis
    (MDR-TB), 374
multiple sclerosis (MS), 191–195, 192t
multi-tasking, 46
Mu opioid agonists, 686–692
muscle fasciculation, 202
muscle relaxants, 146–150
muscles
    anatomy and physiology of, 120–122f,
        120–123
    relaxants, 146–150
    spasms, 145–146, 146f
    types of, 120–121, 121f
musculoskeletal system
    anatomy and physiology of, 120–122f,
        120–123
    complementary and alternative
        therapies for, 154–155
    gouty arthritis, 137–140, 138f
    inflammation and swelling,
        151–154, 151f
    muscle relaxants, 146–150
    muscle spasm, 145–146, 146f

osteoarthritis, 123–130, 124f
osteoporosis, 140–145
rheumatoid arthritis, 130–137, 130f
mutagenic, 781
myasthenia gravis, 201–202, 202t
Mycobacterium tuberculosis, 371
myocardial infarction, 306–307
causes of, 306
nitrates, 307t, 308–309
overview of drug therapy for, 307t
symptoms of, 306
treatment of, 306–307
myoclonic seizure, 169

N

naked virus, 632
nalbuphine, 693–694
naloxone, 696, 712
naltrexone, 697
narcolepsy, 245t, 248–250
narrow-angle glaucoma, 265
narrow therapeutic index, 329
nasal irrigation, 396
nasal route, 68
National Association Boards of
    Pharmacy (NABP), 28
National Healthcareer Association
    (NHA), 28
National Institutes of Health (NIH),
    30, 54
National Pharmacy Technician
    Association (NPTA), 28, 80
national waiting list, kidney
    transplantation and, 568
nausea and vomiting, 443–449
    antihistamines and antic
        holinergics, 444–445t, 445
    dopamine receptor antagonists,
        447–448
    neurokinin-1 receptor antagonists,
        448–449
    serotonin receptor antagonists, 446
nebulizer, 349, 349f
needles, size of, 67
negative feedback, 464
negative margin, 771
neoadjuvant chemotherapy, 772
neostigmine, 712
nephrons, 70, 539
nephrotoxicity, 543, 609
nervous system
    afferent and efferent system, 162, 162f
    Alzheimer's disease, 195–197
    amyotrophic lateral sclerosis
        (ALS), 203
    anatomical divisions of, 162, 162f
    anatomy of, 162–164, 162f, 163f, 164f
    attention deficit hyperactivity disorder
        (ADHD), 197–200
    autonomic, 162, 162f
    central, 162
    complementary and alternative
        therapies for, 204–205

fibromyalgia, 204
functional divisions of, 162–163,
    162f, 163f
Huntington's disease, 203–204
major neurotransmitters,
    164–166, 165t
multiple sclerosis (MS), 191–195
myasthenia gravis, 201–202, 202t
neurons and neurotransmitters,
    163–164, 164f
Parkinson's disease, 183–191
peripheral, 162
physiology of, 164–166, 165t
restless legs syndrome (RLS), 204
seizure disorders, 166–183, 170–172t
somatic, 162, 162f
sympathetic and parasympathetic,
    163, 163f
neuraxial anesthesia, 698
neurokinin-1 receptor antagonists,
    448–449
neuroleptic drugs, 229
neuromuscular blockade, 603
neuromuscular blocking agents,
    709–710
neurons, 163–164, 164f
    seizures and, 166
neuropathic pain, 679
neurotransmitters
    action of major, 164–166, 165t
    defined, 163
    depression and drug therapy, 212
    neurons and, 163–164, 164f
    seizures and, 167
neutral protamine hagedorn (NPH)
    insulin, 482
New Drug Application (NDA), 29–30
niacin, 735
nicotine, 392
    supplements, 393–394
    withdrawal, 392–393, 392t
nitazoxanide, 430
nitrates, 307t, 308–309
nitrofurantoin, 594
nitroimidazole, 606
nitrous oxide (N₂O), 702
NKA (no known allergies), 73
NKDA (no known drug allergies), 73
nociceptive pain, 678–679
nociceptors, 678
nodular acne, 92
nonadherence, 27, 72
noncompetitive inhibition, 10
nondihydropyridine calcium channel
    blockers, 293
noninstitutional setting, 59
nonnarcotic analgesics, 123–126
nonnucleoside reverse transcriptase
    inhibitor (NNRTI), 648
nonpathologic, 69
nonproprietary name, 5
nonspecific immunity, 583
nonsteroidal anti-inflammatory drugs
    (NSAIDs), 124–125t, 126–129
    photosensitivity and drugs

treating, 90t
side effects and drug interactions, 128,
    129
tips for users of, 127
nonsteroid hormone, 464
nonvirilized males, 502
norepinephrine, 164, 165t
    serotonin-norepinephrine reuptake
        inhibitor (SNRI), 213–214t,
        218–220
normal saline (NS), 620
Norwalk virus, 425
nosocomial infection, 587
nosocomial pneumonia, 371
nucleoside reverse transcriptase inhibi-
    tor (NRTI), 643

O

obesity, 750–754, 751–752t
    lipase inhibitors, 752
    opioid antagonist and bupropion, 754
    sympathomimetic drugs, 753–754
obsessive-compulsive disorder
    (OCD), 216
off-label use, 30
olive oil, 277
omega-3 fatty acids, 319
oncogenes, 769, 769f
on-off phenomenon, 186
open-angle glaucoma, 265
ophthalmic antibiotics, 610–611t
ophthalmic glaucoma agents,
    265–266t, 265–267
ophthalmic ointments, 270–273,
    271–272t
ophthalmic route, 68
opiate, 681
opiates, 268t
opioid analgesics, 681–683, 682–683t
opioid antagonists, 696–697
    and bupropion, 754
opioids, pain management and, 681–694
    antagonists, 696–697
    cautions and considerations, 684t,
        685–686
    disorder and treatments, 694–697, 695t
    dosing and administering,
        683–684, 683t
    mixed opioid agonists, 692–694
    Mu opioid agonists, 686–692
    opioid analgesics, 681–683, 682–683t
    side effects, 684
opioid toxicity, 696
opioid use disorder, 685
optic nerve, 264f, 265
oral candidiasis, 620
oral contraceptive (OC), 513, 516
oral herpes, 637
oral iron supplement, 561
oral route, 66–67, 66t
oral thyroid supplementation, 470
Orange Book, 36
    as study aid, 52

order, 59

organ of Corti, 274, 274*f*

orthostatic hypotension, 221–222, 295

osmolarity, 739

osmosis, 738

osmotic laxatives, 436–437

osteoarthritis (OA), 123–130, 124*f*

osteoblast, 122, 122*f*

osteoclast, 122, 122*f*

osteomalacia, 733

osteoporosis, 140–145

   risk factors for, 141

otic medications, 275–277, 275*t*

otic route, 68

otitis externa, 275–277, 275*t*

otitis media, 274–277, 275*t*

ototoxicity, 781

otoxicity, 609

oval window, 273, 274*f*

overactive bladder.

      See urge incontinence

overflow incontinence, 545

over-the-counter (OTC) drug, 29, 37–38

   children and, 73

   for colds and allergies, 377

   medication management and, 74–75

oxazolidinone, 607

oxycodone, 691

oxytocic agent, 527

P

package insert

   defined, 52

   organization of, 52*t*

   as study aid, 52

pain

   anesthesia and, 697–715, 698–701*t*

   complementary and alternative therapies, 722–723

   defined, 677

   mechanisms, 678–679

      centralized, 679

      neuropathic, 679

      nociceptive, 678–679

   migraine headaches, 715–722, 717–718*t*

   nonnarcotic analgesics, 123–126

   opioids and, 681–694

      antagonists, 696–697

      cautions and considerations, 685–686

      disorder and treatments, 694–697, 695*t*

      dosing and administering, 683–684, 683*t*

      mixed opioid agonists, 692–694

      Mu opioid agonists, 686–692

      opioid analgesics, 681–683, 682–683*t*

      side effects, 684

   pathway in tissue injury, 151, 151*f*

   physiology of, 677–680

   response to, 680

salicylates, 151–153, 152*t*, 154*t*

   sources of, 678*t*

   timing of, 679–680

palliative chemotherapy, 773

pancreas, 407, 467

pancreatic enzyme supplements, 369

panic disorders, 241–242

pantothenic acid, 736

Paracelsus, 23

parasites, lice and scabies, 108–110, 108*f*, 108*t*, 109*f*, 110*f*

parasympathetic nervous system, 163, 163*f*

parenteral iron supplements, 561

parenteral nutrition, 757–760, 759–760*t*

parenteral route, 66*t*, 67

Parkinson's disease, 183–191

   characteristic signs of, 183

   commonly used agents for, 185–186*t*, 186–191

   pathology of, 183–184

paroxysmal seizure, 166

partial seizure, 167–168, 168*f*

passive immunity, 662

Pasteur, Louis, 111

patent, 36

pathogen, 582

pathogenic, 584

pathologic, 69

patient-controlled analgesia (PCA) pump, 685

patient counseling, 27

patient education for medication management, 74–76

peak expiratory flow rate (PEFR), 346

peak flow meter, 346, 346*f*

pediculosis, 108

pellagra, 736

penicillins, 595

peptic disease, 416–419

   H. Pylori agents, 417–419

   ulcers, 416*f*, 417*t*

peptic ulcers, 416

percussion, 367

percutaneous coronary intervention (PCI), 324

perimenopause, 503

peripheral nervous system, 162

peripheral neuropathy, 781

peripheral vascular resistance (PVR), 287

peristalsis, 427

peritoneal dialysis, 564, 565*f*

peroral (PO) route, 66

personal protective equipment (PPE), 805

petit mal seizure, 168–169

phagocytosis, 583

pharmacist, role of, 26

pharmacodynamics, 3, 6–7

   mechanisms of drug action, 6–7

   messengers and receptors, 6

pharmacognosy, 4

pharmacokinetics, 3, 7–10

   absorption, 8–9

   aging and, 69

   distribution, 9

   elimination, 10

   metabolism, 9–10

   modeling, 12–13

   parameters for, 10–12

pharmacologic effect, 4

pharmacology

   contemporary pharmacy practice, 25–28

   defined, 3

   historical perspective on, 24

pharmacopoeia, 23

Pharmacopoeia of the United States, 24

pharmacy-specific study aids, 47–51

   identifying drugs utilizing generic drug stems, 48–49, 48*f*, 49–50*t*

   learning by drug class, 47–48

   mnemonic devices, 50–51, 51*t*

pharmacy technician

   certification and, 28

   responsibilities of, 26–27

Pharmacy Technician Accreditation Commission (PTAC), 28

Pharmacy Technician Certification Board (PTCB), 28, 80

Pharmacy Technician Educators Council (PTEC), 28

pharmakon, 22

phlebitis, 175

phophodiesterase 4 inhibitors, 366

phosphate binders, 566

phosphate (PO_4^{3-}), 747–748

phosphodies terase-5 (PDE-5) inhibitor, 508

photosensitivity, 89, 90*t*

pH value, 610

phylloquinone, 734

phytoestrogen, 529

phytonadione, 734

PI3K/AKT/mTOR pathway agents, 800

pimple, 91

pink eye, 270

placebo, 30

plant sterol esters, 333

plasma cell, drug binding to plasma protein, 9

pneumonia, 371

   community-acquired pneumonia (CAP), 371

   nosocomial pneumonia, 371

polycarbophil, 435

polyenes, 620–621

polyethylene glycol 3350, 437

polypharmacy, 72

pooling, 758

positive feedback, 464

postexposure prophylaxis (PEP), 662

postmarketing surveillance, 32

post-traumatic stress disorder (PTSD), 212

potassium, K-BANK Mnemonic, 51, 51*t*

potassium channel blockers, 300*t*, 302–303, 303*t*

potassium (K^+), 744–745

potassium-sparing diuretic, 556

potentiation, 15t
precaution, 13
preexposure prophylaxis (PrEP), 662
pregnancy, 524–527, 524t
    drug classification for, 32
    induce labor, drugs used to, 526–527
    slow labor, drugs used to, 526
    tests, 525
premature atrial contraction, 299t
premature ventricular contraction, 299t
premenstrual dysphoric disorder
        (PMDD), 216
preparation error, 807
presbycusis, 273
Prescribers' Digital Reference (PDR), 53
prescribing error, 807
prescription
    abbreviations on, 62, 62t, 63t
    defined, 59
    elements of, 60, 60t, 61f
Prescription Drug User Fee Act, 31
priapism, 226
primary chemotherapy, 772
priming, 390
probiotics, 456, 760, 761t
prodrug, 637
progesterone, 499, 505
progestin hormone therapy products, 505
progestins, 499
programmed death pathway, 801–802
prokaryotic, 614
prophylactic drug, 4
prophylaxis, 13
propofol, 706
proprietary name, 5
prostaglandin, 6, 123, 151, 151f
prostaglandin agonists, 265t
prostaglandin E1 analogs, 415
protamine sulfate, 327
protease, 369
protease inhibitor (PI), 651–655
proton pump inhibitor (PPI), 413
proto-oncogene, 769
protozoan, 429
provoked pain, 680
pruritic, 96
pruritus, 14
Pseudomonas aeruginosa, 369
pseudoparkinsonism, 232
psoriasis, 96–102, 98–99t
psychiatric and related drugs
    alcohol dependence, 251–255
    anxiety, 240–244
    bipolar disorder, 226–228
    complementary and alternative
        therapies, 255–256
    depression and mood disorders,
        212–226
    schizophrenia and psychosis, 229–240
    sleep and sleep disorders, 244–251
psyllium, 435
ptosis, 201
Public Health Agency, Canada, 665
pulmonary embolism (PE), 319

pulmonary function tests, 346
pulse dosing, 616
pupil, 263, 264f
Pure Food and Drug Act, 29
purified protein derivative (PPD), 373
Purple Book, 37
    as study aid, 53
pyelonephritis, 543
pyridostigmine, 712
pyridoxine, 736

Q

QT prolongation, 595
quick-relief medications, 347
quinolones, 271t, 275t. *See* fluoroquino-
        lones

R

radiation therapy, 771
radioiodine ablation, 470
rapid-acting insulin, 479
R-CHOP, 784, 785t
rDNA, 4
reabsorption, 541
rebound congestion, 384
receptor, 6, 6f
rectal route, 68
rectum, 406
red yeast rice, 333
reflux, 408
regular insulin U-100, 482
regurgitation, 408
renal artery, 539
renal cortex, 539
renal medulla, 539
renal system, 537–576
    advanced chronic kidney disease,
        564–568
    anatomy and physiology, 538–542, 538f
        kidneys, 539–540f, 539–541
        ureter, 541–542
        urinay bladder, 541–542, 541f
    anemia, 559–564, 560t
    benign prostatic hyperplasia,
        548–551, 548t
    chronic kidney disease, 551–559, 551t
    complementary and alternative
        therapies, 571
    dialysis, 564–568
    end-stage chronic kidney disease,
        568–571
    kidney transplantation, 568–571
    pharmakinetics and, 542–543
        nephrotoxicity and renal dosing, 543
        renal function, assessment of,
            542–543
        renal system dysfunction, 542
    urinary incontinence, 545–546t,
        545–547
    urinary tract infection,
        543–545, 544t

renal transplant drug, 568
renal vein, 539
renin-angiotensin system, 287
repolarization, 286, 286f
reproductive system, 497–534
    childbirth and, 524–527
    complementary and alternative
        therapies, 529–530
    contraception, 511–524
    growth disorders, 527–529
    hormone replacement therapy,
        499–507, 500–501t
    pregnancy and, 524–527, 524t
    related hormones, 497–499, 498f
    sexual dysfunction, 507–511, 508t
rescue medicine, 351
respiratory acidosis, 748
respiratory alkalosis, 748
respiratory distress syndrome (RDS),
        371–372
respiratory system
    anatomy and physiology of,
        343–345, 344f
    asthma, 345–356
    chronic obstructive pulmonary disease
        (COPD), 356–367, 357f
    complementary and alternative
        therapies, 396
    coughs, colds and allergies, 376–390
    cystic fibrosis, 367–370
    exchange of oxygen/carbon dioxide in
        lungs, 343–344, 344f
    histoplasmosis, 376
    lungs' natural defense system, 358, 358f
    pneumonia, 371
    respiratory distress syndrome (RDS),
        371–372
    smoking cessation, 391–395
    tuberculosis, 372–376, 373–374t
restless legs syndrome (RLS), 204
retina, 263, 264f
retinoids, 268t
retrieval practice, 45
retrovirus, 642
reverse transcriptase, 642
Reye's syndrome, 154
rheumatoid arthritis, 130–137, 130f
    drug therapy for, 131–137
rhinitis medicamentosa, 384
riboflavin, 735
rickets, 733
rifaximin, 430
rights of medication administration,
        64, 65f
ringworm, 105
Risk Evaluation and Mitigation Strategy
        (REMS) programs, 79
robo-tripping, 383
rod cells, 263
Rosacea, 91–96
rotavirus, 425
routes of administration. *See* dosage
        routes
RxList, 53

S

saccharomyces boulardii (S. boulardii), 456
safety. *See* medication safety
Safety Data Sheet (SDS), 806, 806*f*
salicylates, 151–153, 152*t*, 154*t*
saliva, 407
salivary glands, 407
Salix alba, 155
salmonella, 425
satiety, 484
scabies, 108–110, 108*f*, 109*f*
schizophrenia, 229
Schmiedeberg, Oswald, 25
sclera, 263, 264*f*
seasonal affective disorder (SAD), 212
sebaceous glands, 88, 88*f*
seborrheic dermatitis, 96
sebum, 91
secondary cancers, 781
secondary diabetes, 475
second-phase insulin secretion, 484
secretion, 541
sedation (drowsiness), 681
seizure disorders, 166–183, 170–172*t*
  calcium channel blockers, 170*t*,
    177–178, 178*t*
  GABA enhancers, 170*t*,
    178–179, 180*t*
  glutamate inhibitors, 170–171*t*,
    180–183, 182*t*
  overview of drug therapy for, 169–170
  sodium channel blockers, 170–172*t*,
    173–177
  synaptic vesicle protein binder, 171*t*,
    182–183, 183*t*
seizure(s)
  causes of, 166–167
  defined, 166
  focal (partial), 167–168, 168*f*
  generalized, 168–169, 168*f*
  overview of, 166–167
  paroxysmal, 166
  seizure threshold, 177
selective estrogen receptor modulators
  (SERMs), 142*t*, 143–144
selective serotonin reuptake inhibitor
  (SSRI), 213–218, 213*t*
  serotonin syndrome, 213
self-injector pen, 479
self-testing study method, 45
semicircular canals, 274, 274*f*
Semmelweis, Ignaz Philip, 25
serotonin, 164, 165*t*
  schizophrenia and, 229
  selective serotonin reuptake inhibitor
    (SSRI), 213–218, 213*t*
  serotonin-norepinephrine reuptake
    inhibitor (SNRI), 213–214*t*,
    218–220
serotonin (5-HT) receptor
  antagonists, 446
serotonin-norepinephrine reuptake
  inhibitor (SNRI), 213–214*t*,
  218–220
  serotonin syndrome, 213

serotonin syndrome, 213
serum creatinine (SCr), 542
serum plasma lab values, 26*t*
sevoflurane, 704
sexual dysfunction, 507–511, 508*t*,
  510–511
  erectile dysfunction, 508–510
sexually transmitted infections,
  611–613, 614*t*
  agents for, 613–614, 614*t*
  chlamydia, 611
  gonorrhea, 612
  nongonococcal urethritis, 613
  syphilis, 612–613
  vaginitis, 613
Shiatsu acupressure, 456
short-acting beta-agonists (SABAs),
  349*t*, 351–352
short-acting insulin, 479
side effects
  defined, 13
  noncompliance and, 75
signa, 60*t*
signal transduction inhibitors, 798–799
simple focal seizure, 167
sinoatrial (SA) node, 286, 286*f*, 297–299,
  298–299*f*
sinus rhythm, 297
skeletal muscles, 121, 121*f*, 122–123
skin
  acne, 91–96
  anatomy and physiology, 87–88, 88*f*
  antiseptics and disinfectants,
    111–113, 111*t*, 112*t*
  bacterial infections, 102–107
  complementary and alternative
    therapies, 113
  dandruff, 97, 102, 102*f*
  dermatitis, 96–102
  drug therapies for sun exposure,
    90–91, 90*t*
  eczema, 96–102
  fungal infections, 103*t*, 105–107
  infections of, 102–107
  lice and scabies, 108–110
  photosensitivity, 89, 90*t*
  psoriasis, 96–102
  Rosacea, 91–96
  skin cancer, 89
  sun exposure and drug treatments,
    88–91
  topical corticosteroids, 98–99*t*, 100
  viral infections, 107
  warts, 107
  wrinkles, 91–96
sleep, stages of, 244
sleep disorders
  insomnia, 244–245
  narcolepsy, 245*t*, 248–250
  therapy for, 244–251, 255–256
  Z-drugs, 246–248
slow viral infection, 634
small intestine, 406
  drug absorption in, 8–9
    grapefruit and, 15, 15*f*

small molecules, 4
smoking cessation, 225, 391–395
  benefits of, 391, 391*t*
  drug therapy for, 393–395
  planning to stop smoking, 392–393
  symptoms of nicotine withdrawal,
    392–393, 392*t*
smooth muscle, 121, 121*f*
sodium bicarbonate, 748
sodium channel blockers, 170–172*t*,
  173–177
sodium-glucose linked transporter-2
  (SGLT-2) inhibitor, 487
sodium (Na⁺), 743–744
sodium phosphate, 440
solubility, 7
solutions, 68
somatic nervous system, 162, 162*f*
spacer, 347–348
spacing study method, 44
specificity, 6
spectrum of activity, 587
spermicide, 512
SPF (sun protection factor), 89
spill kit, 806
spleen, 582
squamous cell carcinoma, 89
stable angina, 305
stapes, 273, 274*f*
Staphylococcus aureus, 104
statins, 314*t*, 315–316
status asthmaticus, 347
status epilepticus, 168
steatorrhea, 369
Stedman's Medical Dictionary, 55
steroid hormone, 464
Stevens-Johnson syndrome, 594
stimulant laxatives, 437–438
stomach, 406
stop orders, 64
stress ulcer, 416
stretch receptor, 377
stroke, 321–333
  hemorrhagic, 321–322, 321*f*
  ischemic, 321, 321*f*
  overview of, 321–322
  risk factors for, 322
  stroke management, 322
  symptoms of, 321
  types of, 321–322, 321*f*
study skills, 43–54
  drug information resources, 52–54
    electronic and drug resource apps,
      53–54
    FDA Orange, Purple and Green
      books, 52–53
    package inserts, 52
  evidence-based study methods, 43–47
    contiguity principle, 45
    eliminating distractions, 46
    growth mindset, 46–47
    interleaving *vs.* blocking, 44–45
    self-testing, 45
    spacing, 44
  health information resources

governement healthcare websites, 54–55

medical dictionaries and encylclopedia, 55

pharmacy-specific study aids, 47–51

identifying drugs utilizing generic drug stems, 48–49, 48f, 49–50t

learning by drug class, 47–48

mnemonic devices, 50–51, 51t

subcutaneous injection, 67

subcutaneous tissue, 88, 88f

sublingual route, 67

substance P, 179

substantia nigra, 184, 184f

succinylcholine, 709–710

sulfasalazine, 421–422

sulfonamide, 271t, 593

sulfonylurea, 487

sun protection factor (SPF), 89

sunscreen, 89

suppositories, 68

suppuration, 111

surfactant, 371

surfactant laxative, 436

suspensions, 68

Susrutas, 22

sweat glands, 88, 88f

sympathetic nervous system, 163, 163f

sympathomimetic drugs, 753–754

sympathomimetics, 753

synapse, 163, 164f

synaptic vesicle protein binder, 171t, 182–183, 183t

synergism, 15t

synergistic drug therapy, 602

synergistic effect, 780

syphilis, 612

systemic effect, 13, 68

systole, 284

systolic blood pressure, 287–288

T

tachycardia, 297, 299t

tachypnea, 357

tapentadol, 691–692

tardive dyskinesia, 232

target, hormone, 463

target activation, 390

targeted anticancer therapies, 793–880, 794–795t

angiogenesis inhibitors, 795–796

Bruton's tyrosine kinase (BTK) inhibitor, 799

monoclonal antibodies, 796–798

PI3K/AKT/mTOR pathway agents, 800

signal transduction inhibitors, 798–799

tech-check-tech, 27

testosterone, 498

tetracyclic antidepressants, 214t, 222–223

tetracyclines, 604

The Book of Life (Sushruta), 22

therapeutic agent, 4

therapeutic effect, 13

therapeutic level, 12

therapeutic range, 11, 12f

thiamine, 735

thiazide diuretics, 297

thiazolidinediones (TZD), 488

threshold dose, 785

thrombin, 319

thrombocytopenia, 326

thrombolytic agents, 322, 324t, 333

thrush, 105

thyroid disorders, 467–471

hyperthyroidism, 470–471

hypothyroidism and thyroid replacement therapy, 468–469

thyroid gland, 465–466, 466f

thyroid storm, 470

thyrotoxicosis. *See* hyperthyroidism

thyroxine (T$_4$), 465

tinea, 105

tocolytic agent, 526

tocopherol, 734

tolerance, 14

tonic-clonic seizure, 168

tonicity, 739

tophus, 137

topical corticosteroids, 98–99t, 100, 269t

topical route, 66t, 68

topoisomerase I enzyme, 784

topoisomerase II enzyme, 784

topoisomerase inhibitors, 784–786

total body water (TBW), 738

total cholesterol, 313

total nutrient admixture (TNA), 758

total parenteral nutrition (TPN), 757

trade name, 5

tramadol, 692

transcription error, 807

transdermal contraceptive, 519–520

transgender, 506

transient ischemic attack (TIA), 321

traveler's diarrhea (TD), 429

travel immunization clinic, 665

travel vaccine, 665

treatment as prevention (TasP), 661

tricyclic antidepressants (TCAs), 214t, 220–223

triglycerides, 313

triiodothyronine (T$_3$), 465

T-score, 141

tuberculosis, 372–376, 373–374t

multidrug-resistant tuberculosis (MDR-TB), 374

overview of, 372–373

treatment for, 373–374t, 373–376

tumor burden, 770

tumor cell proliferation, 770

tumor necrosis factor-alpha (TNF-alpha) inhibitors, 98

tumor suppressor gene, 769, 769f

tympanic membrane, 273, 274f

type 1 diabetes, 474

type 2 diabetes, 474

U

ulcer, 416

ulcerative colitis and Crohn's disease, 419–423

aminosalicylates, 421–422

biologic therapies, 422–423

corticosteroids, 420–421

immunosuppressants, 423

unstable angina, 306

ureter, 541–542

urethral sphincter

external, 542

internal, 542

urge incontinence, 545

uric acid, 137

uricosuric agents, 139

urinary analgesics, 544–545

urinary incontinence, 542, 545–546t, 545–547

anticholinergics (antimuscarinics), 546–547

beta-3 adrenergic agonist, 547

urinary retention, 70, 542

urinary system. *See* renal system

aging and, 70

urinary tract infection, 543–545, 544t

antibiotics, 544

urinary analgesics, 544–545

urinay bladder, 541–542, 541f

urticaria, 14

USAN (United States Adopted Name), 5

US National Library of Medicine, 30

USP Dictionary of USAN and International Drug Names, 5

US Pharmacopoeia-National Formulary (USP-NF)

purpose of, 32

US Pharmacopoeia (USP), 24

V

Vaccine Information Statement (VIS), 669

vaccines. *See* immunizations

vaginal contraceptives, 520

vaginal route, 68

vancomycin, 608

variant angina, 306

vasodilators, 308

vasomotor, 503

vein, 283, 284f

ventricular fibrillation, 298, 299t

verbal orders, 64

vertigo, 274, 444

vesicant, 786, 786t

vial, 479

viral infections, 631–674, 633f, 635–636t, 644–645t, 660t

antiretroviral agents, 642–662, 644–645t

antiviral agents, 635–636t, 635–642

classification of, 634

complementary andalternative therapy, 670

viral *(continued)*
   HIV/AIDS agents, 642–662, 660*t*
   and host-cell interaction, 634–635
   immunity and immunization,
      662–670, 664*t*, 666–667*f*
   latent, 634
   significant, 632–633
   skin, 107
   stages of, 632
viral load, 651
virilization, 502
virion, 632
virus, 631
Vitamin A, 277
Vitamin B$_{12}$, 563
Vitamin D, 101, 566
vitamin E, 334
vitamin K, 329
   antagonists, 323*t*, 328–330
vitamins, 732–738, 732*t*
   defined, 732
   fat-soluble vitamins, 732–734
      vitamin A, 732–733
      vitamin D, 733–734
      vitamin E, 734
      vitamin K, 734–735
   water-soluble vitamins, 735–738

vitamin B1, 735
vitamin B2, 735
vitamin B3, 735–736
vitamin B5, 736
vitamin B6, 736
vitamin B7, 736–737
vitamin B9, 737
vitamin B12, 737
vitamin C, 737–738
vitreous humor, 264, 264*f*

W

warfarin antidote, 323*t*
warts, 107
washout period, 221
water-soluble vitamins, 735–738
   vitamin B1, 735
   vitamin B2, 735
   vitamin B3, 735–736
   vitamin B5, 736
   vitamin B6, 736
   vitamin B7, 736–737
   vitamin B9, 737
   vitamin B12, 737
   vitamin C, 737–738

Wernicke-Korsakoff syndrome, 735
wheals, 14
wheat dextrin, 435
wheezing, 345
white blood cells (WBCs), 634
Willow bark *(Salix alba)*, 155
withdrawal
   alcohol, 252–253, 253*t*
   nicotine, 392–393, 392*t*
wrinkles, 91–96

X

xanthine derivatives, 351*t*, 356
xanthine oxidase inhibitor, 139–140

Y

yeast infection, 105
yoga, 396

Z

Z-drugs, 245*t*, 246–248
zero-order elimination, 12

PHOTO CREDITS

Cover © istock/Roel Smart, istock/Sylvain LAgarA, shutterstock/hin255, shutterstock/umiberry;

Preface © Paradigm Education Solutions;

Unit 1 Opener page 1, © Shutterstock/Waraporn Wattanakult;

Chapter 1 page 6, © Shutterstock/Kateryna Kon; page 7, © Paradigm Education Solutions; page 8, © Paradigm Education Solutions; pages 10–12 © Paradigm Education Solutions; page 14, © Istock/gokhanilgaz; page 15, © Istock/YinYang; page 16, © Paradigm Education Solutions; page 17 (top) © Istock/Olivier Le Moal, (bottom) © Istock/Mantonature;

Chapter 2 page 22, © iStockphoto/PhilSigin; page 24, public domain; page 25 © Istockphoto/HultonArchive; page 27, © Istock/ stevecole images; page 30, © Shutterstock/Serdar Tibet; page 31, © Paradigm Education Solutions; page 33, (top) © Shutterstock/Atomazul, (bottom) © Paradigm Education Solutions; page 36, © Paradigm Education Solutions;

Chapter 3 page 44, © Shutterstock/wavebreak media; page 46, © Shutterstock/Macrovector; page 47, © Shutterstock/Solis Images; page 48 (both) © Paradigm Education Solutions; page 53, © Shutterstock/Pixel-Shot; page 54 © Shutterstock/AnnaStills;

Chapter 4 page 61, (both) © Paradigm Education Solutions; page 62, © Istock/ stevecoleimages; page 65, (both) © Paradigm Education Solutions; page 67, (top) © Shutterstock/Somnuek saelim, (bottom) © Istock/valeriopardi; page 68, (top) © Shutterstock/bikeriderlondon, (bottom) © Istock/mady70; page 69, © Istock/gpointstudio; page 72, © Istock/Suzifoo; page 74 © Paradigm Education Solutions; page 75, © Paradigm Education Solutions;

Unit 2 Opener page 85, © Shutterstock/Licvin;

Chapter 5 page 88, © Paradigm Education Solutions; page 92, © istock/lzf; page 95, © istock/Lisa Thornberg; page 96, © Shutterstock/Juergen Faelchle; page 97, Wikipedia; page 102, © Shutterstock/ Roblan; page 104, © Staph-Infection-Pictures.com; page 106, © Shutterstock/carroteater; page 107, © Shutterstock/Berents; page 108, © Wikipedia/Kalumet; page 109,

© Paradigm Education Solutions; page 110, (left) Wikipedia/Gilles San Martin, (right) Wikipedia/public domain; page 113 © Istock/Watcha;

Chapter 6 page 120, (left) © Shutterstock/SciePro; (right) Shutterstock/SciePro; page 121, (both) © Paradigm Education Solutions; page 122, (both) © Paradigm Education Solutions; page 124, © Paradigm Education Solutions; page 130, © istockphoto/WILLSIE; page 138, Wikipedia/Hellerhoff; page 146, © Paradigm Education Solutions; page 151, © Paradigm Education Solutions; page 155, (top) © Shutterstock/Studio 72, (bottom) © Shutterstock/n_defender;

Chapter 7 page 162, © Paradigm Education Solutions; page 163, © Paradigm Education Solutions; page 164, © Paradigm Education Solutions; page 166, © istock/dblight; page 168, © Paradigm Education Solutions; page 175, © Istock/watanyou; page 184, © Paradigm Education Solutions; page 185, © Paradigm Education Solutions; page 190, © istock/franckreporter; page 201, © Paradigm Education Solutions; page 205, © istock/Elenathewise;

Chapter 8 page 212, Shutterstock/Photographee.eu; page 214, © Paradigm Education Solutions; page 219, © Paradigm Education Solutions; page 222, © istock/CrazyD; page 226, © Shutterstock/loreanto; page 237, © Wikipedia; page 240, © istockphoto/mediaphotos; page 247, © istock/Roel Smart; page 248, © istock/Vadko80;

Chapter 9 page 264, © Paradigm Education Solutions; page 269, © Paradigm Education Solutions; page 272, © Paradigm Education Solutions; page 274, © Paradigm Education Solutions; page 277, © Paradigm Education Solutions; page 278, © Shutterstock/baibaz;

Chapter 10 page 284, © Shutterstock/Olga Bolbot; page 285, (both) © Paradigm Education Solutions; page 286, © Paradigm Education Solutions; page 287, © Paradigm Education Solutions; page 298, © Paradigm Education Solutions; page 299, © Paradigm Education Solutions; page 306, © Shutterstock/pixelheadphoto digitalskillet; page 314, © Custom Medical Stock Photos; page 317, © Shutterstock/MedstockPhotos; page 321, © Paradigm Education Solutions; page 322, © Shutterstock/Elen Bushe; page 331, © Shutterstock/Enlightened Media;

Chapter 11 page 344, (top) © Paradigm Education Solutions, (bottom) © Shutterstock/ Steve Cymro; page 345, © Paradigm Education Solutions; page 346, © istock/abalcazar; page 347, © istock/esolla; page 348, © istock; page 349, © istock/7409185; page 357, © Paradigm Education Solutions; page 358, © Shutterstock/Alila Medical Media; page 359, © istock/Johnrob; page 363, © Paradigm Education Solutions; page 366, © Paradigm Education Solutions; page 373, © Shutterstock/Puwadol Jaturawutthichai; page 377, © shutterstock/wavebreakmedia; page 378, © istock/DRB Images, LLC; page 384, © istockphoto; page 386, © istock/Jitalia; page 387, © istock/evemilla; page 389, © istock/MarkHatfield; page 392, © istock / Freila; page 396, © istock/yogesh_more; page 397, © shutterstock/antoniodiaz;

Chapter 12 page 406, © Paradigm Education Solutions; page 407, © Paradigm Education Solutions; page 408, (top) © Paradigm Education Solutions, (bottom) © istock/yanyong; page 409, © Paradigm Education Solutions; page 413, © Shutterstock/edstockPhotos; page 416, © Paradigm Education Solutions; page 424, © Paradigm Education Solutions; page 427, © Shutterstock/Keith Homan; page 429, © istock/ Eraxion; page 431, © Paradigm Education Solutions; page 432, © (top) istock/Karisssa, (bottom) Paradigm Education Solutions; page 435, © istock/21691240; page 439, © istock/mtreasure; page 441, © Paradigm Education Solutions; page 443, © John Bavosi / Science Source; page 446, © Shutterstock/Sarayut Hyongsit; page 456, © (top) istock/AlexRaths, (bottom) istock/fcafotodigital;

Chapter 13 page 464, © Paradigm Education Solutions; page 465, © Paradigm Education Solutions; page 466, (both) © Paradigm Education Solutions; page 467, © Paradigm Education Solutions; page 468, © (top) istock/Marilyn Haddrill, (bottom) © Paradigm Education Solutions; page 470, © Custom Medical Stock Photo, Inc; page 474, © Shutterstock/Syda Productions; page 479, © (both) Paradigm Education Solutions; page 480, (top) © Shutterstock/Dmitry Lobanov, (middle and bottom) © Paradigm Education Solutions; page 481, © Shutterstock/Orawan Pattarawimonchai; page 482, © Paradigm Education Solutions; page 490, © istock/burwellphotography;

Chapter 14 page 498, © Paradigm Education Solutions; page 504, (top) © Shutterstock/Image Point Fr; (bottom) Courtesy of Estrogel; page 508, © istock/ jfmdesign; page 511, © Shutterstock/Image Point Fr; page 513, (top) © istock/Jenny Swanson; (bottom) © istockphoto/Eau Claire Media; page 518, © Martin Shields / Science Source; page 520, © istock/ PrimeTime_Productions; page 522, © istock/ EduardoLuzzatti; page 530, © istock/botamochi;

Chapter 15 pages 538–540, © Paradigm Education Solutions; page 541, © Shutterstock/Blamb; page 548, © Paradigm Education Solutions; page 555, © Paradigm Education Solutions; page 557, © Paradigm Education Solutions; page 565, (both) © Paradigm Education Solutions; page 568, © Shutterstock/Luuuusa; page 571, © iStock.com/ Boogich;

Unit 3 Opener page 579 © iStock/nullko;

Chapter 16 page 582, © Science Source; page 585, © istock/sturti; page 586, Courtesy of Med-health; page 594, (top) © Paradigm Education Solutions, (bottom) © Dr. M.A. Ansary / Science Source; page 598, © Shutterstock/ Denis Tabler; page 604, Courtesy of Chalet Dental; page 608, © Paradigm Education Solutions; page 609, © Shutterstock/ Evikka; page 615, © Wikipedia; page 620, © Paradigm Education Solutions; page 622 © istock/fotolinchen;

Chapter 17 page 633, © Shutterstock/Designua; page 634, © Shutterstock/Christoph Burgstedt; page 643, © Paradigm Education Solutions; page 646, © Paradigm Education Solutions; page 658, © Shutterstock/IVASHstudio; page 661, © istock/ Frances Twitty; page 665, © istock/Christopher Futcher; page 666, © public domain (cdc.gov); page 667, © public domain (cdc.gov); page 668, © istock/dra_schwartz; page 669, © istock/ KarenMower; page 670, (top) © Shutterstock/ LightCooker, (bottom) ©Phototake;

Chapter 18 page 681, © Shutterstock/Jearu; page 684, © Wikipedia/DiverDave; page 687, © Wikipedia; page 702, © Shutterstock/Roman Zaiets; page 713, © Paradigm Education Solutions; page 722, © istock/ luamduan;

Chapter 19 page 733, © istock/&#169 Ana Amorim; page 734, (top) © Shutterstock/Oleg Zaslavsky, (bottom) © istock/Serg_Velusceac; page 736, © Shutterstock/ Dionisvera; page 737, © Shutterstock/monticello; page 739, © Paradigm Education Solutions; page 740, © Paradigm Education Solutions; page 741, © Paradigm Education Solutions; page 744, © istock/svetikd; page 745, © istock/John_Lerskau; page 750, © Paradigm Education Solutions; page 756, © Paradigm Education Solutions; page 757, © Shutterstock/Chaikom; page 758, © Burger/ Phanie / Science Source;

Chapter 20 page 768, © Shutterstock/Africa Studio; page 769, (both) © Shutterstock/ Anastasiia Okhrimenko; page 770, © Paradigm Education Solutions; page 771, © Shutterstock/ Mark_Kostich; page 772, © Shutterstock/Monkey Business Images; page 774, © (top) Shutterstock/

DKN0049, (bottom) Shutterstock/LaksamonBut; page 778, © (top) Shutterstock/Felix Miznoznikov, (bottom) Paradigm Education Solutions; page 787, © (top left) Shutterstock/Sodel Vladyslav, © (top right) Shutterstock/Hane Street, © (bottom left) Shutterstock/chromakey_sketch, © (bottom right) Shutterstock/Rawpixel.com; page 797, © Paradigm Education Solutions; page 801, © Shutterstock/joshya; page 806, © Paradigm Education Solutions; page 807, © Paradigm Education Solutions